KU-555-305

Difficult Diagnosis

Robert B. Taylor, M.D.

Professor and Chairman
Department of Family Practice
Oregon Health Sciences University School of Medicine
Portland, Oregon

W.B. Saunders Company
Philadelphia / London / Toronto / Mexico City / Rio de Janeiro / Sydney / Tokyo

W. B. Saunders Company: West Washington Square
Philadelphia, PA 19105

1 St. Anne's Road
Eastbourne, East Sussex BN21 3UN, England

1 Goldthorne Avenue
Toronto, Ontario M8Z 5T9, Canada

Apartado 26370—Cedro 512
Mexico 4, D.F., Mexico

Rua Coronel Cabrita, 8
Sao Cristovao Caixa Postal 21176
Rio de Janeiro, Brazil

9 Waltham Street
Artarmon, N.S.W. 2064, Australia

Ichibancho, Central Bldg., 22-1 Ichibancho
Chiyoda-Ku, Tokyo 102, Japan

Library of Congress Cataloging in Publication Data

Main entry under title:

Difficult diagnosis.

1. Diagnosis. I. Taylor, Robert B. [DNLM: 1. Diagnosis. WB 141 D569]

RC71.D53 1985 616.07′5 83–19071

ISBN 0–7217–1058–7

Difficult Diagnosis ISBN 0-7216-1058-7

Last digit is the print number: 9 8 7 6 5 4 3 2

CONTRIBUTORS

JONATHAN ABRAMS, M.D.
Professor, Department of Medicine (Cardiology), The University of New Mexico School of Medicine, Albuquerque, New Mexico.
Cardiomegaly

M. ELIZABETH ARCHER, M.D.
Department of Dermatology, University of Texas Medical Branch, Galveston, Texas.
Urticaria, Chronic

B. LEWIS BARNETT, Jr., M.D.
Walter M. Seward Professor and Chairman, Department of Family Medicine, University of Virginia Medical School, Charlottesville, Virginia.
Hypercalcemia

WILBUR BENSON BASSETT, Jr., M.D.
Volunteer Faculty, Department of Medicine, Emory University School of Medicine, Atlanta, Georgia; Attending Physician, Medical Center, St. Francis Hospital, Doctor's Hospital, Columbus, Georgia; Attending Physician, Cobb Hospital, Phenix City, Alabama.
Cancer, Metastatic from Unknown Site

JOHN A. BELIS, M.D.
Associate Professor, Department of Urology, West Virginia University School of Medicine, Morgantown, West Virginia.
Priapism

GEORGE S. BENSON, M.D.
Associate Professor, Department of Surgery (Urology), University of Texas Medical School at Houston, Houston, Texas.
Hematuria

RICHARD E. BLACKWELL, Ph.D., M.D.
Associate Professor, Department of Obstetrics and Gynecology, University of Alabama in Birmingham School of Medicine, Birmingham, Alabama.
Puberty, Precocious

EILEEN D. BREWER, M.D.
Assistant Professor, Department of Pediatrics, University of Texas Medical School at Houston, Houston, Texas.
Hematuria

JOSEPH L. BYRNE, M.D.
Clinical Instructor, Department of Surgery, Upstate Medical Center, State University of New York, Syracuse, New York.
Abdominal Pain, Acute

JOHN J. CALABRO, M.D.
Professor of Medicine and Pediatrics, Departments of Medicine and Pediatrics, University of Massachusetts Medical School; Director of Rheumatology, St. Vincent Hospital, Worcester, Massachusetts.
Erythema Nodosum

ROBERT R. CARROLL, M.D.
Private Practice, Albany, Georgia.
Purpura

JOHN E. CARTER, M.D.
Assistant Professor, Department of Medicine (Neurology), University of Texas Health Sciences Center at San Antonio, San Antonio, Texas.
Visual Field Defect

LAWRENCE T. CHOY, M.D.
Department of Medicine, Nassau Hospital, Mineola, New York.
Hirsutism and Hypertrichosis

MICHAEL G. CORBETT, M.D.
Assistant Clinical Professor, Department of Internal Medicine (Pulmonary), University of California, Davis, School of Medicine, Sacramento, California.
Pulmonary Nodule, Solitary

RICHARD A. DEVAUL, M.D.
Dean, School of Medicine, and Professor, Department of Psychiatry and Behavioral Medicine, West Virginia University, Morgantown, West Virginia.
Delirium

JAMES R. DINGFELDER, M.D.
Instructor, Duke University School of Medicine, Durham, North Carolina.
Infertility

BERNARD J. D'SOUZA, M.D.
Associate Professor, Division of Pediatric Neurology, Duke University Medical Center, Durham, North Carolina.
Seizures, Recent Onset

EDWARD R. EICHNER, M.D.
Professor, Department of Medicine, University of Oklahoma Health Sciences Center, Oklahoma City, Oklahoma.
Splenomegaly

SHERMAN ELIAS, M.D.
Associate Professor, Department of Obstetrics and Gynecology, Northwestern University Medical School, Chicago, Illinois.
Prenatal Detection of Genetic Disorders

STANLEY FAHN, M.D.
H. Houston Merritt Professor, Department of Neurology, Columbia University Colleges of Physicians and Surgeons; Attending Neurologist, Presbyterian Hospital and Neurological Institute of New York, New York, New York.
Dystonia

PAUL M. FISCHER, M.D.
Assistant Professor, Department of Family Practice, Medical College of Georgia, Augusta, Georgia.
Alkaline Phosphatase, Elevated

ALBERT B. GERBIE, M.D.
Professor, Department of Obstetrics and Gynecology, Northwestern University Medical School, Chicago, Illinois.
Prenatal Detection of Genetic Disorders

BARBARA A. GILCHREST, M.D.
Associate Professor, Department of Dermatology, Tufts University School of Medicine, Boston, Massachusetts.
Pruritus, Generalized

ROBERT A. GOLDENBERG, M.D.
Associate Professor and Chairman, Department of Otolaryngology, Wright State University School of Medicine, Dayton, Ohio.
Vertigo

LEE GOLDMAN, M.D.
Associate Professor, Department of Medicine, Harvard Medical School, Boston, Massachusetts.
Chest Pain, Atypical

IRWIN GOLDSTEIN, M.D.
Assistant Professor, Department of Urology, Boston University School of Medicine; Director of Urology, Boston City Hospital, Boston, Massachusetts.
Impotence

MARC B. GOLDSTEIN, M.D.
Professor, Department of Medicine, University of Toronto, Toronto, Ontario, Canada.
Oliguria

JOSEPH W. GRIFFIN, Jr., M.D.
Associate Professor, Department of Medicine, Medical College of Georgia, Augusta, Georgia.
Dysphagia

HOWARD D. GROVEMAN, M.D.
Assistant Professor, Department of Community and Family Medicine, University of California, San Diego, La Jolla, California.
Gynecomastia

ROBERT W. GUYNN, M.D.
Professor, Department of Psychiatry and Behavioral Sciences, The University of Texas Medical School at Houston, Houston, Texas.
Delirium

JOHN T. HARRINGTON, M.D.
Professor, Department of Medicine, Tufts University School of Medicine; Chief, General Medicine Division, New England Medical Center, Boston, Massachusetts.
Polyuria

ROBERT S. HILLMAN, M.D.
Professor, Department of Medicine, University of Vermont, Burlington, Vermont; Chief of Medicine, Maine Medical Center, Portland, Maine.
Anemia, Megaloblastic

JACK HIRSH, M.D.
Professor and Chairman, Department of Medicine, McMaster University, Hamilton, Ontario, Canada.
Calf Pain

JOHN E. HOCUTT, Jr., M.D.
Instructor, Department of Family Medicine, Jefferson Medical College of Thomas Jefferson University, Philadelphia, Pennsylvania; Associate, Department of Family Practice, Wilmington Medical Center, Wilmington, Delaware.
Unconscious Patient

W. KEITH HOOTS, M.D.
Assistant Professor, Departments of Pediatrics and Internal Medicine, University of Texas Medical School at Houston; Assistant Professor and Pediatrician, University of Texas System Cancer Center, M. D. Anderson Hospital and Tumor Institute, Houston, Texas.
Eosinophilia

RUSSELL D. HULL, M.D.
Associate Professor, Department of Medicine, McMaster University, Hamilton, Ontario, Canada.
Calf Pain

WILLIAM L. JAFFEE, M.D.
Clinical Assistant Professor, Department of Medicine, Jefferson Medical College of Thomas Jefferson University, Philadelphia, Pennsylvania; Head, Section of Endocrinology and Metabolism, Wilmington Medical Center, Wilmington, Delaware.
Short Stature

JONAS T. JOHNSON, M.D.
Assistant Professor, Department of Otolaryngology, University of Pittsburgh School of Medicine, Pittsburgh, Pennsylvania.
Salivary Gland Enlargement

JAMES R. JONES, M.D.
Professor and Chairman, Department of Obstetrics and Gynecology, University of Medicine and Dentistry of New Jersey, Rutgers Medical School, New Brunswick, New Jersey.
Hyperprolactinemia

JOSEPH L. JORIZZO, M.D.
Associate Professor, Department of Dermatology, University of Texas Medical Branch, Galveston, Texas.
Urticaria, Chronic

D. M. KAJI, M.D.
Assistant Clinical Professor, Department of Medicine, Mt. Sinai School of Medicine, New York; Assistant Chief, Renal Section, Veterans Administration Medical Center, Bronx, New York.
Hyponatremia and Hypernatremia

WISHWA N. KAPOOR, M.D.
Assistant Professor, Department of Medicine, University of Pittsburgh School of Medicine, Pittsburgh, Pennsylvania.
Syncope

COLLIN S. KARMODY, M.D.
Professor, Department of Otolaryngology, Tufts University School of Medicine, Boston, Massachusetts.
Smell and Taste Disturbances

MICHAEL KARPF, M.D.
Falk Associate Professor, Department of Medicine (General Internal Medicine), University of Pittsburgh School of Medicine, Pittsburgh, Pennsylvania.
Syncope

THEODORE E. KEATS, M.D.
Professor and Chairman, Department of Radiology, University of Virginia Medical School, Charlottesville, Virginia.
Lytic Lesions in Bone

EKKEHARD KEMMANN, M.D.
Associate Professor, Department of Obstetrics and Gynecology, University of Medicine and Dentistry of New Jersey, Rutgers Medical School, New Brunswick, New Jersey.
Hyperprolactinemia

CRAIG S. KITCHENS, M.D.
Associate Professor, Department of Medicine, University of Florida College of Medicine, Gainesville, Florida.
Purpura

HERBERT S. KUPPERMAN, M.D., Ph.D.
Associate Professor, Department of Medicine, New York University Medical Center, New York, New York.
Puberty, Delayed

ANDREW S. LEVEY, M.D.
Assistant Professor, Department of Medicine (Nephrology), Tufts University School of Medicine; Director, Dialysis Unit, New England Medical Center, Boston, Massachusetts.
Polyuria

GERALD S. LEVEY, M.D.
Professor and Chairman, Department of Medicine, University of Pittsburgh School of Medicine, Pittsburgh, Pennsylvania.
Syncope

HOWARD LEVINE, M.D.
Department of Otolaryngology and Communicative Disorders, Cleveland Clinic Foundation, Cleveland, Ohio.
Neck Mass

GLEN A. LILLINGTON, M.D.
Professor, Department of Internal Medicine (Pulmonary), University of California, Davis, Sacramento, California.
Pulmonary Nodule, Solitary

STEVEN B. LIPPMANN, M.D.
Associate Professor, Department of Psychiatry and Behavioral Sciences, University of Louisville School of Medicine, Louisville, Kentucky.
Dementia

L. KEITH LLOYD, M.D.
Professor, Department of Surgery (Urology), University of Alabama Medical Center in Birmingham, Birmingham, Alabama.
Urinary Incontinence

JERRE F. LUTZ, M.D.
Associate Professor, Department of Medicine (Cardiology), Emory University School of Medicine; Director, Cardiac Catheterization/Cardiac Function Laboratories, Grady Memorial Hospital, Atlanta, Georgia.
Cyanosis

ROBERT THOMAS MANNING, M.D.
Professor, Department of Internal Medicine, University of Kansas School of Medicine–Wichita; Director of Internal Medicine Education, Wesley Medical Center, Wichita, Kansas.
Jaundice

E. WAYNE MASSEY, M.D.
Associate Professor, Department of Neurology, Duke University Medical Center, Durham, North Carolina.
Tremor

JANICE M. MASSEY, M.D.
Associate in Medicine, Department of Neurology, Duke University Medical Center, Durham, North Carolina.
Tremor

RICHARD W. McCALLUM, M.D.
Associate Professor, Department of Internal Medicine (Gastroenterology), Yale University School of Medicine, New Haven, Connecticut.
Gastric Stasis Syndromes

JOHN A. McCURDY, Jr., M.D.
Assistant Clinical Professor, Department of Surgery, University of Hawaii, John A. Burns School of Medicine, Honolulu, Hawaii.
Tinnitus

KAY F. McFARLAND, M.D.
Professor, Department of Obstetrics and Gynecology, University of South Carolina School of Medicine, Columbia, South Carolina.
Amenorrhea

ROBERT McLELLAN, M.D.
Department of Obstetrics and Gynecology, St. Agnes Hospital, Baltimore, Maryland.
Pelvic Pain in Women

WARREN C. MILLER, M.D.
Director, Humana Pulmonary Center, Webster, Texas.
Respiratory Failure, Acute

JEROME V. MURPHY, M.D.
Clinical Professor, Department of Pediatrics, Medical College of Wisconsin, Milwaukee, Wisconsin.
Seizures, Recent Onset

DANIEL M. MUSHER, M.D.
Professor, Departments of Medicine and Microbiology and Immunology, Baylor College of Medicine; Chief, Infectious Disease, Veterans Administration Medical Center, Houston, Texas.
Fever of Unknown Origin

LUIZ NASCIMENTO, M.D.
Assistant Professor, Department of Medicine, University of Illinois; Veterans Administration West Side Medical Center, Chicago, Illinois.
Hyperkalemia and Hypokalemia

D. MELESSA PHILLIPS, M.D.
Associate Professor, Department of Family Medicine, University of Mississippi School of Medicine, Jackson, Mississippi.
Hyperhidrosis

SUSAN K. PINGLETON, M.D.
Associate Professor, Department of Internal Medicine (Pulmonary), University of Kansas Medical Center, Kansas City, Kansas.
Pleural Effusion

THOMAS LEE POPE, Jr., M.D.
Clinical Assistant Professor, Department of Radiology, University of North Carolina School of Medicine, Chapel Hill, North Carolina.
Lytic Lesions in Bone

NICHOLAS W. READ, M.A., M.D.
Senior Lecturer, Departments of Physiology and Medicine, University of Sheffield; Consultant Gastroenterologist, Royal Hallamshire Hospital, Sheffield, United Kingdom.
Diarrhea, Chronic

L. RAYMOND REYNOLDS, M.D.
Consulting Endocrinologist, Department of Medicine, Lexington Clinic, Lexington, Kentucky.
Hypocalcemia

DOMINICK RICCI, M.D.
Private Practice, Solana Beach, California.
Gastric Stasis Syndromes

ANTONIO R. RODRIGUEZ, M.D.
Private Practice; Attending Physician, Medical Center, St. Francis Hospital, Doctor's Hospital, Columbus, Georgia; Attending Physician, Cobb Hospital, Phenix City, Alabama.
Cancer, Metastatic from Unknown Site

RONALD M. ROTH, M.D.
Assistant Professor, Department of Medicine, University of New Mexico School of Medicine, Albuquerque, New Mexico.
Cardiomegaly

ALEXANDER SCHIRGER, M.D.
Associate Professor, Division of Hypertension Diseases and Internal Medicine, Mayo Medical School; Consultant, Division of Hypertensive Diseases and Internal Medicine, Mayo Clinic, Rochester, Minnesota.
Edema, Peripheral

BRIAN P. SCHMITT, M.D.
Assistant Professor, Department of Medicine, University of Illinois at Chicago, Chicago, Illinois.
Erythrocyte Sedimentation Rate, Elevated

JUDD SHELLITO, M.D.
Assistant Professor, Department of Medicine, University of California, San Francisco, San Francisco, California.
Hemoptysis

FRANK C. SNOPE, M.D.
Professor, Department of Family Medicine, University of Medicine and Dentistry of New Jersey, Rutgers Medical School, New Brunswick, New Jersey.
Weight Loss

ELLEN F. SOEFER, M.D.
Assistant Professor, Departments of Pediatrics and Family Practice and Community Health, Temple University School of Medicine; St. Christopher's Hospital for Children, Philadelphia, Pennsylvania.
Failure to Thrive, Infant

STUART JON SPECHLER, M.D.
Assistant Professor, Department of Medicine, Boston University School of Medicine, Boston, Massachusetts.
Gastrointestinal Bleeding of Unknown Origin

MICHAEL R. SPENCE, M.D.
Associate Professor, Department of Gynecology and Obstetrics, The Johns Hopkins University School of Medicine, Baltimore, Maryland.
Pelvic Pain in Women

JOHN A. SPITTELL, Jr., M.D.
Mary Lowell Leary Professor, Division of Cardiovascular Diseases and Internal Medicine, Mayo Medical School; Consultant, Division of Cardiovascular Diseases and Internal Medicine, Mayo Clinic, Rochester, Minnesota.
Edema, Peripheral

DAVID E. SWEE, M.D.
Assistant Professor, Department of Family Medicine, University of Medicine and Dentistry of New Jersey, Rutgers Medical School, Piscataway, New Jersey.
Weight Loss

ROBERT B. TAYLOR, M.D.
Professor and Chairman, Department of Family Practice, Oregon Health Sciences University, School of Medicine, Portland, Oregon.
Headache, Acute

JERRY TEMPLER, M.D.
Associate Professor, Department of Surgery (Otolaryngology), University of Missouri Health Sciences Center, Columbia, Missouri.
Facial Pain

JACK E. TETIRICK, M.D.
Associate Clinical Professor, Department of Surgery, The Ohio State University College of Medicine; Director of Medical Affairs, Grant Hospital, Columbus, Ohio.
Breast Discharge

EDWARD TSOU, M.D.
Associate Professor, Department of Medicine (Pulmonary), Georgetown University School of Medicine, Washington, D.C.
Pneumonia, Poorly Resolved

MARK T. TSUANG, M.D.
Assistant Professor, Department of Surgery (Urology), University of Cincinnati College of Medicine, Cincinnati, Ohio.
Scrotal Mass

ARTHUR A. VERCILLO, M.D.
Clinical Professor, Department of Surgery, Upstate Medical Center, State University of New York, Syracuse, New York.
Abdominal Pain, Acute

RICHARD F. WAGNER, Jr., M.D.
Teaching Fellow, Department of Dermatology, Boston University School of Medicine, and Department of Dermatology, Tufts University School of Medicine, Boston, Massachusetts.
Hirsutism and Hypertrichosis

NANETTE K. WENGER, M.D.
Professor, Department of Medicine (Cardiology), Emory University School of Medicine; Director, Cardiac Clinics, Grady Memorial Hospital, Atlanta, Georgia.
Cyanosis

MICHAEL R. WILLS, M.D., Ph.D.
Professor, Departments of Pathology and Internal Medicine, University of Virginia Medical School, Charlottesville, Virginia.
Hypercalcemia

GARY L. WOLF, M.D.
Instructor, Department of Medicine, University of Massachusetts Medical School, Worcester, Massachusetts.
Erythema Nodosum

PEAK WOO, M.D.
Assistant Professor, Department of Otolaryngology, Upstate Medical Center, State University of New York, Syracuse, New York.
Smell and Taste Disturbances

J. BENJAMIN YOUNGER, M.D.
Professor, Department of Obstetrics and Gynecology, University of Alabama in Birmingham School of Medicine, Birmingham, Alabama.
Puberty, Precocious

SYED N. ZAMAN, M.D.
Clinical Assistant Professor, Department of Surgery, Upstate Medical Center, State University of New York, Syracuse, New York.
Abdominal Pain, Acute

PREFACE

A book entitled *Difficult Diagnosis* was written by H. J. Roberts, M.D., and published by W. B. Saunders Company in 1958. This new book differs from the previous work in two important ways: First of all, medicine is now, a quarter-century later, so much more complex that no single author could write an authoritative, comprehensive volume spanning virtually all specialty areas. Second, whereas Roberts discussed literally hundreds of clinical entities, it has now become necessary to limit the number of topics in order to discuss each in adequate depth.

Roberts' original preface stated one reason why he undertook the writing: "I needed a book like this in my own practice." So do I. This work describes the diagnostic approach to a selected group of challenging clinical problems. The topics of the chapters that follow have been chosen to represent the most enigmatic clinical presentations, without regard for the frequency of their occurrence in practice. The topic list represents areas—amenorrhea, purpura, jaundice, chronic urticaria, and delayed puberty are just a few—that have frequently prompted me to make a trip to the library or seek consultation. In each instance, the chapter has been written by an expert on that topic, with data recorded more or less according to a standard format. The approach is one that I have found useful in practice: an overview of the problem, a directed medical history with high-payoff questions, a physical examination focused on specific areas, laboratory investigations that include the latest technology, and a systematic, sometimes algorithmic, analysis of clinical data.

Difficult Diagnosis is intended for use by the primary care physician and by the specialist who encounters patients with problems outside his or her field of expertise. The problems discussed in this book transcend traditional specialty lines; that is, the patient with facial pain may be seen by the neurologist, neurosurgeon, otolaryngologist, or oral surgeon, as well as by the family physician. For this reason, the topics are listed alphabetically rather than by specialty or organ system. The focus is on diagnosis, and information regarding therapy is included only when it may facilitate diagnosis, e.g., the use of a trial of progesterone in amenorrhea.

I am grateful to W. B. Saunders Company for the opportunity to compile and edit this work, and extend special thanks to: Albert E. Meier, Editor-in-Chief; Robert C. Butler, Production Manager; Janet E. Macnamara, Senior Copy Editor; and Terri Siegel, Designer. My wife, Anita D. Taylor, M.A.Ed., participated in all phases of planning, author recruitment, manuscript editing, and proofreading. Finally, I extend heartfelt appreciation to the 95 authors who, by contributing their specialized talents and considerable effort, have made this textbook possible.

ROBERT B. TAYLOR, M.D.

CONTENTS

ABDOMINAL PAIN, ACUTE

JOSEPH L. BYRNE ☐ ARTHUR A. VERCILLO ☐ SYED N. ZAMAN

☐ SYNONYMS: Pain in the abdomen, belly pain

BACKGROUND

Definition and Origins

Abdominal pain describes a sensation of malaise or discomfort related to the abdominal cavity. Difficulty in establishing a precise diagnosis arises from the fact that an enormous number of disease entities produce abdominal pain. Abdominal pain can be caused by any of three broad categories of disease: intra-abdominal disease, referred pain from localized extra-abdominal disease, and systemic disease.

Intra-abdominal Disease

Critical to the establishment of the diagnosis of abdominal pain is an understanding of the mechanisms of abdominal pain. There are essentially two types of abdominal pain, which derive from the neurologic anatomy of the abdomen.

Visceral Pain. The abdominal viscera and the visceral peritoneum that envelops them are supplied by a paucity of nerve endings mediated through the splanchnic nerves. In addition, the innervation is multisegmental and overlapping, so that visceral pain is not well localized. The visceral pain fibers respond to increased intraluminal pressure and not to direct stimuli such as crushing and burning. Owing to the poor localization, obstruction or distension of almost any hollow viscera initially manifests as vague discomfort in the central portion of the abdomen. An example of this vagueness is the periumbilical pain produced by initial distension of the appendiceal lumen in early appendicitis.

Parietal Pain. The parietal peritoneum is supplied by somatic afferent nerves that can precisely localize adjacent inflammatory processes. For example, as appendicitis progresses to transmural inflammation, precise localization of pain to the right lower quadrant occurs as the parietal peritoneum is irritated.

Referred Pain from Extra-abdominal Disease

Abdominal pain due to extra-abdominal disease is common because central pathways for afferent neurons are shared. Thus, severe angina and other primary thoracic diseases may manifest as abdominal pain. Similarly, severe retroperitoneal disease, such as rupture of an aortic aneurysm, often causes abdominal pain. Table 1 presents the most common causes of referred abdominal pain.

Embryologic considerations are also important in the diagnosis of abdominal pain. For example, the common origin of the testicle and kidney explain the presentation of ureteral colic as sharp testicular pain.

Systemic Disease

Presenting symptoms of a variety of systemic illnesses include acute abdominal pain. These illnesses are listed in Table 2.

Incidence and Causes

Abdominal pain was the chief presenting complaint in one out of every 20 emergency room patients seen recently in a large medical center.[3] Interestingly, the most common final diagnosis in this study was abdominal pain of unknown cause (41.3 per cent). The next three most common diagnoses were also nonsurgical: gastroenteritis (6.9 per cent), pelvic inflammatory disease (6.7 per cent), and urinary tract infection (5.2 per cent). The most common surgical disease, appendicitis, was observed in only 4.3 per cent of cases. This study highlights the facts that the majority of patients presenting with abdominal pain have nonsurgical disease and that often no specific

Table 1. MOST COMMON CAUSES OF REFERRED ABDOMINAL PAIN

Location	Disorders
Cardiothoracic	Pericarditis Pleuritis Pneumonia Acute myocardial infarction
Abdominal wall	Rectus sheath hematoma Muscle strain
Retroperitoneal	Renal colic Renal infarct Ruptured abdominal aortic aneurysm
Pelvic	Mittelschmerz Endometriosis

Table 2. SYSTEMIC ILLNESSES CAUSING ABDOMINAL PAIN

Metabolic	Acute porphyria Uremia Diabetic ketoacidosis Addisonian crisis
Hematologic	Sickle cell anemia Leukemia
Toxic	Heavy metal poisoning Bacteria (staphylococcus, tetanus) Drug effects Insect bite reactions

diagnosis is made. Statistics, however, are no consolation to the individual patient, and the burden of proof lies on the diagnostician first to exclude a life-threatening, surgically treatable illness as the cause of abdominal pain. The challenge, therefore, in diagnosis of the acute abdomen is to separate those patients with conditions that require diagnosis in a matter of minutes if treatment is to be successful such as leaking aortic aneurysms, from the overwhelming number of patients with benign conditions for which the diagnostic process can proceed in a leisurely fashion.

HISTORY

A carefully taken history remains the cornerstone of diagnosis of the acute abdomen. Table 3 summarizes the key points to address in history taking. The history should record the exact time of onset. Pain that awakens the patient from sleep is often of serious import. Of similar importance is the subsequent temporal pattern of the pain. For example, as illustrated in Figure 1, one can often separate the pain caused by obstruction of a hollow viscus, which recurs in waves, from that caused by perforation of a viscus, in which a crescendo of severe pain is often followed by regression. The waxing-and-waning pattern of pain from obstruction of a hollow viscus can often

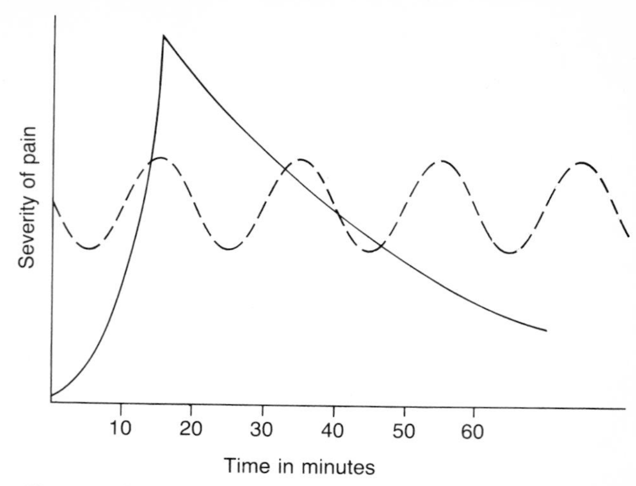

Figure 1. Temporal sequence of abdominal pain as a guide to diagnosis. *Solid line* indicates pattern in perforated viscus. *Dotted line* indicates pattern in obstruction of hollow viscus.

be quite similar, whether the viscus involved is part of the gastrointestinal tract, the biliary tract, or the genitourinary tract. The interval of freedom from pain may be helpful in localizing the site of obstruction in the gastrointestinal tract, because the interval between cramping pains is longer if the site of obstruction is more distal.[4]

The pattern of radiation of pain is another key feature in the history. Radiation to the shoulder implies irritation of the diaphragm with pain referred via the phrenic nerve. It may suggest perforated ulcer with diaphragmatic irritation, splenic rupture or infarct, or liver abscess. Pain radiating to the back is typical of pancreatitis, penetrating peptic ulcer, and rupture of abdominal aortic aneurysms.

The character of the pain may be helpful. For example, the dull, fixed pain of pyelonephritis may often be distinguished from the tearing pain of a leaking aortic aneurysm.

Provocative and palliative features are noteworthy. For example, biliary colic and intestinal angina are typically aggravated by eating, whereas the pain of peptic ulcer is relieved by the neutralizing effect of a meal. Pain aggravated by urination may suggest appendicitis irritating the right ureter or a pelvic abscess in proximity to the bladder.

The timing and character of associated emesis are important. In appendicitis, pain almost invariably precedes emesis. Emesis of gastric contents with bile staining may occur with biliary colic, ureteral colic, or proximal small bowel obstruction. The emesis of feculent material is virtually pathognomonic of distal small bowel obstruction.

Syncope in association with abdominal pain may suggest hypotension and severe blood volume loss as seen in ruptured aortic aneurysms, ectopic pregnancy, or ruptured spleen. A menstrual history is critical in women; amenorrhea suggests

Table 3. KEY POINTS OF HISTORY IN ACUTE ABDOMINAL PAIN

Pain:
Time of onset
Pattern of recurrence
Pattern of radiation
Character
Provocative and palliative features
Character of emesis?
Syncope?
Menstrual history

ectopic pregnancy, and pain in midcycle suggests mittelschmerz.

Previous medical history should be completely evaluated. Alcohol abuse is important in gastritis, peptic ulcer, and pancreatitis. Prior abdominal surgery is of obvious importance. It is worth noting that adhesions from previous surgery are one of the three most common causes of bowel obstruction in the adult, hernia and neoplastic lesions being the remaining two causes.

PHYSICAL EXAMINATION

General observation of the patient is critical to the rapid assessment of the severity of the illness. Pallor, lethargy and cool, cyanotic extremities may suggest imminent hypovolemic shock from blood loss. Likewise, a patient with diffuse peritonitis usually lies extremely still because of pain with any motion, but a patient with ureteral colic often is writhing in pain.

Routinely, the temperature, pulse, and respiratory rate should be recorded, although they are highly variable as indices of the severity of acute abdominal pain. Abnormal vital signs are helpful in targeting patients with significant disease. However, it is not uncommon to see perforated appendicitis, for example, with entirely normal vital signs, including temperature.

The abdominal examination should include the traditional activities of inspection, palpation, percussion, and auscultation. *Inspection* may reveal the restricted respiratory motion seen in advanced peritonitis or, occasionally, the visible pulsation of an aortic aneurysm. Maintenance of thigh flexion indicates psoas abscess or appendicitis. *Palpation* should detect areas of maximal tenderness, muscle guarding, and masses. Organomegaly should be sought, and special attention should be directed to the inguinal rings and femoral triangles for hernial defects or incarcerated masses. Table 4 suggests diagnoses that may be suggested by localization of findings on palpation. *Percussion* of the abdomen is valuable in assessing whether abdominal distension is liquid, as in ascites, or tympanitic, as in the presence of bowel obstruction or perforated viscus. Loss of the liver dullness usually noted in the right upper quadrant suggests free intraperitoneal air from a perforated viscus. Exquisite tenderness to light percussion is a reliable indicator of peritonitis and should replace more heavy-handed methods of searching for "rebound" tenderness. A distended bladder, which should be detected by percussion, may establish that the abdominal pain is secondary to prostatic obstruction, a not uncommon diagnosis in the elderly male. *Auscultation* is probably the least helpful mode of examination. Traditionally, the silent abdomen has been considered pathognomonic for diffuse peritonitis, and the high-pitched borborygmi of peristalsis pathognomonic for mechanical intestinal obstruction. In reality, active peristalsis often persists despite extensive peritonitis, and the late stages of mechanical obstruction may be associated with a silent abdomen. Auscultation of an abdominal bruit may suggest arterial insufficiency, but ruptured aneurysms and ischemic bowel are often found in the absence of bruit.

Table 4. DIAGNOSES OF THE ACUTE ABDOMEN ACCORDING TO LOCALIZATION OF FINDINGS ON PALPATION

Localization	Likely Diagnoses
Right upper quadrant	Acute cholecystitis
	Hepatitis
	Hepatomegaly due to congestive heart failure
	Peptic ulcer
	Retrocecal appendicitis
	Right lower lobe pneumonia
	Carcinoma of hepatic flexure of colon
	Right pyelonephritis
	Hepatic abscess
Left upper quadrant	Gastritis
	Splenic rupture
	Left pyelonephritis
	Myocardial ischemia
	Left lower lobe pneumonia
	Splenic infarct
Right lower quadrant	Appendicitis
	Regional enteritis (Crohn's)
	Ectopic pregnancy
	Torsion or rupture of right ovarian cyst
	Meckel's diverticulitis
	Psoas abscess
	Endometriosis
	Cecal carcinoma
Left lower quadrant	Diverticulitis
	Carcinoma of left colon
	Ectopic pregnancy
	Torsion or rupture of left ovarian cyst
	Psoas abscess
	Endometriosis

Certain physical signs used traditionally in the abdominal examination may be helpful. They are as follows.

Psoas test: With the patient lying on the left side, forced extension of the right hip will cause pain if the psoas muscle is irritated by an inflamed appendix.

Obturator test: With the patient supine, rotation of the hip joint with the thigh flexed may cause pain if the obturator muscle is irritated by a pelvic appendicitis.

Murphy's sign: Deep inspiration during deep palpation in the right upper quadrant will cause pain if the gallbladder is distended or inflamed.

Grey Turner's sign: Flank discoloration by subcutaneous hematoma may be seen in advanced cases of hemorrhagic pancreatitis.

Careful pelvic and rectal examinations are mandatory in all cases of acute abdominal pain.

DIAGNOSTIC STUDIES

Complete blood count and urinalysis are the first-line tests useful in acute abdominal pain. It should be emphasized that a normal hematocrit is the rule in early hemorrhage, even of extensive proportions, because equilibration takes hours to occur.

The white blood cell (WBC) count is notoriously inaccurate for identifying acute surgical conditions in the abdomen. In a representative sample of surgical explorations focusing on appendicitis, patients with appendicitis or another surgical condition did have, on the average, higher white blood cell counts than patients with nonsurgical disease, but significant numbers of patients in both surgical groups had white blood cell counts less than 10,000 cells/mm^3.[5] On the other hand, 55 per cent of the patients with nonsurgical disease had white blood cell counts exceeding 10,000 cells/mm^3.

Urinalysis may confirm a diagnosis of urinary tract infection. Red cells are usually, but not invariably, present in cases of ureteral calculi. Urinalysis for human chorionic gonadotropin (hCG) is helpful if ectopic pregnancy is suspected.

Amylase determinations may be made if pancreatitis is suspected, but normal amylase levels may be seen in advanced pancreatitis, usually in the setting of chronic pancreatitis with an extensively damaged pancreas. Many other acute abdominal conditions, including cholecystitis, ischemic bowel, and perforated or obstructed bowel, may cause elevations in the serum amylase level. The urine amylase level may be elevated even in the face of normal serum amylase levels; however, amylase elevations are seen in such a wide variety of diseases that their diagnostic value is limited.

Radiographs of the abdomen should be taken in two planes, one either decubitus or upright, so that air-fluid levels can be detected. Air-fluid levels suggest mechanical bowel obstruction but are also found in paralytic ileus due to other abdominal disorders. Free air from a perforated viscus may be better seen on an upright chest film. Calcification noted in the region of the pancreas indicates chronic pancreatitis. Blunting of the psoas shadows is seen in massive hemorrhage or abscess formation. Gallstones, appendicoliths, and ureteral calculi should be sought.

It should not be inferred that every patient with abdominal pain needs radiography. Patients clearly suffering from abdominal catastrophes should undergo prompt surgical exploration without the hazardous delays imposed by these additional tests. Also, as noted previously, the majority of patients with abdominal pain prove not to have serious illness, and the cost effectiveness of routine abdominal films has been demonstrated to be quite low.[6] Often a simple trial of observation and careful follow-up can avoid the costs of multiple radiographs.

Special radiographic studies have a limited role in diagnosis of the acute abdomen. An intravenous pyelogram may be used to confirm the diagnosis of ureteral calculus if suggested by the history, physical findings, and urinalysis results. Barium studies in the setting of acute abdominal pain should be discouraged, because they may be dangerous if a viscus is already perforated and they may obscure the findings of subsequent, urgent evaluations such as ultrasonography and angiography. Ultrasonography may be useful to demonstrate gallstones and has the advantages of being safe and simple and of not introducing contrast media into the abdomen.

Radioisotopic scanning of the biliary tree is being used increasingly to determine whether the cystic duct is blocked, a better sign of acute cholecystitis than the mere presence of gallstones, which may in fact be asymptomatic. Intravenous cholangiography has virtually disappeared from the diagnostic armamentarium.

Arteriography may be useful if superior mesenteric artery embolus or thrombosis is suspected. Ischemic bowel, which is being recognized more often as the elderly population increases in size, is a difficult diagnosis to make. Again, the premature administration of barium precludes the use of arteriography. This procedure is not necessary in cases of suspected ruptured abdominal aortic aneurysm, and the best diagnostic measure if such a diagnosis is suspected is emergency laparotomy.

Laparoscopy has been suggested as a useful diagnostic tool, particularly in menstruating females, in whom it is often difficult to distinguish between appendicitis and pelvic disease.[7] This procedure, however, has not gained widespread popularity in the diagnosis of acute abdominal pain, even in the female population. The distinction between appendicitis and pelvic disease can usually be made via combined surgical and gynecologic consultation and occasionally by the addition of pelvic ultrasonography or barium enema. Barium enema is most helpful if it demonstrates a filling defect in the cecum, suggesting an appendiceal mass, but the disadvantages of any barium study in the setting of acute abdomen are real and must be weighed carefully before the procedure is ordered.

Upper gastrointestinal endoscopy has undoubtedly increased the accuracy of diagnosis of peptic ulceration. Unfortunately, it is expensive and uncomfortable. Often in cases of acute peptic ulcer, the patient can be treated empirically initially, and when the condition has proved to be stable over the course of 48 to 72 hours, the diagnosis can be made by barium swallow.

Although rare, Meckel's diverticula often contain ectopic gastric mucosa that will specifically take up certain radioisotopes. This test may be useful in cases of obscure, recurrent abdominal pain.

ASSESSMENT

An accurate diagnosis is essential in acute abdominal pain because so many of the diseases involved are treated quite safely if diagnosed early yet have catastrophic consequences if there is undue delay in diagnosis. In a study of 1,000 consecutive emergency room evaluations for abdominal pain, 11 patients were erroneously discharged and on return were found to have acute surgical problems.[3] Eight of the 11 were found ultimately to have acute appendicitis, and three to have intestinal obstruction. In this section, discussion focuses on these two problem areas of diagnosis and also on selected other diagnoses that are troublesome to the clinician.

Acute Appendicitis

As noted, appendicitis remains the most common cause for error in diagnosis of acute abdominal pain. The diagnosis is most often missed in three specific groups:

1. Children 1 to 14 years of age, in whom the diagnosis at surgery is usually mesenteric adenitis, a syndrome of abdominal pain caused by mesenteric lymph node enlargement usually on the basis of an upper respiratory viral illness. Yaijko and Steel[8] noted that 50 per cent of patients found to have mesenteric adenitis at surgery gave a history of recent upper respiratory infection, and that the WBC count was less than 12,500 cells/mm^3 in 75 per cent of cases. The peak incidence of mesenteric adenitis was between 11 and 20 years of age in the study, whereas the peak incidence of appendicitis is between 16 and 25 years of age.
2. Women 10 to 29 years of age, in whom the diagnostic error is most often made by confusing appendicitis with pelvic inflammatory disease.
3. The elderly, who demonstrate a less dramatic physiologic response to serious illness. Many elderly patients with advanced appendicitis have no fever or leukocytosis and only minimal abdominal tenderness.

How, then, can one best avoid overlooking appendicitis? One should pay careful attention to the history, which in appendicitis begins with crampy periumbilical pain (visceral pain) and is followed by localization to the right lower quadrant as transmural inflammation proceeds, irritating the parietal peritoneum (parietal pain). The pain should be followed by nausea, emesis, or, at the least, anorexia. Localized tenderness in the right lower quadrant remains the key physical finding. Normal urinalysis and the presence of leukocytosis are confirmatory signs, but as emphasized before, a normal WBC count by no means excludes the diagnosis. Rarely will the plain film of the abdomen demonstrate a fecalith. Perhaps the key point is that diagnostic laparotomy in cases of strongly suspected appendicitis remains the most reasonable course. Hospitals that maintain rates for negative exploration results for appendicitis that are less than 10 per cent are probably overconservative in the use of laparotomy and may well expose their patient population to the hazards of perforated appendicitis.

Bowel Obstruction

This diagnosis probably accounts for a common cause of error in diagnosis owing to its wide variety of clinical presentations. Silen[9] analyzed the causes of bowel obstruction by incidence; his results are summarized in Table 5. Careful questioning regarding a change in bowel habit (common in colonic neoplasms) and identification of previous abdominal surgery are the two key points in history taking. Physical examination may not demonstrate abdominal distension if the obstruction is high and the bowel is decompressed by vomiting. Again, palpation of all hernial orifices and a careful rectal examination with stool guaiac test for occult blood are necessary. The plain films of the abdomen also can be unremarkable in proximal obstruction.

Laparotomy

A good summary of common diagnostic pitfalls is given in the study by Yaijko and Steel[8] of 178 patients in whom laparotomy revealed no abnor-

Table 5. CAUSES OF BOWEL OBSTRUCTION

Cause	Incidence (%)
Hernia	41
Adhesions	29
Intussusception	12
Cancer	10
Volvulus	4
Miscellaneous	4

(Data from Silen W. Cope's early diagnosis of the acute abdomen. 15th ed. New York: Oxford University Press, 1979:149. Reprinted with permission.)

Table 6. PREOPERATIVE AND POSTOPERATIVE DIAGNOSES IN PATIENTS UNDERGOING LAPAROTOMY FOR ACUTE ABDOMINAL PAIN IN WHOM NO SURGICAL DISEASE WAS FOUND

Diagnosis	Percentage of Patients
Preoperative	
Appendicitis	56
"Acute surgical abdomen"	13
Acute cholecystitis	7
Ectopic pregnancy	4
Perforated viscus	3
Small bowel obstruction	3
Postoperative	
No final diagnosis made	39
Mesenteric adenitis	15
Pelvic inflammatory disease	11
Gastroenteritis	7
Acute pyelonephritis	4
Pancreatitis	3

Data from Yaijko RD, Steel G. Exploratory celiotomy for acute abdominal pain. Am J Surg 1976; 128:773–6.

malities. The population consisted of patients with abdominal pain and no history of trauma. The results are given in Table 6. It is interesting to note that even after laparotomy and subsequent follow-up, no definite cause for the abdominal pain could be found in 39 per cent of the patients. Again, mesenteric adenitis and pelvic inflammatory disease were the two leading entities prompting surgical exploration for suspected appendicitis with a negative result.

CONCLUSION

Precise diagnosis of acute abdominal pain rests primarily on carefully taken history and physical examination supplemented by a few simple laboratory and radiographic studies. Because laparotomy is the definitive mode of diagnosis and therapy in many patients, it should be carried out promptly if a surgical disease is strongly suspected.

REFERENCES

1. Sleisenger MH, Fordtran JS. Gastrointestinal disease. Philadelphia, W. B. Saunders, 1978;398.
2. Schwartz SI. Principles of surgery. 3rd ed. New York: McGraw-Hill, 1979; 1043.
3. Brewer RJ, Golden GT, Hitch DC, et al. Abdominal pain. An analysis of 1000 consecutive cases in a university hospital emergency room. Am J Surg 1976;131:219–23.
4. Beal JM. The acute abdomen. In: Sabiston DC, ed. Davis-Christopher Textbook of Surgery. 12th ed. Philadelphia: W. B. Saunders, 1982;875–95.
5. Chang FC, Hogle HH, Welling DR. The fate of the negative appendix. Am J Surg 1973;126:752–54.
6. Eisenberg RL, Heincken P, Hedgcock W, et al. Evaluation of plain abdominal radiographs in the diagnosis of abdominal pain. Ann Intern Med 1982;97:257–61.
7. Barnes AB, Welch JP, Malone LJ. Initial experience with laparoscopy for gynecologic patients in a teaching hospital. Arch Surg 1972;105:734–7.
8. Yaijko RD, Steel G. Exploratory celiotomy for acute abdominal pain. Am J Surg 1974;128:773–6.
9. Silen W. Cope's early diagnosis of the acute abdomen. 15th ed. New York: Oxford University Press, 1979;149.

ALKALINE PHOSPHATASE VALUE, ELEVATED

PAUL M. FISCHER

□ SYNONYMS: Elevated ALP, hyperphosphatasemia

BACKGROUND

Clinical Setting

It is not uncommon in clinical practice to come across an unexpectedly elevated serum alkaline phosphatase (ALP) value. This is an increasingly frequent finding because of the availability of inexpensive multiple-test biochemical profiles. The rationale for including the ALP measurement in such a battery of laboratory tests is that it may be useful in screening for skeletal or hepatobiliary disease. Several studies have evaluated the use of biochemical screening tests in large populations of "healthy" patients. In one study of patients being seen for "multiphasic health checkups," 3.9 per cent had abnormally high ALP values.[1] A second study documented a 4.3 per cent rate of elevated ALP values on a 15-test screening chemistry panel.[2] Physicians were later asked about these ALP abnormalities; 86.4 per cent of the elevated values were previously unknown and 91.2 per cent were found in patients with no obvious clinical reason for hyperphosphatasemia. In that setting, it is the clinician's responsibility to decide whether the unexplained abnormal value indicates disease and, if so, what further evaluation or treatment is indicated. Abnormal screening test results can point the clinician to an unexpected and potentially treatable disease. They can also lead to time-consuming and unnecessary investigations. The physician must thoroughly understand a laboratory test in order to make appropiate clinical decisions on the basis of its results.

Enzymology

Alkaline phosphatase is a family of enzymes found in nearly all body tissues, where its general action is to catalyze the hydrolysis of phosphate esters in an alkaline medium.[3] The specific function of these enzymes in vivo is unclear and may well vary for different tissues. The ALP isoenzymes can be differentiated by electrophoresis and heat sensitivity. The serum ALP that is measured clinically in adult patients consists of an approximately 50-50 mixture of the liver- and bone-derived isoenzymes.[4] Other ALP isoenzymes that can be measured and have some clinical usefulness come from the placenta, kidneys, leukocytes, and intestines.

The ALP derived from bone correlates with osteoblastic activity, i.e., the production of new bone. It is most significantly elevated in conditions such as Paget's disease. The ALP value is usually normal or only slightly elevated in diseases with osteoclastic (i.e., osteolytic) activity, such as multiple myeloma.

The elevation of ALP in biliary disease is due to an increased synthesis of the enzyme by hepatobiliary cells.[5] It is used clinically as a marker for "obstructive" or "cholestatic" biliary disease. In contrast, the ALP value may be normal or only slightly elevated in illnesses that result in direct hepatocellular damage (i.e., a "nonobstructive pattern"). Although this clinical rule of thumb does hold when examining groups of diseases, it may not hold true for the individual patient with a specific hepatobiliary disease.

Alkaline Phosphatase Testing

The optimal laboratory conditions for the ALP assay are a subject of considerable debate. As a result, there are variations in the test procedures between clinical laboratories. The variations include the choice of enzyme substrate, the choice of buffer system, and the temperature at which the test is performed.[6] There are no universally agreed upon normal ranges for this enzyme. Each laboratory creates its own "reference range" and reports this value with the test result. The reference range is usually chosen so that it includes 95 per cent of the ALP values for healthy adults obtained under the specific test conditions used in the particular laboratory. One must be careful not to compare the ALP values from different laboratories unless their reference ranges are known.

Serum is the usual specimen used for ALP measurement. A regular "red top" or serum separator tube is preferred. The blood should not be collected in a tube with citrate, EDTA, or oxalate.[7] Values may be falsely elevated if the blood sample is collected from a limb on which a tourniquet has been used for longer than 30 seconds.[8] Sample hemolysis does not effect the ALP value. There is little change in the ALP activity with storage at room temperature for up to 4 days.[5] Properly handled specimens mailed from the physician's office to a reference laboratory are therefore suitable for ALP testing.

There is no need for special patient preparation before drawing blood for ALP determination. Test values have been shown to be largely unaffected by the time of day, exercise, prolonged bed rest, and recent alcohol consumption. A meal high in fat may result in a 25 per cent elevation in the serum ALP value in some patients.[7] Fasting is not required for most routine ALP testing, but the patient should fast when the test is repeated to follow up a previously elevated result.

The reference values for ALP vary greatly with age. Children normally have an ALP value of 2–3 × URL (two to three times the upper reference limit) for the adult reference range, owing to the rapid deposition of bone in a child's skeleton. During the adolescent growth spurt, the ALP value increases to 3–4 × URL for adults. The ALP value falls to the adult level by age 20 in women and age 30 in men. The adult reference range then remains unchanged until age 50. There is disagreement about the reference range in older adults. Some authors have found a slight increase in the serum ALP value in normal populations of healthy older patients. Others believe that this increase is due to the inclusion for study of patients with subclinical hepatic or skeletal disease.[9, 10]

The serum ALP value rises during pregnancy as a result of the production of a placental ALP isoenzyme, to 1.5 × URL by the third trimester. Markedly elevated ALP values have been reported in pregnancy but are uncommon.[5] The ALP values return to pre-pregnancy levels by the end of the first month postpartum. An elevated ALP value in pregnancy is not clinically useful in assessing either maternal or fetal health.

ALP Isoenzyme Increases

The majority of serum ALP elevations are due to an increase in either the skeletal or the biliary isoenzyme. It is often clinically useful to determine which is increased. Clinical laboratories separate these isoenzymes by either electrophoresis or heat stability testing. The bone isoenzyme is relatively heat labile compared with the hepatic isoenzyme. Alternatively, one may measure the serum glutamyl transpeptidase (GGT) level, which is a sensitive indicator of biliary obstruction but is not affected by bone disease. If the ALP value is elevated but the GGT value is normal, the ALP elevation is likely to be due to an increase in the skeletal isoenzyme.

Drugs That Cause ALP Elevations

A wide variety of drugs has been reported to result in elevations of the serum ALP (Table 1). A complete list of drug effects on ALP values has recently been published.[8] It should be emphasized that only a small percentage of patients taking any of the implicated drugs will have elevated ALP values. Classes of drugs that have frequently been reported to increase the ALP include estrogens, progestogens, phenothiazines, antidepressants, and nonsteroidal antiinflammatory agents. Because some commercially prepared albumin is made from placental tissue, the use of intravenous albumin may lead to a marked elevation in the serum ALP value. Most of the other drugs listed produce ALP elevation by their action on the liver. Some drugs have classically been reported to produce either a "cholestatic" or "hepatotoxic" effect, as indicated by liver enzyme measurements. For other drugs the effect is "mixed." The individual case may not follow the classic pattern for the specific drug.

Table 1. DRUGS ASSOCIATED WITH AN ELEVATED ALKALINE PHOSPHATASE VALUE

Acetohexamide	Levodopa
Albumin	Methotrexate
Allopurinol	Methyldopa
Amantadine	Methyltestosterone
Barbiturates	Naproxen
Chloramphenicol	Norethandrolone
Chlorpromazine	Norethindrone
Colchicine	Oxacillin
Erythromycin estolate	Phenytoin
Estradiol	Procainamide
Estriol	Propranolol
Ethionamide	Sulfonamides
Halothane	Tetracycline
Indomethacin	Tolbutamide
Isoniazid	

Diseases That Cause ALP Elevations

Diseases in which ALP elevations are seen are listed in Table 2.

Hepatobiliary Diseases

Liver function tests have traditionally been interpreted as indicating either a "hepatic" or a "cholestatic" process. The former is also referred to as "nonobstructive." It is indicated by elevation in the aminotransferase and unconjugated bilirubin levels with a normal or only slightly increased ALP value. The cholestatic or obstructive process is indicated by a normal aminotransferase level but elevated ALP, GGT, and conjugated bilirubin values.

Complete biliary obstruction results in an ALP value of 3–10 × URL. Obstruction is most commonly due to a common bile duct stone; less common causes include tumors of the pancreas, biliary tree, or gallbladder, primary biliary cirrhosis, acute pancreatitis, and chronic relapsing pancreatitis. With complete obstruction there is often an associated elevation in the bilirubin level.

Incomplete biliary obstruction produces an elevated ALP but normal bilirubin value, because the obstruction causes the hepatocytes to produce an increase in ALP, which passes into the circulation, but the bilirubin is handled by the unobstructed portions of the liver and its level therefore does not rise in the serum. Incomplete obstructions may be due to a hepatic duct stone or to a space-occupying lesion in the liver, such as primary hepatic tumor, metastatic tumor, or abscess.

Several infections are responsible for elevations in ALP level. It is usually elevated to 2–3 × URL in viral hepatitis. Dramatic increases such as those seen in serum aminotransferase levels are uncommon. Infectious mononucleosis usually results in an elevated ALP when the liver is involved; the bilirubin level is usually normal in this disease. Cytomegalovirus infections with hepatitis may also produce an elevated ALP value.

Infiltrative diseases of the liver, such as sarcoidosis and amyloidosis, may result in an increase in the ALP value. When such disorders do not involve the liver, the ALP value is normal.

The ingestion of even large quantities of alcohol has little effect on the serum ALP value in most patients. In cases of acute alcoholic hepatitis, the value may transiently rise to 3 × URL. Most patients with alcoholic cirrhosis have a normal ALP value. Even patients with end-stage cirrhosis and hepatic coma usually have ALP elevations of only 2–3 × URL. A variety of drugs and hepatotoxins other than alcohol causes ALP elevation (see Table 1).

Patients with cholelithiasis and no biliary ob-

Table 2. CAUSES OF ALKALINE PHOSPHATASE ELEVATION AND THEIR CHARACTERISTICS

Cause	Characteristics
Nonpathogenic Causes	
Pregnancy	Third trimester
Age	Men younger than 30 yr and women younger than 20 yr
Albumin use	Infusion of albumin produced from placental tissues
Hepatobiliary diseases	
Cholelithiasis with obstruction	Fever, nausea, vomiting, abdominal pain
Hepatic abscess	Fever, nausea, vomiting, abdominal pain, right shoulder pain
Biliary cirrhosis	Itching, dark urine, jaundice, diarrhea, bone pain
Alcoholic hepatitis	Alcohol use, nausea, vomiting, abdominal pain, fever
Primary or metastatic hepatic tumor	Weight loss, abdominal pain, fever, jaundice
Pancreatitis	Nausea, vomiting, abdominal pain, weight loss, steatorrhea
Hepatotoxic drug	Medication use, nausea, vomiting, jaundice
Viral hepatitis	Anorexia, vomiting, fatigue, myalgias, headache, fever, jaundice
Infectious mononucleosis	Headache, fatigue, fever, sore throat, adenopathy
Sarcoidosis	Fever, weight loss, dyspnea, cough, pruritus
Amyloidosis	History of multiple myeloma, rheumatoid arthritis, tuberculosis, or osteomyelitis
Severe cirrhosis	Jaundice, edema, abdominal distention, bleeding
Skeletal Diseases	
Paget's disease	Backache, bone pain, increased hat size, bone swelling, headache
Osteomalacia	History of gastrectomy, anticonvulsant use, renal failure, antacid abuse
Primary hyperparathyroidism	Kidney stones, muscle weakness, duodenal ulcer
Primary or metastatic tumor	Bone pain, bone swelling
Other Diseases	
Congestive heart failure	Edema, fatigue, dyspnea, orthopnea
Breast cancer with metastases	Nipple discharge, breast lump, bone pain
Lymphoma/leukemia	Fatigue, weight loss, bone pain, night sweats, abdominal fullness
Lung cancer with metastases	Smoking history, cough, dyspnea, weight loss
Renal carcinoma	Hematuria, flank pain, weight loss, fatigue
Prostatic cancer	Back pain, nocturia, bone pain, weak urinary stream
Renal failure	Prior history of renal failure
Hyperthyroidism	Weight loss, nervousness, tremor, diarrhea, heat intolerance
Diabetes mellitus	Prior history of diabetes mellitus

struction have normal ALP values. Likewise, patients with either acute or chronic cholecystitis have normal serum ALP values unless there is accompanying obstruction.

Skeletal Disorders

The serum alkline phosphatase level is elevated in disorders in which there is increased osteoblastic activity, i.e., new bone formation. Paget's disease is the prototype illness in which new bone is formed, and 90 per cent of patients with this disease have elevated ALP values. In Paget's disease, the ALP elevation parallels the urinary hydroxyproline excretion and also the radiographic findings of the disease. Some patients may have normal ALP values, but most patients with active disease have values elevated to 3–20 × URL.

Osteomalacia is another skeletal disease associated with an elevated ALP value. This disease is due to the failure to calcify bone, which results in uncalcified osteoid. For poorly understood reasons, osteomalacia is accompanied by an increase in osteoblastic activity and therefore an ALP elevation. Osteomalacia is found in particular clinical settings, such as in phosphate depletion from abuse of antacids containing aluminum hydroxide, following gastrectomy, after long-term anticonvulsant use, with renal failure, and with vitamin D deficiency. Some patients with osteomalacia have elevated ALP values, but many do not. This measurement is therefore a poor screening tool for osteomalacia in patients with pre-existing risk factors for the disease. It is important to note that patients with osteoporosis generally have normal or only mildly elevated ALP values.

Primary hyperparathyroidism may result in an elevated ALP, but most patients have values within the normal range. Those patients with an elevated ALP also are found to have radiographic evidence of parathyroid osteopathy.

Benign bony tumors such as chondromas and osteomas are associated with normal ALP levels. Some patients with osteogenic sarcomas have ALP elevations, and this subgroup has a worse prognosis than those patients whose ALP values are normal. Malignancies with skeletal metastases may result in ALP elevations, but the test is much less sensitive than a bone scan for detection of metastases.

Fractures uncommonly produce minimal and transient elevations in ALP value.

Other Diseases

Congestive Heart Failure. Ten to 46 per cent of patients with congestive heart failure have a mild elevation of ALP.[8] Rarely greater than 2 × URL, the elevation is believed to be due to passive congestion of the liver.

Breast Cancer. Elevations of ALP in patients with breast carcinoma are most likely due to hepatic or skeletal metastases. Rarely, the cancer itself may produce an ALP isoenzyme that is electrophoretically distinct from the usual ALP isoenzymes.

Lymphoma/Leukemia. ALP values have been reported to be elevated in these two diseases. Both skeletal and liver infiltration by the tumor may be the cause.

Lung Cancer. Most patients with carcinoma of the lung have normal ALP values. Elevations are likely to be due to hepatic or skeletal metastases.

Hypernephroma. The patients with a kidney tumor may have an elevated ALP, which is believed to be due to ectopic ALP production by the tumor.

Renal Failure. Most patients with end-stage renal disease have normal ALP values. An elevated value usually represents azotemic osteodystrophy.

Prostatic Cancer. A high percentage of patients with prostatic carcinoma and skeletal metastases have ALP elevations. The ALP value may be elevated before the acid phosphatase value in metastatic disease.

Hyperthyroidism. Thirty per cent of patients with hyperthyroidism have elevated ALP values.[8] The increase usually represents an increase in the skeletal ALP isoenzyme.

Diabetes Mellitus. Some studies have indicated a mild elevation in the serum ALP in diabetic populations, which is probably due to diabetes-related liver disease.

HISTORY

As previously noted, the majority of patients with elevated ALP values have no history of the abnormality and no obvious clinical cause. Elicitation of patient history should be directed specifically at those disorders that have been associated with hyperphosphatasemia (see Table 2).

PHYSICAL EXAMINATION

Uncovering the reason for an elevated alkaline phosphatase value in a "routine" physical examination is unusual. It is therefore important during the examination to look carefully for clinical signs of those diseases that result in ALP elevations. These findings are listed in Table 3.

Table 3. CLINICAL FINDINGS IN DISEASES LIKELY TO CAUSE ALP ELEVATION

Region or Aspect Examined	Sign(s) of Disease
General	Fever, lymphadenopathy
Eyes	Pale conjunctiva, exophthalmos, diabetic retinopathy
Neck	Thyroid nodule, thyroid enlargement, jugular venous distention
Mouth	Tonsil exudate, palatine petechiae
Chest	Gynecomastia, breast mass, breast dimpling
Lungs	Rales, effusion
Heart	Cardiomegaly, gallop rhythm
Abdomen	Right upper quadrant tenderness, palpable gallbladder, hepatomegaly, splenomegaly, liver edge tenderness, ascites, liver friction rub, flank mass
Rectal area	Prostate nodule
Extremities	Edema, clubbing, tremor, bone tenderness
Neurologic	Hyperreflexia, tremor, neuropathy
Skin	Jaundice, spider angiomas, palmar erythema, xanthomas, loss of body hair, hyperpigmentation

ASSESSMENT

The most common setting in which the clinician encounters an elevated alkaline phosphatase level is its unexpected discovery in a routine biochemical screening panel. The patient may have had such testing as a part of an annual examination or because of a specific but unrelated clinical problem. The ALP determination is often included because of its potential for identifying unsuspected hepatic or skeletal disease, but it has marked limitations as a screening tool, for several reasons. First, it is not at all *specific* for any particular disease. The clinician is therefore faced with the problem of where to turn next to evaluate an elevated ALP. Second, the test is not at all *sensitive* in identifying all of the patients with any single disease. As discussed previously, many of the patients with those diseases most commonly associated with ALP elevations have normal serum alkaline phosphatase levels. Finally, the diseases most strongly associated with an elevated ALP value have low incidences in the general population.

These factors have led many physicians to ignore the unexpected finding of a mildly elevated ALP value, dismissing it as "a laboratory error," "borderline normal," or "clinically insignificant." In one study of elevated ALP values on screening panels, 52 per cent of the elevated levels were interpreted to be "normal" by the attending physician, and 20 per cent received no comments at all in the patient's chart; only 28 per cent were noted to be abnormal.[11] Of those noted to be abnormal, one-third were accorded no explanation in chart notes and no further testing, one-third had an explanation noted on the chart, and one-third prompted a repeat determination. Of the 118 elevated ALP values examined in this study, only one led to a new diagnosis, that of viral hepatitis. In a second study of similar design, 42 per cent of the elevated ALP values were interpreted as clinically insignificant, 32 per cent had no chart explanation, 17 per cent were not noted on the chart, 9 per cent prompted repeat determinations that were normal, and 4 per cent prompted repeat determinations that were elevated.[12] In this study, the degree of ALP elevation appeared to have no bearing on physician response.

The usual physician response to an elevated ALP value on routine screening seems to be to arbitrarily discount it. Can we use this information more effectively? A series of guidelines are suggested in the algorithm. These steps must be individualized for each patient on the basis of the clinician's knowledge of the patient and those diseases for which the patient is at greatest risk.

The first step is to decide whether the patient falls into a group for whom the adult reference range is inappropriate. Women who are younger than 20 years, are pregnant, or have given birth a month or less before, and men younger than 30 years may have ALP values higher than the upper reference limits for healthy adults.

The second step is to review any medications that the patient is taking. More than 200 drugs have been associated with ALP elevations (see Table 1). The *Physician's Desk Reference* is a handy starting point for such a review. If one of the medications the patient is taking has been implicated in ALP elevation, a drug-free trial period can be helpful in proving the association. A drug that appears to elevate the ALP in a particular patient should probably be discontinued because of the risk of liver damage.

The third step is to review the patient's history and physical findings, particular attention being paid to those signs and symptoms described earlier in the chapter. If an adequate explanation cannot be found through review of the chart, the patient should return to the office for further questioning and examination. The right question or physical finding may save the patient further testing or alternatively may point to an important, previously missed diagnosis.

The other laboratory values on the original screening panel should be carefully examined. Were any of the other liver function tests elevated? Was the calcium level elevated? Do the BUN and creatinine values indicate renal impairment? Is the thyroxine level elevated? The test values that fall just within the reference ranges may no longer be considered "normal" in light of the elevated ALP value.

It is also important to consider the degree of elevation. The higher the value, the more significant it is likely to be. A value of 3 × URL usually represents disease, even if it is as yet asymptomatic.

Elevated ALP values between 1 and 1.5 × URL are common and in most cases do not indicate disease. If a single value falls in this mildly elevated range, the next step would be to repeat the determination. The patient should be fasting for the repeat test, and the person who draws the blood should be sure not to leave the tourniquet on for longer than 30 seconds before taking the sample. If the second value is within the reference range and the patient is asymptomatic, no further testing is usually indicated. If the second test value falls in the 1–1.5 × URL range, it is usually sufficient to repeat the test again at a later time to follow the trend. One should be sure to enter "Elevated ALP, cause undetermined" on the problem list in the patient's chart. It is inappropriate to discount the test results as "clinically insignificant" when the clinical significance is as yet unknown.

If the original ALP value is higher than 1.5 × URL with no explanation, further testing is in order. The ALP determination should be repeated with the patient fasting. At the same time, either ALP isoenzymes or GGT should be measured to determine which ALP fraction is elevated (skeletal or biliary). In particular patients, other blood work may be indicated, such as a slide test for infectious mononucleosis (Monospot), viral hepatitis studies, thyroid function tests, amylase determination, complete blood count, and calcium or phosphate measurements.

If the blood work results indicate an elevation in the hepatic fraction of the ALP, the next step is to visualize the hepatobiliary system. Ultrasonography, computerized tomography, or radionuclide scanning can be used. Each of these imaging techniques has its own advantages and should be chosen with the particular clinical situation in mind.

If the blood work results indicate an elevation in the skeletal fraction of the ALP, only a few diseases are likely to be the cause. Radiographs of the pelvis and femur often show the changes associated with Paget's disease or osteomalacia. Likewise, the urinary excretion of hydroxyproline is elevated in these two diseases. Metastatic bone disease is best visualized using a bone scan. Hyperparathyroidism is diagnosed by means of parathyroid hormone immunoassay.

An orderly approach to evaluating an elevated ALP has three desirable results: the few patients with disease will be distinguished from the large number who are normal; the patients at little risk for skeletal or biliary disease will be spared unnecessary testing; and the clinician will benefit from having carefully thought through a clinical

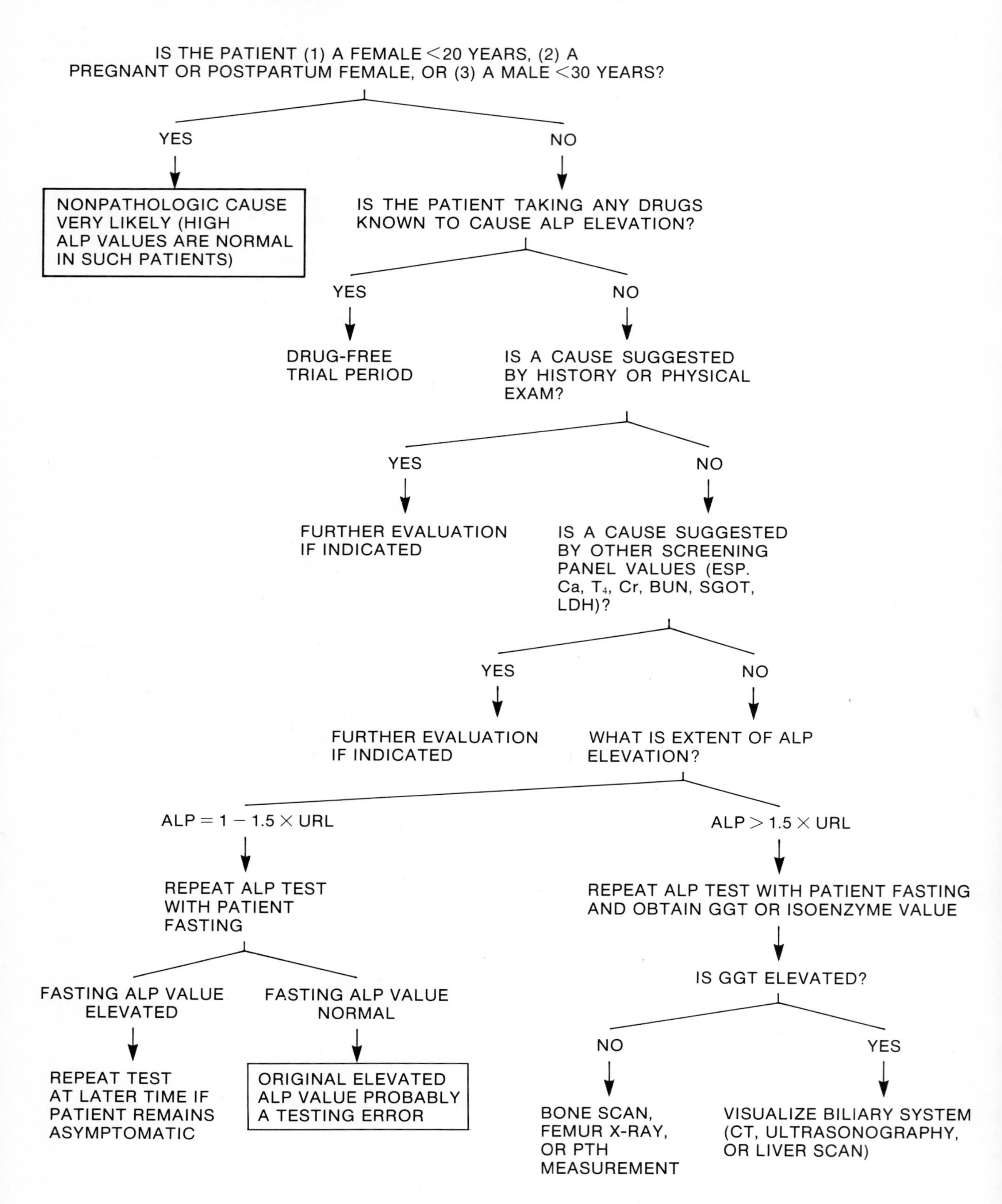

DIAGNOSTIC ASSESSMENT OF UNEXPECTEDLY ELEVATED ALP VALUE
IS THE PATIENT (1) A FEMALE <20 YEARS, (2) A PREGNANT OR POSTPARTUM FEMALE, OR (3) A MALE <30 YEARS?
YES
NO
NONPATHOLOGIC CAUSE VERY LIKELY (HIGH ALP VALUES ARE NORMAL IN SUCH PATIENTS)
IS THE PATIENT TAKING ANY DRUGS KNOWN TO CAUSE ALP ELEVATION?
YES
NO
DRUG-FREE TRIAL PERIOD
IS A CAUSE SUGGESTED BY HISTORY OR PHYSICAL EXAM?
YES
NO
FURTHER EVALUATION IF INDICATED
IS A CAUSE SUGGESTED BY OTHER SCREENING PANEL VALUES (ESP. Ca, T4, Cr, BUN, SGOT, LDH)?
YES
NO
FURTHER EVALUATION IF INDICATED
WHAT IS EXTENT OF ALP ELEVATION?
ALP = 1 − 1.5 × URL
ALP > 1.5 × URL
REPEAT ALP TEST WITH PATIENT FASTING
REPEAT ALP TEST WITH PATIENT FASTING AND OBTAIN GGT OR ISOENZYME VALUE
FASTING ALP VALUE ELEVATED
FASTING ALP VALUE NORMAL
IS GGT ELEVATED?
REPEAT TEST AT LATER TIME IF PATIENT REMAINS ASYMPTOMATIC
ORIGINAL ELEVATED ALP VALUE PROBABLY A TESTING ERROR
NO
YES
BONE SCAN, FEMUR X-RAY, OR PTH MEASUREMENT
VISUALIZE BILIARY SYSTEM (CT, ULTRASONOGRAPHY, OR LIVER SCAN)

problem rather than arbitrarily discounting an unexpectedly abnormal test result.

REFERENCES

1. Friedman GD, Goldberg M, Ajuha JN, Siegelaub AB, Bassis ML, Collen MI. Biochemical screening tests—effect of panel size on medical care. Arch Intern Med 1972;91–7.
2. Bates B, Yellin JA. The yield of multiphasic screening. JAMA 1972;222:74–8.
3. McNeely MD. Liver function. In: Sonnenwirth AC, Jarett L, eds. Gradwohl's clinical laboratory methods and diagnostics. 8th ed. St. Louis: C. V. Mosby, 1980;537–51.
4. Wolf PL. Interpretation of increased and decreased serum alkaline phosphatase. In: Griffiths JC, ed. Clinical enzymology. New York: Masson, 1979;111–21.
5. Posen S, Doherty E. Serum alkaline phosphatase in clinical medicine. Adv Clin Chem 1981;22:163–245.
6. Tietz NW. Alkaline phosphatase: general comments. In: Griffiths JC, ed. Clinical enzymology. New York: Masson, 1979;69–79.
7. Ladenson JH. Nonanalytical sources of variation in clinical chemistry results. In: Sonnenwirth AC, Jarett L, eds. Gradwohl's clinical laboratory methods and diagnostics. 8th ed. St. Louis: C. V. Mosby, 1980;149–92.
8. McComb RB, Bowers GN, Posen S. Alkaline phosphatase. New York: Plenum, 1979;525–786.
9. Kampmann JP, Sinding J, Moller-Jorgensen I. Effect of age on liver function. Geriatrics 1975;30(8):91–5.
10. Hodkinson HM, McPherson CK. Alkaline phosphatase in a geriatric inpatient population. Age Ageing 1973;2:28–33.
11. Amberg JM, Schneiderman LJ, Berry CC, Zettner A. The abnormal outpatient chemical panel serum alkaline phosphatase: analysis of physician response, outcome, cost and health effectiveness. J Chron Dis 1982;35:81–8.
12. Schneiderman LJ, DeSalvo L, Baylor S, Wolf PL. The "abnormal" screening laboratory result—its effects on physician and patient. Arch Intern Med 1972;129:88–90.

AMENORRHEA

KAY F. McFARLAND

□ SYNONYM: Absence of menses

BACKGROUND

Definition and Origins

Menstruation is the spontaneous, periodic shedding of the outer one-third of the mucosa that lines the uterine cavity. The monthly cycle of growth and breakdown of the endometrium is regulated by complex mechanisms involving hypothalamic releasing hormones, pituitary gonadotropins, and ovarian hormones.[1] An abnormality at any level—the hypothalamus, pituitary, ovary, uterus or outflow tract—may be responsible for abnormalities of menstruation and for amenorrhea.

In ovulatory menstrual cycles, vaginal bleeding usually occurs every 24 to 35 days and lasts 2 to 8 days. However, anovulatory cycles with long intervals between periods are so frequent after menarche,[2] in the perimenopausal years, and even during the mid-reproductive years that bleeding must be absent for 3 months before the term amenorrhea is used. The absence of menses for three or more normal cycle lengths in a woman who previously menstruated is called secondary amenorrhea. The term primary amenorrhea refers to the failure of menses to begin by age 16 or simply the absence of menses in a woman who has never menstruated.

Although amenorrhea is often physiologic, e.g., due to pregnancy, the absence of menses may be a sign of female reproductive dysfunction and, thus, deserves careful evaluation. If a systematic plan is followed, the cause of amenorrhea usually can be determined quickly and economically. In most instances, only two or three office visits and less than a half a dozen tests and procedures are needed to establish the etiology.

Incidence

Amenorrhea is listed as the 94th most common problem encountered by family physicians.[3] However, it is of greater significance than this rank might indicate, because absence of menses is of concern only to a subgroup of the general population, specifically women between ages 16 and 40. The magnitude of the problem is considerable in light of one report that infrequency or absence of menses was the chief complaint in 11 per cent of college students seen in a university health center.[4] In another study, the 1-year incidence rate of secondary amenorrhea in young women was estimated to be 3.3 per cent.[5]

Causes

There are a number of ways to classify amenorrhea. In order to provide a systematic approach to the evaluation of a patient with primary or secondary amenorrhea, three major categories of amenorrhea should be considered.[6] *Physiologic* causes should be dealt with first. If they are not present, then *anatomic* abnormalities should be excluded. Finally, *genetic and endocrinologic* causes should be considered.

Physiologic Causes

Physiologic Delay. Breast buds and pubic hair, the first signs of maturation, tend to appear around age 11½ and to precede menses by 1 year or so.[7] A growth spurt occurs at the same time that breast buds appear, and maximum linear growth per unit time precedes menses by about 6 months. In the United States, the mean age of menarche is 12½ to 13 years. Growth slows markedly after the onset of menses, and most young women grow less than 4 inches after menarche.[8] Although the ages of development of the secondary sex characteristics and menarche vary considerably, the range can be estimated by adding or subtracting 3 years from the mean. A delay in the onset of puberty is indicated by the absence of breast development and pubic hair by age 14, the failure to menstruate by age 16, or the failure to begin menses within 3 years after breast buds appear.

There is considerable evidence that body weight has a significant influence on the timing of puberty and menarche.[9] Most young women are at or above the 10th percentile in weight for their height[10] or weigh more than 90 lb when menses begin. Heavy girls, who obtain this critical weight at a younger age, menstruate earlier than thin girls. Improved nutrition and an increase in the average weight of young women may be responsible for the decrease in the mean age of menarche that has been observed in many industrialized countries during the last decade.[11]

Pregnancy and Lactation. Pregnancy is the most common cause of secondary amenorrhea and may cause primary amenorrhea as well. Most women resume menses 2 months after giving birth, and 90 per cent of nonlactating women have a return to menses within 3 months of delivery. On the other hand, amenorrhea often persists for 10 months or longer in women who breast-feed their infants.[12] Because the duration of amenorrhea during lactation can be quite variable, the absence of menses in a woman who is nursing should be considered physiologic.

Menopause. The age range for the normal occurrence of menopause is considerably greater than that of menarche. The mean age of menopause is around 50 years, but spontaneous cessation of menses may occur 10 years earlier or later. Amenorrhea after the age of 40 usually is physiologic.

Anatomic Causes

Anatomic abnormalities without associated genetic or endocrine disorders are rare causes of amenorrhea. Those that may cause primary amenorrhea include imperforate hymen, labial fusion, transverse vaginal septum, and vaginal agenesis.[13] Secondary amenorrhea may result from destruction of the endometrium by an infection such as tuberculosis or, more frequently, from a curettage following delivery or an abortion. If the endometrium fails to regenerate, amenorrhea ensues, and intrauterine scarring may occur with formation of synechiae that obliterate the uterine cavity (Asherman's syndrome).

Genetic and Endocrinologic Causes

Hypothalamic Disorders. Nearly one-fourth of cases of amenorrhea may be related to weight loss or a low percentage of body fat.[14] Amenorrhea that occurs with weight loss is thought to be due to hypothalamic dysfunction, although the exact mechanism is not clear. Usually, weight loss precedes the cessation of menses, but there have been documented reports of amenorrhea occurring before weight loss in patients who subsequently developed anorexia nervosa. Amenorrhea associated with exercise and chronic disease also may be related to the effect of low body weight on the hypothalamus. Hypothalamic pituitary function also may be altered in women who are extremely obese. Anovulation causing oligomenorrhea and occasionally amenorrhea may occur with marked obesity. In some of these women, restoration of menses may follow weight loss.

A number of other hypothalamic disorders cause amenorrhea. For example, systemic diseases such as sarcoidosis may involve the hypothalamus and produce amenorrhea. In addition, isolated gonadotropin deficiency, often a result of deficiency or absence of gonadotropin-releasing hormone secretion, is another rare cause. Both LH and FSH may be deficient, or only one of the gonadotropins may be involved. Stress, which has also been implicated as the cause of amenorrhea, may be related to changes in hypothalamic function. It is thought that hypothalamic mechanisms are involved in many cases of amenorrhea for which no cause can be found.[15]

Pituitary Disorders. Elevated prolactin levels occur in 15 to 20 per cent of women with amenorrhea and may be found in association with pituitary tumors of all sizes as well as in patients without a demonstrable tumor. The percentage of patients with hyperprolactinemia and amenorrhea who have pituitary tumors differs in various series, ranging from 25 to 75 per cent.[16, 17] Other lesions that cause amenorrhea by damaging the hypothalamic pituitary connections or by directly affecting the pituitary include postpartum pituitary necrosis, craniopharyngioma,[18] and the empty sella syndrome.[19]

Gonadal Dysfunction. Ovarian dysfunction resulting in either low or high estrogen and androgen levels may cause amenorrhea. In ovarian dysgenesis, estrogen production is so low that the secondary sex characteristics fail to develop, the uterine endometrium is not stimulated, and menarche does not occur. Gonadal dysgenesis often is associated with a 45,X karyotype, but may be found with a normal 46,XX pattern and with a number of other chromosome karyotypes, including 45,X/46,XX; 45,X/46,X,i(Xq); and 46,XY.[20]

Menstrual irregularities, including amenorrhea, frequently are found in patients with polycystic ovarian disease (Stein-Leventhal syndrome).[21] Anovulation is common and may be due to the effect of the ovarian hormones estrogen and androgen on the hypothalamus-pituitary regulation of the gonadotropins. Prolactin levels are elevated in up to 25 per cent of patients with this disorder.

Patients with the genetic disorder testicular feminization often present with a chief complaint of amenorrhea. Although the genotype is 46,XY and testosterone levels are in the male range, phenotypically these patients are unmistakably female. The feminization is due to androgen insensitivity, which is most commonly caused by deficiency of an intracellular receptor protein specific for testosterone and dihydrotestosterone.

Adrenal Disorders. Primary and secondary amenorrhea rarely may be caused by adrenal disease. Women who have deficiency of the 17-hydroxylase enzyme do not produce normal levels of estrogen and, therefore, do not develop secondary sex characteristics or menstruate. Those with congenital adrenal hyperplasia due to deficiency of either the 21- or 11-beta-hydroxylase enzyme may present with amenorrhea and hirsutism due to androgen excess. Amenorrhea may also be a presenting symptom in patients with Cushing's syndrome.

Thyroid Disorders. Hypothyroidism may be associated with abnormalities in menstruation.[22] Irregular heavy bleeding is more common than prolonged amenorrhea in patients with primary thyroid failure. Absence of menses is more frequently seen in those with hypothyroidism due to pituitary failure.

Drugs

There are a number of ways that drugs can cause amenorrhea. Phenothiazines, tricyclic antidepressants, and many of the centrally acting antihypertensive medications such as reserpine and methyldopa cause amenorrhea through their effect on hypothalamic function. Chemotherapeutic agents, such as cyclophosphamide, may cause ovarian failure and thereby amenorrhea.

Oral contraceptives with a low estrogen content may produce amenorrhea, owing to inadequate stimulation of the endometrium. Whereas most patients elect to switch or stop oral contraceptives when amenorrhea occurs, those who decide to continue may have absence of menses as long as they take the low-estrogen pills. Also, there are numerous reports of amenorrhea occurring after discontinuation of oral contraceptive pills.[23, 24] The real significance of post-pill amenorrhea is difficult to determine, because most studies have not had a control group and some controlled studies have failed to demonstrate a statistical relationship between the use of the pill and subsequent amenorrhea.[25]

HISTORY

General. The emphasis of the history varies somewhat depending on whether or not the patient has ever menstruated. For example, in primary amenorrhea, the initial questioning centers on the patient's growth pattern and the time of attainment of each stage of development. Reviewing a growth chart is helpful, because maximum linear growth usually precedes menarche by about 6 months and most girls grow 5 to 9 cm during the year preceding menarche.

In secondary amenorrhea, the previous menstrual history is of prime importance. The age of onset of menses, the cycle length, the duration and amount of flow, and the exact date of the last menstrual period should be noted. The obstetric history, especially the date of the patient's last delivery, and whether or not and for how long lactation persisted should be recorded. Whether or not the patient has had an abortion or curettage also may be significant.

The next questioning generally centers on the most likely causes of amenorrhea, which include pregnancy, hypothalamic-pituitary dysfunction related to weight change, and drugs. The type of birth control used should be recorded, and questions should be asked regarding early symptoms of pregnancy, such as the presence of tenderness or enlargement of the breasts, nausea, and increased facial pigmentation. Patients with primary amenorrhea who have normal breast development are asked these same questions, as one can assume by the presence of breast development that the ovary is producing estrogen and that pregnancy is possible.

Changes in weight and a patient's exercise pro-

Table 1. PHYSICAL FINDINGS AND THEIR SIGNIFICANCE IN AMENORRHEA

Aspect of Examination	Finding	Suggested or Associated Disorder(s)
Height	Less than 58 in.	Turner's syndrome
Weight	Lower than 10th percentile for height	Hypothalamic dysfunction
Blood pressure	Elevated	Congenital adrenal hyperplasia, Cushing's syndrome, Turner's syndrome
Skin	Pale or sallow	Hypothyroidism, renal failure
	Dry and thick	Hypothyroidism
Breasts	No development	Absence or greatly diminished levels of estrogen
	Galactorrhea	Hyperprolactinemia
Pubic hair	Absent	Testicular feminization, pituitary failure
	Sparse	Turner's syndrome, pituitary failure
	Male or diamond-shaped distribution	Polycystic ovarian disease, congenital adrenal hyperplasia, other adrenal disorder
Pelvic exam	Vagina not visualized	Labial fusion, vaginal agenesis, intact hymen
	Clitoris large	Increased androgen levels
	Cervix not visualized	Uterine agenesis, transverse vaginal septum
	Cervix bluish red	Pregnancy
	Uterus enlarged	Pregnancy
Reflexes	Slow relaxation phase	Hypothyroidism

gram may be significant. Athletes who have a relatively low percentage of body fat frequently have irregular menses or amenorrhea. For example, ballet dancers, who tend to be extremely thin and exercise vigorously, are prone to delayed menarche as well as secondary amenorrhea.[26] Amenorrhea is more common in athletes who have a history of menstrual dysfunction or delayed menarche and in those who are nulliparous, young, and under stress.[27] Menses frequently will return with an increase in weight or a decrease in exercise.[28]

Other questions asked to exclude concurrent illness or to establish the etiology of amenorrhea should concern a change in heat or cold tolerance, change in the hair, nails or skin, or mental or physical "slowing up" (hypothyroidism), fullness or swelling of the face (hypothyroidism, Cushing's disease), inability to concentrate (hypothyroidism), headaches (pituitary tumor), change in sense of smell (hypogonadotropic hypogonadism, Kallmann's syndrome), abdominal cramps (imperforate hymen), and hot flashes (menopause).

Family History. It is often assumed that a family history is important in assessing the likelihood of delayed menarche in a young woman. In fact, however, it does not significantly influence the evaluation. Nevertheless, it is usually noted for completeness, as there is a correlation in age of menarche between mother and daughters. This correlation may be related to the pattern of body weight within families as much as or more than to other genetic or inherited factors that could affect the timing of puberty.

Social History. Irregularity of menses and, occasionally, amenorrhea are associated with stress. Again, this association may be quite closely related to weight loss.

Previous Medical History. Patients should be asked if they have had sarcoidosis, as this disorder may directly involve the hypothalamus, producing deficiencies in gonadotropin-releasing hormones and other releasing hormones. Other chronic medical disorders should be noted, because the weight loss associated with chronic disease may cause hypothalamic dysfunction and amenorrhea. Interestingly, a history of paralytic poliomyelitis and migraine has been associated with delayed menarche. Oophorectomy and ovarian irradiation are such obvious causes of amenorrhea that although these should be noted, it is unlikely that a patient who has had significant pelvic irradiation or surgery would present with a complaint of amenorrhea without already realizing that these factors are responsible for the lack of menstruation.

High-Payoff Queries

The following questions are especially likely to elicit valuable historical data:

1. *Do you think you are pregnant? What kind of birth control method do you use?* Pregnancy should be considered a possibility on the initial visit and every time a patient is seen subsequently. It is the most common cause of amenorrhea.
2. *Have you gained or lost weight lately? If so, how much?* Weight loss, especially with vigorous exercise, is a very common cause of amenorrhea. Excessive body weight also has been associated with amenorrhea.
3. *Do you have any milk or other discharge from your breasts?* Galactorrhea secondary to increased prolactin may be associated with a pituitary adenoma or drug use, or may occur without a known cause.
4. *What medications are you taking? Did you take any medications the month that your menses stopped? If so, which ones?* Phenothiazines, antihypertensives, oral contraceptives, and intramuscular progester-

one are commonly used drugs that can produce menstrual irregularity or amenorrhea.

5. *Have you noticed any increase in body hair?* A positive response suggests the possibility of ovarian or adrenal disease.

6. In primary amenorrhea, one should ask: *At what age did you develop breast buds, pubic hair, and underarm hair, and grow especially rapidly?* Development of secondary sex characteristics increases the likelihood that the cause of primary amenorrhea involves a system other than the ovaries, although the appearance of secondary sex characteristics does not exclude a primary ovarian abnormality.

PHYSICAL EXAMINATION

The physical examination should determine if there is an anatomic cause for the amenorrhea, should establish the stage of development of the secondary sexual characteristics in patients with primary amenorrhea, and may give a clue to an underlying genetic or systemic process causing amenorrhea.

Physical findings and their significance are listed in Table 1.

ASSESSMENT AND DIAGNOSTIC APPROACH

The clinical features that are most helpful in diagnosing and assessing the disorders that cause amenorrhea are described in Table 2.

The diagnostic approaches to the evaluation of primary and secondary amenorrhea are shown step-by-step in the algorithms. Actually, the evaluations of primary and secondary amenorrhea are similar, with just a little shift in emphasis. For example, in those with primary amenorrhea, it is important to assess the level of endogenous estrogen secretion by means of the history and physical examination. This determination is based primarily on the degree of breast development, the amount of pubic hair, and the growth pattern. In patients with normal sexual development, special attention is given to looking for signs of early pregnancy and hyperprolactinemia, the common causes of secondary amenorrhea. A serum pregnancy test will be needed to exclude early pregnancy; the urine slide test for pregnancy may not be positive until 4 or more weeks after fertilization and therefore cannot be relied on for early diagnosis.

On physical examination, if the cervix is visualized, most of the anatomic causes of amenorrhea can be excluded. Withdrawal bleeding after a course of progesterone or estrogen plus progesterone verifies that the endometrium is intact and responsive to hormonal stimulation. Bleeding after a course of progesterone alone indicates that estrogen levels are adequate to stimulate endometrial growth and that the problem is anovulation. If bleeding occurs only after estrogen has been added to progesterone, the amenorrhea is due to endogenous estrogen deficiency. Low or normal levels of FSH and LH in a patient with low endogenous estrogen secretion indicate that the problem is pituitary-hypothalamic dysfunction. High FSH and LH levels, on the other hand, indicate that the estrogen deficiency is related to ovarian failure.

The most common laboratory tests used to evaluate amenorrhea are prolactin, serum thyroxine (T_4), T_3 uptake, and the free thyroxine index (FTI). If the results are normal, a karyotype and FSH and LH determinations generally are the only other tests needed to establish a diagnosis. A TSH measurement is ordered if the T_4 is low, and tomograms or computerized tomography scan of the sella may be needed if the prolactin is elevated. Already in some medical centers, CT scanning has replaced tomography for evaluation of the sella,[29] and it will be more widely used in the future. If only the size of the sella is in question, a coned-down radiograph of the sella may be used as a screening test in lieu of tomography or CT scanning, in order to avoid the high doses of radiation to the eyes in tomography and to reduce the cost of evaluation. The tests used to assess amenorrhea and their specific indications are shown in Table 3.

Basically, the evaluation of primary and secondary amenorrhea involves only a few steps. If the history and physical examination do not reveal the cause of amenorrhea, then pregnancy must be excluded, usually with the use of a pregnancy test. If a diagnosis is not established with this procedure, a T_4, T_3 uptake, and prolactin measurements are made. Depending on whether the results are normal or not, a lateral coned-down view, CT scan, or tomograms of the sella are ordered. TSH, LH, and FSH determinations and diagnostic trial of progesterone or progesterone plus estrogen may be needed in some cases. Occasionally a karyotype will be diagnostic. Procedures should be done systematically, excluding physiologic, anatomic, and endocrine-genetic causes. Even with careful evaluation, a definite cause is not found in as many as 15 per cent of patients with secondary amenorrhea.[15]

Implications of Amenorrhea

Fortunately, amenorrhea is not a life-threatening disorder. Generally the causes of primary amenorrhea are more serious than those of secondary amenorrhea, because the absence of menses at age 16 increases the possibility of a genetic or endo-

Table 2. COMMON CAUSES OF AMENORRHEA

Cause	Clinical and Laboratory Features
Physiologic	
Delayed menarche	Age ≥16 years or no menses 3 years after breast development is noted Weight below 10th percentile for height Pregnancy test result negative Prolactin, FTI, FSH, LH, coned-down view of sella, and karyotype all normal
Pregnancy	No birth control method used; nausea, vomiting, excessive fatigue, breast tenderness Uterus enlarged, soft, pulsatile; cervix bluish red; pigmentation of face Pregnancy test result positive
Lactation	Nursing or recent pregnancy Galactorrhea No laboratory tests needed
Menopause	Age usually >40 years; hot flashes, inability to sleep, emotional lability Dryness of vaginal vault ↑ FSH and LH
Anatomic	
Genital tract obstruction	Diagnosed on physical examination
Failure of development of vagina/uterus	Diagnosed on physical examination
Endometrial destruction	History of curettage, especially following an abortion or delivery; history of tuberculosis; no withdrawal bleeding after course of estrogen plus progesterone FSH, LH levels normal
Genetic or Endocrinologic	
Turner's syndrome	Height 58 in. or less, lack of breast development, sparse pubic hair, low hairline, webbed neck, broad chest with widely spaced nipples, short fourth metacarpal, decreased hearing, low-set ears, multiple nevi, high arched palate, strabismus, absence of femoral pulses, cubitus valgus Karyotype 45,X
Gonadal dysgenesis with normal karyotype	Prepubertal; no somatic abnormalities Karyotype 46,XX
Testicular feminization	Often tall stature, normal breast development, absence of pubic hair and uterus, occasionally mass in inguinal canal (testes) Testosterone in male range Karyotype 46,XY
Ovarian failure	Hot flashes ↑ FSH and LH
Polycystic ovarian disease	Hirsutism, male pattern escutcheon, obesity Ovaries enlarged
Pituitary tumor	If tumor develops before puberty: Short stature, lack of development of secondary sex characteristics, appearance younger than chronologic age If tumor develops after puberty: sparse pubic hair, abnormal sella on x-ray or CT scan, visual field defect ↓ FSH, LH, T_3, FTI, TSH, and GH; ↑ prolactin
Postpartum pituitary necrosis	History of intrapartum hemorrhage, hypotension, failure to lactate postpartum Sparse pubic hair, clinical signs of hypothyroidism, ↓ FSH, LH, T_3, FTI, TSH, GH, and prolactin Sella x-rays or CT scan normal
Empty sella syndrome	Obese, multiparous Sella x-rays and CT scan abnormal
Hyperprolactinemia	Galactorrhea Sella CT scan and x-rays normal or abnormal
Other hypothalamic causes	History of weight loss; vigorous exercise; sarcoidosis Other clinical findings of sarcoidosis
Hypothyroidism, primary	Mental and physical slowness, cold intolerance, constipation, sallow appearance, dry, thick skin, slow reflexes, goiter, facial fullness in cheek area, periorbital edema ↓ T_4, T_3 uptake, and FTI; ↑ TSH
Congenital adrenal hyperplasia (21- or 11-B-hyroxylase deficiency)	Hirsutism, normal or ↑ BP, enlarged clitoris, muscular physique, short adult stature ↑ 17-ketosteroids, and pregnanetriol; suppression 17-ketosteroids by glucocorticoids
Cushing's syndrome	Depression, weakness, ↑ BP, moon facies, truncal obesity, acne, striae, purpura, thin skin, buffalo hump, hirsutism Abnormal GTT, failure to suppress plasma cortisol with dexamethasone, 0.5 mg q6h x 8 doses
Drugs	History of recent use of oral contraceptives, phenothiazines, antihypertensives, progesterone, chemotherapeutic agents

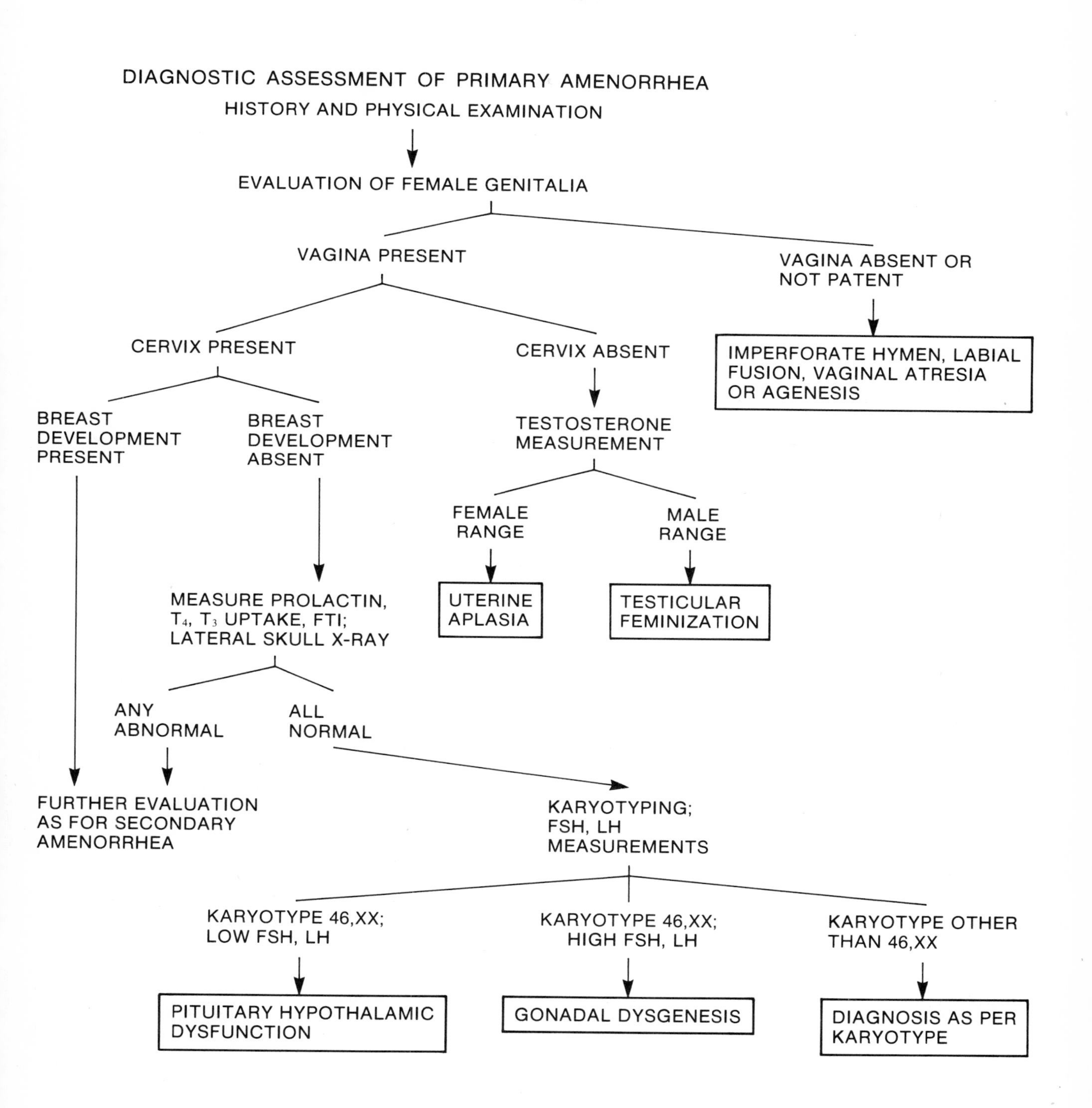
DIAGNOSTIC ASSESSMENT OF PRIMARY AMENORRHEA
HISTORY AND PHYSICAL EXAMINATION
EVALUATION OF FEMALE GENITALIA
VAGINA PRESENT
VAGINA ABSENT OR NOT PATENT
IMPERFORATE HYMEN, LABIAL FUSION, VAGINAL ATRESIA OR AGENESIS
CERVIX PRESENT
CERVIX ABSENT
TESTOSTERONE MEASUREMENT
FEMALE RANGE
MALE RANGE
UTERINE APLASIA
TESTICULAR FEMINIZATION
BREAST DEVELOPMENT PRESENT
BREAST DEVELOPMENT ABSENT
MEASURE PROLACTIN, T_4, T_3 UPTAKE, FTI; LATERAL SKULL X-RAY
ANY ABNORMAL
ALL NORMAL
FURTHER EVALUATION AS FOR SECONDARY AMENORRHEA
KARYOTYPING; FSH, LH MEASUREMENTS
KARYOTYPE 46,XX; LOW FSH, LH
KARYOTYPE 46,XX; HIGH FSH, LH
KARYOTYPE OTHER THAN 46,XX
PITUITARY HYPOTHALAMIC DYSFUNCTION
GONADAL DYSGENESIS
DIAGNOSIS AS PER KARYOTYPE

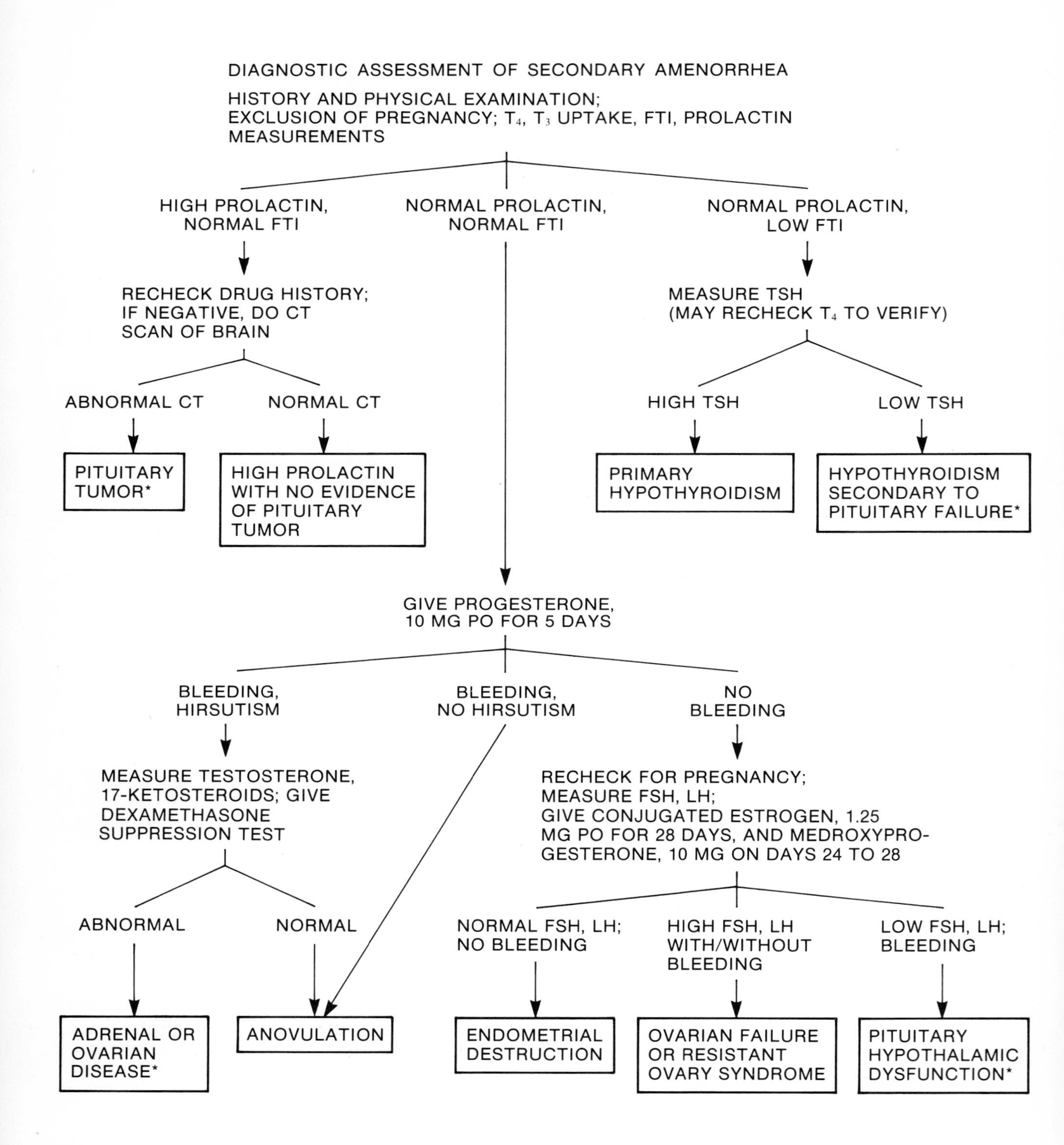

*Further tests usually indicated (see Hyperprolactinemia chapter.—Ed.)

Table 3. TESTS INDICATED TO EVALUATE AMENORRHEA

Test(s)	Indication(s)
Pregnancy test	The first and most important test in secondary amenorrhea; also important in primary amenorrhea if the patient has developed secondary sex characteristics (e.g., breasts)
Prolactin determination	In primary or secondary amenorrhea in all patients who are not on a medication known to increase prolactin (e.g., phenothiazines, oral contraceptive pills)
Lateral skull x-ray or coned-down view of sella	To evaluate the size of the sella turcica in patients with primary or secondary amenorrhea in whom prolactin levels are normal and there is no other obvious cause of amenorrhea
CT scan of the sella	High prolactin level or an abnormal sella on x-ray; also whenever an intracerebral lesion is suspected
Measurements of 17-ketosteroids and plasma testosterone, dexamethasone suppression test	Hirsutism
FSH, LH levels	In primary amenorrhea, if all the preceding tests give normal results. In secondary amenorrhea if the patient has failed to have withdrawal bleeding after a course of progesterone. Gonadotropin levels will be high if estrogen deficiency is due to ovarian failure
Karyotype	Primary amenorrhea and rarely also in secondary amenorrhea in patients with high FSH and LH levels in whom a chromosomal abnormality is suspected
Administration of medroxyprogesterone, 10 mg orally for 5 days	In secondary amenorrhea to assess endogenous estrogen levels. If bleeding occurs 1–7 days after stopping progesterone, one can conclude that the endometrium has been primed by endogenous estrogen and that the problem is anovulation and not estrogen deficiency. If no bleeding occurs, a course of estrogen plus progesterone is prescribed.
Administration of conjugated estrogen, 1.25 mg orally for 28 days, and medroxyprogesterone, 10 mg orally on days 24–28	In secondary amenorrhea, if bleeding did not occur after progesterone alone, but follows a course of progesterone and estrogen, one may conclude that the problem is estrogen deficiency

crine abnormality. On the other hand, pregnancy and anovulation are much more common in patients with secondary amenorrhea. Nevertheless, every patient must be evaluated in a very systematic manner in order to avoid overlooking a treatable abnormality.

REFERENCES

1. Fritz MA, Speroff L: The endocrinology of the menstrual cycle: the interaction of folliculogenesis and neuroendocrine mechanisms. Fertil Steril 1982;38:509–29.
2. Apter D, Viinikka L, Vihko R: Hormonal pattern of adolescent menstrual cycles. J Clin Endocrinol Metab 1978;47:944–54.
3. Marsland DW, Wood M, Mayo F: Rank order of diagnoses by frequency. J Fam Pract 1976;3(1):16–8.
4. Singh KB: Menstrual disorders in college students. Am J Obstet Gynecol 1981;140:299–302.
5. Petersson F, Fries H, Nillius SJ: Epidemiology of secondary amenorrhea. Am J Obstet Gynecol 1973;117:80–6.
6. McFarland KF: Amenorrhea. Am Fam Physician 1980;22:95–100.
7. Zacharias L, Wurtman RJ, Schatzoff M: Sexual maturation in contemporary American girls. Am J Obstet Gynecol 1970;108:833–46.
8. Fried RI, Smith EE: Postmenarcheal growth patterns. J Pediatr 1962;61:562–5.
9. Fishman J: Fatness, puberty, and ovulation. N Engl J Med 1980;303:42–3.
10. Frisch RE, McArthur JW: Menstrual cycles: fatness as a determinant of minimum weight for height necessary for their maintenance or onset. Science 1974;185:949–51.
11. Wyshak G, Frisch RE: Evidence for a secular trend in age of menarche. N Engl J Med 1982;306:1033–5.
12. El-Minawi MR, Foda MS: Postpartum lactation amenorrhea. Am J Obstet Gynecol 1971;111:17–21.
13. Leduc B, Campernhout JV, Simard R: Congenital absence of the vagina. Am J Obstet Gynecol 1969;100:512–20.
14. Knuth UA, Hull MGR, Jacobs HS: Amenorrhoea and loss of weight. Br J Obstet Gynaecol 1977;84:801–7.
15. Radwanska E: Secondary amenorrhea. Obstet Gynecol Annu 1982;11:203–51.
16. Jacobs HS: Prolactin and amenorrhea. N Engl J Med 1976;295:954–6.
17. Badawy SZA, Nusbaum ML, Omar M: Hypothalamic-pituitary evaluation in patients with galactorrhea-amenorrhea and hyperprolactinemia. Obstet Gynecol 1980;55:1–7.
18. Kapcala LP, Molitch ME, Post KD, Biller BJ, Prager RJ, Jackson IMD, Reichlin S: Galactorrhea, oligo/amenorrhea, and hyperprolactinemia in patients with craniopharyngiomas. J Clin Endocrinol Metab 1980;51:798–800.
19. Shreefter MJ, Friedlander RL: Primary empty sella syndrome and amenorrhea. J Clin Endocrinol Metab 1975;46:535–8.
20. Mashchak CA, Kletzky OA, Davajan V, Mishell DR: Clinical and laboratory evaluation of patients with primary amenorrhea. Obstet Gynecol 1981;57:715–21.
21. Raj SG, Thompson IE, Berger MJ, Taymor ML: Clinical aspects of the polycystic ovary syndrome. Obstet Gynecol 1979;49:552–6.
22. Boroditsky RS, Faiman C: Galactorrhea-amenorrhea due to primary hypothyroidism. Am J Obstet Gynecol 1973;116:661–5.

23. Shearson RP: Amenorrhoea after treatment with oral contraceptives. Lancet 1966;2:1110–1.
24. Hull MGR, Bromham DR, Savage PE, Barlow TM, Hughes AO, Jacobs HS: Post-pill amenorrhea: a causal study. Fertil Steril 1981;36:472–6.
25. Tolis G, Ruggere D, Popkin DR, et al: Prolonged amenorrhea and oral contraceptives. Fertil Steril 1979;32:265–8.
26. Frisch RE, Wyshak G, Vincent L: Delayed menarche and amenorrhea in ballet dancers. N Engl J Med 1980;303:17–19.
27. Baker, ER: Menstrual dysfunction and hormonal status in athletic women: a review. Fertil Steril 1981;36:691–6.
28. Warren MP: The effects of exercise on pubertal progression and reproductive function in girls. J Clin Endocrinol Metab 1980;51:1150–7.
29. Nachtigall RD, Monroe SE, Wilson CB, Jaffe RB: Prolactin secreting pituitary adenomas in women. Am J Obstet Gynecol 1981;140:303–8.

ANEMIA, MEGALOBLASTIC

ROBERT S. HILLMAN

☐ SYNONYMS: Macrocytic anemia, nuclear maturation disorder, pernicious anemia, vitamin B_{12} deficiency anemia, folic acid deficiency anemia, refractory macrocytic anemia (di Guglielmo's syndrome)

BACKGROUND

Definition and Origins

The distinctive finding of unusually large red cells, *macrocytes,* in circulation together with megaloblasts in the marrow is the recognized hallmark of the megaloblastic anemias. Pathophysiologically, this combination reflects a defect in DNA synthesis, chromosome replication, and cell division. Any organ with a high turnover of cells will demonstrate the abnormality. For example, patients with folic acid or vitamin B_{12} deficiency, two common causes of megaloblastic anemia, demonstrate megaloblastic changes involving gastric and intestinal mucosa and cervical epithelium as well as the marrow. The hematologic system, however, by nature of its very rapid cell turnover, is most sensitive to any disturbance of DNA synthesis. It is also the system most readily sampled for detection of the characteristic megaloblastic change. Detection has been made even easier by the development of automated cell counters, which accurately measure the volume of circulating erythrocytes and provide a numerical value for the macrocytosis, thereby offering the primary care physician a routine screening measurement for the early detection of megaloblastic anemia.

Recognition of this abnormal pattern of hematopoiesis more than 100 years ago stimulated a series of investigations that led to the discovery of many of the major steps in DNA synthesis. One dramatic aspect of this research was the discovery of the vitamins folic acid and B_{12}. On the basis of Whipple's observation in 1925 that liver appeared to stimulate hematopoiesis, Minot and Murphy carried out their Nobel prize–winning experiment showing the effectiveness of liver therapy in patients with pernicious anemia.[1] Soon after this, Castle characterized the role of intrinsic factor, the carrier protein secreted by gastric parietal cells that is required to promote the absorption of the extrinsic factor (vitamin B_{12}) present in liver.[2] The extrinsic factor was subsequently isolated and its structure was determined using the new technique of x-ray diffraction by Hodgkin; for this effort in characterizing vitamin B_{12}, she also was awarded a Nobel prize.

Even before vitamin B_{12} was fully purified, Wills and associates[3] identified a second factor, present in crude liver extract, that cured a macrocytic anemia in Indian women but was ineffective in pernicious anemia patients. This factor was later isolated from leafy vegetables, and its structure was defined as the vitamin folic or pteroylglutamic acid. The subsequent growth of knowledge concerning the roles of these two vitamins (folic acid, B_{12}) in DNA synthesis has been dramatic. As depicted in Figure 1, both folic acid and vitamin B_{12} are involved in essential steps in purine and pyrimidine metabolism and the conversion of deoxyuridylate to thymidylate, a required path-

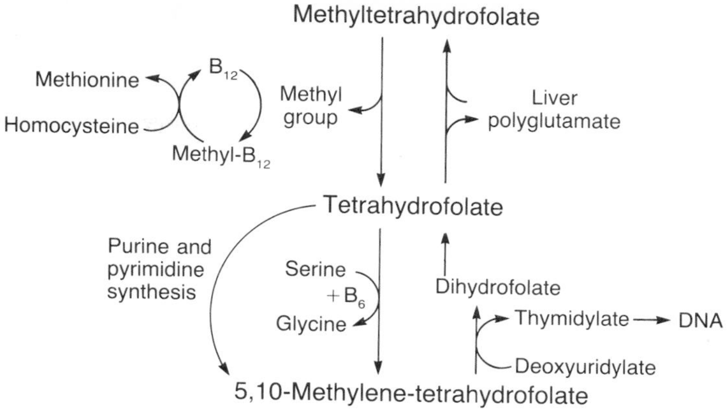

Figure 1. Metabolic pathways and interrelationships of folic acid and vitamin B_{12}; see text for discussion.

way in DNA synthesis.[4, 5] Two active forms of vitamin B_{12} have now been defined. The deoxyadenosyl B_{12} congener is involved in the isomerization of L-methylmalonyl CoA, whereas the methyl B_{12} congener acts as a methyl donor in the conversion of homocysteine to methionine. The latter reaction is closely tied to the intracellular metabolism of folic acid. *N*-5-Methyltetrahydrofolate acts as a methyl donor for vitamin B_{12}, and the product of this reaction, tetrahydrofolate, becomes the substrate for a number of important metabolic pathways, including conversion of serine to glycine, purine and pyrimidine metabolism, and thymidylate synthesis.

The roles of vitamin B_{12} and folic acid are inextricably connected. If either vitamin is in short supply, a common defect in DNA synthesis is produced. For example, a dietary deficiency of folic acid causes the availability of *N*-5-methyltetrahydrofolate for the donation of a methyl group to vitamin B_{12} to be reduced, resulting in both a failure of methionine synthesis and a reduction in supply of tetrahydrofolate for all subsequent steps in folate metabolism. The production of 5, 10-methylenetetrahydrofolate is crippled, and normal thymidylate synthesis cannot occur. Thus, abnormal DNA synthesis is a natural outcome of folate deficiency. In the case of vitamin B_{12} deficiency, a block in the conversion of *N*-5-methyltetrahydrofolate to tetrahydrofolate occurs because of the inability of methyltetrahydrofolate to transfer its methyl group to vitamin B_{12}. New folate from the diet is trapped as methyltetrahydrofolate, and those pathways served by tetrahydrofolate suffer for lack of adequate substrate.[5] The outcome is the same as that of folate deficiency: a major defect in DNA synthesis.

Primary and secondary defects in DNA synthesis are also produced by drugs that interfere with steps in folate metabolism or directly inhibit DNA assembly.[6] For example, chemotherapeutic agents that act as dihydrofolate reductase inhibitors disrupt the normal intracellular metabolic pathways of folate and produce a megaloblastic defect. Through inhibition of the reduction of dihydrofolate to tetrahydrofolate, the recycling of folate and its involvement in thymidylate synthesis is prevented. Agents that interfere with purine and pyrimidine metabolism and thymidylate synthetase itself can also produce a megaloblastic anemia. Other agents directly attack DNA assembly. Finally, megaloblastic morphology is observed in patients with inborn errors of metabolism of folic acid and vitamin B_{12} and in malignant diseases in which there is an acquired defect in DNA synthesis and cell maturation.

Incidence and Causes

The incidence of megaloblastic anemia in any population is a function of nutritional behavior, frequency of specific gastrointestinal disorders and surgical procedures, the use of chemotherapeutic drugs that act against folate metabolism and DNA synthesis, and, to a lesser extent, the incidence of primary malignant processes. Disorders of folic acid and vitamin B_{12} metabolism are still leading causes of megaloblastic anemia in western societies. However, for selected populations of patients, such as those receiving chemotherapy, a defect in DNA synthesis secondary to use of a specific drug can be a much more important etiologic factor.

Disorders of Folate Metabolism

The common disorders of folate metabolism are summarized in Table 1. Although the inborn errors of folate metabolism are quite rare, they must be regarded as likely possibilities in the differential diagnosis of a megaloblastic anemia in an infant.[7] Inherited defects involving an intracellular metabolic folate pathway are almost always associated with severe, progressive mental retardation, whereas defects in absorption or cellular uptake of folate are amenable to pharmacologic doses of the vitamin.

Table 1. DISORDERS OF FOLATE METABOLISM

Inborn errors	Congenital malabsorption
	Impaired cellular uptake
	Formiminotransferase deficiency
	Methyltransferase deficiency
Acquired metabolic defects	Alcoholism
	Vitamin B_{12} deficiency
	Vitamin C deficiency
	Ingestion of folate antagonists
	Dihydrofolate reductase inhibitors (methotrexate, triamterene, trimethoprim, pyrimethamine)
	Anticonvulsants
	Oral contraceptives
Deficiency states	Inadequate intake
	Malnutrition
	Alcoholism
	Malabsorption
	Tropical sprue
	Celiac disease
	Intestinal lymphoma
	Increased requirement
	Pregnancy
	Hemolysis
	Neoplasia

In adults, both acquired metabolic defects and folate deficiency states are quite common. Severe alcoholism is a leading cause of folate-deficient megaloblastic anemia in many western societies. At least two mechanisms appear to be involved. Not only do chronic alcoholics have an inadequate intake of dietary folic acid, which in time leads to depletion of folate stores and a true deficiency state, but also alcohol interferes with in vivo metabolic pathways for folate supply to tissues. Sustained alcohol ingestion has been shown to block the normal recirculation of folate through the enterohepatic cycle so as to acutely depress the level of folate in serum and reduce the supply to rapidly dividing tissues such as the marrow.[3] This process helps explain the observation that a megaloblastic anemia can develop in an alcoholic within a few weeks despite the continued presence of adequate liver folate stores. At the same time, dietary folate can prevent the effect of alcohol on folate metabolism by circumventing the block in the folate enterohepatic cycle. Alcoholics whose diets are supplemented with folic acid do not develop megaloblastic anemia.

Megaloblastic anemia secondary to a defect in folate metabolism is also seen when the chemotherapeutic agent methotrexate is administered. This drug acts as a dihydrofolate reductase inhibitor and prevents the recycling of dihydrofolate to tetrahydrofolate for support of the thymidylate synthetase pathway.[7] Other drugs, including triamterene, trimethoprim, and pyrimethamine, are weaker inhibitors of dihydrofolate reductase but can produce a similar defect in patients with marginal folate status. Anticonvulsants and oral contraceptives also interfere with folate metabolism, although the exact mechanism of their effect has not been determined.

Both vitamin B_{12} and vitamin C are essential to normal folate metabolism. As previously described, severe vitamin B_{12} deficiency deprives cells of sufficient tetrahydrofolate to carry out the steps of purine, pyrimidine, and thymidylate synthesis. Thus, the vitamin B_{12}–deficient patient is functionally folate-deficient. Vitamin C may also play an important role in folate metabolism. Some patients with scurvy demonstrate a megaloblastic anemia that is only partially responsive to folic acid; treatment with vitamin C is required for full recovery.[9] However, the mechanism of this interaction is still poorly understood.

Absolute folate deficiency can develop because of poor dietary intake, a defect in intestinal absorption, or a marked increase in requirement. Folate malnutrition is seen in newborns who are fed goat's milk or a formula that is deficient in folate. Dietary deficiency of folate is also common in chronic alcoholics. Malabsorption of folate occurs in patients with tropical sprue, celiac disease, and widespread intestinal lymphoma. Because folic acid is absorbed throughout the small intestine, extensive disease must occur before a deficiency state evolves, in contrast to vitamin B_{12}, malabsorption and deficiency of which can be produced by disease limited to the ileum. Perhaps the most dramatic evolution of folate deficiency is in patients with tropical sprue.[10] In this condition, the mucosal absorption of folate appears to be uniquely affected, so that the symptoms and signs of a severe megaloblastic anemia may overshadow gastrointestinal complaints.

In a state of increased cell turnover, such as pregnancy, severe hemolytic anemia, or the dramatic growth of a tumor, the folate requirement may exceed the supply available in a normal diet.[11] In pregnancy, the fetus has a clear advantage over the mother, in that the placenta extracts folate at the expense of maternal tissues. The mother may therefore devleop megaloblastic anemia without depriving the fetus of adequate folate for normal development.

Disorders of Vitamin B_{12} Metabolism

The more important clinical disorders of vitamin B_{12} metabolism are listed in Table 2. As with the folate defects, inborn errors of vitamin B_{12} metabolism are quite rare. Their diagnosis can be extremely important, however, because even a limited period of vitamin B_{12} deficiency in a newborn results in a neurologic deficit that could be prevented by adequate therapy. Of the acquired metabolic defects and vitamin B_{12} deficiency states, those conditions that produce malabsorption of vitamin B_{12} are the most important. The original studies of patients with pernicious anemia showed

Table 2. DISORDERS OF VITAMIN B_{12} METABOLISM

Inborn errors	Congenital intrinsic factor deficiency Familial vitamin B_{12} malabsorption Transcobalamin II deficiency
Acquired metabolic defects	Intrinsic factor deficiency Pernicious anemia Folate deficiency N_2O exposure
Deficiency states	Inadequate intake Veganism Malabsorption Intrinsic factor deficiency Zollinger-Ellison syndrome Intestinal lymphoma Ileitis Ileal resection Tropical sprue Celiac disease Parasitic infestation Blind loop syndrome Small-intestinal diverticulosis with bacterial overgrowth Increased requirement Pregnancy Neoplasia

the importance of intrinsic factor in the absorption of dietary vitamin B_{12}.[2] This protein, which is secreted by the parietal cells located in the fundus of the stomach, is essential for absorption of vitamin B_{12} by the mucosal cells of the ileum. Inadequate production of intrinsic factor can result from a congenital defect in secretion or from a loss of parietal cells, as in pernicious anemia, progressive gastric atrophy, or gastric surgery. Malabsorption of the intrinsic factor–vitamin B_{12} complex is seen in patients with autoimmune disease, Zollinger-Ellison syndrome, intestinal lymphoma, ileitis, surgical resection of the ileum, tropical sprue, celiac disease, parasitic infestation, blind loop syndrome, and intestinal diverticulosis with bacterial overgrowth. Mechanisms include disruptions of the normal pH, transit time, and mucosal cell function and, in parasitism and bacterial overgrowth, competition for the vitamin B_{12} prior to absorption.

Inadequate dietary intake can also produce vitamin B_{12} deficiency and megaloblastic anemia. Because vitamin B_{12} is present in most foods containing animal by-products, dietary B_{12} deficiency occurs only in persons who keep to a strict vegetarian diet and do not use vitamin supplements. The likelihood of developing vitamin B_{12} deficiency during pregnancy is also considerably less than with folic acid, probably because of the higher level of vitamin B_{12} stores maintained in normal liver. Available stores of folate can sustain a fasting individual for only 1 to 3 months, but sufficient vitamin B_{12} stores are available to supply tissues for 2 to 3 years.

Finally, acquired metabolic defects in vitamin B_{12} metabolism are seen both with folate deficiency and with exposure to anesthetic levels of nitrous oxide.[12] As discussed previously, an adequate supply of methyltetrahydrofolate is required as a methyl donor for the homocysteine-to-methionine reaction. The clinical importance of such a defect is uncertain, however, because adequate amounts of methionine can be provided by the diet. Developing a megaloblastic anemia during nitrous oxide anesthesia is of clinical importance only with the use of continuous anesthesia for periods of 12 to 24 hours in patients with tetanus. The infrequent use of such therapy makes this clinical complication unlikely.

Primary Disorders of DNA Synthesis

Primary disorders of DNA synthesis that cause megaloblastic anemia are listed in Table 3. Several inborn errors of metabolism, including hereditary orotic aciduria, Lesch-Nyhan syndrome, and thiamine-responsive megaloblastic anemia, need to be considered in the differential diagnosis of megaloblastic anemia in a newborn.[7] Acquired metabolic defects include those associated with drugs that inhibit purine, pyrimidine, and thymidylate synthesis and DNA assembly. Generally, these are chemotherapeutic agents used in treatment of leukemia and lymphoma, so the development of megaloblastosis can be anticipated in this setting. Megaloblastic morphology of bone marrow cells is also seen in patients with acquired, idiopathic sideroblastic anemia and so-called refractory macrocytic anemia, or di Guglielmo's syndrome. Both of these conditions are now understood to be preleukemic states and examples of clonal malignancies.

HISTORY

Even though the first clue to a megaloblastic anemia is usually the finding of macrocytosis on a complete blood count, a carefully obtained his-

Table 3. PRIMARY DISORDERS OF DNA SYNTHESIS

Inborn errors	Hereditary orotic aciduria Lesch-Nyhan syndrome Thiamine-responsive megaloblastic anemia
Acquired metabolic defects	Ingestion of metabolic inhibitors of: Purine synthesis (6MP, 6GT) Pyrimidine synthesis (6-azauridine) Thymidylate synthesis (5-fluorouracil) DNA assembly (hydroxyurea) Neoplastic states Acquired, idiopathic sideroblastic anemia Refractory macrocytic anemia (di Guglielmo's syndrome)

tory and thorough physical examination can provide important information regarding the etiology of the anemia.

History of the Present Illness. The symptoms and signs of anemia generally correspond to its relative severity, that is, to the relationship of the defect in oxygen transport with the age and physical condition of the patient. Mild anemia in an otherwise healthy individual can be completely asymptomatic or can be associated with little more than a slight increase in exertional dyspnea, tachycardia, and sweating with physical exercise. As the anemia becomes more severe, these symptoms increase proportionately, and the patient complains of excessive fatigue with even moderate exertion. Elderly patients have greater difficulty. For example, in the presence of cerebrovascular disease, mild anemia can produce significant regional ischemia. Therefore, exertional angina, peripheral vascular insufficiency, and cerebrovascular ischemia are common problems in elderly patients with anemia.

The rate of onset is also important in determining symptoms. For example, a major hemorrhage with both blood volume and red cell mass depletion is associated with marked symptoms and signs of anemia and vascular insufficiency. Losses of more than 20 to 25 per cent of the circulating blood volume are accompanied by generalized weakness, dizziness, and, in some patients, syncope. An attempt at exercise results in noticeable tachycardia, a pounding headache, and palpitations. If volume loss exceeds 25 to 30 per cent of the patient's original blood volume, symptoms and signs of acute hypovolemic shock become manifest.

Patients with megaloblastic anemia do not generally present with symptoms or signs of acute volume loss. Rather, they complain of the insidious onset of tiredness, easy fatigability, and ischemic pain on exercise, often extending back 6 to 12 months. In addition, they may report problems such as insomnia, nightmares, and sleep interrupted by a disturbed breathing pattern, and, during the day, an inability to concentrate. When the anemia is severe, symptoms and signs of congestive heart failure may appear.

Vitamin B_{12}–deficient patients may also have neurologic complaints, including numbness and dysesthesias of the hands and feet, impairment of fine finger movements, unsteadiness of gait, weakness or stiffness of the lower extremities, and, in males, impotence and difficulty urinating.[13] Irritability, memory loss, and mild depression or swings in mood are common. Major psychiatric problems are less common, although acute confusion, severe impairment of memory and judgment, and, in some instances, marked depression or manic psychosis are seen.

In eliciting the history, one should document the rapidity and pattern of onset and identify any tendency to exacerbation or remission. Vitamin B_{12} deficiency develops insidiously, with symptoms waxing and waning over 6 to 12 months. Folic acid deficiency usually evolves in a much shorter time and is frequently associated with chronic alcoholism. A careful and detailed history regarding the patient's nutritional status and any problems with alcohol abuse is therefore important.

Complaints relative to the gastrointestional tract are very common. Anorexia and weight loss are present most of the time, and a complaint of a sore mouth and tongue is likely. The patient may also describe a loss of taste. Diarrhea is common and may suggest a primary gastrointestinal illness. Any detailed review of the gastrointestinal history should include questions regarding surgery, changes in bowel function that might suggest malabsorption, and recent travel or a gastronomic adventure that could result in parasitic infestation.

Family History. Multiple cases of pernicious anemia may be seen in a single family, but a clear inheritance pattern has not been established. Pernicious anemia or elevated levels of parietal cell antibodies have been reported in 20 to 25 per cent of siblings of affected patients but are present in less than 10 per cent of parents and children.

Social and Occupational History. A pure nutritional deficiency of vitamin B_{12} is seen in patients who maintain a strict vegetarian diet without vitamin supplementation. However, this is a very uncommon cause of a megaloblastic anemia. The more common social problem in western societies is alcoholism, which has a high incidence, and the concurrent problem it causes in folate nutrition.

Drug History. A careful history of drug use is extremely important. Megaloblastic anemia is a predictable complication with many of the chemotherapeutic agents, including the inhibitors of dihydrofolate reductase and the metabolic inhibitors that impair purine, pyrimidine, and thymidylate synthesis and DNA assembly.

Previous Medical History. A history of gastrointestinal surgery or a major medical illness that impairs gastrointestinal function and nutrition is extremely important. The removal of a major portion of the stomach or the establishment of a Billroth II anastomosis impairs intrinsic factor secretion and, within 1 to 5 years, produces vitamin B_{12} deficiency. The predictable impact of surgery has led to the prophylactic treatment of affected patients with both vitamin B_{12} and iron. Patients with a history of regional ileitis or an ileal resection will also have a defect in vitamin B_{12} absorption despite normal intrinsic factor secretion. Although folic acid absorption does not require a special carrier protein and is not confined to a single portion of the small intestine, folate malabsorption is seen in patients with widespread intestinal disease such as celiac disease and tropical sprue. Inasmuch as western diets provide only marginally adequate levels of folate, any increase in demand for folate such as occurs in pregnancy and hemolytic anemia also places the patient at risk for developing a folate-deficient megaloblastic anemia.

PHYSICAL EXAMINATION

The physical examination can be very helpful in guiding diagnosis and management. Detection of both hematologic and neurologic abnormalities, so-called combined system disease, immediately focuses attention on vitamin B_{12} deficiency as the most likely cause. In contrast, organ damage secondary to chronic alcohol ingestion makes folic acid deficiency more likely. Key features to look for in any patient with megaloblastic anemia include the following.

General Appearance. Patients with pernicious anemia often have a sallow appearance as the result of the pallor of the anemia together with a slight increase in bilirubin. They also are said to be predominantly fair-skinned, fair-haired or prematurely gray, and blue-eyed. Patients with folic acid deficiency may show the signs of poor general hygiene and organ damage associated with chronic alcoholism. However, cirrhosis need not be advanced in order for the patient to have severe megaloblastic anemia.

Head and Neck Examination. Slight scleral icterus is common in patients with severe anemia. In addition, patients with long-standing vitamin B_{12} deficiency show cheilosis and glossitis with a smooth, red, shiny tongue.

Cardiopulmonary Examination. As a part of normal compensation for anemia, there may be widened pulse pressure, increased stroke volume, and tachycardia with exercise. With severe anemia, biventricular failure can appear, with cardiac enlargement, signs of pulmonary congestion, jugular venous distension, and peripheral edema. Systolic flow murmurs are common, and in patients with vitamin B_{12} deficiency, orthostatic hypotension and cardiac arrhythmias may be seen.

Abdominal Examination. Slight enlargement of the liver and spleen is occasionally seen with pernicious anemia. Marked hepatosplenomegaly with signs of liver damage, such as ascites, severe jaundice, spider, angiomata, and gynecomastia, suggests severe alcoholic cirrhosis and concomitant folic acid deficiency.

Neurologic Examination. Peripheral neuropathies may be seen both in alcoholics with folate deficiency and in patients with pernicious anemia. With progression, however, the distinctive features of vitamin B_{12} peripheral neuritis should become apparent, including the impairment of vibration sense, the loss of position sense, and increasing difficulty with coordination. The combination of numbness in the lower extremities, impairment of fine finger movements, ataxia, Romberg's sign, and loss of both position and vibration senses that is most marked in the lower extremities is indicative of the dorsal column lesion of vitamin B_{12} deficiency. Other neurologic abnormalities that may be appreciated are major deficits in mental status, spasticity or stiffness of the extremities, an extensor plantar reflex with either increased or decreased ankle jerks, dysesthesias or loss of cutaneous sensation, and, in the rare case, ophthalmoplegia. Impairment of vision in pernicious anemia patients is most likely secondary to a retinal hemorrhage or retrobulbar neuritis. The major problem in differential diagnosis is the peripheral neuropathy with impairment of cerebellar function that can occur in patients with severe, chronic alcoholism.

DIAGNOSTIC STUDIES

The definitive diagnosis of megaloblastic anemia occurs in the laboratory. It involves accurate interpretation of the values obtained from the complete blood count, the correct use of marrow aspirate examination findings to confirm megaloblastic morphology, and the appropriate ordering of specific measurements of vitamin levels or vitamin absorption to determine etiology.

Interpreting the Routine Blood Count

The initial clue to megaloblastic anemia is generally the detection of macrocytosis from the mean cell volume (MCV) or the appearance of the peripheral smear. The sensitivity and specificity of any rise in the mean cell volume depend on several factors, including the nature of the DNA synthesis defect and the severity and duration of the anemia. In the case of the vitamin deficiencies, the mean cell volume rises to levels in excess of 120 fl in those patients who have had severe anemia (hematocrit less than 25 to 30 per cent) for several months. Chronicity of disease is extremely important, because it allows the normal cells in circulation to be replaced by abnormal macrocytic cells. In the patient with an anemia of shorter duration or less severity, the MCV is within the upper normal range or only slightly elevated. In this situation, other causes also must be considered (Table 4).

Slight to moderate macrocytosis is a common finding in patients who are receiving chemother-

Table 4. PATTERNS OF MACROCYTOSIS

Disorder	MCV (f1)	Morphology
Megaloblastic anemia (Hematocrit <30%)	100–130	Macro-ovalocytes, poikilocytosis
Reticulocytosis (Cell count >10%)	100–110	Polychromatophilic macrocytes (shift cells)
Liver disease	90–110	Uniform macrocytosis, target cells

apeutic drugs or have advanced liver disease independent of a specific vitamin deficiency state. A predictable macrocytosis also accompanies reticulocytosis, because reticulocytes produced under the stress of anemia are macrocytic. This occurrence depends on the level of the reticulocyte count, so the macrocytosis of a high reticulocyte count (greater than 10 per cent) should not cause confusion. With liver disease, the MCV is rarely greater than 110 fl, and the peripheral smear demonstrates a relatively uniform increase in cell diameter. This finding is quite different from the macrocytosis of vitamin B_{12} and folic acid deficiency, in which there are both marked red cell poikilocytosis and the appearance of multilobed neutrophils on peripheral smear. The latter finding is the white cell equivalent of macrocytosis; however, unlike with macrocytosis, it is difficult to provide a quantitative measure of this change. An obvious increase in the number of neutrophils with five to six nuclear lobes suggests a megaloblastic anemia, since less than 3 to 5 per cent of neutrophils normally have more than five lobes.

Bone Marrow Aspirate Examination

Traditionally, the diagnosis of a megaloblastic anemia depends on the demonstration of megaloblastic morphology in marrow aspirate. As with the degree of macrocytosis, the full expression of megaloblastic morphology depends on the severity and duration of the anemia and the specific etiology. The severity is extremely important. In the earliest states of a vitamin deficiency state, the megaloblastic change can be quite subtle. Only when anemia becomes severe and erythropoietin stimulation of the marrow is very high does full-blown megaloblastosis appear.

Early changes are usually limited to a few nuclear aberrations in late orthochromatic normoblasts. With progression, the typical findings of marked erythroid hyperplasia and ineffective erythropoiesis develop. Moreover, the distinctive morphologic pattern of increased numbers of immature megaloblasts with fine nuclear chromatin and a lack of progression to adult polychromatophilic and orthochromatic normoblasts becomes established. This is a visual demonstration of the ineffective erythropoiesis that is so typical of all megaloblastic anemias. Many of the early precursors fail to reach maturation and die within the marrow, so the number of reticulocytes produced is far lower than the total number of precursors in the marrow (Table 5).

The effective production of neutrophils and platelets is also disrupted. With a severe deficiency state or a primary defect in DNA synthesis, neutropenia and thrombocytopenia are common. As in the erythroid defect described earlier, an increased number of megaloblastic white cell precursors, giant myelocytes and metamyelocytes, are

Table 5. ERYTHROKINETIC PROFILES OF VITAMIN DEFICIENCY STATES AND PRIMARY DISORDERS OF DNA SYNTHESIS

	Vitamin Deficiency States		
Study or Determination	***Folate Deficiency***	***Vitamin B_{12} Deficiency***	**Primary Disorders of DNA Synthesis**
Peripheral smear	Macrocytosis that increases with severity of anemia (>120 fl)		Variable macrocytosis (90–120 fl)
Marrow aspirate examination			
Morphology	Megaloblastic		Variable—megaloblastic/leukemia transformation
E/G ratio	>1:1 (erythroid hyperplasia)		1:3 to 1:1 (variable cellularity)
Reticulocyte index	<1.0		<1.0
Iron studies			
Serum iron/TIBC	Increased/normal		Increased/normal
Iron stores	Appear increased		Appear increased
Sideroblasts	Normal or slight increase in number		Abnormal/ringed sideroblasts
Vitamin studies			
Serum folate concentration (normal = 3 ng/ml)	<3 ng/ml	Usually increased (>10–20 ng/ml)	
Serum B_{12} concentration (normal = 100 pg/ml)	Usually increased (>200 pg/ml)	<100 pg/ml	
Schilling test	Normal	Usually abnormal	

observed in the marrow along with a decrease in production of mature neutrophils. Moreover, the neutrophils that are produced often contain more than five nuclear lobes. When thrombocytopenia is present, it is also the result of ineffective thrombopoiesis.

The pattern of serum iron level and iron stores in the marrow is another marker of the defect in erythropoiesis of the megaloblastic patient. Typically, as red cell production becomes increasingly ineffective, the serum iron level increases to full saturation of the total iron binding capacity. In addition, the amount of reticuloendothelial cell iron visible on Prussian blue stain of the marrow increases out of proportion to the total available body iron stores. Both findings reflect the rapid turnover of hemoglobin iron secondary to premature death of erythroid precursors.

Once therapy is initiated, the serum iron level falls to normal within a few days as ineffective erythropoiesis ceases. Furthermore, as effective production of red cells proceeds, marrow iron stores are quickly depleted, even to the point of iron deficiency in patients with vitamin B_{12} or folate deficiency secondary to malabsorption. In such situations, total body iron stores may be inadequate to support a full recovery unless iron supplementation is provided.

The morphologic pattern of iron deposits in erythroid precursors can also be diagnostically helpful. Normally, 50 to 60 per cent of developing erythroid precursors show to one to five fine ferritin granules in their cytoplasm. The number of granules and the coarseness of their structure can be seen to increase in patients with megaloblastic anemia. With pure vitamin B_{12} or folic acid deficiency, the number of granules per cell and the number of cells showing granules increase slightly, although the changes are not dramatic. In chronic alcoholics with folate deficiency, precursors often show increased numbers of large iron granules together with a defect in nuclear maturation. In some patients, such deposits create the appearance of ringed sideroblasts, in which the iron granules form perinuclear halos. Ringed sideroblasts are also seen in patients with idiopathic, acquired sideroblastic anemia and di Guglielmo's syndrome.

Special Tests

A number of special laboratory tests can help identify the cause of megaloblastic anemia.[14] The most important of these are the measurements of serum vitamin levels and of the absorption of vitamin B_{12} (the Schilling test). Accurate measurements of serum vitamin B_{12} levels and serum and red cell folic acid levels are now routinely available from clinical laboratories. The method most commonly used employs a radioisotope dilution technique, which avoids the problem of assay interference in patients taking antibiotics or other drugs. However, as with any assay system, the clinician must be careful to interpret the result in light of the patient's condition. Some commercial kits used to measure vitamin B_{12} levels have come under criticism because of problems with falsely high results. In the case of serum folate levels, the timing of specimen collection is critical. The rate of recovery of serum folate levels following the cessation of alcohol ingestion can be very rapid, especially once the patient begins to eat. Thus, blood for vitamin assays should be drawn as soon as a megaloblastic anemia is appreciated.

Because of the lability of the serum folate level, the red cell folate value has been recommended as a better measure of overall folate status. The red cell folate value is not in dyamic equilibrium with the serum folate level, so a low red cell folate value can be detected for days or weeks after therapy has been initiated. The red cell folate value is less accurate, however, and is also less sensitive to the early onset of folate deficiency. For example, in the acute alcoholic, folate deficiency and mild anemia may occur without a significant fall in the red cell folate simply on the basis that insufficient time has passed for the circulating red cells to be replaced by deficient cells. Difficulty of interpretation is less with vitamin B_{12} levels. Recovery from a vitamin B_{12}–deficient state is slow and cannot occur simply on the basis of a change in diet. Thus, the serum vitamin B_{12} level is valid as long as the patient has not received pharmacologic doses of vitamin B_{12} by injection. In the evaluation of a newborn with a megaloblastic anemia, an evaluation of the vitamin B_{12}–binding proteins, transcobalamin I and II, is essential. A congenital deficiency of transcobalamin II in the newborn produces a B_{12}-deficient megaloblastic anemia even though the serum vitamin B_{12} level is in the normal range.[15] Vitamin B_{12} is bound to transcobalamin I, which has a low turnover rate and therefore does not release adequate amounts of the vitamin for proliferating tissues. Studies of transcobalamin-binding proteins are of less importance in adults. Very high vitamin B_{12} levels are observed in patients with liver disease and myeloproliferative disorders secondary to the release of abnormal binding proteins. A selective deficiency in transcobalamin II has not been reported in adults.

The clinical diagnosis of vitamin B_{12} malabsorption is possible despite replacement therapy. The Schilling test uses radiolabeled vitamin B_{12} in combination with purified intrinsic factor to permit accurate identification of vitamin B_{12} malabsorption.[16] A commercial kit is now available that combines two isotopes, one free and the other bound to intrinsic factor, to measure simultaneously the presence and character of malabsorption.

Demonstration of poor absorption of free vitamin B_{12} that is corrected by the presence of intrinsic factor suggests pernicious anemia, whereas malabsorption of both isotopes indicates a primary process involving the small intestine.

Other Tests

A number of other laboratory measurements have been described for use in characterizing defects in DNA synthesis. They include measurements of the excretion of methylmalonic acid in urine, the formiminoglutamic acid (FIGLU) test, and the direct demonstration of abnormal thymidylate synthesis in marrow by the deoxyuridine suppression test. Although these tests are of significant value in research studies of megaloblastic anemia, they do not have routine clinical importance.

ASSESSMENT

In evaluation of any patient with a megaloblastic anemia, the timing of the work-up is extremely important. Many of the findings described in the erythropoietic profile—including the characteristics of marrow morphology, the disparity between marrow erythroid hyperplasia and the reticulocyte count (ineffective erythropoiesis), the increase in the serum iron level and iron stores, and the finding of abnormal sideroblasts on marrow iron stain—change rapidly once effective therapy is begun. In addition, specific measurements of vitamin levels are of virtually no value unless they are obtained prior to a change in diet or the institution of vitamin therapy. This is most dramatic for the alcoholic, in whom a rapid correction of the megaloblastic defect occurs with cessation of alcohol intake. In such a circumstance, accurate diagnosis requires that a *full* hematologic work-up be performed without delay. Drawing samples at different times can engender an even greater dilemma. For example, a delay of even 24 to 48 hours in performing a bone marrow aspiration after drawing blood will make it impossible to compare morphologic findings to the mean cell volume, reticulocyte count, and serum iron determined from the blood sample.

When one is armed with a full laboratory evaluation, the differential diagnosis of the megaloblastic anemias is relatively straightforward (see Table 5). The pattern of peripheral blood smear and marrow morphology and the erythrokinetic profile should permit accurate separation of the vitamin deficiency states from the primary defects in DNA synthesis. In this separation, clues from the marrow morphology and the marrow iron stain are especially important. Uncomplicated vitamin B_{12} and folic acid deficiency states show a progressive megaloblastic defect, with increasing macrocytosis and ineffective erythropoiesis, that correlates with the severity of the anemia. Abnormal forms of sideroblasts appear only in patients with severe and prolonged alcoholism. In contrast, patients with acquired, idiopathic sideroblastic anemia or di Guglielmo's syndrome show variable macrocytosis, irregular changes in marrow morphology, and highly abnormal sideroblast patterns on Prussian blue stain of the marrow. Their erythrokinetic profiles can range from ineffective to hypoproliferative in association with marked pancytopenia. Finally, with any of the primary disorders of DNA synthesis, leukemic transformation is common.

The separation of folic acid from vitamin B_{12} deficiency is usually possible on the basis of serum vitamin levels as long as specimens are drawn promptly, before a change in diet or the start of a specific treatment. When these measurements are unavailable, a therapeutic trial with small amounts of parenterally administered folic acid or vitamin B_{12} can be used to make the diagnosis; however, many factors interfere with the results of such a trial. For example, the patient's response may be independent of the therapy given, or a concurrent illness may blunt the reticulocyte response to appropriate therapy. In a similar fashion, multiple deficiency states, especially the presence of iron deficiency, can effectively prevent reticulocytosis despite adequate amounts of folic acid or vitamin B_{12}; this occurrence is not uncommon in patients with tropical sprue or long-standing malabsorption. Finally, a good therapeutic trial takes more than a week to perform and, if carried out in the hospital, can be extremely expensive.

The alternative approach, and in the extremely ill patient the preferred approach, is to administer full amounts of both folic acid and vitamin B_{12} to guarantee correction of any vitamin deficiency state and to use the vitamin levels obtained prior to therapy for diagnosis. If these are unavailable, the Schilling test can still characterize vitamin B_{12} malabsorption after therapy. If double-vitamin therapy fails to help the patient, a primary disorder of DNA synthesis should be considered, and the bone marrow aspirate examination should be repeated. Persistence of megaloblastic morphology in such a patient is virtually diagnostic of a refractory macrocytic anemia as seen in di Guglielmo's syndrome.

REFERENCES

1. Kass L. Pernicious anemia. Vol II. Philadelphia: WB Saunders Co, 1976.
2. Castle WB. Development of knowledge concerning the

gastric intrinsic factor and its relation to pernicious anemia. N Engl J Med 1953;249:603–14.
3. Wills L, Clutterbuck PW, Evans PDF. A new factor in the production and cure of macrocytic anaemias and its relation to other haemopoietic principles curative in pernicious anaemia. Biochem J 1937;31:2136–47.
4. Hillman RS. Vitamin B_{12}, folic acid, and the treatment of megaloblastic anemias. In: Gilman AG, Goodman LS, Gilman A, eds. The pharmacological basis of therapeutics. 6th ed. New York: MacMillan, 1980;1331–46.
5. Das KC, Herbert V. Vitamin B_{12} folate interrelations. Clin Haematol 1976;5:697–725.
6. Stebbins R, Bertino JR. Megaloblastic anaemia produced by drugs. Clin. Haematol., 1976;5:619–30.
7. Cooper BA. Megaloblastic anaemia and disorders affecting utilization of vitamin B_{12} and folate in childhood. Clin Haematol 1976;5:631–59.
8. Hillman RS, McGuffin R, Campbell C. Alcohol interference with the folate enterohepatic cycle. Trans Assoc Am Physicians 1977;90:145–56.
9. Jandl JH, Gabuzda GJ. Potentiation of pteroylglutamic acid by ascorbic acid in the anemia of scurvy. Proc Soc Exp Biol Med 1953;84:452–5.
10. O'Brien W. Acute military tropical sprue in South East Asia. Am J Clin Nutr 1968;21:1007–12.
11. Lindenbaum J. Folic acid requirement in situations of increased need. In: Folic acid: proceedings of a workshop on human folate requirements, 1975. Washington, DC: National Academy of Sciences, 1977;256–76.
12. Amess JA, Burnan JF, Mancekievill DG, Mollin DL. Megaloblastic hemopoiesis in patients receiving nitrous oxide. Lancet 1978; ii:339–42.
13. Herbert V, Tisman G. Effects of deficiencies of folic acid and vitamin B_{12} on central nervous system function and development. In Gaull G, ed. Biology of Brain Dysfunction. Vol I. New York: Plenum Press, 1973;373–92.
14. Carmel R. The laboratory diagnosis of megaloblastic anemia. West J Med 1978;128:294–304.
15. Schilling RF. Instrinsic factor studies. II. The effect of gastric juice on the urinary excretion of radioactivity after the oral administration of radioactive vitamin B_{12}. J Lab Clin Med 1953;42:860–6.
16. Hakami N, Nieman PE, Canellos GP, Lazerson J. Neonatal megaloblastic anemia due to inherited transcobalamin II deficiency in two siblings. N Engl J Med 1971;285:1163–70.

BREAST DISCHARGE

JACK E. TETIRICK

SYNONYMS: Galactorrhea, bloody nipple discharge

BACKGROUND

Milk, the physiologic secretion of the breast, is defined as a lactose-containing substance secreted from breast tissue.[1] The appearance of the discharge is not enough to identify it as milk in a difficult case.[2] The inappropriate secretion of milk is *galactorrhea*. Other abnormal breast discharges may be serous, cloudy, serosanguinous, and bloody nipple discharges. Purulent discharges may appear from the fistulae of chronic breast abscesses. Exudates are derived from surface lesions of the nipple or elsewhere on the breast.

Discharges Containing Milk (Galactorrhea)

Galactorrhea persisting after childbirth and associated with amenorrhea has been named Frommel's disease or the Chiari-Frommel syndrome.[3] The amenorrhea-galactorrhea syndrome may or may not relate to pregnancy and may or may not be associated with hyperprolactinemia. Nonpuerperal galactorrhea, if associated with a pituitary tumor, is known as the Forbes-Albright syndrome.[4, 5] When the condition is without evidence of pituitary tumor, it is called the Argonz–del Castillo syndrome.[6] These descriptive titles are mostly of historic interest. It is now known that varied presentations result from impairment of hypothalamic and pituitary function, and the mistake of confusing a clinical description with a diagnosis should be avoided.[7, 8]

Epidemiology

Meningiomas of the suprasellar region, craniopharyngiomas, and other brain tumors may be associated with galactorrhea.[9, 10] Diffuse cerebral diseases such as post-traumatic coma and tuberous sclerosis can be also causally related.[11, 12]

There are widely scattered case reports of galactorrhea appearing in relation to diseases and irritations of the chest and thoracic skin, including sarcoidosis, herpes zoster, and removal of skin tattoos, following thoracotomy or laparotomy, and even with axillary stimulation secondary to the use of a crutch.[13–17]

Galactorrhea is commonly associated with diseases of the endocrine system. A prolactin-secreting adenoma of the pituitary is the most frequently associated pituitary tumor, but chronophobe adenomas, thyroid-stimulating hormone (TSH)–secreting adenomas, and Cushing's disease are also

Table 1. DRUGS THAT MAY CAUSE GALACTORRHEA

Generic Name	Trade Name(s)	Mechanism
Phenothiazines and other antipsychotics		Dopaminergic receptor blockade
Chlorpromazine	Thorazine, Promapar	
Prochlorperazine	Compazine	
Trifluoperazine	Stelazine	
Fluphenazine	Prolixin, Permitil	
Trimeprazine	Temaril	
Thioridazine	Mellaril	
Haloperidol	Haldol	
Molindone	Moban	
Antidepressants		
Imipramine	Tofranil, Janimine, SK-Pramine	Unclear
Amoxapine	Asendin	Possibly dopaminergic receptor blockade
Amitriptyline	Elavil, Endep, Amitid	Unclear; not well documented
Doxepin	Sinequan, Adapin	Unclear; not well documented
Benzodiazepines		
Chlordiazepoxide	Librium SK/Lygen, A-Poxide	Unclear; not well documented
Diazepam	Valium	Unclear, not well documented
Amphetamines		
Amphetamine	Benzedrine	Not well documented; better documented for causing gynecomastia
Dextroamphetamine	Dexedrine	
Methamphetamine	Desoxyn	
Amphetamine complex	Biphetamine	
Antihypertensives		
Methyldopa	Aldomet	Unclear
Reserpine	Serpasil, Sandril, Reserpoid	Dopamine depletion
Rauwolfia	Raudixin	Dopamine depletion
Hormonal Agents		
Estrogens	Premarin Ogen	Stimulation of prolactin synthesis and release shown in male
Tamoxifen	Nolvadex	Unclear; seen in premenopausal patient with breast carcinoma
Oral Contraceptives	(Various)	Unclear; with use and after stopping
Medroxyprogesterone	Depo-Provera	Unclear
Other drugs		
Metoclopramide	Reglan	Dopaminergic receptor blockade
Meprobamate (anti-anxiety agent)	Equanil, Miltown, SK-Bamate	Not well documented
Verapamil (calcium channel–blocking agent)	Calan	Possibly intracellular hypocalcemia
Cimetidine (histamine$_2$ receptor–blocking agent)	Tagamet	Unclear
Isoniazid (antitubercular agent)	Nydrazid, Niconyl	Unclear

reported.[18–20] Other endocrine tumors, including feminizing adrenal tumors and granulosa cells tumors, may produce galactorrhea.[21, 22] Rare causes are the "paraendocrine" tumors, which produce hormonally active substances or receptor site–blocking substances, e.g., oat cell carcinoma, choriocarcinoma, hypernephroma, hydatidiform mole, ovarian teratoma, and myeloma.[23–25] Galactorrhea is frequently associated with syndrome of polycystic ovaries, either as a presenting symptom or following treatment with medroxyprogesterone acetate.[26]

Thyroid function has a profound effect on lactation.[27, 28] Spontaneous hypothyroidism of long standing in a premenopausal woman may be finally diagnosed when galactorrhea appears.[29] Hyperthyroidism, particularly TSH pituitary thyrotoxicosis, has been noted to cause galactorrhea.[19]

Galactorrhea in the male is an ominous finding. Males with pituitary tumors are less likely to demonstrate galactorrhea early in the disease; hence, when such a discharge is present, the outlook is unfavorable.[30] Galactorrhea in the male may be the first sign of acromegaly. Testicular failure, either primary or the result of chemotherapy, may produce galactorrhea.[31, 32] Virtually the only harmless settings for galactorrhea in males are following recovery from starvation with or without hyperalimentation and in association with medication (Table 1).

Galactorrhea in children is also an indicator of serious endocrine disease. Significant amounts of both estrogen and prolactin are needed to produce milk secretion before adolescence. In infants the phenomenon is known as witch's milk *(hexenmilch)*. A transient effect related to the maternal and placental hormones, it should cease several weeks after birth.

Physiology

The breast has properly been called a mirror of the endocrine system.[23] Prolactin, the principal hormone influencing breast tissue, is phylogenetically the most ancient of the polypeptide hormones. It would be better named a "life-style" hormone that influenced nurture and reproduction before breasts evolved. Amphibians require prolactin to adapt between aquatic and terrestrial life. Fish require prolactin for nest building and egg farming.

In human physiology, the effects of prolactin are subtle, widely distributed, and sometimes contradictory. Prolactin secretion varies with the time of day, shows a large burst during rapid eye movement (REM) sleep, and is markedly elevated by stress.[16] Prolactin is elevated at the onset of lactation but often falls to a normal range as lactation continues. Its effect on breast tissue is influenced by "priming" by other hormones, particularly estrogen. Pregnancy causes marked hyperplasia of pituitary lactotropes, as do birth control pills and other chronic stimulators of the system. Whether or not these prolactin-producing stimuli cause pituitary prolactin adenomas, and, if so, whether the phenomenon is reversible, is unproven.

Most investigators look at the hypothalamus for an understanding of galactorrhea, particularly when obvious cause is absent. Certainly this gland is the common source for most pituitary stimuli. The neuroendocrine transmitter dopamine influences prolactin production paradoxically, presumably by stimulating the release of prolactin-inhibitory substance (PIF) by the hypothalamus, which is then transmitted to the pituitary gland via the pituitary portal circulation. Interference with PIF secretion or transmission by non–prolactin-producing pituitary tumors may explain prolactin elevation in these cases as well as in cases of craniopharyngioma, "empty sella" syndrome, and other enigmas.[33] Drugs such as the phenothiazines and tricyclic amines block dopamine receptors in the hypothalamus, producing galactorrhea.[34] Reserpine and related compounds deplete central dopamine stores. Degradation products of drugs such as digitalis may block receptor sites for dopamine (see Table 1).

The instances of galactorrhea following childbirth and lactation or resulting from stress or skin stimulation are thought to be due to perturbations of the neuroendocrine equilibrium in the hypothalamic-pituitary axis. They often spontaneously resolve or can be "reset" by a trial of bromocriptine or other agents that stimulate dopaminergic receptors in the hypothalamus.[35, 36]

Nonmilk Discharge

Nipple discharge of a nonmilk substance usually indicates benign disease. The diagnosis of localized nipple discharge requires careful screening and considerable common sense. The principal breast diseases producing nipple discharge are cystic mastitis, ductal ectasia, intraductal papillomatosis, and carcinoma. On the basis of collected series of patients with nipple discharge, the incidence of malignancy associated with the discharge seems to be 10 per cent or higher.[37] Most such reports suffer from high selectivity, being from institutions specializing in cancer treatment or including patients with obvious breast tumor in which a discharge can be elicited. If such a bias is removed, and particularly if the large number of women with breast discharge who are treated only in the physician's office are included, the incidence of cancer as the cause of the discharge is less than 1 per cent. Therefore, panic and overtreatment should be avoided. At the same time the possibility of cancer must always be kept in mind and each patient with discharge must be carefully studied to rule it out.

Purulent Breast Discharge

True purulent breast discharges characteristically occur from a drainage site other than the nipple. Cloudy, thick nipple discharges usually are not truly purulent i.e., they contain not pus cells but inspissated cellular debris from ductal ectasia. Chronic purulent breast discharge typically occurs at the areolar margin or close to it, representing the draining sinus of a small chronic abscess that has become epithelialized. Sebaceous adenomas elsewhere on the breast, particularly in the inframammary fold, may become infected, drain, and form recurrent chronic purulent fistulas to the surface.

Breast Exudates

Most exudates (surface discharges) occur from lesions of the breast skin that are not different from dermal lesions elsewhere. The unique and important disease producing an exudate is Paget's disease of the nipple, in which the exudate comes from the surface of the nipple owing to the loss of integrity of the epithelium secondary to invasion by malignant cells. The underlying tumor, usually a ductal breast carcinoma, may be clinically undetectable.

HISTORY

The important elements of the history are shaped by the bicameral nature of the diagnostic problem—general endocrine disorder versus local breast disease.

History of the Present Illness. The exact character of the discharge—color, consistency, and frequency—is of fundamental importance. Does it come from one or both nipples? Does it appear from the same *duct* on the nipple? Is the discharge spontaneous or does it appear only with pressure or stimulation? Does the discharge change in volume or character in concert with the menstrual cycle? What is the *exact sequence* of the onset of the discharge in relation to pregnancy, lactation, illness, surgery, or medication? What is the history of present or past breast disease, including treatment?

Are there any other breast symptoms? Is there history of frequent breast skin or nipple stimulation, such as exercising or working in rough clothing, vigorous or habitual sexual foreplay, or unusually frequent self-examination or "testing" for the discharge?

History Regarding the Neuroendocrine System. Is there any difficulty with thinking or concentration? Headaches? Any impairment of sight, hearing, or smell? Any change of balance, gait disturbance, or dizziness? Can the patient walk about in his or her bedroom in the dark?

The patient should be asked for symptoms associated with endocrine diseases, e.g., recent change in hat or glove size, intolerance to cold or heat, or change in the skin texture or hair distribution. He or she should also be asked about unexplained episodes of tachycardia, flushing, pounding pulse, emotional lability, change in sexual desire or function, appetite, weight change, and urinary frequency. A careful history of conception, birth, and lactation and any difficulty with any of these functions is needed. The menstrual history is critical.

Emotional and Drug History. This category may seem a peculiar combination of the usual anamnesis, but there is good reason for it. First of all, many patients under treatment for depression and other emotional disorders conceal their medication history unless specifically questioned. Second, many of the endocrine diseases, particularly thyroid disease, produce emotional states that make factual histories difficult (an occurrence that in itself should increase the suspicion of the examiner). Finally, in a few patients chronic stress may be the cause of galactorrhea.[38, 39] Also, some women maintain galactorrhea by frequently expressing the fluid from their nipples, and some receive frequent stimulation and sucking of the breasts from a sexual partner.

High-Payoff Queries

1. *What are the exact color, location, and frequency of your nipple discharge?* Discharges are usually milky but may be clear and viscous. Bloody, serosanguineous, and copiously watery discharges indicate serious local disease processes. Minimal amounts of bilateral greenish discharge usually indicate cystic mastitis. Thick gray discharge usually indicates ductal ectasia. Reproducible discharges in single locations mean local disease processes. Frequency usually correlates reasonably well with the seriousness of the problem; profuse, frequent discharges demand vigorous investigation.

2. *Have you ever noted any discharge from the other nipple?* Bilateral discharge practically rules out breast cancer as a possible cause.

3. *Have you found anything wrong with your breasts other than the discharge?* If there is an associated lump, the patient is a cancer suspect. If he or she has had many lumps in both breasts for many years and if the discharge is minimal and green, chronic cystic mastitis is probable.

4. *Did you have any difficulty with your breasts before the discharge appeared?* Severe mastodynia or a history of breast engorgement may precede the onset of prolactin-induced galactorrhea. Breast cancers that produce a discharge are otherwise asymptomatic, as are the intraductal papillomas. Patients with ductal ectasia may have a history of expressing large amounts of the material followed by relief of pain and reduction of a central mass or engorgement.

5. *What medicines are you taking?* A correct drug history may avoid an expensive endocrine workup (see Table 1).

6. *Are your menstrual periods normal?* Galactorrhea associated with amenorrhea is likely to be caused by a pituitary tumor. Long-standing secondary amenorrhea without childbearing may reflect a syndrome of polycystic ovaries. Menorrhagia may represent an ovarian tumor.

7. *What is your history of pregnancy and nursing?* The examiner must be certain the patient is not pregnant or lactating. Pregnancy may produce or cause hypertrophy of a small pituitary adenoma, and galactorrhea may date from an episode of pregnancy and lactation. Pregnancy and lactation also produce a "benign" type of galactorrhea in which no anatomic lesion is ever demonstrated and spontaneous resolution is common.

8. *If you didn't have this discharge, would you feel just fine?* Localized breast diseases, even serious ones, usually do not produce systemic symptoms. Galactorrhea secondary to drugs or hormone diseases usually is found in patients who do not "feel just fine."

9. *How often do you check this discharge?* Benign, inconsequential bilateral discharge can be maintained for years by an anxious patient expressing the fluid daily.

PHYSICAL EXAMINATION

Important local findings in the breast itself can be the key to diagnosis. The breasts are carefully examined in both the supine and sitting positions,

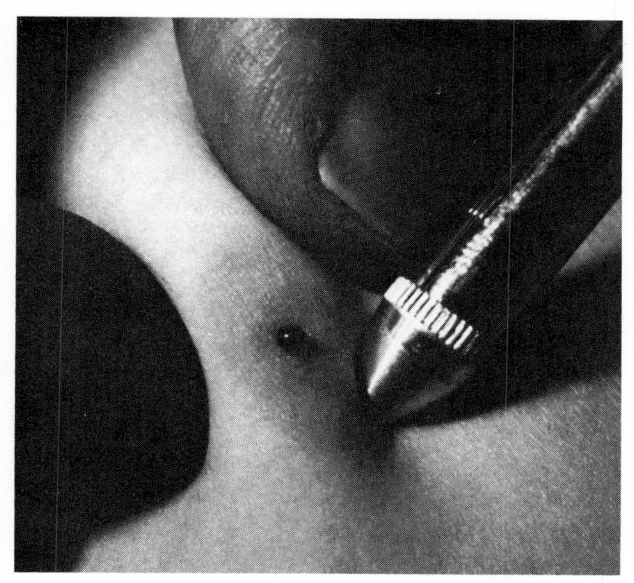

Figure 1. The patient is a 4-year-old child with a complaint of a left nipple discharge. A blunt instrument is used to search the areolar margin to localize the exact pressure point that produces this single duct discharge.

with and without the arms extended. (It is an error to examine the breasts with the patient's hands resting on top of the head; the idea of arm extension is to *stretch* the breast tissue, placing the suspensory ligaments between breast tissue and dermis on maximum tension.)

While the patient is in the supine position, the clinician should use a magnifying lens to observe the appearance and character of the discharge. Appearance of an isolated bloody or serosanguinous discharge only at a single duct is almost pathognomonic of an intraductal papilloma. This close inspection is supplemented by a careful circumferential examination of the areolar margin to search for a "pressure point" (Fig. 1). Reproducible discharge from a single pressure point localizes a papilloma; nearly all papillomas lie within 20 mm of their duct orifice.

The examination of exudates (surface discharges) under magnification is done after careful debridement of any crusting of the nipple. The examiner then searches for any change in the beaded appearance of the surface epithelium. If the surface is broken, is "bright" (smooth), or has granulations between the beads, the examiner should introduce a drop of lidocaine (Xylocaine) and remove a tiny sliver of surface tissue for pathologic examination for suspected Paget's disease.

Frequently the physical findings consist of a bilateral, minimal, clear or light-greenish discharge and bilateral, irregularly distorted lumpy breast tissue typical of chronic cystic mastitis.

When there is abundant bilateral galactorrhea, the local findings usually do not contribute to the diagnosis, and the examiner must begin an extensive physical examination. Frequently, in the instance of a benign perturbation of prolactin secretion, such an examination yields nothing, but in the case of a major endocrine disorder, there is great likelihood that some exotic physical finding may lead to the diagnosis.

Patients with suprasellar tumors (craniopharyngioma and meningioma) frequently exhibit paralysis of the extraocular muscles.[9, 10] If there is suspicion of such a tumor or of a pituitary lesion, the visual fields must be tested. The eyegrounds must be examined for evidence of increased intracranial pressure and the patient should be carefully observed for proptosis or ocular signs of thyrotoxicosis. Strength, agility, coordination, and balance should be at least briefly assessed.

The classic findings of acromegaly, Cushing's syndrome, myxedema, or thyrotoxicosis are obvious if the possibility is considered, as are the findings of feminism in the male and pelvic tumors in the female. Children should be carefully examined for flank and pelvic tumors.

DIAGNOSTIC STUDIES

A small subset of patients with nipple discharge require extensive, costly laboratory procedures. Only careful history taking and physical examination avoid unnecessary inconvenience and expense.

Laboratory Studies

All patients with nipple discharge should have a serum assay of prolactin, TSH, and T_4. Patients with hyperprolactinemia and abnormal sellar anatomy as seen on diagnostic imaging, those with persistent and worsening hyperprolactinemia despite normal sellar anatomy, and, finally, even normoprolactinemic patients with prolonged galactorrhea (more than 2 years) may be candidates for pituitary hormonal stimulation tests.[40, 41] TSH stimulation acts directly on the pituitary gland to release prolactin. L-Dopa administration suppresses prolactin by hypothalamic stimulation of prolactin inhibitory factor (PIF). Chlorpromazine administration blocks PIF release. In theory, results of these tests are lower in the presence of an autonomous prolactin-secreting tumor. In practice, the results are seldom sufficiently specific to stand alone in dictating management.

Bromocriptine administration is used as a "therapeutic test" in certain patients with borderline or moderately elevated prolactin in whom no evidence of pituitary tumor can be demonstrated. If there is prompt reversal of galactorrhea without recurrence after bromocriptine administration, the condition is considered to have been a benign perturbation of prolactin production induced by drugs, pregnancy, exogenous hormones, or even starvation. The risk associated with this maneuver lies in masking the presence of a small adenoma, particularly if the bromocriptine therapy also reverses infertility and pregnancy occurs. In this latter situation, rapid enlargement of the adenoma is likely.[41, 42]

An elevated TSH level may indicate myxedema (in the presence of reduced T_4) or, rarely, TSH thyrotoxicosis produced by a TSH-producing pituitary tumor (with elevated T_4).

Thin-layer chromatography analysis of the discharge for lactose, a simple and exact procedure, is indicated particularly in the instance of prolonged clear discharge if there is a question whether the secretion is milk.[1]

Imaging

Lateral Skull Films. Every patient with nipple discharge should have a lateral skull film for visualization of the sella turcica and clinoid processes. This is useful only to find large pituitary and hypothalamic tumors without further delay.

CT Scan. Patients with definite hyperprolactinemia (prolactin level more than 100 ng/ml) should undergo contrast-reinforced computed tomography of the head. The specificity of this modality for small adenomas far surpasses that of pneumoencephalography and polycycloidal tomography.

Mammography. Xeromammography should be performed in all patients with nipple discharge. A normal xeromammogram coupled with normal physical findings essentially rules out carcinoma of the breast as a possible source of the discharge.

Galactogram. A contrast study of the breast duct system is a useful adjunct to mammography. It requires skill and experience of the radiologist as well as proper instruments and patient preparation.[43, 44] Patients with breast discharge from a single duct orifice or with very thick brown or gray discharge should have a galactogram (Fig. 2).

Fistulogram. Fistulous orifices can be studied by retrograde injection of contrast material in a manner similar to ductal injection. Fistulas can thus be traced to a parent chronic abscess cavity for complete anatomic diagnosis.

Tissue Analysis

Any patient with a palpable breast tumor or positive mammogram findings must undergo tissue analysis according to the management principles for breast carcinoma. Nipple biopsy is indicated in the presence of abnormal surface epithelium. Analysis of the discharge fluid itself is of such low sensitivity and specificity as to be useless and is therefore not recommended. Analysis of the specific secretions of endocrine tumors has been greatly enhanced by modern intracellular immunofluorescent stain tehniques.[20]

ASSESSMENT: CONSTELLATIONS OF FINDINGS

The principal difficulty in assessment of breast discharge is not the aggregation of all the possibilities or even the elimination of many of them by careful history taking and physical examination, but in the use of common sense in the process of validating the diagnosis.

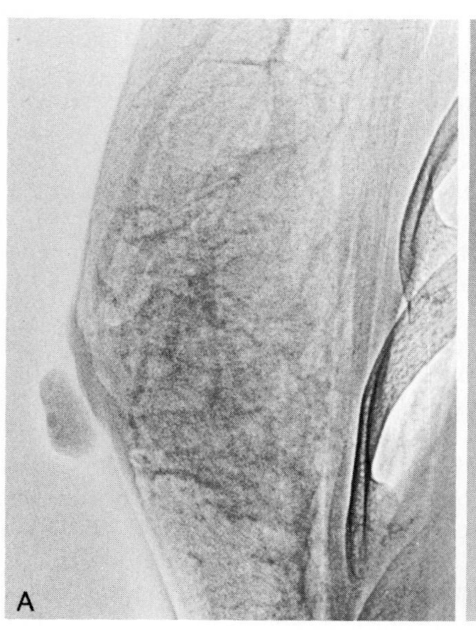

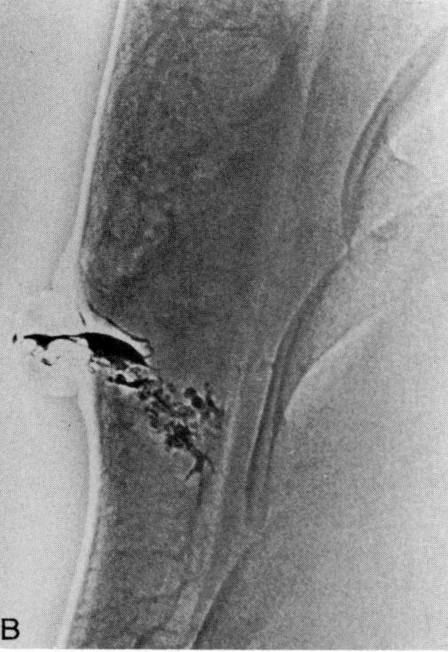

Figure 2. The patient is a 43-year-old woman with a complaint of a bloody discharge from the left nipple for 1 year. The mammogram *(A)* was interpreted as normal. The galactogram *(B)* demonstrates a large intraductal papilloma and marked distal ectasia of the obstructed duct system.

The Cancer Constellation

If a tumor is found on breast examination, the nipple discharge should be regarded as secondary in importance to the breast mass, which should receive prompt attention leading to diagnosis and treatment.[45] If there is no palpable tumor mass in the breast, the likelihood that the discharge is a symptom of breast cancer is very much reduced. Localized breast discharge signals the presence of localized breast disease (Fig. 3). The finding of a dominant breast tumor on physical examination or mammogram immediately indicates management for breast cancer.

A bloody or serosanguineous discharge with a "pressure point" usually signifies the presence of an intraductal papilloma (Fig. 4) and occasionally of a carcinoma.[46] The galactogram demonstrates the size and location of the lesion and whether it is multiple, and may even enable diagnosis of an occult malignancy to be made.[43, 47]

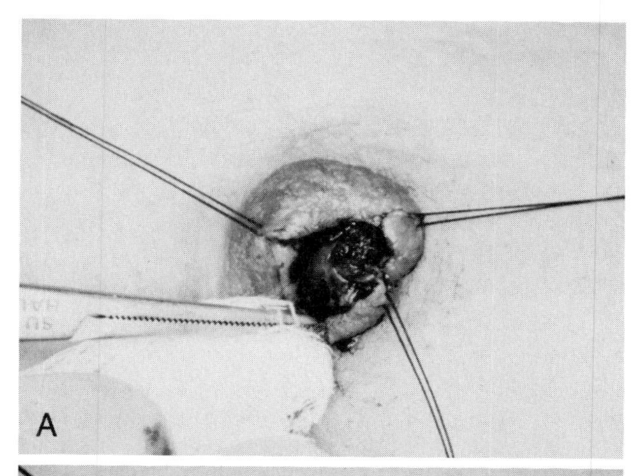

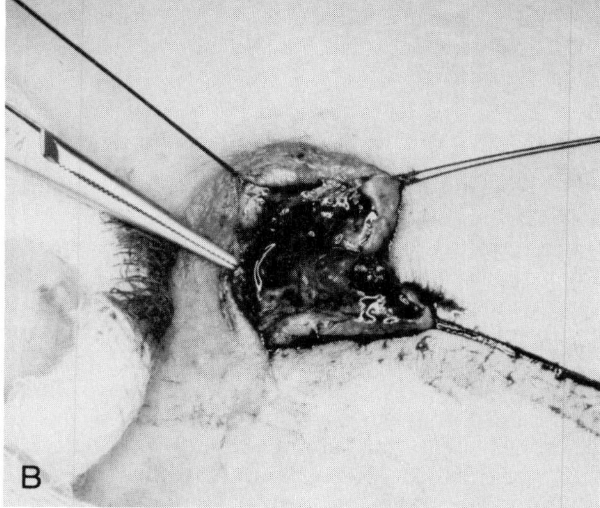

Figure 3. *A,* The beginning dissection of the nipple of the left breast of the patient whose galactogram appears in Figure 2*B*. The inferior suture transfixes the margin of the duct from which the bleeding occurred. *B,* The extent of this papilloma in the further distal dissection of the duct is shown.

A thick, paste-like gray discharge from one or several duct orifices is typical of ductal ectasia. This is an uncommon breast disease occurring chiefly in older women, usually after menopause, that may manifest as only a discharge or as a subareolar mass that decompresses on pressure to release the inspissated material. If there is rupture of such a duct, an inflammatory reaction with foreign body giant cells, edema, and induration occurs. The patient then presents with a central breast mass, often with nipple retraction on arm elevation and, not infrequently, enlargement of one or several axillary nodes. Such patients are understandably considered to have breast carcinoma until a tissue biopsy examination proves the diagnosis of ductal ectasia with rupture and granuloma formation.

Inverted nipples may produce a similar purulent discharge secondary to intermittent chronic infection due to epithelial desquamation with poor hygiene and drainage. The benign nature of this process is confirmed by the rapid and complete response to débridement and cleansing.

Other purulent discharges require surgical management to excise the area of chronic sepsis for final diagnosis as well as treatment.

A small amount of greenish cloudy discharge is a common finding in patients with a long-standing, chronic cystic mastitis. The other findings of this disease are sufficient validation of the diagnosis in the absence of a new mass or mammographic change. Nonoperative management of this disease requires a patient who is faithful to follow-up and who understands that such management cannot, by definition, eliminate the possibility of a malignancy.

Exudates from Paget's disease of the breast are serosanguinous. The ductal cancer that produces the cells growing upward along the ducts to the nipple surface may be too small to be noted on breast examination and too centrally located in dense breast tissue to be seen on mammography. The clue is the change in the character of the nipple in comparison with its mate—it may become less convoluted, slightly more erect, and, finally, ulcerated. The exudate appears during this process, a faint serosanguinous staining of the clothing often before any gross break in the surface epithelium. After such rupture occurs, granulations appear, and the exudate is bloody. In women, crusted nipples are common, but they do not bleed after careful débridement and the surface is not seen to be broken under magnification. Any doubt should be resolved by excising a sliver of nipple tissue—a simple office maneuver—and submitting the tissue for histologic study.

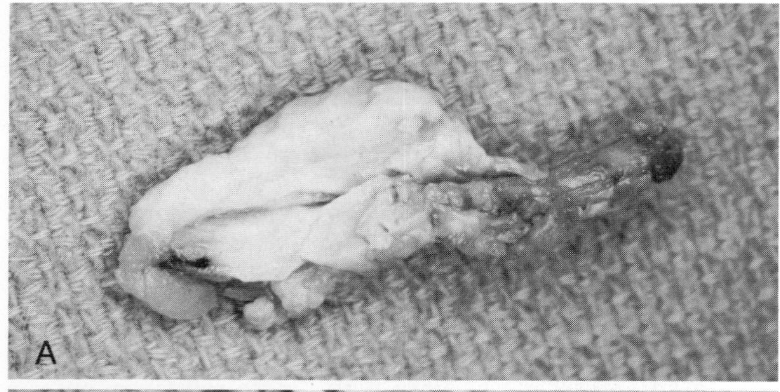

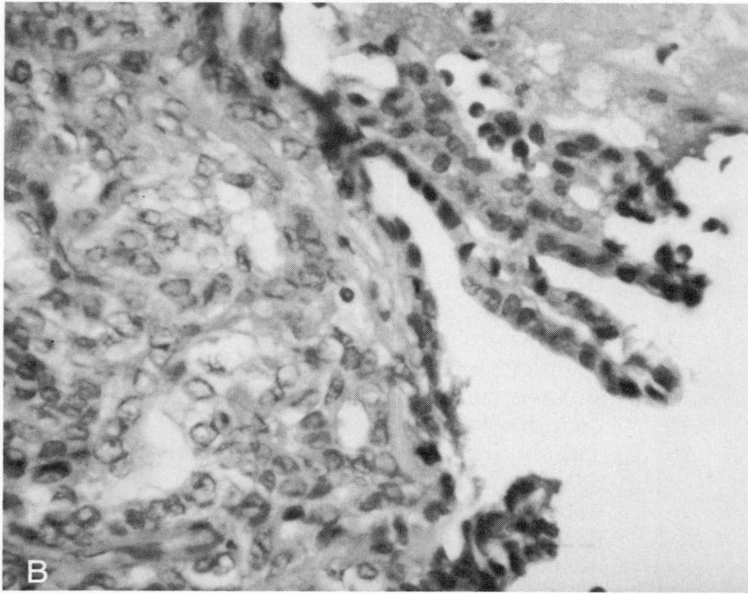

Figure 4. The gross surgical specimen from the patient described in Figure 2. The compressed elongated papilloma can be easily displaced from the duct except at its attached base. *B,* Photomicrograph of a section of this benign tumor.

The Pituitary Tumor Constellation

Elevated Serum Prolactin Value. Assessment of serum prolactin values is the best guide to the diagnosis of pituitary tumor.[39] The assessment requires consideration of two other important variables, secondary amenorrhea and drug use.

Patients with *secondary amenorrhea* in addition to galactorrhea are more likely to harbor pituitary adenomas. In a series reported by March and coworkers,[46] 40 per cent of 75 patients with this clinical combination had radiographic evidence of tumor. If the secondary amenorrhea followed the use of birth control pills, galactorrhea was more common but the tumor incidence was the same.

In addition to a history of contraceptive medications, the use of *lactogenic agents* must be determined. Prolactin values in patients using lactogenic drugs should be normal or, if borderline, should return to normal within 30 days of discontinuation of the agent. Galactorrhea should cease within 3 months. If continued use of the drug is necessary, serial prolactin determinations should be made to ensure that the level remains stable. A rising concentration dictates study of sellar anatomy. Galactorrhea as a side effect of the use of neuroleptic drugs usually appears with the first year of use; appearance at a later date may signal the development of a pituitary adenoma.

All patients with serum prolactin values greater than 100 ng/ml should have contrast-enhanced CT scanning of the sella turcica. Patients with borderline prolactin elevation plus other high-risk factors (amenorrhea plus galactorrhea, failure of resolution after drug withdrawal, rising concentration, unresolved galactorrhea lasting more than 12 months) should also undergo such study. There is evidence that therapeutic effectiveness in the treatment of pituitary adenomas may be related to early diagnosis and intervention. Abnormal sellar anatomy may take the form of "empty sella syndrome," a rare and benign artifact requiring no intervention,[39] or of a clinoid bone or pituitary soft tissue defect indicative of tumor.

If the sellar anatomy appears normal, the decision to use bromocriptine as a therapeutic test must be made. If the bromocriptine response results in lowering of prolactin levels and cessation of galactorrhea, the presumption of a benign perturbation of prolactin release is validated. Patients so treated should have follow-up breast examination four times yearly and a repeat prolactin determination in 1 year. Any recurrence of hyperprolactinemia or galactorrhea is an indication for assessment for pituitary adenoma.

Those hyperprolactinemic patients who fail to respond to bromocriptine therapy need yearly study of the sella to rule out a developing adenoma, unless spontaneous reduction of prolactin value and cessation of galactorrhea occur.

Hyperprolactinemia in conjunction with other elevated pituitary hormones is evidence of a pituitary tumor. The pituitary tumors associated with Cushing's syndrome and sellar enlargement are the most invasive and malignant of all pituitary adenomas.[8]

Normal Serum Prolactin Value. Normoprolactinemic patients with galactorrhea should be observed. Thyroid disease, particularly hypothyroidism, must be ruled out. Follow-up for women with normal menses can be accomplished with quarterly breast examination and yearly prolactin testing. In most cases the galactorrhea ceases spontaneously, the prolactin levels or menses become abnormal, or another endocrine disease is diagnosed. Women with abnormal menses and infertility may be considered for bromocriptine trial, particular care being taken to avoid pregnancy during the trial and for 6 months after return to normal menstrual cycles without bromocriptine support. A CT scan to verify normal pituitary anatomy should precede this "therapeutic test." If pregnancy does occur during the bromocriptine trial, a CT scan should be performed in the second trimester to rule out the presence of an adenoma, and postpartum lactation should be suppressed with bromocriptine.[41]

Males with normoprolactinemic galactorrhea should undergo growth hormone analysis, sex hormone analysis, and a careful search for ectopic production of hormonally active steroids as well as pituitary CT scanning.

Women with prolonged normoprolactinemic galactorrhea (longer than 3 years) should receive CT scanning of pituitary anatomy. A recheck of thyroid function should precede this evaluation. A small residual cohort of women remain undiagnosed and they should have quarterly breast examinations and annual mammography and prolactin studies.

Diagnostic Considerations

The diagnosis of nipple discharge is not a trivial task. The physician must be prepared to be patient, to use time wisely, and to have the discipline to live with a degree of uncertainty. The patient with localized breast discharge can be overtreated if there is a panic to find a carcinoma. The patient with a pituitary or hypothalamic tumor can be undertreated unless the indolence of these lesions is appreciated, particularly if the powerful pharmacologic agents available to lower serum prolactin are improperly used. It is the fear of some serious disease, not the discharge itself, that causes most patients to seek the physician's advice. What is ironic about this problem is that anxiety itself may be responsible for some of the instances of galactorrhea.[38] Some patients with small amounts of clear discharge and in whom all else is normal remain undiagnosed. They tend to be anxious and unhappy. They need counseling, consideration, and frequent reassurance, to which they appear to respond favorably. Whether this represents a diagnosis of anxiety, a placebo effect, or just a desire for comfort is unclear; the hypothalamus does not yield its secrets readily.

REFERENCES

1. Hagler L, Coppes RI, Block MB, Hofeldt FD, Herman RH. Clinical implications of lactose-positive breast secretions in nonpuerperal females. Obstet Gynecol 1975;46:302–7.
2. Kulski JK, Hartmann PE, Gutteridge DH. Composition of breast fluid of a man with galactorrhea and hyperprolactinaemia. J Clin Endocrinol Metab 1961;51:581–2.
3. Lippard CH. The Chiari-Frommel syndrome. Am J Obstet Gynecol 1961;72:724–6.
4. Forbes AP, Henneman PH, Griswold GC, Albright, F. Syndrome characterized by galactorrhea, amenorrhea and low urinary FSH: comparison with acromegaly and normal lactation. J Clin Endocrinol Metab 1954;14:265–71.
5. Canfield CJ, Bates RW. Nonpuerperal galactorrhea. N Engl J Med 1965;273:897–902.
6. Argonz J, del Castillo EB. A syndrome characterized by estrogenic insufficiency, galactorrhea and decreased urinary gonadotropin. J Clin Endocrinol Metab 1953;13:79–87.
7. Kleinberg DL, Noel GL, Frantz AG. Galactorrhea: a study of 235 cases, including 48 with pituitary tumors. N Engl J Med 1977;296:589–600.
8. Young RL, Bradley, EM, Goldzieher JW, Myers PW, Lecocq FR. Spectrum of nonpuerperal galactorrhea: report of two cases evolving through the various syndromes. J Clin Endocrinol 1967;27:461–6.
9. Shah RP, Leavens ME, Samaan NA. Galactorrhea, amenorrhea, and hyperprolactinemia as manifestations of parasellar meningioma. Arch Intern Med 1980;140:1608–12.
10. Naskau Y, Satoshi N, Handa J, Takeuchi J. Amenorrhea-galactorrhea syndrome with craniopharyngioma. Surg Neurol 1980;12:154–6.
11. deLeo R, Petruk KC, Crockford P. Galactorrhea after prolonged traumatic coma: case report. Neurosurgery 1981;9:177.
12. Bloomgarden ZT, McLean GW, Rabin D. Autonomous hyperprolactinemia in tuberous sclerosis. Arch Intern Med 1981;141:1513–15.
13. Caro JF, Israel HL, Glennon JA. Galactorrhea in sarcoidosis: dynamic studies of prolactin, growth and gonadotropic hormone levels. Am J Med Sci 1979;277:289–94.

14. Arora NS, Oblinger MJ, Feldman PS. Chronic pleural blastomycosis with hyperprolactinemia, galactorrhea, and amenorrhea. Am Rev Resp Dis 1979;120:451–5.
15. Sandler MP, Forman MB, Lopis R, Kalk WJ. Galactorrhoea, amenorrhoea and hyperprolactinaemia after an operation on the breast: a case report. S Afr Med J 1980;57:95–6.
16. MacFarlan IA, Rosin MD. Galactorrhoea following surgical procedures to the chest wall: the role of prolactin. Postgrad Med J 1980;56:23–5.
17. Freeman D, Jennings J. Crutch-induced galactorrhea and amenorrhea. Arch Intern Med 1981;141:1847–8.
18. Cohen GH, Dorfman S, Norwood C. Tomographic diagnosis of pituitary microadenomas in Forbes-Albright syndrome (amenorrhea-galactorrhea). Am J Obstet Gynecol 1978;130:822–4.
19. Benoit R, Pearson-Murphy BE, Robert F, et al. Hyperthyroidism due to a pituitary TSH secreting tumour with amenorrhoea-galactorrhoea. Clin Endocrinol 1980; 12:11–9.
20. Kalyanaraman UP, Halmi NS, Elwood PW. Prolactin-secreting pituitary oncocytoma with galactorrhea-amenorrhea syndrome. Cancer 1980;46:1584–9.
21. Drop SL, Bruining GJ, Visser HK, Sippell WG. Prolonged galactorrhoea in a 6-year-old girl with isosexual precocious puberty due to a feminizing adrenal tumour. Clin Endocrinol 1981;15:37–43.
22. Hatjis CG, Polin JI, Wheeler JE, Hayes JM. Amenorrhea-galactorrhea associated with a testosterone-producing, solid granulosa cell tumor. 1978:131:226–7.
23. Emerson K. The mammary gland; a mirror of the endocrine system. Med Times 1980;108:35–45.
24. Wahba MH. Cure of postpartum hyperprolactinaemia galactorrhoea-amenorrhoea by removal of benign ovarian teratoma. Br J Obstet Gynaecol 1980;87:631–3.
25. Tatsumi N, Wada Y. IgA Myeloma with lactation. Acta Haematol 1981;65:132–7.
26. Wortsman J, Hirschowitz JS. Galactorrhea and hyperprolactinemia during treatment of polycystic ovary syndrome. Obstet Gynecol 1980;55:460–3.
27. Shahshanhani MN, Wong ET. Primary hypothyroidism, amenorrhea, and galactorrhea. Arch Intern Med 1978;138:1411–2.
28. Check JH, Adelson HG. Amenorrhea-galactorrhea associated with hypothalamic hypothyroidism. Am J Obstet Gynecol 1981;139:736–8.
29. Contreras P, Generini G, Michelsen H, Pumarino H, Campino C. Hyperprolactinemia and galactorrhea: spontaneous versus iatrogenic hypothyroidism. J Clin Endocrinol Metab 1981;53:1036–9.
30. Carter JN, Tyson JE, Tolis G, VanVliet S, Faiman C, Friesen HG. Prolactin-secreting tumors and hypogonadism in 22 men. N Engl J Med 1978;299:847–52.
31. Draznin B, Maman A. Estrogen-induced galactorrhea in man. Arch Intern Med 1979;139:1059–60.
32. Hulugalle RS, Shetty SP, Gollapudi MG. Galactorrhea in a man with normal testicular function. JAMA 1978; 240:2565.
33. Bryner JR, El Gammal T, Acker JD, Asch RH, Greenblatt RB. Intrasellar subarachnoid herniation or empty sella associated with galactorrhea. Obstet Gynecol 1978; 51:198–203.
34. Zeitner RM, Frank MV, Freeman SM. Pharmacogenic and psychogenic aspects of galactorrhea: case report. Am J Psychiatry 1980;137:111–2.
35. Cohen MR. Galactorrhea and the factors behind symptom production. Am J Psychiatry 1980;137:1277–8.
36. Donald RA, Espiner EA, Livesey JH. Treatment of amenorrhoea, galactorrhoea and hypogonadism with bromocriptine. Aust NZ J Med 1978;8:262–6.
37. Callaghan JT, Cleary RE, Crabtree R, Lemberger L. Clinical response of patients with galactorrhea to pergolide, a potent, long-acting dopaminergic ergot derivative. Life Sci 1981;28:95–102.
38. Murad TM, Contesso G, Mouriesse H. Nipple discharge from the breast. Ann Surg 1982;195:259–64.
39. Naguib YA, Shaarawy DM, Nagui AR, Thabet SM, Azim SA. Endocrinologic and psychologic aspects of galactorrhea associated with normal menstrual cycles. Int J Gynaecol Obstet 1981;19:285–90.
40. Badawy SZ, Nusabum ML, Omar M. Hypothalamic-pituitary evaluation in patients with galactorrhea-amenorrhea and hyperprolactinemia. Obstet Gynecol 1980;55:1–7.
41. Turksoy RN, Farber M, Mitchell GW. Diagnostic and therapeutic modalities in women with galactorrhea. Obstet Gynecol 1980;56:323–9.
42. Shewchuk AB, Adamson GD, Lessard P, Ezrin C. The effect of pregnancy on suspected pituitary adenomas after conservative management of ovulation defects associated with galactorrhea. Am J Obstet Gynecol 1980;136:659–66.
43. Ansari AH, Pearson OH. Recent advances in diagnosis and management of galactorrhea. Int J Fertil 1978;23: 262–9.
44. DiPietro S, DeYoldi GC, Bergonzi S, Gardani G, Saccozzi R, Clemente C. Nipple discharge as a sign of preneoplastic lesion and occult carcinoma of the breast: clinical and galactographic study in 103 consecutive patients. Tumori 1979;65:317–24.
45. Kindermann G, Paterok E, Weishaar J, et al. Early detection of ductal breast cancer: the diagnostic procedure for pathological discharge from the nipple. Tumori 1979;65:555–62.
46. March CM, Mishell DR, Kletzky OA, Israil R, Davajan V, Nakamura RM. Galactorrhea and pituitary tumors in postpill and non-postpill secondary amenorrhea. Am J Obstet Gynecol 1979;134:45–8.
47. Murad TM,Contesso G, Mouriesse H. Papillary tumors of large lactiferous ducts. Cancer 1981;48:122–3.

CALF PAIN

JACK HIRSH □ RUSSELL D. HULL

□ SYNONYM: Leg pain

BACKGROUND

The patient with calf pain poses a perplexing clinical problem, because calf pain is a common presenting symptom not only of venous thrombosis, a potentially serious condition, but also of less serious disorders. In most clinical settings, it is likely to be caused by one of the more benign disorders. Calf pain is the presenting symptom of venous thrombosis in more than 50 per cent of symptomatic patients with venographically proven thrombosis, but it is highly nonspecific and its severity and extent correlate poorly with the size (and hence potential danger) of the venous thrombus.[1, 2] The dilemma facing the physician is to decide when calf pain should be investigated for venous thrombosis using more objective tests and when is it safe to conclude that the pain is not caused by venous thrombosis.

This chapter contains a discussion of the various causes of calf pain and describes a practical approach to its diagnosis through specific and objective tests.

Causes

Most tissues in the calf, including muscle, bone, subcutaneous tissue, ligaments, tendons, and vascular and perivascular tissue, contain pain-sensitive fibers. Inflammation of any of these structures can produce calf pain like that of deep venous thrombosis, which is produced by inflammation of the vessel wall or perivascular tissues. Calf pain may therefore be caused by a variety of other disorders (Table 1).[1, 2]

Table 1. CAUSES OF CALF PAIN

Venous thrombosis
Muscle strain, cramp, or trauma
Muscle tear
Direct muscle or leg trauma
Spontaneous muscle hematoma
Arterial insufficiency (muscle ischemia)
Neurogenic pain
Ruptured popliteal (Baker's) cyst
Arthritis of the knee or ankle
Achilles tendinitis
Inflammation of other tissues in the lower limb
Bone lesions
Varicose veins
Superficial venous thrombosis
Pregnancy or use of oral contraceptives
Postphlebitic syndrome
Cellulitis
Tendon injury

Venous Thrombosis

The majority of patients who develop venous thrombosis have no clinical manifestations.[4] When symptoms or signs do occur, they are caused either by obstruction to venous outflow, by inflammation of the vessel wall or perivascular tissue, by a combination of these two factors, or by embolization of the thrombus into the pulmonary circulation. The common clinical symptoms and signs of venous thrombosis are pain, tenderness, and swelling.[1, 2] It should be emphasized, however, that these are highly nonspecific and may be caused by any of the conditions listed in Table 1. The time-honored Homans sign is also nonspecific and can be elicited in many of the conditions that simulate venous thrombosis. Thus, although these clinical features may lead to suspicion of venous thrombosis, they should not be used to make a definitive diagnosis or as a basis for therapeutic decisions. Less common manifestations of venous thrombosis are venous distension; discoloration, including pallor, cyanosis, and redness; and a palpable cord.

Pain and Tenderness. Pain and tenderness are probably caused by local inflammation of a vein wall and perivascular tissue and, in the case of proximal vein thrombosis, by venous distension. The pain and tenderness associated with calf vein thrombosis are usually localized to the calf, whereas the pain and tenderness associated with proximal vein thrombosis may be localized to the calf or may occur in the thigh or iliac region. Patients with proximal vein thrombosis may also have more diffuse calf pain and tenderness when these symptoms and signs are associated with marked swelling.

The pain of venous thrombosis is not characteristic. It may be either an ache or a cramp, sharp or dull, and severe or mild. It is often aggravated by movement and weight-bearing and is associated with local tenderness. The pain may improve with bedrest with leg elevation and heparin therapy, but these features also are not specific for venous thrombosis.

Associated Features. Swelling due to edema frequently accompanies the leg pain and tenderness caused by venous thrombosis. Typically, the edema pits on pressure, but sometimes it is mild and can be detected only as an increased turgor of calf muscles, which is best appreciated by carefully palpating the relaxed calf. When swelling is due to obstruction of a large proximal vein, it usually occurs distal to the site of obstruction and may be relatively painless. On the other hand, swelling due to inflammation is usually localized to the site of thrombosis and is associated with pain and tenderness. Swelling usually subsides when the leg is elevated.

Venous dilatation is a relatively uncommon manifestation of acute venous thrombosis. When it occurs, it is an early feature of obstruction to venous drainage and usually disappears when the leg is elevated or new collateral channels form. Discoloration is also a relatively uncommon manifestation of venous thrombosis. The leg may be pale, cyanotic, or reddish blue. Cyanosis, which is caused by impaired venous return and stagnant anoxia, occurs in patients with proximal vessel obstruction. Rarely, the leg may be diffusely red, hot, and inflamed owing to marked perivascular inflammation; this clinical picture may be difficult to differentiate from that of cellulitis. Pallor is uncommon but may be seen in the early stage of acute iliofemoral vein thrombosis and is thought to be caused by arterial spasm.

When an easily palpable vessel becomes thrombosed, it may be felt as a tender cord, and if the vein is very superficial, it may be obviously warm.

Muscle Strain or Trauma

Muscle ache may occur after jogging, hiking, tennis, squash, or walking in ill-fitting shoes. The discomfort may commence soon after the episode of unusual muscular activity or may be delayed for 12 to 24 hours. Pain usually occurs in the calf but also may involve the thigh. There may be tenderness, which at times can be quite severe. There may be no swelling, but the leg muscles may feel tense, heavy, and turgid. In some patients, the pain may be associated with considerable swelling due to edema.

The correct diagnosis is made relatively easily if there is an obvious history of unaccustomed exercise and if the pain and tenderness are in both legs or involve muscle groups in the anterior tibial compartment. However, if pain and tenderness are unilateral and involve the calf muscles, it may be impossible to distinguish muscle strain from venous thrombosis without objective testing.

Muscle Tear

Fibers of the gastrocnemius muscle or, less commonly, the plantaris muscle may be torn as a result of sudden strong stretching of contracting calf muscles during plantar flexion. Usually, only a small part of the muscle is torn at the musculotendinous junction, but occasionally there may be a large tear or even separation of muscle from tendon or avulsion of the tendon. Typically, the muscle tear occurs when the foot is suddenly flexed against resistance, for example, when the individual stands or begins to run. There is a sudden severe pain at the back of the leg that may feel like a direct blow to the calf muscles. It may temporarily subside and then be followed by a constant pain that becomes rapidly more severe as a hematoma forms and the calf muscles go into spasm. Examination reveals local tenderness, and it may be possible to palpate the localized swelling caused by hematoma. If there is a complete tear or avulsion of the muscle at its attachment to the tendon (a complete tendon rupture), one may be able to palpate the gap produced by the tear.

After several days, an ecchymosis may appear either in the posterior aspect of the medial malleolus or in the anteromedial part of the leg, but this occurrence is not invariable. Pain and tenderness may continue for days or even weeks and may be very severe, particularly during any activity involving plantar flexion.

In most patients with muscle tear, the diagnosis is clinically obvious and further investigations are unnecessary. In some patients, however, symptoms do not develop for a number of hours after injury, and objective testing is required to rule out complicating deep venous thrombosis.

Direct Muscle or Leg Trauma

Direct muscle trauma sustained during a vigorous sporting activity or an accident may produce delayed pain and swelling due to hematoma and inflammation. It can present considerable diagnostic difficulty because venous thrombosis is a well-recognized complication of leg trauma.

Spontaneous Muscle Hematoma

Occasionally, patients who are treated with anticoagulants develop pain and swelling of the leg either without obvious trauma or following mild trauma. It may be difficult to decide whether these symptoms are caused by hemorrhage or recurrent venous thrombosis, particularly if the patient is being treated with anticoagulants for venous thrombosis. Differentiation between these two causes by means of objective testing is important, because if a diagnosis of recurrent venous thrombosis has been made in error and anticoagulant therapy is continued in a patient with hematoma, the consequences may be disastrous.

Arterial Insufficiency

Arterial insufficiency is not usually confused with venous thrombosis because the clinical features of the two conditions are sufficiently distinctive. The pain of acute arterial occlusion is sudden in onset and may be associated with some tenderness. The limb is cold and pale, the pulses are nonpalpable, and there is usually no swelling. Occasionally in the early stages of acute iliofemoral vein thrombosis, the limb may be very pale owing to arterial spasm and the clinical picture may resemble that of arterial thrombosis, but the two conditions can usually be readily differentiated within a few hours of onset of symptoms.

Neurogenic Pain

Compression of the sciatic nerve or lateral cutaneous nerve of the thigh produces leg pain that is easily differentiated from the pain of venous thrombosis by its characteristic distribution. Neurogenic pain is not associated with swelling, is sudden in onset, and is aggravated by maneuvers that stretch the nerve. There may be evidence of a neurologic deficit, but even in its absence, differentiation between the two conditions can usually be made through careful history taking and examination.

Ruptured Popliteal Cyst

When a popliteal cyst (Baker's cyst) ruptures, the fluid contents track down the tissue planes between the calf muscles and produce an inflammatory response with pain, tenderness, heat, and swelling that may simulate the clinical features of acute venous thrombosis. In most cases, there is a history of arthritis of the knee or of traumatic or operative injury to the knee. Occasionally, popliteal cyst rupture may occur without a history of knee trauma or arthritis, or the episode of calf pain and swelling may be preceded by intermittent pain or swelling in the region of the popliteal fossa by months or years. On examination of the knee, there may be evidence of arthritis or previous surgery or trauma and a fullness in the popliteal fossa on the affected side. The diagnosis can be readily established by arthrography, but because venous thrombosis and popliteal cyst rupture may occur in the same patient, it is necessary to exclude venous thrombosis specifically before attributing the acute clinical features to the ruptured cyst.

Arthritis of the Knee or Ankle or Achilles Tendinitis

Acute pain and swelling produced by arthritis of the knee or ankle joint or by inflammation of the Achilles tendon may occasionally be confused with those of venous thrombosis. Careful history and examination reveals that the pain, tenderness, and swelling are localized mainly to the affected joint, so that in most cases, these conditions can be readily differentiated from venous thrombosis. Confusion sometimes arises in patients with systemic lupus erythematosus, who may develop acute arthralgia of the ankle or knee with pleuritis that is mistaken for venous thrombosis with pulmonary embolism. However, the two conditions are readily differentiated by careful history taking and examination.

Inflammation of Other Tissues in the Lower Limb

Lower limb cellulitis, lymphangitis, vasculitis, myositis, and panniculitis may each produce pain and tenderness of the lower limb. These conditions can usually be differentiated from venous thrombosis on clinical grounds alone when they are fully developed but may occasionally be confused with it in their early stages or if they are atypical. Atypical cellulitis or lymphangitis can be difficult to differentiate from phlebitis with marked perivascular inflammation; there may be pain, tenderness, and swelling of the calf as well as pain and tenderness in the femoral triangle in all three conditions. Myositis produces diffuse muscular pain and involves muscle groups that are not specifically localized over the deep veins of the calf. The clinical features of vasculitis and panniculitis are distinctive and should not produce diagnostic problems.

Bone Lesions

Lesions affecting the bones of the leg, including tumors, subperiosteal hematoma, and fractures, produce pain, tenderness, and swelling that may sometimes superficially resemble venous thrombosis. Diagnostic problems may arise when confused, elderly patients sustain a fracture of the femoral neck, because they often have swelling of the thigh due to bleeding. It may be difficult to obtain a history of trauma. The diagnosis of hip fracture is usually obvious after careful clinical examination, although coexisting venous thrombosis is common.

Varicose Veins

Patients with varicose veins often have pain and tenderness in the calf after they have been standing for a while. Occasionally, an obvious superficial varicose vein becomes inflamed and thrombosed and the pain is more severe. When these clinical features occur in association with more diffuse pain in the calf or with edema of the leg, it may be difficult to exclude associated deep vein thrombosis without performing objective diagnostic tests.

Superficial Venous Thrombosis

In most patients with thrombosis of a superficial calf vein, the diagnosis is obvious. The pain and tenderness are localized to an easily palpable superficial vein. In some cases, however, the pain and tenderness may extend beyond the area of superficial thrombosis and may be accompanied by swelling; in these instances, associated deep vein thrombosis should be excluded by objective testing.

Pregnancy and Oral Contraceptive Ingestion

Pain and tenderness in the leg may occur in a patient who is pregnant or is taking an estrogen-containing oral contraceptive pill. Occasionally, these symptoms in pregnant patients are associated with considerable swelling of the calf or thigh that may be unilateral. In many cases, the symptoms and signs are not due to venous thrombosis. The cause of pain and tenderness is uncertain but may be venous dilatation caused by estrogens, inflammation of the vein wall without associated thrombosis, or, in pregnant patients, muscle cramps. Compression of the iliac vein by the enlarged uterus may also contribute to the unilateral leg swelling seen in pregnancy.

Postphlebitic Syndrome

Typically, patients with the postphlebitic syndrome have long-standing symptoms of swelling associated with an ache in the calf that occurs on standing or leg exercise. Some of these patients present with repeated episodes of more severe swelling and pain, possibly in association with calf tenderness. The majority of the acute episodes are not caused by a recurrence of venous thrombosis and do not require anticoagulant treatment, but it is often difficult to exclude acute venous thrombosis without objective testing. Such exacerbations are probably caused by progressive venous dilatation, which produces further valvular incompetence and a sudden increase in calf venous pressure.

DIAGNOSTIC STUDIES (OBJECTIVE TESTING)

Invasive Studies

Venography

Venography is the reference method against which all other diagnostic procedures for venous thrombosis are assessed. In ascending venography, the deep and superficial venous systems are opacified by injection of radiopaque dye into a dorsal foot vein. If adequately performed and interpreted, this procedure can be relied on to confirm or exclude the diagnosis in patients with clinically suspected venous thrombosis.[5, 6]

With good technique, ascending venography outlines the deep venous system of the legs, including the external and common iliac veins, in most patients.[6] Common femoral or iliac venography, however, may be required if external and common iliac veins are not adequately visualized by the ascending technique or if the inferior vena cava needs to be outlined. The current methods of ascending venography are not reliable for visualizing the deep femoral or internal iliac veins.

The interpretation of venography requires an understanding of the dynamics of venous flow, the physical properties of the water-soluble radiopaque contrast media used in venography, and the anatomy of the venous system.[6] In the upright position, the veins of each lower extremity hold more than 300 ml of blood. At rest, the flow in these veins is under the influence of low pressure gradients. Because the water-soluble radiopaque contrast media used in venography differ significantly in their physical properties from blood, layering and incomplete mixing of contrast medium with blood may occur. When the patient is supine, the radiopaque medium tends to stream and can produce artifacts, which can be minimized if the patient is examined in a semi-upright position. In this position, the blood is displaced by the heavier contrast medium injected into a superficial vein of the dorsal arch of the foot. In order to obtain complete filling, the extremity should be completely relaxed. Relaxation can be achieved by ensuring that the limb is bearing no weight at the time of injection.

Venography has a number of disadvantages: it is invasive, produces pain in approximately 50 per cent of patients, and induces clinically significant phlebitis in 1 to 2 per cent of patients.[2, 5] It is also expensive and time-consuming. For these reasons, many diagnostic centers have replaced or supplemented venography with noninvasive testing for clinically suspected venous thrombosis.

^{125}I-Fibrinogen Leg Scanning

^{125}I-fibrinogen leg scanning detects thrombi that are actively accreting fibrin in veins of the calf and distal thigh.[4] Falsely positive results occur if scanning is performed over a hematoma, a large wound area, or an area of inflammation, but in the absence of these conditions, leg scanning is both sensitive and specific for acute thrombosis of calf and lower thigh veins.[11] Leg scanning should not be used as the only diagnostic test in patients with clinically suspected venous thrombosis because it fails to detect thrombi in approximately 30 per cent of patients and because there may be a delay before a sufficient amount of the fibrinogen accumulates in the thrombus for the test result to register as positive. In many patients with acute venous thrombosis, the leg scanning result becomes positive within 24 hours of injection of ^{125}I-fibrinogen. In some patients with symptomatic acute venous thrombosis, however, it may take 48 hours or even 72 hours for enough radiolabeled fibrinogen to accumulate in the thrombus to allow a positive diagnosis.[1] ^{125}I-fibrinogen scanning is valuable when used to complement IPG in patients with clinically suspected venous thrombosis.

Noninvasive Studies

Impedance Plethysmography

Impedance plethysmography (IPG) is used to detect changes in blood volume in the calf in response to intermittent venous obstruction. This test is sensitive and specific for proximal vein thrombosis in symptomatic patients with clinically suspected venous thrombosis.[1, 2] A positive IPG result can be used to make therapeutic decisions in the vast majority of such patients.[2] A negative result essentially excludes a diagnosis of proximal vein thrombosis[2] but does not exclude calf vein thrombosis. Falsely positive results may occur with disorders that interfere with arterial inflow or venous outflow, including severe congestive cardiac failure, constrictive pericarditis, severe arterial insufficiency, hypotension, and external compression of veins.[6–8] Most of these disorders are readily recognized clinically. Falsely positive results may also occur if the technician performs the test incorrectly or if the patient is not relaxed. The test cannot be performed in a patient who has a plaster leg cast or cannot be properly positioned because of immobilization or pain.

Doppler Ultrasound Scanning

Like IPG, Doppler ultrasound scanning is sensitive to symptomatic proximal vein thrombosis but relatively insensitive to calf vein thrombosis.[9, 10] Its major drawbacks are that its interpretation is subjective and that it requires considerable skill and experience to perform reliably. In skilled hands, however, it is almost as sensitive for detection of symptomatic proximal vein thrombosis as is the IPG. Doppler ultrasonography is more specific than IPG in the patient with raised venous pressure or arterial insufficiency and can be used in the patient in traction with a plaster leg cast.

Other Studies

Other plethysmographic techniques, such as strain gauge plethysmography and air-cuff volume plethysmography, may be interchangeable with IPG. Because their value as diagnostic tests for venous thrombosis has not been as well studied as that of IPG, however, these techniques are not discussed further.

DIAGNOSTIC APPROACH FOR A FIRST EPISODE OF CALF PAIN

Through a carefully taken history and thorough physical examination, it should be possible to rule out many of the causes of calf pain other than acute venous thrombosis (Table 2). The dilemma facing the clinician is that even after such a process, only about 20 per cent of the ambulatory patients and 50 per cent of the bedridden patients in whom other conditions have been ruled out actually have venous thrombosis.[1, 2] If venography is the only objective test available, it should be performed on all patients with leg symptoms or signs compatible with venous thrombosis. If noninvasive tests are available and their results are applied appropriately, they can supplant venography in the majority of patients. See the algorithm, "Diagnostic Assessment of Calf Pain (First Episode)."

A clinical suspicion of venous thrombosis can be either confirmed or denied by performing serial impedance plethysmography or Doppler ultrasonography alone or by combining IPG with ^{125}I-fibrinogen leg scanning or venography.[1, 2] If the IPG result is positive in the absence of conditions known to produce falsely positive results, a diagnosis of venous thrombosis can be confidently made and proper treatment instituted. If, however, the IPG result is negative, the clinician has

Table 2. DIFFERENTIAL DIAGNOSIS OF ACUTE LEG PAIN

Signs and Symptoms	Probable Diagnosis
Pain and tenderness localized in the calf	Venous thrombosis
Tenderness in the popliteal fossa along anteromedial aspect of thigh in the groin	Venous thrombosis
Pain and tenderness over the tibia or anterior compartment of leg	Venous thrombosis highly unlikely
Previous knee surgery, evidence of arthritis of knee, or soft mass in popliteal fossa	Ruptured popliteal (Baker's) cyst
Inflamed or thrombosed varicose veins	Superficial venous thrombosis
Localized tender mass in calf	Torn calf muscle
Ecchymoses in region of calf or below medial malleolus	Torn calf muscle
Onset of pain preceded by sudden plantar flexion of foot	Torn calf muscle
Recent history of unusual exercise or activity	Muscle strain

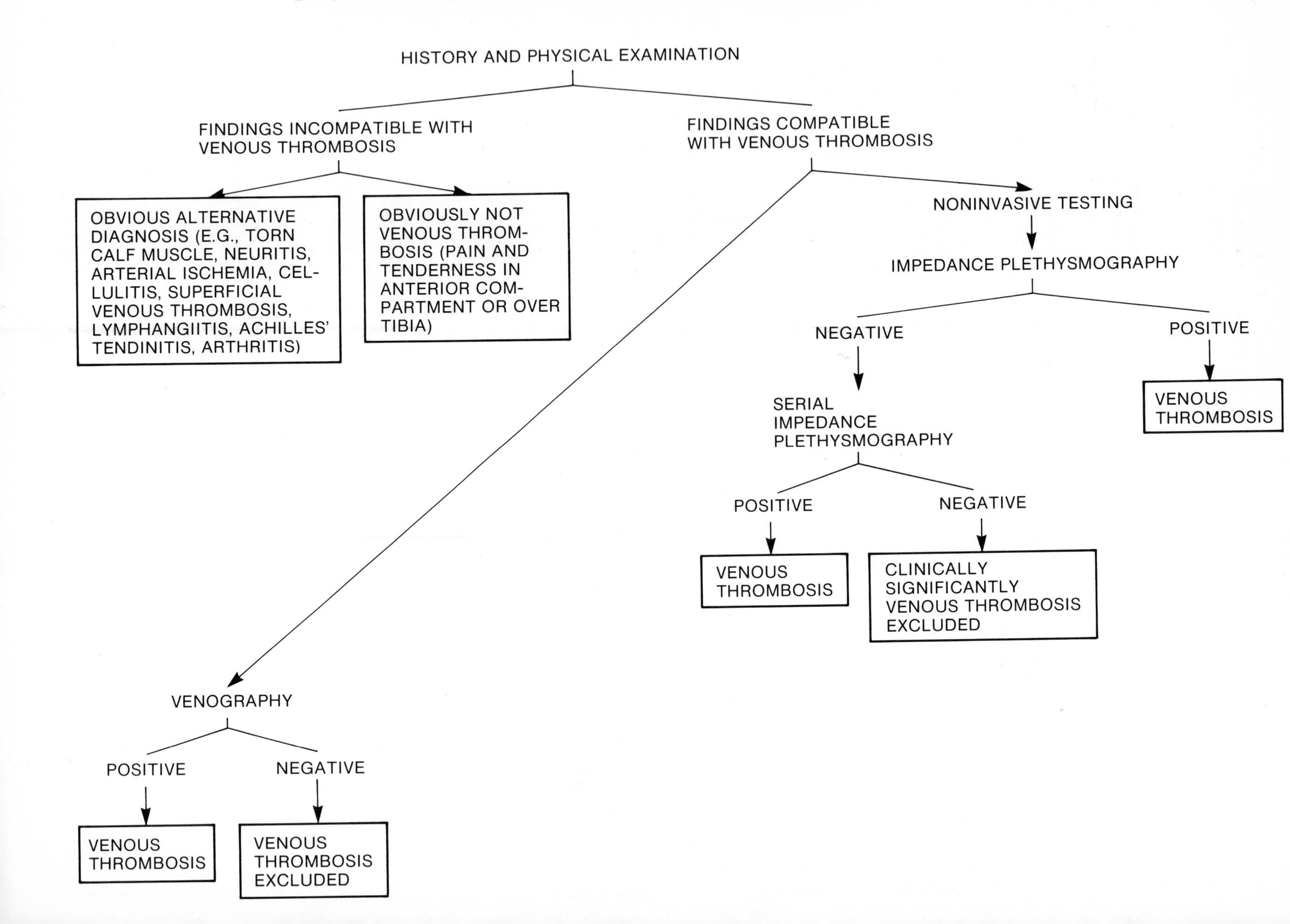
DIAGNOSTIC ASSESSMENT OF CALF PAIN (FIRST EPISODE)
HISTORY AND PHYSICAL EXAMINATION
FINDINGS INCOMPATIBLE WITH VENOUS THROMBOSIS
OBVIOUS ALTERNATIVE DIAGNOSIS (E.G., TORN CALF MUSCLE, NEURITIS, ARTERIAL ISCHEMIA, CELLULITIS, SUPERFICIAL VENOUS THROMBOSIS, LYMPHANGIITIS, ACHILLES' TENDINITIS, ARTHRITIS)
OBVIOUSLY NOT VENOUS THROMBOSIS (PAIN AND TENDERNESS IN ANTERIOR COMPARTMENT OR OVER TIBIA)
FINDINGS COMPATIBLE WITH VENOUS THROMBOSIS
NONINVASIVE TESTING
IMPEDANCE PLETHYSMOGRAPHY
NEGATIVE
POSITIVE
VENOUS THROMBOSIS
SERIAL IMPEDANCE PLETHYSMOGRAPHY
POSITIVE
NEGATIVE
VENOUS THROMBOSIS
CLINICALLY SIGNIFICANTLY VENOUS THROMBOSIS EXCLUDED
VENOGRAPHY
POSITIVE
NEGATIVE
VENOUS THROMBOSIS
VENOUS THROMBOSIS EXCLUDED

three alternatives: (1) repeated IPG examinations to detect extending calf vein thrombosis,[8] (2) ^{125}I-fibrinogen leg scanning to detect calf vein thrombosis,[1] or (3) venography.

Use of Serial IPG Examinations

The use of repeated examination by impedance plethysmography has been advocated by a number of experienced investigators and has been shown to be safe.[8] The rationale for this approach is based on the supposition that calf vein thrombi that are not detected by IPG do not require treatment unless they extend. Extension can be detected by performing IPG examinations on the third and fifth days after the first one. The reason for the effectiveness of this approach can be readily appreciated if one considers the risks of proximal vein thrombosis in patients who have a negative IPG result. In approximately 800 of 1,000 ambulatory patients with clinically suspected venous thrombosis, the IPG results are negative and venography (if performed) would confirm that proximal vein thrombosis is not present. Of the 170 patients with positive IPG results, 160 would have proximal vein thrombosis and 10 would have calf vein thrombosis. Thirty patients would have a negative IPG result even though they do have calf vein thrombosis. Assuming that all 30 are not confined to bed because of an associated condition and, therefore, remain ambulatory, the calf thrombi in about six patients would extend into the proximal venous segment; these six patients could be readily identified by serial impedance plethysmography examinations.

Use of ^{125}I-Fibrinogen Leg Scanning

Results of ^{125}I-fibrinogen leg scanning are positive in most untreated patients with acute calf vein thrombosis even though there may be no extension of the thrombus, because the radioactive fibrinogen diffuses into the thrombus and is laid down as radioactive fibrin.[1] If this approach is preferred, the radiolabeled fibrinogen is injected intravenously after the results of the IPG have been shown to be negative, and the leg is scanned within 24 hours and again at 72 hours.

Use of Venography

If venography were performed in all patients with negative IPG results, invasive testing would be done in approximately 80 per cent of symptomatic patients, most of whom do not have thrombosis. For this reason, venography is considered to be the least desirable of the three primary approaches.

Use of Doppler Ultrasound Scanning

In comparison with IPG, Doppler ultrasonography has similar but somewhat lower sensitivity and specificity for proximal vein thrombosis and slightly higher sensitivity for calf vein thrombosis. It could be used instead of IPG or in combination with ^{125}I-fibrinogen leg scanning for symptomatic patients, but such an approach would require formal evaluation before it could be recommended.

DIAGNOSIS OF RECURRENT LEG PAIN

The diagnostic approach is illustrated in Table 3 and the algorithm, "Diagnostic Assessment of Recurrent Leg Pain." Usually, two possible causes must be considered.

Acute Recurrent Venous Thrombosis

Most patients with venous thrombosis or pulmonary embolism who receive adequate treatment with anticoagulants do not develop recurrence.[12, 13, 14] Venous thrombosis rarely recurs during adequate anticoagulant treatment but may do so after therapy has been stopped if there is a continuing risk factor (such as immobilization or carcinoma) or if the patient requires surgery or

Table 3. INVESTIGATION OF CHRONIC LEG PAIN

Question	Comment
Is there long saphenous vein incompetence?	Diagnosis made by inspection of leg, venous tourniquet, and demonstration of reflux on Doppler ultrasound scanning.
Are varicose veins present?	Nonspecific sign that does not differentiate between primary varicose veins and varicosities secondary to deep vein obstruction or incompetence.
Is there deep vein incompetence?	Diagnosed by demonstrating reflux with Doppler ultrasound probe placed over posterior tibial vein.
Is there obstruction to venous outflow?	Demonstrated by plethysmography or ultrasound scanning.

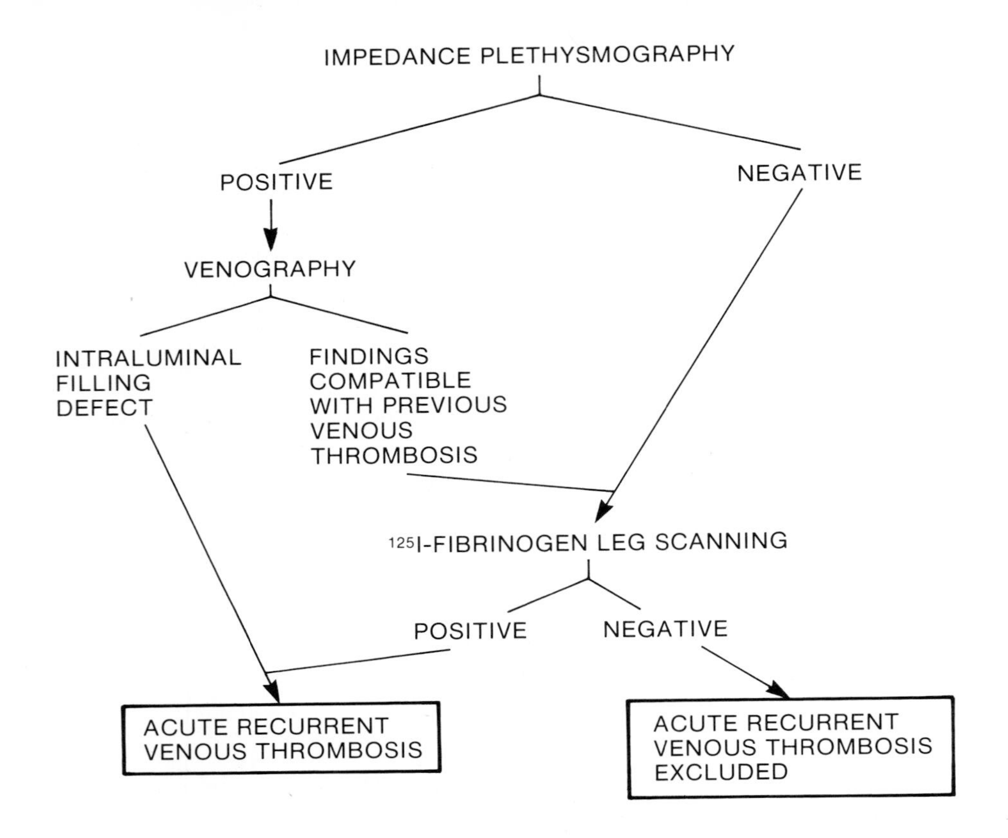

becomes bedridden with a medical illness. Recurrence also is seen in patients with an underlying predisposing cause such as antithrombin III or protein C deficiency.

If clinical features suggestive of recurrence do appear, it is important to ensure that they are not manifestations of the initial episode of venous thrombosis, so that the patient is not exposed unnecessarily to the risk and expense of a second course of anticoagulants. Patients may develop symptoms of pain and swelling in the involved leg soon after the acute episode, when they become mobile. In most cases, these symptoms are due not to acute recurrent venous thrombosis but to inflammation of venous and perivascular tissues or to venous obstruction.[15]

Patients may also present with symptoms of pain, tenderness, or swelling of the leg months or years after the original acute venous thrombotic event. If the symptoms occur as an acute exacerbation after a long asymptomatic interval, a diagnosis of acute recurrent venous thrombosis should be considered and the investigation should proceed accordingly. If the symptoms occur as repeated exacerbations against a background of chronic leg pain, they are likely to be caused by nonthrombotic complications of chronic venous insufficiency, and in most cases further investigation is not required. Some patients with chronic leg pain develop subacute exacerbations that may or may not be due to recurrent venous thrombosis and require objective testing.

The first step in the investigation of a patient with clinically suspected recurrent venous thrombosis is to determine whether the diagnosis of acute venous thrombosis had been made in the past using acceptable objective tests. If such a diagnosis has not been made, the patient should undergo venography to determine the state of the deep venous system. If the findings are completely normal, a diagnosis of venous thrombosis as the cause of the patient's symptoms can be excluded. If an intraluminal filling defect is found, it is reasonable to attribute the patient's recent symptoms to an acute episode of venous thrombosis (obliteration of the deep venous system, recanalization of the deep venous system with valvular destruction, or obstruction of the deep venous system with formation of collaterals). ^{125}I-fibrinogen leg scanning should be done, because such a finding does not exclude a recent acute episode of venous thrombosis.

If a previous episode of deep venous thrombosis is confirmed by venography, the present symptoms can be investigated by either venography or impedance plethysmography. If the venogram shows a new intraluminal filling defect, the patient should be treated as for acute recurrent venous thrombosis. If the venographic findings are compatible with previous disease, ^{125}I-fibrinogen leg scanning should be done. If the leg scan result is positive, a diagnosis of acute recurrent venous thrombosis can be made. If, on the other hand, the result of IPG is negative, a diagnosis of acute recurrent venous thrombosis can be excluded and the patient does not require treatment.

Chronic Venous Insufficiency

Chronic calf pain varying in intensity from a mild intermittent ache to severe bursting, incapacitating pain on exertion occurs when venous return of blood from the lower limbs is impaired. In the erect position, venous return from the lower limbs largely depends on the competence of the venous valves of the lower limb and the patency of the major venous channels.[16]

Chronic venous insufficiency may occur when there is disease of any of the four classes of leg veins: the outflow tract, consisting of the popliteal, superficial femoral, common external, and common iliac veins; the deep veins of the calf (intramuscular veins); the superficial veins of the calf, which communicate with the deep veins through connecting veins; and the long and short saphenous veins, which communicate directly with the major deep veins in the outflow tract and have no direct connection with the veins within the calf muscle pump.

When the calf muscles contract, there is an increase in pressure within the intramuscular veins, which normally forces blood into the outflow tract and toward the heart because of the numerous valves within the veins that permit only unidirectional flow. During muscle relaxation, the pressure within the intramuscular veins is lower than the pressure in the superficial veins, so the deep venous system is refilled by blood flowing from the superficial veins through the communicating veins.

With valvular incompetence confined to the long saphenous vein, there is retrograde blood flow in that vein during exercise, but if the remainder of the venous system is normal, the calf pump can cope with the extra load and the symptoms are relatively minor. With valvular incompetence of the communicating veins, high pressures generated within the calf pump during exercise are transmitted directly into the superficial veins and the symptoms are more serious. The patient complains of aching pains, night cramps, some ankle edema, and skin pigmentation, and in some cases there is ulceration of the skin overlying the incompetent communicating veins.

The most severe symptoms occur with either obstruction or valvular incompetence of the major outflow tract. In valvular incompetence, the calf does not empty of blood during muscle contraction, and high pressures are generated within the deep veins of the calf, causing dilatation in the communicating veins and secondary valvular incompetence. An increase in pressure within the superficial veins during exercise results. Signs and symptoms include constant aching pain in the calf, skin pigmentation, eczema, lipodermatosclerosis, and, in extreme cases, ulceration. With obstruction to the major outflow tract, the patient also complains of severe bursting pains during exercise (venous claudication).

REFERENCES

1. Hull R, Hirsh J, Sackett DL, Powers P, Turpie AGG, Walker I. Combined use of leg scanning and impedance plethysmography in suspected venous thrombosis: an alternative to venography. N Engl J Med 1977;296:1497–1500.
2. Hull R, Hirsh J, Sackett DL, et al. Replacement of venography in suspected venous thrombosis by impedance plethysmography and 125I-fibrinogen leg scanning. Ann Intern Med 1981;94(1):12–5.
3. Katz RS, Zizic TM, Arnold WP, Stevens MB. The pseudothrombophlebitis syndrome. Medicine 1977;56:151–4.
4. Kakkar VV. The diagnosis of deep vein thrombosis using the 125I fibrinogen test. Arch Surg 1972;104:152–9.
5. Bettmen MA, Paulin S. Leg phlebography: the incidence, nature and modification of undesirable side effects. Radiology 1977;122:101–4.
6. Hull R, Taylor DW, Hirsh J. Impedance plethysmography: the relationship between venous filling and sensitivity and specificity for proximal vein thrombosis. Circulation 1978,58:898–902.
7. Hull R, van Aken WG, Hirsh J, et al. Impedance plethysmography using the occlusive cuff technique in the diagnosis of venous thrombosis. Circulation 1976;53:696–700.
8. Wheeler HB, O'Donnell JA, Anderson FA, Penney BC, Peura RA, Benedict C. Bedside screening for venous thrombosis using occlusive impedance phlebography. Angiology 1975;26:199–210.
9. Sumner DS, Lambeth A. Reliability of Doppler ultrasound in the diagnosis of acute venous thrombosis both above and below the knee. Am J Surg 1979;138:205–10.
10. Barnes RW, Russell HE, Wu KK, Hoak JC. Accuracy of Doppler ultrasound in clinically suspected venous thrombosis of the calf. Surg Gynecol Obstet 1976;143:425–8.
11. Hirsh J, Gallus AS. 125-I-labeled fibrinogen scanning: use in the diagnosis of venous thrombosis. JAMA 1975;233:970–3.

12. Hull R, Delmore T, Genton E, et al. Warfarin sodium versus low-dose heparin in the long-term treatment of venous thrombosis. N Engl J Med 1979;301:855–8.
13. Hull R, Delmore T, Carter C, et al. Adjusted subcutaneous heparin versus warfarin sodium in the long-term treatment of venous thrombosis. N Engl J Med 1982;306:189–94.
14. Hull R, Hirsh J, Jay R, et al. Different intensities of anticoagulation in the long term treatment of proximal vein thrombosis. N Engl J Med 1982;307:1676–81.
15. Hull R, Carter C, Jay R, et al. The diagnosis of acute recurrent deep vein thrombosis. A diagnostic challenge. Circulation 1983; 67:901–6.
16. Browse NL, Clemenson G, Lea Thomas M. Is the postphlebitic leg always postphlebitic? Relation between phlebographic appearances of deep-vein thrombosis and the late sequelae. Br Med J 1980;281:1167–70.

CANCER, METASTATIC, FROM UNKNOWN PRIMARY SITE

ANTONIO R. RODRIGUEZ □ WILBUR B. BASSETT, JR.

□ SYNONYMS: CUP (cancer of unknown primary) syndrome, cancer of unknown origin, metastasis of undetermined source, metastatic carcinoma from occult primary tumor

BACKGROUND

Metastatic cancer from an unknown primary site is a fascinating diagnostic challenge. Despite the vast array of diagnostic techniques now available, this disorder has been rated as high as the eighth (8th) most common type of cancer.[1] Reports in the medical literature repeatedly emphasize that even after extensive studies, the site of origin is often not identified antemortem—or even at autopsy.[2] Indeed, this disorder presents a uniquely difficult diagnostic problem; the physician knows what to search for but cannot find the origin.

Definition

The cancer of unknown primary (CUP) syndrome can be defined as a malignancy manifesting as biopsy-proven metastatic disease without an obvious source. This definition is rather vague. How extensive is the evaluation before the decision is made that the primary source cannot be found? There is no consensus in the literature as to the exact definition of this disorder.[2] A practical definition might be one of metastatic cancer in any patient in whom a thorough history, physical examination, and routine laboratory studies (complete blood count, urinalysis, biochemical profile, and chest x-ray) do not reveal the primary origin.

Incidence

Metastatic cancer from an unknown primary site is more common than often realized. About 10 to 15 per cent of all cancer patients have been noted to present with occult primary lesions.[3] Thus, it may be more common than other well-known malignancies such as leukemia, myeloma, and Hodgkin's disease.

Tumor Biology

Cancer from an unknown primary exhibits atypical behavior. Often, the pattern of metastatic sites is unusual. For example, liver metastases without bone involvement may be the first manifestation of prostatic cancer.

Another peculiarity of this disorder is the incidence of organ primary sites. Cancer of the pancreas accounts for only 3 per cent of all cancers, yet it is the most common cause of metastatic carcinoma of unknown origin.[4, 5]

HISTORY AND PHYSICAL EXAMINATION

The importance of a complete history and physical examination cannot be overemphasized in the diagnostic evaluation of carcinoma of unknown primary site. Many times, the physical examination must be repeated several times over a number of weeks before the primary malignancy can be determined. The information obtained from history and physical examination may be the principal clues leading to the primary site initially or guiding one to order the proper diagnostic tests to find the primary. The following discussion begins with the metastatic presentation and details the rationale for excluding carcinoma of unknown primary syndrome.

Cervical Node Presentation

The patient presents with a nodal enlargement that may or may not be painful, representing a tumefaction in the cervical area. Such a mass should be considered malignant until proven otherwise.

A careful history, including any hoarseness, dysphagia (pointing toward a primary laryngeal or lung cancer), heavy cigarette smoking or alcohol intake, and the treatment of prior skin conditions, in particular moles or malignant melanomas, should be solicited. The examination should include the larynx, oral cavity, nasopharynx, hypopharynx, oropharynx, external auditory canals, and nasal passages. Often topical anesthesia or sedation and sometimes general anesthesia are required for a thorough examination.

Most of the primary tumors found on aforementioned examination are histologically proven to be either squamous cell or undifferentiated type "head and neck" carcinomas. If the histologic analysis shows adenocarcinoma, the thyroid, lungs, salivary gland, breast, and gastrointestinal tract should be considered as the possible source, and each of these areas should be examined carefully. Primary tumors of the parotid and salivary glands are usually apparent on physical examination. Detection of a Delphian node, located along the midline of the neck between the isthmus of the thyroid and the cricoid cartilage, warrants a careful scrutiny of the thyroid gland. Any information about discharge from the breast, abdominal pain or masses, change in bowel habits, and bleeding from the gastrointestinal tract should be elicited when an adenocarcinoma is found. A stool specimen for occult blood analysis should be part of every complete physical examination.

Supraclavicular Node Presentation

In an occasional patient with supraclavicular adenopathy, especially an undifferentiated cancer, the primary site is in the head and neck region; therefore, a careful search as noted previously is indicated. Most commonly, such malignancies are metastases from the lung or gastrointestinal tract. A Virchow's or Troisier's node (left medial supraclavicular area) suggests an intra-abdominal origin. When involved by metastatic tumor, such nodes can be felt by deep palpation beneath the clavicle. A right supraclavicular node metastasis suggests a primary tumor of the lung or prostate gland. Involvement of nodes in the subclavian triangle suggests lung or breast cancer. This knowledge prompts one to take a thorough history in relation to the lung, prostate, or gastrointestinal tract. Does the patient have any pulmonary symptoms? If the patient is male, is there hematuria or symptoms of prostatism? Have there been any changes in bowel habits or any bleeding? Does the patient have a breast mass or a history of breast malignancy? These are examples of questions that may lead to the primary cancer.

Inguinal Node Presentation

Metastases in this region may arise from squamous cell carcinoma of the anogenital region, melanomas of the lower trunk, lower extremity, or anogenital region, or adenocarcinoma of the ovary or gastrointestinal tract. Involvement of nodes in the femoral triangle often indicates a lower limb primary site. Cancerous medial triangle nodes indicate a primary lesion of the genitourinary or anorectal region (bladder, ovary, or rectum).

Axillary Node Presentation

Isolated axillary lymphadenopathy proves to be nonmalignant in most patients.[1] In the female, metastasis to the axilla often comes from a primary site in the breast or lung. A careful examination of these organs is indicated. In the search for the primary tumor, the upper limbs must be closely inspected, particularly for subungual or palmar lesions, because melanomas and even epidermoid carcinoma may originate in these sites.

Intrathoracic Presentations

The lung is the most favored extralymphatic site for metastasis in the carcinoma of unknown primary syndrome.[5] It is often difficult to determine whether a pulmonary lesion is primary or is a metastasis from another organ. Symptoms such as cough, shortness of breath, wheezing, hemoptysis, and chest pain should be sought. Physical findings of effusion, pneumonia, or atelectasis may be present. An occasional patient with malignancy in the lung may present with clubbing or hypertrophic pulmonary osteoarthropathy. It is important to note that either metastatic or primary lung cancer may be associated with this syndrome.

In the superior vena cava syndrome, swelling of the head, neck, arm, or supraclavicular region may be noted. Approximately 75 per cent of patients with this syndrome have lung cancer, 15 per cent have lymphomas, and 7 per cent have metastasis to the lung and mediastinum.

In pericardial involvement, either pericardial rub or signs and symptoms of pericardial effusion with or without tamponade may be present. By far the most common neoplastic causes are, in order of diminishing frequency, bronchogenic carcinoma, breast cancer, lymphoma, leukemia, melanoma, and gastrointestinal neoplasms.

Bone Presentations

Bone is the second most frequent extralymphatic site of metastasis. Metastasis to the bone usually presents with a painful lesion, although a fracture or mass may be the first symptom. Metastasis is most commonly found in those bones containing the largest amount of red marrow, i.e., pelvis, ribs, and spine. Pertinent questions should be asked in regard to the breast, thyroid, skin, and lung.

Intra-Abdominal Presentations

The liver is the third most common extralymphatic site of metastatic lesions.[5] Pain, masses, or ascites may be the presenting picture. Jaundice may be present if there is obstruction or enough damage to liver parenchyma. In patients who have the CUP syndrome in the form of liver metastasis, the primary is usually subdiaphragmatic.[6]

Other signs characteristic of cancer include abdominal masses, rectal shelf, frozen pelvis, ascites, ovarian masses, and Sister Mary Joseph nodules (cancerous umbilical nodes usually indicating an intra-abdominal malignancy). A wide variety of neoplasms manifest in this manner, and a thorough evaluation via history and physical examination of the GI tract, GU tract, breast, and lung should be considered.

Central Nervous System Presentations

Metastatic tumors to the brain manifest in many ways, but most patients have signs and symptoms of increased intracranial pressure, such as headache with nausea or vomiting and personality changes. Next to the carcinoma of the lung, the most common source for a brain metastasis is an undetermined primary site.

Epidural tumors may manifest as localizing neurologic defects with or without accompanying pain. The primary sites to consider include breast, lungs, prostate, and kidney as well as myelomas and malignant lymphomas.

Bone Marrow Presentations

Bone marrow involvement is most often without symptoms, but leukoerythroblastic pancytopenia may result in anemia or infectious or hemorrhagic complications manifesting their respective signs and symptoms. Prostate, lung, GI tract, and thyroid are common primary malignancies in bone marrow metastasis. In the CUP syndrome, a pancreatic primary must be considered.

Paraneoplastic Presentations

In CUP syndrome, the neoplasm is recognized by its remote dissemination. Tumors may also become symptomatic through their indirect or remote metabolic effects on remote organs, which are known as "paraneoplastic syndromes." The variety of endocrine, rheumatologic, neurologic, and other systemic symptoms that have been described often provide clues to specific types of occult neoplasm. Although not technically part of the CUP syndrome, paraneoplastic syndromes also represent a clinical state that is more symptomatic than the primary tumor itself. For example, if inappropriate antidiuretic hormone syndrome is seen, oat cell carcinoma should be sought.

Subcutaneous and Soft Tissue Presentations

Wtih few exceptions, patients who demonstrate skin metastases have easily detected primaries. Cancer of the kidney has the greatest tendency to metastasize to the skin, often over the low extremities, whereas cancers of the colon and bladder have the peculiar tendency to metastasize to skin over the abdominal wall and upper extremity.[7]

DIAGNOSTIC STUDIES

Diagnostic studies in metastatic cancer from an unknown primary site should be directed toward the abnormalities detected through the history and physical examination. In addition, metastatic cancer with known effective therapy should be considered and excluded. Table 1 is a list of potentially treatable systemic malignancies.

Table 1. METASTATIC CANCERS IN THE ADULT FOR WHICH THERAPY MAY BE USEFUL

Adenocarcinoma (breast, prostate, endometrium, ovary, or stomach)
Squamous cell carcinoma (head and neck)
Leukemia
Lymphoma
Myeloma
Germ cell tumors
Sarcoma
Small cell cancer of the lung
Medullary carcinoma of the thyroid
Islet cell tumors of pancreas

Basic Laboratory Tests

The finding of microcytic anemia on complete blood count should prompt the clinician to evaluate the GI tract for the primary source. Microscopic hematuria on routine urinalysis might be the only clue to renal cell or bladder cancer. Routine serum chemistry values may indicate that further investigation should be done and may point to specific organ involvement. An elevated total protein value is suggestive of multiple myeloma. In the patient with a normal liver function profile, nuclear scan of the liver is rarely positive.[8]

Tumor Markers

A few specific laboratory tests may identify specific tumor types. The carcinoembryonic antigen (CEA) level is elevated in certain gastrointestinal malignancies, although not exclusively. Acid phosphatase is a specific marker for prostatic cancer. Alpha-fetoprotein and beta-subunit of human chorionic gonadotrophin are characteristic of germ cell neoplasms. Alpha-fetoprotein is also a marker for hepatoma. A monoclonal protein in the serum or the urine may be seen in myeloma, lymphoma, and Waldenström's macroglobulinemia.

Histologic Examination

Histologic analysis of the metastasis may give a clue as to the original site involved. Squamous cell carcinoma in a cervical node biopsy specimen usually indicates that the primary is in the head and neck region. Adenocarcinoma in a cervical node may come from a lung or gastrointestinal malignancy. A precise histologic diagnosis is essential in the investigation of CUP syndrome. It has been noted that in as many as 35 to 45 per cent of cases, the histologic diagnosis in CUP syndrome is undifferentiated carcinoma.[9] Thus, the clinician is often faced with the task of searching for the primary site of an undifferentiated malignancy.

Performing special procedures on the tissue specimen may be helpful in identifying undifferentiated malignancies. Electron microscopy studies may identify oat cell cancer by demonstration of dense granules; this differentiation is important, because oat cell cancer responds well to chemotherapy. Epithelial characteristics such as the presence of desmosomes can rule out lymphoma.

Special stains such as mucin stains have been employed to identify adenocarcinoma. More recently, immunocytochemistry with specific tumor markers has been used to identify the tissue of origin. Immunoglobulin staining may identify lymphoma, glucagon will indicate pancreatic islet cell tumor, and the presence of factor VIII antigen in the cells is characteristic of angiosarcoma.[10] Assay of estrogen or progesterone receptors is helpful in identifying breast, ovarian, and uterine cancer.[11]

Imaging

Extensive radiographic studies (barium enema study, upper GI series, and intravenous pyelogram) are usually part of the investigation of cancer from an unknown primary. On close analysis, however, Neumann and Nystrom[2] found a very low diagnostic yield for these procedures. In addition, positive results are misleading, because they are as likely to be falsely as truly positive. However, when organ dysfunction, such as the presence of melena or hematuria, is proven, such radiographic studies are helpful. Endoscopy is indicated to confirm suspicious lesions seen on these studies. More recently, computerized axial tomography has been reported to improve considerably our ability to locate unknown primary cancer.[12] Gallium scanning may be helpful in locating occult primary lung cancer; it has also been noted that lung lesions revealed by gallium scanning are primary cancers 95 per cent of the time, whereas 75 per cent of lung lesions not demonstrated by gallium scanning are metastatic.[13] Mammography, although of low diagnostic yield, should be done in all female patients with metastatic adenocarcinoma because of the possibility that the source is treatable breast cancer.

Skeletal x-rays and bone scans may determine lytic or blastic lesions. Pure lytic lesions suggest myeloma or kidney, thyroid, or lung cancer. Blastic lesions suggest breast cancer in women and prostatic cancer in men.

DIAGNOSTIC APPROACH

Because physicians are trained to find the diagnosis, they often feel personally challenged to locate an occult primary cancer "at all costs." Such an effort is usually futile. A primary site is ultimately identified in no more than 50 per cent of patients with CUP syndrome, even after autopsy.[4] Many of the diagnostic procedures are costly, time-consuming, and uncomfortable. Often, prolonged investigation paralyzes therapeutic decisions and causes the patient to be frustrated, angry, and uncooperative during later treatment, as well as magnifying the psychosocial problems that normally affect a patient with cancer.

The philosophy of care for patients with CUP syndrome should include the recognition that many have an incurable disease with short survival time and that the primary site is often never identified. Any prolonged effort toward diagnosis may impair not only the quantity but also the quality of life left to these patients. Therefore the diagnostic work-up should be efficient rather than exhaustive. A detailed history, careful physical examination, and simple but selective laboratory investigations are appropriate. The physician who recognizes these facts will then be able to give better care and comfort to the particularly unfortunate patient with cancer of unknown primary.

REFERENCES

1. Krementz ET, Cerise EJ, Foster DS, Morgan LR Jr. Metastases of undetermined source. Curr Probl Cancer 1979;4:1–37.
2. Neumann KH, Nystrom JS. Metastatic cancer of unknown origin: non–squamous cell type. Semin Oncol 1982;9:427–34.
3. Moertel CG, Reitemeier RJ, Schutt AJ, Hahn RG. Treatment of the patient with adenocarcinoma of unknown origin. Cancer 1972;30:1469–72.
4. Nystrom JS, Weiner JM, Wolf RM, Bateman JR, Viola MV. Identifying the primary site in metastatic cancer of unknown origin. JAMA 1979;241:381–3.
5. Nissenblatt, MJ. The CUP syndrome (carcinoma unknown primary). Cancer Treat Rev 1981;8(4):211–24.
6. Schneider JR, Nystrom JS. How to handle metastatic adenocarcinoma with an unknown primary site. Your Patient and Cancer 1982;45–50.
7. Richardson RG, Parker RG. Metastases from undetected primary cancers. West Med 1975;123(4):337–9.
8. Stewart JF, Tattersall MH, Woods RL, Fox RM. Unknown primary adenocarcinoma: incidence of overinvestigation and natural history. Br Med J 1979;1:1530–33.
9. Grosbach AB. Carcinoma of unknown primary site. A clinical enigma. Arch Intern Med 1982;142:357–9.
10. MacKay B, Ordonez NG. The role of the pathologist in the evaluation of poorly differentiated tumors. Semin Oncol 1982;9:396–415.
11. Kiang DT, Kennedy BJ. Estrogen receptor assay in the differential diagnosis of adenocarcinomas. JAMA 1977;238:32–4.
12. Karsell PR, Sheedy PF, O'Connell MJ. Computed tomography in search of cancer of unknown origin. JAMA 1982;248:340–3.
13. Golomb HM, DeMeesser TM. Lung cancer: a combined modality approach to staging and therapy. Cancer 1979;29:258–75.

CARDIOMEGALY

RONALD M. ROTH □ JONATHAN ABRAMS

□ SYNONYMS: Enlarged heart, big heart, cardiac enlargement, macrocardia, megacardia, cardiomegalia

BACKGROUND

Definition

Cardiomegaly is the general term for enlarged heart. An abnormal increase in cardiac size may involve any or all of the four chambers. It is not always easy to determine which chambers of the heart are enlarged, and specialized techniques are often necessary. The size and configuration of the heart are quite variable among normal individuals because of differences in body build, geometry of the chest, asymmetric position of the heart within the thorax, the phase of respiration when evaluated, posture, and method of evaluation. A small heart does not necessarily imply cardiac normality, nor does an "enlarged heart" automatically imply disease of the myocardium or cardiac valves. The diagnosis of cardiomegaly is often more subjective than commonly realized, because the upper limits of cardiac size are ill defined.

Cardiomegaly is detected on physical examination or chest roentgenography, usually the latter. Typically, an enlarged heart is discovered only after intracardiac chambers dilate. Considerable ventricular hypertrophy without dilatation can be concealed in a heart of "normal size." An increase in left ventricular wall thickness from the normal

10 mm to 20 mm signifies important hypertrophy, but the extra 1 cm may not be detectable on physical examination or radiography. In addition, a single chamber (e.g., left atrium or right ventricle) may be definitely enlarged without producing abnormalities that can be demonstrated on physical examination or chest x-ray.

Once increased heart size or specific chamber enlargement is identified, the physician is obligated to determine why it has occurred and to assess the physiologic consequences. Thus, the diagnosis of cardiomegaly should stimulate a systematic cardiovascular evaluation.

A complete differential diagnosis for cardiomegaly is beyond the scope of this chapter. Table 1 lists the majority of conditions that may lead to cardiac enlargement. In general, cardiomegaly is more likely to be found in the subacute or chronic phase of a disease process than in the acute or early phase. Symptoms or clinical signs of cardiac disease are not necessarily present when an enlarged heart is first discovered. In time, however, the vast majority of subjects with overt cardiomegaly will manifest additional clinical evidence of heart disease.

HISTORY

Obtaining a detailed history may not always be helpful in elucidating a case of unexplained cardiomegaly. Often when a routine x-ray report or, less commonly, an electrocardiogram suggests cardiac chamber enlargement, the patient is totally asymptomatic. Even careful questioning may yield no useful clues.

Symptoms of Cardiovascular Disease

Patients with enlarged hearts frequently have symptoms of cardiac disease. Because most instances of cardiomegaly in adults are associated with an enlarged left or right ventricle, the history should focus on obtaining evidence of ventricular dysfunction or overt congestive heart failure (CHF), which may not have been previously diagnosed. Patients should be carefully questioned about a history of dyspnea, either at rest or during exertion. Symptoms of orthopnea, paroxysmal nocturnal dyspnea, or nocturnal asthma may not have been elicited in the past. Patients often adjust to chronic cardiac conditions without noticing major limitation. Easily induced fatigue or a nonspecific decrease in effort tolerance may be important clues to underlying cardiac disability.

Isolated left ventricular failure manifests predominantly as orthopnea and dyspnea on exertion, less commonly as paroxysmal nocturnal dyspnea. Right ventricular or biventricular failure results in systemic venous hypertension. Therefore, the patient should be carefully questioned about swelling of the ankles or feet, particularly at the end of the day. In more advanced cases, intermittent or sustained abdominal swelling may be noted, which is usually a result of hepatomegaly or ascites. Unless massive jugular venous distension or tricuspid insufficiency is present, patients usually do not notice swelling of the jugular veins. Palpitations represent a nonspecific symptom not clearly related to an enlarged heart.

Chest Pain. Although cardiomegaly is not a common presenting sign of coronary artery disease, it is clear that a history of myocardial infarction or clear-cut ischemic symptoms consistent with stable or unstable angina should focus attention on the presence of coronary atherosclerosis, the most common adult cardiac condition. Thus, myocardial ischemic pain is an important symptom to elicit. Angina per se does not cause cardiac enlargement, but previous episodes of infarction leading to myocardial fibrosis may result in cardiac hypertrophy and dilatation; patients with significant left ventricular dysfunction usually have some degree of cardiomegaly, although striking abnormalities of wall motion and a markedly depressed ejection fraction may occasionally be seen in a patient with coronary artery disease who has a normal cardiac silhouette. If a left ventricular aneurysm results from a previous myocardial infarction, cardiomegaly is the rule, often manifesting as a distinctive bulge in the cardiac roentgenographic silhouette.

Acute pericarditis is often associated with pericardial fluid, and mild to moderate "cardiomegaly" may occasionally be present in such cases. In some types of chronic pericarditis, pericardial effusion may be present, and the cardiac silhouette can be quite large. Pericardial tamponade, a rare and dramatic syndrome, may occur in a number of settings, including trauma, uremia, and collagen vascular disease. Chest pain is usually present, but not always. The heart is typically only mildly enlarged. Pericardial pain is classically pleuritic, is frequently made worse or better with different body positions, and may be increased by swallowing and relieved by leaning forward.

Pertinent Previous History

Patients with suspected or proven cardiomegaly should be carefully questioned regarding a previous heart murmur or a prior episode of acute rheumatic fever. Although rheumatic fever is uncommon, many individuals remember being told that they had a murmur as a child or young adult. A history of hypertension, even labile, may be significant; many individuals with long-standing mild hypertension have left ventricular hypertrophy. The Framingham Study documented that hypertension is the most common cause of conges-

Table 1. CAUSES OF CARDIAC ENLARGEMENT

Condition	Frequency	Comments
Normal Physiologic States		
Pregnancy	Common	Increased blood volume; increased cardiac output and stroke volume. Elevated diaphragms in late pregnancy.
Athletic heart	Common	Increased end-diastolic volume; physiologic ventricular hypertrophy and/or enlargement; increased stroke volume; vagotonic bradycardia.
Cardiomyopathies (primary diseases of myocardium)		
Hypertrophic Cardiomyopathy	Uncommon	Cardiac "muscular dystrophy" with disproportionate or asymmetric ventricular hypertrophy with or without obstruction (IHSS). Cardiac enlargement, if present, is usually mild.
Restrictive/infiltrative Cardiomyopathies	Uncommon	"Stiff heart" with impaired ventricular filling. Cardiac enlargement is typically mild.
Amyloidosis	Rare	Usually primary and associated with hepatomegaly and macroglossia. Occasionally related to multiple myeloma.
Hemochromatosis	Rare	"Iron heart," congestive heart failure, diabetes, cirrhosis, and skin pigmentation.
Carcinomatosis	Uncommon	Infiltration of myocardium and/or pericardium by melanoma, leukemia, lymphoma, carcinoma of lung or breast.
Radiation carditis	Uncommon	Myocardial fibrosis; chamber dilatation. Previous history of thoracic irradiation.
Loeffler's myocarditis	Rare	Eosinic infiltration and endomyocardial fibrosis.
Sarcoid	Rare	Granulomatous infiltration of the myocardium.
Congestive Cardiomyopathies	Common	"Dilated cardiomyopathies." Moderate to marked cardiomegaly, often with congestive failure.
Alcoholism	Common	May account for some "idiopathic cardiomyopathies." Long history of heavy drinking.
Infections		
Viral	Probably common	Any virus may be responsible; mostly Coxsackie, influenza, echovirus.
Bacterial		
Streptococcus	Uncommon	Acute rheumatic fever and active carditis.
Bacterial endocarditis	Uncommon	Enlargement due to severe aortic or mitral regurgitation.
Protozoal		
Chagas' disease	Common	South America
Toxoplasmosis	Uncommon	May account for some idiopathic cardiomyopathies.
Endocrine disorders		
Hyperthyroidism	Uncommon	Increased heart rate, stroke volume, and cardiac output.
Hypothyroidism	Uncommon	Bradycardia and pericardial effusion.
Diabetes	Common	Perivascular infiltrates and focal myocardial fibrosis.
Electrolyte disturbances		
Phosphate deficiency	Rare	High-dosage antacid therapy.
Magnesium deficiency	Rare	Secondary to GI loss, diuretics, parathyroid disease, alcohol.
Nutritional cause		
Thiamine deficiency	Rare	Vitamin B_1, beriberi. High-output congestive heart failure, usually in alcoholics.
Drugs		
Adriamycin and daunorubicin	Common	Cardiotoxic antineoplastic agents; dose-related.
Cyclophosphamide	Uncommon	Hemorrhagic myocarditis.
Sulfonamides	Rare	Eosinophilic myocarditis.
Connective tissue disorders (collagen vascular diseases)		
Rheumatoid arthritis	Uncommon	Most commonly pericarditis and pericardial effusion.
Systemic lupus erythematosus	Uncommon	May involve any area of the heart: valves, pericardium, myocardium, coronary arteries, conduction tissue.
Progressive systemic sclerosis (scleroderma)	Rare	Myocardial fibrosis.
Neuromuscular disorders		
Friedreich's disease	Rare	Ataxia, speech defects.
Muscular dystrophy	Rare	Muscle weakness, pseudohypertrophy of calf muscles.
Peripartum cardiomyopathy	Uncommon	Last month of pregnancy or first 5 months following pregnancy.
Ischemic cardiomyopathy	Common	Severe coronary artery disease; diffuse or focal ventricular aneurysm also possible.

Table continued on opposite page

Table 1. CAUSES OF CARDIAC ENLARGEMENT *Continued*

Condition	Frequency	Comments
Idiopathic cardiomyopathy	Common	Diagnosis of exclusion; many cases may have alcoholic or viral etiology.
Hypertension	Common	Chronic pressure overload leads to hypertrophy and ultimately cardiac enlargement and failure.
Valvular Heart Disease		Chronic volume and/or pressure overload
Aortic stenosis	Common	Pressure overload of the left ventricle with left ventricular hypertrophy. Only moderate cardiac enlargement is present.
Aortic insufficiency	Common	Volume overload of the left ventricle. Can lead to massive left ventricular enlargement.
Mitral stenosis	Common	Left atrial and, often, right heart enlargement. Cardiomegaly is usually moderate. Pulmonary vascular congestion usually present.
Mitral regurgitation	Common	Volume load of the left atrium and ventricle with left atrial and ventricular enlargement.
Tricuspid insufficiency	Uncommon	Volume load of right heart results in right ventricular and atrial enlargement (in adults, usually secondary to pulmonary hypertension resulting from left heart disease).
Congenital Heart Disease		
Without Shunt		
Right-sided disease		
Pulmonic stenosis	Uncommon	Right ventricular and right atrial enlargement.
Ebstein's anomaly	Rare	Displaced tricuspid valve with tricuspid insufficiency and right atrial and right ventricular enlargement.
Left-sided disease		
Coarctation of aorta	Uncommon	Upper body hypertension; left ventricular enlargement.
With Shunt		
Acyanotic		
Atrial septal defect	Common	Right heart enlargement; pulmonary plethora.
Patent ductus arteriosus	Common in infants	Left heart enlargement with large shunts, pulmonary plethora.
Ventricular septal defect	Common	Cardiac enlargement proportional to size of shunt; pulmonary plethora.
Cyanotic		
Tetralogy of Fallot	Uncommon	Heart size inversely proportional to severity of lesion.
Eisenmenger's syndrome	Rare	Right heart enlargement secondary to severe pulmonary hypertension from intracardiac shunt.
Pericardial Effusion	Common	Enlarged "water bottle heart" may simulate congestive heart failure but lung fields are usually clear.
High-Output States		Increases in cardiac work and blood volume lead to enlargement of left and right heart. May result in gross cardiac enlargement and heart failure.
Arteriovenous fistula	Uncommon	Congenital or traumatic.
Severe anemia	Common	Decreased systemic vascular resistance; increased blood volume
Renal insufficiency	Common	Exacerbated by hypervolemia, hypertension, and anemia.
Pulmonary disease	Uncommon	Hypoxia; polycythemia; increased blood volume.
Polycythemia vera	Rare	Markedly increased blood volume and increased viscosity.
Cor Pulmonale	Common	Right heart enlargement secondary to pulmonary hypertension. May be underestimated owing to hyperinflated, emphysematous lungs.
Tumors		
Cardiac	Rare	May involve pericardium, myocardium, or valves.
Metastases	Uncommon	Lung, breast, and lymphoma are the usual sources.
Sarcomas	Rare	Most common primary cardiac malignancy.
Myxoma	Rare	Most common benign cardiac tumor. Left atrial myxoma simulates mitral stenosis.
Mediastinal tumor	Rare	Lymphoma, thymoma, etc. May simulate cardiac enlargement.
Myocardial Infarction	Common	If extensive, leads to left heart and later right heart enlargement and failure. Left ventricular aneurysm also possible.
Complete Heart Block	Uncommon	Slow heart rate; large stroke volume. Cardiomegaly accentuated if radiograph is taken at end of long diastolic pause.

tive heart failure in an adult population.[1] Cardiomegaly with left ventricular dilatation typically precedes overt heart failure symptoms by months to years.

A history of diabetes or abnormal glucose tolerance may be important. There is suggestive evidence that long-standing diabetes may lead to myocardial dysfunction and a "diabetic cardiomyopathy."[2] The incidence of congestive heart failure in older diabetics, particularly women, is extremely high.[3] In addition, diabetics have an increased prevalence of coronary artery disease and commonly develop clinical manifestations of coronary disease in adult life. One must remember that diabetics have a high incidence of "silent" myocardial infarction, and there may be no history of chest pain or a diagnosed heart attack when electrocardiography demonstrates a transmural infarct. The combination of diabetes and hypertension is particularly detrimental and frequently results in an enlarged heart.

A general medical history should include a careful evaluation for previous viral illnesses or a bad case of "flu" for which a patient may have sought medical attention. In many cases, so-called idiopathic cardiomyopathy is a result of a previous viral infection of the heart. Patients with acute or subacute viral myocarditis may have had concomitant symptoms of productive cough, fever, malaise, and weakness.

Social History

An important potential cause of cardiomegaly is alcoholic cardiac muscle disease. Individuals who drink heavily for 10 years or more may occasionally develop alcoholic cardiomyopathy, in which cardiomegaly is universally present. Alcohol should be suspected as an etiologic factor in cardiomegaly in anyone who drinks appreciably, even if there are no signs and symptoms of congestive heart failure. The key factor is large ethanol intake over many years. Cirrhosis is not usually found in such patients.

Medication History

Patients who are taking hydralazine or procainamide are at risk for drug-induced lupus syndrome, in which pericarditis with pericardial effusion could produce cardiomegaly. Methyldopa (Aldomet) can rarely cause an autoimmune myocarditis. Of increasing importance in cardiomegaly is treatment with adriamycin or other anthracycline compounds for various malignancies; these drugs produce cumulative dose-related cardiac toxicity, and cardiomegaly may occur before symptoms of CHF appear.

High-Payoff Queries

In a patient who has cardiomegaly without any symptoms, one is most likely to be dealing with a cardiomyopathic process or left ventricular enlargement resulting from chronic hypertension. In the symptomatic patient with cardiomegaly, information regarding possible symptoms of congestive heart failure is important. Obviously, anything in the history that suggests coronary artery disease would be an important diagnostic clue.

The first eight questions listed here deal with possible causes of the cardiomegaly; the remaining questions help establish the status of cardiovascular function.

1. *Have you ever had a heart murmur or rheumatic fever?*
2. *Have you ever had or been told you have high blood pressure?*
3. *Do you drink? How much?*
4. *Have you had a virus or "flu" recently that seemed to go to your lungs?*
5. *Have you recently been pregnant?* In the young woman with cardiomegaly, a pregnancy history is important, particularly with respect to symptoms of fatigue and shortness of breath late in the third trimester or after delivery, during which a clinically undiagnosed peripartum cardiomyopathy may have occurred.
6. *Do you or does anyone in your family have diabetes?*
7. *Have you ever had a heart attack or chest pains?*
8. *Can you remember what medications you are taking now or have taken recently?*
9. *Do you tire easily?*
10. *Has it become harder lately to do energetic things?*
11. *Do you feel short of breath during or after exertion?*
12. *Is it harder to breathe when you are lying down than when you are sitting or standing?*
13. *Do you cough or wheeze sometimes at night?*
14. *Have you noticed that your ankles swell, particularly at the end of the day?*

PHYSICAL EXAMINATION

General Appearance. A patient with unsuspected cardiomegaly often looks completely healthy. On the other hand, if there is severe underlying heart disease the patient may appear to be chronically ill. With advanced cardiac dysfunction, dyspnea or tachypnea is often evident, especially in the supine position. A patient in overt congestive heart failure is usually unable to lie flat and has peripheral edema. Ascites as well as peripheral edema is present with severe right-sided cardiac failure.

Pulmonary Examination. Examination of the lungs for rales and pleural effusions is useful in patients with overt congestive heart failure; in the uncommon patient who has cor pulmonale secondary to intrinsic lung disease, evidence of chronic bronchitis and emphysema is found upon examination of the lungs.

Cardiac Examination. A careful and complete cardiac examination is mandatory in any individual with an enlarged heart. It should begin with careful inspection of the venous pulse for jugular venous distension. In individuals who are able to lie flat without dyspnea but who have an elevated venous pressure, right-sided heart disease (cor pulmonale) and constrictive pericarditis should be considered. Occasionally, patients with cardiomyopathy manifest dominant right heart failure and are quite comfortable lying supine in spite of elevated systemic venous pressure.

The arterial pulse may be of diagnostic importance if the carotid pulsations show a slow upstroke, a shudder, and a small volume, a pattern consistent with aortic stenosis. In aortic regurgitation, which is commonly associated with cardiomegaly, the carotid pulses have an abnormally increased amplitude and may be bounding, often with a bisferious (double) impulse. Obviously, careful blood pressure measurements should be made, and if hypertension is detected (even if noted for the first time), it may be an important clue to the etiology of the heart enlargement.

The most important part of the physical examination in suspected cardiomegaly is assessment of precordial motion.[4–6] It is essential to attempt corroboration of a clinically enlarged heart with careful precordial examination. The normal supine apical impulse is produced by the left ventricle and the left interventricular septum. The impulse is usually found at the midclavicular line or medial to it in the fourth or fifth interspace. Percussion is not useful unless the point of maximal impulse (PMI) cannot be felt. If this is the case, percussion should be employed in an attempt to define the left cardiac border. In tall thin subjects, the normal PMI may occasionally be in the fifth or sixth interspace but should be located well within the midclavicular line. If the supine apical impulse is displaced laterally into the outer left chest, the heart is likely to be enlarged. Usually, when the apical impulse is more than 10 cm from the midsternal line, the heart is abnormal. The impulse itself should be no larger than a quarter and is usually smaller. It is typically felt in only one interspace. In the left lateral decubitus position, a PMI larger than 3 cm in diameter strongly suggests cardiac enlargement.

The normal apical impulse (PMI) has an early outward impulse with definite retraction during the second half of systole (Fig. 1*A*). An apex impulse that is sustained or heaving, with outward motion continuing into the second half of systole, is likely to reflect underlying left ventricular dilatation or a pressure overload state (Fig. 1*B*). Presence of a sustained systolic impulse in the supine position may actually be more reliable in detecting cardiac enlargement than that of a lateral displacement of the PMI, which may be affected by extracardiac factors such as body habitus, intrathoracic abnormalities, and pulmonary disease. A high-amplitude, hyperdynamic PMI with normal contour suggests a left ventricular volume overload, e.g., aortic or mitral regurgitation (Fig. 1*C*).

Right ventricular enlargement is detected by carefully palpating for a parasternal lift. Normally, precordial motion is not palpable at the lower left sternal border except in young or thin individuals.

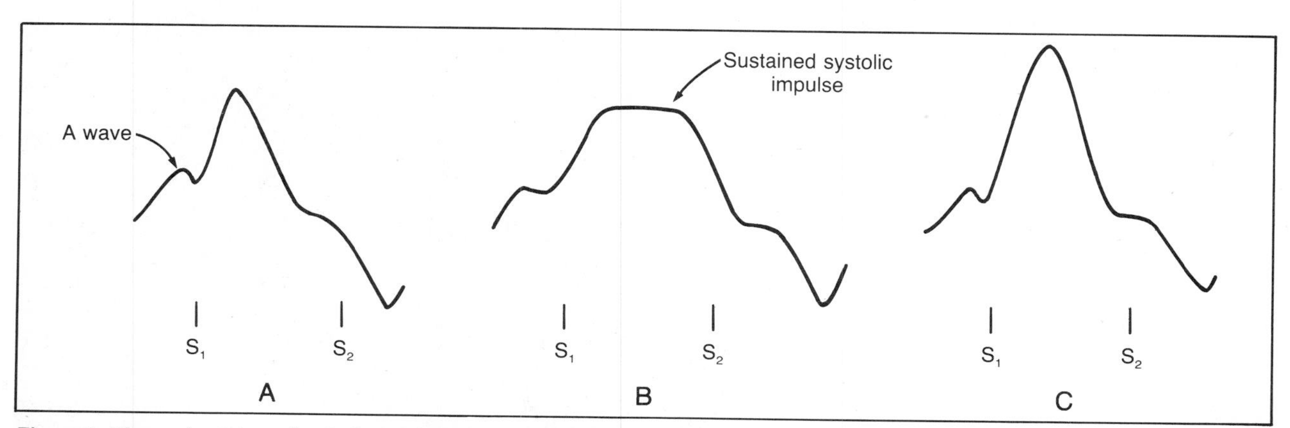

Figure 1. The major types of apical impulse: normal *(A)*, sustained *(B)*, and hyperkinetic *(C)*. These diagrams represent the three basic variants of the LV apex impulse. In patients with suspected or proven cardiomegaly, the contours of the PMI may take on any of these forms, or the apical impulse may be absent. The most important diagnostic finding on precordial palpation is that of a sustained or protracted systolic impulse (LV lift or heave), which correlates with an increase in LV muscle mass, whether there is a pressure overload state or a dilated, spherical LV cavity with depressed systolic function. In the normal subject, the A wave cannot be felt.

Examination for a parasternal or right ventricular lift should be done with the patient holding his or her breath in midexpiration, and the examiner using firm pressure with the palm of the hand pushing downward along the third to fifth interspaces at the lower left sternal edge. Right ventricular dilatation or hypertrophy typically produces a gentle thrusting anterior motion that is often better seen than felt.

The detection of left or right ventricular enlargement on physical examination confirms the diagnosis of cardiomegaly. However, the apical impulse is not always easily felt; in the absence of a clear-cut, palpable PMI, one may not conclude that the heart is of normal size. In older persons, the apical impulse is commonly absent. Right ventricular enlargement is frequently present in the absence of a detectable parasternal or right ventricular heave.

Heart Sounds and Murmurs. The presence of an "organic" heart murmur or abnormal heart sounds confirms the presence of heart disease and may unequivocally indicate the etiology of the cardiomegaly. Any systolic ejection murmur of long duration (well heard into late systole) is probably abnormal. A true holosystolic murmur is abnormal and suggests mitral or tricuspid regurgitation. Diastolic murmurs are always abnormal and usually connote aortic regurgitation or mitral stenosis. Detection of ejection clicks or an opening snap also corroborates the presence of underlying valve disease.

Causes of Pseudocardiomegaly

Before pursuing a diagnostic work-up for an enlarged heart, one must be certain that a real increase in cardiac dimensions is present. A number of conditions, some relatively common, can mimic cardiac enlargement.

Straight Back Syndrome. In individuals with a relatively narrow anteroposterior chest diameter, loss of the normal thoracic kyphosis, or abnormalities of the sternum, such as pectus excavatum, the cardiac silhouette on x-ray may be increased in the PA view (Fig. 2).[7] This phenomenon has been referred to as the "pancake effect"; the heart is literally compressed between the vertebral column and sternum. The pulmonary artery often appears enlarged as well, and cardiac murmurs may be present. The straight back syndrome should be considered when, on the chest x-ray, the distance between the sternum and the eighth thoracic vertebra is 11 cm or less in a man or 9 cm or less in a woman, or the ratio between the transthoracic and the AP thoracic dimensions is less than 38 per cent.[7]

Pericardial Effusion. An increase in pericardial fluid may result in a larger cardiac silhouette.

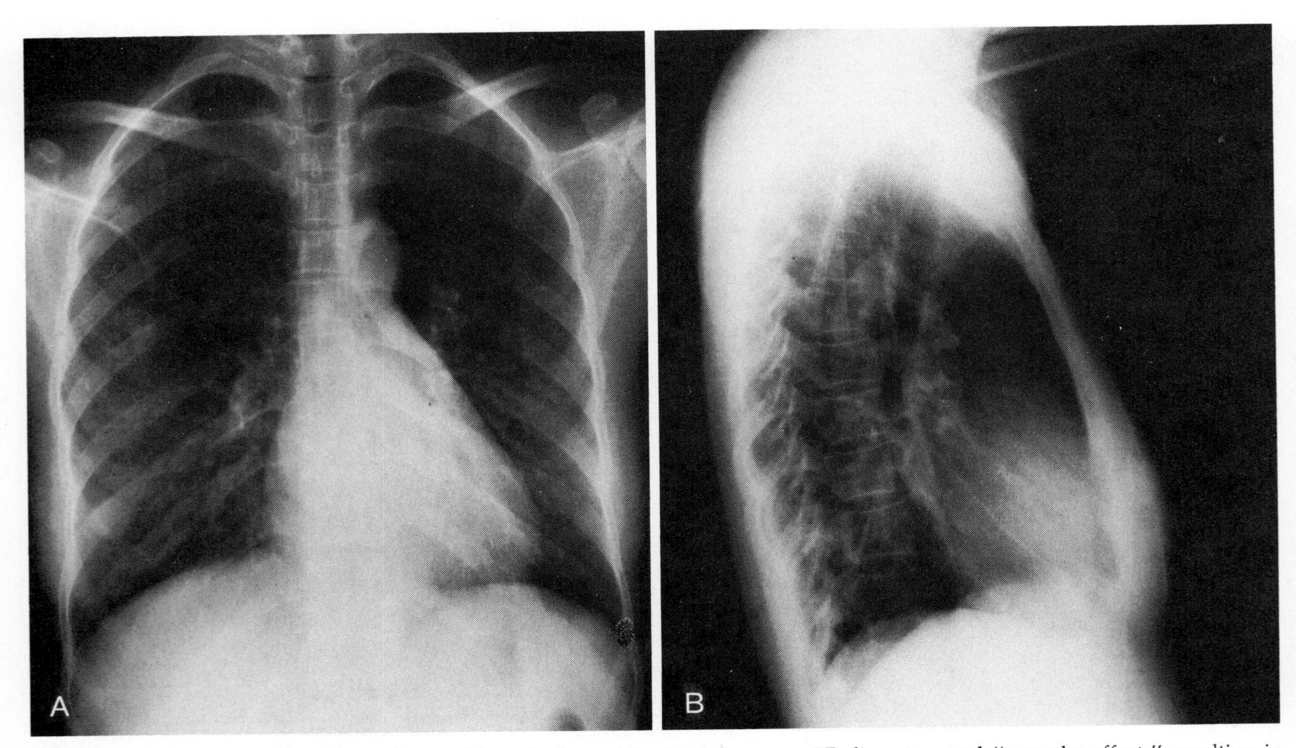

Figure 2. *A* and *B*, Straight back syndrome. Note the loss of kyphosis, narrow AP diameter, and "pancake effect," resulting in an appearance of cardiomegaly on the PA view. This is a common cause of pseudocardiomegaly.

Pericardial effusions may be found in fluid overload states, myxedema, and intrinsic pericardial disease, resulting in mild to moderate cardiomegaly. Rarely, huge pericardial effusions are seen, particularly in patients who have metastatic tumor implants on the pericardium. Whenever pleural effusions are prominent and the heart is enlarged, one must consider that a large pericardial effusion may be present. M-mode echocardiography and two-dimensional echocardiography, both essential to the diagnosis of increased pericardial fluid, also provide an assessment of the actual cardiac dimensions, which may be normal or increased.

Apical or Epicardial Fat Pad. When the epicardial fat pad is usually prominent, the apical cardiac silhouette may appear to be enlarged.

Congenital Absence of the Pericardium. In this unusual condition, pseudocardiomegaly may be produced by eventration of the heart into the lateral chest.

Large Pleural Effusions. When large left or right pleural effusions are present, the cardiac silhouette may appear to be enlarged. Decubitus chest x-rays are quite useful in such situations.

Ascites, Abdominal Distension, or Marked Hepatomegaly. Whenever the abdominal contents are increased in volume, the diaphragm may be elevated and pseudocardiomegaly can appear. Even with vigorous attempts to obtain a full inspiration, many patients with abdominal disease are unable to lower their diaphragm sufficiently, and their cardiac silhouettes appear to be abnormally large.

Technical Factors. Poor inspiratory effort or faulty radiographic technique may occasionally cause "cardiomegaly." This problem can be solved by obtaining a repeat x-ray with careful attention to technique.

DIAGNOSTIC STUDIES

The evaluation of patients with cardiomegaly is far more sophisticated in the 1980s than in the past, when a work-up consisted of electrocardiography (ECG) and four-way radiographic views of the chest with a barium swallow. With the use of a combination of electrocardiography, chest x-ray, cardiac isotope studies, echocardiography, and angiography, the rate of accuracy in diagnosing the cause of cardiomegaly approaches 100 per cent. Only in cardiomyopathic processes does the precise etiology often remain elusive (even after myocardial biopsy in some cases).

Roentgenography

A chest x-ray report is often the first indication of cardiomegaly and possible cardiac disease. Roentgenography is also very useful in the diagnostic evaluation of an enlarged heart. The conventional posteroanterior chest film is the simplest means of appraising heart size. Although there are elaborate methods for "mensuration" of the cardiac silhouette (transverse diameter, long diameter, broad diameter, the area of the frontal cardiac silhouette, etc.),[8–12] the conclusion that a particular heart is enlarged is more commonly reached through a subjective visual impression based on the physician's experience of what constitutes the normal range. The cardiothoracic (CT) ratio is frequently used as a semiquantitative yet rough guide to estimating cardiac enlargement. This ratio reflects the relationship of the transverse diameter of the heart to the internal diameter of the chest at its widest point (Fig. 3). This ratio does not exceed 50 per cent in the vast majority of healthy adults.[13] However, the roentgenographic impression of cardiomegaly is complicated by a number of factors (described in following discussion), some of which are not necessarily related to heart size or function. *It is important to realize that cardiac enlargement can be present despite a normal cardiothoracic ratio and that, conversely, actual heart size may be normal in the presence of an increased cardiothoracic ratio.*

Several common sources of variation may affect the assessment of radiographic heart size (see also discussion of pseudocardiomegaly). A thin, asthenic body habitus with a long thoracic cavity, low diaphragms, and a vertically oriented heart tends to minimize the appearance of cardiac enlargement. In contrast, a stocky, sthenic habitus with elevated diaphragms and a horizontally oriented heart may result in apparent cardiomegaly.

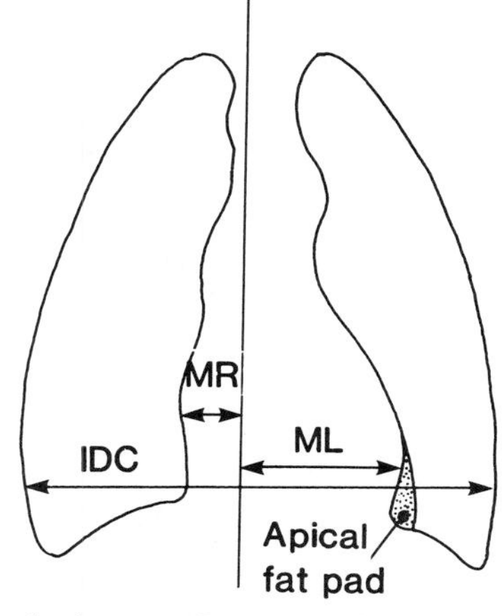

Figure 3. Cardiothoracic (CT) ratio. The CT ratio relates the transverse diameter of the heart (MR + ML), excluding the apical fat pad, to the internal diameter of the chest (IDC): CT ratio = (MR + ML) ÷ IDC, where *MR* is the distance from the midsternal line to the right border of the cardiac silhouette, and *ML* is the distance from the midsternal line to the left border of the cardiac silhouette.

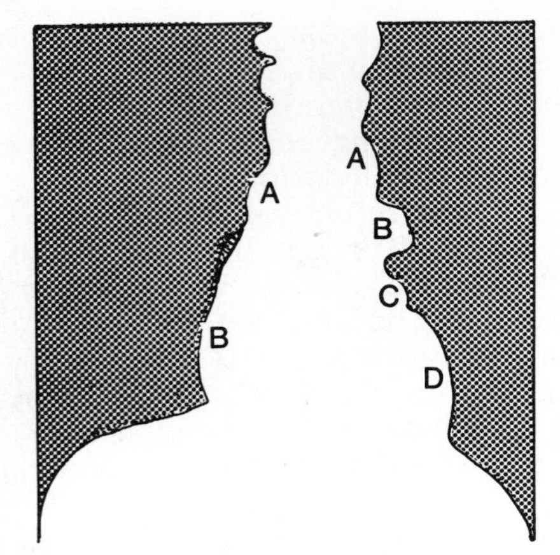

Figure 4. Segments of the normal cardiac silhouette (PA view). Right heart border: *A,* superior vena cava; *B,* right atrium. Left heart border: *A,* aortic knob; *B,* pulmonary artery; *C,* left atrium; *D,* left ventricle.

Similarly, an inadequate inspiratory effort during x-ray or diaphragm elevation from any cause, such as abdominal distension, orients the heart horizontally and tends to exaggerate heart size. On the other hand, a hyperinflated chest (chronic lung disease) may mask cardiomegaly. Patient positioning can also influence the interpretation of heart size. When the subject is placed correctly in the PA position, the sternal manubrium is centered directly over the vertebral bodies. If the patient is rotated even slightly, the cardiac configuration and impression of heart size will be altered. Inclusion of the pericardial or apical fat pad within the heart border can lead to an overestimation of heart size.[14] The heart may also be displaced by atelectasis, pneumothorax, and eventration or herniation of the diaphragm, causing an alteration of cardiac configuration and apparent heart size. Finally, differences in technique (x-ray distance less than 6 ft, portable filming, anteroposterior view) may magnify the heart size. Serial radiographs with identical technique demonstrating a progressively enlarging heart offer the best evidence of true cardiomegaly.

Cardiac enlargement as estimated radiographically occurs primarily as a result of chamber dilatation. As previously mentioned, considerable ventricular hypertrophy can be concealed in a heart of radiographically normal size. It is often difficult to accurately assess specific chamber enlargement from the standard PA and lateral chest films. In the normal PA x-ray of the heart, the radiographic right heart border consists of the superior vena cava, the right atrium, and occasionally the inferior vena cava, and the left heart border is composed of the aortic knob, the main and left pulmonary arteries, the left atrium, and the left ventricle (Fig. 4). In an enlarged heart, however, these relationships can be unpredictably altered. What appears to be an enlarged left heart border may actually be due to right heart enlargement causing posterior displacement of the left heart, and vice versa. The traditional four-way views of the chest with barium swallow can give more accurate information about specific chamber enlargement than a standard chest film (Figs. 5 and 6). This technique is less widely used today and has been largely supplanted by echocardiography, which yields considerably more precise information, such as the presence or absence of myocardial hypertrophy, wall motion abnormalities, and pericardial fluid.

Chamber Enlargement

Assessment of specific cardiac chamber enlargement may often be inferred from the standard PA and lateral films of the chest.

Left atrial enlargement is suggested by a double density along the right heart border and elevation of the left main stem bronchus. Rarely, massive left atrial dilatation encroaches on and actually forms the right heart border. On a lateral film, a very large left atrium may be seen to be enlarged posteriorly. The left atrium is prominent in mitral valve disease, ventricular septal defect, patent ductus arteriosus, left ventricular failure, and any generalized cardiac enlargement (Fig. 7).

Left ventricular dilatation may be suspected when there is a high take-off from the central cardiac

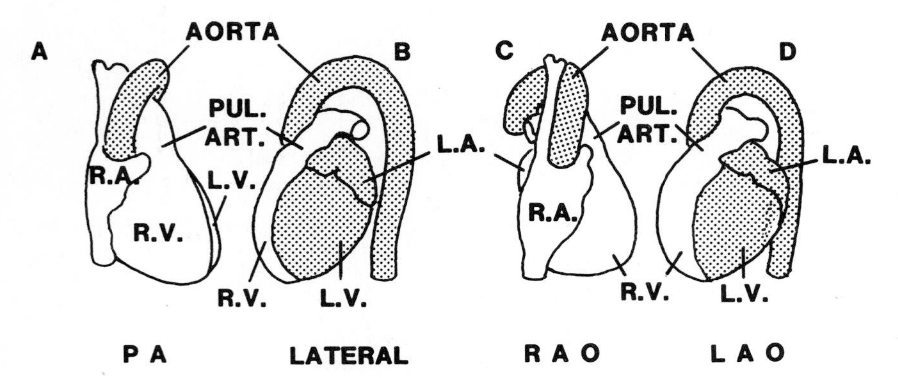

Figure 5. Diagrammatic representation of the cardiac silhouette in the four standard views. *A,* Posteroanterior view shows the left ventricle, right ventricle, and right atrium. *B,* Lateral view demonstrates the right ventricle anteriorly, left atrium and left ventricle posteriorly. *C,* Right anterior oblique view shows the right ventricle anteriorly and left atrium posteriorly. *D,* Left anterior oblique view demonstrates the right ventricle anteriorly and left ventricle posteriorly.

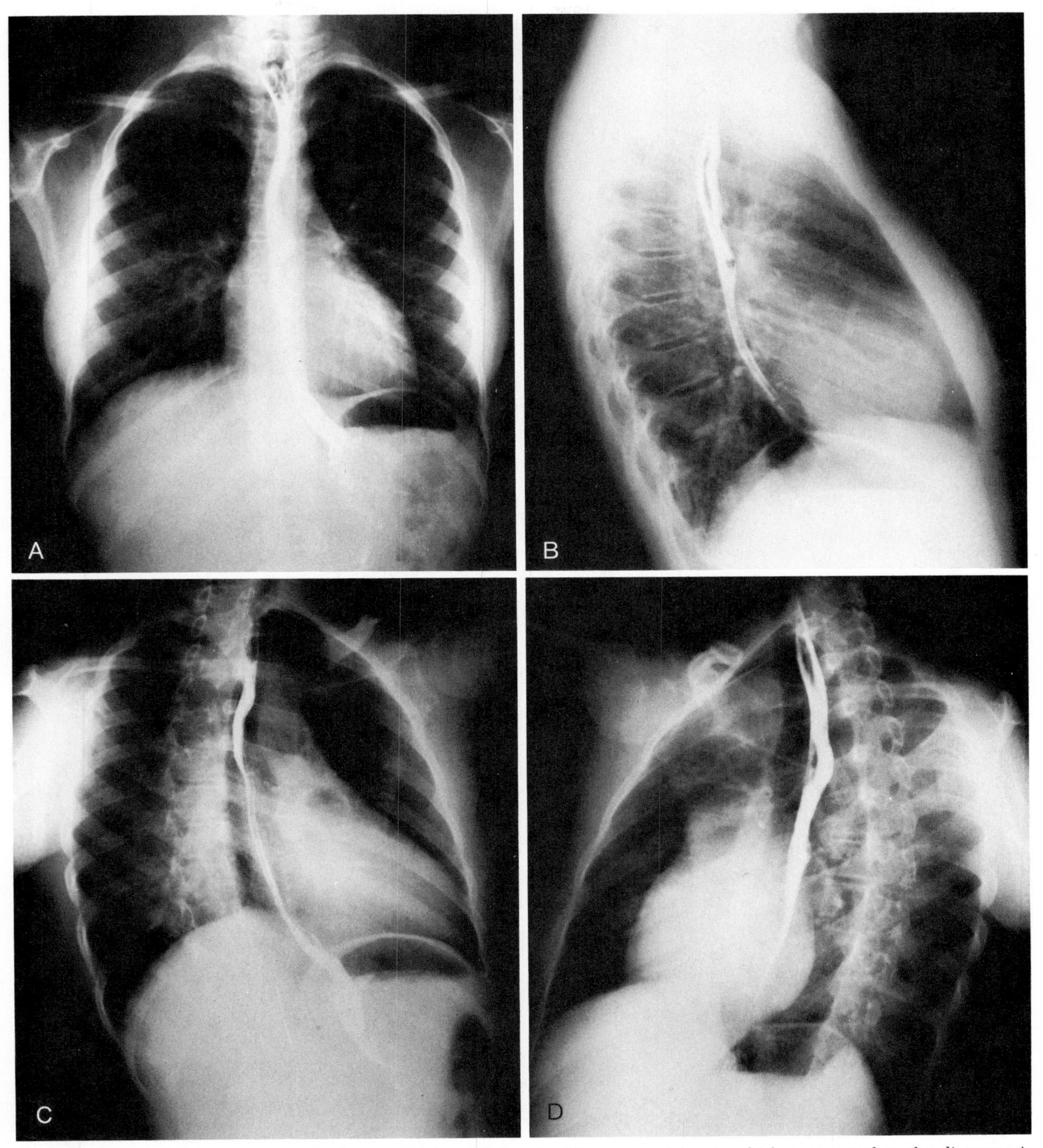

Figure 6. The conventional four-way radiographic views of the chest in a normal heart, which correspond to the diagrams in Figure 5. *A*, Posteroanterior view. *B*, Lateral view. *C*, Right anterior oblique view. *D*, Left anterior oblique view.

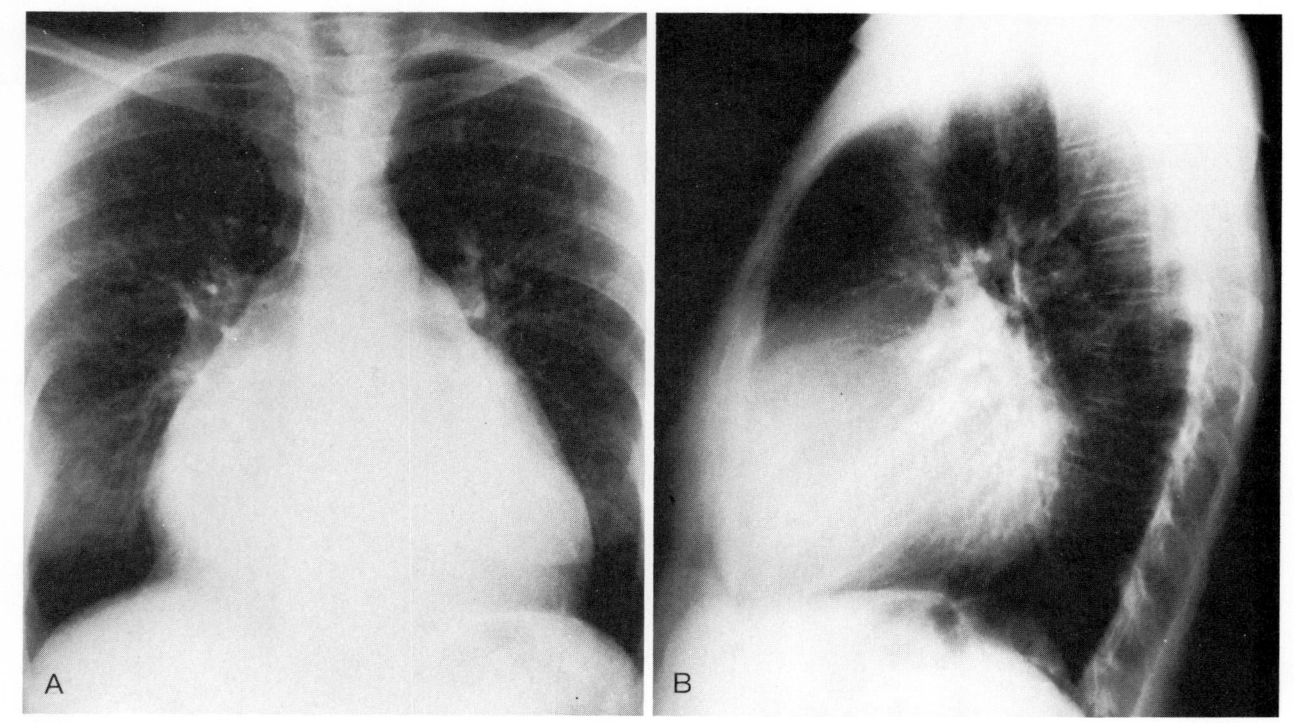

Figure 7. Marked cardiomegaly due to severe long-standing mitral stenosis. *A,* Left atrial enlargement is represented on the PA film by a double-density shadow on the right, convexity of the upper left heart border, and elevation of the left mainstem bronchus. The central pulmonary vasculature is also prominent. *B,* On the lateral film there is evidence for right ventricular enlargement with loss of the retrosternal clear space. Note the prominent posterior extension of the dilated left atrium.

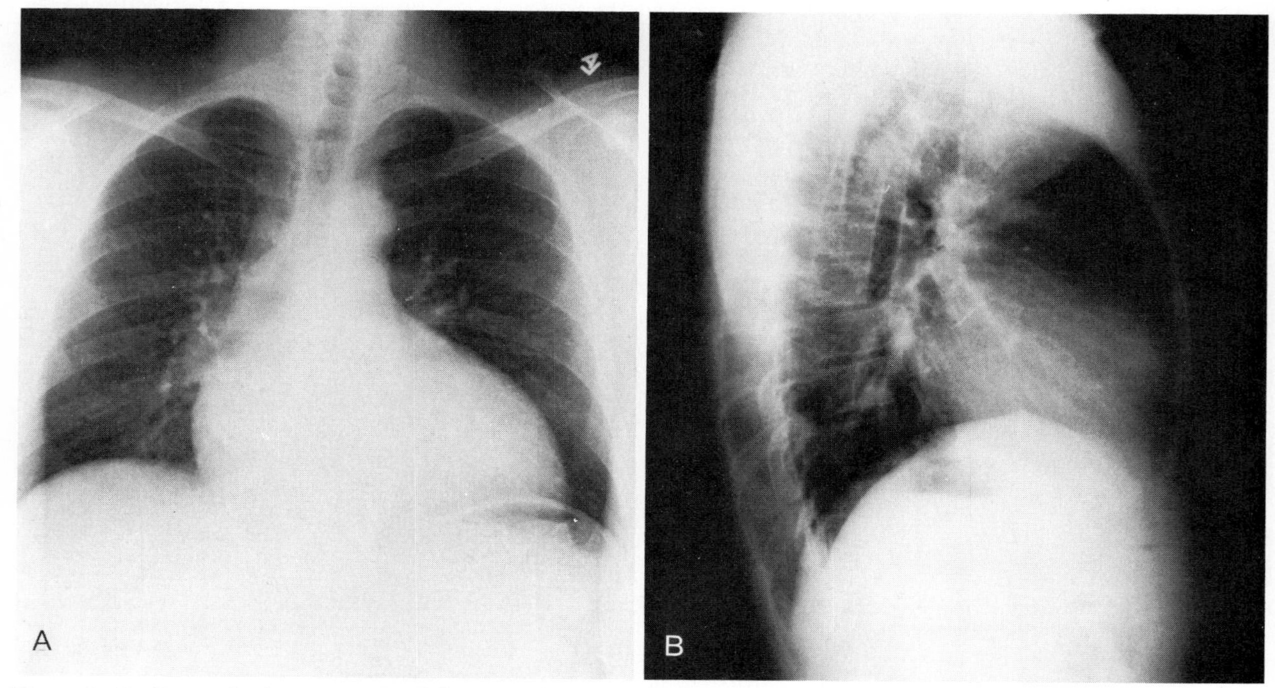

Figure 8. Cardiomegaly due to massive left ventricular enlargement from severe long-standing aortic insufficiency. Note the prominent left ventricular contour on the PA film *(A)* and the posterior displacement of the left ventricle beyond the inferior vena cava shadow on the lateral film *(B)*.

silhouette or increased convexity of the left ventricular contour, or when the cardiac apex is displaced downward and outward in the PA projection. Right heart enlargement, however, may simulate this radiographic configuration. In the lateral view, the enlarged left ventricle projects posteriorly behind the inferior vena cava. Normally the left ventricle should "clear" the shadow of the inferior vena cava (Fig. 8*B*). Left ventricular enlargement occurs with hypertension, aortic valve disease, mitral regurgitation, hypertrophic cardiomyopathy (IHSS), coarctation of the aorta, ventricular septal defect, patent ductus arteriosus, coronary artery disease, and cardiomyopathy (Fig. 8).

Right atrial enlargement is difficult to determine radiographically but may give an elongated curve to the right heart silhouette. The right atrium is prominent in atrial septal defect, Ebstein's anomaly, and tricuspid valve disease.

Right ventricular dilatation may cause elevation of the cardiac apex above the diaphragm in the PA projection and prominent retrosternal cardiac convexity (diminished retrosternal space) in the lateral view (see Figs. 7 and 9). The right ventricle may enlarge as a result of pulmonary hypertension (pulmonary embolus, mitral valve disease, cor pulmonale, left ventricular dysfunction, etc.), tricuspid valve disease, and pulmonic valve disease.

Pulmonary Vasculature

The pulmonary vasculature can also provide useful information in the evaluation of an enlarged heart. Redistribution or encephalization of pulmonary veins, hilar haziness, peribronchial cuffing, Kerley B lines (horizontal lines near the costophrenic angles), and pleural effusions suggest pulmonary venous hypertension (e.g., mitral valve disease, left ventricular failure). On the other hand, oligemia (in which the lung fields are radiographically clear) in the presence of cardiomegaly may suggest obstruction to pulmonary outflow with secondary right-to-left shunting (congenital heart disease). Clear lung fields associated with a large, smoothly outlined heart without specific chamber prominence may suggest pericardial effusion, Ebstein's anomaly (tricuspid valve disease and right-to-left shunt), or, rarely, severe pulmonic stenosis. Cardiomyopathy may also be associated with a large heart of nonspecific configuration, but there is usually an increase in pulmonary vascularity or "congestion" (Fig. 10).

Other Factors

Radiographic enlargement of the heart can also be simulated by pericardial and mediastinal masses, such as pericardial cysts, thymomas, and

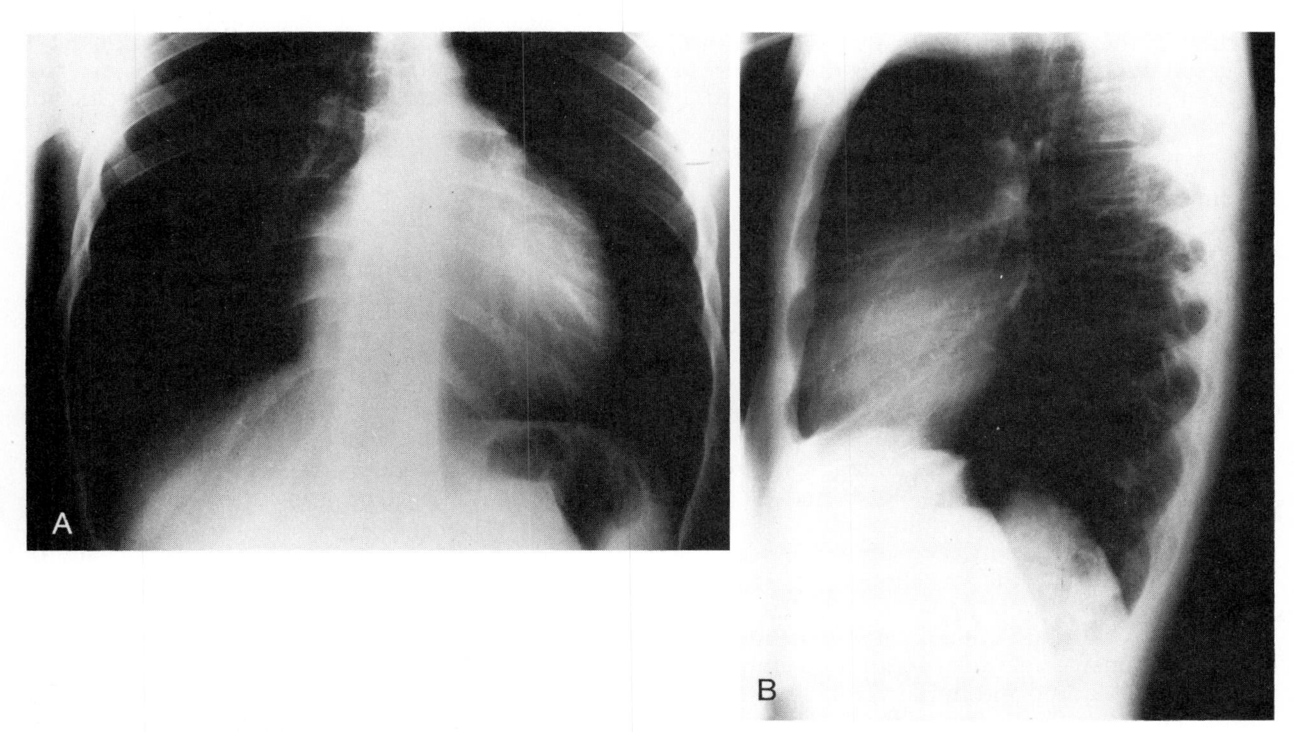

Figure 9. Cardiac enlargement due to Ebstein's anomaly and tricuspid regurgitation. The PA projection *(A)* demonstrates right atrial enlargement and elevation of the left heart border. The lateral film *(B)* discloses loss of the retrosternal space due to right ventricular enlargement and resultant posterior displacement of the left heart.

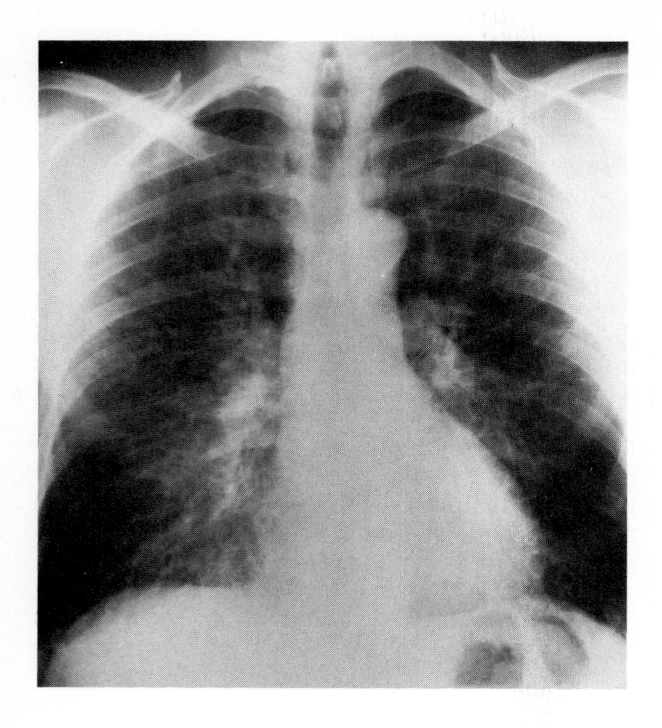

Figure 10. Borderline cardiomegaly with evidence of left heart failure: encephalization of the pulmonary veins, hilar haziness, and Kerley B lines in the lower lung fields.

lymphomas, which may give the false impression of general cardiac enlargement or even specific chamber dilatation.

Calcification, although best visualized on cardiac fluoroscopy, can occasionally be seen on a plain chest film. If it is present, localization of the calcium to the aortic or mitral valve, pericardium, or coronary arteries may help to determine the cause of the heart enlargement.

Electrocardiography

The standard 12-lead electrocardiogram (ECG) indirectly aids in the diagnosis of cardiomegaly. Criteria are well established for the electrocardiographic diagnosis of right and left ventricular hypertrophy as well as for abnormalities of the right and left atria. The electrocardiographic diagnosis of chamber hypertrophy or dilatation does not necessarily mean that cardiomegaly or specific chamber enlargement will be identified on chest roentgenography or echocardiography.

The electrocardiogram can support or suggest clinical clues as to the etiology of an enlarged heart. Evidence of definite left ventricular hypertrophy and/or left atrial enlargement is consistent with hypertensive heart disease, hypertrophic cardiomyopathy, aortic and mitral valve disease, and cardiomyopathy (Fig. 11). Evidence of right ventricular hypertrophy and/or right atrial abnormality on ECG can be associated with certain types of congenital heart disease, pulmonary hypertension, and cor pulmonale. Ischemic changes or electrocardiographic evidence of infarction suggests coronary artery disease. The "athletic heart" has characteristic features on ECG, including sinus bradycardia, first-degree block, early repolarization, and nonspecific T wave changes.[15] Hypothyroid heart disease may manifest as low voltage and bradycardia. Axis shifts, nonspecific ST-T changes, and other ECG abnormalities are frequently associated with but are not specific for cardiomegaly.

Echocardiography

Although the combination of clinical examination, chest roentgenography, and electrocardiography may greatly narrow the differential diagnosis in a patient with cardiomegaly, the exact cause may remain uncertain. With the use of M-mode and two-dimensional (2-D) echocardiography, both cardiac anatomy and function can be precisely evaluated, a specific diagnosis usually can be made, and prognosis frequently can be determined.

Echocardiography utilizes a focused beam of ultrasound alternately emitted and received by a transducer placed over the precordium. This sound wave can be "aimed" at the various cardiac structures. The information received is displayed and recorded in motion on paper (M-mode) or on video (2-D). A normal M-mode echocardiogram taken at the level of the mid–left ventricular body is shown in Figure 12. Note the normal chamber sizes and the normal systolic motion of the septum and posterior left ventricular wall.

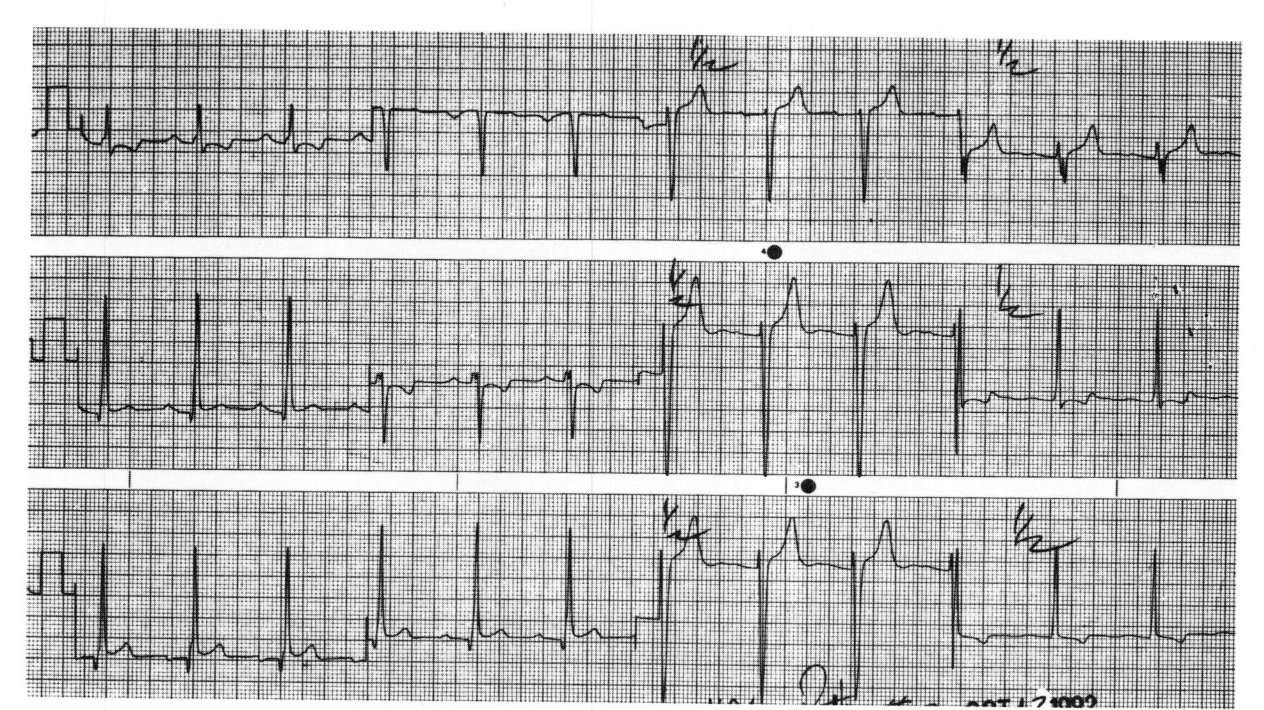

Figure 11. ECG in a patient with long-standing aortic valve disease. Note the increased voltage, especially in the precordial leads (half standard). There are typical secondary ST-T changes of left ventricular strain. This ECG is consistent with marked left ventricular hypertrophy.

Information Obtained

A combination of M-mode and 2-D echocardiography yields several important pieces of information in a patient with cardiomegaly.[16]

Cardiac Valves. All four cardiac valves can usually be visualized on an echocardiogram. Abnormalities of valve motion, leaflet thickening, and calcification can readily be determined. Often, the etiology of a particular valve abnormality (rheumatic heart disease, congenital heart disease, bacterial endocarditis) can be elucidated. Subtle changes in valve motion may also imply abnormal hemodynamics such as pulmonary hypertension or elevation of left ventricular end-diastolic pressure.

Chamber Dimensions. All four cardiac chambers are usually well displayed by ultrasound, and the presence of specific chamber enlargement or generalized cardiomegaly can be determined. Accurate measurement of the left ventricle and left atrium in centimeters can be made in most cases. Anatomy of the right ventricle and right atrium is typically somewhat less well visualized.

Hypertrophy. Wall thickness of both ventricles and the septum is accurately measured on an echocardiogram. Hypertrophy, if present, may be concentric (often owing to pressure overload) or

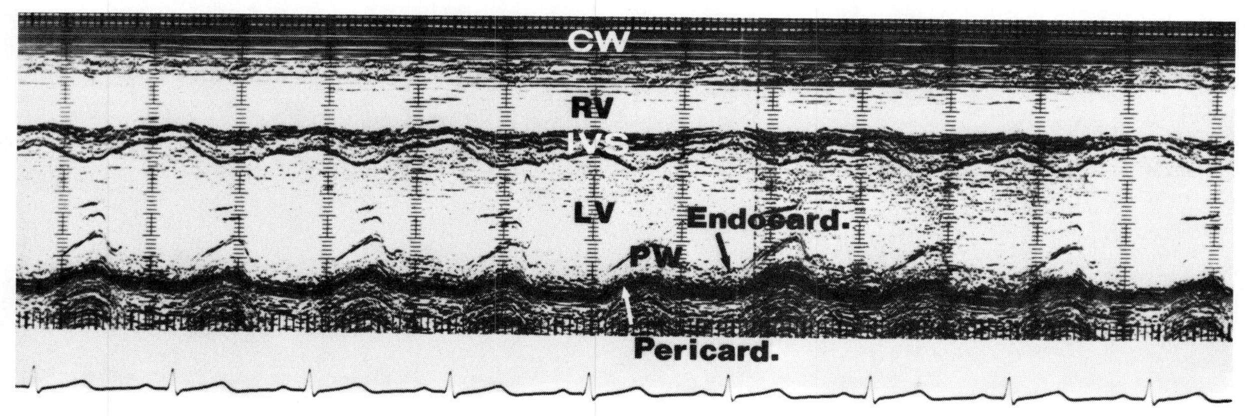

Figure 12. Normal M-mode echocardiogram. *CW*, chest wall; *RV*, right ventricle; *IVS*, interventricular septum; *LV*, left ventricle; *PW*, posterior wall; *Endocard.*, endocardium; *Pericard.*, pericardium.

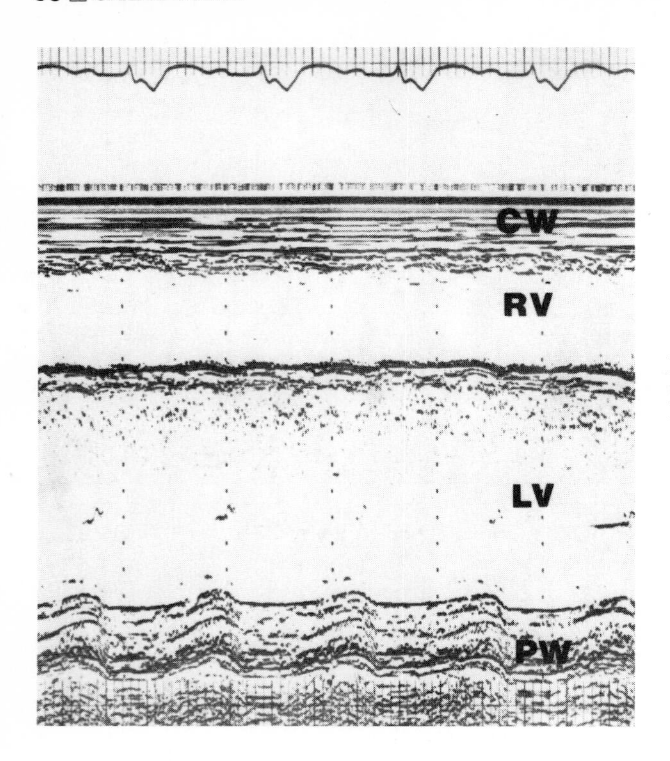

Figure 13. M-mode echocardiogram of a severe cardiomyopathy due to viral myocarditis. *CW*, chest wall; *RV*, right ventricle; *LV*, left ventricle; *PW*, posterior wall.

asymmetric (suggestive of hypertrophic cardiomyopathy).

Wall Motion. Patterns of ventricular wall motion can be well visualized using 2-D and M-mode techniques. A segmental or focal contraction abnormality suggests ischemic (coronary) heart disease, whereas a diffuse contractile abnormality implies chronic valvular heart disease, hypertension, or cardiomyopathy. Figure 13 shows an example of severe cardiomyopathy. Note the large cavity of the left ventricle and the diminished wall motion.

Pericardial Disease. The presence or absence of a pericardial effusion, which appears as an echo-free space, can be easily assessed on electrocardiogram, and the amount of fluid can be roughly quantitated. Pericardial thickening and calcification may also be suggested, as well as subtle signs of abnormal hemodynamics due to pericardial compression (cardiac tamponade). Figure 14 is an

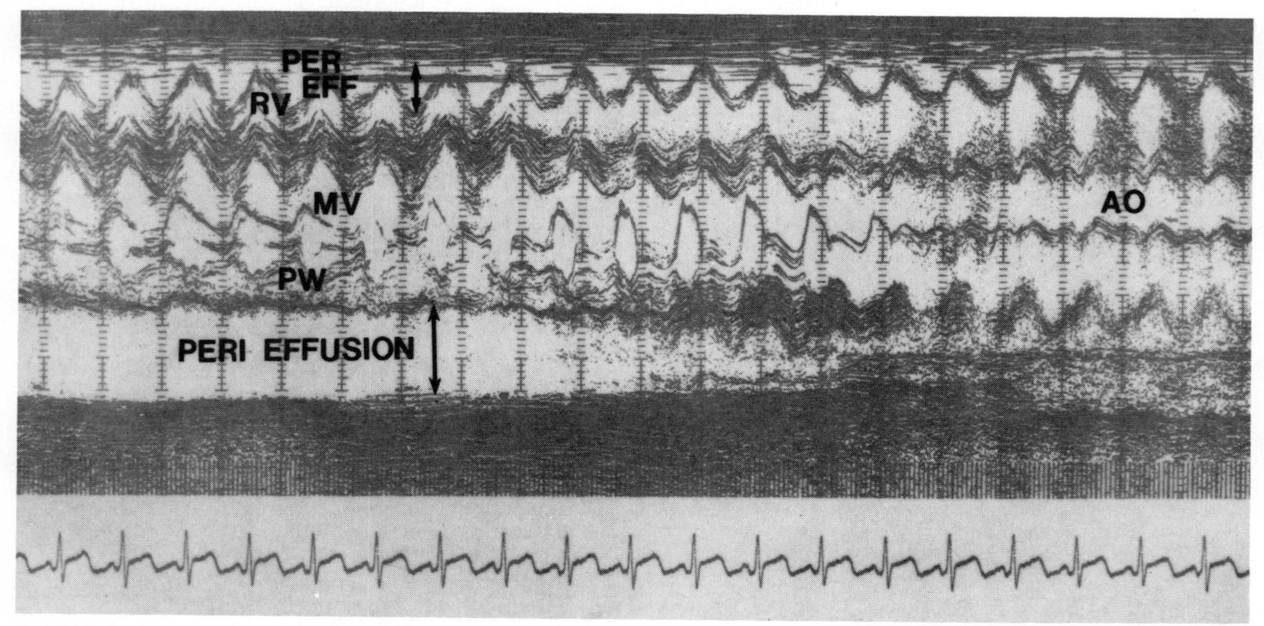

Figure 14. M-mode echocardiogram of a large anterior and posterior pericardial effusion. *RV*, right ventricle; *MV*, mitral valve; *PW*, posterior wall; *AO*, aorta; *PER EFF (PERI EFFUSION)*, pericardial effusion.

example of a large anterior and posterior pericardial effusion. Note that as the ultrasound beam scans from the left ventricle to the level of the aorta and left atrium, the effusion disappears; this is a classic echocardiographic feature of pericardial fluid.

Tumors. Cardiac and mediastinal tumors can simulate cardiomegaly on radiography. Intracardiac tumors are best visualized by ultrasound, by which they can be localized to a specific area of the heart. On the other hand, apparent cardiomegaly on chest x-ray with a normal cardiac ultrasound study would suggest an extracardiac (mediastinal) mass.

Use of Echocardiographic Information

Using the information obtained from echocardiography and from the physical examination, one can usually determine the etiology of cardiac enlargement. For example, a dilated left ventricle with good wall motion (and appropriate murmurs) suggests aortic or mitral insufficiency, whereas a dilated left ventricle with poor wall motion suggests a cardiomyopathy, ischemic damage, or, less commonly, end-stage valvular heart disease; prognosis is poor for all three. A hypertrophied left ventricle with thickened, calcified, and poorly moving aortic valve leaflets is characteristic of aortic stenosis. Isolated left atrial enlargement in the presence of a thickened and abnormally moving mitral valve suggests mitral stenosis. A dilated left ventricle with good posterior wall motion but hypokinesis of the septum and anterior wall implies prior anterior myocardial infarction due to coronary artery disease.

Echocardiography has significantly contributed to the noninvasive diagnosis of cardiomegaly. In particular, ultrasonography readily differentiates cardiac enlargement due to pericardial effusion, valvular heart disease, coronary disease, and primary disease of the myocardium.

Cardiac Catheterization

Cardiac catheterization is the "gold standard" against which all other cardiac studies are judged. It is generally regarded as a combined hemodynamic and angiographic procedure undertaken to confirm a suspected diagnosis, to prepare for cardiac surgery, or to sort out confusing cardiac problems.[17]

Cardiac catheterization provides precise information concerning pressures of the right and left heart (pulmonary hypertension, elevated left ventricular end-diastolic pressure, etc.), quantification of regurgitant and stenotic valve lesions, assessment of left and right ventricular volumes and function, patency of coronary arteries, hemodynamic significance of pericardial disease (cardiac tamponade, constrictive pericarditis), and evaluation of congenital heart disease and shunts.

Other Studies

A number of additional tests, if used selectively, may be useful in the evaluation of cardiomegaly. They are outlined in Table 2.[18, 19]

ASSESSMENT

In most instances cardiomegaly is not a questionable diagnosis. When an enlarged heart is first discovered, the clinician must carefully determine which chambers are dilated and whether ventric-

Table 2. ANCILLARY TESTS USEFUL IN THE EVALUATION OF CARDIOMEGALY

Test	Indication(s)
CBC	Evaluation of severe anemia, polycythemia (COPD), or elevated white count suggesting an inflammatory process (endocarditis, myocarditis)
Blood chemistry profile	Evaluation of chronic renal failure, liver disease, diabetes, parathyroid disease, phosphate or magnesium deficiency
Serum lipid measurements	Coronary artery disease
Urinalysis	Renal disease, diabetes
T_3, T_4, TSH determinations	Hyperthyroidism, hypothyroidism
Erythrocyte sedimentation rate	Inflammatory process
ANA and rheumatoid factor	Connective tissue disease
VDRL	Syphilitic aortic valve disease
Iron and iron binding capacity	Anemia, hemochromatosis
Blood cultures	Bacterial endocarditis
ASO titer	Acute rheumatic fever
Arterial blood gases	Chronic lung disease, cor pulmonale, cyanotic congenital heart disease
Treadmill test	Assessment of coronary disease, determination of functional class
Gated nuclear scan	Ejection fraction gives quantification of global left ventricular function
Thallium scan	Coronary artery disease
Phonocardiogram	Timing of abnormal heart sounds
Vectorcardiogram	Differentiating confusing ECG patterns (conduction abnormality, bundle branch block, infarct, hypertrophy)

ular hypertrophy is present. When the diagnosis of cardiomegaly is suspected or unclear, it is imperative that the situation be clarified. The finding of an enlarged heart is of major importance, as it suggests a decreased life expectancy and possible disability from cardiovascular disease. Repeat chest radiography with careful attention to technique or high-quality M-mode and two-dimensional echocardiography should be performed in all questionable cases.

Symptoms

Many individuals with cardiomegaly are asymptomatic or have no history of a cardiovascular disorder. Some patients, however, may have fatigability and dyspnea on exertion (often for years) that they have attributed to a sedentary existence, smoking, or other health problems. Many people are simply not aware that they have significant effort limitations because of their inactive lifestyles. Thus, careful questioning about shortness of breath on effort, orthopnea, and fatigue is mandatory when cardiomegaly is discovered. A treadmill test for functional capacity often clarifies situations in which the pathophysiologic implications of an enlarged heart are uncertain.

Common Causes of Cardiomegaly

Although the list of potential causes of an enlarged heart is quite large (see Table 1), a relatively small group of disorders account for the vast majority of adult patients with cardiomegaly in clinical practice. These are listed in Table 3, along with the most useful diagnostic criteria and procedures for establishing them.

Work-up for Cardiomegaly Patients

The approach outlined here is useful in the evaluation of an enlarged heart.

I. Document or confirm the presence of cardiomegaly.
   A. Identify which chambers are enlarged.
   B. Dilatation and/or hypertrophy present?
   C. Quantify the degree (i.e., the severity) of the chamber enlargement.

II. Establish the cause of cardiomegaly.

III. Assess the functional significance of cardiomegaly.
   A. Symptoms of dyspnea, fatigue, etc.
   B. Status of ventricular function, congestive heart failure, etc.
   C. Determine New York Heart Association Functional Class.

IV. Establish a therapeutic plan.
   A. Preventive measures when appropriate, e.g., control of high blood pressure, modification of coronary risk factors, cessation of alcohol ingestion.
   B. Medical therapy: digitalis, diuretics, beta blockers, nitrates, calcium channel blockers, antihypertensive drugs.
   C. Surgical therapy: valve replacement, mitral commisurotomy, coronary artery bypass surgery, repair of atrial septal defect.

Implications of Cardiomegaly

Cardiomegaly is a very important finding. It may be the first evidence of significant cardiovascular disease or an obvious accompaniment of generalized cardiac dysfunction. In general, dilatation of cardiac chambers in the absence of a volume overload (mitral or aortic regurgitation) is more ominous than hypertrophy and is more likely to be associated with contractile or systolic impairment of cardiac function.

Obviously, cardiomegaly is only a marker for cardiovascular abnormality, and its ultimate significance depends on the functional status of the heart, the underlying cause of the cardiac disorder,

Table 3. THE MOST COMMON CAUSES OF HEART ENLARGEMENT

Cause	Important Diagnostic Criteria and Procedures
Hypertension, hypertensive heart disease	Documented high blood pressure, especially of long duration ECG or echocardiographic evidence of left ventricular hypertrophy
Valvular heart disease or intracardiac shunt	Abnormal cardiac sounds and murmurs on physical examination Echocardiographic confirmation of abnormal valvular structure or function and appropriate chamber enlargement Cardiac catheterization
Coronary artery disease	Documentation of prior myocardial infarction(s) by history or ECG History of angina pectoris Routine treadmill or radionuclide isotope scan stress testing Coronary arteriography
Cardiomyopathy	No evidence of valvular, coronary, or hypertensive heart disease Evidence of cardiac muscle dysfunction on echocardiography, radionuclear angiogram, or cardiac catheterization Identification of a possible etiologic agent: viral titer rise, acute myocarditis, heavy chronic alcoholic intake Absence of a specific causative agent does not preclude cardiomyopathy

and the degree of potential for reversibility or stabilization. It is incumbent upon the primary physician to make a complete and accurate assessment of each individual with an enlarged heart and to provide follow-up on a regular basis, utilizing all appropriate medical and surgical therapy indicated.

REFERENCES

1. Kannel WB, Castelli WP, McNamara PM, McKee PA, Feinleib M. Role of blood pressure in the development of congestive heart failure. The Framingham Study. NEJM 1972; 187:781–7.
2. Ahmed SS, Regan TJ. Diabetic cardiomyopathy: diagnosis and clinical significance. Pract Cardiol 1982;8:76–84.
3. Kannel WB, McGee DL. Diabetes and cardiovascular disease. The Framingham Study. JAMA 1979;241:2035–8.
4. Abrams J. Precordial motion in health and disease. Mod Cardiovasc Dis 1980;49:55–60.
5. Mounsey JPD. Inspection and palpation of the cardiac impulse. Prog Cardiovasc Dis 1967;10:187–206.
6. Stapleton JF, Groves BM. Precordial palpation. Am Heart J Dis 1971;81:409–27.
7. de Leon A, Perloff JK, Twigg H, Majd M. The straight back syndrome. Clinical cardiovascular manifestations. Circulation 1965;32:193–203.
8. Meszaros WT. Cardiac enlargement. In: Cardiac roentgenology. Springfield, Ill: Charles C Thomas, 1969;54–74.
9. Davies H, Nelson WP. Understanding cardiac radiology. In: Cardiology. Boston: Butterworths, 1978;372–98.
10. Rushmer RF. The size and configuration of the heart and blood vessels. In: Cardiovascular dynamics, 4th ed. Philadelphia: WB Saunders, 1976;382–410.
11. Simon G. The normal heart shadow. In: Principles of chest x-ray diagnosis, 4th ed. Boston: Butterworths, 1978; 10–6.
12. Simon G. Cardiovascular abnormalities. In: Principles of chest x-ray diagnosis, 4th ed. Boston: Butterworths, 1978;180–214.
13. Felson B. A review of over 40,000 normal chest roentgenograms. In: Chest roentgenology. Philadelphia: WB Saunders, 1973;494–8.
14. Tucker DH, Gaylor DH, Jacoby WJ, Sumner RG. Prominence of the left epipericardial fat pad: a cause of apparent cardiomegaly. Am J Med 1965;38:268–73.
15. Raskoff WJ, Goldman S, Cohn K. The "athletic heart." JAMA 1976;236:158–62.
16. Abbasi AS. Echocardiography in the differential diagnosis of the large heart. Am J Med 1976;60:677–86.
17. Grossman W. Cardiac catheterization and angiography. Philadelphia: Lea & Febiger, 1976;3–9.
18. Collins RD. Dynamic differential diagnosis. Philadelphia: JB Lippincott, 1981;2:106–12.
19. Collins RD. Dynamic differential diagnosis. Philadelphia: JB Lippincott, 1981:487.

CHEST PAIN, ATYPICAL

LEE GOLDMAN

□ SYNONYMS: Atypical angina, chest pain of uncertain etiology

BACKGROUND

Definition

Before embarking on a detailed discussion of the evaluation of the patient with atypical chest pain, we should determine what is commonly meant by *typical chest pain*. Typical chest pain, or pain that is considered absolutely classic for ischemic heart disease, implies typical angina pectoris. Typical angina pectoris is commonly described as a heaviness, a sense of constriction, a pressure, or a squeezing that is located principally in the substernal area and that often radiates to the neck, to the left shoulder, and down the ulnar aspect of the left arm. Some patients may deny pain but then describe a pressure or discomfort that is unlike any pain that they have previously encountered. Other patients may not be able to describe their discomfort in words, but instead may use the classic clenched-fist gesture in an attempt to describe the sensation.

In addition to the character and location of the discomfort, typical angina pectoris has several other key features. First and foremost, it is classically provoked by exercise and disappears within a matter of minutes when the patient rests. Excitement, anger, fright, and other strong emotions may precipitate the discomfort, which is also felt with exertion. Second, classic anginal pain is usually relieved by nitroglycerin within 5 minutes or less; nitroglycerin should also cause the pain to disappear more rapidly than it would with rest alone. Of patients with the classic anginal syndrome, cardiac catheterization will document coronary artery disease in approximately 90 per cent.[1, 2] When the history is classic, no single diagnostic test or combination of diagnostic tests (other than a normal coronary arteriogram) can be sufficient to rule out the probability that the pain is caused by coronary artery disease.

In clinical practice, however, the difficult diagnosis concerns the patient whose history does not include all the classic features of angina pectoris.

The chest pain may be atypical for angina pectoris in terms of the words used to describe it; for example, some patients may use the word sharp as a synonym for severe, and other patients may describe the pain as an aching sensation or as indigestion. The description may also be atypical in terms of location; some patients with angina pectoris will complain of pain chiefly in the neck, arms, shoulder, or even jaw and teeth. Chest pain may also be atypical in terms of the kinds of activities that provoke it. It is characteristic for chest pain to be precipitated by the same activities each day; some patients, however, can do very little physical activity in the morning without having severe angina pectoris yet can engage in rather vigorous activity later in the day. Also, in some patients with angina pectoris, chest pain occurs early during physical activity, but if they continue to exercise the pain will actually go away. Other patients note angina pectoris principally after a large meal, presumably because the large demand for splanchnic blood flow increases cardiac stress. In some elderly or debilitated patients who are not very active, chest pain may be provoked principally by emotional stress rather than any discernible activity.

Because of the many atypical features of pain that is truly attributable to coronary artery disease, it is not surprising that a number of other conditions can be confused with atypical angina pectoris. Included are costochondral conditions, musculoskeletal abnormalities of the chest wall and shoulder, neurologic conditions, abnormalities of the lung and pleura, esophageal and other gastrointestinal disorders, and a number of cardiac conditions other than coronary artery disease (Table 1). Just as one can describe a syndrome of typical angina pectoris, one can also describe sets of symptoms that are typical for each of these other conditions. Of course, the most difficult problem in differential diagnosis occurs when the clinical syndrome is not typical for any of these conditions.

Table 1. CAUSES OF CHEST PAIN THAT IS NOT TYPICAL OF ANGINA PECTORIS

Musculoskeletal disorders	Costochondritis, including Tietze's syndrome Muscle or ligament damage Intercostal muscle cramp Bursitis or tendinitis
Neurologic disorders	Ruptured cervical disc Cervical arthritis
Pulmonary disorders	Pneumothorax Pleurisy (viral, etc.) Tracheobronchitis Lung tumor
Gastrointestinal disorders	Hiatal hernia Ulcer disease Gallbladder disease
Cardiac disorders	Aortic stenosis Idiopathic hypertrophic subaortic stenosis Mitral valve prolapse Pericarditis Coronary artery spasm Nocturnal angina

HISTORY AND CAUSES

As is true for most conditions causing chronic pain, the differential diagnosis of atypical chest pain is strongly dependent on a detailed and accurate history. Because pain that engenders suspicions of but is atypical of angina pectoris is caused by noncardiac conditions in at least 50 per cent of cases,[1, 2] it is important to understand what features of the history might point to noncardiac causes.

Musculoskeletal Disorders

Musculoskeletal chest pain disorders include those related to costochondral or chondrosternal joints, to the ligaments or muscles of the anterior chest, to the bursae of the shoulder, to osteoarthritis of the dorsal or thoracic spine, to cervical discs, and to the brachial plexus.

The classic costochondral or chondrosternal disorder, Tietze's syndrome, is characterized by swelling, redness, and warmth of an anterior chest joint articulation. However, such objective, visible signs are found only in severe disease, and this diagnosis cannot be eliminated because of their absence. Rather, the diagnosis is suggested by a history of minor trauma or a new or unusually vigorous physical activity. The pain may actually be precipitated by movements of the chest wall, but it is not at all uncommon for patients to complain of aching, sharp, or stabbing chest pain that is most notable after the activity is completed. A similar history is usually noted in patients in whom ligamentous or muscular abnormalities provoke musculoskeletal pain. Commonly, sharp or knife-like pains originating from these latter abnormalities are described as being fleeting, often lasting for a second or less. By comparison, in Tietze's syndrome, the dull ache that often follows exercise may last for many hours and it is commonly relieved by heat, anti-inflammatory drugs, or analgesics.

Severe musculoskeletal problems, such as torn muscles, generally are abrupt in onset. By comparison, most other musculoskeletal causes of chest pain have subacute onset, over a period of days or weeks, and may often occur in patients who have had similar episodes of discomfort at earlier times in their lives.

Another common musculoskeletal syndrome is the intercostal muscle cramp. This pain, which may be similar to the muscle cramps that many patients notice in their calves at night, is commonly related to tension. The patient often describes the pain as an ache but may also complain that it is difficult to expand his or her chest; this latter feature may be confused with the constriction or pressing quality commonly associated with angina pectoris. However, like other musculoskeletal causes of subacute chest pain and unlike angina pectoris, intercostal cramps are most commonly noted while the patient is at rest, especially when lying in bed trying to fall asleep.

A good general point to remember is that angina pectoris commonly interferes with a patient's activities, often causing him or her to stop or alter daily activities. By comparison, musculoskeletal chest pains are often noted during periods of inactivity and tend to be ignored when the patient is actively pursuing interesting activities.

Many types of musculoskeletal pain are also clearly pleuritic in nature, or they may be obviously precipitated by movements of the trunk or chest wall. Such characteristics are very uncommon for angina pectoris. Inflammation of the subacromial bursae, the supraspinatus tendon, or less commonly the deltoid tendon can cause pain in the shoulder or clavicular area that radiates to the anterior chest. This pain usually has many of the same characteristics as other musculoskeletal causes of chest pain.

Neurologic Disorders

Cervical arthritis or rupture of a cervical disc may occasionally be manifested as chest pain. However, in most such cases the patient has neck and occasionally shoulder pain as well.

Pulmonary Disorders

The historical hallmark of pulmonary causes of chest pain is their pleuritic nature. The pain of a spontaneous pneumothorax is usually sudden in onset and intensely pleuritic. The chest pain that accompanies or follows many viral infections, especially coxsackie B viruses, is also pleuritic. Commonly, affected patients describe an ongoing or a recently resolved upper respiratory infection. Tracheobronchitis, which may manifest as chest pain because of either localized irritation or muscle soreness due to repeated coughing, is usually easy to distinguish from angina pectoris.

An additional hallmark of pulmonary causes of chest pain is their recent onset. By comparison, on detailed questioning, many patients with angina pectoris, even if they are presenting to a physician for the first time, recall previous episodes of pain that were milder or that came on only with more severe exertion.

Gastrointestinal Diseases

Although classic gastrointestinal pain should be easily distinguishable from classic angina pectoris, atypical presentations of disorders in the two organ systems may be distressingly similar. Burning discomfort beneath the sternum is the hallmark of a hiatal hernia, and the same sensation in the epigastrium is typical of a gastric or duodenal ulcer. A significant minority of patients with angina pectoris, however, also describe their pain as burning or as feeling like indigestion. Prompt relief by antacids is the hallmark of acid-induced gastrointestinal pain, but spontaneous resolution of angina pectoris may also occur coincidentally with administration of antacids. Thus, one must be sure that the response to antacids is prompt and that similar relief is not equally likely to occur spontaneously. Fortunately, many patients with acid-induced symptoms have a long history of such complaints, and the onset of the symptoms may antedate their entry into the age group prone to coronary artery disease.

Occasionally, cholecystitis may also manifest as pain that is epigastric or substernal. This pain, which is more of an ache than a burning sensation, classically follows a large meal by 1 or more hours. Acute cholecystitis may be exceptionally difficult to distinguish from acute myocardial infarction. In chronic cholecystitis, however, the occurrence of pain after meals rather than with exertion is usually sufficient to make the distinction. In fact, the relation of pain to activity is usually the basis for differentiating gastrointestinal from cardiac complaints. The discomfort of ulcer disease or hiatal hernia is likely to be provoked by aspirin, alcohol, and certain foods and to be relieved somewhat by the ingestion of bland foods or antacids. Hiatal hernia pain commonly is at its worst when the patient lies down or wakes up in the morning. Ulcer disease commonly flares in the early morning hours, when the stomach is empty but still secreting acid, and is less severe during waking hours, when acid secretion is at its nadir. Gastrointestinal pain is virtually never precipitated by exercise, with the rare exception of esophageal pain caused by activities that increase intra-abdominal pressure and severely exacerbate esophageal reflux.

Although the relationship of pain to eating and exercise is usually adequate for differential diagnosis, problems arise in two particular situations. First, as noted previously, sudden and severe gastrointestinal pain occurring at rest may be very difficult to distinguish from the pain of acute myocardial infarction; because an acute myocardial infarction may be the first clinical evidence of ischemic heart disease,[3] this presentation is often difficult to diagnose. Second, in some patients, angina pectoris may be provoked by a large meal, and its pain may be very difficult to distinguish from that of gallbladder disease or even ulcer disease or hiatal hernia, especially in a patient who does not exercise sufficiently for one to be sure that such activity would not also cause angina pectoris. It should be emphasized that angina pectoris provoked by eating a large meal is usually fairly severe, so the patient who is physically active usually also reports similar pains brought on by activity at other times. However, in the very sedentary patient, the cardiovascular response to a large meal may actually be a larger myocardial stress than imposed by any of the patient's other activities of daily living.

It is important to emphasize that hiatal hernia pain may actually have two forms. First, classic substernal burning related to esophageal reflux and acid irritation of the esophagus usually occurs while the patient is lying down. Second, severe reflux may on occasion precipitate esophageal spasm and produce pain that is virtually indistinguishable from that of myocardial ischemia. Furthermore, esophageal spasm may respond promptly to nitroglycerin, much as angina pectoris does. The relationship of the pain to exercise is again the most useful point to establish.

Cardiac Disorders Other Than Angina Pectoris

Several cardiac conditions may cause ischemic cardiac symptoms that are identical to those produced by angina pectoris. Classic examples are valvular aortic stenosis and idiopathic hypertrophic subaortic stenosis. The pain caused by these two conditions is indistinguishable by means of history from the pain caused by coronary artery disease.

Mitral valve prolapse, on the other hand, is commonly associated with atypical chest discomfort.[4] As usually described, the pain of mitral valve prolapse has many characteristics of musculoskeletal chest pain, and it commonly occurs in patients who are young, female, and asthenic.

Pericarditis, whether caused by viral infections, uremia, bacterial infections, or other inflammatory conditions, may cause several different pain syndromes. Because the pericardium has little if any pain fibers of its own, most of the pain associated with pericarditis is related to inflammation of the adjacent parietal pleura. Thus, the most common type of pericardial pain is pleuritic, and it is related to respiration, coughing, or deep inspiration, much like pulmonary causes of chest pain. Such pain is commonly described as sharp and stabbing, and its most severe component will last for seconds at most. However, pain related to severe inflammation of the relatively insensitive visceral pericardium or afferent cardiac nerve fibers may sometimes cause a more typical cardiac pain, which is often described as steady, aching, or even crushing or pressing. It tends to be constant, to last for many hours, and to be unrelated to physical exertion. In patients with viral pericarditis, a classic viral infection syndrome in the prior weeks is often elicited. In patients with systemic lupus erythematosus, rheumatoid arthritis, or uremia, a meticulous history usually reveals other evidence of the generalized disease.

Several unusual manifestations of coronary artery disease must also be included in the general category of atypical chest pain. First, angina that occurs at night may be termed angina decubitus or nocturnal angina. Angina decubitus, which typically occurs within an hour or so after assuming the recumbent position, is ischemic heart disease provoked by blood redistribution and increased venous return. Nocturnal angina may also involve ischemic chest pain that occurs later during sleep, at times provoked by the sympathetic response to REM dreaming.

Finally, one must consider the syndrome of coronary artery spasm with or without superimposed underlying coronary artery stenosis. Coronary artery spasm occurs at rest in the absence of a prior increase in heart rate or blood pressure, and the pain it causes is usually described as otherwise typical of angina pectoris. Patients who have spasm superimposed on underlying atherosclerotic lesions are commonly men in the fifth decade or older, whereas those with spasm of otherwise normal coronary arteries more typically are young women.[5]

PHYSICAL EXAMINATION

Although the history is the cornerstone of evaluation for the patient with atypical chest pain, several key aspects of the physical examination should be emphasized. Most patients with musculoskeletal chest pain have localized tenderness to palpation, so full palpation of the anterior chest wall is essential. The subacromial bursae and the supraspinatus tendon, inflammation of which can cause left shoulder and anterior chest discomfort, should also be palpated. Pain related to bursitis or tendinitis is commonly exacerbated by abduction of the shoulder more than 90 degrees. Patients with classic Tietze's syndrome have objectively detectable swelling, but absence of this sign should not eliminate the possibility of a musculoskeletal origin for the chest pain.

If chest pain is produced by local palpation, it

is especially important to determine whether the pain produced is identical to the pain the patient complains of. Many patients with true angina pectoris have some degree of chest tenderness in addition, and it is imperative that the physician not be misled into assuming that all patients with chest tenderness have musculoskeletal disorders.

In the patient with cervical arthritis or rupture of a cervical disc, rotation of the neck usually exacerbates the pain. In addition, spasm of the neck muscles is often found.

Patients with systemic arthritis manifested as chest wall pain should have systemic signs of arthritis.

Patients in whom pulmonary disorders are causing the pain may have rales, rhonchi, or a pleural friction rub. However, many patients with viral pleuritis do not have audible rubs.

In patients with gastrointestinal causes of atypical chest pain, there are rarely any important physical findings. However, patients with ulcer disease or gallbladder disease may have localized tenderness in the epigastrium or right upper quadrant, especially during acute episodes.

Patients with valvular aortic stenosis or idiopathic hypertrophic subaortic stenosis commonly have characteristic murmurs, which in the latter condition are especially exacerbated by the Valsalva maneuver.[6] The patient with mitral valve prolapse has a midsystolic click or late systolic murmur. The patient in whom pericarditis is causing chest pain commonly has a percardial rub, which is usually best heard with the patient in the sitting position at full expiration. It should be noted that by comparison, the pain of pericarditis is most commonly felt with the patient supine and is exacerbated by respiration.

Between episodes of acute pain, the patient with angina pectoris rarely has any definitive physical findings. The presence of hypertension, a fourth heart sound, or skin signs of hypercholesterolemia may increase the suspicion of coronary artery disease, but they are by no means diagnostic of angina pectoris. If the patient is examined during the acute episode of pain, however, increases in heart rate and blood pressure are commonly found. In addition, a fourth or third heart sound may develop during acute ischemia, and in some patients a transient murmur of papillary muscle dysfunction also develops. During episodes of acute pain, patients with angina pectoris commonly appear diaphoretic and ill at ease, whereas many patients with atypical chest pain from other causes do not appear to be ill at all.

DIAGNOSTIC STUDIES

In many patients, a presumptive diagnosis of the cause of atypical chest pain can be made without any laboratory tests. Blood tests are rarely helpful, although an elevated sedimentation rate may point to a diagnosis of arthritis or other inflammatory processes, iron deficiency anemia may raise the suspicion of a hiatal hernia or ulcer disease, and glucose intolerance or hypercholesterolemia may increase the suspicion of coronary artery disease. A chest x-ray rarely reveals diagnostic abnormalities, but it is usually obtained to eliminate the possibilities of pneumothorax, a malignant process that may cause chest irritation or pain, and congestive heart failure.

The Electrocardiogram

One cannot definitively diagnose angina pectoris on the basis of the resting electrocardiogram, but some ECG abnormalities would certainly increase one's suspicion that the pain is related to coronary artery disease. For example, Q waves indicative of a prior myocardial infarction are virtually diagnostic for coronary artery disease. However, if the patient is sure that the present pain is totally unlike the pain he or she felt during a myocardial infarction, the present pain is unlikely to be angina pectoris. Conversely, if the pain feels like the pain of an earlier myocardial infarction, it is likely to be caused by ischemic heart disease regardless of how atypical it seems to be. Finally, if the electrocardiogram results are diagnostic of an old myocardial infarction in a patient without a clinical history of a previously diagnosed infarction, one must also be aware that long-standing atypical chest pain may represent a myocardial infarction followed by angina pectoris.

Electrocardiographic findings of left ventricular hypertrophy or ST-T wave changes of ischemia or strain are often present in patients with hypertension who have no coronary artery disease and do not have angina pectoris. Nevertheless, demonstration of left ventricular hypertrophy by electrocardiogram was a major risk factor for coronary artery disease in the Framingham Study[7] and this finding must increase the suspicion that an episode of atypical chest pain represents myocardial ischemia.

Exercise Tests

In many cases, the history and physical examination leave the physician wishing for a diagnostic test capable of assisting in the differential diagnosis of atypical chest pain. For many years, the exercise test was thought to be such a tool. Recently, however, extensive research has indicated that the exercise test result, much like that of any other diagnostic test, may be dramatically related to the probability of coronary artery disease but is

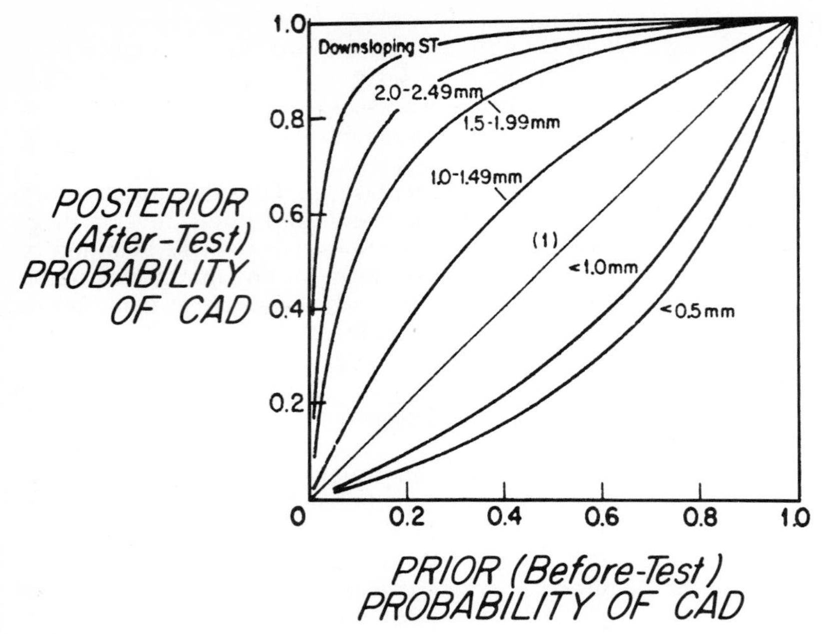

Figure 1. These curves show the posterior (after-test) probability as a function of prior (before-test) probability for different results of the exercise electrocardiogram. Note that 1.0 mm or more of ST-segment depression increases the probability of disease, whereas less than 1.0 mm of ST-segment depression is associated with a modest reduction in the probability of disease. *CAD*, coronary artery disease. (Adapted from Rifkin RD, Hood WB: Bayesian analysis of electrocardiographic exercise stress testing. N Engl J Med **297**:681, 1977, with permission.)

not so perfectly accurate as to be predictive in all patients.[1, 2, 8, 9] Using Bayes's theorem, one can calculate a change in probability of disease if one knows the pretest probability of disease and the accuracy of the diagnostic test, as long as one assumes that the information provided by the new test is no more associated with the prior information than would be expected by chance.[9] As shown in Figure 1, a given exercise test result has a different meaning depending on the prior (before-test) probability that the patient has coronary artery disease. In patients with atypical angina, a negative exercise test result reduces the probability of coronary artery disease to about 25 per cent, a moderately positive result (1 to 2 mm of ST depression) increases the probability to about 75 per cent, and a strongly positive result (more than 2 mm of ST depression) increases it to about 95 per cent (Fig. 2).[10]

In addition to the standard exercise electrocardiogram, there are two other types of exercise tests that have been useful in predicting the presence or absence of coronary artery disease, the exercise thallium scan and the exercise radionuclide ventriculogram.[11–14] The former test involves injection of radioactive thallium at peak exercise. Thallium, which is a potassium analog, will flow to areas of myocardium that have adequate blood supply. Thus, in the absence of coronary artery stenosis, the exercise thallium scan shows good thallium uptake in all areas of the left ventricular myocardium. In contrast, thallium up-

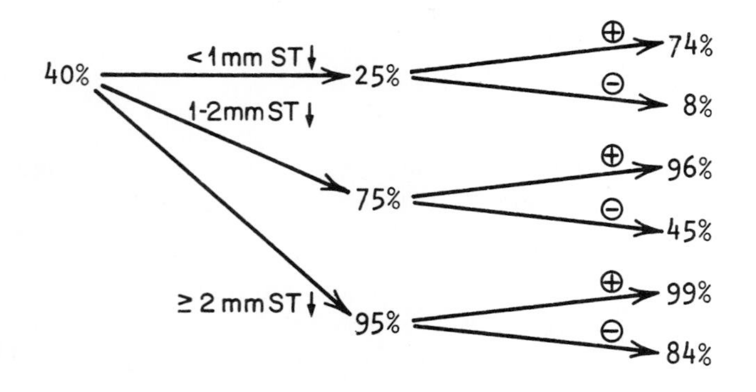

Figure 2. These percentages demonstrate how an exercise electrocardiogram and an exercise thallium test may affect the probability of coronary artery disease (CAD) in a patient with atypical anginal symptoms. (From Goldman L: Non-invasive evaluation of chest pain. Urban Health **9**:29, 1980. Reprinted by permission.)

take is diminished or absent in an area that does not have adequate blood supply because of coronary artery stenosis. If the patient has had a myocardial infarction, the area of diminished uptake is evident both with exercise and at rest. Conversely, if the patient has transient ischemia related to exercise, which is the pathophysiologic equivalent of angina pectoris, the thallium uptake in an area of myocardium is reduced or absent with exercise but normal at rest.

Because the information obtained from an exercise thallium scan is reasonably independent of that obtained from a standard exercise electrocardiogram, the same Bayesian analyses that have been applied to the information content of exercise ECGs have been applied to the information content of exercise thallium scans. As shown in Figure 2, the sequential use of an exercise thallium scan after an exercise electrocardiogram may further refine the probability of coronary artery disease in the patient with atypical chest pain. If results of both tests are positive, the probability of coronary artery disease is above 95 per cent; if one is positive and one negative, the probability is somewhere between 45 and 85 per cent; and if both are negative, the probability is 8 per cent.

More recently, the use of exercise radionuclide ventriculograms has been shown to yield information approximately as accurate as that given by exercise thallium scanning. In brief, a radionuclide ventriculogram is performed by injecting radioactive material and then observing the left ventricular ejection fraction as averaged over many beats using computerized techniques that integrate or "sum" the number of radioactive counts in the area of the left ventricle during many systoles and diastoles. In normal persons, exercise results in an increase in the left ventricular ejection fraction, although this response is blunted in patients over age 60.[14] In patients with coronary artery stenosis, the left ventricular ejection fraction tends to decline with exercise. This decline, which is related to ischemia in patients with coronary artery disease, is rarely found in normal patients but may be found in a number of cardiac conditions other than coronary artery disease. In terms of diagnostic decision-making, the results of an exercise radionuclide ventriculogram have about the same impact on the probability of coronary artery disease as those of an exercise thallium scan. The one major advantage of an exercise thallium scan is that it may show an additional area of transient ischemia in a patient with a fixed area of diminished uptake from a prior myocardial infarction. By comparison, a reduction in exercise ejection fraction in a patient wih a prior myocardial infarction may not indicate major areas of new ischemia but may rather be related to the effects of the previous myocardial infarction.

Predictive Value of Exercise Tests

Although recent elegant analyses have used Bayes's theorem to determine the incremental value of the various cardiologic diagnostic tests, many of these analyses have assumed that relatively little is known about the patient prior to the diagnostic test. Recently, my colleagues and I have shown that a combination of information, including the typicality of the chest pain, the presence or absence of a prior myocardial infarction, the patient's gender, the patient's age, the cholesterol level, and a history of smoking, could result in far more accurate predictions of coronary artery disease than can be made on the basis of the typicality of the chest pain alone.[15] In essence, this analysis combined the historical features related to the chest pain with a variety of epidemiologic risk factors to derive predictions that were 84 per cent accurate about whether patients with chest pain would be shown to have significant coronary artery disease at cardiac catheterization. When such detailed analysis was available, the additional information provided by the exercise electrocardiogram had very limited incremental predictive power, the percentage of patients correctly classified increasing only to 87 per cent.

These findings suggest that when the physician knows a lot about the patient, the results of the exercise test are associated with the previous data to a much greater degree than would be expected by chance. Therefore, the calculations made according to Bayes's theorem may overestimate the true incremental information provided by the exercise test. In other words, the more the physician knows about the patient in terms of history, risk factors, and physical findings, the less new information is provided by the exercise test. In such patients, an exercise test result that contradicts the clinical impression is almost as likely to be misleading as it is to be helpful.

The limited value of the exercise test and of other diagnostic tests can be further demonstrated by what has been termed threshold analysis.[16] In brief, this concept suggests that a diagnostic test result is helpful mainly when it changes the probability of disease enough to move it across a therapeutic threshold. In other words, a change in the probability of disease has clinical relevance only when some decision would be based on the change. For example, a statistician might be very impressed if the probability of coronary artery disease were changed from 75 to 50 per cent, but a physician may say that no decisions about therapy would be altered by the change.

When we analyzed the value of the exercise test in this way, we found that in no more than about 20 per cent of patients would the probability of coronary artery disease be moved across a clinically important threshold by an exercise test result. In addition, in one-third of patients whose probabilities were moved across clinically relevant thresholds, the results of the exercise tests were misleading. Thus, the net correct yield of the exercise test was small, causing the probability of coronary artery disease to move correctly across any of a variety of clinically important thresholds that a physician might choose in only about 6 per cent of patients.

These data from a variety of investigations leave the practicing physician in somewhat of a dilemma. The exercise test, exercise thallium scan, and exercise radionuclide ventriculogram can all provide useful diagnostic information, but the more the physician knows about the patient the less reliance should be placed on such results when they conflict with the clinical impression. A battery of consistently negative cardiologic test results can reduce the probability of coronary artery disease to less than 10 per cent in an average patient with atypical chest pain. Such a reduction is reassuring for the patient and physician, but both must realize that a probability of less than 10 per cent does not absolutely rule out the possibility. In many instances, patients and physicians alter their approach even when the probability of a serious condition is a good deal less than 50 per cent. Thus, patients whose probability of coronary artery disease is less than 50 per cent may also be given a therapeutic trial of anti-anginal medications. If the chest pain responds clinically to such a trial, the likelihood that the symptoms are related to coronary artery disease increases, although there are no good experimental data to quantify the likelihood precisely.

Coronary Angiography

When either the patient or the physician must know definitively whether coronary artery disease is present, there is no substitute for a coronary angiogram. Such a test is considered the "gold standard" for the diagnosis of coronary artery disease. Unfortunately, the presence of coronary artery disease is not necessarily a guarantee that an atypical chest pain syndrome is caused by the anatomic lesions seen on angiography. In such cases, it may be helpful to demonstrate that activities that cause chest pain also cause measurable hemodynamic abnormalities. Thus, cardiologists sometimes recommend left atrial pacing during cardiac catheterization in patients with atypical chest pain syndromes.[17] The left atrium is paced at rates of 150 beats/min or more in an attempt to provoke myocardial ischemia. A result is positive when the patient's chest pain is precipitated and is accompanied by objective signs of myocardial ischemia such as electrocardiographic changes, increases in left ventricular end diastolic pressure, or evidence of altered lactate metabolism. If no objective abnormalities are found at catheterization, it is usually concluded that the coronary artery stenoses are not the cause of the chest pain, particularly if the pain is especially atypical.

Another technique sometimes used during cardiac catheterization is the injection of ergonovine in an attempt to precipitate coronary artery spasm in patients whose pain is suggestive of this diagnosis.[18] In the classic positive result, injection of ergonovine causes marked spasm of the coronary artery, accompanied by chest pain and typical ECG changes. Although a small number of normal patients may have some degree of spasm after the injection, the results of this provocative test are usually reliable.

Echocardiography

An echocardiogram is usually not very helpful in diagnosing coronary artery disease, unless it shows segmental wall motion abnormalities. Because such abnormalities are usually found in patients with a history of myocardial infarction or with obvious electrocardiographic abnormalities, using echocardiography to screen for left ventricular segmental wall motion abnormalities is not recommended. However, the echocardiogram may be important in diagnosing valvular aortic stenosis, idiopathic hypertrophic subaortic stenosis, or mitral valve prolapse, three noncoronary but cardiac causes of chest pain. In patients with suspicious murmurs or clicks, the echocardiogram therefore may be helpful in elucidating the cause of atypical chest pain.

Other Tests

For the diagnosis of gastrointestinal complaints, a barium swallow, upper gastrointestinal series, oral cholecystography, abdominal ultrasonography, or hepatic iminodiacetic acid (HIDA) scanning may often be useful. In especially difficult cases, a Bernstein test—the passage of a tube into the esophagus, followed by the instillation of concentrated acid into the distal esophagus—may be crucial.[19] In a positive result, the patient's chest pain, which may involve heartburn or esophageal spasm, will be precipitated. Although the test is especially useful, one must remember the relative implications of coronary disease versus gastrointestinal disease; the physician should be certain or virtually certain that coronary disease is not present before performing a Bernstein test in a patient with atypical chest pain.

REFERENCES

1. Diamond GA, Hirsch M, Forrester JS, et al. Application of information theory to clinical diagnostic testing: the electrocardiographic stress test. Circulation 1981;63:915–21.
2. Weiner DA, Ryan TJ, McCabe CH, et al. Exercise stress testing: correlations among history of angina, ST-segment response and prevalence of coronary artery disease. N Engl J Med 1979;301:230–5.
3. Kannel WB, Feinleib M. Natural history of angina pectoris in the Framingham Study: prognosis and survival. Am J Cardiol 1972;29:154–63.
4. Devereux RB, Perloff JK, Reichek N, Josephson ME. Mitral valve prolapse. Circulation 1976;54:3–14.
5. Luchi RJ, Chahine RA, Raizner AE. Coronary artery spasm. Ann Intern Med 1979;91:441–9.
6. Dohan MC, Criscitiello MG. Physiological and pharmacological manipulations of heart sounds and murmurs. Mod Concepts Cardiovasc Dis 1970;9:121–7.
7. Kannel WB. Prevention of cardiovascular disease. In: Harvey WP, et al., eds. Current problems in cardiology. Chicago: Year Book Medical Publishers, Inc., 1976;13–68.
8. Epstein SE. Implications of probability analysis on the strategy used for noninvasive detection of coronary artery disease: role of single or combined use of exercise electocardiographic testing, radionuclide cineangiography and myocardial perfusion imaging. Am J Cardiol 1980;46:491–9.
9. Rifkin RD, Hood WB. Bayesian analysis of electrocardiographic exercise stress testing. N Engl J Med 1977;297:681–6.
10. Goldman L, Adams JB. Cost-effectiveness in medical decision making: cardiac nuclear medicine and exercise electrocardiograms. Cardiovasc Rev Rep 1981;2:45–53.
11. Ritchie JL, Zaret BL, Strauss HW, et al. Myocardial imaging with thallium-201: a multicenter study in patients with angina pectoris or acute myocardial infarction. Am J Cardiol 1978;42:345–50.
12. Melin JA, Piret LJ, Vanbutsele RJM, et al. Diagnostic value of exercise electrocardiography and thallium myocardial scintigraphy in patients without previous myocardial infarction: a Bayesian approach. Circulation 1981;63:1019–24.
13. Berger HJ, Reduto LA, Johnstone DE, et al. Global and regional left ventricular response to bicycle exercise in coronary artery disease: assessment by quantitative radionuclide angiocardiography. Am J Med 1979;66:13–20.
14. Port S, Cobb FR, Coleman RE, Jones RH. Effect of age on the response of the left ventricular ejection to exercise. N Engl J Med 1980;303:1133–7.
15. Goldman L, Cook EF, Mitchell N, et al. Incremental value of the exercise test for diagnosing the presence or absence of coronary artery disease. Circulation 1982;66:945–53.
16. Pauker SG, Kassirer JP. The threshold approach to clinical decision making. N Engl J Med 1980;302:1109–17.
17. Waters DD, Forrester JS. Myocardial ischemia: detection and quantitation. Ann Intern Med 1978;88:239–50.
18. Heupler FA, Proudfit WL, Razavi M, Shirey EK, Greenstreet R, Sheldon WC. Ergonovine maleate provocative test for coronary arterial spasm. Am J Cardiol 1978;41:631–40.
19. Davies HA, Jones DB, Rhodes J. "Esophageal angina" as the cause of chest pain. JAMA 1982;248:2274–8.

CYANOSIS

JERRE F. LUTZ □ NANETTE K. WENGER

BACKGROUND

Definition

Cyanosis is a bluish discoloration evident on physical examination that is imparted to the skin and mucous membranes by the underlying capillary network.

Pathophysiology

Clinical evidence of cyanosis correlates with the presence of 5 gm or more of unsaturated (reduced) hemoglobin per 100 ml of capillary blood.[1] The absolute amount of unsaturated hemoglobin seems to be more important than the percentage. Cyanosis is most evident on the fingernails, tongue, lips, ears, nose, cheeks, hands, and feet.

A normal individual with hemoglobin AA can develop cyanosis at high altitudes, where the inspired air has a low partial pressure of oxygen.[2] Cyanosis with pulmonary disease results from blood flow into hypoaerated areas of the lungs; the resultant ventilation-perfusion mismatch increases the amount of circulating unsaturated hemoglobin. Cyanosis in congenital heart disease, as postulated by DeSenac[3] in 1794, generally results from the intracardiac admixture of venous (unoxygenated) blood with arterial (oxygenated) blood (a right-to-left shunt). Peripheral cyanosis may occur as a result of diminished peripheral blood flow; increased oxygen extraction by the tissues increases the amount of unsaturated hemoglobin in the capillary bed.

Cyanosis may occur with a normal arterial pO_2 in patients with abnormal hemoglobins, such as hemoglobin Beth Israel and hemoglobin Kansas, which have a significantly lower oxygen affinity than hemoglobin AA.[2] Methemoglobin, whether occurring as a congenital defect or due to drug ingestion, is characterized by a central iron atom in the ferric rather that the ferrous form; cyanosis is clinically apparent with as little as 1.5 gm of methemoglobin per 100 ml of capillary blood.[4] Cyanosis has occasionally been described in patients with severe intravascular hemolysis and is due to the increased amounts of circulating methemoglobin and methemalbumin. Sulfhemoglobin may likewise alter the hemoglobin molecule, resulting in a lower oxygen affinity; only 0.5 gm of sulfhemoglobin per 100 ml of blood is required for cyanosis to be clinically evident.[4]

Problems In Recognition

Perception of cyanosis is influenced by the capillary density in the underlying surface, the amount of cutaneous blood flow, the thickness of the skin, and the extravascular skin pigments. Recognition of cyanosis is more difficult in black and oriental as well as suntanned and icteric patients.[1]

Cyanosis may be difficult to discern in severely anemic patients (serum hemoglobin level less than 7 gm/100 ml) even with a significant percentage of desaturated hemoglobin; cyanosis is unlikely to be appreciated with a hemoglobin level less than 5 gm/100 ml.[1] Detection of cyanosis may also be difficult in polycythemic patients, who may have elevated levels of both saturated and desaturated hemoglobin. The individual physician's ability to detect cyanosis also varies widely; some physicians may identify cyanosis at an arterial saturation of 85 per cent, whereas others can do so only at a 75 per cent saturation.[1, 5]

Some laboratories report an oxygen saturation derived from the pO_2 (assuming hemoglobin AA) rather than obtained by direct measurement; therefore, the physician must know the method used to avoid being deceived by a normal "derived" saturation with a normal pO_2, when the measured saturation would actually be low.

Carboxyhemoglobinemia due to carbon monoxide inhalation may be confused with cyanosis; it is characterized by a cherry red flush, whereas polycythemic patients have a ruddy complexion, so-called red cyanosis. The slate-blue discoloration of argyria may mimic cyanosis but the abnormal skin pigmentation due to the deposition of silver does not blanch with pressure. Brownish skin discoloration can be due to Addison's disease or hemochromatosis.

HISTORY

Acutely Ill Cyanotic Patients

Cyanosis is typically recognized when the patient is initially seen. Chest pain and dyspnea are the most common accompanying symptoms. The most likely causes in this subset of patients include pulmonary embolism, pneumothorax, acute pulmonary edema, and acute upper airway obstruction. Hemoptysis may accompany pulmonary infarction. Concomitant inability to speak indicates upper airway obstruction in an alert cyanotic patient. Several patients have presented with an acute illness after consuming food into which cooling fluid had leaked; ingestion of sodium nitrite, used an an anticorrosive agent, caused severe methemoglobinemia and cyanosis.[6]

Chronically Ill Cyanotic Patients

A patient with chronic cyanosis may or may not be symptomatic and may or may not be aware of the cyanosis. The family should also be questioned as to the duration of the cyanosis. A patient with cyanosis from childhood should be suspected of having congenital heart disease or congenital methemoglobinemia. A history of squatting as a child may be further indicative of congenital heart disease. The presence of clubbing of the fingers and toes in association with cyanosis makes a long-standing process highly likely.

In the asymptomatic or minimally symptomatic chronically cyanotic patient, methemoglobinemia, sulfhemoglobinemia, or acrocyanosis should be suspected. A family history of such a disorder or a history of drug ingestion (especially nitrite compounds, sulfonamides, or aniline derivatives)[4, 7] strongly suggests the diagnosis of methemoglobinemia or sulfhemoglobinemia. Mild fatigue, dyspnea on exertion, and headaches on a chronic basis are occasionally reported by patients with abnormal hemoglobins.

Chronically symptomatic cyanotic patients usually describe chest pain or dyspnea, which is generally due to a cardiopulmonary disorder. This etiologic subset includes patients with chronic bronchitis, emphysema, interstitial pulmonary fibrosis, pulmonary arteriovenous fistulae, congenital heart disease, and hypoventilation secondary to morbid obesity.

PHYSICAL AND LABORATORY EXAMINATIONS

Cyanosis can be characterized on physical examination as localized, peripheral, differential, or generalized.[8]

Localized Cyanosis

Patients with localized cyanosis have retardation of blood flow, typically to an extremity, with resultant increased oxygen extraction by the tissues. Arterial thromboembolism, venous stasis, or application of a tourniquet can create a cyanotic extremity. A greater degree of arterial occlusion causes markedly diminished flow and a pale extremity.

Acrocyanosis is a benign condition; greater distal cyanosis of the upper than of the lower extremities may be related either to differential capillary density or to local changes in capillary flow. Placing a cyanotic extremity in warm water increases the local blood flow, causing the cyanosis to disappear temporarily.

Peripheral Cyanosis

Vasoconstriction and increased oxygen extraction are also the mechanisms underlying peripheral cyanosis. The peripheral type may occur in normal extremities exposed to severe cold, in extremities of patients with Raynaud's phenomenon or disease, and in the cool, clammy extremities of patients who are in shock, have congestive heart failure, or are receiving dopamine (Intropin) or other vasoconstrictor drugs.

Differential Cyanosis

Cyanosis that is greater in the hands than the feet suggests transposition of the great arteries with either preductal coarctation of the aorta or interruption of the aorta; pulmonary hypertension has reversed the shunt through a patent ductus arteriosus, so that more oxygenated blood is carried to the legs. Clubbing and cyanosis that are greater in the toes than the left hand, with a relatively pink right hand, suggest the diagnosis of pulmonary hypertension with reversed shunting of blood via a patent ductus arteriosus; unoxygenated blood is delivered to the lower extremities.[9]

Generalized Cyanosis

A truly asymptomatic patient with generalized cyanosis in whom findings on physical examination, chest roentgenogram, and electrocardiogram are normal and arterial blood gas analysis reveals a normal pO_2 and a normal measured arterial oxygen saturation probably has acrocyanosis.

Acute Cyanotic Disorders

In an acutely ill patient with generalized cyanosis, the physical examination, chest roentgenogram, and electrocardiogram will help differentiate among the following most likely diagnostic possibilities.

Pulmonary Embolism. Respiratory distress or tachypnea is common. A prominent A wave in the jugular venous pulse, distended neck veins, a loud and widely split pulmonic component of the second heart sound, and occasionally a right ventricular (parasternal) lift are evident. The electrocardiogram may show sinus tachycardia or atrial fibrillation, occasionally a P pulmonale and an $S_1Q_3T_3$ pattern, and commonly nonspecific ST-T changes. The findings on chest roentgenography may be normal or there may be areas of hypoperfusion or atelectasis.

Arterial hypoxemia and a decrease in oxygen saturation severe enough to cause cyanosis should be present on blood gas analysis.

Pneumothorax. Respiratory distress is prominent in patients with cyanosis due to a pneumothorax. Typically, increased intrathoracic tension with a tracheal and mediastinal shift are evident on physical examination. The electrocardiogram reveals sinus tachycardia; a low arterial pO_2 and oxygen saturation are revealed by arterial blood gas analysis.

Café Coronary. Upper airway obstruction should be suspected in an alert cyanotic patient who is unable to converse. Laboratory data are not likely to be available.

Pulmonary Edema. Respiratory distress is characteristic, often accompanied by pink, frothy sputum. A third heart sound or summation gallop and systemic arterial hypotension suggest pulmonary edema of cardiac origin. The chest roentgenogram reveals interstitial or alveolar infiltrates; arterial pO_2 and oxygen saturation are diminished.

Subacute Cyanotic Disorders

A cyanotic patient presenting with a subacute illness that has progressed over several days is likely to have pneumonia or sepsis. Fever, rales, and evidence of consolidation on chest examination further substantiate the diagnosis of pneumonia. The chest roentgenogram often reveals pulmonary infiltrates, and arterial blood gas analysis (with the patient breathing room air) shows a low pO_2. A generalized rash in conjunction with fever and cyanosis suggests the toxic shock syndrome.[10]

Chronic Cyanotic Disorders

A chronically symptomatic patient with cyanosis usually has one of several cardiopulmonary disorders. The most likely causes and their respective objective findings are as follows.

Bronchitis-Emphysema. The patient exhibits respiratory distress, wheezing, or evidence of expiratory obstruction to air flow. The chest roentgenogram reveals hyperinflated lungs, occasionally with bleb formation. The electrocardiogram may show sinus tachycardia and evidence of right ventricular hypertrophy; arterial blood gas analysis demonstrates a low oxygen saturation, with or without carbon dioxide retention.

Pulmonary Interstitial Fibrosis. Respiratory distress, diffuse rales, and restricted chest wall movement are evident on physical examination. There are also bilateral interstitial infiltrates accompanied by low arterial pO_2 and oxygen saturation.

Pulmonary Arteriovenous Fistulae. Patients with pulmonary arteriovenous fistulae generally have a systolic murmur on physical examination; diastolic or continuous murmurs are unusual. The chest roentgenogram may show single or multiple lung masses. Peripheral telangiectases (especially on the mucous membranes) are found in patients with associated hereditary hemorrhagic telangiectasia.

Congenital Heart Disease. A cyanotic patient with some respiratory distress, an abnormal chest wall configuration (left chest more prominent than the right), and cardiac murmurs and thrills should be considered to have congenital heart disease until proven otherwise. The chest roentgenogram generally shows cardiomegaly (although occasionally the heart size can be surprisingly normal), an abnormal cardiac silhouette, or abnormal pulmonary blood flow patterns; the electrocardiogram is usually abnormal, often with evidence of right ventricular hypertrophy.[11, 12] Arterial blood gas analysis reveals decreases in pO_2 and oxygen saturation. A child with cyanotic congenital heart disease who is old enough to walk most likely has tetralogy of Fallot.

ASSESSMENT

Diagnostic Approach

In all patients with cyanosis a careful physical examination, a chest roentgenogram, an electrocardiogram, a serum hemoglobin determination, and arterial blood gas analysis for pO_2 and oxygen saturation should be performed. In patients with arterial or venous occlusive diseases (including Raynaud's disease) in whom the diagnosis can be made on the basis of history and physical examination, only the blood gas analysis is not clearly beneficial for evaluation. The algorithm summarizes the diagnostic approach to a patient with generalized cyanosis.

Therapeutic Approach

Acrocyanosis is a benign condition requiring no treatment other than reassurance.

Methemoglobinemia can be congenital or drug-induced. The drugs most commonly implicated are nitrites, sulfonamides, and aniline derivatives. Drug-induced methemoglobinemia can be rapidly reversed by discontinuation of the drug. Oral methylene blue, 100 to 300 mg daily, restores the oxygen-carrying capacity in all forms of methemoglobinemia, whereas ascorbic acid, 100 to 500 mg daily, is effective only in congenital methemoglobinemia.[4] Sulfhemoglobinemia can be due to nitrite-forming bacteria or to drug ingestion. Despite discontinuation of the offending drug (the same compounds are most frequently implicated), reversal of the problem typically takes months, because sulfhemoglobin is irreversibly bound, and methylene blue is ineffective in speeding up the restoration of the oxygen-carrying capacity.[4]

When acute upper airway obstruction is due to ingested food, a cricothyroidotomy is the treatment of choice. When upper airway obstruction is due to acute epiglottitis or tumor, tracheostomy may be necessary to assure adequate ventilation.

Heparin or streptokinase therapy is indicated for the treatment of acute pulmonary embolism. Oxygen administration and respiratory support are generally necessary if cyanosis is due to pulmonary embolism.

Sepsis and pneumonia resulting in cyanosis require oxygen administration, ventilatory support, and administration of the appropriate antibiotics.

A pneumothorax sizable enough to produce cyanosis requires a thoracotomy tube, oxygen administration, and respiratory support.

The treatment of pulmonary edema depends on its etiology.[13] Cardiac pulmonary edema is generally characterized by an elevated pulmonary capillary wedge pressue (measured via Swan-Ganz catheterization) and responds to diuretic drugs and afterload reduction. Noncardiac pulmonary edema is often due to altered alveolar capillary integrity; the pulmonary capillary wedge pressure is normal. Ventilatory support in these patients is most important, whereas diuretic drugs and afterload reduction may be harmful because they decrease the cardiac output.

Bronchitis and emphysema are treated with ventilatory support, bronchodilator drugs, and control of any superimposed infection. Corticosteroid hormones may be indicated in selected patients with reactive airway disease.

Surgery may be indicated for pulmonary arteriovenous fistulae; however, multiple fistulae or fistulae with extensive pulmonary involvement may not be resectable.

Guidelines for the treatment of cyanotic congen-

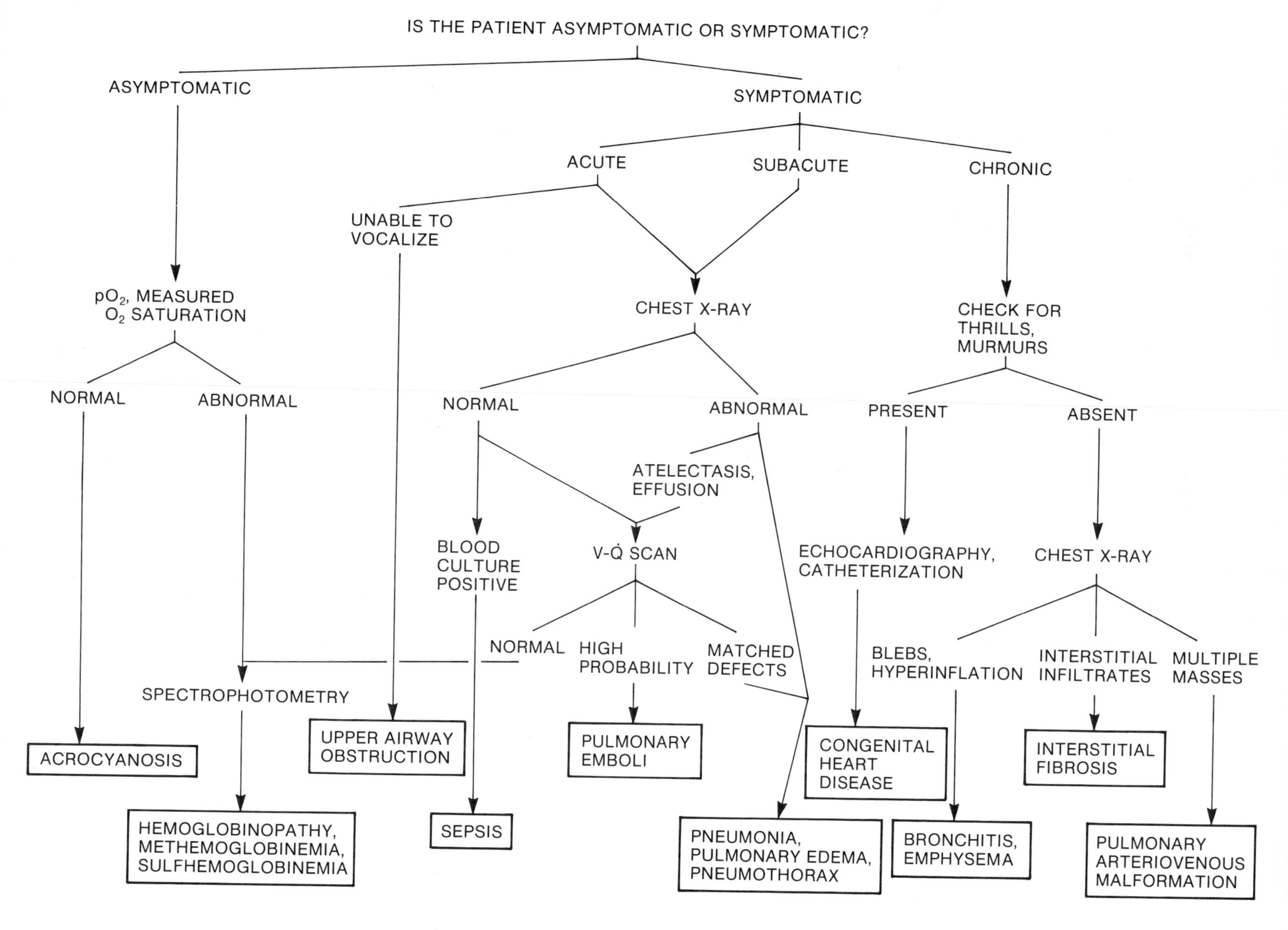
DIAGNOSTIC ASSESSMENT OF GENERALIZED CYANOSIS
IS THE PATIENT ASYMPTOMATIC OR SYMPTOMATIC?
ASYMPTOMATIC
SYMPTOMATIC
ACUTE
SUBACUTE
CHRONIC
UNABLE TO VOCALIZE
pO_2, MEASURED O_2 SATURATION
CHEST X-RAY
CHECK FOR THRILLS, MURMURS
NORMAL
ABNORMAL
NORMAL
ABNORMAL
PRESENT
ABSENT
ATELECTASIS, EFFUSION
BLOOD CULTURE POSITIVE
V-Q̇ SCAN
ECHOCARDIOGRAPHY, CATHETERIZATION
CHEST X-RAY
NORMAL
HIGH PROBABILITY
MATCHED DEFECTS
BLEBS, HYPERINFLATION
INTERSTITIAL INFILTRATES
MULTIPLE MASSES
SPECTROPHOTOMETRY
ACROCYANOSIS
UPPER AIRWAY OBSTRUCTION
PULMONARY EMBOLI
CONGENITAL HEART DISEASE
INTERSTITIAL FIBROSIS
HEMOGLOBINOPATHY, METHEMOGLOBINEMIA, SULFHEMOGLOBINEMIA
SEPSIS
PNEUMONIA, PULMONARY EDEMA, PNEUMOTHORAX
BRONCHITIS, EMPHYSEMA
PULMONARY ARTERIOVENOUS MALFORMATION

ital heart disease include establishment of the correct diagnosis, control of any superimposed pulmonary infection, protection against infective endocarditis, and management of the polycythemia. Adolescent males at puberty are at greatest hazard from polycythemia; a hematocrit in excess of 70 per cent is generally poorly tolerated, and erythropheresis may be needed to reduce symptoms and thromboembolic risk. Thrombosis, migraine headaches, gout, and hypertension are also potential problems.[14]

REFERENCES

1. Lundsgaard C, Van Slyke DD. Cyanosis. Medicine 1923;2:1–76.
2. Braunwald E. Cyanosis, hypoxia, and polycythemia. In: Isselbacher KS, Adams RD, Braunwald E, Petersdorf RG, Wilson J, eds. Harrison's textbook of medicine, 9th ed. New York: McGraw-Hill, 1980:166–8.
3. DeSenac JB. Traité de la structure du coeur, de son action, et de ses maladies. Paris, 1794:II:404.
4. Finch CA. Methemoglobinemia and sulfhemoglobinemia. N. Engl J Med 1948;239:470–7.
5. Barrett HR, Holland JG, Josenhans WT. When does central cyanosis become detectable? Clin Invest Med 1982;5:39–43.
6. Ten Brink WA, Wiezer JH, Luijpen AF, Van Heijist AN, Pikaan SA, Selderrijk R. Nitrite poisoning caused by food contaminated with cooling fluid. J Toxicol Clin Toxicol 1982;19:139–47.
7. Bower PJ, Peterson JN. Methemoglobinemia after sodium nitroprusside therapy. N Eng J Med 1975;293:865.
8. Francis PB. Cyanosis. In: Walker HK, Hall WD, Hurst JW, eds. Clinical methods, 2nd ed. Boston: Butterworths, 1980:733–6.
9. Silverman ME, Hurst JW. Inspection of the patient. In: Hurst JW, ed. The heart, arteries, and veins, 5th ed. New York: McGraw-Hill, 1982:165–82.
10. Chesney PJ, Crass BA, Prlyak MB, et al. Toxic shock syndrome: management and long-term sequelae. Ann Intern Med 1982;96:847–51.
11. Perloff JK. Congenital heart disease. In: Wyngaarden JB, Smith LH, eds. Cecil's textbook of medicine, 16th ed. Philadelphia: WB Saunders, 1982:168–89.
12. Kelly MJ, Jaffe CD, Shown SM, Kleinman CS. A radiographic and echocardiographic approach to cyanotic congenital heart disease. Radiol Clin North Am 1980;18:411–40.
13. Schlant RC, Sonnenblick EH. Pathophysiology of heart failure. In: Hurst JW, ed. The heart, arteries, and veins, 5th ed. New York: McGraw-Hill, 1982:382–407.
14. Plauth WH, Nugent EW, Schlant RC, Edwards JE, Williams WH, Kirklin JH. Congenital heart disease. In: Hurst JW, ed. The heart, arteries, and veins, 5th ed. New York: McGraw-Hill, 1982:643–853.

DELIRIUM

RICHARD A. DEVAUL □ ROBERT W. GUYNN

□ SYNONYMS: Acute organic brain syndrome, acute cerebral insufficiency, febrile delirium, acute confusional state, acute organic psychosis, toxic confusional state, toxic delirious reaction, reversible dementia, metabolic encephalopathy, toxic encephalopathy.[1,2]

BACKGROUND

Definition

Lipowski[3] has defined delirium as a transient mental disorder reflecting acute brain failure due to widespread derangement of cerebral metabolism. This definition was advanced following a demonstration by Engel and Romano[4] that delirium is a manifestation of cerebral metabolic insufficiency. As such, it is a nonspecific syndrome indicating a threshold phenomenon of physiologic impairment of the brain similar to the medical syndromes of cardiac, renal, and hepatic insufficiency.

Historical Considerations

In his discussion of the etymology of the word delirium, Lipowski[5] notes references to its use as long ago as the time of Hippocrates. The term probably was introduced into the medical literature by Celsus in the first century A. D. It is derived from the Latin word *delirare,* which means literally "to go out of the furrow." Since its introduction, however, delirium has been synonymous with derangement, craziness, or insanity. It also has been used to describe a transient mental syndrome accompanying medical illness, particularly febrile episodes. Delirium has been called acute organic brain syndrome in the psychiatric literature and diffuse or toxic encephalopathy in the neurologic literature, and it has been considered synonymous with delirium tremens or febrile delirium in the general medical literature.

Engel and Romano[4] comment on the curious fact that although physicians are strongly biased toward the organic origin of mental disorders, they have little interest in delirium, which is the one mental disorder known to be caused by derangement of cerebral metabolism. These incongruities in usage, physician attitudes and behaviors, and association with psychiatry as opposed to the rest of medicine have perpetuated the general medical neglect of this important syndrome.

Clinical Description

Delirium may be induced experimentally by a wide variety of drugs such as alcohol, barbiturates, and anesthetics, as well as by hypoxia, sleep deprivation, and withdrawal from chemical addiction.[1, 3, 5, 6, 7] Additionally, delirium commonly is a complication of medical disorders such as renal failure, hepatic failure, hyperthyroidism, and hyperglycemia and of postsurgical recovery.[7, 8] However, the underlying pathophysiologic processes have yet to be defined. The brain is composed of neuronal tissue that is very sensitive to changes in its physiologic environment. Blood glucose levels, blood perfusion, pH balance, and metabolic by-products such as ammonia all may dramatically affect the metabolic activity of the brain.

Clinically, the syndrome of delirium always involves the following impairments of global cognitive function:

1. *An inability to perceive and process new information from the environment.* This impairment is commonly manifested as disorientation to time and place, deficiencies in short-term memory and recall, tendency to misidentify new surroundings or people as familiar ones (familiarization), and tendency for disjointed, muddled, or illogical thinking. The patient often will appear "confused," an adjective frequently found in nurses' notes that should signal the possibility of delirium as the diagnosis.

2. *Disorders of attention.* The patient exhibits varying levels of awareness ranging from hyperarousal to stupor. The ability to focus, shift, or sustain attention is impaired. The patient may be easily distracted, may be unable to react to changes in questioning, or may simply "phase" in and out of a coherent state.

3. *Disturbances of sleep.* A disturbance of normal sleep pattern always is present. Interrupted or fragmented sleep, insomnia, and stupor all may be characteristic. Insomnia, the most frequently cited disturbance, may be described by the recovered patient as a dream-like state. Conversely, the hypoaroused patient may be stuporous, appearing to sleep a great deal of the time. Nurses' notes documenting changes in the sleep pattern may offer another valuable clue to the early diagnosis of delirium. Return to the normal sleep pattern frequently heralds recovery.

Delirium is characterized by an acute onset, in contrast to functional psychoses, which invariably are preceded by a period of weeks to months of increasingly bizarre behavior. Also typical of delirium are fluctuations between cognitive impairment and lucidity. Initially this condition is reversible, but if it is not identified and the underlying cause corrected, delirium may progress to permanent brain damage or death. It may last a few hours to many months, depending upon the etiology. Secondary symptoms may be psychotic. Delusions and hallucinations are common, placing the delirious patient at risk of a misdiagnosis of functional psychosis and subsequent inappropriate treatment.

Subtypes

Lipowski[5] suggests that there are two clinical variants of the delirium syndrome, the hypoactive and the hyperactive (Steinhart[6] uses hypoaroused and hyperaroused). A patient may conform to either subtype throughout the syndrome's clinical course or may shift from hypoactive to hyperactive or vice versa. Hypoactivity, owing to the passivity induced by a semistuporous state, runs a great risk of going unnoticed. Only when the condition progresses to stupor or shifts to the hyperactive state is the patient likely to be identified as having a problem. A hyperactive patient generally comes to the attention of the health care team as a "management problem." Agitation, uncooperativeness, and lability of mood are characteristic of the hyperactive state. The patient is more likely to suffer from hallucinations and delusions, therefore risking being labeled as a psychiatric patient. Once this appellation has been attached, an alarming phenomenon occurs in most medical treatment units: Because the nursing staff no longer feels capable of dealing with the patient, the physician is compelled to act, usually by administering an antipsychotic or sedative as symptomatic treatment. Such treatment usually worsens the condition and distracts attention from the underlying cause.

Case Reports. The following case illustrates the hypoactive subtype:

Mrs. Y, a 62-year-old white mother of three, was admitted to a university hospital medical service for evaluation of chest pain of acute onset. Initial medical evaluation revealed bronchitis (probably of viral origin), a mild urinary tract infection, slight obesity, and adult-onset diabetes under reasonable control. On the fifth hospital day the patient became increasingly lethargic and disinterested in food. The attending physician requested psychiatric consultation for Mrs. Y's apparent depression. A review of her chart revealed additional data, notably borderline liver function readings and nurses' notes indicating an increasing number of hours of sleep and one episode of confusion. When the psychiatric examiner introduced himself to Mrs. Y and inquired whether she had ever seen him before, she responded that she thought he was a family friend. The patient was disoriented as to time and place, had fluctuating attention, and exhibited nondirectional thinking. Further medical evaluation, including liver function tests, revealed acute liver failure.

In many respects this is a typical case of hypoactive or stuporous delirium. The patient was not perceived as a "management problem" until she failed to improve, at which time consultation was sought for what was thought to be a severe depression. Also notable was the response to the consultation by the attending physician, who believed strongly that the patient could not have a medical problem. It was only after insistence by the psychiatric consultant that the patient be further medically evaluated that liver failure was diagnosed.

Illustrative of the hyperactive subtype is the following case:

Mr. N, A 67-year-old retired professional, was admitted to the surgical service of a university hospital for prostate surgery to relieve benign prostatic hypertrophy. He was in excellent health prior to surgery and the procedure went well. Mr. N's postoperative course was complicated by infection, which responded promptly to antibiotic treatment. However, he became restless and agitated and was regarded as a "nursing problem." He was discharged in the care of his daughter, who was a nurse. Amitriptyline (Elavil), 50 mg q.i.d., was prescribed, and he and his family were told that nothing more could be done. For 3 months the patient slept approximately 2 hours a night, and his waking periods were characterized by restlessness, agitation, and intermittent confusion. The patient's family physician eventually referred him to the psychiatric inpatient unit for treatment of agitated depression. Initial evaluation revealed disorientation, fluctuating alertness, and illogical associative thought. An EEG showed generalized slowing consistent with the diagnosis of delirium. A thorough medical evaluation revealed no underlying disease. Discontinuation of amitriptyline resulted in a complete return to presurgical function after 14 days.

In this case, a patient with postoperative delirium was discharged from the hospital because he was a "management problem." The clinical course of the condition paralleled the administration of amitriptyline, although delirium typically is a temporary condition that either progresses in severity or clears spontaneously. Again, a psychiatric disorder was diagnosed, even though there was documented evidence (primary symptoms and characteristic EEG) for a diagnosis of delirium.

Predisposing Factors

Certain patients are at an increased risk of developing delirium. Three predisposing factors generally agreed upon are age, history of brain damage, and addiction to alcohol or drugs.[1] Vulnerability to delirium seems to increase with advancing age, although the underlying mechanism is unknown. Because widely varying incidence rates have been reported, they can only be estimated.[1, 3, 5] For example, in a review of reported incidence rates for delirium in older patients on general medical and surgical wards, Liston[1] found a range of 14 to 30 per cent. The association of brain damage with delirium is well-documented.[1–3, 5, 6] Delirium frequently occurs with alcohol or drug addiction and with withdrawal from addiction, thereby complicating the management of a substance-dependent patient.[1–3, 5, 6] In addition to these specific predisposing factors, others have been associated with an increasing vulnerability to delirium; namely, postoperative recovery status, sensory input, sleep deprivation, psychological stress, and personality make-up.[1, 3, 5, 6, 8] For example, rigid, controlled personalities are probably less vulnerable to delirium than are normal individuals. An awareness of these associated factors also will aid in the early identification of delirium-prone patients.

HISTORY

Delirium is diagnosed by simply documenting the presence of the primary symptoms, which are memory impairment, attention disorders, and sleep pattern disturbance, either by observation or inquiry (direct or indirect questions). Orientation to time, place, and person may be quickly tested at the bedside. Disorientation to time is a more sensitive measure than disorientation to place. Many individuals normally may not be able to name the exact date, but errors of more than several days and confusion of weekdays and weekends are significant. If disoriented to place, a patient may misidentify the surroundings as being familiar. For example, the patient may state that he or she is on the front porch at home and that members of the health care team are relatives or friends. This tendency of delirious patients to make an alien and incomprehensible environment seem familiar is called *familiarization.* Disorientation to person does not occur in acute delirium if one means disorientation to self; the delirious person may, however, not recognize others in his environment. A test of short-term recall involves asking the patient to recall three unrelated words or concepts, such as *red, flag,* and *1944,* after a lapse of 2 or 3 minutes.

It is important to test cognitive functions in addition to simple memory because the delirious patient often is inconsistent in the degree of deficits of several cognitive functions. The patient may well do very poorly on one intellectual function task yet perform normally on others. Therefore, the finding of a reasonably normal response to one task does not prove the absence of delirium. Several tasks must be given. A normal person of average intelligence and education should be able to abstract a proverb never heard before, do simple arithmetic tasks without paper and pencil, subtract serial sevens from 100 or serial threes from 20, and repeat five to seven random digits given at 1-second intervals (or repeat three to five digits in reverse order). Ironically, the nondelirious depressed patient may claim to have a poor memory or that he or she "can't think." On specific testing with appropriate gentle encouragement, however, the depressed patient should be able to accomplish satisfactorily the tasks of memory and cognition, although perhaps at a speed slower than normal.

Often a patient exhibits wandering and nondirectional thinking, making it difficult to obtain a coherent history. Medical students and house officers have been known to spend hours with a mildly delirious patient, obtaining disjointed histories of dubious validity without ever questioning the patient's mental state. The patient often is noted to drift in and out of wakefulness or to attend to some inquiries but not to others. The fluctuating level of awareness and distractibility frequently are labeled "confusion" in nurses' notes.

The delirious patient may show mood and affective disturbances, especially lability. The patient may laugh and cry in rapid succession or may be alternatingly angry and friendly. If one mood persists, it tends to be depression. Depression may well be the most common reason for psychiatric referral of a patient not suspected to have an organic delirium. The two case examples already given illustrate this point. Often, in such cases time is lost that should be used to correct or treat the organic deficit. It is too easy to explain depression in a hospitalized medical patient and therefore to ignore it or even consider it normal. Emotional blunting or torpor, also seen in the delirious state, may be mistaken for depression, again resulting in failure to recognize the real problem. The patient may manifest intense anxiety and agitation. Once frightened, he or she may flee or become combative, and acute disorientation or paranoid ideation may erupt.

Typically, delirium shows diurnal variation, being worse at night. The changes may occasionally be extreme, the patient being psychotic at night and showing few or no cognitive deficits during the day. In addition, an obvious change in the patient's sleep pattern usually is evident. It is important to remember that regardless of uncooperativeness or evidence of psychotic symptoms, the presence of the primary symptoms indicates that the patient is suffering from delirium. Too often, a patient who begins to hallucinate or who develops delusions is assumed automatically to be schizophrenic.

Several researchers have experimented with long and complicated mental status evaluations and physical examinations in diagnosis of organic brain syndromes.[9–11] Most, however, have tailored the list of questions and tests to several reliable items for ascertaining cognitive function. The "mini mental state" examination is a good example of a simple bedside screening tool.[11] It employs simple questions to determine orientation and recent memory function.

Once delirium is diagnosed, a concerted effort to identify the underlying cause or causes should be undertaken. The nonspecific nature and the seriousness of the condition of delirium (which should be considered a medical emergency) require a thorough assessment of the patient's medical status. Often a single cause cannot be identified, but the patient's deterioration can be explained by multiple factors, such as overmedication, marginal pulmonary function, and an electrolyte imbalance. In determining the reason for delirium, it is helpful to approach the problem from the perspective of the following three broad categories of probable causes: acute drug intoxication, withdrawal syndromes, and central nervous system (CNS) disease or systemic illness (Table 1).

Acute Drug Intoxication. This is a major cause of delirium. Drugs that affect the CNS, such as alcohol, anticholinergics, barbiturates, minor tranquilizers, sedatives, and steroids, have the greatest potential for causing delirium.[1, 6, 7, 12, 13] Hospitalized patients particularly are prone to drug-induced delirium because of the number of medications administered to them. When drug-induced delirium is suspected, all nonessential medications should be stopped in a diagnostic as well as therapeutic maneuver. It is important to note that following discontinuation of the offending medication, the patient may not recover for 10 days to 3 weeks.[2]

Withdrawal Syndromes. If the onset of delirium occurs 48 to 72 hours after hospital admission, withdrawal from drug dependency or addiction should be a prime consideration. The substances most commonly associated with withdrawal delirium are alcohol, narcotics, and barbiturates as well as sedatives and minor tranquilizers taken in large doses. A test for withdrawal delirium consists of administering a maintenance dose level (average daily dose) of the same drug, or one of the same family, with subsequent improvement of the patient's condition.

Table 1. COMMON CAUSES OF DELIRIUM

Drugs	
Acute intoxication	Most commonly, those with direct effects on brain metabolism and function: Alcohol Minor tranquilizers Psychedelics Barbiturates Sedatives L-Dopa Anticholinergics (particularly implicated)
Withdrawal	Alcohol Barbiturates Narcotics Minor tranquilizers and sedatives in large doses
Systemic disorders	
Endocrine	Hypothyroidism Hypoglycemia Parathyroidism Adrenal dysfunction Hyperthyroidism Hyperglycemia
Nutritional	Vitamin deficiencies Alcoholism
Neoplastic	(Secondary effects of carcinoma)
Metabolic	Uremia Hepatic failure Pulmonary insufficiency Cardiac failure Electrolyte imbalance Anemia Porphyria
Vascular	Hypertension Collagen vascular disease
Infection	(Secondary to systemic infection)
Drug- or chemical-induced	Bromides Carbon monoxide Steroids
Diffuse CNS disorders	
Inflammatory	Meningitis Encephalitis Syphilis Collagen vascular disease
Tumor	Brain abscess Subdural hematoma Primary carcinoma Metastatic carcinoma
Trauma	Concussion Post-traumatic hemorrhage
Vascular	Hemorrhage Embolism
Other	Ischemia Hydrocephalus Seizures

CNS Disease or Systemic Illness. Any systemic or diffuse CNS disease can cause delirium. Systemic disorders precipitating delirium may be of an endocrine, nutritional, metabolic, or vascular nature. Secondary infections and neoplasms also may be causes. Inflammatory or traumatic CNS disorders may underlie delirium. Tumors or diffuse cerebral disorders of a vascular nature also should be considered. It is important to note that the development of delirium may be a signal that a recognized disorder is not responding to treatment or that secondary complications have arisen. Often, delirium is the result of a combination of physiologic problems instead of a single identifiable illness. An example of this situation would be delirium in an older patient caused by marginal pulmonary function together with excessive medication.

PHYSICAL EXAMINATION

A thorough physical examination of a delirious patient is imperative. It may be difficult to conduct a physical examination in a hyperactive patient who is uncooperative and paranoid. With such a patient, it is crucial to resist the temptation to medicate, because medication frequently aggravates the delirious state and ultimately interferes with the diagnostic process. The fluctuating nature of delirium usually provides lucid intervals that prove favorable for orienting the patient and proceeding with the examination. Occasionally, psychiatric consultation and, rarely, physical restraints may be required.

Physical findings vary with the underlying causes and should be compared with those of the initial physical examination, if available. One study on delirium in children found that the symptoms and course of delirium were virtually the same as in adults.[10] A notable difference was that delirium in children may be followed for days to months by evidence of minor learning disabilities. The same researchers discovered a number of "soft" neurologic signs in children, elicited by the face-hand stimulation test and the subtraction of serial sevens test. Hysterical conversion symptoms of various types also may occur during the course of delirium.[14]

DIAGNOSTIC STUDIES

The diagnosis of delirium can be confirmed by the use of an electroencephalograph (EEG). Engel and Romano[4] have documented that bilateral diffuse abnormality of EEG background activity is an almost invariable feature of delirium. The abnormality typically consists of a relative slowing with or without superimposed fast activity. In their review of the use of the electroencephalograph in the diagnosis of delirium, Pro and Wells[13] confirmed these findings and also found that the superimposed fast activity usually is associated with the hyperactive subtype and may be seen in cases of delirium induced by acute intoxications and drug withdrawal.[13] Owing to the fluctuating nature of delirium, a single EEG may not suffice for a diagnosis. A normal EEG may be recorded during a lucid interval; therefore, serial EEGs usually are required.

The diagnostic use of the amobarbital sodium interview also has been documented.[3, 5, 15] If a patient truly is suffering from delirium, cognitive impairment is likely to be accentuated while he or she is under sedation. A psychotic patient is less inhibited and exhibits improved cognitive function during the interview. In addition, a patient suffering from a disorder of organic etiology has a lower tolerance for the drug.

ASSESSMENT

A simple algorithm for assessment emphasizes the importance of one's awareness of delirium, particularly in certain patients and settings. Generally, the diagnosis of delirium is obvious and is easily verified by serial EEGs. However, it may be useful to consider the differential diagnosis of dementia and functional psychoses in detail. The importance of differentiating delirium from dementia and the functional psychoses is stressed here in light of a recent study by Rabins and Folstein,[16] who found that delirious patients had a higher mortality rate than demented, cognitively impaired, and depressed patients. This finding held true after a 1-year period in the study subjects.

Once evidence of global cognitive impairment has been established, the primary diagnostic concern is the differential diagnosis between delirium and dementia (see also the chapter on dementia). Dementia also produces signs of global cognitive impairment but is caused by permanent brain damage.

Although there is a diminution in intellectual function, often with evidence of memory defect and other cognitive dysfunction, dementia differs from delirium in that it is a stable, nonfluctuating condition to which the patient has made adjustments over time. In dementia, sleep pattern disturbance is uncommon and the patient is usually elderly. By the time dementia is clinically apparent, a careful history reveals long-standing and progressive social impairment. At times, delirium may be superimposed on dementia; the EEG is helpful for such a determination. The EEG shows characteristic changes in delirium but is normal in dementia.

Dramatic secondary psychotic symptoms and irrational paranoid behavior put delirious patients at risk for a diagnosis of functional psychosis. Misdiagnosis can be avoided through careful consideration of the onset, symptoms, and course of the condition. Delirium has an acute onset, but functional psychosis is characterized by history of increasingly bizarre behavior. Onset of a functional psychiatric illness generally occurs at a fairly early age; it would be unusual for a patient with such an illness not to have a psychiatric history prior to most medical hospitalizations. The symptoms of a functional psychosis, such as schizophrenia or manic-depressive psychosis, occur with a clear sensorium. The patient is oriented, memory is intact, and there is a perception of reality simultaneous with the psychotic symptoms. The patient with a functional psychosis may exhibit sleep pattern disturbance and agitation, but symptoms do not follow the fluctuating course characteristic of delirium. Rarely, a patient with a functional psychosis may become delirious. The presence of the primary symptoms of delirium requires management of the medical problem before the secondary diagnosis of functional psychosis can be determined. The EEG is a reliable laboratory aid in this situation.

The kinds of hallucinations and delusions a patient experiences are usually different in delirium and functional psychosis.[17] Visual and mixed hallucinations are generally organic in origin. Auditory hallucinations are generally seen in functional psychosis. Hallucinations of the delirious patient often are emotionally neutral or even positive experiences ("A train went through my window." "What are the children doing on the curtains?" "I had a nice visit with my grandmother"). The acutely schizophrenic individual usually reports frightening or unpleasant hallucinations. Hallucinations secondary to delirium are reported as part of the actual environment ("I see bugs on the wall." "There are little men under my bed"). The schizophrenic reports hallucinations while retaining the ability to report reality accurately ("I noticed when my grandfather clock struck one that God spoke to me"). Finally, the hallucinations of delirium show diurnal variations, being worse at night and often remembered as "vivid dreams." Schizophrenia is far less susceptible to diurnal changes.

The delusions of the delirious patient usually are paranoid and generally relate to his or her immediate situation. They are "understandable" given the patient's disorientation. For example, such a patient may believe that the nurses are trying to hurt him or her. It is rare for delirious

DIAGNOSTIC ASSESSMENT OF DELIRIUM

AWARENESS OF DELIRIUM

↓

HIGH-RISK FACTORS:
- Uncooperative, belligerent patient
- Observation that patient is confused
- Signs of decreased awareness
- History of alcohol or drug abuse
- History of CNS trauma or disease
- Changes in sleep pattern
- Diffuse or rambling speech
- Presence of hallucinations or delusions

↓

ASSESSMENT OF ORIENTATION, AWARENESS, AND SLEEP PATTERN

↓

EEG

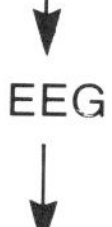

CLINICAL ASSESSMENT OF UNDERLYING CAUSES

patients to be concerned about worldwide plots, the FBI, or Martians. The paranoid schizophrenic, on the other hand, is more likely to worry about such expansive, global ideas.

In summary, delirium can be distinguished from functional psychosis by inquiry and documentation of the primary symptoms of global cognitive impairment (disorientation, memory loss, variation in levels of awareness) and is confirmed by EEG.

REFERENCES

1. Liston EH. Delirium in the aged. Psychiatr Clin North Am 1982;5:49–66.
2. DeVaul RA, Jervey FL. Delirium: a neglected medical emergency. Am Fam Physician 1981;24:152–7.
3. Lipowski ZJ. Delirium updated. Compr Psychiatry 1980;21:190–6.
4. Engel GL, Romano J. Delirium, a syndrome of cerebral insufficiency. J Chron Dis 1959;9:260–77.
5. Lipowski ZJ. Delirium: acute brain failure in man. Springfield, Ill: Charles C Thomas, 1980.
6. Steinhart MJ. Treatment of delirium—a reappraisal. Int J Psychiatry Med 1978–79;9:191–7.
7. Summers WK. A clinical method of estimating risk of drug induced delirium. Life Sci 1978;22:1511–6.
8. Dubin WR, Field HL, Gastfriend DR. Post cardiotomy delirium; a critical review. J Thorac Cardiovasc Surg 1979;77:586–94.
9. Jenkyn LR, Walsh DB, Culver CM, Reeves AG. Clinical signs in diffuse cerebral dysfunction. J Neurol Neurosurg Psychiatry 1977;40:956–66.
10. Prugh DG, Wagonfeld S, Metcalf D, Jordan K. A clinical study of delirium in children and adolescents. Psychosom Med Suppl 1980;42:177–95.
11. Anthony JC, LeResche L, Niaz V, Van Korff MR, Folstein MF. Limits of the "mini-mental state" as a screening test for dementia and delirium among hospital patients. Psychol Med 1982;12:397–408.
12. Tune LE, Holland A, Folstein MF, Damlouji NF, Gardner TJ, Coyle JT. Association of postoperative delirium with raised serum levels of anticholinergic drugs. Lancet 1981;2:651–3.
13. Pro JD, Wells CE. The use of the electroencephalogram in the diagnosis of delirium. Dis Nerv System 1977;38:804–8.
14. DeVaul RA. Hysterical symptoms. In: Hall RCW, ed. Psychiatric presentations of medical illness—somatopsychic disorders. New York: SP Medical & Scientific Books, 1980;105–16.
15. Santos AB, Manning DE, Waldrop WM. Delirium or psychosis? Diagnostic use of the sodium amobarbital interview. Psychosomatics 1980;21:863–4.
16. Rabins VP, Folstein MF. Delirium and dementia: diagnostic criteria and fatality rates. Br J Psychiatry 1982;140:149–53.
17. DeVaul RA, Hall RCW. Hallucinations. In: Hall RCW, ed. Psychiatric presentations of medical illness—somatopsychic disorders. New York: SP Medical & Scientific Books, 1980;91–103.

DEMENTIA

STEVEN B. LIPPMANN

□ SYNONYMS: dementing illness, organic brain syndrome (OBS), chronic organic brain syndrome, degenerative brain disease (related term), senility (improper usage)

Definition

Dementia is an acquired condition of diminished mental capacity. Declining intellectual performance produces a clinical syndrome resulting from diffuse or disseminated cerebral dysfunction.[1, 2] The word dementia is derived from the Latin roots: *de* ("from" or "out of"), *ment* ("mind"), and *ia* ("pathologic condition").[3] It implies disease that adversely affects brain neuronal function. Short-term memory impairment and disorientation are the main clinical features.

Numerous different and distinctive disorders have been established as causes for dementing illnesses.[1–7] Despite varied causation, the clinical presentations have similarities. Dementia is *not* a diagnosis; it designates a syndrome of mental deterioration that requires identification of the specific cause and design of an individualized treatment plan.[1–10] Contrary to popular belief, some dementing disorders are treatable.[1–7] Other processes are subject to suppression of disease, and therapies are available for symptom palliation.[10]

BACKGROUND

A search for curable and arrestable causes of dementias is foremost in the approach to patients with diminished mental capacity.[1–7] Early diagnosis dramatically improves prognosis in selected cases.[11] Despite the many chronic, progressive, and incurable dementias, a favorable prognosis in dementia can also be observed. Frequently, older demented patients are not given adequate work-up or medical attention. Classified as "incurable" or "senile, with hardening of the arteries," they are dismissed as individuals who cannot be helped and are sent to nursing homes where they receive still less medical care. Without access to the health services available to others, these patients have increased morbidity and mortality rates. Such a situation could lead to a lifetime of sedation to calm behavioral signs of an undetected but diagnosable and treatable dementing ailment.

Dementia, though not an inevitable consequence of aging, is more common in geriatric populations, approximately 15 per cent of which is affected.[4, 12] The shift in population demographics to an older society increases physician exposure to the problems of cognitive dysfunction.[13] Approximately 12 per cent of our population is 65 years of age or over. In the first three-quarters of this century, the relative number of persons beyond the age of 65 has tripled and the absolute number has increased seven- to eight-fold.[13] A similar trend is projected for the future.

Dementia, the major psychiatric disorder of old age, is not a normal state of mind.[1, 2] Healthy older people usually do not exhibit significantly diminished mental capacity. *Benign senescent forgetfulness* refers to the mild memory impairments found in many aged people.[14] In dementia, the degree of cognitive dysfunction is abnormal.[8] Functional ability is preserved in senescent forgetfulness but is lost in dementias.[4]

The use of *senility* in referring to dementia in the elderly is to be avoided, because it *erroneously* implies age-conferred normality to a disease state. It also falsely implies irreversibility of a condition sometimes caused by treatable illnesses. Dementia does not include mental retardation, because it assumes normal development prior to the loss of function. The term organic brain syndrome is also not used here because it lacks specificity. Dividing patients into "pre-senile" and "senile" dementia categories, which simply delineates the age of symptom onset as before and after 65 years, is arbitrary and without clinical value.[2]

The enlarging proportion of our population that is aged fosters interest in geriatrics and intellectual dysfunction. There are at least 50 established medical, neurologic, and psychiatric causes for dementing illnesses (Table 1).[1–7, 14] Alzheimer's disease and conditions that can simulate it clinically (e.g., depression, residual effects of chronic alcoholism, Pick's disease) are the most common causes; they account for well over 60 per cent of cases.[1–4, 8, 12] The other causes are a host of diverse disorders, including metabolic, traumatic, neoplastic, and infectious processes.

Table 1. CAUSES OF DEMENTIA CLASSIFIED BY TREATABILITY AND TYPE*

	Causes Potentially Treatable by Specific Therapy	Less Treatable Causes†
Metabolic	Hypothyroidism and other endocrinopathies Wilson's disease	Hypoglycemia and/or anoxia
Traumatic	Subdural hematoma Normal-pressure hydrocephalus	Cerebral damage
Neoplastic	Intracranial tumor (primary or metastatic)	Remote effect of systemic malignancy
Deficiency	Pernicious anemia Folate deficiency Pellagra	Wernicke-Korsakoff's syndrome sequelae‡
Infective	Cerebral abscess Tertiary CNS lues Normal-pressure hydrocephalus Meningitides and encephalitides Subacute bacterial endocarditis	Jakob-Creutzfeldt disease Meningitides and encephalitides sequelae (e.g., herpes simplex encephalitis)
Vascular	Poly-infarct dementia (multiple CVA, e.g., frequent emboli)	
Toxic	Chronic alcohol abuse Heavy metal poisoning	
Degenerative		Alzheimer's disease Pick's disease
Hereditary		Huntington's disease

*Only a *partial* listing with somewhat arbitrary classification; some conditions may fit both categories.
†Symptomatic therapies are applied in many cases.
‡An example of a *treatable* and preventable delirium when acute, but potentially a chronic, less treatable dementia later. Therapy and prevention of Wernicke-Korsakoff's syndrome are a medical emergency in both alcoholic and other malnourished patients, who should be given all the B complex vitamins, particularly vitamin B_1 (thiamine).

Approximately 15 per cent of patients receiving a diagnostic work-up for dementia have an illness that is *potentially* correctable by a specific intervention.[1–7] The range of disorders is wide; hypothyroidism, pernicious anemia, folate deficiency, emotional depression, toxicities, normal-pressure hydrocephalus (NPH), subdural hematoma, intracranial tumor, vascular diseases, and various organ failures (e.g., heart, lung, kidney, liver) are examples. Additionally, one-fourth of such patients have conditions for which therapeutic measures can be helpful, including syphilis, hypertension (in stroke-prone individuals), and alcoholism. Therefore, more than one-third of the patients can benefit from specific therapies, even if they are not cured.[1, 3, 5] Besides therapy for treatable and arrestable ailments, a symptomatic approach is prescribed whenever specific treatments are unavailable or ineffective. For example, symptomatic therapies may be applied to patients with a poly-infarct dementia, after control of diabetes and hypertension has been achieved. Appropriate therapy, derived from the correct diagnosis, can vastly improve the quality of life.[10]

After recognizing disordered cognition, the physician must initiate a thorough work-up to identify the exact etiology.[8] Combining a complete history and physical examination with today's technology makes discovery of the cause feasible. Treatment depends on the cause, and therapeutic plans are based on the findings of the work-up.

HISTORY

Because of recent improvements in our ability to recognize the causes of dementia and because of expansion among therapeutic options, the diagnostic work-up should receive great emphasis. One should vigorously investigate the illness to avoid having to generalize by using the term dementia. The work-up includes a careful diagnostic review of all systems, with emphasis on detection of reversible, arrestable, or contributing illness. Consider each standard differential diagnostic category: toxic, metabolic, neoplastic, infective, inflammatory, vascular, traumatic, degenerative, hereditary.[8]

A detailed history is necessary for diagnostic precision.[11] Emphasize the cardiopulmonary and neurologic systems. Define the onset and course of illness. Record every medication taken, including over-the-counter agents and illicit drugs. Obtain data on alcohol consumption.[8] Inquire about other substance abuses, depression, and metabolic disease. Ask about diet and allergies. Use the standard format for obtaining a previous medical history and review of systems. The family history can provide diagnostic clues.

A thorough clinical history may strongly implicate a diagnostic entity. Alzheimer's disease, for example, is characterized by a slow, gradual progression over many years. A poly-infarct dementia, however, is suggested by stepwise deterioration, often associated with contributing factors such as diabetes, hypertension, hyperlipidemia, heart disease, obesity, and smoking. A history of alcohol abuse may help to identify alcohol-related brain diseases. Diagnostic "tip-offs" can, for example, be found if mental deterioration followed a head injury or meningitis, heightening one's suspicion for NPH.

Evaluate both *intracranial* disease such as a mass lesion (e.g., tumor, hematoma, abscess, gumma) and *extracranial* illnesses that influence brain function, such as remote effects of malignancies and endocrinopathies. Seek information about specific neurologic symptoms, such as incontinence, seizures or asymmetries in function, and weakness. Consider common systemic ailments like uremia and more rare ones, like dialysis-induced dementia, sarcoid, and Wilson's disease. Unrelated problems might be discovered, treatment of which may improve general health. Other disorders (e.g., hip fracture) and social stressors (e.g., grief) can exacerbate the symptoms of dementia (Table 2).[4] Therapy for such contributing factors, as in correction of an anemia, can greatly diminish the dysfunction.

Social History. Evaluate personal and environmental factors, including the social or family support system. Knowledge about the patient's life circumstances is immensely beneficial in planning remediation. Medical treatments are more effectively employed when social factors are considered. Nonmedical therapies likewise are applied as needed. Inquire about the adequacy of housing, diet, and health care delivery, and review issues such as family dysfunction. Consider patient needs for help from community agencies like Meals On Wheels and the Visiting Nurses Association. Also assess the family's reaction to, knowledge of, and need for education about the patient's illness.[15]

PHYSICAL EXAMINATION

A thorough physical examination is required. Pay special attention to cardiovascular, respiratory, neck, and neurologic aspects. The examination includes routine maneuvers and the special ones for the systems of greatest emphasis (e.g., carotid artery auscultation). Visual and auditory screening is performed. Genital, pelvic, and rectal examinations are indicated and should not be "deferred." A Pap smear and stool specimen for occult blood are always obtained.

The neurologic system requires a complete evaluation.[1–4] A cursory examination, assessing only

Table 2. CONDITIONS THAT COMMONLY INCREASE CLINICAL EXPRESSION OF DEMENTIA DYSFUNCTIONS

Medications, alcohol or drug abuses, and their withdrawal states
Polypharmacy (especially drug interactions)
Dehydration, anemia, and fever
Pneumonia and other infections
Hemodynamically significant cardiac arrhythmias
Hepatic, pulmonary, renal, and cardiac failures

some cranial nerves and deep tendon reflexes, may yield normal findings. A *thorough* neurologic evaluation frequently reveals signs of diffuse brain dysfunction. For example, one might evoke a sucking, rooting, snout, grasp, palmomental, or glabellar-tap reflex. These reflexes, called "frontal release signs," are common to many abnormalities of the frontal lobes.[1, 3] Frontal release signs are an abnormal re-emergence of primitive reflexes. Their presence does not diagnose dementia, and their absence does not rule it out. In focal cerebral lesions or advanced dementias, abnormal neurologic signs may be pronounced. A sucking reflex is an exaggerated movement of the lips as they are touched anteriorly by the examiner. Elicit the rooting or snout reflex by stroking the cheek near the lips. Lip movement is pathologic. These signs are observed in frontal lobe diseases and also with bilateral corticobulbar lesions.[3] A grasp reflex is obtained by manual stroking of the patient's palm. The abnormal response is a grasping maneuver by the patient. The palmomental reflex involves observation of the ipsilateral mentalis muscle at the chin when stroking the palm with objects such as a key; small facial-muscle movements are abnormal. The glabellar-tap refers to an inability to accommodate (i.e., stop) the eye blink reflex to the examiner's repeatedly tapping the glabella. Unilateral presence of the reflexes described suggests contralateral cerebral disease.

The jaw-jerk is a related sign. Testing is done by tapping the jaw with the mouth partially opened. A hyperactive jaw-jerk confirms bilateral disease. Focal lesions can be responsible for dementias; however, most such encephalopathies evidence bilaterally diffuse involvements.

One may find other neurologic dysfunctions, such as paratonia or flexion posture.[1–4, 7, 16] Certain dementing illnesses may be expressed as more overtly abnormal signs. The myoclonus of Jakob-Creutzfeldt's disease is an example. Evaluation of station and gait helps detect strokes, posterior column diseases, and other disorders. Walking in small, measured steps is common in frontal-lobe brain diseases.[4, 14] Observe the patient for movement disturbances (e.g., rigidity or chorea), speech defects (e.g., perserveration or aphasia), and impaired sensory perception. Focus especially on cortical sensory evaluations such as graphesthesia, stereognosis, two-point discrimination, and double simultaneous stimulation.[16] These parietal lobe findings may also be accompanied by dyspraxia and right-left confusion. Further discussions of sophisticated neurologic findings are available elsewhere.[1–4]

Mental Status Examination

A spectrum of characteristic intellectual deteriorations and personality changes occur in dementias.[1–8] The mental status examination should reveal disorientation and impairment of short-term memory. Poor judgment, inability to cope with rapid changes, psychosis, and behavioral abnormalities are also common findings.

Orientation refers to the correct recognition of person, place, and time. In demented patients, disorientation varies from subtle to profound. Without specifically testing orientation, one might overlook disorientation to time. Disorientation to person is rare, but not being oriented to place is common in moderate to severe encephalopathies.

Short-term memory dysfunction is the most sensitive sign of dementia.[1] It is distinct from immediate recall and long-term memory, which are not critical in dementia assessments. *Immediate recall* refers to the patient's ability to "parrot back" newly supplied data. *Short-term memory* refers to recall of new information *after a brief interval. Long-term memory* refers to retaining older memories and involves events that occurred before the onset of illness. There are several ways to test short-term memory. One method is to ask patients to remember three unrelated words after a short interval and to ask about verifiable events that happened just previous to the examination ("Where were you seated in the waiting room?"). Frequent testing of these functions provides experience in discerning what is normal for subjects of various ages and educational backgrounds.

Personality alterations include irritability, impulsiveness, suspiciousness, mood swings, and loss of social graces as indicated by inappropriateness, impoliteness, and poor self-care. Apathy is common, with diminished interest, vigor, and motivation. Delusional ideation is often expressed, especially with paranoia or grandiosity, and other psychotic features, such as visual hallucinations, may be present. One may also observe aggressivity or combative behavior not typical of the premorbid state.

ASSESSMENT

The first step in the differential diagnosis of a demented patient is to decide whether the presentation is due to a functional or organic cause.[1, 3–8, 17, 18] Impairments of memory, attention, and concentration can be presenting symptoms in functional and organic disorders. The two types of conditions share symptoms and can coexist or mask each other. Erroneous diagnosis stems partly from the false assumption that all memory-impaired older persons are demented. Many of these patients are actually depressed, and diagnostic confusion with other psychiatric disturbances can also occur.[7] If a functional etiology is suspected, psychiatric information is elicited following standard protocol.

Pseudodementia

Functional illnesses with a clinical pattern similar to dementias are called "pseudodementias." Depression, the most common pseudodementia, often mimics and is mistaken for a dementing illness. Geriatric patients are the group most likely to be misdiagnosed. Depression may be obvious, with complaints of sadness, helplessness, suicidal ideas, insomnia, and weight loss. The diagnosis can also be more difficult to determine. The typical physiologic concomitants of depression (e.g., suppression of sleep and appetite) can be helpful to detect depression that mimics, coexists with, or masks a dementia.

The distinction between brain disease and psychiatric disturbance may be made from the history.[1–4] Record of past emotional illness is common in psuedodementia, whereas normal psychiatric histories and predisposing medical disorders typify many true dementias. In elderly people, mental dysfunction is generally assumed to be organic, without appropriate consideration first being given to functional causes. Encephalopathy can also be mistaken for depression. Differential diagnosis can be vexing when dementia and a depressive illness coexist, and such combinations are common (Table 3).

Because of the frequency with which depression simulates dementia and the times that dementias are mistaken for depression, a diagnostic aphorism has been coined: "If elderly patients complain of sadness, also consider a dementia; however, if they complain of memory dysfunction, rule out depression." The chief complaint seems to be incongruous with the diagnosis.[1, 3–8, 17, 18]

Organically impaired individuals are usually less troubled by and less aware of memory dysfunctions. Demented patients also may conceal their disability. Yet, they often are sad because they realize that their intellectual skills are deteriorating, and they may have "depression-like" complaints. Demented people, who are unaware of, minimize, or deny having intellectual problems, therefore less commonly speak about failing memory. Brain disease patients, despite significant cognitive loss, say little about it. They usually provide inadequate medical histories. In spite of their disability, organically demented patients make active efforts to answer challenges. They "try too hard" to perform tasks that previously were simple.

Table 3. DIFFERENTIAL DIAGNOSTIC TIPS—DEMENTIA OR DEPRESSION?

Organic Dementia	Depressive Pseudodementia
Cognitive deterioration precedes depression (if the latter occurs)	Depression precedes cognitive deterioration
History of a predisposing medical illness is common	History of depression is common
May complain more about sadness than poor memory	Often complains about poor memory and sadness
Poor historian	Fair historian
Often answers questions incorrectly	May avoid answering questions
Denies or conceals problems	Exaggerates problems
Less bothered by dysfunction	Appears upset by dysfunction
Patient "tries too hard" on simple tasks	Patient gives up too easily
Worse at night	Worse in the morning
Self-esteem more intact	Poor self-esteem
Appetite normal	Diminished appetite
Sleep varies from normal to restless	Early morning awakening is a common problem
DST negative (suppressed cortisol levels; a normal test)	DST often positive (cortisol not suppressed; an abnormal result)

On the other hand, depressed patients are prone to pessimism and complaints. They report poor memory and other handicaps. Because of dysphoric mood and anxiety, depressed patients fail to attend to environmental cues and genuinely, although incorrectly, report intellectual deficits. Usually such depressed, pseudodementia patients, despite vociferous memory dysfunction complaints, elaborate detailed historical data. They emphasize difficulties and appear upset. They make little effort to complete tasks or respond to questions. They answer inquiries with statements like "I don't know."

Distinguish between these two states before beginning the work-up or treatment. Depression is one of the diagnosable and treatable conditions that occur with memory dysfunctions. Even in elderly people, depression has a good prognosis.

Dexamethasone Suppression Test

The dexamethasone suppression test (DST), developed for hypothalamic–pituitary–adrenal axis evaluations, has been found to be effective in establishing an objective physiologic criterion for diagnosing depression.[19–21] It is therefore helpful in detection of possible pseudodementias, and is indicated for instances of difficult differential diagnosis. It may help to distinguish a dementia from a depression-induced pseudodementia. One should perform a DST when this differentiation is not clear. If the diagnosis is obvious, a DST is not required.

The dexamethasone suppression test involves the administration of *exogenous* glucocorticoid (dexamethasone) followed by monitoring of the *endogenous* cortisol level the next day.[19–21] Normally, administration of the exogenous hormone suppresses adrenal cortisol production via pituitary gland feedback. In major depression, however, dexamethasone usually does *not* produce the typical cortisol suppression. Many depressed subjects therefore exhibit cortisol hypersecretion, as evidenced by nonsuppressed cortisol levels.

There are several methods for the DST. A suggested protocol follows: Administer 1 mg dexamethasone orally at 11 P.M. The next day, assay serum cortisol levels at 8 A.M., 4 P. M., and 11 P.M. The first and last levels can be omitted, but their inclusion increases precision.

A normal response is for cortisol levels to be below 5 μg/100 ml. Such a *negative* result indicates that steroid production is suppressed. An abnormal response, or *positive* result, occurs when a cortisol level is greater than 5 μg/100 ml. Failure to suppress hormone output is, of course, abnormal and also consistent with Cushing's disease or syndrome, but such a diagnosis can be eliminated on the basis of clinical and other laboratory findings. Depressed patients with a positive DST result would most likely respond to antidepressant treatments. The test is valid in elderly people.[19]

False-positive results of the DST are rare.[20–21] A positive result is precise and may be a reliable diagnostic determinant of depression. False-negative results, however, occur often.[20–21] A negative DST result therefore does not rule out depression. One out of three depressed patients has a negative DST result. Suppressed cortisol levels are a negative result in endocrine disorders, but could be a false-negative result in evaluating for depression.

A false-positive DST result occurs in Cushing's disease or syndrome, malnutrition, pregnancy, hepatic enzyme induction states, uncontrolled diabetes mellitus, fever, acute substance withdrawal syndromes, major systemic illnesses, trauma, dehydration, and possibly other conditions. False-positive results can also follow drug administrations. High-dose estrogen ingestion can invalidate the test result, but oral contraceptives or estrogen replacement appears not to impair reliability. False-negative DST results occur in Addison's disease and hypopituitarism and with corticosteriod therapy. DST results might be invalidated by other endocrinopathies or spironolactone or benzodiazepine therapy.

Psychological Testing

If it is not clear whether the etiology of the dementia is functional or organic, request psychological testing for confirmation. Usually a clinical psychologist performs the evaluation. This procedure is very effective in differentiating pseudodementia from organic mental disease. It can also identify many potential functional disorders. Psychological testing can be ordered at any time, especially if the diagnosis is elusive. Repeated studies can be an objective index for following the course of illness or establishing mental competency.

Ruling Out Delirium

Once functional illness is ruled out and organic processes are being considered, one must differentiate between dementia and delirium. Often this is easy. Delirium is a clinical designation for another form of organic encephalopathy (see chapter on delirium). There are many varied causes for this type of brain dysfunction.[1–3, 11] Deliria are characterized by conspicuous changes in levels of consciousness.[1–3] Patients are often agitated and irritable, or somnolent and withdrawn, or rapidly vacillating. In dementia, the level of consciousness is stable. Delirious patients commonly have certain typical neurologic features. Autonomic nervous system signs, such as those of abnormal pupil size and heart rate, are frequently observed; also typical are movement disturbances such as tremor and asterixis.[1–3, 9] Such signs occur but are more rare in dementing processes. The chorea of Huntington's disease and the resting tremor of Parkinson's disease are more common examples of movement disturbance in demented patients.

Many, but not all, deliria are acute, and most dementias are chronic. The distinction between acute and chronic is not always reliable, e.g., a subacute delirium may mimic dementia. Impaired intellectual function occurs with each condition, alone or in combination. Consider both delirium and dementia until one is ruled out.[8]

Elderly persons are highly susceptible to delirium. The condition is frequently superimposed on another brain disorder of a functional or organic nature. Deliria commonly result from medicine use or abuse, withdrawal states (especially from alcohol), dehydration, infection, and cardiopulmonary dysfunction. Postictal states and fluid-electrolyte imbalance should be considered. New *acute* cognitive disturbance in an older person is considered a delirium until proven otherwise. When delirium is likely, the need for evaluation is urgent; the work-up focuses on intoxications, drug withdrawal, metabolic disturbance, and acute infective or deficiency states.[1–3, 11] The dementia work-up, however, attends more to anatomic, metabolic, and chronic infective states.

DIAGNOSTIC STUDIES

Initial Laboratory Evaluation

When a specific etiology for a dementing process is suspected or obvious, the laboratory evaluation should be appropriate only to that condition. Further work-up awaits negative results.

More commonly, no specific cause for the dementia is implicated. In such presentations, the initial laboratory battery for *all* patients is as listed in Table 4. These studies are performed to screen the body for abnormalities that may induce dementia. Serologic tests for syphilis—the Veneral Disease Research Laboratory (VDRL) or rapid plasma reagin (RPR) test *and* the fluorescent treponemal antibody (FTA) test—are ordered in the geriatric patient. All are done because of the frequency of a seronegative VDRL or RPR result in central nervous system (CNS) syphilis, in which the FTA result remains positive. A lumbar puncture is then indicated to obtain cerebrospinal fluid (CSF). A positive VDRL test result in CSF would establish the diagnosis of tertiary lues, an arrestable condition.

Table 4. LABORATORY WORK-UP FOR SUSPECTED DEMENTIA

Indication(s)	Procedure(s)
Performed in all patients	Urinalysis
	Biochemical survey
	VDRL or RPR *and* FTA tests
	CBC with indices and ESR measurement
	Serum B_{12} and RBC folate determinations
	Thyroid function tests (usually T_4, RT_3U, T_7; TSH as indicated)
	CAT or CT scan of the head*
	EEG
	Electrocardiogram and chest x-ray
	Pap smear and stool specimen for occult blood detection
Other studies	Lumbar puncture and CSF examination
	Psychological testing
	Dexamethasone suppression test
	Heavy metal screening
Tests performed for specific clinical suspicions†	
Normal-pressure hydrocephalus	Isotope lumbar cysternogram
	Ventricular pressure monitoring
Neoplastic disease	Sigmoidoscopy
	Barium enema study
	Skull series
	Bone scan
Toxic disease	Toxicology screening
	Plasma drug level testing
Vascular disorders	Arteriography
	Ultrasonography
Miscellaneous	Arterial blood gases
	Intravenous pyelography
	Upper GI series

*In the future, nuclear magnetic resonance (NMR) could prove superior to CT scanning for evaluation of intracranial morphology.

†These are only some examples of the other possible diagnostic investigations for the cause of dementia. They are obtained only for specific indications and are individualized in each case.

The biochemical survey consists of those standard automated laboratory profiles of blood that include evaluations of electrolytes, glucose, calcium, phosphate, uric acid, and renal and liver function. The complete blood count (CBC), especially with indices, helps identify potential anemias. Determination of the erythrocyte sedimentation rate (ESR) is an inexpensive, simple screening for collagen vascular disease and other inflammatory conditions.

A serum vitamin B_{12} determination is recommended. Pernicious anemia, a well-known cause of dementia, can manifest subtle cerebral disease prior to the development of its typical hematologic or neurologic aspects. The megaloblastic disease assessment is completed by a red blood cell (RBC) folate determination. Folate deficiency is a possible but less established cause of dementia. The RBC folate level is preferred to the serum level because the former more accurately reflects the averaged, long-term folic acid supply.

Thyroid function tests are always ordered, especially because hypothyroidism can cause a treatable dementia yet remain subclinical otherwise. The T_4 (thyroxine) assay combined with the RT_3U (resin-triiodothyronine uptake) and the calculated T_7 (free thyroid index, or FTI) tests is recommended. A thyroid-stimulating hormone (TSH) level is obtained whenever hypothyroidism is considered because it is the most sensitive test for this disorder. Further endocrine assessments may be chosen according to clinical indicators or laboratory abnormalities. In addition to discovery of the cause for the dementia, such a complete work-up may uncover an unsuspected yet contributing ailment.

The Electroencephalogram

The need to obtain an electroencephalogram (EEG) is somewhat controversial. There is a tendency to avoid requesting an EEG without specific indications. However, the test is safe, noninvasive, and sensitive in the detection of toxic or abnormal metabolic processes. Minimal degrees of diffuse EEG slowing can be normal in geriatric patients, and EEG findings can be normal in some demented persons. This investigation is not likely to detect unsuspected, treatable, focal CNS disease that was not noted on physical examination or CT scan.

An EEG is always ordered for specific evaluations of seizures or syncope, and when the diagnosis is enigmatic. An EEG may also be beneficial in other circumstances. For example, a normal tracing recorded in a very gravely ill patient makes the clinician conscious of potential diagnostic errors. Pseudodementia can have such a pattern. The EEG has become, therefore, a routine part of the dementia work-up.

Profound diffuse EEG slowing with normal CT scanning and physical findings (e.g., no detectable anatomic disease) raises the possibility of an undetected toxic exposure or metabolic abnormality. Diffuse slowing is consistent with diffuse dementing processes. In conjunction with other clinical or laboratory findings, the EEG may be a confirmatory yet nondiagnostic test. Serial tracings can provide objective evidence in following disease progression. As cerebral illness advances, the background rhythm should document further slowing. At periodic retesting, for comparison purposes, one should use the same laboratory or provide the electroencephalographer with old EEG recordings or at least their reports.

The CT Scan

Computed tomography (CT or CAT scanning) of the head is probably the most informative single tool for evaluating demented patients (Figs. 1 to 3). It contributes dramatically to the correct identification of many disease processes. Most significantly, CT scanning depicts the morphology of many remediable forms of dementia. Subdural hematoma, normal-pressure hydrocephalus (NPH), and intracranial tumors are sometimes accurately detected on CT scans. The scan may not always be definitive, but it is an excellent screening instrument, and it may indicate the need for further studies such as angiography and cysternography. For example, when the CT findings suggest NPH, isotope lumbar cysternography may be indicated, and neurosurgical consultation is obtained.

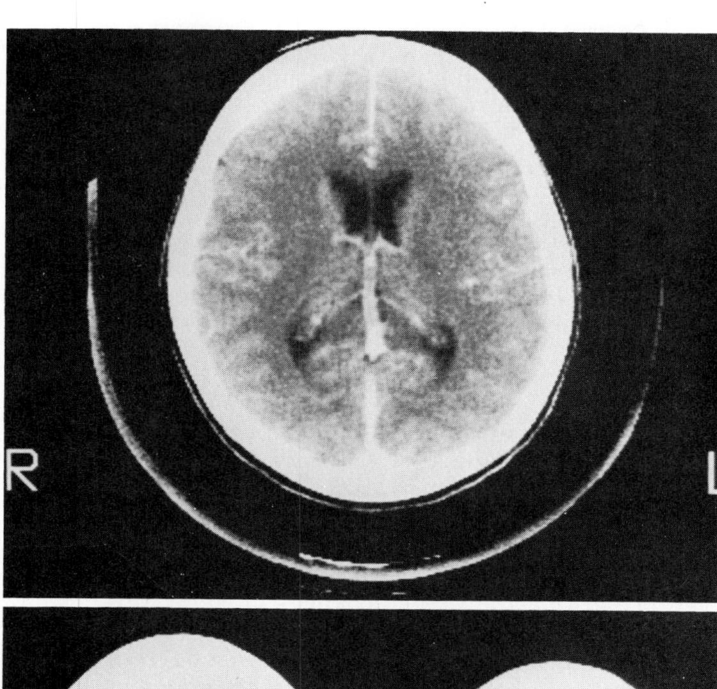

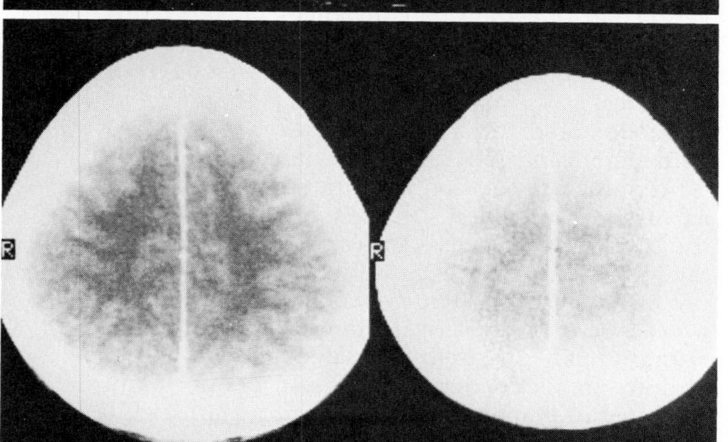

Figure 1. A normal CT scan from a healthy 32-year-old adult.

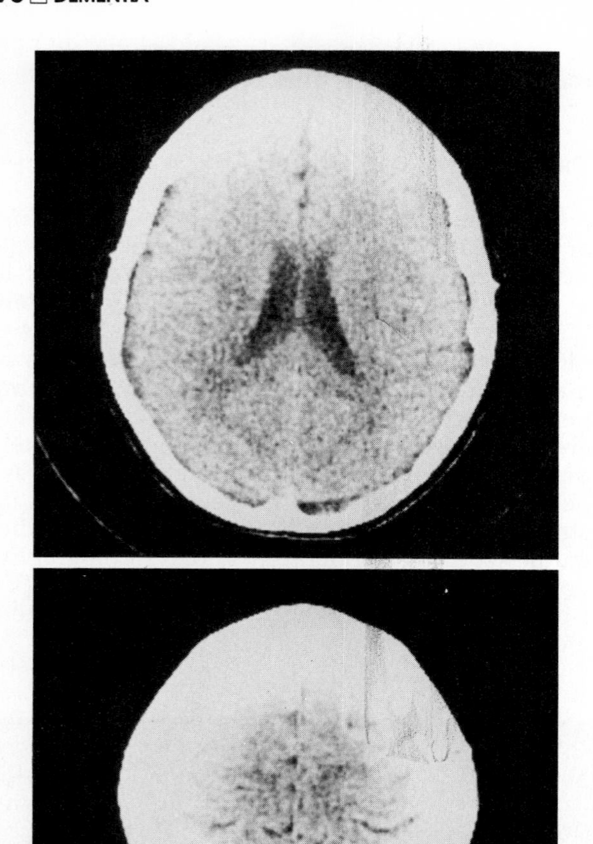

Figure 2. A normal CT scan from a 70-year-old healthy male without dementia. Ventricle and sulci size are normal for the patient's age.

CT scanning can aid in the presumptive, though not definitive, diagnosis of Alzheimer's disease. The typical expectation in Alzheimer's disease is that a CT scan will demonstrate profound, diffuse cerebral atrophy (Fig. 4). The cortical atrophy is evidenced by widened sulci, shrunken gyri, and ventricular dilatation. Such changes must be considered markedly advanced for the patient's age before being used diagnostically. Lesser degrees of cortical atrophy are not clinically relevant. Mild to moderate cortical atrophy does not correlate with significant CNS disease or dementia.

Scanning can also confirm other diagnoses, such as cerebral infarction. NPH is considered when the scan demonstrates significant ventricular dilatation without cortical atrophy. Specific changes on CT scan may identify other disorders. The procedure may reveal caudate nucleus atrophy in Huntington's disease or isolated frontal region atrophy in Pick's disease. Because of the many extracranial etiologies of dementia, a normal CT scan does not rule out a dementia.

Nuclear Magnetic Resonance

Nuclear magnetic resonance (NMR) is a new technique being developed for evaluation of cerebral morphology. In the future NMR may replace CT scanning. The new technique appears to have promise as an accurate diagnostic tool, and its use of a magnetic field, rather than radiation, could also make it safer than CT scanning.

Second Laboratory Battery

Lumbar Puncture

Whenever the results of studies already noted are not diagnostic, a lumbar puncture is performed for analysis of cerebrospinal fluid. The indications are not uniformly agreed upon, but this investigation is always done when called for by specific indications, such as suspicion of tertiary lues. A lumbar puncture is also always performed when the results of initial laboratory studies are normal

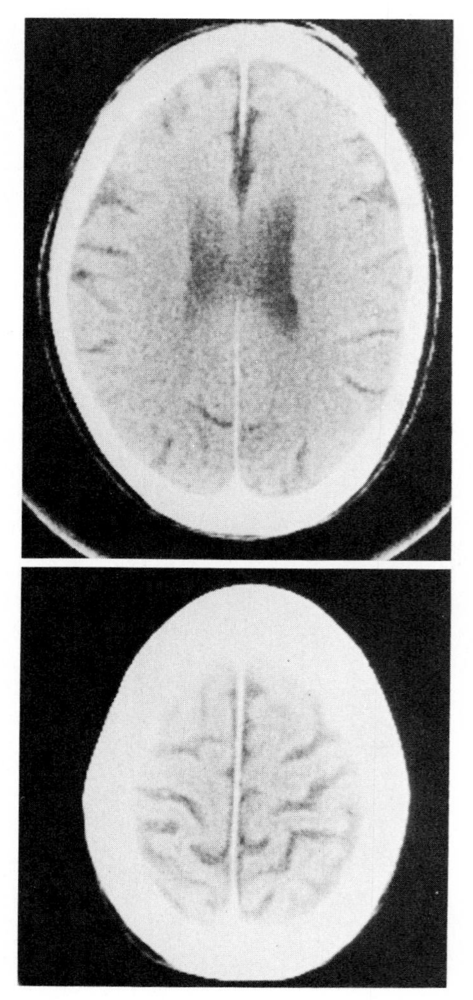

Figure 3. A 74-year-old patient with CT scan evidence of cortical atrophy.

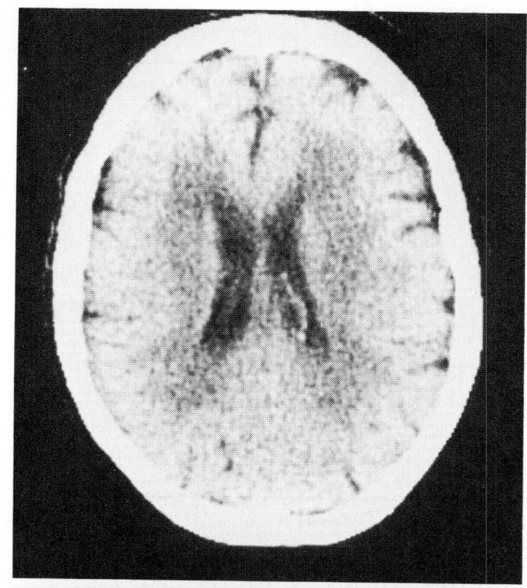

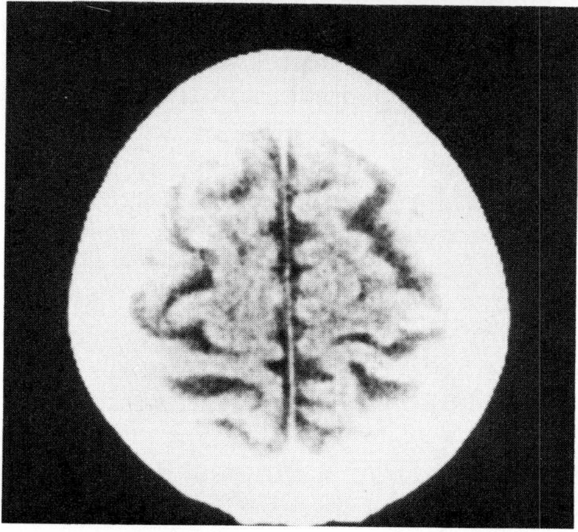

Figure 4. Advanced cortical atrophy is noted on this CT scan from a 63-year-old demented woman. Sulci are grossly enlarged.

in a rapidly progressing, unexplained dementia. Clinicians sometimes omit this procedure in patients of advanced age with many years of prolonged, stable dementia in whom CT scanning reveals diffuse cortical atrophy. The consensus, however, would be to perform a lumbar puncture whenever the previous investigations are not clearly diagnostic. All routine CSF studies are requested. Emphasis should also be placed on detection of chronic, subtle processes such as basilar tuberculous meningitis and fungal infections by ordering of acid-fast smears and cultures and an India-ink preparation of the CSF. Abnormal findings, such as pleocytosis, mandate further evaluations—repeat lumbar puncture, a cryptococcal antigen test, and neurologic consultation.

Psychological Testing

When dementia is obvious, psychological testing is not required. If the diagnosis is not clear at this point in the investigation, however, the need for psychological testing should be reevaluated; such a nondiagnostic picture could, for example, be the result of a pseudodementia. Psychological evaluations are obtained when no diagnosis can be confirmed and are always ordered when a diagnostic error is suspected. Furthermore, they can aid in localization of brain lesions and quantification of disease. Testing can be used for specialized examinations, such as screening for aphasias and dyspraxias. Aphasias can, in rare cases, be mistaken for dementias; the fluent, yet meaningless speech associated with lesions in Wernicke's cerebral area is an example of such a confusing sign.

Further Work-up

If the diagnosis still remains elusive, a review of the case from the beginning is suggested. Screening the urine for heavy metals is also recommended. If no etiology emerges from the review, hospitalization of the patient and discontinuation of all possible medications is considered. In the hospital, the physician gains more control of the patient's medications, diet, and potential drug abuses, and nursing observations and procedural evaluations are enhanced. A drug-free period is worthwhile, when feasible, even if the medicines the patient has been taking are not considered encephalopathogens. Depending on clinical judgment, certain other intoxications may be considered, such as with drugs or poisons. One should also consider unrelated problems that could exaggerate expression of a dementia. If the drug-free period does not provide a diagnosis, one should consider neurologic consultation.

Further work-up then follows *only* according to specific indications. If a neoplastic lesion is suspected, studies such as sigmoidoscopy are obtained. Arterial blood gas assessments might be used to quantify disease in cardiopulmonary conditions. Suspicion about vascular disease, such as raised by a carotid artery bruit, might indicate need for a vascular evaluation. The work-up for a bruit (e.g., arteriography or ultrasonography) in such cases is controversial. Studies may not be done if cerebral infarctions have already occurred or if the patient is otherwise not a surgical candidate. If a collagen vascular disease is likely, an antinuclear antibody test or related tests are ordered. Any other laboratory procedures are obtained only for reasons individualized to each patient. In some patients with dementing illnesses, a diagnosis cannot be confirmed during life. Before one makes the determination "dementia of unknown etiology," however, the complete assessment previously described must have been performed.

PROGRESSION OF ILLNESS

Early dementia presentations may be difficult to recognize or may suggest psychiatric dysfunction rather than neurologic disease. The onset is often insidious and not readily discernible.[14] Patients generally are poor historians. Reliable information is more frequently gained from others. Short-term memory impairment is often denied by the patient but can be seen to be present when one views daily life dysfunctions, such as getting lost or going shopping and forgetting why. Mildly demented persons have problems in decision-making, task completion, and understanding new situations. Adaptive abilities are impaired. Affected persons might do well at familiar tasks yet have difficulty with new situations.

With progression of dementia, memory dysfunction and disorientation become obvious. Periods of general confusion and sundowning may occur. *Sundowning* is a form of sensory deprivation consisting of nocturnal confusion with agitation because visual orientation cues are less present in the dark. Sufferers have poor concentration, attention, and judgment. Thinking becomes concrete and anxiety heightens. These factors worsen cognitive processes. Psychotic signs can appear, especially those of a delusional nature, paranoia being the most common. Hallucinations and illusions can also develop. Neurologic abnormalities and personality changes may become apparent. At this stage, recognition of a dementia generally presents little difficulty.

Late in the course of dementing illnesses, the differential diagnosis may be difficult. Patients who are apathetic, mute, bedridden, and withdrawn give no history and are difficult to examine. The diagnosis can erroneously appear to be functional or an unrelated systemic condition. Neurologic signs may be pronounced and could aid in recognition; they commonly include signs of diffuse cerebral dysfunction but may only be of focal deficits. One can observe parietal lobe impairment, frontal release signs, and language disturbances such as aphasia, loss of vocabulary, and rambling speech.

Advanced dementia patients are often psychotic, with bizarre behavior and personality deterioration. They are regressed and withdrawn. Eventually they become bedridden with contractures, decubitus ulcers, dehydration, malnutrition, and related physiologic failures. This stage leads to pulmonary embolism, pneumonia, and death. Dementia is, therefore, one of the most common indirect causes of death.[1, 4]

SPECIFIC DEMENTIAS

Alzheimer's Disease (and Pick's Disease)

Alzheimer's disease is the most common cause of dementing illness, accounting for over half of cases.[2] Occurring with equal frequency in both sexes, it currently affects 3 million persons in the USA over age 65.[12] It is a chronic, progressive, diffuse disorder of premature CNS neuronal loss, usually in older people, but with an onset as early as midlife. Etiology is unknown. Possible causes include genetic sources, viral diseases, and neurochemical disorders, such as cholinergic system failure and raised concentration of manganese or aluminum.[1–4, 12]

Diffuse neurologic dysfunctions are common in Alzheimer's disease. The CT scan reveals profound diffuse cortical atrophy (see Fig. 4). Histopathologic examination demonstrates neurofibrillary tangles, senile plaques, and granulovacuolar degeneration in proportion to the clinical expression of disease. Brain biopsy or autopsy examination determines the definitive diagnosis. The laboratory findings are otherwise normal. A presumptive diagnosis may be suggested by clinical and laboratory findings. Pick's disease is a rare disorder with a sometimes similar presentation, causing severe cortical atrophy confined to the anterior aspects of the cerebrum.[2]

No treatment reverses or retards the progression of either disease. Symptomatic therapies may cause behavioral improvements. Patients with Alzheimer's and Pick's diseases exhibit a progressive decline in mental function, dying in a bedridden state owing to medical complications.[12]

Vascular Disease

Blood vessel disease is another cause of dementia. Previously, arteriosclerotic disease was virtually always yet erroneously considered the major cause of dementia in older persons. Actually, vascular disease causes dementia in only a minority of demented individuals. Arteriosclerosis may be a factor in up to 20 per cent of cases.[1, 3] Arteriosclerotic disease in one set of arteries does not correlate well with disease in other arteries.[1] The presence of coronary or peripheral arteriosclerosis does not imply such change in cerebral arteries. Autopsy-proven cerebrovascular disease does not correlate with clinical degrees of dementia. A vascular dementia typically is of the poly-infarct type.

Poly-infarct dementias are caused by multiple cerebral infarcts (Fig. 5). Affected patients have a history of stepwise deterioration with periods of acute dysfunction and partial remission. Each relapse represents another infarction. Large strokes,

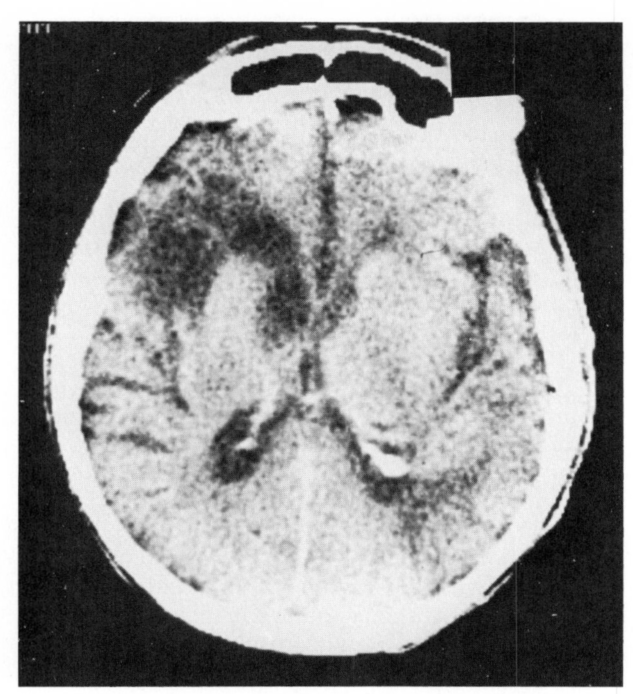

Figure 5. Several cerebral infarcts are demonstrated on CT scan of an elderly man with a diagnosis of polyinfarct dementia. Infarctions of different ages are seen in both hemispheres and in both white matter and gray matter.

because of overt asymmetries on examination, rarely provide diagnostic problems or receive dementia evaluations. Poly-infarct dementia presentations can be subtle but may have the typical features of infarction, such as pseudobulbar palsies and lateralizing signs. The examiner should evaluate for contributing factors such as hypertension, diabetes, hyperlipidemia, carotid artery disease, and embolic foci. Subacute bacterial endocarditis is one of several emboli-producing conditions that can result in a poly-infarct dementia.

Normal-Pressure Hydrocephalus

Clinically, NPH is recognized via a classic triad: dementia, gait disturbance, and urinary incontinence.[1–7, 16] This condition often follows intracranial trauma, infection, or hemorrhage but can occur idiopathically. Progressive ventricular dilatation is the hallmark of the disease. The etiology is unclear. Ventricular enlargement may compress the cerebral cortex against the skull. Demonstration of dilated ventricles without cortical atrophy on CT scanning provides suggestive evidence for NPH (Fig. 6). This finding necessitates further investigation.

A lumbar cysternogram is usually the next step. A radioisotope-labeled vehicle is injected into the lumbar subarachnoid space. Patterns of CSF flow are then monitored. Normally, isotope does not enter the ventricles. In NPH or other forms of communicating hydrocephalus, CSF flow is disordered; isotope is found within the ventricles and remains there protractedly.[1, 4] In Alzheimer's disease, isotope also enters the ventricles but remains only transiently. The study helps determine which NPH patients might benefit from surgical treatment (CSF shunt drainage). Neurosurgical consultation is requested. Further work-up includes placing of pressure monitors within the ventricles to guide decisions about definitive treatment. Surgical CSF shunt placement is most effective in patients with classically recognized NPH. In the absence of the classic triad, shunting is not likely to be effective.

Other Considerations

Various toxic products may be responsible for diminished mental capacity. Encephalopathy often follows abuse of multiple medicines or polydrug interactions. Dementia is notably common in alcoholic subjects, but the mechanism is unknown. Clinical dementia presentations in alcoholics simulate those of Alzheimer's disease, and the CT scans are indistinguishable (Fig. 7). Wernicke-Kor-

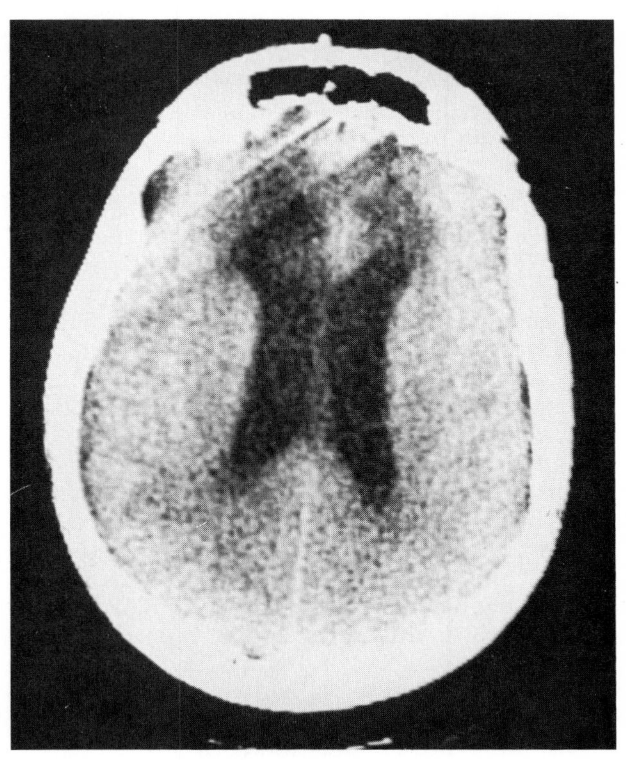

Figure 6. Ventricular enlargement is seen on CT scan of a patient with normal-pressure hydrocephalus.

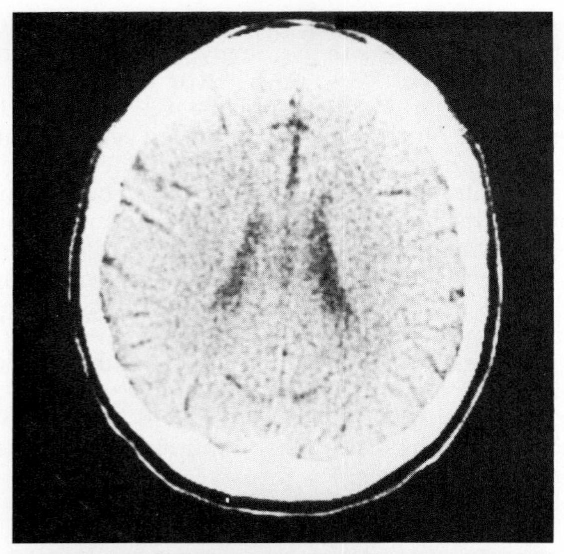

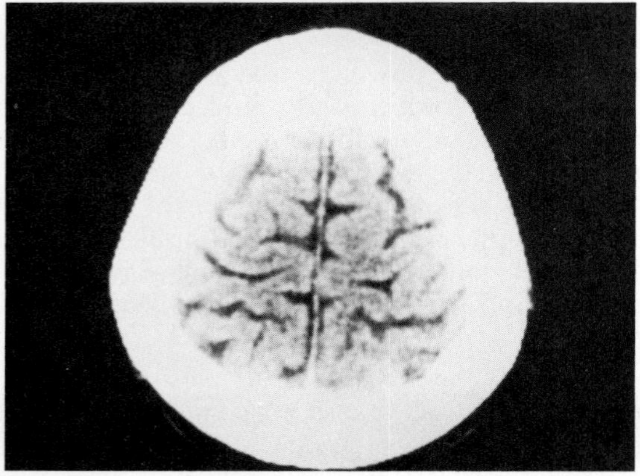

Figure 7. Advanced cortical atrophy seen on CT scan in a 34-year-old, cognitively impaired alcoholic man. For a person of this age, the sulci show massive enlargement.

sakoff's syndrome may also result in dementia. The CT scan in a Wernicke-Korsakoff patient is nonspecific. The diagnosis is based on the alcohol and dietary history and the physical findings or past records of lateral nystagmus. Less often, other toxicities or poisonings may occur. Heavy metal screening or similar procedures may be employed, as needed.

Numerous other diagnostic classifications are associated with dementia. Emotional depression is often detected during the evaluation. Hypothyroidism, pernicious anemia, brain tumor, cerebral injury, and other illness all cause dementias. In elderly people, lesions such as a subdural hematoma may be difficult to detect, especially when there is no history of trauma and the patient presents with only subtle changes in mentation (Fig. 8). Subcortical processes, which may also result in intellectual deterioration, include Parkinson's, Huntington's and Wilson's diseases. Still other encephalopathies exist; these and other illnesses are discussed in standard references.[1–4, 11]

There is no easy method to predict accurately the course of such disorders. Indications in the patient history or family history, if present, may be reliable. Dementing illnesses are often progressive, but all do not inevitably result in profound cerebral dysfunction. Clinical severity in most dementias is generally proportional to the quantity of cerebral tissue damaged. There is a close relation between clinical signs and degree of histopathologic abnormality.[16] The location of the cerebral damage can also be functionally relevant. For example, memory deficits are greater in a dominant temporal lobe injury than in a nondominant frontal lobe process.

The "undiagnosed dementia" category includes only those cases in which full evaluation as described could determine no specific cause. In some such patients the diagnosis is never confirmed, but work-up is worthwhile because of the number of patients identified as having treatable etiologies. Other ailments, related or unrelated to the dementia, may also be discovered that require specific treatment. The evaluation also determines whether a patient may benefit from symptomatic treatment.

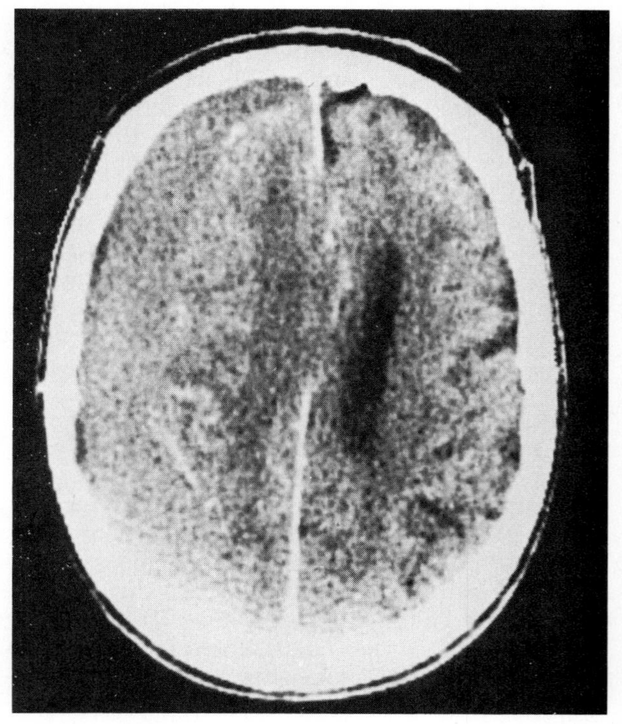

Figure 8. This CT scan reveals a left-sided subdural hematoma with compression of the brain substance and distortion of the left hemisphere, subcortical structures, and ventricles. Note that the brain tissue is medially displaced from the skull on that side.

REFERENCES

1. Wells CE, ed. Dementia, 2nd ed. Philadelphia: FA Davis, 1977.
2. Gilroy J, Meyer JS. In: Medical neurology, 3rd ed. New York: Macmillan, 1979.
3. Wells CE, Duncan GW. Neurology for psychiatrists. Philadelphia: FA Davis, 1980.
4. Ropper AH. A rational approach to dementia. CMA J 1979; 121:1175–90.
5. Wells CE. Chronic brain syndrome: an overview. Am J Psychiatry 1978;135:1–12.
6. Wells CE. Diagnosis of dementia. Psychosomatics 1972; 20:517–22.
7. Seltzer B, Sherwin I. Organic brain syndromes: an empirical study and critical review. Am J Psychiatry 1978; 135:13–21.
8. Lippmann S. Recognition and initial evaluation of dementia. Resident Staff Physician 1981;27:88–96.
9. Lippmann S. Work-up and diagnosis of dementia. Resident Staff Physician 1982;28:50–7.
10. Lippmann S. The treatment of dementia. Resident Staff Physician 1982;28:89–96.
11. Isselbacher KJ, et al., eds. Harrison's principles of internal medicine, 9th ed. New York: McGraw-Hill, 1980.
12. Schneck MK, Reisberg B, Ferris SH. An overview of current concepts of Alzheimer's disease. Am J Psychiatry 1982;139:165–73.
13. Aging and medical education. Washington, DC: National Academy of Sciences, 1978.
14. Kosik KH, Growdon JH. Aging, memory loss, and dementia. Psychosomatics 1982;23:745–51.
15. Rabins PV, Mace NL, Lucas MJ. The impact of dementia on the family. JAMA 1982;248:333–7.
16. Pincus JH, Tucker GJ. Behavioral neurology, 2nd ed. New York: Oxford University Press, 1978.
17. Dubovsky SL. Psychiatric problems in primary practice, No. 5. Nutley, NJ: Roche Products, Inc., 1982.
18. Wells CE. Refinements in the diagnosis of dementia. Am J Psychiatry 1982;139:621–2.
19. Tourigny-Rivard M, Raskind M, Ricard D. The dexamethasone suppression test in an elderly population. Biol Psychiatry 1981;16:1177–84.
20. Carroll BJ. The dexamethasone suppression test: an interview. In: Depression dialogue. Cincinnati: Merrell Dow Pharmaceuticals, 1982.
21. Carroll BJ, Feinberg M, Greeden JH, et al. A specific laboratory test for the diagnosis of melancholia. Arch Gen Psychiatry 1981;38:15–22.

DIARRHEA, CHRONIC

N. W. READ

BACKGROUND AND PATHOPHYSIOLOGY

To the clinician, *diarrhea* implies the passage of abnormally large watery bowel movements. Approximately 9 liters of fluid normally enter the gut every day. Usually no more than 2 liters come from the diet; the rest is composed of secretions from the salivary glands, stomach, biliary tree, pancreas, and intestine. About 8 liters of this fluid is absorbed in the small intestine, and the remainder (0.5 to 1.5 liters) passes through the ileocecal valve into the large intestine, where most is absorbed, yielding a stool of approximately 100 gm. When fluid intake or secretion increases, the absorptive capacity of the gut may adapt to accommodate the extra fluid load. Diarrhea occurs when fluid intake or secretion has been so great as to overwhelm the normal absorptive capacity of the intestine, or when absorption is impaired so that the intestine cannot cope with the normal fluid load.

Increased Intake or Secretion

Diarrhea caused by excessive fluid intake is rare but has been described in compulsive water drinkers and may also occur in heavy beer drinkers. Excessive fluid secretion from the salivary glands, pancreas, or biliary tree sufficient to cause diarrhea has not been described, probably because the absorptive capacity of the small intestine is more than enough to cope with excess fluid from these sources. Abnormally high gastric secretion occurs in the Zollinger-Ellison syndrome, but the diarrhea observed in this condition is related as much to the effect of acid on digestion and fluid transport in the small intestine as to the increased gastric secretion.[1] Thus, excessive secretion sufficient to result in diarrhea almost always comes from the small or large intestine. Excessive small intestine secretion may be produced by tumors secreting polypeptide hormones, such as vasoactive intestinal polypeptide (VIP); by infection with enterotoxigenic organisms, such as *Escherichia coli*, staphylococcus, *Vibrio cholerae*, and possibly many others; and by ingestion of irritant laxatives. The most common cause of excessive colonic secretion is the malabsorption of either long-chain fatty acids or bile acids in the small intestine. These agents are converted by colonic bacteria to potent secretogogues.[2]

Diminished Fluid Absorption

Most fluid and electrolyte absorption in the gut takes place secondary to the absorption of solutes such as sugars and amino acids in the small intestine. It follows that any condition that impairs solute absorption by the small intestine also impairs fluid and electrolyte absorption. Such conditions include chronic pancreatic insufficiency and malabsorption (e.g., celiac disease, or sprue) and possibly also disturbances in intestinal motility resulting in excessively rapid transit of food through the small intestine, which may inhibit absorption by reducing the time during which material is in contact with the epithelium. In all of these conditions, the unabsorbed solute retains fluid in the intestinal lumen by virtue of its osmotic activity. Rarely, defects in fluid and electrolyte absorption may occur independent of any abnormality in solute absorption; an example is congenital chloridorrhea, in which there appears to be a defect in chloride-bicarbonate exchange in the distal ileum.[3]

Colonic Salvage

The ability of the colon to absorb material entering from the ileum is much greater than is usually required. The colon can, for example, absorb between 4 and 7 liters per day of plasma-like solution infused into the cecum at a steady rate. The colon can also accommodate the residues of a meal, containing between 40 and 60 gm of carbohydrate, before the appearance of carbohydrate in the stool and onset of diarrhea. The carbohydrate is converted by anaerobic bacteria to volatile fatty acids (VFA), mainly acetate, propionate, and butyrate.[4] These substances are absorbed rapidly by the colonic epithelium, and the ensuing reduction in luminal osmolality facilitates the absorption of water. The efficiency of carbohydrate salvage may help to explain why many patients with lactase deficiency can drink milk without getting diarrhea and why patients with active celiac disease do not necessarily present with diarrhea.

It seems logical to propose that diarrhea occurs only when the absorptive capacity of the colon is inadequate to cope with the amount of ileal effluent.[5] The inadequacy can result from one of two situations: Either the amount or composition of ileal effluent overwhelms the *normal* capacity for colonic salvage or abnormal colonic function or colonic disease prevents salvage of a normal load (Fig. 1).

Factors that impair the colon's ability to salvage and absorb even a normal amount of ileal effluent include (1) disease or destruction of the colonic epithelium, as in ulcerative colitis, (2) an abnormal pattern of colonic motility, leading to a rapid transit of colonic contents and inadequate time for fermentation and absorption, (3) abnormal colonic secretion, and (4) an inadequate pool of fermentative bacteria, which would slow the conversion of carbohydrate to volatile fatty acids and secondarily impair fluid absorption. A reduction in bacterial population may be important in the diarrhea experienced after ingestion of broad-spectrum antibiotics. Impaired absorption of fat or bile acids in the small intestine may also inhibit colonic salvage, because bile acid and fat are converted by colonic bacteria to potent laxative agents that increase colonic secretion and propulsion.

HISTORY

A carefully taken history of factors relating to defecation is of major importance in elucidating the cause of a patient's diarrhea.

Nature of Stool. Patients complain of diarrhea when they have abnormally frequent movements (more than three per day), abnormally bulky movements, or stools that are soft or liquid, or when bowel action is giving rise to such symptoms as urgency and incontinence. These symptoms do not necessarily all occur together and do not imply the same pathogenesis. It is therefore important

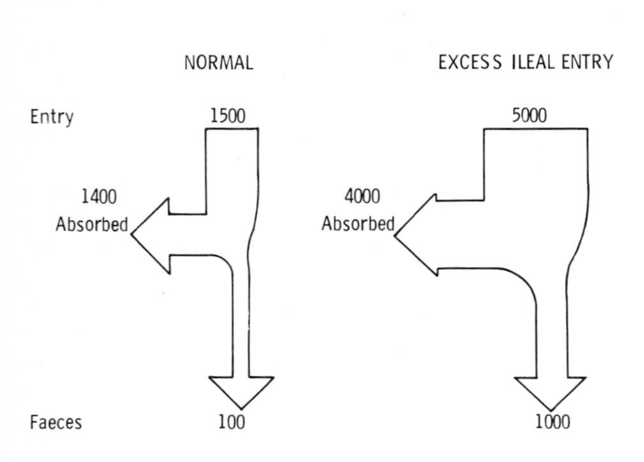

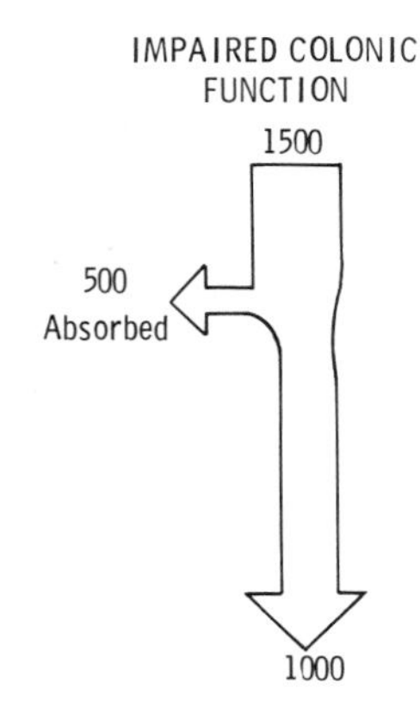

Figure 1. A diagram of the average volumes of fluid entering and leaving the colon under normal conditions and when diarrhea is caused by excessive ileal entry of fluid or impaired colonic absorption.

to find out exactly what the patient means by "diarrhea."

Diarrhea that is of large volume and very watery may suggest abnormal intestinal secretion, which can be caused by bacterial toxins, laxatives, or polypeptide-secreting tumors. Large-volume stools that are frothy, soupy, or greasy, light in color, and foul-smelling strongly indicate malabsorption; passage of formed stools that are unusually bulky may also suggest malabsorption. The presence of free oil in the stool indicates pancreatic disease.

Small-volume, frequent stools are more suggestive of colonic disease. Stools that are hard and resemble rabbit or sheep droppings strongly suggest irritable bowel syndrome (IBS). Blood or blood-stained mucus in the stools usually indicates an inflammatory, infectious, or neoplastic disease, although it is important not to overlook the possibility of ischemic colitis, particularly in the elderly, arteriopathic, or seriously ill patient. Passage of blood excludes the diagnosis of irritable bowel syndrome.

The passage of pus and mucus in the stool strongly suggests inflammatory bowel disease, although pelvic inflammatory disease caused by gynecologic conditions may occasionally also be associated with the frequent and often urgent passage of mucus per anum. Passage of particularly large amounts of mucus, especially in combination with solid stool, is characteristic of villous adenoma of the rectum. In a patient who is well, the passage of mucus is sometimes a manifestation of the irritable bowel syndrome and it may also be produced by laxative ingestion or the use of suppositories.

Timing. Chronic diarrhea commencing with an attack of gastroenteritis, often occurring on vacation, is common and is often diagnosed as irritable bowel syndrome. In such cases it is important to rule out giardiasis and infection by agents such as Campylobacter and Yersinia, which may linger several weeks, and to carry out investigations for lactase deficiency, which is common after an attack of gastroenteritis. Chronic diarrhea commencing after a recent trip to the tropics may be caused by amebiasis or worm infestation.

Diarrhea that occurs in episodes or attacks lasting a few days, especially alternating with periods of constipation, is thought by many to indicate the irritable bowel syndrome, although intermittent or episodic diarrhea may be found in many other conditions, particularly inflammatory bowel disease. Intermittent diarrhea is characteristically associated with facial flushing in the rare carcinoid syndrome.

Diarrhea that is exacerbated by ingestion of food is a common finding and does not help to determine the diagnosis, unless the patient can relate the complaint to a particular type of food.

Watery diarrhea that persists even while the patient is fasting indicates abnormal intestinal secretion due to laxatives, toxigenic bacteria, or polypeptide-secreting tumor. Conversely, diarrhea that stops when the patient stops eating suggests impairment of absorption or digestion.

Nocturnal diarrhea is unlikely in patients with irritable bowel syndrome but occurs quite commonly in patients with celiac disease and may be frequently associated with fecal soiling in patients with neurologic problems, particularly those with diabetic neuropathy.

The association of diarrhea with stressful events suggests irritable bowel syndrome but may also be noted in ulcerative colitis and other conditions.

Associated Features

Pain. Griping lower abdominal pain or tenesmus that is relieved by a bowel movement or the passage of flatus is found in a variety of colonic diseases, particularly diverticular disease, Crohn's disease, irritable bowel syndrome, and neoplasm. It is also common in malabsorption, presumably because of colonic irritation induced by unabsorbed fats or bile acids. Upper abdominal pain radiating through to the back and relieved by sitting up suggests pancreatic disease. Epigastric, ulcer-like pain may suggest Zollinger-Ellison syndrome. Crampy central abdominal pain may be found in Crohn's disease. Ulcerative colitis and pseudomembranous colitis[6] are often associated with painless diarrhea.

Urgency and Incontinence. Urgency and incontinence are commonly experienced by patients with diarrhea but infrequently reported to the doctor.[7] Many physicians regard the presence of incontinence or urgency as a sign of particularly severe diarrhea. Although this may be true in the occasional case, stool weight is normal or near normal in the majority of sufferers. In these patients, urgency and incontinence are related more to a weak anal sphincter, and extensive investigation for diagnosis of diarrhea may be inappropriate.

Drug History. A large number of drugs may cause diarrhea.[8] Some of the more common agents are listed in Table 1. The possibility of drug-induced diarrhea should be carefully considered before laboratory investigations are performed, even if the patient is not taking a drug commonly associated with diarrhea. In fact, before one carries out stool collection, it is important whenever possible to stop all medications.

The most common cause of drug-induced diarrhea is undoubtedly ingestion of antibiotics. Usually the diarrhea is mild, is dose-related after oral administration, and lasts for only a short time after the course of treatment is completed. The cause may be a direct irritant effect on the bowel or the reduction in numbers of fermentative colonic bacteria, or, occasionally, replacement by organisms

Table 1. DRUGS KNOWN TO CAUSE DIARRHEA

Drugs that commonly cause diarrhea	Antibiotics Magnesium salts Colchicine Chenodeoxycholic acid Neostigmine Neomycin (steatorrhea) Laxatives

Drugs that occasionally cause diarrhea	Antihypertensive agents
	  Methyldopa
	  Beta-blockers
	  Bethanidine/guanethidine
	Antirheumatic agents
	  Mefenamic acid
	  Flufenamic acid
	  Flurbiprofen
	  Indomethacin
	  Gold (colitis)
	Oral hypoglycemic agents
	  Biguanides (phenformin)
	  Sulfonylureas (chlorpropamide)
	Oral contraceptive agents
	Cholestyramine (steatorrhea)
	Diuretics

such as Salmonella, Pseudomonas, Staphylococcus, or *Candida albicans*. Oral sulfonamides, tetracyclines, and penicillins are the most familiar causes. It is important to distinguish this common, antibiotic-associated diarrhea, which may be little more than a mild inconvenience, from severe and potentially fatal pseudomembranous colitis, which is thought to be caused by overgrowth of toxigenic *Clostridium difficile*. The antibiotics most commonly implicated in this severe condition are clindamycin, ampicillin, and lincomycin, but no antibiotic is above suspicion. The patient is ill, with a fever and tachycardia, and may be passing mucoid or watery stools.[6] Usually the diarrhea is painless, but abdominal distension and tenderness are common findings. The passage of blood is uncommon in this condition. The diagnosis can be established by colonoscopy and biopsy when the typical white membrane is obvious, and by the identification of toxin in the stool. Finally, it is important to remember that neomycin may induce a mild malabsorption syndrome, and tetracycline may cause steatorrhea.

Intake of diuretics, laxatives, or the analgesic anti-inflammatory agent mefenamic acid (Ponstel) is often overlooked as a cause of particularly severe watery diarrhea. Some patients may be taking diuretics or laxatives in an attempt to lose weight without realizing that these agents will, in fact, cause diarrhea. Finally, it is worth remembering that even drugs used to treat diarrhea, such as salazosulfapyrine and opiates, can actually induce or exacerbate the condition in susceptible individuals. In the elderly or immobile patient, opiates may cause fecal impaction and spurious diarrhea.

Diet. We have found that many causes of troublesome diarrhea may be detected by a careful dietary history. Overindulgence in beer or coffee and the excessive intake of fruit, spicy food, curries, milk, vegetables, or bran may commonly cause diarrhea or may exacerbate diarrhea from other causes. Some patients may have an allergy or intolerance to even small amounts of certain dietary constituents. Early recognition of putative agents and exclusion of them from the diet may avoid extensive investigation.

Family History. The incidence of Crohn's disease, ulcerative colitis, or celiac disease may be high within a family or kinship, whereas a strong family history is present in rare diarrheagenic conditions such as hereditary pancreatitis, medullary carcinoma of the thyroid, and multiple endocrine adenomatosis.

Previous History. A history of abdominal surgery is very important. Vagotomy, cholecystectomy, gastric resection, intestinal resection, and jejunoileal bypass may all cause very troublesome diarrhea. Resection of the ileum more frequently results in diarrhea than resection of the same length of jejunum. Resection of the proximal colon is associated with diarrhea more commonly than resection of the distal colon. The combination of cholecystectomy with vagotomy is particularly troublesome. Polya's operation may cause bacterial overgrowth in the afferent loop. The overgrowth is thought to result in diarrhea by deconjugating and dehydroxylating bile acids, which are poorly absorbed in the ileum and exert a laxative action on the colon. Adhesions from previous operations may cause a partial small bowel obstruction with concomitant bacterial overgrowth of the small intestine. Radiotherapy for such conditions as carcinoma of the cervix may also cause severe diarrhea that usually lasts only a few weeks but can continue for months, perhaps years.

PHYSICAL EXAMINATION

A complete physical examination may often reveal important clues with regard to the diagnosis (Table 2).

Abdominal Examination. The presence of an abdominal mass suggests neoplasm, Crohn's disease, or a diverticular abscess. An enlarged, knobby liver may be caused by metastatic carcinoma of the colon or malignant carcinoid. Guarding and tenderness particularly suggest Crohn's disease or diverticulitis. When a patient with diarrhea complains of gaseous distension of the abdomen, one should consider malabsorption or ingestion of large amounts of unabsorbable polysaccharides, although tender gaseous distension of the abdomen in an ill patient should alert one to the possibility of a toxic megacolon complicating inflammatory bowel disease. A careful rectal ex-

Table 2. PHYSICAL FINDINGS THAT MAY AID DIAGNOSIS IN PATIENTS WITH CHRONIC DIARRHEA

Finding	Possible Diagnoses
Fever	Crohn's disease, ulcerative colitis, lymphoma, amebiasis, pseudomembranous colitis, Whipple's disease
Tachycardia, sweating	Anxiety (IBS), salt and water depletion, thyrotoxicosis
Postural hypotension	Salt and water depletion (? secretory diarrhea), diabetic diarrhea, Addison's disease
Weight loss	Malabsorption, pancreatic disease, neoplasm
Anemia	Malabsorption, neoplasm
Finger clubbing	Crohn's disease, ulcerative colitis, Whipple's disease
Jaundice	Inflammatory bowel disease (sclerosing cholangitis), neoplasm
Hypopigmentation or hyperpigmentation	Addison's disease, celiac disease, diabetes mellitus, Whipple's disease
Arthritis	Crohn's disease, ulcerative colitis, Whipple's disease, amyloidosis
Proteinuria	Amyloidosis
Facial flushing	Malignant carcinoid syndrome
Lymphadenopathy	Lymphoma, Whipple's disease
Neuropathy	Diabetic diarrhea, amyloidosis, Whipple's disease
Scleroderma	Stasis and bacterial overgrowth of the small intestine

amination may reveal decreased anal sphincter tone or a rectal mass or impaction causing spurious diarrhea. Villous adenomas of the rectum are soft and may not be detected by digital examination. Perianal fistulae or fissures in a patient with diarrhea are suggestive of Crohn's disease.

Proctosigmoidoscopy. This is a very important part of the physical examination that must not be overlooked in a patient with diarrhea. The mucosa should be carefully examined for ulceration, friability, contact bleeding, polyps, and tumors. The diffuse inflammatory changes in ulcerative colitis are obvious but may be mimicked by other conditions, such as amebic or bacillary dysentery, Crohn's disease, lymphogranuloma venereum, and gonorrhea. Aphthous-type ulcers are very suggestive of Crohn's disease but may resemble the ulcers seen in amebic colitis. The thick, pale yellow, tenacious membrane of pseudomembranous colitis is typical, although in up to 70 per cent of patients with this disease the membrane may be seen only after endoscopic examination of the colon.[9] The crocodile-skin pigmentation of melanosis coli is diagnostic of the recent heavy use of anthracene laxatives. The microscopic examination of mucosal smears for pus has been emphasized by many authors.[10] An increase in white cells is said to be suggestive of inflammatory bowel disease (including diverticulitis), even if the rectal mucosa appears normal, and to be against the diagnosis of irritable bowel syndrome. Sigmoidoscopy also provides an opportunity to examine the stool and rectal contents. The presence of solid or pellet-like stools may signal irritable bowel syndrome. Pale stools that stick to the mucosa indicate steatorrhea, and the presence of free oil in stool signifies pancreatic insufficiency.

DIAGNOSTIC STUDIES

In most patients, chronic diarrhea can be diagnosed quite readily on the basis of a combination of history, physical examination, sigmoidoscopy, and possibly a barium enema. However, in difficult cases undiagnosed by these methods, further investigations can be planned on the basis of stool measurement and analysis. The algorithm demonstrates the assessment approach.

Stool Weight

Stool collections can be made easy by providing the patient with a disposable plastic collection unit (e.g., Specipan, from Kendall, Boston, Mass.), which can fit over the posterior half of the lavatory pan so that the patient can pass stools into it uncontaminated by urine (Fig. 2). The specimens can then be transferred to an airtight preweighed metal can or plastic bucket that holds at least 3 liters. This container is best kept in a refrigerator. To find out how much feces a patient is passing, the whole container is weighed, the weight of the empty container is subtracted, and the weight of feces is divided by the number of days of collection. It is useful to measure stool weight over at least 3 days while the patient is eating a normal hospital diet and then for 3 days more while the patient is fasting with fluid requirements being supplied by an intravenous infusion.

The majority of people eating a Western diet pass between 50 and 225 gm of stool per day. The common finding that stool weight is normal while the patient is collecting samples in hospital is very useful, as it excludes further investigations aimed at identifying a cause for excessive secretion or impaired absorption. It should not necessarily be taken to indicate that the patient has been deliberately falsifying the history. It could mean that he or she is passing abnormally frequent or urgent motions that are not watery or bulky, suggesting irritable bowel syndrome or anal sphincter dysfunction. Alternatively, diarrhea may cease in the hospital because the patient was ingesting some drug (either laxative or diuretic) or food substance at home that is not available in hospital or because

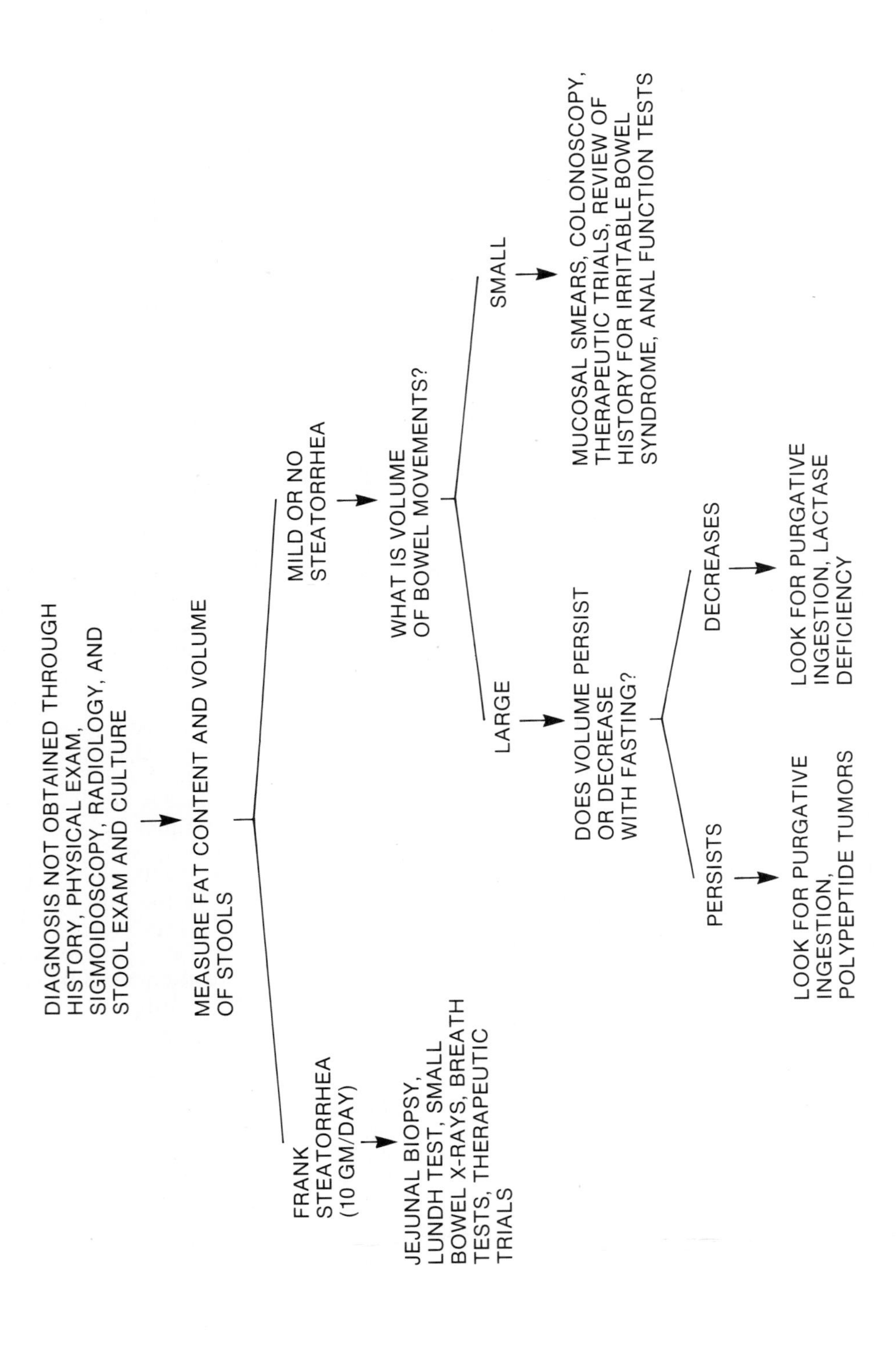
DIAGNOSTIC ASSESSMENT OF CHRONIC DIARRHEA
DIAGNOSIS NOT OBTAINED THROUGH HISTORY, PHYSICAL EXAM, SIGMOIDOSCOPY, RADIOLOGY, AND STOOL EXAM AND CULTURE
MEASURE FAT CONTENT AND VOLUME OF STOOLS
FRANK STEATORRHEA (10 GM/DAY)
JEJUNAL BIOPSY, LUNDH TEST, SMALL BOWEL X-RAYS, BREATH TESTS, THERAPEUTIC TRIALS
MILD OR NO STEATORRHEA
WHAT IS VOLUME OF BOWEL MOVEMENTS?
LARGE
DOES VOLUME PERSIST OR DECREASE WITH FASTING?
PERSISTS
LOOK FOR PURGATIVE INGESTION, POLYPEPTIDE TUMORS
DECREASES
LOOK FOR PURGATIVE INGESTION, LACTASE DEFICIENCY
SMALL
MUCOSAL SMEARS, COLONOSCOPY, THERAPEUTIC TRIALS, REVIEW OF HISTORY FOR IRRITABLE BOWEL SYNDROME, ANAL FUNCTION TESTS

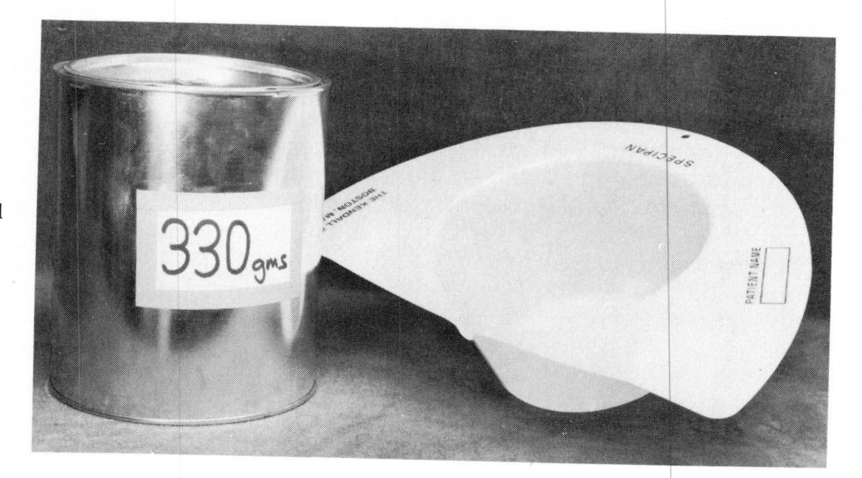

Figure 2. Equipment for quantitative stool collection.

he or she is removed from a stressful home situation. The latter reason suggests irritable bowel syndrome.

The finding of large-volume, watery diarrhea (more than 500 gm/day) that persists while the patient fasts indicates abnormally high intestinal secretion due to polypeptide-secreting tumor, surreptitious drug ingestion, or toxigenic bacteria. Large-volume diarrhea that stops when the patient fasts implies that the diarrhea is related to the intake of food, because of impaired absorption or digestion or food intolerance, or possibly to a drug that the patient ingests only when eating.

Steatorrhea

By far the most useful aspect of stool analysis is the identification of steatorrhea (passage of more than 7 gm of fat per day). In order to obtain accurate quantitative estimates, it is important that the patient is consuming a diet containing approximately 100 gm of fat per day and that stool is collected for at least 5 days.

The presence of steatorrhea indicates impairment of digestion or absorption.[11] Gross steatorrhea (greater than 35 gm/day) is more suggestive of pancreatic disease than of malabsorption. Steatorrhea is not found in diarrhea of colonic origin. If tests of intestinal or pancreatic function fail to yield a diagnosis, it is worth remembering that mild steatorrhea is particularly common in postvagotomy diarrhea and may also be present in secretory diarrheas caused by laxatives or polypeptide-secreting tumors, particularly in the Zollinger-Ellison syndrome. Finally, ingestion of large amounts of peanuts or liquid paraffin (for constipation) may produce severe steatorrhea.

Osmotic Gap

It has been suggested that measurement of the fecal osmotic gap, calculated with the formula Osmolality $-2\,([Na^+] + [K^+])$, is a useful way of distinguishing between secretory diarrheas and osmotic diarrheas caused by impaired absorption or digestion.[12] In secretory diarrheas, it is said, the osmolality of stool water is composed almost entirely of the sum of the electrolytes, whereas in osmotic diarrheas, there is an osmotic gap in the stool water, which contains the unabsorbed solute. This distinction is valid only if the stool volume is large (more than 750 ml/day), and only if the specimens are examined fresh. Moreover, even patients with secretory diarrhea may demonstrate large osmotic gaps if stool samples are collected on days when they are eating normally, presumably because the rapid flow through the small intestine flushes out food material. A more reliable diagnostic criterion for secretory diarrhea is the passage of large volumes of watery diarrhea during a fast. I have found the osmotic gap of value as an indicator of osmotic diarrhea only in the diagnosis of surreptitious ingestion of an osmotic laxative such as magnesium sulfate or lactulose.

Electrolyte Concentrations and pH in Stool

Measurements of pH or concentrations of sodium and potassium in the stool are also of limited value. Normal stool has a high potassium concentration and a low sodium concentration because sodium is absorbed and potassium is secreted in the lumen during passage through the colon. The combination of high sodium and low potassium concentrations may therefore reflect rapid transit of liquid stool through the colon, allowing little time for electrolyte transfer to take place, and would be associated with large stool volumes. However, patients with abnormal colonic secretion induced by villous adenomas of the rectum or ulcerative colitis or malabsorption of bile or fat may pass large volumes of stool rich in potassium.

Stool pH is usually an indicator of fermentation. Stool is normally slightly acidic (pH 5 or 6) because of colonic fermentation of the normal amounts of carbohydrate to volatile fatty acids. A neutral or slightly alkaline pH may be found in patients with secretory diarrheas who are not ingesting food, patients with enhanced alkaline secretion in the colon due to colitis or villous adenoma, and, in theory, patients whose colonic fermentation is inhibited by antibiotics. Patients with impairment of absorption or digestion may tend to pass large, sloppy stools of acidic pH (around 4 or 5), indicating excessive fermentation to volatile fatty acids.

Practical Guide To Further Investigations

Steatorrhea

Patients with frank steatorrhea (fat content more than 10 gm/day) have impairment of either digestion or absorption. The diagnosis can usually be established through a small number of diagnostic investigations, such as a jejunal biopsy, a Lundh test of pancreatic function,[13] x-rays of the small bowel for evidence of celiac disease, Crohn's disease, tumors, fistulae, stasis, and blind loops, and tests to elucidate bacterial overgrowth in the small intestine.

It is important to realize that bacterial overgrowth in the small intestine can cause quite troublesome diarrhea, even in patients in whom no obvious cause for stasis is demonstrated by small-bowel x-ray. This situation is particularly common in the elderly. The new breath tests have made the diagnosis considerably easier. An abnormally high yield of labeled CO_2 after ingestion of a liquid test meal containing ^{14}C-glycocholate[14, 15] and increased excretion of breath hydrogen following a drink of glucose or xylose[15, 16] are said to be diagnostic of bacterial overgrowth. These test results, however, only suggest contact between a large amount of unabsorbed substrate and the bacterial pool. Thus, results may be positive in patients with ileal resection or excessively rapid small bowel transit. False-negative results may occur if the small intestine bacteria cannot metabolize the substrate. When access to breath tests is lacking, bacterial overgrowth in the small intestine may be diagnosed by carrying out a Schilling test of vitamin B_{12} absorption and subsequently measuring the response of both the Schilling test result and steatorrhea to therapeutic trials of a broad-spectrum antibiotic such as metronidazole, trimethoprim, or tetracycline. In steatorrhea in which these tests yield normal or borderline results, therapeutic trials of pancreatic enzymes, antibiotics, or even a gluten-free diet are often very useful.

Large-Volume Secretory Diarrheas

Watery diarrheas of more than a liter in volume that persist on fasting are thought to be due to polypeptide-secreting tumors, to surreptitious ingestion of irritant laxatives, or to infection with enterotoxigenic bacteria.[12] The last is often discounted as a cause of chronic diarrhea of more than 10 days' duration. However, we recently described five patients in whom exhaustive investigation for surreptitious laxative ingestion and polypeptide-secreting tumors yielded no diagnosis.[17] In four of these patients spontaneous remission occurred between 6 weeks and 10 months after onset. The cause in these patients remains obscure but may have been infective.

Surreptitious Laxative Ingestion. Surreptitious laxative ingestion can be investigated in two ways.[18] The first is to carry out a biochemical screening of the urine and feces for laxatives. Phenolphthalein can be detected by alkalinization of the stool or urine, which turns red if it contains the drug. Bisocodyl can be identified by a chromatographic method, and there are chemical methods for detecting anthracene derivatives (senna, cascara, danthron). Magnesium and sulfate in the stool can be detected by chemical assays, and ingestion of magnesium sulfate and lactulose may be indicated by a large fecal osmotic gap. One patient known to me was drinking bath salts containing magnesium sulfate; the diagnosis was established by aspiration of perfumed liquid from the small intestine during intestinal perfusion.[18] Perhaps the most successful investigation for diagnosing surreptitious drug ingestion is a search of the patient's possessions, which can save a considerable amount of time and effort in further investigation. In a recent study my colleagues and I found that of 27 patients who were referred to our unit with chronic diarrhea after extensive diagnostic investigations carried out at other institutions failed to reveal a diagnosis, no fewer than eight had been surreptitiously taking laxatives or diuretics.[19] Several of these patients had undergone mutilating surgery (colectomy, pancreatectomy) for their diarrhea. It is most important for the physician to maintain a healthy index of suspicion with regard to patients with severe diarrhea. The most plausible and apparently genuine people may hide the fact that they are taking laxatives. Some patients may fool the doctor into believing they have diarrhea by adding water or urine to the stool sample. This practice can be easily detected by demonstrating an abnormally low osmolality of stool water. (The normal osmolality of stool water is, in our experience, never less than 260 mOsm/kg.)

Polypeptide/Secreting Tumors. If the patient is not ingesting laxatives, and particularly if the diarrhea is long-standing and has resulted in dehydration and hypokalemia, it may be necessary to carry out further tests in search for a tumor producing intestinal secretogogues. There are so many potential intestinal secretogogues that it is impossible to obtain plasma values for all of them. However, it is important to send plasma samples for VIP, gastrin, and possibly also calcitonin determinations, and to measure 5-hydroxyindoleacetic acid (5-HIAA) in the urine to rule out carcinoid syndrome. The results of these assays must be treated with a degree of caution and should always be confirmed by sending a second sample and by investigations such as angiography, lymphangiography, and ultrasonography to look for a polypeptide-secreting tumor and intestinal perfusion studies to prove that the patient has abnormal intestinal secretion. A further observation, which may be of value in the diagnosis of patients with large-volume diarrhea caused by the Zollinger-Ellison syndrome, is that the diarrhea abates upon continuous aspiration of gastric contents. At the present state of the art, blood should be taken for polypeptide assay only if the patient has large-volume secretory diarrhea proven by stool measurements and if surreptitious laxative ingestion has been ruled out.

Small-Volume Diarrhea (less than 500 ml) With No Steatorrhea

Most cases of diarrhea fall into this category. Although moderate or small-volume diarrhea may suggest colonic disease, many if not all of the conditions mentioned in the preceding categories can cause only moderate diarrhea in their less severe forms.

Colonoscopy has little advantage over a good double-contrast barium enema in investigating colonic causes of diarrhea, except perhaps in the differential diagnosis of Crohn's disease and ulcerative colitis and in the diagnosis of pseudomembranous colitis.

In many patients with diarrhea there is an increase in white cells in the rectal or colonic biopsy specimen. In the absence of other diagnostic histologic features, white cell infiltration probably represents a nonspecific response to irritation (from fatty acids, bile acids, laxatives, etc.) and should not be taken automatically to indicate inflammatory bowel disease. When the diagnosis is in doubt, a therapeutic trial of salazosulfapyridine may be of some help, although a trial of steroids is of little diagnostic value because they may ameliorate diarrhea of almost any cause by inducing a nonspecific increase in salt and water absorption.

My colleagues and I have recently found therapeutic trial of cholestyramine (Questran) particularly helpful in two patients who presented with diarrhea and severe urgency. Presumably, these patients had increased entry of bile acid into the colon or enhanced sensitivity to bile acids.

Irritable Bowel Syndrome. Many patients with small-volume diarrhea and no steatorrhea have the irritable bowel syndrome (IBS). The disorder may be diagnosed by means of a careful history and normal findings on physical examination and routine clinical investigation. A patient who has had recurrent bouts of small-volume diarrhea possibly alternating with constipation and usually associated with pain, but does not appear ill, has not lost weight, and does not have anemia or an elevated erythrocyte sedimentation rate is very likely to have IBS. It is of interest that diarrhea is a more common presentation of IBS in men than in women.

Manning and colleagues[20] reviewed 109 unselected patients referred to gastroenterology or surgical clinics. Symptoms that helped to discriminate patients with IBS from patients with organic disease were distension, relief of pain with bowel movement, and looser and more frequent bowel movements with the onset of pain. A sensation of incomplete evacuation, urgency, and the passage of mucus were also common in IBS. One criticism of this study was that very few patients with organic colonic disease were included, so it is possible that the symptoms "characteristic" of IBS merely discriminated "colonic disease" from disease elsewhere in the abdomen.

Food Intolerance. In one recent study, approximately two-thirds of patients with diarrhea diagnosed as having IBS could be shown to be intolerant to specific food materials because their symptoms returned when these foods were reintroduced into their diets.[21] Thus, food intolerance may well be a more common cause of moderate diarrhea than previously realized. One particularly well-documented food intolerance is caused by lactase deficiency, in which the unabsorbed lactose overwhelms the capacity for colonic salvage. Most people lose their lactase enzyme shortly after weaning; in such patients, ingestion of milk products may produce a mild diarrhea. Moreover, a relative lactose intolerance may develop de novo after a nonspecific gastroenteritis. Lactase deficiency is simply diagnosed by carrying out an oral lactose tolerance test or by measuring the increased breath hydrogen response to an oral lactose load.[22] An increase in intake of nonstarch polysaccharides as part of a slimming regimen (the "F Plan" diet) may increase the colonic load of carbohydrate and lead to diarrhea in susceptible individuals. A colleague of mine has investigated a fitness fanatic whose 700-gm stool was composed almost entirely of undigested bran. Other workers have reported diarrhea related to overingestion of sorbitol, a poorly absorbed sweetener often added to chewing gum and diabetic confections.

Anal Sphincter Dysfunction. Urgency and fecal incontinence are extremely common symptoms in patients with diarrhea, although they will not often volunteer this information spontaneously. Failure to appreciate this common problem and failure to measure stool weight may result in extensive and inappropriate investigation. We have found that measuring the leakage during rectal infusion of 1500 ml of saline provides a useful objective index of the efficiency of the anal continence mechanism in patients with diarrhea.[7]

REFERENCES

1. Rambaud JC, Modigliani R, Emonts P, et al. Fluid secretion in the duodenum and intestinal handling of water and electrolytes in Zollinger-Ellison syndrome. Am J Dig Dis 1978;23:1089–97.
2. Binder HJ. Pathophysiology of bile acid and fatty acid–induced diarrhea. In: Field M, Fordtran JS, Schultz SG, eds. Secretory diarrhea (American Physiological Society. Clinical Physiology Ser. No. 707). Baltimore: Williams & Wilkins, 1980; 159–78.
3. Bieberdorf FA, Gorden P, Fordtran JS. Pathogenesis of congenital alkalosis and diarrhoea. Implications for the physiology of normal ileal absorption and secretion. J Clin Invest 1972;51:1958–64.
4. Cummings JA. Short chain fatty acids in the human colon. Gut 1981;22:763–79.
5. Read NW. Diarrhoea. The failure of colonic salvage. Lancet 1982;2:481–3.
6. Mogg GAG, Keighley MRB, Burdon DW, et al. Antibiotic associated colitis—a review of 66 cases. Br J Surg 1979;66:738–42.
7. Read NW, Harford WV, Schmulen AC, Read MG, Santa-Ana CA, Fordtran JS. A clinical study of patients with fecal incontinence and diarrhea. Gastroenterology 1979;76:747–56.
8. Holdsworth CD. Drug-induced diarrhoea. Prescribers J 1980;20:131–6.
9. Seppala K, Hyelt L, Sipponen P. Colonoscopy in the diagnoses of antibiotic associated colitis. Scand J Gastroenterol 1981;16:465–8.
10. Anthonisen P, Riis P. A new diagnostic approach to mucosal inflammation in proctocolitis. Lancet 1961;2:81–4.
11. Losowsky MS, Walker BE, Kelleher J, eds. Malabsorption in clinical practice. Edinburgh and London: Churchill Livingstone, 1974.
12. Krejs GT, Fordtran JS. Diarrhea. In Sleisenger MH, Fordtran JS, eds., Gastrointestinal disease. 3rd ed. Philadelphia: WB Saunders, 1983;257–77.
13. James O. The Lundh test. Gut 1973;14:582–91.
14. James OFW, Agnew JE, Bouchier IAD. Assessment of the ^{14}C glycocholic acid breath test. Br Med J 1973;111: 191–5.
15. King CE, Toskes PP, Guilarte TR, Lorenz E, Welkos SL. Comparison of the one-gram d (^{14}C) xylose breath test with the (^{14}C) bile acid breath test in patients with small intestine bacterial overgrowth. Dig Dis Sci 1980;25:53–8.
16. Metz G, Gassull MA, Drasar BS, Jenkins DJA, Blendis LM. Breath hydrogen test for small intestinal colonisation. Lancet 1976;1:668–9.
17. Read NW, Read MG, Krejs GJ, Hendler RS, Davis G, Fordtran JS. A report of five patients with large-volume secretory diarrhea but no evidence of endocrine tumour or laxative abuse. Dig Dis Sci 1982;27:193–201.
18. Morris AI, Turuberg LA. Surreptitious laxative abuse. Gastroenterology 1979;77:780–6.
19. Read NW, Krejs GJ, Read MG, Sant-Ana CA, Morawski SG, Fordtran JS. Chronic diarrhea of unknown origin. Gastroenterology 1980;78:264–71.
20. Manning AP, Thompson WG, Heaton KW, Morris AF. Towards a positive diagnosis of the irritable bowel. Br Med J 1978;2:653–4.
21. Alun-Jones V, McLaughlan P, Shorthouse M, Workman E, Hunter JO. Food intolerance a major factor in the pathogenesis of irritable bowel syndrome. Lancet 1982;2:1115–7.
22. Metz G, Jenkins DJA, Peters TJ, Newman A, Blendis LM. Breath hydrogen as a diagnostic method for hypolactasia, Lancet 1975;1:1155–7.

DYSPHAGIA

JOSEPH W. GRIFFIN, JR.

□ SYNONYM: Swallowing dysfunction

BACKGROUND

Dysphagia, simply defined as "difficulty in swallowing," may arise from interference with the swallowing act due to multiple causes, including disease at any site from the oropharynx to the esophagogastric junction. Dysphagia is always related to the swallowing act, and the complaint indicates a pathologic process, either intrinsic or extrinsic to the oropharynx and esophagus. Thus, thorough evaluation is mandatory.

The act of swallowing is a very complex physiologic event with both voluntary and involuntary components. The oral phase is voluntary and consists of positioning and delivering a bolus of mouth contents to the oropharynx. As the bolus arrives at the back of the throat, the involuntary phase is activated by sensory receptors, resulting in deglutition and the initiation of the esophageal primary peristaltic wave.[1] Detailed review of the control and function of pharyngoesophageal neuromuscular activity is beyond the scope of this chapter, but a basic understanding of anatomy and physiology of the esophagus is necessary to interpret clinical signs and symptoms.

Anatomy

The esophagus is a muscular tube extending an average of 20 to 22 cm from the inferior border of the cricopharyngeus muscle through the posterior mediastinum to the gastric cardia at or just below the diaphragmatic hiatus. The proximal esophageal muscle is a continuation of pharyngeal striated muscle, with a transition to smooth muscle occurring at the approximate junction of the upper and middle thirds of the esophagus. At the most proximal border of the esophagus is the upper esophageal sphincter (UES), composed primarily of the cricopharyngeus muscle. The UES is a 2- to 4-cm segment of contracted muscle with a basal pressure of about 100 mm Hg in the anterior posterior direction, which keeps the entrance into the esophagus closed in the resting state. Upon swallowing, the upper sphincter promptly relaxes and allows the swallowed bolus to be propelled into the esophagus. The primary peristaltic wave initiated by swallowing reaches the lower esophageal sphincter (LES) in 5 to 6 seconds. At rest the LES is also closed, creating a zone of high pressure extending a length of 2 to 4 cm with an average pressure of 15 to 25 mm Hg. The LES is a much less distinct anatomic muscular structure than the UES, but the high-pressure zone of the LES is easily detected by manometry. Upon swallowing the LES relaxes, reducing pressure to intragastric levels, and remains relaxed for 5 to 10 seconds, allowing the propelled bolus to progress through the sphincter. The LES contracts with the arrival of the peristaltic wave, which delivers the bolus into the stomach, and then completes the cycle by resuming its basal state of elevated pressure.[2]

The mucosa of the esophagus is stratified squamous epithelium with no secretory activity except for a scant amount of mucus produced from scattered small mucus glands in the submucosa.

Function

The esophagus serves as a conduit for swallowed secretions, liquid, and food to be transported from the pharynx to the stomach. The esophagus has no absorptive or significant secretory function and differs from all the other alimentary tract structures in humans in that it has a single, yet complex muscular transport function.

CLASSIFICATION OF DYSPHAGIA

Table 1 divides conditions producing dysphagia into two basic categories: (1) transfer or oropharyngeal and (2) transport or esophageal disorders. The likelihood that a specific disease process is the cause of the patient's dysphagia depends on multiple factors, especially age, sex, coexistent disease, duration of symptoms, and concomitant symptoms. However, it is important to know what diseases one should consider in the differential diagnosis when evaluating patients with dysphagia.

Table 1. CLASSIFICATION OF CAUSES OF DYSPHAGIA

Transfer-Oropharyngeal Causes	
Neuromuscular disorders	Cerebrovascular disease
	Multiple sclerosis
	Amyotrophic lateral sclerosis
	Parkinson's disease
	Pseudobulbar syndrome
	Bulbar poliomyelitis
	Myasthenia gravis
	Myotonic dystrophy
Collagen vascular disorders	Dermatomyositis-polymyositis
	Mixed disorders
Inflammatory disorders	Infectious pharyngitis
	Mass lesions of pharynx/larynx
	Acute thyroiditis
	Radiation injury
Myopathies of metabolic and endocrine disorders	Myxedema
	Thyrotoxicosis
	Alcoholism
	Diabetes
	Amyloidosis
Structural abnormalities	Zenker's diverticulum
	Cricopharyngeus dysfunction
	Tracheostomy
	Cervical osteophyte formation
Transport-Esophageal Causes	
Motility disorders	Achalasia
	Scleroderma
	Diffuse esophageal spasm
	Nonspecific motor dysfunction:
	Diverticuli
	Reflux esophagitis
	Systemic diseases
	Presbyesophagus
Mechanical narrowing	Tumors:
	Squamous carcinoma
	Adenocarcinoma (association with Barrett's epithelium)
	Gastric fundal carcinoma
	Benign tumors
	Peptic strictures
	Rings and webs
	Vascular lesions
Miscellaneous causes	Infectious esophagitis
	Caustic ingestion
	Systemic diseases
	Postoperative conditions:
	Truncal vagotomy
	Antireflux surgery
	Metastatic carcinoma

Conditions Producing Transfer Dysphagia

Neuromuscular Disorders

A wide variety of neurologic and neuromuscular conditions can affect swallowing. Weakness of the striated musculature involved in initiating swallowing, failure of closure of the nasopharynx and larynx, or failure of UES relaxation may result from such conditions. Usually the primary condition is evident. Dysphagia, as one of the manifestations of the listed disorders, may occur with a frequency of 50 per cent or greater.[3]

Collagen Vascular Disorders

Dermatomyositis and polymyositis predominantly involve the striated muscles; therefore, pharyngeal and upper esophageal muscular weakness is responsible for transfer dysphagia in affected patients. The mixed collagen vascular or "overlap" syndromes may affect both striated muscle and smooth muscle, producing both transfer and transport dysphagia.

Inflammatory Disorders

Acute infectious pharyngitis is common and may produce sufficient pain and edema to interfere temporarily with swallowing. Carcinoma of the larynx, peritonsillar abscess, mumps, acute thyroiditis, and radiation injury are less common causes of inflammatory conditions leading to transfer dysphagia.

Myopathies

Chronic metabolic and endocrine diseases may cause transfer dysphagia similar to that caused by neuromuscular disorders. Frequently, smooth muscle activity is also found to be affected when these patients are studied manometrically. Diabetics and alcoholics may show significant manometric disorders of esophageal motility in conjunction with neuropathies, but these patients may not complain of swallowing difficulties.

Structural Disorders

Dysphagia is associated with a hypopharyngeal diverticulum (Zenker's diverticulum) that occurs in elderly patients (average age more than 70 years). However, such patients may also complain of a throat irritation, a recurrent cough, or a bulge at the side of the neck that decreases in size in association with regurgitation of food and mucus. Aspiration may occur, and if the pouch enlarges sufficiently, obstruction of the proximal esophagus develops. Idiopathic dysfunction of the cricopharyngeus muscle with inadequate or incomplete opening results in dysphagia and is suspected when typical transfer dysphagia is present and no associated neurologic, degenerative, or inflammatory conditions are found. The term cricopharyngeal achalasia is used (by radiologists usually) to describe an incomplete relaxation of the muscle with a horizontal indentation or esophageal bar. Manometric studies frequently do not correlate with the radiographic findings because they do not document abnormal pressures, failure of relaxation on swallowing, or any other abnormalities.[4] Patients with previous tracheostomy or severe cervical osteophyte formation may have dysphagia, which is clinically indistinguishable from cricopharyngeal dysfunction.

Conditions Producing Transport (Esophageal) Dysphagia

Transport dysphagia is caused by abnormal progression of swallowed liquids or solids through the esophagus and into the stomach. Two major classes of diseases are motility disorders and lesions that mechanically narrow the esophageal lumen.

Motility Disorders

Achalasia is the classic primary esophageal motor disorder. It occurs at all ages, most commonly between 20 and 40 years, and affects men and women equally. Achalasia is not a common disease, having an incidence of 1 to 2 per 100,000 population, but referral centers may diagnose five to ten new cases per year. The features of achalasia that lead to dysphagia are: (1) absence of peristalsis due to lack of ganglion cells, (2) elevation of LES pressure above 30 mm Hg (usually three to five times normal), producing a functional obstruction and giving the condition the older name of cardiospasm, and (3) failure of the LES to relax adequately with swallowing.[5]

Patients with primary systemic sclerosis (scleroderma) frequently have involvement of the smooth muscle of the distal esophagus and develop a motor disorder characterized by absence of peristalsis in the lower two-thirds of the esophagus and an abnormally low LES pressure. Skin changes and Raynaud's phenomenon are often present when the esophagus is involved in scleroderma.[6] Affected patients develop dysphagia after a significant history of heartburn from chronic gastroesophageal reflux and failure to clear refluxed gastric acid because of loss of peristalsis. A peptic stricture is the usual cause of the dysphagia, but symptoms are aggravated by the abnormal distal peristalsis.

Diffuse esophageal spasm (DES) is a motility disorder of unknown cause characterized by abnormal segmental contractions of the esophageal muscle, which interfere with normal peristalsis and produce functional obstruction of the esophagus. Several patterns of abnormal muscular contractions are reported in DES, including repetitive contractions after a single swallow or spontaneously occurring repetitive contractions; simultaneous, nonperistaltic waves; and contractions of excessive amplitude (>200 mm Hg) or of excessively long duration (>7 seconds). About one-third of DES patients may also have abnormally elevated pressures in the lower esophageal sphincter and may also demonstrate incomplete relaxation of the LES, findings similar to those in achalasia. The latter variant of diffuse spasm has been termed vigorous achalasia.[7] An unusual form of esophageal spasm associated with syncope on swallowing is believed to be due to vagotonia and bradycardia. Long-term follow-up of patients with motility disorders has shown a few instances of transition from diffuse spasm to achalasia with corresponding changes in symptoms. This observation has led some authors to propose that symptomatic motility disorders represent a broad group of related esophageal motor disorders, with achalasia and diffuse spasm representing the opposite ends of the spectrum.[8]

Nonspecific motility disorders are frequently suspected in patients with epiphrenic (at or just above the esophagogastric junction and commonly known as pulsion type) or midesophageal (more commonly referred to as traction type) esophageal diverticuli. Patients may be asymptomatic or may have pain and dysphagia related to the underlying motor disorder, which is most commonly diffuse spasm or a variant of DES. Multiple diseases, including reflux esophagitis, diabetes, alcoholism, and senile dementia, may cause nonspecific abnormalities such as low-amplitude contractions and nonperistaltic tertiary waves commonly called presbyesophagus. The significance of these nonspecific motility abnormalities in patients without dysphagia is unknown, and certainly no diagnosis can be made in asymptomatic patients.

Mechanical Narrowing

Conditions that anatomically compromise the esophageal lumen may be intrinsic or extrinsic. Squamous carcinoma of the esophagus is the most serious of the obstructing lesions, accounting for 95 per cent of all esophageal cancers. Cancer occurs predominantly in men (ratio 3:1), and the 5-year survival rate is only 4 per cent.[9] Worldwide there are marked variations in the incidence of esophageal cancer; rates of 50 to 130 per 100,000 population are reported in parts of China, Russia, and Iran, but only 15 per 100,000 for black males and four per 100,000 for white males in the United States.[10] Alcohol, smoking, lye strictures, and achalasia are predisposing factors. Barrett's epithelium, an area of gastric-type mucosa in the esophagus associated with long-standing gastroesophageal reflux, predisposes to adenocarcinoma of the esophagus. A malignancy that occurs in the gastric cardia may cause dysphagia by obstructing the esophagogastric junction or by spreading submucosally up the esophagus, destroying the ganglion cells. In the latter case, the esophagus will become aperistaltic and distally dilated, and the clinical presentation and radiographic appearance closely resemble those of achalasia.

Benign tumors of the esophagus are uncommon. Even leiomyoma, the most common of these conditions, is relatively rare. Dysphagia occurs infrequently even in large tumors (3 to 4 cm) because of their submucosal location. Leiomyomas are detected in asymptomatic patients when an upper GI series or endoscopy is performed for other indications. Hemorrhage from leiomyoma of the esophagus is most unusual, and malignant degeneration is no real concern.

Peptic strictures develop in the esophagus owing to fibrosis and scarring after long-term inflammation and ulceration due to chronic reflux of gastric secretions onto the esophageal squamous mucosa. The major factor in the pathogenesis of gastroesophageal reflux is an incompetent lower esophageal sphincter.[11] The sliding hiatal hernia, although not causing gastroesophageal reflux, is very commonly associated with it. Many patients have been told that they have a hiatal hernia that is causing symptoms when, in fact, no gastroesophageal reflux is present. The LES may be very competent even when displaced several centimeters into the thorax by hiatal hernia. Reflux may induce esophageal spasm, and dysphagia can be present without fixed luminal narrowing in peptic esophagitis. Another factor in the development of benign strictures is the use of nasogastric tubes, which increases gastroesophageal reflux and potentiates acid-pepsin mucosal injury. As the dysphagia becomes more severe in patients with stricture formation, the heartburn may improve significantly as the stricture forms a barrier for both refluxed and swallowed material.

Periodic dysphagia for solids is a primary characteristic of luminal narrowing due to a mucosal ring at the anatomic esophagogastric junction. A hiatal hernia is also invariably associated. The lesion, known best as a Schatzki's ring, produces episodes of obstruction when the internal diameter of the lumen at the ring is less than 12 to 13 mm. Rings are a rather common finding on upper GI x-rays, occurring in 6 to 14 per cent of reported series,[12] but symptomatic rings are much less common. Dysphagia due to webs is also intermittent and only for solids. The postcricoid web associated with chronic iron and other nutritional deficiencies is known as Plummer-Vinson or Paterson-Kelly syndrome. It is decreasing in frequency in the

United States as women have fewer pregnancies and are routinely given prenatal vitamins and minerals. Plummer-Vinson syndrome is important primarily because it is associated with an increased risk of squamous carcinoma of the esophagus and hypopharynx. The dysphagia may often disappear with iron therapy and repletion of other nutritional deficiencies without disrupting the web. Thus, the genesis of dysphagia in Plummer-Vinson syndrome is unclear. Asymptomatic webs do occur, and one series reported a 5.5 per cent detection rate for postcricoid webs in 1,000 consecutive cineradiographic studies. Only six patients had symptoms thought to be related to the web, and one fulfilled the criteria necessary for the diagnosis of Plummer-Vinson syndrome.[13]

Dysphagia may occur because of extrinsic pressure from vascular structures when an aberrant right subclavian artery or other vascular anomaly compresses the esophagus. The lesion is known as dysphagia lusoria, and as a rule other cardiovascular abnormalities are present.[14] The first manifestation of a thoracic aortic aneurysm rarely is dysphagia due to compression of the esophagus. Exsanguinating hemorrhage with rupture of the aneurysm into the esophagus can occur.

Miscellaneous Conditions

Infectious esophagitis is an important cause of dysphagia, especially monilial and herpetic infections. The onset is abrupt, with odynophagia (painful swallowing) predominating. The patient may complain of oral lesions or may not have any extra-esophageal involvement. Prime candidates for candida esophagitis include patients who are immunosuppressed, those on antibiotics or corticosteroids, and diabetics. The candida infection disrupts the esophageal mucosa with invasion of organisms.[15] Herpes simplex esophagitis can coexist with candida infection or can occur alone in patients with similar underlying diseases. Herpes simplex esophagitis can produce severe symptoms in otherwise healthy young adults, and dehydration may develop because of the severe odynophagia.[16] Complications of infectious esophagitis are uncommon but include systemic dissemination of the infection, bleeding, and esophageal obstruction or perforation.

Ingestion of caustic agents, either accidental or suicidal, produces intense burning of the mouth and chest. An inability to swallow ensues, and extensive esophageal injury leads to bleeding, necrosis, and possibly death. Diagnosis is usually not a problem, but determination of the caustic agent and extent of injury is of paramount importance. The patient surviving the acute insult frequently develops strictures, and dilatation with mercury-filled bougies is performed early in an attempt to prevent stricture formation.

The esophagus can be involved in numerous systemic illnesses causing dysphagia. Crohn's disease, sarcoidosis, Behçet's disease, pemphigoid, and epidermolysis bullosa are conditions that have primary manifestations in other organ systems but can affect the esophagus.[17, 18] An occasional patient who has undergone truncal vagotomy will experience dysphagia in the immediate postoperative period. Symptoms are similar to those of strictures, and distal narrowing may be demonstrated on x-rays. Usually the dysphagia is temporary and responds to bougienage. Disorders of motility have been documented in the postvagotomy state and may contribute to the dysphagia. Similarly, patients who have undergone fundoplication operations for reflux esophagitis may have postoperative dysphagia because of narrowing of the very distal esophageal lumen by the gastric wrap. The dysphagia typically is temporary and usually responds to bougienage.

The esophagus can occasionally be the site of metastatic malignancy with dysphagia resulting from significant obstruction by intraluminal masses or extrinsic encircling growths. The most common sources of esophageal metastasis are breast, lung, and oat cell carcinoma and the leukemias and lymphomas.

HISTORY

Diseases of the esophagus produce characteristic symptoms that usually allow the physician to form a correct initial "impression" and to localize the disease site. In development of the present illness, careful questioning will reveal the presence of one symptom or, more usually, a constellation of symptoms, that allows the physician to "fit" the case into one of the two major classifications of dysphagia, transfer and transport. Often, further categorization into one of the subgroups is possible because of rather specific symptoms produced by particular lesions.

Symptoms of Transfer Dysphagia

The disruption of orderly transfer of mouth contents into the upper esophagus may result in misdirection of the bolus with nasal or oral regurgitation, often with a forceful spraying of the mouth contents. Aspiration into the upper trachea is common, and the patient gags, sputters, and then coughs. Aspiration pneumonia may occur and may actually be the reason that the patient seeks medical care. Liquids are more likely to be aspirated in oropharyngeal dysphagia than solids. Another symptom of transfer dysphagia may be a frank inability to initiate swallowing or the need to make repeated efforts prior to a successful swallow. Patients may carry a cup in which to spit their saliva when transfer dysphagia is severe. Because of the nature of the problem, weight loss and malnutrition are common. The underlying neuromuscular or cerebral disease is obvious in many of these patients, but the relationship of dysphagia to the primary disease process may not be appreciated. The patient with an organic brain syndrome may be unable to give an adequate history, and the presenting complaint may be weight loss or aspiration pneumonia, with the patient and family not initially reporting that there is difficulty swallowing.

Symptoms of Transport Dysphagia

Transport (esophageal) dysphagia results when there is abnormal progression of swallowed liquids or solids down the esophagus and into the stomach. The swallowing act is initiated normally, but shortly thereafter (2 to 5 seconds), the bolus "sticks," "catches," "doesn't go down right," or "just stops." Substernal fullness without severe pain is usual except in diffuse spasm, in which the pain may be the predominant symptom.

Motility Disorders

Characteristically, motor disorders such as achalasia cause liquid and solid food dysphagia. Achalasia patients do not complain of heartburn, whereas scleroderma patients have a long history of severe heartburn. Regurgitation in motor disorders is frequent. Patients may report finding their pillows or nightclothes soiled during the night by regurgitated food eaten many hours previously. In achalasia, aspiration and weight loss may develop as the dysphagia slowly worsens. The esophageal colic seen in diffuse esophageal spasm may be a severe pressure or a crushing substernal chest pain similar to the pain of angina or myocardial infarction. The location, pattern of radiation, and duration of esophageal colic also mimics cardiovascular pain. Diffuse esophageal spasm is frequently associated with eating, and the patient may be aware of certain triggering factors such as iced alcoholic or carbonated drinks. Stress may also be an important predisposing factor.[19]

Mechanical Narrowing

Obstructing lesions such as cancer and strictures produce progressive dysphagia. The initial complaint is difficulty in swallowing meats, dry breads, and apples, and then the dysphagia progresses to include all solids. Cancers cause rapid progression of symptoms over weeks to a few months, whereas benign strictures may progress so slowly that patients are unable to recall the onset of symptoms. Again, the history of heartburn is an important differential point, as it is generally much more prominent in the patient with a peptic stricture. Sensitivity to acidic foods or liquids such as citrus and tomato juices is common in patients with peptic esophagitis and is usually absent in patients with malignant obstruction. Weight loss occurs in progressive dysphagia from both malignant and benign causes but is much more pronounced in the patient with cancer.

Intermittent dysphagia for solids only is characteristic of esophageal rings. The patient classically experiences difficulty while eating steak, so the condition has been labeled the "steakhouse syndrome."[12] He or she will note that a bolus is stuck or lodged in the subxiphoid area and will attempt to relieve the obstruction by straightening or arching the back, standing, or drinking water. If unsuccessful, the patient may leave the table, induce regurgitation in the restroom, and then return to finish the meal without difficulty. The next episode may not occur for weeks or months, and because of the intermittent nature of the symptoms, progressive dysphagia and weight loss are most unusual in patients with Schatzki's ring. When the episodes become more frequent and begin to interfere with the patient's lifestyle, he or she reports to the physician appearing quite healthy but often very anxious about having underlying cancer. Dysphagia due to webs is also intermittent and only for solids.

Painful swallowing is characteristic of infectious esophagitis because of disruption of the mucosa. The onset is generally abrupt; the pain is worse for solids than for liquids, but the patient may refuse to swallow anything because of severe discomfort. In these conditions, the esophagus may be extremely sensitive to acidic substances. Although patients who have been taking broad-spectrum antibiotics are very likely to have candida esophagitis, the sudden onset of dysphagia or odynophagia in the patient taking tetracycline may be caused by an esophageal ulcer. Ascorbic acid has also been reported to cause an isolated esophageal ulcer with dysphagia and odynophagia. In these medication-induced ulcers, the patient commonly reports that the pills are swallowed while in bed with only a sip of water, and delayed passage through the esophagus with prolonged mucosal contact time has been documented.[20]

On the basis of three characteristics—liquid or solid dysphagia, intermittent or progressive symptoms, and presence or absence of heartburn—it is often possible to decide which of the major causes of transport dysphagia is the likely diagnosis. Furthermore, if a patient is able to localize a site of difficulty to some point along the sternum, there is very good correlation with the anatomic

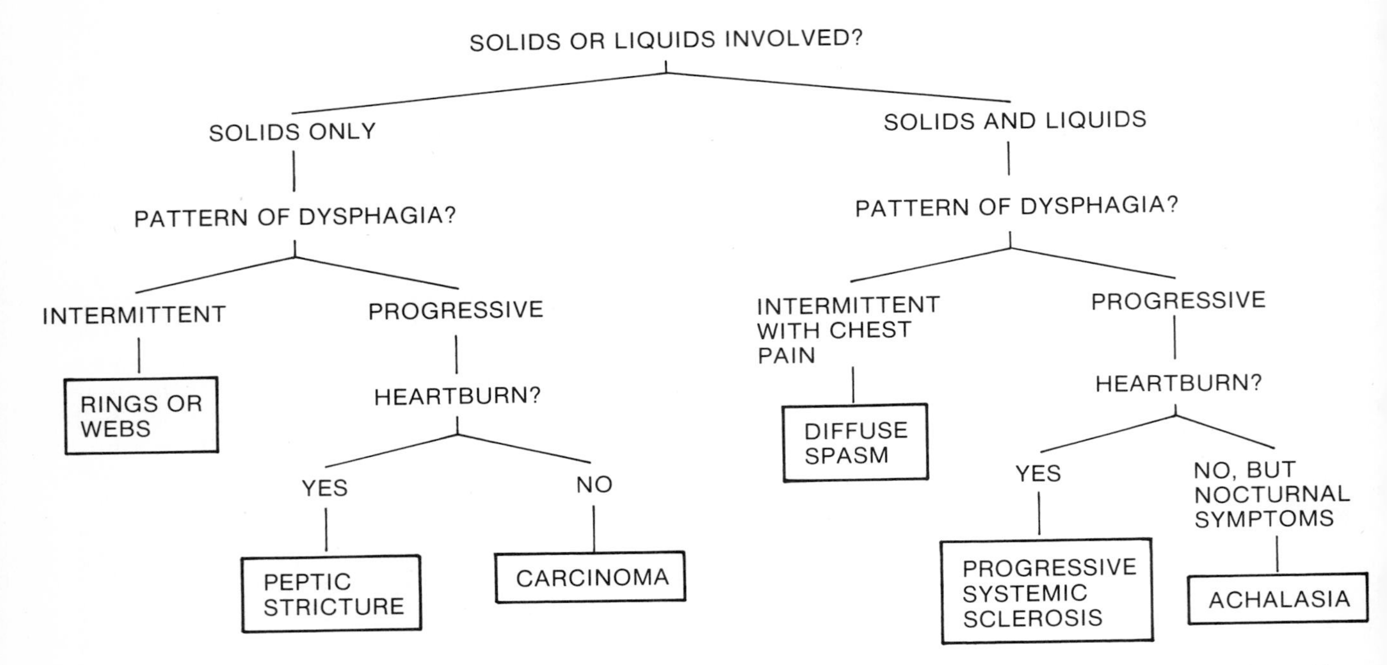

site of the disease process. Lesions arising from any location in the esophagus may produce symptoms that are referred to the suprasternal notch, however, and there is no correlation with the site of obstruction.

The algorithm demonstrates diagnosis based on historic aspects of the more common causes of transport dysphagia.*

Symptoms That Do Not Indicate Esophageal Disease

There are numerous presenting symptoms that do not arise from the esophagus, although patients may interpret them as difficulty in swallowing. The most common is a persistent lump in the throat that may be exaggerated by swallowing, known as globus hystericus. The fact that the lump is always present clearly differentiates the patient with this disorder from the patients with symptoms occurring only with or within a few seconds of swallowing. Likewise, a continuous "knot" type of discomfort under the sternum or at the xiphoid that is not associated with dysphagia is unlikely to be of esophageal origin. Excessive belching is rarely associated with esophageal or gastric stasis and usually is a manifestation of aerophagia. Other symptoms that a patient may relate to the upper GI tract but that do not have any specificity (and usually no clinical significance) include hypersalivation, a burning tongue, halitosis, and a bitter taste in the mouth.[22]

*The algorithm is adapted from Cattau EL, Castell DO. Symptoms of esophageal dysfunction. Adv Intern Med 1982; 27:151–81.

PHYSICAL EXAMINATION

The patient with dysphagia should be examined thoroughly, but the yield of diagnostic findings is not high. General appearance and weight for comparison with those on previous examination are obviously important. A careful palpation for cervical and supraclavicular nodes and thyromegaly is performed, as well as testing of the full range of neck motion. Careful auscultation is done for neck bruits, and facial muscle and cranial nerves are examined in patients with symptoms suggesting neuromuscular causes of dysphagia. The chest examination is important to exclude pulmonary complications. The most important aspect of the physical examination in patients with dysphagia is observing the patient's swallow. Having the patient drink water will suffice when transfer dysphagia is suspected, but watching a patient eat solid food may be necessary to gain some better understanding of transport dysphagia. Examination for occult blood in the stool is also necessary.

ASSESSMENT

The diagnostic modalities available for assessment of dysphagia include radiology, manometry, and endoscopy. Routine laboratory testing is not helpful in the evaluation of dysphagia per se, but suspicion of a systemic disease requires hematologic, chemical, or immunologic studies to adequately define such a disorder and confirm its presence.

Diagnostic Imaging

Radiologic evaluation is the initial method of investigation in patients with dysphagia, and the radiologist should be completely informed of the suspected pathology. The primary physician must assume the responsibility of properly informing the radiologist either by providing complete information on the x-ray request form or by speaking to the consultant. The diagnostic yield of a barium esophagogram is significantly diminished when a technologist perfunctorily performs the studies and the radiologist views the films only at the completion of the examination. Chest, cervical spine, and soft tissue x-rays of the neck can be extremely important studies in selected cases, but usually the barium swallow is the examination initially requested. Stewart[23] recommends that esophageal x-rays routinely accomplish the following: direct observation of pharyngeal and esophageal motility; some assessment of both the upper and the lower esophageal sphincters; morphologic evaluation of the esophagus for stricture, dilatation, mass, and displacement; detection of the presence or absence of hiatal hernia; and observation of gastroesophageal reflux and its order of magnitude. In transfer dysphagia and motility disorders, cine or video recording of the barium swallow allows repeated viewing of the swallowing mechanism, cricopharyngeal function, and peristaltic activity. Lateral projections of the hypopharynx and cervical area are especially helpful in the evaluation of transfer dysphagia. Figure 1 demonstrates cricopharyngeal dysfunction in a patient with severe transfer dysphagia.

Transport dysphagia requires study of the peristaltic striping waves and careful attention to the passage of the barium column in both recumbent and upright positions. The use of a solid bolus such as a marshmallow or a 12-mm compressed barium tablet adds significantly to the assessment of normal or abnormal esophageal motility. The solid bolus also tends to impact or catch on a narrowing or intraluminal growth, allowing vivid demonstration of malignant and benign structures, rings, and webs, although liquid barium may pass rapidly and unhindered.[23] Radiographic findings can be diagnostic in both motility disorders and mechanical obstruction, but superficial or small mucosal lesions may go undetected. Double-contrast techniques in the esophagus result in an increased rate of diagnosis of these smaller lesions.[24] The correlation of the radiographic findings with the patient's symptoms remains the responsibility of the primary physician, and often a "nonstenotic" or "nonspecific" abnormality demands further investigation because of the clinical presentation. Figures 2 to 5 demonstrate typical radiographic findings in achalasia, cancer, a long benign stricture, and Schatzki's ring. Radiographic studies performed meticulously and with careful attention to subtle changes remain the primary means of assessing dysphagia.

Manometry

If motility disorders are suspected on the basis of the history or are demonstrated radiographically, esophageal manometry is the next step in assessment. The patient usually must be referred to a gastroenterologist for this study. Current catheter assembly and transducer technology allow excellent assessment of the pressures and integrity of the upper and lower esophageal sphincters, peristalsis in both striated and smooth muscle segments of the esophagus, and pressure generated by muscular contractions.[25] Manometry is the preferred method of confirming the diagnosis in achalasia, scleroderma involving the esophagus, and diffuse esophageal spasm. Characteristic findings have been discussed previously and are summarized in Table 2. Manometry is

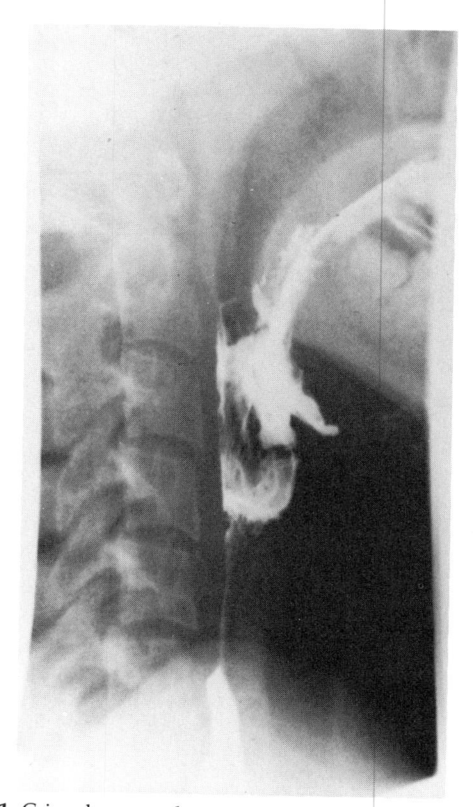

Figure 1. Cricopharyngeal spasm (UES "achalasia") in a patient with transfer dysphagia.

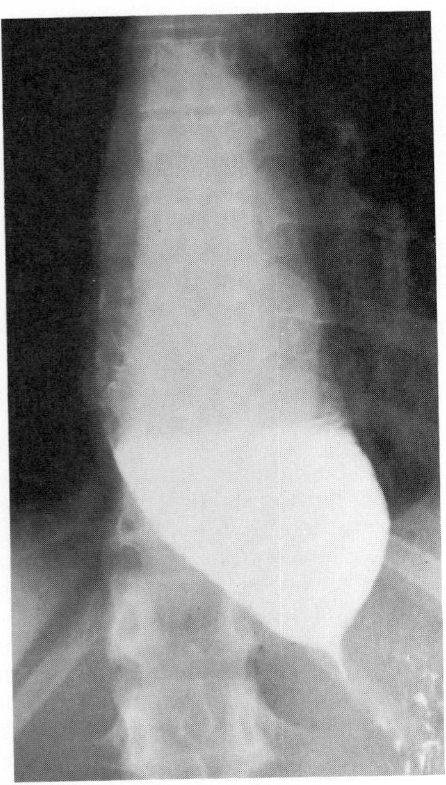

Figure 2. Grossly dilated aperistaltic esophagus with terminal beaking, classic for achalasia.

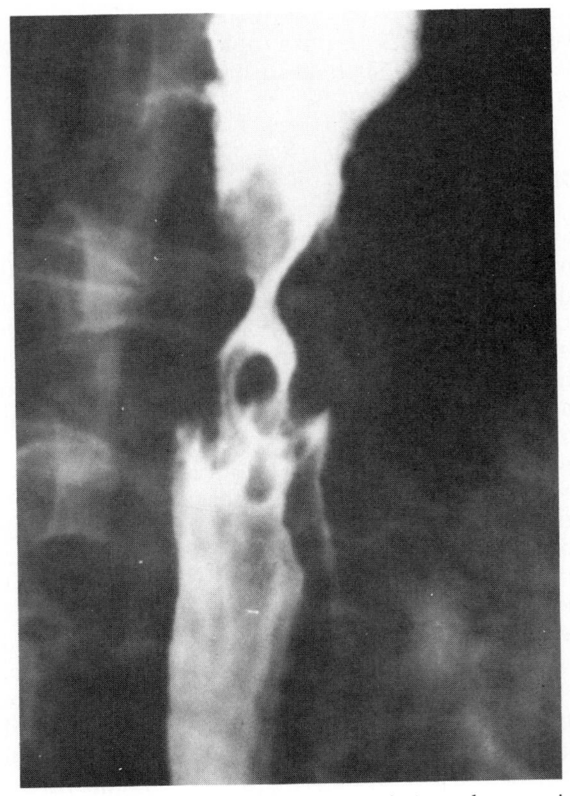

Figure 3. Cancer in midesophagus with irregular margins, destruction of mucosa, and narrowing of the lumen by the mass.

Table 2. MANOMETRIC AND RADIOGRAPHIC FEATURES OF COMMON MOTILITY DISORDERS

Disorder	Peristalsis	Lower Esophageal Sphincter	Response to Pharmacologic Agents	Radiologic Features
Achalasia	Absent throughout	Pressure elevated above 30 mm Hg, often 3–5 × normal Failure to completely relax with swallowing	Cholinergic drugs: classic "denervation response"	Chest x-ray: widened mediastinum with air-fluid level, no gastric air bubble Barium swallow: dilatation, no peristalsis, terminal beaking No GE reflux
Scleroderma	Absent or of low amplitude in distal ⅔	Very low pressure, perhaps undetectable	Cholinergic drugs: none to minimal increase in distal contractions and LES pressure	Barium swallow: normal proximal motility No peristalsis in lower ⅔ Free GE reflux Distal stricture
Diffuse esophageal spasm	Variable; very disordered; simultaneous, repetitive, or spontaneous contractions High amplitude (above 200 mm Hg) Long duration (more than 7 sec)	Variable; elevated in "vigorous achalasia"	Cholinergic drugs: variable, similar to that in achalasia Nitrates: decrease in amplitude and duration of contractions	Barium swallow: segmental tertiary contractions or generalized "corkscrew" appearance with pseudodiverticula No dilatation or terminal beaking

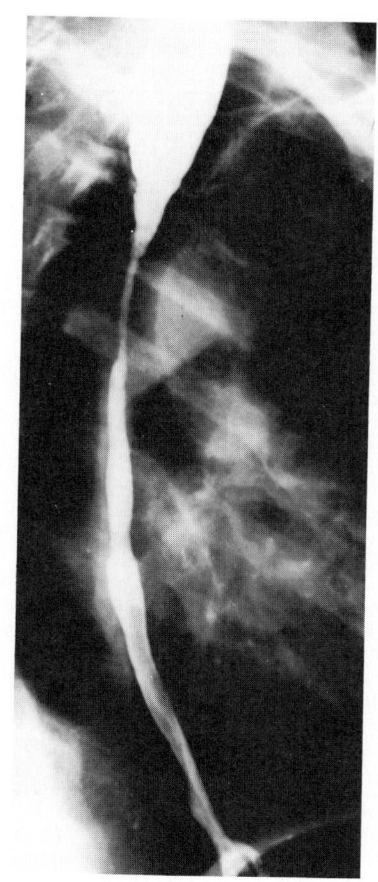

Figure 4. Upper esophageal narrowing of a long benign stricture from caustic ingestion with smooth tapering margins. There is no evidence of a mass.

frequently of substantial benefit in detecting motility disorders in patients with Zenker's diverticulum and in symptomatic patients found to have midesophageal or epiphrenic diverticula. Therapeutic decisions regarding surgical resections of the diverticulum and myotomy can be made more rationally if an associated motor disturbance is demonstrated.

Patients undergoing manometry can also have additional tests to assist with diagnosis and to assess therapeutic efforts. The diagnosis of patients with angina-type chest pain of unclear etiology even after cardiac evaluation may be aided with the combination of acid perfusion of the esophageal body with 0.1N HCl (the Bernstein test) and manometry. In a study of 58 such patients given the Bernstein test, the esophagus was strongly implicated as a source of pain in 20 patients, suspected in 18 others, and cleared in 7.[26] Other pharmacologic provocative tests include the injection of bethanechol, edrophonium, ergonovine, and pentagastrin in selected instances. The effects of nitrates on motility and pain can be recorded at manometry and can be of significant assistance in diagnostic and therapeutic decisions.[27]

Endoscopy

Fiberoptic endoscopy is widely available, is easily performed, and is the best means of direct visual examination of the esophageal mucosa. It is particularly useful in transport dysphagia and odynophagia, even when barium esophagograms are normal. Biopsy, brush cytology, and aspiration of secretions and washings for culture or cytology are easily accomplished to confirm diagnoses of cancer, peptic esophagitis, benign strictures, Barrett's epithelium, and infections. Diagnostic accuracy exceeds 95 per cent in malignancy.[28] Improving survival in patients with esophageal cancer requires earlier diagnosis, and older individuals with recent onset of solid food dysphagia should undergo endoscopic evaluation regardless of x-ray findings. The patient with a stricture that prevented passage of the endoscope into the stomach must undergo repeat endoscopy following dilatation if a malignancy was not confirmed on the initial examination.

It is also recommended that endoscopy be performed in all patients with achalasia, even in cases with classic radiographic and manometric features. An occasional patient has a fundic malignancy that completely mimics the classic motor disorder.[29] Endoscopy is indicated early in caustic injury to evaluate the extent of esophageal damage. Can-

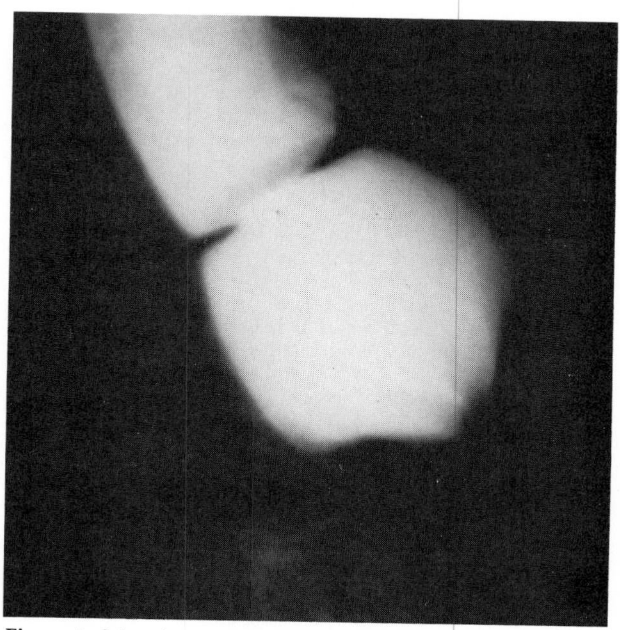

Figure 5. Schatzki's ring: symmetrical narrowing by concentric mucosal ring at esophagogastric junction. Note the associated hiatal hernia. A 12-mm barium tablet demonstrated significant delay in passing into the stomach.

cer surveillance in premalignant lesions such as Barrett's esophagus, lye stricture, and achalasia is best performed by endoscopy with multiple biopsies and cytology to assess premalignant microscopic changes in the mucosa. Occasionally, patients who exhibit classic globus hystericus require endoscopy for total reassurance that the esophagus is normal. Endoscopy yields less information than radiology about esophageal motility and extrinsic masses.

Fiberoptic endoscopy of the upper gastrointestinal tract is a very safe examination when performed by experienced endoscopists, but complications do occur at the rate of approximately 0.2 per cent. Many of the complications are related to pre-endoscopy medications, which usually consist of some combination of meperidine and diazepam. Rate of perforation of the hypopharynx or esophagus and hemorrhage was reported in one large survey to be 0.06 per cent; the mortality rate in perforation was 0.6 per cent.[30] With use of the pediatric or "skinny" endoscopes, skillful physicians perform endoscopy with minimal or no physical or emotional trauma to patients. Except in the most critically ill or uncooperative (unwilling) patient, endoscopy is usually required in the evaluation of dysphagia.

REFERENCES

1. Goyal RK, Cobb BN. Motility of the pharynx, esophagus and esophageal sphincters. In: Johnson LR, Christensen J, Grossman MI, Jacobsen ED, Schultz SG, eds. Physiology of the gastrointestinal tract. New York: Raven Press, 1981;1:359–91.
2. Hurwitz AL, Duranceau A, Haddad JK. Normal esophageal motility. In: Disorders of esophageal motility. Philadelphia: WB Saunders, 1979;14–26.
3. Hellemans J, Pelemans W, Vantrappen G. Pharyngoesophageal swallowing disorders and the pharyngoesophageal sphincter. Med Clin North Am 1981;65:1149–71.
4. Hurwitz AL, Nelson JA, Haddad JK. Oropharyngeal dysphagia: manometric and cine esophagographic findings. Am J Dig Dis 1975;20:313–24.
5. Pope CE II. Motor disorders. In: Sleisenger MH, Fordtran JS, eds. Gastrointestinal disease. 3rd ed. Philadelphia: WB Saunders, 1983;424–45.
6. Hurwitz AL, Duranceau A, Postlethwait RW. Esophageal dysfunction and Raynaud's phenomenon in patients with scleroderma. Am J Dig Dis 1976;21:601–6.
7. Castell DO. Achalasia and diffuse esophageal spasm. Arch Intern Med 1976;136:571–9.
8. Vantrappen G, Janssens J, Hellemans J, Coremans G. Achalasia, diffuse esophageal spasm, and related motility disorders. Gastroenterology 1979;76:450–7.
9. Silverberg E. Cancer statistics, 1983. CA 1983;33:9–25.
10. Day NE. Some aspects of the epidemiology of esophageal cancer. Cancer Res 1975;35:3304–7.
11. Cohen S, Snape WJ Jr. The pathophysiology and treatment of gastroesophageal reflux disease. Arch Intern Med 1978;138:1398–401.
12. Goyal RK, Glancy JJ, Spiro HM. Lower esophageal ring. N Engl J Med 1970;282:1298–350, 1355–62.
13. Nosher JL, Campbell WL, Seaman WB. The clinical significance of cervical esophageal and hypopharyngeal webs. Radiology 1975;117:45–7.
14. Berenzweig H, Baue AE, McCallum RW. Dysphagia lusoria: report of a case and review of the diagnostic and surgical approach. Dig Dis Sci 1980;25:630–6.
15. Kodsi BE, Wickremesinghe PC, Kozinn PJ, Iswara K, Goldberg PK. Candida esophagitis—a prospective study of 27 cases. Gastroenterology 1976;71:715–9.
16. Springer DJ, DaCosta LR, Beck IT. A syndrome of acute self-limiting ulcerative esophagitis in young adults probably due to herpes simplex virus. Dig Dis Sci 1979;24:535–9.
17. Mukhapadhyay AK, Graham DY. Esophageal motor dysfunction in systemic diseases. Arch Intern Med 1976;136:583–7.
18. Pope CE II. Involvement of the esophagus by infections, systemic illnesses, and physical agents. In: Sleisenger MH, Fordtran JS, eds. Gastrointestinal disease. 3rd ed. Philadelphia: WB Saunders, 1983;495–501.
19. Vantrappen G, Hellemans J. Oesophageal spasm and other muscular dysfunction. Clin Gastroenterol 1982;11:453–77.
20. Seaman WB. The case of the antibiotic dysphagia. Hosp Pract 1979;14:206–8.
21. Cattau EL, Castell DO. Symptoms of esophageal dysfunction. Adv Intern Med 1982;27:151–81.
22. Spiro HM. Clinical gastroenterology. 3rd ed. New York: Macmillan, 1983;19–21.
23. Stewart ET. Radiographic evaluation of the esophagus and its motor disorders. Med Clin North Am 1981;65:1173–94.
24. Montagne JP, Moss AA, Margulis AR. Double blind study of single and double contrast upper gastrointestinal examinations using endoscopy as a control. Am J Roentgenol 1978;130:1041–5.
25. Dodds WJ. Instrumentation and methods for intraluminal esophageal manometry. Arch Intern Med 1976;136:515–23.
26. Brand DL, Martin D, Pope CE II. Esophageal manometrics in patients with angina-like chest pain. Am J Dig Dis 1977;22:300–4.
27. Swamy N. Esophageal spasm: clinical and manometric response to nitroglycerine and long acting nitrates. Gastroenterology 1977;72:23–7.
28. Winawer SJ, Melamed M, Sherlock P. Potential of endoscopy, biopsy and cytology in the diagnosis and management of patients with cancer. Clin Gastroenterol 1976;5:575–95.
29. Tucker HJ, Snape WJ Jr, Cohen S. Achalasia secondary to carcinoma: manometric and clinical features. Ann Intern Med 1978;89:315–8.
30. Shakmir M, Schumen BM. Complications of fiberoptic endoscopy. Gastrointest Endosc 1980;26:86–91.

DYSTONIA

STANLEY FAHN

☐ SYNONYMS: Torsion dystonia, dystonia musculorum deformans

BACKGROUND

Definitions

Dystonic Movements and Dystonic Postures. There are several types of abnormal involuntary movements, including tremor, chorea, athetosis, tics, myoclonus, and dystonia. *Dystonic movements* are abnormal involuntary motions of a twisting nature (hence the use of the term torsion dystonia)[1] in which the peak of the movement is sustained for a second or longer.[2] If the duration of sustained contraction is minutes or longer, the ensuing posture is referred to as a *dystonic posture.* Such postures can last hours or days and may even be present during the entire waking day. Subsequent contractures and ankyloses can render the postures permanent. When severe, dystonic postures are present during sleep. Otherwise, sleep eliminates the involuntary movements in dystonia as it does in other types of movement disorders.

Action Dystonia. When dystonic movements occur in a part of the body only when that body part is voluntarily moving, the disorder is *action dystonia.* This is usually the manner by which primary dystonia first manifests itself, and it represents the earliest and mildest form of dystonic movement. Examples include twisting movements of a leg when the patient is walking but not sitting, abnormal contractions of the arm during handwriting but not when the arm is at rest, and abnormal contractions of the vocal cords when the patient is speaking. A more severe form of action dystonia is the development of dystonic movements elsewhere in the body during a voluntary movement of a body part. For example, during handwriting or while speaking, there may be dystonic movements of the trunk, neck, face, or legs. Such spread of dystonia is referred to as overflow.

Generalized, Segmental, and Focal Dystonias. Dystonic movements and postures can occur in all parts of the body. If only a single body part is involved, the disorder is labeled a *focal dystonia.* If more than one body part is involved and if these parts are contiguous (such as neck, arm, and trunk), *segmental dystonia* is used. If there is involvement of at least one arm and the opposite leg, *generalized dystonia* is appropriate. Primary dystonia usually begins in only one body part, i.e., as a focal dystonia. As the disorder progresses, it becomes segmental and then generalized. Generally, the younger the age at onset, the more likely for dystonia to progress to become generalized.[3] In contrast, the older the age at onset, the more likely it will remain a focal dystonia. There are a variety of focal dystonias, and most of them have been given specific names. They are discussed separately later in the chapter.

Paroxysmal Dystonia. Dystonic movements or postures that occur suddenly and unexpectedly and last for only a transient period are referred to as *paroxysmal dystonia* or paroxysmal dystonic choreoathetosis. Such a movement or posture may be triggered by emotion, by fatigue after exercise, or after drinking alcohol or caffeine.[4] The dystonic postures last up to several hours. Paroxysmal dystonia should be differentiated from other paroxysmal movements, such as seizures, paroxysmal ataxia, and paroxysmal kinesigenic choreoathetosis. The last entity is induced by sudden movement, lasts only a few seconds to a few minutes, and consists of choreic rather than dystonic movements.

Tardive Dystonia. Dystonic movements can be the result of chronic exposure to antipsychotic drugs. This form of dystonia, referred to as *tardive dystonia,*[5] is related to tardive dyskinesia, which is a more rapid, repetitive type of movement disorder caused by such agents. In contrast to tardive dyskinesia, tardive dystonia can affect children as well as adults. The dystonic movements can be focal, segmental, or generalized, just as in classic primary dystonias.

Variety of Focal Dystonias

Cranial Dystonias. *Blepharospasm* is forceful closure of the eyelids due to sustained contractions of the orbicularis oculi muscles. It may be accompanied by contractions of other muscles innervated by the facial nerve, such as the frontalis and zygomatic muscles. The contractions can spread to involve muscles in the lower part of the face.

Oromandibular dystonia consists of contractions involving muscles around the mouth and jaw. The jaw can be pulled upward to cause clenching of the teeth, or downward to produce sustained opening of the mouth. These mandibular muscles are innervated by the trigeminal nerve. Muscles of the lower face innervated by the facial nerve, such as orbicularis oris, platysma, and mentalis, may be contracting simultaneously.

The combination of blepharospasm and oromandibular dystonia is referred to as the *Meige syndrome,* in honor of the French neurologist who first described the condition.

These three cranial dystonias are usually present

at rest. In fact, specific actions tend to reduce them. For example, talking, singing, humming, and eating usually suppress oromandibular dystonia and blepharospasm. Probably less than 10 per cent of the cranial dystonias manifest as action dystonia rather than at rest. The act of talking is the most common trigger for facial action dystonia.

Lingual Dystonia. *Lingual dystonia* indicates involuntary contractions of the tongue. Rather than sustained protrusions of the tongue, which are relatively uncommon, lingual dystonia usually occurs as an action dystonia. The tongue protrudes inappropriately when the patient is talking, chewing, or swallowing. Lingual dystonia can be a part of the oromandibular dystonia spectrum.

Spastic Dysphonia. Laryngeal dystonia presents as dysphonia. The most common form is spastic dysphonia, in which the voice is raspy and broken into fragments owing to action dystonia of the vocal cords, which may be accompanied by pharyngeal muscle contractions as well. The vocal cords have abnormally moved closer together with action, thereby restricting the flow of air passing between them. As a result, the patient can utter very prolonged "sssss . . ." or "zzzzz . . ." sounds.

Breathy Dysphonia. A less common form of laryngeal dystonia is breathy dysphonia. In this condition the vocal cords are too far apart; the sound is soft and the patient can say only a few words before needing to breathe again. Too much air passes through the larynx, so that the "sssss . . ." and "zzzzz . . ." sounds can be sustained only briefly.

Torticollis. Dystonia of the neck region is referred to as *torticollis.* The head is usually turned, with the chin deviated toward one shoulder. Not uncommonly that shoulder is elevated, and sometimes it is also anteriorly displaced. The head can assume other postures, such as extension (retrocollis), flexion (anterocollis), and tilting to either shoulder. Regardless of the head positioning, the term torticollis is used. Because there can be increased spasms at times, or because there may be irregular pulling movements of the head, the term spasmodic torticollis is sometimes employed. Often associated with torticollis is tremor of the head, usually in the horizontal plane.

Writer's Cramp (Graphospasm) and Occupational Cramps. Focal dystonia of the arm usually begins in the form of action dystonia while the patient is carrying out a skilled activity such as writing. Although this disorder is referred to as writer's cramp or graphospasm, other acts requiring the use of the arm and hand can be affected. Musicians appear to be particularly affected, as well as people with other occupations.[6] The muscles of the fingers, hand, and arm contract abnormally during the voluntary action, causing the limb to move in abnormal directions. With progression, the abnormal dystonic movements that were initially present only with action can also occur at rest and can involve more proximal muscles of the arm.

Scoliosis, Kyphosis, and Lordosis. In the trunk, focal dystonia can present as scoliosis, kyphosis, lordosis, or leaning of the body to one side. These abnormal postures initially may be present only when the patient is standing. If it progresses, it can also be seen when the patient is sitting and even lying down.

Club Foot. No special name has been applied to focal action dystonia of the leg, perhaps because this is the most common initial site of involvement in children. However, once fixed dystonia has developed in the foot, it is colloquially referred to as *club foot.* Much more common than fixed dystonia is action dystonia of the leg, which occurs when the child is walking. The foot usually has an unusual twisting or kicking motion as the affected leg comes forward during a stride. Many children have this dystonic movement only when walking forward, not when running or walking backward. With progression, the abnormal movements are seen in these other activities and then may be present even with the leg at rest, such as during sitting or lying.

Genetics of Primary Dystonia

That torsion dystonia can occur in several members of a family has been known since the first report on dystonia by Schwalbe[7] in 1908, although he thought that such an occurrence represented psychologic problems in the family. There were several subsequent reports about the hereditary nature of torsion dystonia, but this concept seems to have been largely ignored until Zeman[8, 9] described families with clear-cut autosomal dominant transmission and pointed out that some affected members in the family may have limited clinical expression of the disorder, such as spasmodic torticollis, blepharospasm, writer's cramp (graphospasm), spastic dysphonia, kyphoscoliosis, or club foot. To this list we possibly can add stuttering. Zeman pointed out that family members and patients may have an associated essential tremor, a phenomenon also seen by others.

Eldridge[12] noted the high prevalence of torsion dystonia in individuals of Ashkenazi Jewish descent, particularly in patients in whom the dystonia begins in childhood. He explained this finding on the basis of an autosomal recessive mode of inheritance. From their survey, Eldridge and Gottlieb[13] calculated that the gene frequency in this population is 1 in 65 and that the disease affects 1 in 17,000 in this ethnic group. Recently, Korczyn and colleagues[14] have challenged the autosomal recessive inheritance hypothesis, claiming

Table 1. CAUSES OF SECONDARY DYSTONIA*

Other hereditary neurologic disorders	Wilson's disease Huntington's disease (Westphal variant) Hallervorden-Spatz disease GM_1 gangliosidosis Hexosaminidase A and B deficiency Juvenile dystonic lipidosis Glutaric acidemia Joseph's disease
Environmental causes	Perinatal cerebral injury Infection (either concomitant or sequela) Reye's syndrome Head trauma Focal cerebral vascular injury Brain tumor Toxins (carbon monoxide, manganese) Drugs (levodopa, antipsychotics, metoclopramide, anticonvulsants)
Hysteria	

*Discussions of each of these causes are cited by Fahn.[17]

that their survey of torsion dystonia in Israel indicates that the disorder in Ashkenazi Jews is inherited via autosomal dominant transmission with a low rate of penetrance. This theory is based on the presence of torsion dystonia in two successive generations in some of their families. The issue remains unsettled, because as Eldridge[15] points out, involvement in two successive generations could occur when an affected individual marries a carrier, thus giving rise to affected offspring in a pattern resembling autosomal dominance, so-called quasi-dominance. Quasi-dominance would be expected to occur when the gene frequency within a population is high and marriage takes place within it. Thus, there is no consensus on the nature of genetic transmission in the Ashkenazi population.

Another genetic form of torsion dystonia that has been reasonably well described is a sex-linked recessive form that occurs on Panay Island in the Philippines.[16] Twenty-three of the known 28 cases of torsion dystonia in the Philippines have come from Panay.

Causes

Dystonia can be divided etiologically into primary and secondary categories. Within the primary category are cases with a known familial pattern of the disorder, the genetics of which were discussed previously. Also in the primary category are cases without either a known familial pattern or any other known etiologic factor to account for the dystonia; this is the largest group of cases, and the form can be referred to as sporadic or idiopathic dystonia. The smaller category of secondary dystonia consists of both recognized hereditary neurologic disorders and environmental factors that cause dystonia (Table 1).[17]

Incidence and Prevalence

Little is known about the demographics of dystonia. No epidemiologic surveys have been carried out, so the prevalence and incidence are unknown. Although considered an uncommon condition, dystonia in its many forms is more common than generally realized. In our Movement Disorder Clinic, my colleagues and I have seen approximately 400 patients with a large variety of dystonic movements and postures; they can be divided into the categories listed in Table 2. The largest group has adult-onset focal dystonias.

HISTORY

Although the diagnosis of dystonia depends primarily on the physical inspection of the patient and differentiation of the observed abnormal movements and postures from other types of dyskinesias, the history provides valuable information regarding the etiology of the disorder. It can also furnish clues as to whether the abnormal

Table 2. DISTRIBUTION OF PATIENTS PRESENTING WITH DYSTONIA TO A LARGE MOVEMENT DISORDER CLINIC*

	Primary Dystonia		Secondary Dystonia	
Category†	*Number*	%	*Number*	%
Childhood-onset				
Focal	7	1.8	1	0.3
Segmental	9	2.3	10	2.5
Generalized	55	13.9	13	3.3
Unilateral	3	0.8	13	3.3
Subtotal	74	18.7	37	9.3
Adult-onset				
Focal	173	43.7	3	0.8
Segmental	34	8.6	0	0
Generalized	9	2.3	5	1.3
Unilateral	0	0	3	0.8
Subtotal	216	54.5	11	2.8
Paroxysmal dystonia	14	3.5		
Tardive dystonia			33	8.3
Hysterical dystonia			11	0.3
Total	304	76.8	92	23.2

*A total of 396 patients with dystonia were seen by the Movement Disorder Group between Sept. 1, 1973, and Feb. 1, 1983, at Columbia-Presbyterian Medical Center, New York City.

†*Childhood onset* for this tabulation is defined as onset of dystonia before age 18; adult onset, at age 18 or older. The categories of paroxysmal, tardive, and hysterical dystonia are explained in the text; no distinction was made as to age at onset for these three forms.

movements are dystonia or some other type of dyskinesia.

History of the Present Illness. The medical history should record the onset of the abnormal movement, its location in the body, and what type of action brought it on. Was it preceded by any trauma, infection, or ingestion of drugs (particularly the antipsychotic agents such as the phenothiazines and butyrophenones)? Was there any exposure to carbon monoxide or manganese? One should ask the patient to describe the nature of the abnormal movement when it first occurred and any changes that have taken place over time. Was it present with only a specific action or with several types of action? Did it appear with the affected body part at rest and without action? Have the abnormal movements spread to other parts of the body? If so, the patient should describe the spread chronologically. How severe are the abnormal movements? What functions are interferred with? Is walking affected? Can the hand grasp and carry out tasks such as writing, dressing, buttoning, shaving, combing hair, cutting food, and handling eating utensils? Is speech or swallowing affected? If there are movements of the head or face, around the mouth, or in closure of the eyelids, are they exacerbated or reduced by walking, talking, driving, chewing, exposure to sunlight, watching movies or television, sewing, resting the head against the wall or the high back of a chair, or placing the hand on the chin or face?

Family History. The family history provides information on whether the dystonia seen in the patient could have an hereditary basis. However, it should be noted that a history of dystonia in the family can be missed if one depends only on information obtained from the patient. One needs to examine the parents and other relatives, because many individuals deny anything is wrong, even if they have difficulties with handwriting. It is important to inquire specifically if anyone has ever had wryneck (torticollis), club foot, hunchback (kyphosis), scoliosis, stuttering, tremor, writer's cramp, problems with handwriting, tics, or facial movements. Because autosomal dominant dystonia is not completely penetrant, it may skip generations. In taking the family history, one needs to inquire about the ethnic background of the patient to determine whether the dystonia could be associated with the Ashkenazi Jewish variety.

Previous History. One should obtain details about the birth history and developmental milestones. About 26 per cent of patients with supposed primary dystonia have a history of birth injury or delayed development. These patients could have secondary dystonia, known as delayed-onset dystonia, secondary to static encephalopathy.[18] One should learn about the patient's healthy history, including psychiatric history. Has the patient been depressed or nervous, requiring medications? If so, were any of these drugs major tranquilizers?

High-Payoff Queries

1. *When the abnormal movements began, were they present all the time or only with certain activities?* Primary dystonia of the limbs almost always begins with action dystonia. Secondary dystonias and hysterical dystonias commonly begin with a fixed dystonia.

2. *In what part of your body did the abnormal movements begin?* In children, dystonic movements frequently begin in the legs. In adults, they usually begin in the neck, face, or arms.[3]

3. *Have you previously experienced head trauma, infection, or stroke, or have you taken drugs or been exposed to toxins recently?* A positive answer may suggest a secondary dystonia.

4. *Was there anything unusual about your development as a child?* A positive answer would suggest delayed-onset dystonia secondary to a static encephalopathy.

5. *What is your ethnic and religious background?* There is a higher incidence of dystonia in Ashkenazi Jews.

6. *Did anyone in your family ever have a similar problem?* A positive response would suggest a hereditary basis for the dystonia.

7. *Has anyone in your family ever had tremor, writer's cramp, scoliosis, hunchback, torticollis, club foot, abnormal facial movements, tics, or stuttering?* A positive response would suggest a hereditary basis for the dystonia.

8. *What factors exacerbate the abnormal movements and what reduces them?* Characteristically, dystonic movements rather than other types of abnormal movements are influenced by changes in body posture and activity. Placing a hand on the chin usually lessens torticollis, for example. Talking usually relieves the movement of Meige's syndrome, and walking usually aggravates it. Lying down usually reduces most dystonias, although tardive dystonia can be aggravated by lying down in some patients. Sleep usually causes all movement disorders to disappear, including dystonia.

9. *Are the abnormal movements worse at certain times of the day?* Dystonia with marked diurnal fluctuation has been described by Segawa and colleagues.[19] In this variant, the patient has dystonia in the afternoon and evening, but little abnormal movement in the morning. The familial occurrence of this disorder fits an inherited transmission pattern of autosomal dominance with low penetrance.

10. *Do the abnormal movements occur all of a sudden, "out of the blue"?* A positive response suggests that the problem may be paroxysmal dystonia.

PHYSICAL EXAMINATION

The diagnosis depends upon observation of dystonic movements. Patients with paroxysmal dystonia, however, may not have abnormal movements at the time of examination.

General Physical Examination

The general physical examination usually does not provide many clues as to the etiology of the dystonia. However, the eyes should be inspected for Kayser-Fleischer rings in the cornea; a slit-lamp examination is required to be certain that they are not present. Their presence is pathognomonic of the diagnosis of Wilson's disease. Is there a curvature of the spine, and are any joints fixed with contractures? If so, these findings could be the end result of severe dystonic postures.

General Neurologic Examination

The general neurologic findings, aside from the presence of abnormal involuntary movements, are normal in primary dystonia but can be abnormal in secondary dystonia. The presence of weakness, abnormal reflexes, sensory loss, cerebellar signs, and cranial nerve abnormalities indicates a secondary form of dystonia. The absence of these signs does not exclude secondary dystonia, however. Muscle tone can be either hypertonic or hypotonic in patients with dystonia, depending on whether the limbs are manipulated during a dystonic contraction or in between abnormal movements.

Because the findings of a general neurologic examination are normal—i.e., there is no weakness, sensory loss, or reflex changes—it is not uncommon for diagnosis of conversion reaction to be made. In fact, approximately 40 per cent of all patients eventually diagnosed as having torsion dystonia are misdiagnosed at one time as having a conversion reaction.[20] On the other hand, the presence of false weakness, inappropriate sensory loss, or pain or tactile stimulation could be the first clue that one is dealing with dystonic movements that are also of a psychologic nature (see "Differentiation from Hysteria").

Evaluation of Involuntary Movements and Postures

Positions and Activities of the Patient. Inspection for abnormal involuntary movements must be carried out with the patient sitting at rest, lying supine, lying prone, standing, walking, writing with each hand, and performing the finger-to-nose maneuver and other special activities that might influence the severity of disease. These include placing the head against a wall if the patient has torticollis, dressing and undressing if there is dystonia of the arms, and walking backwards and running if the patient has dystonia of the legs. Inspection should also be carried out when the patient is talking and also when listening. If the patient has special tactile or proprioceptive "tricks" that lessen the dystonic movements, he or she should be asked to demonstrate them. They may include placing hands on the chin to reduce torticollis, adducting the arms to reduce dystonia when eating, and standing when writing.

Observing the Distribution of Abnormal Movements and Postures. One should determine which body parts are affected by checking the face (eyelids and mouth), jaw, tongue, neck, shoulders, both arms, curvature of the spine, pelvis, and both legs. These body parts are inspected in each of the positions and activities listed in the preceding paragraph. If dystonic movements are restricted to just one side of the body (hemidystonia), the dystonia is probably secondary to some cerebral insult rather than primary.

Observing the Speed, Duration, and Pattern of Abnormal Movements. The speed of the dystonic movement is more often rapid than slow, leading the clinician to mislabel such rapid movements as chorea or even myoclonus. The repetitive and twisting pattern of dystonia should suggest the proper diagnosis. A useful term for very rapid and continual movement is *dystonic spasms.* In part, these rapid, repetitive contractions are the result of the patient's attempts to overcome the involuntary contraction. A useful approach is to ask the patient to let the muscles contract and allow the limbs to move where they want to go. In this way, the movements may become sustained, and the diagnosis becomes more obvious.

A variant of dystonic spasms is *dystonic tremor.* These rhythmic oscillations develop as the patient attempts to voluntarily overcome the abnormal contractions, and instead of a sustained contraction, the movements are broken up owing to grouping of the action potentials.[21] Again, having the patient allow the limb to move to the posture desired by involuntary dystonic movements can eliminate the tremor in most situations.

When the dystonic movements are slow, they merge into athetosis. *Athetotic dystonia* is a convenient label for these types of movements. Athetosis is the most common form of dystonia with onset in infancy.

Observing for Severity of Abnormal Movements. Several factors must be considered in evaluating the severity of dystonic movements: forcefulness of the dystonic movements, presence of fixed dystonic postures, presence of pain from the constant muscle contractions, and the effect on the function of each affected body part. Is the primary function affected? For example, in blepharospasm, during how much of the day can the patient see? In arm dystonia, can the patient grasp? In leg dystonia, can the patient walk? Another factor to consider when assessing severity is whether the abnormal movements are present when the affected body part is at rest or only during active voluntary movement. Dystonia is considered more severe if present at rest than if present only with action.

Differentiating Dystonic Movements from Other Types of Movement Disorders. As mentioned, athetosis is probably just a form of dystonia that begins in infancy. Choreic movements flow from one part of the body to another. In contrast, dystonic movements recur in the same body part in a more repetitive pattern. Myoclonus, whether arrhythmic or rhythmic, is "lightning-like" in speed. Occasionally, some dystonic spasms can be this rapid. The twisting nature of dystonic spasms and their continual nature should suggest the correct diagnosis. Tics are patterned sequences of coordinated movements that occur irregularly, in contrast to dystonic movements, which are constant or occur with action of the involved body part. Some tonic tics contain prolonged contractions that can sometimes be confused with dystonia; however, the patterned sequence of the tic movement, its intermittent occurrence, and its frequent accompaniment by vocalizations should distinguish it. Furthermore, many patients with tics know when a tic is about to occur and can even suppress it temporarily. Tremors, which are oscillations about a body plane, usually present no problem in identification. Essential tremor can, however, be present in patients with dystonia,[11, 12, 22] and its presence should not distract from a diagnosis of dystonia. Head tremor is often present in patients with torticollis.

DIAGNOSTIC STUDIES

The history and neurologic examination are the major bases for establishing the diagnosis and etiology in most cases of dystonia. Few laboratory tests are necessary.

Laboratory Studies

The diagnosis of Wilson's disease can be made or excluded on the basis of 24-hour urine copper, serum copper, and serum ceruloplasmin levels. If necessary, a liver biopsy for copper concentration can also be done. Assay for organic acids in the urine can determine glutaric acidemia, a rare metabolic disorder. Other routine laboratory tests are rarely helpful except to rule out some other concurrent disorder.

Imaging

Computerized tomography (CT scanning) of the head can be helpful in excluding causes of secondary dystonia such as infarction, brain tumor, Wilson's disease, and other degenerative diseases. Dilated ventricles and atrophic changes can sometimes be seen as a complication of birth injury and other static encephalopathies. Findings of CT scanning are normal in primary dystonia. Plain x-rays of the spinal column can be used to measure the degree of spinal curvature in scoliosis.

Other Tests

Electromyography is sometimes helpful because it can reveal simultaneous contractions of agonist and antagonist muscles, which are a hallmark of dystonic postures and movements.[21] However, the simultaneity is seen in volitional contractions as well, so its presence does not differentiate organic and hysterical dystonia. Neither does an amobarbital interview, because patients with either organic or hysterical dystonia can improve with relaxation techniques. Electroencephalographic findings may be abnormal in secondary dystonia but are normal in primary dystonia.

ASSESSMENT

Diagnostic Approach

With any movement disorder, the diagnostic approach is first to assign the abnormal movements to the proper classification—chorea, athetosis, myoclonus, tics, and dystonia. Only by seeing a large number of patients with various movement disorders can one develop a keen sense of the subtle differences between them. In general, though, there usually is a clear separation between the various types of involuntary movements. Guidelines already mentioned should help. Once the abnormal movements are appropriately recognized, consideration is given to etiology (see Table 1). The history can give the most clues. One should seek genetic factors and any history of brain injury. Selective laboratory tests as outlined can give further assistance.

Prognostic Indicators

A major factor of prognostic importance is the cause of the dystonia. Dystonia due to static encephalopathy tends to plateau and not to progress, whereas that due to a progressive degenerative disorder will worsen over time. One helpful rule for determining whether dystonia is primary or secondary is that most cases of unilateral dystonia (hemidystonia) are secondary rather than primary.

Generally, age at onset is the most important

factor for prognosis and for the distribution pattern of primary dystonia.[3] As discussed, with childhood onset (age less than 11), dystonia commonly begins in the legs; in more than 80 per cent of cases, the dystonia becomes generalized with time, and in 50 per cent, the dystonia causes severe disability. In contrast, adult-onset dystonia commonly begins in the arms or the axial muscles. In fact, in the study by Marsden and colleagues,[3] dystonia with onset after the age of 20 never began in the legs. Such cases also never progressed to become generalized; they either remained focal or progressed only to the segmental type. Dystonia usually remained mild, and only 14 per cent of the patients became severely disabled. From these considerations, one can generalize that adult-onset focal dystonia (blepharospasm, oromandibular dystonia, graphospasm, spasmodic torticollis, spastic dysphonia) usually remains focal, with limited progressive severity or spread to other sites.[23]

Differentiation from Hysteria

Misdiagnosis is more common in dystonia than in any other movement disorder. There are two types of misdiagnoses. The first is mistaking the abnormal movements of dystonia for some other type, most commonly chorea. The second is mistaking primary dystonia for a psychologic problem. Because there is no weakness, sensory loss, or reflex change and because the abnormal movements are altered by changes of posture, by voluntary motor activity of the affected part, and by tactile and proprioceptive "tricks," unsophisticated clinicians may assume that the abnormal movements are the result of a psychologic problem. Instead, the knowing clinician utilizes these typical aspects of primary dystonia to make the correct diagnosis.

The opposite problem, that of making the accurate diagnosis of hysterical dystonia rather than primary dystonia, is more difficult. Documented cases of hysterical dystonia have now been reported.[24] The best clue that one is dealing with a psychologic disorder is inconsistency of neurologic findings. False weakness (strength "gives way"), false sensitivity to stimuli (pain on light touch by the examiner but not by clothes or touch by the patient), and evidence of self-inflicted wounds suggest that one is dealing with a psychologic problem. Another helpful clue is that hysterical dystonia (and some other causes of secondary dystonia) may begin with fixed postures. In contrast, primary dystonia usually begins as an action dystonia and only later may progress to dystonia at rest and, ultimately, dystonic posture or fixed dystonia.

REFERENCES

1. Fahn S, Eldridge R. Definition of dystonia and classification of the dystonic states. Adv Neurol 1976;14:1–5.
2. Herz E. Dystonia. I. Historical review: analysis of dystonic symptoms and physiologic mechanisms involved. Arch Neurol Psychiat 1944;51:305–18.
3. Marsden CD, Harrison MJG, Bundey S. Natural history of idiopathic torsion dystonia. Adv Neurol 1976;14:177–87.
4. Lance JW. Familial paroxysmal dystonic choreoathetosis and its differentiation from related syndromes. Ann Neurol 1977;2:285–93.
5. Burke RE, Fahn S, Jankovic J, et al. Tardive dystonia: late-onset and persistent dystonia caused by antipsychotic drugs. Neurology 1982;32:1335–46.
6. Sheehy MP, Marsden CD. Writer's cramp—a focal dystonia. Brain 1982;105:461–80.
7. Schwalbe W. Eine eigentumliche tonische Krampfform mit hysterischen Symptomen. Inaug Diss, Berlin, G. Schade, 1908.
8. Zeman W, Kaelbling R, Pasamanick B. Idiopathic dystonia musculorum deformans. I. The hereditary pattern. Am J Hum Genet 1959;11:188–202.
9. Zeman W, Kaelbling R, Pasamanick B. Idiopathic dystonia musculorum deformans. II. The formes frustes. Neurology 1960;10:1068–75.
10. Couch J. Dystonia and tremor in spasmodic torticollis. Adv Neuro 1976;14:245–58.
11. Baxter DW, Lal S. Essential tremor and dystonic syndromes. Adv Neurol 1979;24:373–77.
12. Eldridge R. The torsion dystonias: literature review and genetic and clinical studies. Neurology 1970;20(No. 11, Part 2): 1–78.
13. Eldridge R, Gottlieb R. The primary hereditary dystonias: genetic classification of 768 families and revised estimate of gene frequency, autosomal recessive form, and selected bibliography. Adv Neurol 1976;14:457–74.
14. Korczyn AD, Kahana E, Zilber N, Streifler M, Carasso R, Alter M. Torsion dystonia in Israel. Ann Neurol 1980;8:387–91.
15. Eldridge R. Inheritance of torsion dystonia in Jews. Ann Neurol 1981;10:203–4.
16. Lee LV, Pascasio FM, Fuentes FD, Viterbo GH. Torsion dystonia in Panay, Philippines. Adv Neurol 1976;14:137–51.
17. Fahn S. Torsion dystonia: clinical spectrum and treatment. Semin Neurol 1982;2:316–23.
18. Burke RE, Fahn S, Gold AP. Delayed onset dystonia in patients with "static" encephalopathy. J Neurol Neurosurg Psychiatry 1980;43:789–97.
19. Segawa M, Hosaka A, Miyagawa F, Nomura Y, Imai H. Hereditary progressive dystonia with marked diurnal fluctuation. Adv Neurol 1976;14:215–33.
20. Lesser RP, Fahn S. Dystonia: a disorder often misdiagnosed as a conversion reaction. Am J Psychiat 1978;153:349–452.
21. Yanagisawa N, Goto A. Dystonia musculorum deformans: analysis with electromyography. J Neurol Sci 1971; 13:39–65.
22. Marsden CD. Dystonia: the spectrum of the disease. In: Yahr MD, ed. The basal ganglia. New York: Raven Press, 1976;351–67.
23. Marsden CD. The problem of adult-onset idiopathic torsion dystonia and other isolated dyskinesias in adult life (including blepharospasm, oromandibular dystonia, dystonic writer's cramp, and torticollis, or axial dystonia). Adv Neurol 1976;14:259–76.
24. Fahn S, Williams D, Reches A, Lesser RP, Jankovic J, Silberstein SD. Hysterical dystonia: a rare disorder. Report of five documented cases. Neurology 1983;33(Suppl 2):161.

EDEMA, PERIPHERAL

JOHN A. SPITTELL JR. ☐ ALEXANDER SCHIRGER

☐ SYNONYMS: Swelling, elephantiasis, dropsy

BACKGROUND

Edema has been recognized for centuries as indicative of disease. Commonly, because of hearsay, patients are fearful that edema indicates "heart failure" or, when their edema is unilateral, are concerned about the possibility of "blood clots."

Distinguishing edema due to a systemic condition from that due to a regional disorder and then identifying the specific cause of the edema can vary from a straightforward and downright easy clinical exercise to a very difficult and complex diagnostic problem. Correct diagnosis, of course, is vital to proper management not only of the edema, but also of any underlying etiologic condition that itself may be reversible or may require specific therapeutic measures.

Definition and Origin

Simply stated, *edema* is enlargement of a part due to an excess of fluid in the tissues. It can be the result of increased capillary permeability in the involved part, of obstruction of the venous or lymphatic flow from the involved part, or of the increased accumulation of fluid in the tissues because of lowered oncotic pressure of the plasma.[1]

In this chapter, only edema of the extremities is discussed. Although edema of the upper extremity can occur for any of the reasons noted above, edema of the lower extremities is a much more common clinical problem (because of gravitational influence due to our upright posture) and is used as the basis for diagnostic considerations. The differentiation of systemic types of edema from regional types is covered initially. Then the more difficult task of identifying the specific types of regional edema is addressed in detail, because it is these that seem to create the greatest diagnostic problems.

Incidence and Causes

Limb edema is a common complaint—the fourth most frequent reason for visiting a physician's office[2]—because it is readily noted, generally believed to indicate disease, and cosmetically undesirable, particularly for women. Because of these concerns, patients usually do not delay seeking help when they note edema.

A practical classification of the causes of edema is presented in Table 1.

HISTORY

Frequently, an impression that will ultimately prove to be the correct diagnosis can be gained from the medical history of the patient with edema.

The distinction between systemic and regional edema is easy if the patient has edema confined to one extremity (which tends to exclude systemic types) or has symptoms of cardiac, renal, hepatic, or chronic gastrointestinal disease associated with generalized or bilateral lower extremity edema. Idiopathic edema is commonly intermittent and is often generalized in distribution, so that other

Table 1. A CLASSIFICATION OF EDEMA

- I. Systemic edema
  - A. Cardiac disease
  - B. Renal disease
  - C. Hepatic disease
  - D. Nutritional edema (hypoproteinemia)
  - E. Idiopathic edema
- II. Regional edema
  - A. Venous edema
    - 1. Acute deep venous thrombosis
    - 2. Chronic venous insufficiency
    - 3. Venous obstruction
  - B. Lymphedema
    - 1. Idiopathic lymphedema
      - a. Congenital lymphedema
      - b. Lymphedema precox
    - 2. Inflammatory lymphedema
    - 3. Obstructive lymphedema
  - C. Lipedema
  - D. Miscellaneous types
    - 1. Orthostatic edema
    - 2. Arteriovenous anomalies
    - 3. Edema following arterial surgery
    - 4. Edema associated with musculoskeletal disorders
      - a. Muscular problems
      - b. Tenosynovitis
      - c. March fracture
      - d. Baker's cyst
    - 5. Reflex sympathetic dystrophy
- III. Drug-induced edema
  - A. Hormones
  - B. Antihypertensive agents
  - C. Anti-inflammatory agents
  - D. Other drugs

types of edema must be excluded before this diagnosis is made.

For sorting out the various types of regional edema, historical features again can be quite useful. The sudden onset, the common association of a precipitating event (e.g., surgery, fracture, or congestive heart failure), and the frequent occurrence of pain and tenderness in the involved extremity suggest acute deep venous thrombosis. In the patient with chronic limb edema, chills and fever, particularly if recurrent, bring the possibility of an inflammatory type of lymphedema to mind. Otherwise, lymphedema can generally be characterized as chronic, painless, and progressive. Whether the edema is unilateral or bilateral is of some diagnostic value, even in the regional types. The edema associated with lipedema ("fat legs") is always bilateral and does not involve the foot and toes.[3] Orthostatic edema and drug-induced edema are typically bilateral and do involve the foot and toes.[4]

Family history, social history, and occupational history are of relatively little value in the diagnostic evaluation of the patient with edema, but obviously an occupation that involves relative immobility (sitting or standing) for long periods can be a significant aggravating factor.

A drug history should always be taken from the patient with edema, and any drug that is known to cause or aggravate fluid retention or whose use bears a temporal relationship to the onset of the edema should be suspected.

High-Payoff Queries

The following eight questions may elicit particular useful diagnostic information.

1. *When did the swelling begin?* The relationship to other events is particularly useful in deep venous thrombosis, whereas in lymphedema the age of the patient at onset is an important clinical discriminant. Idiopathic lymphedema (nine times as common in women as in men) usually begins before age 40, typically about the time of menarche, and obstructive lymphedema almost always appears after age 40.[5]

2. *Does the involved extremity hurt?* Pain in the swollen extremity suggests thrombophlebitis, inflammatory lymphedema, or a musculoskeletal disorder. Pain should be distinguished from tenderness, because although both are present in the conditions just noted, tenderness without pain is commonly seen in lipedema ("fat legs").

3. *Does the swelling recede overnight?* The edema of chronic venous insufficiency and orthostatic edema does recede with elevation overnight; edema of systemic origin may shift to another body part that is dependent during bed rest (e.g., the back), giving the patient the illusion that it has receded; lymphedema recedes slowly and often incompletely with elevation.

4. *Do you have shortness of breath with usual exertion or when you lie down?* An affirmative answer to this question strongly suggests cardiac disease.

5. *Have you ever had kidney infections or "albuminuria"?* The presence of these historical clues raises the question of a renal basis for the edema.

6. *Have you had hepatitis or jaundice?* Patients with chronic hepatic disease severe enough to cause edema often have had one or both of these. Along the same line, forthright inquiry about alcohol consumption should be included in every history.

7. *Has your appetite, weight, or bowel habit changed?* A change in any of these features may alert the clinician to the uncommon, but important, nutritional types of edema.

8. *Do you take any medication, pills, or capsules?* To avoid the patient's omission of replacement therapy or anovulatory agents, it is best to phrase the query both as "medication" and as "pills." The list of drugs that may cause edema has grown steadily, as shown in Table 2, and this query is particularly salient if the person with edema also has hypertension, pain, depression, menopausal symptoms, or parkinsonism.

Table 2. COMMONLY PRESCRIBED DRUGS THAT CAN CAUSE EDEMA

Hormones	Corticosteroids
	Female hormones
	Estrogen
	Progesterone
	Testosterone
Antihypertensive agents	Rauwolfia agents
	Hydralazine (Apresoline)
	Guanethidine (Ismelin)
	Alpha-methyldopa (Aldomet)
	Beta-adrenergic blocking drugs
	Clonidine (Catapres)
	Minoxidil
	Calcium channel blockers
Anti-inflammatory agents	Phenylbutazone (Butazolidin)
	Naproxen (Naprosyn)
	Ibuprofen (Motrin)
	Indomethacin (Indocin)
Miscellaneous	Antidepressants (monamine oxidase inhibitors)
	Amantadine hydrochloride (Symmetrel)

PHYSICAL EXAMINATION

The person with peripheral edema should have a complete physical examination, in order to avoid overlooking important etiologic or related conditions.

Examination of the skin may provide important clues, such as arterial spider hemangiomata of chronic hepatic disease, venous "stars" due to chronic venous obstruction, facial suffusion of superior vena cava obstruction, stasis pigmentation or dermatitis in the medial distal leg with chronic venous insufficiency, and dermatophytosis in lymphedema due to or complicated by recurrent cellulitis and lymphangitis.

The ocular fundus may show important changes in the patient with edema due to chronic renal disease and/or diabetes mellitus.

Examination of the venous system should include the pulsations of the jugular veins (the patient should be lying with the head raised to 45 degrees above the horizontal) to avoid missing the characteristic prominent "x and y" descent in the patient whose peripheral edema is due to chronic constrictive pericarditis or the elevated venous pressure in the patient with congestive heart failure. If varicose veins are not to be overlooked, the patient must be examined while standing. Likewise, popliteal (Baker's) cysts are best seen with the patient standing.

Careful cardiac examination is essential, of course, to identify features of a failing heart (other than the jugular venous distension just mentioned) such as rapid atrial fibrillation, cardiac enlargement, and a third heart sound. Likewise, the pericardial "knock" of chronic constrictive pericarditis is a significant, diagnostic finding.

The distribution of the edema is an important distinguishing feature. In the patient with lipedema ("fat legs") the feet and toes are not swollen, whereas in other types of lower extremity edema they are. In fact, in lymphedema of long standing, the typical "squaring" of the toes is a helpful clinical finding.

The color and texture of the skin of an edematous limb can give valuable diagnostic help. With venous obstruction the skin is often suffused and may show an increased superficial venous pattern or venous "stars." A hallmark of long-standing venous insufficiency is the brownish pigmentation of venous stasis in the skin of the distal medial leg. The swelling in lymphedema is firm, and the skin feels thickened. The tissue of the legs in lipedema ("fat legs") has the typical soft consistency of adipose tissue. In the patient in whom recurrent lymphangitis is the basis of lymphedema, the red and inflamed lymphatic channels may be seen during an acute episode. When edema is secondary to bleeding within a muscle compartment in the leg, a telltale meniscus-shaped area of ecchymosis appears beneath one or both malleoli in a day or two.

The location of any tenderness is an important aspect in separating the various types of regional edema. Although it is not always associated with tenderness of the calf, popliteal space, over the femoral vein, or in Scarpa's triangle, deep venous thrombosis so often has such a feature that it must be a consideration when such tenderness is present. The various musculoskeletal disorders that cause edema are all tender to palpation in appropriate locations as well.

DIAGNOSTIC STUDIES

When the history and physical examination do not clearly exclude the systemic types of edema, the laboratory evaluation may need to be extensive (Table 3).[6] It should be tailored individually to each patient to confirm the suspicions gained clinically. Several points are worthy of note in regard to the laboratory studies when systemic edema is suspected:

1. The serum protein electrophoresis is most useful to identify hypoproteinemia (usually due to anorexia nervosa or to intestinal malabsorption) and the serum protein abnormalities seen in renal disease, severe hepatic disease, and primary amyloidosis.
2. A normal ECG does not exclude chronic constrictive pericarditis or cardiac amyloidosis; when ECG changes are present they may indicate nothing more than low voltage.
3. In chronic constrictive pericarditis, the heart may be normal in size on chest roentgenograms. CT scanning has been a helpful procedure in many cases, but right heart catheterization may be necessary to confirm or exclude the diagnosis with confidence.
4. When malabsorption is a consideration, additional studies including stool fat content, roentgenograms of the intestine, and even biopsy of the intestinal mucosa may be necessary to determine the basic cause of the nutritional deficiency.

No laboratory studies are diagnostic for idiopathic edema. It is often a diagnosis that is

Table 3. DIAGNOSTIC PROCEDURES IN THE PATIENT WITH EDEMA

Serum protein electrophoresis Liver function tests Serum thyroxine TSH radioimmunoassay
ECG Chest x-ray Echocardiography CT scan of thorax Radionuclide angiogram of heart
Venous Doppler ultrasonography
Impedance plethysmography Ultrasonography
Venography
Renal tomograms CT scan of abdomen
Lymphangiography

(Modified from Schirger A. Diagnosis and management of leg edema in the elderly. Geriatrics 1982;37:26–32.)

suspected clinically and is confirmed by exclusion of other possible causes.

When the edema is believed to be a regional problem, venous Doppler ultrasonography and impedance plethysmography are noninvasive diagnostic procedures of proven value in diagnosing or excluding deep venous thrombosis, but when their results are equivocal or in difficult problems, contrast venography (or isotope venography for the patient allergic to contrast media) is the "gold standard" for diagnosis.[7] The venous Doppler examination is excellent for confirming deep venous incompetence. When obstruction of the popliteal vein by a popliteal (Baker's) cyst or popliteal aneurysm is a possibility, ultrasound examination of the popliteal space is an excellent noninvasive procedure.[8] In the patient with lymphedema, the diagnosis can usually be made with confidence on clinical grounds; in patients in whom obstructive lymphedema due to neoplasm is a consideration and the neoplasm is not evident on physical examination, CT scan of the abdomen and pelvis have been so useful to us that we seldom perform contrast lymphangiography for diagnostic reasons any longer, unless it is indicated for consideration of a specific surgical procedure such as lymphaticovenous anastomosis.

ASSESSMENT

In evaluating the patient with peripheral edema, it is best to try on the basis of history and physical examination to categorize the edema as "systemic" or "regional" in type, as shown on the algorithm. Within these two broad categories, it is most useful clinically to consider the "treatable" and "reversible" types of edema first.

Systemic Edema

When the basis of edema is a systemic process, the edema is generalized and involves at least two if not all of the extremities. Often there is ascites, and the fluid accumulation is great enough that the patient notes a significant weight gain.

In cardiac edema there is usually an associated history of a cardiac event or cardiac symptoms such as dyspnea, orthopnea, palpitation, and chest pain. Important physical findings are abnormalities of cardiac size, rhythm (particularly pulsus alternans), or sounds (particularly the presence of a third heart sound) and jugular venous distension. In examining the jugular venous pulse, one can obtain important clues to the type of cardiac problem by identifying the waves—e.g., the prominent "x and y" descent in chronic constrictive pericarditis, the large "cv" wave in tricuspid valve incompetence, and the slow "y" descent in tricuspid stenosis. In cardiomyopathy there may be associated systemic symptoms, varying from the recent flu-like illness to the nonspecific symptoms of fatigue, anorexia, and weight loss.

In the person with edema due to renal disease there is commonly a history of a recent pharyngitis, a urinary infection, or a noticeable change in the urine. With long-standing renal disease there may be hemorrhages and exudates in the ocular fundi. In the patient with renal vein thrombosis there is often flank pain and recent or associated peripheral venous thrombosis as well as heavy proteinuria. Renal tomograms, ultrasonograms, or CT scans will show abnormalities of renal size, but an excretory urogram is necessary to demonstrate abnormalities of the collecting system or ureters.

When edema has a hepatic basis, the diagnosis is usually not difficult. Antecedent alcoholism, hepatitis, or jaundice is usually present as well as some or all of the physical signs of chronic hepatic disease—arterial "spiders," liver palms (erythema), gynecomastia, and prominent venous collaterals of the abdominal wall; of course, ascites and splenomegaly are usual.

Nutritional edema is uncommon but important. There are usually other signs of nutritional deficiency such as cheilosis, red tongue, and weight loss. The relative frequency of anorexia nervosa currently makes this disease the most common nutritional cause of edema in clinical practice today. In edema due to bowel disease, there is often a history of abdominal cramping or loose stools, and stool fat determinations and gastrointestinal roentgenograms are essential.

Idiopathic edema probably gives more diagnostic difficulty than any other type.[9,10] Typically, affected patients are women who episodically develop edema when up and about during the day; the fluid accumulation during the day causes a progressive gain in weight from morning to evening. In addition to the edema of the lower extremities, the patient may note swelling of the abdomen and breasts. She may have puffiness of the face and hands on arising in the morning, that recedes with ambulation. The fluid retention that occurs during the day (upright posture) tends to lessen at night (recumbency) owing to diuresis. This orthostatic aspect of idiopathic edema, and also determination that it is due to orthostatic sodium retention or orthostatic water retention, can be demonstrated by water excretion tests.[11]

Regional Edema

When edema involves only one extremity it is usually one of the regional types. However, regional edema can involve both lower extremities,

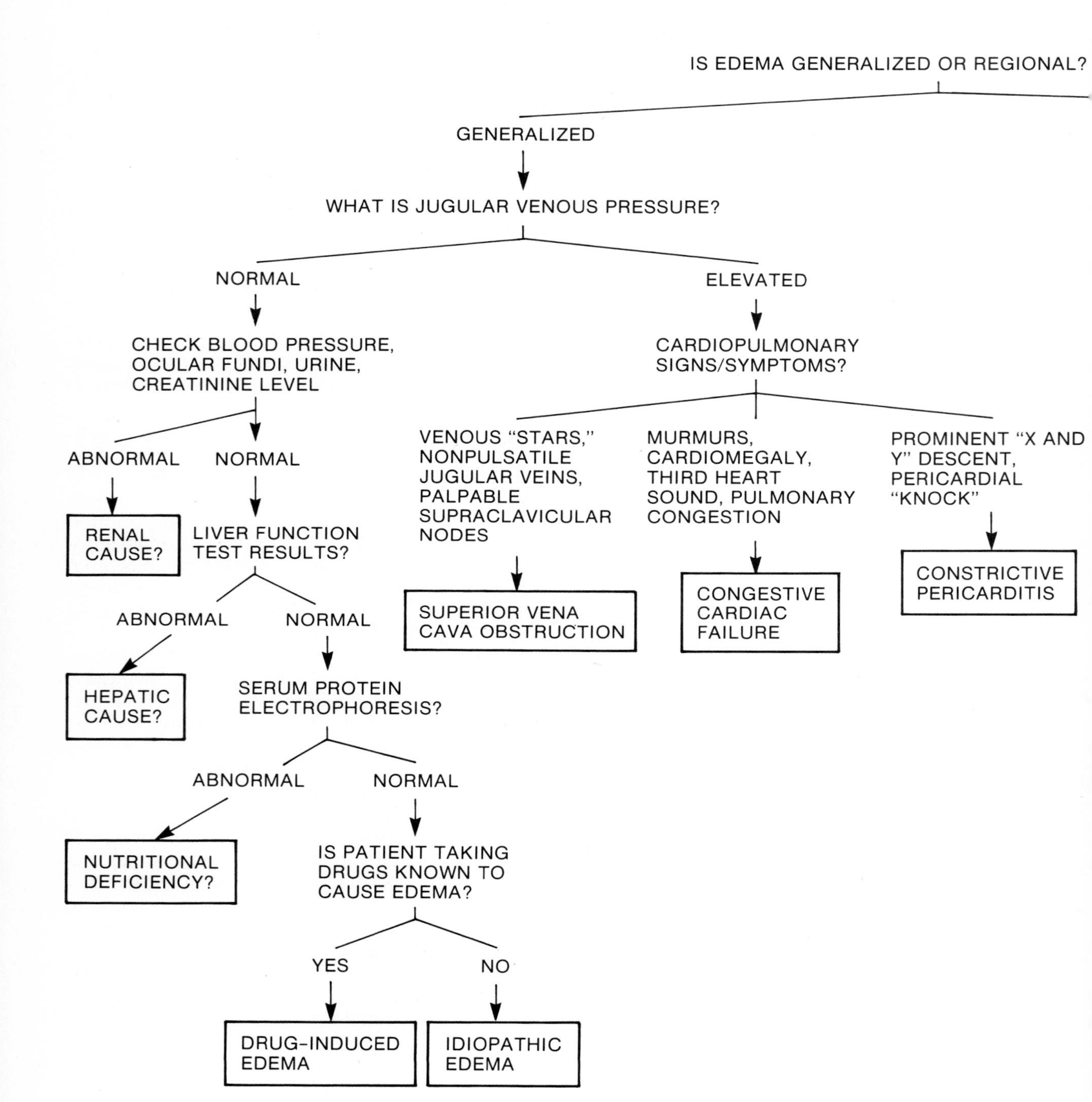
DIAGNOSTIC ASSESSMENT
IS EDEMA GENERALIZED OR REGIONAL?
GENERALIZED
WHAT IS JUGULAR VENOUS PRESSURE?
NORMAL
ELEVATED
CHECK BLOOD PRESSURE, OCULAR FUNDI, URINE, CREATININE LEVEL
CARDIOPULMONARY SIGNS/SYMPTOMS?
ABNORMAL
NORMAL
RENAL CAUSE?
LIVER FUNCTION TEST RESULTS?
VENOUS "STARS," NONPULSATILE JUGULAR VEINS, PALPABLE SUPRACLAVICULAR NODES
MURMURS, CARDIOMEGALY, THIRD HEART SOUND, PULMONARY CONGESTION
PROMINENT "X AND Y" DESCENT, PERICARDIAL "KNOCK"
SUPERIOR VENA CAVA OBSTRUCTION
CONGESTIVE CARDIAC FAILURE
CONSTRICTIVE PERICARDITIS
ABNORMAL
NORMAL
HEPATIC CAUSE?
SERUM PROTEIN ELECTROPHORESIS?
ABNORMAL
NORMAL
NUTRITIONAL DEFICIENCY?
IS PATIENT TAKING DRUGS KNOWN TO CAUSE EDEMA?
YES
NO
DRUG-INDUCED EDEMA
IDIOPATHIC EDEMA

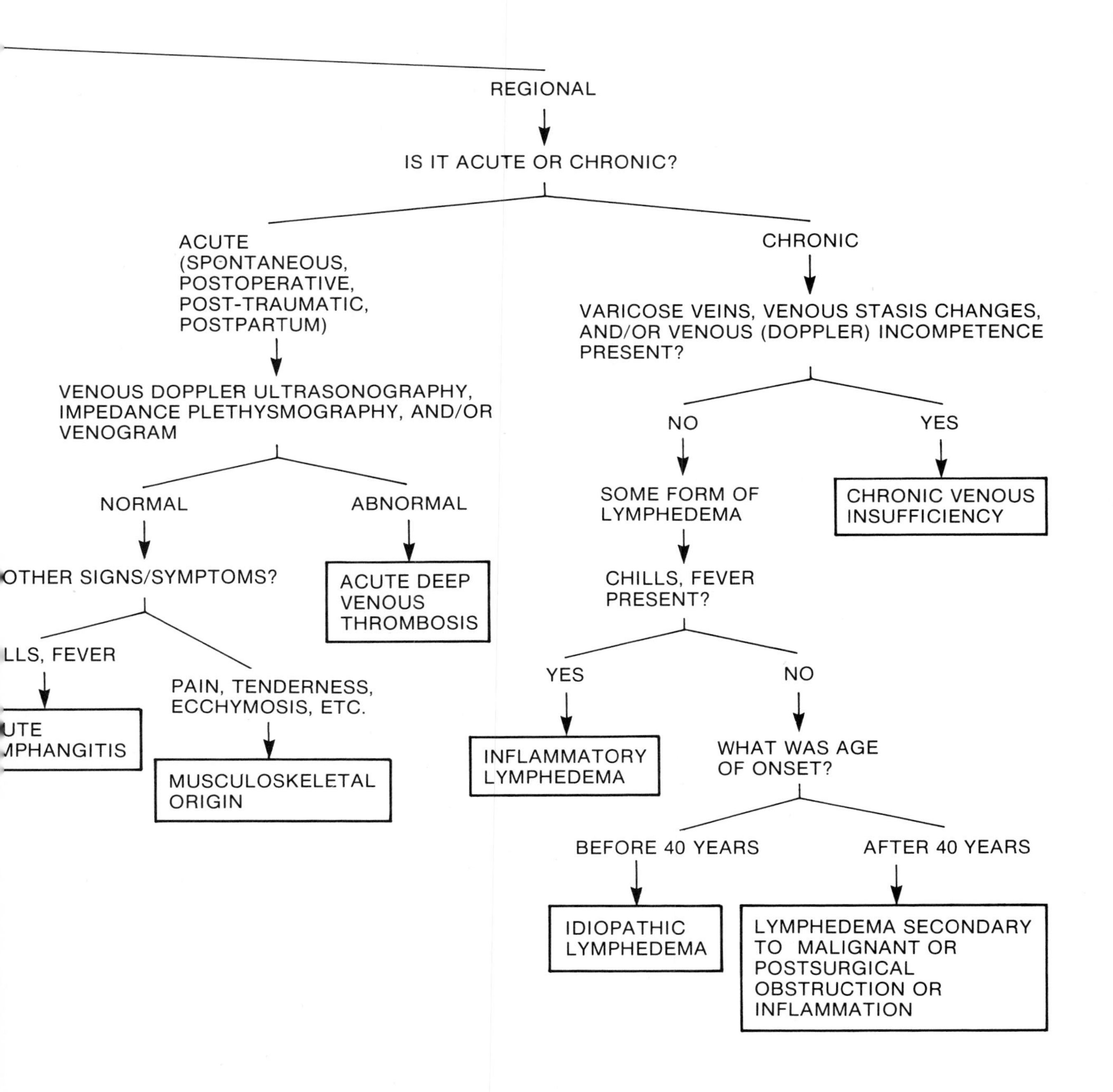

OF PERIPHERAL EDEMA
REGIONAL
IS IT ACUTE OR CHRONIC?
ACUTE (SPONTANEOUS, POSTOPERATIVE, POST-TRAUMATIC, POSTPARTUM)
CHRONIC
VENOUS DOPPLER ULTRASONOGRAPHY, IMPEDANCE PLETHYSMOGRAPHY, AND/OR VENOGRAM
VARICOSE VEINS, VENOUS STASIS CHANGES, AND/OR VENOUS (DOPPLER) INCOMPETENCE PRESENT?
NORMAL
ABNORMAL
NO
YES
OTHER SIGNS/SYMPTOMS?
ACUTE DEEP VENOUS THROMBOSIS
SOME FORM OF LYMPHEDEMA
CHRONIC VENOUS INSUFFICIENCY
LLS, FEVER
PAIN, TENDERNESS, ECCHYMOSIS, ETC.
CHILLS, FEVER PRESENT?
UTE
IPHANGITIS
MUSCULOSKELETAL ORIGIN
YES
NO
INFLAMMATORY LYMPHEDEMA
WHAT WAS AGE OF ONSET?
BEFORE 40 YEARS
AFTER 40 YEARS
IDIOPATHIC LYMPHEDEMA
LYMPHEDEMA SECONDARY TO MALIGNANT OR POSTSURGICAL OBSTRUCTION OR INFLAMMATION

rendering the differentiation from systemic edema more difficult.

Venous edema may be either acute or chronic. In acute deep venous thrombosis, pain and tenderness to palpation over the involved vein are common, in addition to the pitting edema. When the larger deep veins (popliteal, superficial, and common femoral) are occluded by thrombosis, there is usually an increase in the superficial venous pattern as well. When chronic venous hypertension is due to varicose veins or to deep vein (postphlebitic) incompetence, the signs of chronic venous stasis (stasis pigmentation, stasis ulcer) develop in the distal medial leg in addition to the orthostatic edema. In patients with obstruction of a deep vein by an extrinsic process (mass or scarring) the edema may mimic lymphedema in its firmness and slowness to recede with elevation, but the signs of chronic venous obstruction (venous "stars," collateral venous pathways, and the livid skin color) usually aid in the clinical differentiation. The use of a handheld Doppler device can provide immediate confirmation of venous obstruction or venous incompetence in these cases.

Lymphedema is usually painless, progressive, and unaccompanied by the signs of chronic venous stasis. On palpation the edema is firm, with thickening of the skin (pig skin or peau d' orange), and it recedes more slowly with elevation than venous edema. Inflammatory types of edema are seen in all age groups; the most common cause is dermatophytosis; the cracks between the toes serve as the portal of entry for the offending bacteria, usually streptococci. Lymphedema precox can usually be distinguished from obstructive lymphedema on clinical grounds, because it affects women nine times as frequently as men and usually begins before age 40, often about the time of menarche. Obstruction of lymphatics can occur as a result of surgery, scarring from radiation, or neoplastic involvement of nodes. The latter, obstructive lymphedema due to neoplasm, more commonly begins after age 40, has no sex predilection, and usually is secondary to a neoplasm arising in a pelvic structure (GU tract or GI tract) or to lymphoma; the malignant nodes are usually evident on examination or can be demonstrated by CT scan of the pelvis. If doubt exists about deep venous patency in a lymphedematous extremity, the Doppler venous examination is a useful noninvasive way to confirm it.

It is difficult to explain why the patient with lipedema presents so much diagnostic difficulty. Almost always occurring in a woman, the problem is obvious, symmetrically fat legs. The complaint to the physician commonly is "swelling," which indeed does occur and is orthostatic. Like other types of orthostatic edema it is usually worse premenstrually, in warm weather, with long sitting, or after liberal salt intake. The edema is soft, and pits readily (excluding lymphedema), and is unaccompanied by the signs of chronic venous stasis (excluding chronic venous insufficiency); its long-standing nature excludes deep venous thrombosis. When varicose veins coexist, there is a reason for difficulty in diagnosis, but the symmetry and typical contour of fat deposition, with normal feet and toes, should serve to distinguish lipedema.

Orthostatic edema is not a specific entity. Indeed most peripheral edema is orthostatic, but at times the typical soft pitting edema is due primarily to the lack of the muscular pumping action of the legs. This is most often seen in the geriatric patient who sits all day or in the person who sleeps sitting in a chair or with a foot hanging out of the bed (e.g., to try to relieve ischemic rest pain).

When there is an arteriovenous connection, the high arterial pressure is transmitted to the venous circulation distal to the connection. As a result of the venous hypertension the veins enlarge and may become varicose, and the extremity becomes edematous, livid, and warm. If the limb is traumatized, the ensuing ulceration has the appearance of a venous stasis ulcer. The arteriovenous connection should be easy to diagnose by auscultation, which detects the continuous bruit of a congenital fistula or the multiple-pitched systolic and diastolic bruit of an acquired arteriovenous fistula.

Frequently, after restoration of pulsatile flow to an ischemic limb by arterial surgery or percutaneous balloon angioplasty, the distal leg and foot are edematous for a short time. Although there is an orthostatic effect, this form of postoperative edema seems best explained by increased vascular permeability in the ischemic limb; it gradually resolves in one to several weeks without treatment. Venous Doppler ultrasound examination is a convenient bedside tool to differentiate this form of edema from postoperative venous thrombosis.

When edema complicates a musculoskeletal disorder, pain and tenderness are frequently the dominant complaint—often the patient notes the edema only when apprised of it. With calf muscle tears (e.g., plantaris tendon) the sudden pain and the telltale meniscus-shaped ecchymosis beneath the malleoli readily differentiate the edema from other regional types. When edema complicates tenosynovitis or march fracture, the localized tenderness is the most valuable differential feature. A popliteal cyst may cause edema of the distal leg by compressing the popliteal vein in the popliteal space or by herniating beneath the heads of the gastrocnemius muscle; in both cases the picture is one of venous obstruction accompanied by pain and tenderness in the popliteal space or upper calf. As mentioned earlier, ultrasonography is the preferred means of identifying popliteal cysts.[8]

Reflex sympathetic dystrophy is primarily a neurologic disorder but deserves inclusion at this point in a discussion of edema, because it follows some type of trauma and there commonly is a "moist" phase during which the involved extremity is swollen.[12] Generally the extremity is warm and moist but of normal color, and even though swelling is present, the patient complains almost exclusively about the diffuse dysesthesia and pain. With time, or with sympathetic nerve block or administration of ganglion-blocking drugs (e.g., prazosin), the edema recedes, suggesting that an increased vascular permeability is the basis of the edema in reflex sympathetic dystrophy.

REFERENCES

1. Ruschhaupt WF III. Differential diagnosis of edema of the lower extremities. In: Spittell JA, ed. Clinical vascular disease. Philadelphia: FA Davis, 1983.
2. Kaniglaski J. A profile of office practice. Bull Am Col Phys 1977;18:18.
3. Allen EV, Hines EA Jr. Lipedema of the legs: a syndrome characterized by fat legs and orthostatic edema. Proc Staff Meet Mayo Clin 1940;15:184–7.
4. Fairbairn JF II: Clinical manifestations of peripheral vascular disease. In: Juergens JL, Spittell JA Jr, Fairbairn JF II, eds. Peripheral vascular diseases. 5th ed. Philadelphia: WB Saunders, 1980;3–49.
5. Schirger A, Peterson LFA: Lymphedema. In: Juergens JL, Spittell JA Jr, Fairbairn JF II, eds. Peripheral vascular diseases. 5th ed. Philadelphia: WB Saunders, 1980;823–51.
6. Schirger A. Differential diagnosis and management of leg edema in the elderly. Geriatrics 1982;37:26–36.
7. Wheeler HB. A modern approach to diagnosing deep venous thrombosis. Cardiovasc Med 1980;5:217–31.
8. Carpenter JR, Hattery RR, Hunder GG, et al. Ultrasound evaluation of the popliteal space: comparison with arthrography and physical examination. Mayo Clin Proc 1976;51:498–503.
9. Edwards OM, Bayliss RIS. Idiopathic edema of women. Q J Med 1976;177:124–44.
10. Feldman HA, Jayakumar S, Pushett JB. Idiopathic edema: a review of etiologic concepts and management. Cardiovasc Med 1978;3:475–88.
11. Streeten DHP. Differential diagnosis of leg edema. Pract Cardiol 1982;8:159–72.
12. Juergens JL, Pluth JR. Trauma and peripheral vascular disease. In: Juergens JL, Spittell JA Jr, Fairbairn JF II, eds. Peripheral vascular diseases. 5th ed. Philadelphia: WB Saunders, 1980;615–6.

EOSINOPHILIA

W. KEITH HOOTS

□ SYNONYM: Elevated eosinophil count

BACKGROUND

The eosinophil was first described as a distinct cell in blood by T. W. Jones in 1846.[1] In the years since, many diseases have been described in which eosinophilia is a characteristic finding. Within the last decade some of the clinical entities have been grouped into distinct "eosinophilic syndromes" as it has become apparent that this single cell type may, on occasion, be associated with unique pathogenesis. On the other hand, eosinophilia has always been recognized as a hallmark of certain infectious processes. What is so unique about a normal cell that is observed but rarely in human blood, and why does its increase so often imply unusual disease? These are the questions that hematologists continue to ask. The complete cellular physiology of the human eosinophil is yet to be deciphered. Nonetheless, eosinophilia may best be discussed in light of some of the cell's known unique physiology. Therefore, within the context of distinguishing different diseases with eosinophilia, reference is made in this chapter to specialized eosinophil functions as they contribute to clinical symptoms.

Eosinophilia, like many clinical findings, represents the parsimony of human biology to stress and injury; that is to say, myriads of diverse insults may induce eosinophilia. The intriguing task for the clinician is to deduce from subtle differences in degree, rather than kind, what the source is. Appropriate therapy can then be chosen. It is the purpose of this discussion to clarify these subtle differences and thereby to enhance diagnosis.

Definition

By convention, *eosinophilia* exists when the number of eosinophils in the peripheral blood exceeds 350 per μl. Normally, 3.1 per cent of all white blood cells in the circulating blood of an average adult are eosinophils; the normal range in children aged 4 to 12 years is slightly higher. The peripheral blood contains only a small fraction of the total eosinophil pool. For each circulating eosinophil, there are approximately 300 mature and immature eosinophilic cells in the bone marrow and 100 to 300 more in the body tissues.[2]

Morphology and Function of Eosinophils

Cellular Structure and Function. Eosinophils are so named because of the staining characteristics of the granules within the cytoplasm. There are two basic components of the cytoplasm, a core and a matrix. The core is crystalloid, usually fairly electron-dense, and surrounded by the eosinophilic-staining matrix (Fig. 1).

The life span of an eosinophil in the blood stream varies from 5 to 24 hours. A β-adrenergic receptor appears to play a role in the release of eosinophils from the marrow. Within the bone marrow itself, the eosinophilic promyelocyte is the earliest identifiable cell in the eosinophil series. The maturation pattern is nearly identical to that observed in neutrophilic maturation. Recent evidence has shown that lymphocytes may modulate the production of eosinophils within the marrow through the release of lymphokines or lymphocyte-derived regulators.[3] Specific modification of eosinophilic function within the circulation is discussed later in the chapter.

Eosinophils are capable of phagocytizing organisms much as neutrophils do. However, the phagocytic response of eosinophils is less than that of neutrophils, possibly owing to a relative paucity of receptors on human eosinophils. It is therefore unlikely that the eosinophil plays a major role in routine phagocytosis. Studies have shown, however, that the eosinophil functions as a cytotoxic killer cell against certain parasites. As a specific example, eosinophils are the principal effector cells in antibody-dependent killing of schistosoma organisms seen in schistosomiasis. Receptors for human IgG and human complement on the surface of eosinophils may trigger this cytotoxic function.[4]

Eosinophil-Derived Substances. Metazoan and parasitic cytotoxicity and other allergic-type responses that are mediated by eosinophils are dependent on complement binding for recognition. Such recognition leads to secretion of peroxidase,

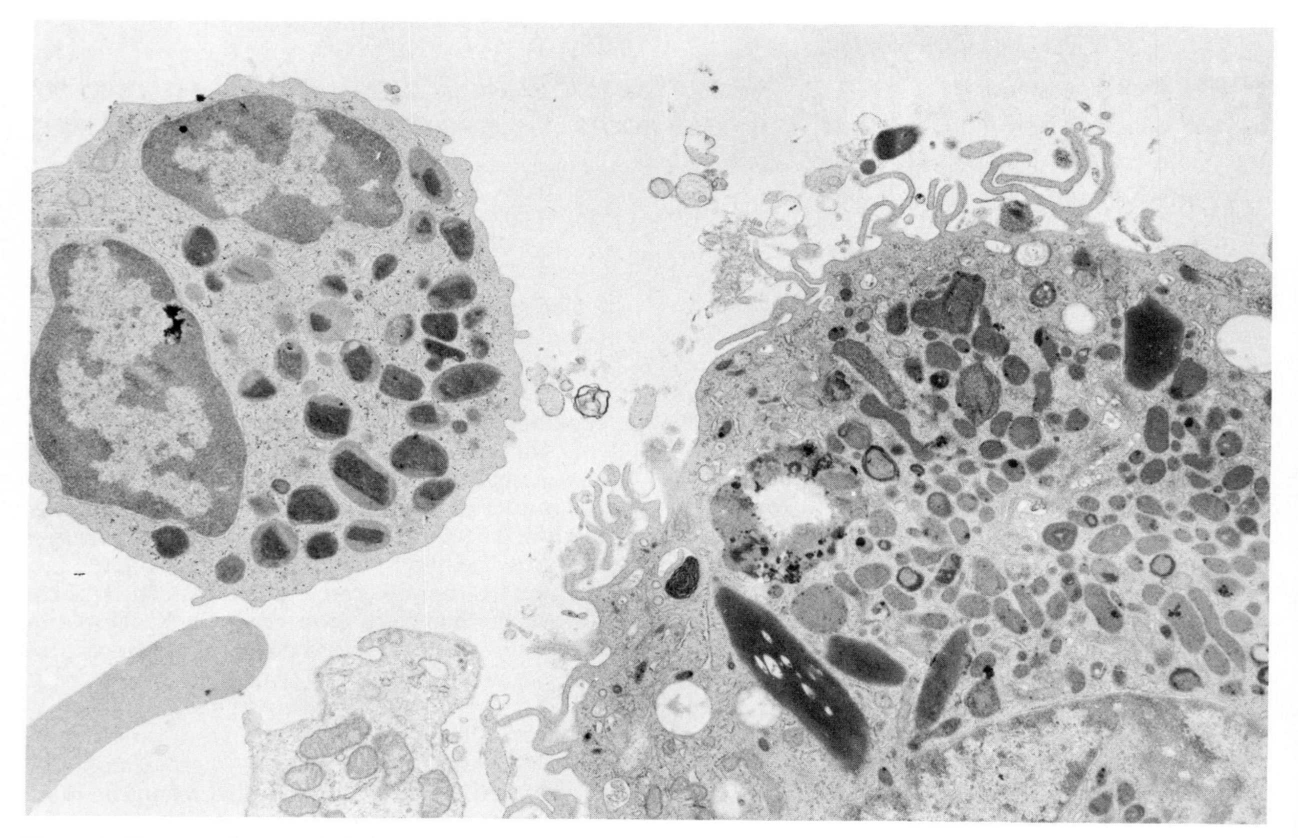

Figure 1. The granulocytic cell *(left)* is an eosinophil that is invading lung parenchyma in a patient with hypereosinophilic syndrome. The cytoplasmic core and matrix can be distinguished by the presence of crystalloid within the core particles. The surrounding matrix is seen as the fine granular area around the crystals.

histamine, and the "major basic protein" (MBP) from the granules, which mediate cytotoxicity. In addition, their presence may be harmful to surrounding tissues via a "bystander" effect.[5]

Eosinophilic Modifiers. The process by which eosinophilia becomes a clinical phenomenon is not well understood; immediate hypersensitivity or activation of the complement cascade appears to provoke release of eosinophils from the bone marrow. Specifically, degranulation of mast cells is important, because it results in a release of both histamine and the proteins eosinophilic chemotactic factor of anaphylaxis (ECFA), eosinophilic chemotactic factor of complement (ECF-C), and an eosinophil stimulator promoter (ESP). Additionally, antigen-antibody complexes may stimulate release of ESP. These factors then interact with lymphocytes to induce further lymphokine release.[5]

CLINICAL SPECTRUM OF EOSINOPHILIA AND DISEASE

The causes of eosinophilia are summarized in Table 1.

Allergic Symptomatology

It has long been known that eosinophilia occurs in patients with allergy. In those individuals who have allergic rhinitis, nasal eosinophilia is a common finding. Similarly, evidence of airway eosinophilia may be demonstrated in respiratory secretions of patients with asthma. Allergic disorders appear to cause eosinophilia by the binding of IgE antigen-antibody complexes to the surface of mast cells. These cells then liberate histamine and eosinophilic chemotactic factor, as described previously. Eosinophils migrate to the site of the allergic reaction and become "selectively" cytotoxic. The presence of foreign organisms such as parasites activates further cytotoxicity.

Autoimmune Symptomatology

Just as eosinophilia is a manifestation of allergic symptoms, it is often seen in autoimmune conditions. A possible prototype eosinophilic autoimmune disease is the hypereosinophilic syndrome (HES). HES is a diagnosis of exclusion, made by ruling out other allergic and autoimmune etiologies. In addition, other systemic diseases of a malignant origin (discussed later) must be considered and discounted. Eosinophilia of over 1,500 eosinophils/μl that persists longer than 6 months, a lack of evidence of allergy or parasitic infection, and signs and symptoms of organ involvement (including hepatosplenomegaly, organic heart murmur, congestive heart failure, diffuse or focal CNS abnormalities, pulmonary fibrosis, fever, weight loss, and anemia) are the triad of criteria necessary for the diagnosis of HES.[6]

Predominantly a disease of young adult males, HES has a variably poor prognosis. Because of the pulmonary manifestations of dyspnea with infiltrates, the differentiation that must be made between this disease and the Loeffler syndrome may be difficult. The latter is a benign self-limited condition, variably ascribed to parasitic infection, that has minimal symptoms, migratory lung infiltrates, and no cardiac involvement. Also, the vasculitis seen with HES may make differentiation from polyarteritis difficult.

Recently, there has been debate about whether HES is an entity distinct from acute eosinophilic leukemia (AEL). No consensus has been reached, but there appears to be an overlapping spectrum of symptoms. The amount of organ involvement and the clinical outcome are bimodal. Those patients having primarily cardiopulmonary symptoms and vasculitis appear to follow a clinical course most consistent with a disseminated vasculitis. On the other hand, those patients with primary hepatosplenomegaly, extraordinarily high eosinophilic count, and rapid clinical deterioration probably have the malignancy, AEL.

Hypereosinophilic syndrome is very rare in children. Variations of the disease may be isolated to specific organ involvement. If the heart is primarily involved, the clinical diagnosis of endocarditis with endomyocardial fibrosis may actually be a variation of HES.

Other autoimmune phenomena associated with eosinophilia include the following: eosinophilic fasciitis, rheumatoid arthritis, polyarteritis nodosa, chronic hepatitis, regional enteritis, eosinophilic cystitis, eosinophilic gastroenteritis, and infection of ventriculoperitoneal shunt (see Table 1). There is a suggestion that the eosinophilia of chronic peritoneal dialysis is a result of an autoimmune phenomenon as well.[7] A complete discussion of each entity is beyond the scope of this discussion; however, individual entities are mentioned subsequently in a differential diagnosis context for the patient in whom eosinophilia is a presenting symptom.

In addition to systemic autoimmune disease, eosinophilia may be observed with local inflammatory lesions that may prove difficult to differentiate from the early HES. A discussion of several such immune-related diseases follows.

Eosinophilic Myositis. This disorder may manifest as a muscle pseudotumor associated with eosinophilia. There may be localized swelling and tenderness in the area of a large muscle group that is very difficult to distinguish from the presentation of parasitic entities that invade muscles,

Table 1. CAUSES OF EOSINOPHILIA*

Type of Disorder	More Frequently Associated with Eosinophilia	Less Frequently Associated with Eosinophilia
Infectious	Metazoan infestations, e.g. hookworm, schistosomiasis, ascariasis, trichinosis Filariasis Echinococcus infection Loeffler's pneumonia due to parasites	Lymphochorionic virus Infection of the CNS Infantile staphylococcal infection Scarlet fever Chorea Erythema multiforme Histoplasmosis
Allergic	Asthma Seasonal rhinitis Urticaria Neonatal eosinophilic colitis	Angioneurotic edema Allergic granulomatosis (Churg-Strauss syndrome)
Dermatologic	Pemphigus, pemphigoid Well's syndrome (recurrent granulomatous dermatitis)	Eosinophilic papillary folliculitis
Malignant	Eosinophilic leukemia Acute lymphoblastic leukemia Acute nonlymphocytic leukemia Chronic myelogenous leukemia Carcinoma (vagina, nasopharynx, thyroid, penis, skin) Adenocarcinoma of the stomach or uterus Malignant histiocytosis	Disseminated glioblastoma Hodgkin's disease Lymphoma Lung cancer Gastrointestinal cancer Fibrous histiocytoma Islet cell tumor of pancreas
Autoimmune	Eosinophilic fasciitis Eosinophilic myositis Eosinophilic gastroenteritis Eosinophilic cystitis Loeffler's endocarditis Chronic hepatitis	Ulcerative colitis Regional enteritis Rheumatoid arthritis Angiitis Polyarteritis nodosa
Idiopathic	The hypereosinophilic syndrome (HES) Pulmonary infiltration with eosinophilia (PIE) Angiolymphoid hyperplasia with eosinophilia	Systemic mastocytosis Postsplenectomy state
Therapy-associated	Infected ventriculoperitoneal shunt	Radiation therapy
Drug-associated	Penicillin Cephalosporins Nitrofurantoins Para-aminosalicylic acid Phenytoin Hydralazine Chlorpromazine	Warfarin Captopril Carbamazine
Congenital and neonatal	Monosomy 7 Familial erythrophagocytic lymphohistiocytosis Eosinophilia of prematurity Hyperimmunoglobulinemia	Cardiovascular defects Thrombocytopenia–absent radius (TAR) syndrome Congenital immune deficiencies (SCIDS and x-linked agammaglobulinemia)

*Causes are listed in order by incidence of eosinophilia.[2, 26]

such as trichinosis and cysticercosis. Usually there is pain and swelling of the extremities, and occasionally dermal involvement is seen. In addition, there may be systemic symptoms of fever and malaise. Eosinophilic myositis may occur as part of HES or, more commonly, as an isolated phenomenon.[8]

Eosinophilic Fasciitis. Eosinophilic fasciitis is a skin and facial disease difficult to distinguish from scleroderma. It differs from scleroderma in being relatively acute in onset, following episodes of unusual physical exertion, and responding to corticosteroids. Usually, eosinophils are found in blood and skin tissue. Also in contrast to scleroderma, degranulating mast cells rather than immune complex deposition mediate the inflammatory pathogenesis of eosinophilic fasciitis.[9]

Eosinophilic Gastroenteritis. An autoimmune mechanism with mast cell activation of the complement cascade also seems to be operative in eosinophilic gastroenteritis. Patients present with postprandial nausea, vomiting, cramping, periumbilical pain, and loose, watery stools. Charcot-Leyden crystals, which are the breakdown products of eosinophils, may be present in the stools. Thickening of the bowel wall is often seen on proctoscopic or rectosigmoid biopsy. The pathogenesis is not completely understood, but an autoimmune mechanism is strongly suggested.[10]

Eosinophilic Cystitis. A bladder irritation mimicking other forms of intractable cystitis such as interstitial cystitis, tuberculosis, and bladder neoplasm has been described as secondary to an allergic or immune disorder. Eosinophilia is invariably seen in the blood and the bladder wall. The disease is usually chronic in duration, and in some patients food allergens have been incriminated.[11]

Hepatitis. Hepatitis may be associated with eosinophilia. In most cases, however, the systemic signs and symptoms point to hepatitis, and isolated eosinophilia without these symptoms would preclude such a diagnosis.

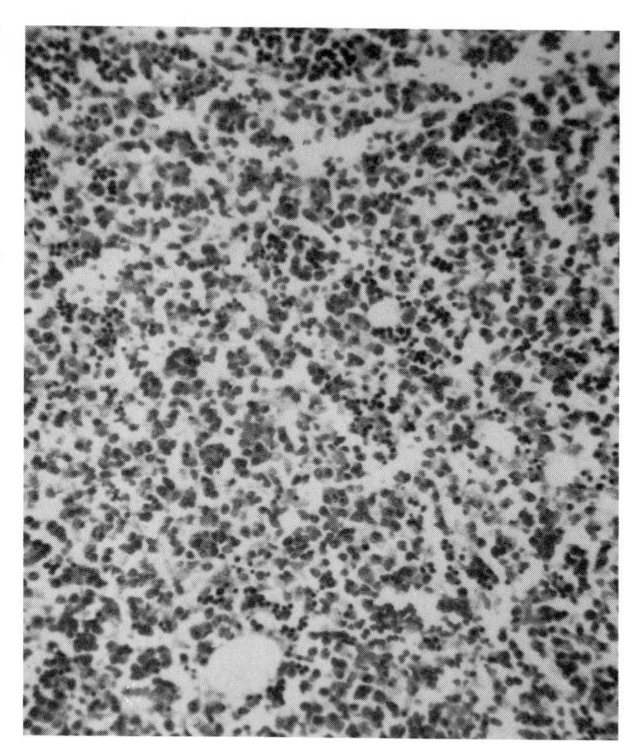

Figure 2. Eosinophilic blast cells infiltrating bone marrow are seen as the predominant cell type in this bone marrow aspirate from a patient with acute eosinophilic leukemia. There is a notable absence of normal bone marrow cells, including megakaryocytes, myeloid precursors, and erythroid precursors.

Eosinophilia Associated with Malignancy

Eosinophilia as a concomitant sign of multiple tumors has been recognized for some time. Eosinophilia has been observed most often in association with carcinoma of the nasopharynx and bronchus, and in adenocarcinoma of the stomach, large bowel, uterus, and thyroid. In addition, it has been seen in Hodgkin's disease and histiocytoma.[12]

The pattern of eosinophilia in malignancy appears to have clinical significance. It has been noted that eosinophilia can be associated with either the tumor tissue or the blood. Malignancies in which eosinophilia is observed in the tumor alone appear to have a better prognosis than those without eosinophilia. However, those tumors associated with blood eosinophilia often demonstrate tumor spread and poor prognosis.[12]

Malignant transformation of eosinophils gives rise to AEL (Fig. 2). Eosinophilia, however, is not uncommon in other leukemias as well, such as acute lymphocytic leukemia (ALL) and acute myelogenous leukemia (AML). At times, it is very difficult to differentiate AEL from the reactive eosinophilia associated with ALL and AML. Specific cell marker studies are the most definitive means of distinguishing types.

The difficulty in differentiating incipient HES from eosinophilia associated with leukemia has been mentioned. In this regard, it is noteworthy that chloromas and blastomas (i.e., masses of eosinophils and blast cells) are very rare in HES but are often seen in the leukemias. In addition, in comparisons of chromosome studies from patients with HES with karyotypes of patients with proven leukemia, HES has usually been associated with no abnormalities; conversely, aneuploidy and polyploidy often are seen in ALL, AML, and AEL.[13] With such similarity in presentation, these specific studies may be crucial in differentiating the entities.

Eosinophilic Response to Parasitic Infection

Eosinophilia, often extreme, is so commonly associated with helminthic infection that physicians should instinctively consider parasitic infestation whenever eosinophilia appears. Certain metazoan infestations are characteristically associated with very high eosinophilic states; these include schistosomiasis, trichinosis, visceral larva migrans, and filariasis. There are an estimated 200 million cases of schistosomiasis alone worldwide.[14] Absolute eosinophil counts are usually greater than 3,000 per μl, often much higher. The lymphadenopathy and hepatosplenomegaly observed in these infections may cause diagnostic confusion with HES. Appropriate diagnostic and culture studies must be performed to make the distinction.

As has been discussed, eosinophils appear to have a special cytotoxicity for helminthic organisms. This property apparently explains the protection that eosinophilia confers to individuals during an infestation with a parasitic infection. As a result of the large amount of eosinophilic infiltration in the areas of local parasitic infestation, however, tissue damage may be caused by the release of the eosinophilic proteins, which are themselves toxic to surrounding tissues. The clinical symptoms arise because of both the destruction by the worm in the midst of surrounding organ tissue and the associated inflammatory destructive process mediated by the eosinophilia.

Eosinophilia in the Pediatric Patient

Eosinophilia is not uncommon in children. In the United States, allergy is probably the most common cause of eosinophilia in the pediatric population. Approximately 85 per cent of children with bronchial asthma have eosinophil counts in excess of 600 per µl. Usually eosinophilia is persistent and its degree does not correlate with the severity of symptoms. Worldwide, the most common cause of eosinophilia is parasitic infestation. As has been noted, eosinophilia is generally seen in helminthic but not protozoan infections. In particular, *Giardia lamblia* infection is associated with an absence of eosinophilia.[2]

Visceral larva migrans, an infection with *Toxocara canis* or *Toxocara cati,* is the most common helminthic disease in children. The eosinophilia seen with it is most marked during the larval development and migration of the disease. Clinically, hepatomegaly, pulmonary infiltrates, anemia, and hypoglobulinemia are also seen. The visceral form is distinct from cutaneous larva migrans and the creeping eruption caused by *Ancylostoma braziliense.* This latter entity presents as a pruritic, serpiginous rash. Although these three are the more common parasites in Western society, the frequency of other types of helminthic infection in children worldwide is quite dependent on cultural practices and endemic species.

Children with certain inherited disorders also may present with eosinophilia. These include familial histiocytosis and severe combined immunodeficiency syndrome, in both of which the absolute eosinophilic count tends to be less than that seen in parasitic infection. In addition, certain genetic and chromosomal anomalies may predispose to malignancy associated with eosinophilia. Monosomy 7 predisposing to eosinophilia and leukemia is an example of this phenomenon.[15]

Eosinophilic gastroenteritis is predominantly a childhood disease, most patients being less than 20 years of age. An allergic history is variably present.

Eosinophilia is commonly seen in premature infants, who often have eosinophilia until they regain their birth weight. Recent evidence has associated the high eosinophil count with the establishment of an anabolic state.[16]

HISTORY

Eosinophilia is most commonly detected during a routine laboratory work-up for a patient with unusual complaints. The physician will have obtained a clinical history prior to the time he discovers that the patient has eosinophilia, unlike those occasions in which the patient is known to have eosinophilia because of prior medical evaluation. The awareness of eosinophilia allows for selective inquiry during history taking by the physician and also aids selection of further laboratory testing.

History of the Present Illness. Eosinophilia may be a manifestation of a myriad of diseases with multiple clinical findings. When a physician is aware of the eosinophilia at the time the history is obtained, this multiplicity of symptoms may conform to certain types of well-described syndromes. To diagnose rare diseases, one must have knowledge of these strange patterns of complaints. The following discussion suggests some pertinent questions that may prove helpful in diagnosing the more common causes of eosinophilia. The algorithm illustrates the categorization of patients according to presenting complaint and laboratory results.

A patient complaining of localized muscle tenderness with pain who has no history of systemic disease should be asked about exercise or exertion just prior to the onset of complaints. Not only would this information be important for diagnosing traumatic injury to the muscle, but in cases of eosinophilic myositis and fasciitis, there often is a preceding muscle injury.

The presence of eosinophilia points the astute dermatologist toward some very characteristic lesions, such as cutaneous larva migrans, described previously. A rarer entity is Well's syndrome, or recurrent granulomatous dermatitis with eosinophilia, which manifests as skin lesions, granulomas, and eosinophilia.[17] It must be distinguished from more systemic diseases such as Hodgkin's disease, which may also manifest as rash and eosinophilia. In addition, inquiries concerning toxic or drug exposure are essential when skin disease is present, since rashes and eosinophilia may be common to both.

DIAGNOSTIC ASSESSMENT OF EOSINOPHILIA

IS THE EOSINOPHILIA CONGENITAL OR ACQUIRED?

- CONGENITAL → ARE THERE BIRTH DEFECTS?
  - NO → CONGENITAL IMMUNE DEFICIENCIES, EOSINOPHILIA WITH PREMATURITY, OR FAMILIAL HISTIOCYTOSIS
  - YES → THROMBOCYTOPENIA WITH ABSENCE OF RADIUS, MONOSOMY 7, OR CONGENITAL HEART DISEASE
- ACQUIRED → STOOL EXAM FOR OVA AND PARASITES
  - NEGATIVE → REPEAT EOSINOPHIL COUNT
    - <3,000 CELLS/μL → HISTORY OF ALLERGY?
      - YES
      - NO → SYSTEMIC COMPLAINTS?
        - NO
        - YES
    - >3,000 CELLS/μL → REPEAT STOOL EXAM FOR OVA AND PARASITES
      - NEGATIVE → CARDIOPULMONARY SYMPTOMS (PNEUMONIA, CARDITIS)?
      - POSITIVE → MICROBIOLOGIC ID OF HELMINTH
  - POSITIVE → MICROBIOLOGIC ID OF HELMINTH

Algorithm continues on following pages

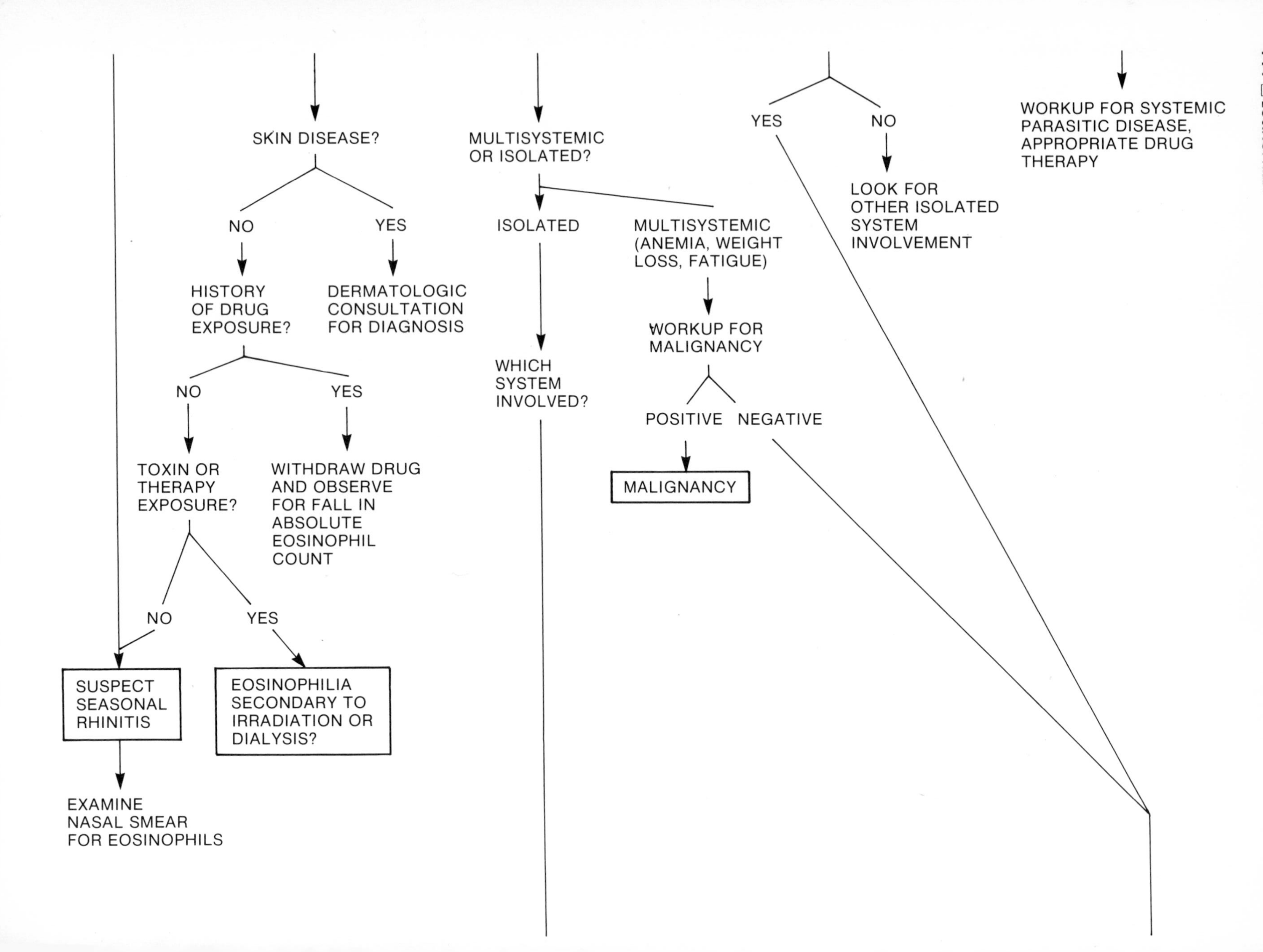
SKIN DISEASE?
NO
YES
HISTORY OF DRUG EXPOSURE?
DERMATOLOGIC CONSULTATION FOR DIAGNOSIS
NO
YES
TOXIN OR THERAPY EXPOSURE?
WITHDRAW DRUG AND OBSERVE FOR FALL IN ABSOLUTE EOSINOPHIL COUNT
NO
YES
SUSPECT SEASONAL RHINITIS
EOSINOPHILIA SECONDARY TO IRRADIATION OR DIALYSIS?
EXAMINE NASAL SMEAR FOR EOSINOPHILS
MULTISYSTEMIC OR ISOLATED?
ISOLATED
MULTISYSTEMIC (ANEMIA, WEIGHT LOSS, FATIGUE)
WHICH SYSTEM INVOLVED?
WORKUP FOR MALIGNANCY
POSITIVE
NEGATIVE
MALIGNANCY
YES
NO
LOOK FOR OTHER ISOLATED SYSTEM INVOLVEMENT
WORKUP FOR SYSTEMIC PARASITIC DISEASE, APPROPRIATE DRUG THERAPY

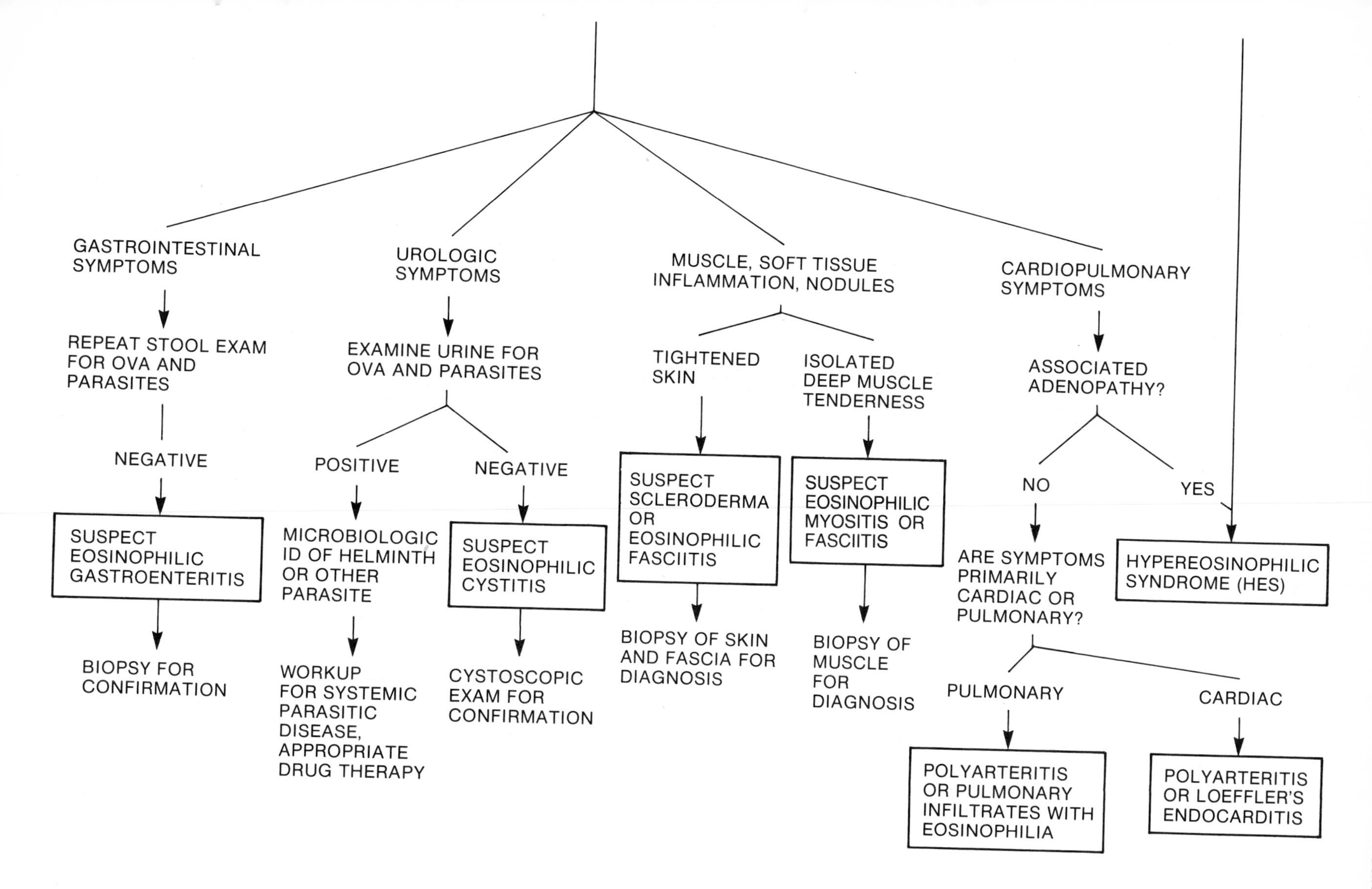
GASTROINTESTINAL SYMPTOMS
REPEAT STOOL EXAM FOR OVA AND PARASITES
NEGATIVE
SUSPECT EOSINOPHILIC GASTROENTERITIS
BIOPSY FOR CONFIRMATION
UROLOGIC SYMPTOMS
EXAMINE URINE FOR OVA AND PARASITES
POSITIVE
MICROBIOLOGIC ID OF HELMINTH OR OTHER PARASITE
WORKUP FOR SYSTEMIC PARASITIC DISEASE, APPROPRIATE DRUG THERAPY
NEGATIVE
SUSPECT EOSINOPHILIC CYSTITIS
CYSTOSCOPIC EXAM FOR CONFIRMATION
MUSCLE, SOFT TISSUE INFLAMMATION, NODULES
TIGHTENED SKIN
SUSPECT SCLERODERMA OR EOSINOPHILIC FASCIITIS
BIOPSY OF SKIN AND FASCIA FOR DIAGNOSIS
ISOLATED DEEP MUSCLE TENDERNESS
SUSPECT EOSINOPHILIC MYOSITIS OR FASCIITIS
BIOPSY OF MUSCLE FOR DIAGNOSIS
CARDIOPULMONARY SYMPTOMS
ASSOCIATED ADENOPATHY?
NO
ARE SYMPTOMS PRIMARILY CARDIAC OR PULMONARY?
PULMONARY
POLYARTERITIS OR PULMONARY INFILTRATES WITH EOSINOPHILIA
CARDIAC
POLYARTERITIS OR LOEFFLER'S ENDOCARDITIS
YES
HYPEREOSINOPHILIC SYNDROME (HES)

A complaint of abdominal cramping and pain, vomiting, and diarrhea with bleeding should immediately arouse the physician's suspicion of an infectious cause. When these symptoms are seen with eosinophilia, helminthic infection and allergic eosinophilic gastroenteritis should be considered. Duration of symptoms and travel history should help distinguish these entities.

Complaints of bladder irritation or painful urination with associated eosinophilia may suggest eosinophilic cystitis. On occasion, symptoms may imitate tuberculosis or a bladder neoplasm. The history and severity of symptoms may not be a clue, although the initial complaints help to point to definitive physical findings and special procedures to diagnose the condition.

Insightful Inquiry. The exacting physician asks specific questions that may narrow the diagnostic choices. Some specific questions that should be asked of patients with known eosinophilia are: Are the symptoms in question of recent onset? If not, how long have they been present, and did they begin in conjunction with travel, known toxic exposure, or drug use or abuse? Do the symptoms pertain chiefly to one area of the body or are they diffuse? If diffuse, are they associated with general changes of health, such as weight loss and chronic fatigue? By asking such questions, the physician can put the correct emphasis on aspects of the physical examination and better choose appropriate laboratory studies.

Previous Medical History and System Review. Information that does not appear germane to the initial presenting complaint is often obtained from a previous medical history. However, further inquiry may suggest an unrelated second disease that is responsible for eosinophilia. An example might be a complaint of anal pruritus in a child with otitis media who has ancillary infection with pinworms. In this case, the eosinophilia relates to a secondary disease rather than the complaint that brought the patient for medical attention.

Through a carefully taken medical history and a meticulous review of systems, the physician may discover the obscure cause for eosinophilia, particularly when it is unrelated to the primary disease.

Family History. A patient with a family history of *allergy* may be predisposed to allergic diseases himself. On the other hand, an absolute eosinophil count greater than 1,000 per μl is unlikely to have an allergic etiology, and a more intensive investigation for other sources must be undertaken.

Since *malignancies* are among the more common causes of eosinophilia, notation of family members with malignancy should raise one's suspicion of eosinophilia secondary to an underlying cancer. Similarly, a family history of autoimmune diseases may predispose to rheumatoid arthritis, polyarteritis, and even HES.

Lifestyle. Details about a patient's lifestyle are quite important. History of travel to a subtropical region point to tropical filariasis, trichinosis, and other endemic helminthic infections as viable differential diagnoses. Accordingly, an awareness of the endemic areas for certain parasites may help the physician differentiate schistosomiasis from tropical filariasis, because the former is more common in Africa, and the latter more common in India and Asia.

Drug and Therapeutic History. Drug exposure history is likewise a vital part of any work-up for eosinophilia. Many drugs have been implicated as primary precipitants of moderate eosinophilia. Penicillin, ampicillin, cephalosporins, nitrofurantoin, para-aminosalicylic acid, phenytoin, hydralazine, and chlorpromazine are most commonly cited.[2] Other implicated drugs include warfarin and carbamazepine.[18, 19] New prescription drugs are continually available, so the prudent clinician is always alert to pharmacologic causes of eosinophilia.

Other exposures may be important in eosinophilia as well. For example, therapeutic doses of ionizing irradiation for localized malignancy can produce eosinophilia. Occupational radiation exposures should also be considered.

Finally, unusual therapeutic methods may themselves cause eosinophilia, in particular, hemodialysis for chronic renal disease.[7] In addition, premature infants undergoing therapy for neonatal lung disease, necrotizing enterocolitis, or other chronic diseases frequently have intrinsic eosinophilia, perhaps because they have a limited capability to respond to different noxious stimuli.

PHYSICAL EXAMINATION

General Evaluation

Careful observation is essential to any good physical examination. In a cachectic, pale patient, cancer may be the underlying cause of eosinophilia. At the other extreme, for the active and vigorous child with an "allergic shiner" no further search may be required to explain mild eosinophilia. Astute observation, in this case, obviates the need for an expensive work-up. However, since eosinophilia is associated with so many diverse diseases, careful organ-by-organ analysis is usually required to determine the source of the proliferation of eosinophils.

Organ System Evaluation

Neurologic Examination. Eosinophilia is not associated with peripheral neuropathies or degenerative neurologic disease. Similarly, it is scarcely seen with acute neurologic infection such as meningitis or encephalitis. When systemic eosinophilia is observed in conjunction with CNS or CSF eosinophilia, however, one must be alert to peculiar presentations of diseases. For example, certain types of viral meningitis, such as lymphocytic choriomeningitis, may present with CSF and systemic eosinophilia.[20] However, nuchal rigidity and meningism associated with eosinophilia may not in themselves be diagnostic of infectious meningitis, because eosinophilia in the CSF has been seen with disseminated glioblastoma and other CNS neoplasia. In one review, only 94 of 10,000 quantitated cytologic examinations of CSF demonstrated CSF eosinophilia; infections and inflammatory diseases were most commonly implicated.[21] Eosinophils may actually be neurotoxic in themselves. That eosinophilia causes CNS tissue damage has been proven definitively in animals and suggested in humans. This eosinophilic neurotoxicity has been called the Gordon phenomenon.[22] It is possible that patients with HES or eosinophilic leukemia may exhibit weakness, hemiplegia, and incoordination owing to eosinophilic infiltration of the CNS.

Eye Examination. Since retinitis and iriditis may be complications of HES, careful ophthalmologic examination is important in patients considered to be at risk for the disorder.

Cardiac Examination. Cardiac symptoms in association with eosinophilia also occur in HES. Signs of congestive heart failure, including hepatosplenomegaly, tachycardia, heart murmur, and hyperdynamic precordium, may be demonstrable. The presence of cardiopulmonary symptoms may help differentiate HES from the eosinophilic myeloproliferative syndromes. Most authors agree that cardiopulmonary symptoms predominate in HES, whereas they are unusual in eosinophilia-associated malignancies.

Less severe heart and lung findings are also seen in other eosinophilic diseases. Specific examples include fibroplastic parietal endocarditis, which is a manifestation of Loeffler's endocarditis. In the latter, eosinophilic infiltration of the heart, lungs, nervous system, and skin is seen along with peripheral eosinophilia.

Pulmonary Examination. Pulmonary infiltrates and eosinophilia often coexist. HES is, of course, an example of such coexistence. The cardinal sign in so-called pulmonary infiltrates with eosinophilia (PIE) is migratory lung infiltrates. In Loeffler's syndrome, an example of PIE, remarkable rales and rhonchi are detected on auscultation. Cardiac signs are usually absent. Hence, isolated rales, wheezes, and rhonchi may imply the PIE of Loeffler's syndrome rather than HES.

Parasitic infections also commonly produce lung disease. For example, patients with filariasis often present with paroxysmal coughing and wheezing. Pulmonary findings mimick a severe asthmatic attack.

Gastrointestinal Examination. Careful palpation and auscultation of the abdomen are essential in differentiating the enteral diseases associated with eosinophilia. For example, hyperactive bowel sounds, borborygmi, and periumbilical tenderness to palpation are common in patients with eosinophilic gastroenteritis. On the other hand, patients with hepatosplenomegaly may have HES. When eosinophilia is seen in conjunction with other abdominal masses such as myeloblastomas or chloromas, leukemia (ALL or AEL) is the etiology. Isolated hepatosplenomegaly and adenopathy with eosinophilia suggest Hodgkin's disease. A rectal examination is indicated in all patients with gastrointestinal symptoms. The presence of bloody diarrhea suggests helminthic infection of the GI tract. Guaiac testing and culture of stool specimens obtained at rectal examination are essential.

Dermatologic Examination. A number of diseases associated with eosinophilia have dermatologic manifestations. The erythematous serpiginous rash of cutaneous larva migrans is a common cause of pruritus in children. Feet, buttocks, arms, hands, and back are common sites of larval invasions.[23]

The tight skin of HES mimics that of scleroderma. Characteristically, it takes the appearance of whitish, hardened skin with indentations.

Musculoskeletal Examination. Just as a careful inquiry about possible muscle pain, weakness, or other findings is important, so is a muscle group examination. The noninflamed muscle pseudotumors of eosinophilic myositis are readily palpable; the presence of erythema and localized tenderness over a muscle, however, suggests trichinosis or cysticercosis.[14] Eosinophilia and morphea-like lesions overlying a tender muscle are practically diagnostic of eosinophilic fasciitis. Weakness and proximal and distal extremity incoordination with or without joint inflammation are variably demonstrable in patients with HES.

Lymphatic Examination. Significant palpable lymphadenopathy with eosinophilia is rare. Axillary, supraclavicular, and inguinal adenopathy associated with hepatosplenomegaly should prompt the clinician to investigate for lymphoid malignancy. However, localized adenopathy in one extremity is more commonly a manifestation of a localized helminthic infection such as trichinosis or cysticercosis. One other rare disease that may manifest as large, slowly progressing papules and nodules that appear around the head and neck is angiolymphoid hyperplasia with eosinophilia.[24] These lesions enlarge by slow extension and are usually limited to the head and neck.

Genitourinary Examination. On most occasions one cannot diagnose an eosinophilia-associated disease on the basis of a genitourinary examination. More commonly, the definitive diagnosis requires intravenous pyelography or cystoscopy. However, eosinophilia in the presence of urethral irritation and tenderness over the bladder area point to eosinophilic cystitis. In the prodrome of HES, mucosal ulceration of the vagina and perineal area in women or of the urethral meatus in men is seen.[25] It must be differentiated from those parasitic infections that involve the bladder, such as *Schistosoma haematobium* infection, in which there may be ureteral obstruction owing to florid granulomatous and inflammatory lesions of both the ureters and the bladder.[14]

DIAGNOSTIC STUDIES

Laboratory Studies

Hematology. By definition, eosinophilia implies a laboratory confirmation of more than 350 eosinophils/µl in the complete blood count. In addition to the CBC, examination of a bone marrow aspirate or biopsy specimen is necessary for certain diagnoses (e.g., AEL), especially to distinguish them from other diseases with anemia and very high eosinophilic count (e.g., HES). The bone marrow in patients with HES also has granulocytic increases with normal megakaryocytes. AEL, on the other hand, is myelophthisic, in that all normal bone marrow cells are replaced by eosinophilic blast forms.

The presence of anemia is also a common finding in several other diseases. Gastrointestinal infections with helminthic parasites produce anemia. In addition, presenting signs of rheumatoid arthritis may include both eosinophilia and anemia. The presence of anemia is often a harbinger of a more significant systemic disease and points toward diseases of multisystemic origin.

In individuals with an allergic history, a Wright-stained smear of nasal secretions showing marked eosinophilia is a helpful diagnostic finding. Although further allergic testing may be indicated, this simple test may obviate the need for expensive laboratory tests to eliminate other possibilities.

Blood Chemistry. Measurements of electrolytes to assess hydration as well as serum transaminase levels to check for liver involvement are intrinsic components of a work-up for gastrointestinal symptoms and eosinophilia. Likewise, a routine urinalysis may demonstrate the presence of red blood cells or protein that is consistent with the possibility of helminthic infestation of the bladder. In rare cases, helminthic eggs such as those of schistosoma may be seen in the urine as well as in feces; either finding provides a definitive diagnosis of infestation. Serum protein quantitation is also important in some diseases, particularly in allergic eosinophilic gastroenteritis and enterocolitis, in which hyperproteinemia is a common manifestation. Specialized immunofluorescent tests such as assays for antinuclear antibody and rheumatoid factor are important for differentiating classic collagen diseases such as systemic lupus erythematosus and rheumatoid arthritis from the rare eosinophilic diseases such as eosinophilic fasciitis and HES.

Microbiology. There is little question that the most important microbiologic examination that can be done in the presence of eosinophilia is a stool examination for ova, parasites, and worms. Even in the United States, where helminthic infestation is not as common as it is worldwide, any significant eosinophilia in which the count is greater than 1,000 eosinophils/µl obligates the clinician to exclude helminthic infection. Diseases such as hookworm are endemic in the southeastern regions particularly. In addition to ova and parasites, Charcot-Leyden crystals should be looked for in a stool specimen. Such eosinophilic-staining material suggests that there is a large eosinophilic infiltration in the GI tract.

Since the presence of one eosinophil in the CSF is pathologic, one must consider eosinophilic infestation of the CNS or unusual viral meningitis on those rare occasions when it is found. Even more rarely, CNS malignancy manifests as CSF eosinophilia.

Imaging

Chest X-Ray. A routine chest x-ray is probably the most important radiograph one can routinely order in a patient with eosinophilia, especially with even minimal pulmonary symptoms. Many helminthic parasites have a pulmonary phase. Loeffler's filariasis and lung flukes cause characteristic radiologic densities; these vary from cysts to dense nodular opacities (Fig. 3). It is beyond the scope of this discussion to differentiate these x-ray findings.

Computed Tomography. In any patient with CNS disease, computed tomographic scanning is indicated for localizing densities or abscesses. In addition, in those patients with diffuse adenopathy and hepatosplenomegaly, a lymphangiogram may differentiate the two possible diagnoses (e.g., HES and AEL). Contrast filling defects are much more characteristic of malignancies.

Specialized Tests

To delineate the cause of disease associated with eosinophilia, an invasive procedure may be re-

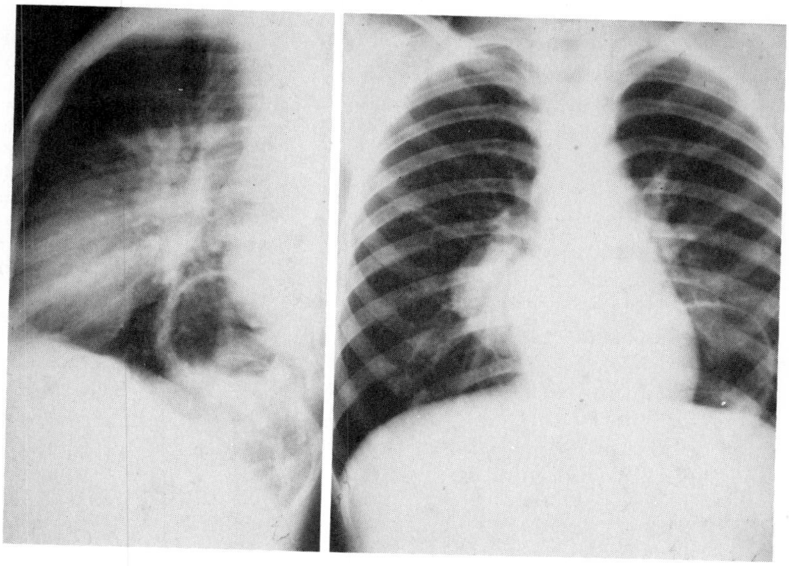

Figure 3. The lateral and AP chest x-rays demonstrate a large cystic mass produced by infection with *Echinococcus granulosus*. Similar findings may be seen in patients with other helminthic infestations of the lung.

quired, such as arthrocentesis of a rheumatoid joint to determine whether there is eosinophilic infiltration, or bronchoscopy with intraluminal biopsy to differentiate the lung infiltrates of HES from those of Loeffler's syndrome. In patients with cardiac symptoms, echocardiography may be helpful in determining the extent of endocarditis or myocarditis. Further, because HES is associated with a tendency to multiple thromboses, such diagnostic procedures as Doppler ultrasound localization of thrombus, ^{125}I-fibrinogen scanning, and venography may prove useful in elucidating particular manifestations of the thromboembolic phenomenon.

For GI lesions, endoscopy or colonoscopy is frequently necessary. Symptoms progressing to intestinal obstruction will naturally require laparotomy for both diagnosis and treatment. Cystoscopy may be indicated for symptoms in the bladder or upper urinary tract.

Pathologic Examination (Tissue Biopsy)

In many cases, definitive diagnosis can be made only by examination of involved tissue. Certainly in a case of eosinophilic myositis, biopsy of muscle with examination of the sarcolemmic membrane for deposition of IgG is the definitive technique for diagnosis. For diagnosis of malignant diseases, biopsy is the *sine qua non*, whether the involved tissue be bone marrow or lymph node. Additionally, skin biopsies are often required to look for parasites in suspected cutaneous larva migrans or for the allergic infiltration seen in allergic dermatitides.

Rectosigmoid biopsy may be needed to look for a sawtooth mucosal pattern with diffuse thickening of the valvulae conniventes, which is pathognomonic for eosinophilic gastroenteritis.

Electron microscopic demonstration in a fascial biopsy specimen of fibroblasts, accumulation of protocollagen fibrils, and numerous degranulating mast cells is definitive for eosinophilic fasciitis.[9]

ASSESSMENT

Synthesis of Clinical Findings

The foregoing discussion demonstrates the great diversity of disease processes that may be associated with eosinophilia. Like neutrophilia, eosinophilia may point to either an acute or a chronic problem. In addition, as with neutrophilia, malignant transformation of eosinophils can also occur to produce leukemia. Just as neutrophilia suggests bacterial infection, eosinophilia suggests parasitic infection. It should be re-emphasized that under all circumstances in which marked eosinophilia is seen (i.e., more than 3,000 eosinophils/μl) it is incumbent upon the physician to rule out parasites. Thereafter, rarer etiologies can be considered.

Clinical Follow-Up

A discussion of the therapy for this wide variety of diseases is beyond the scope of this chapter. However, the response of eosinophilia to treatment may help corroborate a diagnosis or serve as the rationale for further work-up.

It is characteristic for the eosinophil count to rise acutely at the time effective treatment is instituted for parasitic infections. The rise indicates adequate response to therapy. It then takes an extended period for the eosinophil count to return to a normal level after treatment. The increase in eosinophils probably represents a more effective cytotoxicity in the presence of an effective drug. On the other hand, in the patient with eosinophilic leukemia or Hodgkin's disease that has been in remission, a rising eosinophil count may be a harbinger of recurrent disease. Certainly in the case of tumor-associated blood eosinophilia, the return of eosinophilia following effective therapy usually portends imminent relapse or metastatic disease; as such, the eosinophilia may be an indicator of the efficacy of therapy.[26] Such early indication of recrudescence may allow one to alter therapy before the patient becomes quite ill with recurrent disease.

In most nonmalignant disease, a falling eosinophil count implies improvement. The return of the eosinophil count to less than 300 per μl usually obviates the need for further intervention unless symptoms recur.

EOSINOPENIA

Although eosinophilia is common, eosinopenia (less than 50 eosinophils/μl) is rarely described. Even when looked for, it has been seen very infrequently, most often during the use of corticosteroid therapy. Down's syndrome patients may rarely be eosinopenic.[2] In premature infants, eosinopenia is seen in association with sepsis. There is a dearth of information concerning the risk of infestation with parasites in eosinopenic individuals. One might hypothesize that in endemic areas, susceptibility to such deficiency may have been strongly selected *against* in much the same way that sickle trait has been selected *for* in indigenous malarial regions. However, little if any confirmatory data are available to substantiate this view.

REFERENCES

1. Jones TW. The blood corpuscle in its different phases of development in the animal series. Memoir I. Vertebrate Phil Trans R Soc London 1846;136:63.
2. Baehner RL. Disorders of granulopoiesis. In: Miller DR, Pearson HA, Bachner RL, McMillan CW, eds. Smith's blood diseases of infancy and childhood. St. Louis: CV Mosby, 1978;497–556.
3. Basten A, Beeson PB. Mechanism of eosinophilia II. Role of the lymphocyte. J Exp Med 1970;131:1288–1305.
4. Anwar AR, Kay AB. Membrane receptors for IgG and complement (C4, C3b and C3d) on human eosinophils and neutrophils and their relation to eosinophilia. J Immunol 1977;119:976–81.
5. Hesdorff C, Ziady F. Eosinophilic gastroenteritis: a complication of schistosomiasis and peripheral eosinophilia? S Afr Med J 1982;61:591–3.
6. Epstein D, Taromina V. Hypereosinophilic syndrome. Radiology 1981;140:59–62.
7. Voudiclaris S, Kalmantis T, Virvidakis K, Karafoulidou A, Papaspyriou-Zona A. Eosinophilia in patients undergoing dialysis. Br Med J 1982;284:272–3.
8. Agrawal BV, Geisen PC. Eosinophilic myositis: An unusual case of pseudotumor and eosinophilia. JAMA 1981;246:70–1.
9. Cramer S, Kent L, Abromosky C, Moskowitz R. Eosinophilic fasciitis: immunopathology ultrastructure, literature review and consideration of its pathology in relation to scleroderma. Arch Pathol Lab Med 1982;106:85–91.
10. Lucak BK, Sansaricq C, Snyderman SE, Greco A, Fazzini EP, Bazaz GR. Disseminated ulcerations in allergic eosinophilic gastroenterocolitis. Gastroenterology 1982; 77:248–52.
11. Littleton RH, Farah RN, Cerny JC. Eosinophilic cystitis: An uncommon form of cystitis. J Urol 1982;127:132–3.
12. Lowe D, Jorizzo, J, Hertt M. Tumor associated eosinophilia: a review. J Clin Pathol 1981;34:1343–8.
13. Ellman L, Hammond D, Atkins L. Eosinophilic chloromas and chromosome abnormality in a patient with a myeloproliferative syndrome. Cancer 1979;43:2410–3.
14. Mahmoud AAF. Schistosomiasis. In: Wyngaarden JB, Smith LH Jr, eds. Cecil textbook of medicine. 16th ed. Philadelphia: WB Saunders, 1982;1754–60.
15. Humphrey M, Hutter J, Tom W. Hypereosinophilia in a monosomy F myeloproliferative disorder in childhood. Am J Hematol 1981;11:107–10.
16. Gibson E, Vawcheu Y, Corrigan J. Eosinophilia in premature infants: relationship to weight gain. J Pediatr 1979;95:99–101.
17. Burkitt JM. Well's syndrome: recurrent granulomatous dermatitis with eosinophilia. Arch Dermatol 1981; 117:759.
18. Hall D, Link K. Eosinophilia associated with Coumadin. N Engl J Med 1981;304:18.
19. Lee T, Cochrane G. Pulmonary eosinophilia and asthma associated with carbamazepine. Br Med J 1981;282:440.
20. Chesney P, Katcher M, Nelson D, Horowitz S. CSF eosinophilia and chronic lymphocytic choriomeningitis versus meningitis. J Pediatr 1979;94:750–53.
21. Defendini R, Hunter S, Schlesinger E, Leifer E, Rowthaard L. Eosinophilia meningitis in a case of disseminated glioblastoma. Arch Neurology 1981;38:52–3.
22. Durack D, Sani S, Klebanoff S. Neurotoxicity of human eosinophils. Proc Nat Acad Sci 1979;76:1443–7.
23. Weinberg S, Leider M, Shapiro L. Color Atlas of Pediatric Dermatology. New York: McGraw-Hill, 1975:208–9.
24. Gardner JH, Amonette RA, Chesney T. Angiolymphoid hyperplasia with eosinophilia. J Derm Surg Oncol 1981;7:414–8.
25. Leiterman K, O'Duffy D, Perry H, Greip P, Guilani E, Gleich G. Recurrent incapacitating mucosal ulcerations. JAMA 1982;247:1018–20.
26. Killermeyer RW. Eosinophilia. In: Dietschy JM, Lichtman MA, eds. The science and practice of clinical medicine. Vol. VI: hematology and oncology. New York: Grune & Stratton, 1980:131–3.

ERYTHEMA NODOSUM

JOHN J. CALABRO □ GARY L. WOLF

□ SYNONYMS: Erythema nodosum migrans, dermatitis contusiformis

BACKGROUND

The term erythema nodosum was coined by Robert Willan, an English dermatologist, in his classic monograph on erythemas published in 1807.[1] Willan emphasized not only the tenderness of the lesions and their predilection for the shins but also the vivid play of colors, in which bright red spots gradually fade to dark red and blue and finally to purplish yellow "bruises."

Earlier writers believed erythema nodosum (EN) to be a specific disease entity, a view widely held throughout the late 19th and early 20th centuries.[2] Recent experience indicates, however, that erythema nodosum is a hypersensitivity vasculitis resulting from a host of unrelated disorders as well as from use of drugs.

Etiology

The causes of erythema nodosum are multiple and variable, including infectious as well as noninfectious etiologies (Table 1).[2, 3] Currently, sarcoid is one of the three most common causes of EN, along with tuberculosis and streptococcal infections.[4]

Drugs have also been implicated in the etiology of erythema nodosum.[2, 3] These include the salicylates, bromides, iodides, sulfonamides, antibiotics, vaccines and other biologic preparations, and oral contraceptives.[5–7] Familial erythema nodosum has also been reported.[8] Finally, in addition to a number of miscellaneous causes, including pregnancy, many cases are classified as idiopathic because no underlying cause is obvious.[3–5]

Epidemiology

EN is an uncommon syndrome that appears more frequently in females. It can affect all ages but occurs primarily in young adults and children and is rare before 2 years of age.[9] The incidence varies greatly and clearly depends upon factors influencing potential underlying causes.[10]

Variables such as changes in season, which influence the incidence of streptococcal infections, and geographic factors, such as the prevalence of coccidioidomycosis in the southwestern United States, are important epidemiologic determinants. In the past several decades, however, with effective and early treatment of streptococcal and mycobacterial infections, the frequency with which erythema nodosum is associated with these conditions has diminished considerably.[2, 10]

Pathogenesis

Both cell-mediated and immune complex–mediated disease mechanisms have been postulated in the pathogenesis of EN.[10] Immunoglobulin and complement can be demonstrated in vessel walls in some lesions.[11] The disclosure of mycobacterial and streptococcal antigens in biopsies of skin lesions associated with these organisms supports the concept of an immune complex–mediated mechanism.[12]

Evidence for abnormalities of cellular immunity in the pathogenesis of erythema nodosum is only indirect.[10] The similarity between the histologic appearance of EN and that of delayed hypersensitivity reactions has been emphasized.[13] The association of erythema nodosum with diseases that produce a cellular immune response in the host, such as tuberculosis and fungal infections, as well as with diseases in which the cell-mediated response is suppressed, such as sarcoidosis, suggests that cellular components of the immune response are operative.[10]

Table 1. MAJOR CAUSES OF ERYTHEMA NODOSUM

Infectious causes	Streptococcal disease*
	Tuberculosis*
	Psittacosis
	Yersinia infections
	Coccidioidomycosis
	Histoplasmosis
	Blastomycosis
	Leprosy
	Cat-scratch disease
	Lymphogranuloma venereum
	Trichophyton infections
Noninfectious causes	Sarcoidosis*
	Behçet's syndrome
	Inflammatory bowel disease
	Ulcerative colitis
	Regional enteritis
	Neoplasms
	Leukemia
	Hodgkin's disease
	Pregnancy
	Drugs
	Vaccines

*Currently the three most common causes in the United States.

The recent disclosure of a high frequency of the HLA-B8 tissue antigen in erythema nodosum patients is evidence of a genetic predisposition to the syndrome. In one study of 25 patients with EN from varying causes, 15 (60 per cent) had the HLA-B8 antigen, compared with only 22 per cent of 100 healthy controls.[14] From these findings, it has been postulated that microorganisms and drugs represent some sort of antigenic exposure that most individuals can handle without immunologically mediated sequelae. In contrast, individuals carrying the HLA-B8 antigen are predisposed to the syndrome because of some unexplained aberration in antigen disposal.[14]

Histopathology

Erythema nodosum consists of inflammatory lesions that initially involve small blood vessels as well as interlobar septa and fat lobules located at the junction of the reticular dermis and subcutaneous fat. No histopathologic findings are specifically diagnostic of EN, and in fact, the spectrum of changes ranges from vasculitis to panniculitis.[13, 15, 16]

Early lesions (12 to 48 hours old) reveal perivascular inflammation that affects primarily veins and less frequently arteries. Initial changes are characterized by vascular damage with swelling of endothelial cells, edema of the vessel wall, and invasion of both the vessel wall and perivascular tissue by an inflammatory infiltrate composed primarily of polymorphonuclear leukocytes, occasionally of lymphocytes, and only rarely of eosinophils. Hemorrhage into surrounding tissue also occurs, constituting an important pathologic feature. The vascular supply to fat is located in the interlobar septa. Consequently, as the septa are affected, radially organized histiocytes develop around involved vessels and invade the interlobar septa and fat lobules of the panniculus (Fig. 1).

Chronic changes usually evolve within a week after the onset of the cutaneous eruption but can be seen as early as 48 hours. At this stage, lymphocytes dominate the cellular infiltrate, but histiocytes and giant cells may also be present. Vascular occlusion can also be noted at this stage, in conjunction with continued infiltration of fat lobules by chronic inflammatory cells. Granulomatous changes may then ensue, with infiltration by lymphocytes, giant cells, histiocytes, and, rarely, plasma cells. However, caseating granulomas and fat necrosis do not occur. Rarely, microabscesses containing polymorphonuclear or eosinophilic leukocytes can be found. Vascular proliferation may also occur in areas of fibrosis in thickened septa.

Long-standing changes result in septal widening of the subcutaneous fat as the inflammatory infiltrate is converted to fibrous tissue. Generally, the upper dermis and epidermis are not affected, except when the inflammatory changes are marked.

The Clinical Spectrum

EN is often classified as a subtype of erythema multiforme, to which it is closely related. The erythematous nodules that characterize erythema nodosum can arise anywhere that there is subcutaneous fat. Recurrent attacks separated by months or years are not uncommon. However, the chronic form, in which nodules persist for years, is rare.[17]

The onset of an attack is often acute, accompanied by systemic manifestations such as fever and malaise. Myalgia and arthralgia are common, but arthritis may also occur. Hilar adenopathy is another feature, and although its presence is often a clue to underlying sarcoidosis, the simultaneous occurrence of nodose skin lesions and hilar lymph node enlargement may have other causes.[15]

HISTORY

A diagnosis of EN can be made clinically, but the more important task is evaluating the patient for a potential cause, such as an underlying disease or an offending drug. Consequently, a detailed history, including the recent use of drugs, may be revealing. The physician must recognize, however, that the complaints of the patient may be part of the clinical spectrum of erythema nodosum and in no way related to an underlying disease or to exposure to a drug. Fever, chills, malaise, anorexia, weight loss, myalgia, arthralgia, and arthritis may all be due to the EN syndrome itself. Nevertheless, the patient must be questioned for signs and symptoms of potentially associated diseases, since the cutaneous eruption itself will offer no clues as to its cause.

Age and Family History. The age of the patient has considerable relevance to the search for potential causes. In a child with EN, a streptococcal or other upper respiratory infection will more than likely be the primary cause. Rarely is sarcoidosis a major cause of erythema nodosum in children. On the other hand, sarcoidosis ranks as one of the major causes of EN in adults, along with tuberculosis and streptococcal infection. In the elderly, underlying malignancy must always be a major consideration.

There should be inquiry concerning other family members, because erythema nodosum can be familial. In familial cases, no common precipitating cause is obvious.[8]

Geographic Factors. If the patient with erythema nodosum resides in the southwest or in the

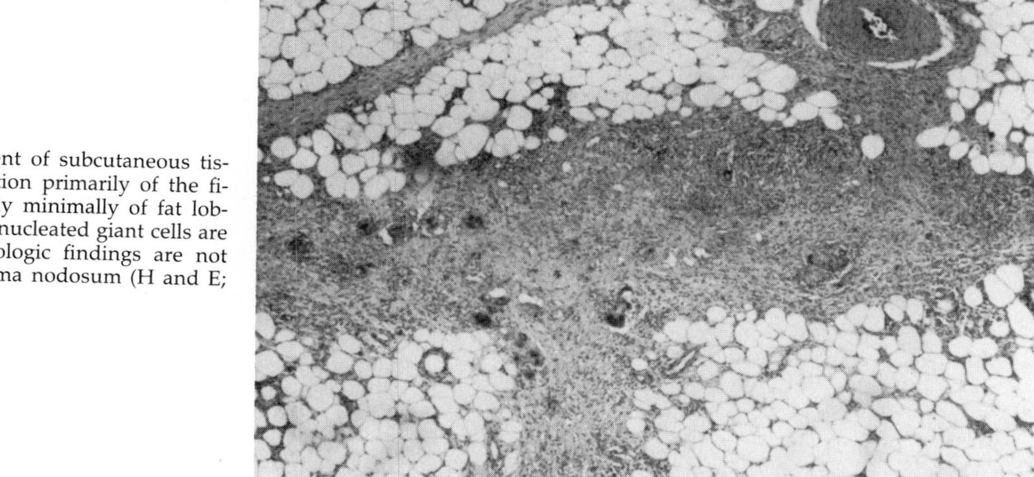

Figure 1. Involvement of subcutaneous tissue, with inflammation primarily of the fibrous septa and only minimally of fat lobules. Scattered multinucleated giant cells are present. These histologic findings are not diagnostic of erythema nodosum (H and E; low power).

Ohio or Mississippi Valley, or has recently visited one of these areas, the cause of the skin lesions may be primary coccidioidomycosis or histoplasmosis. Tuberculosis is more apt to be the primary infection in other parts of the United States and in Europe. The patient should be questioned concerning recent tuberculosis exposure at work and school and during travel. He or she should also be asked about the usual signs and symptoms that characterize tuberculosis. Clearly, in the recognition of tuberculosis, malaise and weight loss may be as important as night sweats and chronic cough as early clues.

Review of Systems. A detailed review of systems may provide clues to an underlying disorder. For example, the patient should be asked about recent upper respiratory infection, since the onset of EN is frequently heralded by streptococcal or other upper respiratory infections. Chronic diarrhea or another bowel complaint may be a clue to underlying inflammatory bowel disease, such as ulcerative colitis or Crohn's disease. More recently, infectious enterocolitis from Campylobacter or Salmonella has been reported to be associated with EN.[4, 18, 19] A history of anterior uveitis signals the possibility of either sarcoidosis or Behçet's syndrome. A history of recurrent aphthous ulcers also points to Behçet's syndrome. Fungal infections of the feet or nails should be considered when no other cause is apparent.[20]

The possibility of uncommon primary causes of erythema nodosum should be considered as well. These include such varied disorders as syphilis, herpes zoster, otitis media, prostatic abscess, dental abscess, peritoneal infection, axillary abscess, and peritonsillar abscess.[2] Rheumatic fever is only rarely associated with EN, even though both disorders represent hypersensitivity reactions to the streptococcus.[15] Much of the early confusion on this issue was based on the incorrect assumption that the arthralgia and arthritis of erythema nodosum represent rheumatic fever.

Drug Exposure. Exposure to drugs or vaccines must be reviewed carefully with the patient. For example, exposure to salicylates is not always obvious because patients are often not aware of their presence in many over-the-counter analgesic preparations. Women should be especially questioned concerning the use of oral contraceptives, and all patients should be screened for recent exposure to sulfonamides and antibiotics.

Less common incriminating agents include estrogens, aminopyrine, phenacetin, arsphenamine, antimony compounds, diphtheria toxoid, bacterial and "flu" vaccines, tuberculin, BCG, and the Frei antigen.[2–5] In fact, in view of the recent association with the HLA-B8, it is quite feasible that any drug can precipitate EN in a genetically predisposed individual.

PHYSICAL EXAMINATION

A careful physical examination will disclose not only the typical cutaneous lesions but also other features of the clinical spectrum of erythema nodosum. The general appearance of the patient often provides clues to the systemic nature of the syndrome.

General Appearance. The appearance of patients with erythema nodosum is quite variable. Some seem entirely well save for the skin eruption. Others appear acutely ill because of fever, chills, anorexia, weight loss, and malaise.

Although the fever is usually low grade, it may be high, reaching levels of 40.5°C (105°F). Fever rarely lasts beyond a week or two; otherwise, an underlying cause other than EN should be sus-

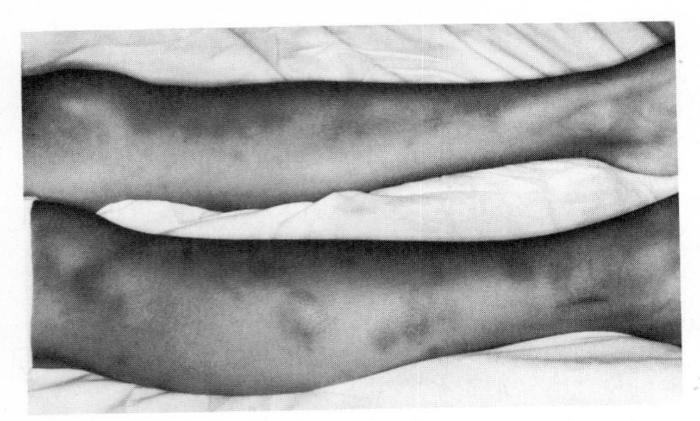

Figure 2. Typical nodules on the shins of a girl with erythema nodosum caused by streptococcal pharyngitis. The nodules are tender to palpation and the skin overlying the lesions is red, smooth, and shiny.

pected. In fact, the features of the primary cause may dominate the clinical presentation as well as the physical findings.

Cutaneous Lesions. The skin eruption usually appears suddenly as crops of erythematous, painful, nonpruritic, slightly raised lesions on the anterior surfaces of both shins (Fig. 2). Occasionally, a single lesion, unilateral crops, or involvement of the extensor surfaces of the forearms may be found. Because lesions can occur wherever subcutaneous fat is present, they may appear almost anywhere, including the calves, thighs, and buttocks, and even obscure areas such as the episclera of the eye. Episcleral nodules pursue the same course as the skin lesions.[15] They usually develop in the palpebral fissure near the insertion of the medial rectus muscle. They are frequently bilateral and are more superficial than other forms of episcleral nodules.

The individual lesions of EN vary in diameter from 0.5 to 5.0 cm. The skin over the nodules is red, smooth, and shiny. Individual lesions may coalesce to form sizable indurations, which may then result in considerable edema of the affected limbs. Resolution without ulceration, scarring, or permanent pigmentary changes usually occurs within 1 to 3 weeks. During this time, lesions progress from a bright red to a darker red or purple, along with intermediate color changes including blue, green, and yellow.

The centrifugal propagation of nodules, the central fading of individual lesions, the spectrum of color changes, and the prompt resolution are distinctive features of erythema nodosum. However, they are not constant features, and variations have been observed.[15, 17] In erythema nodosum migrans, for example, an individual nodule divides and forms separate lesions as it migrates peripherally and clears centrally.[21] Also, whereas most lesions are deep nodules, they may instead develop as superficial, slightly edematous, warm, red, tender areas.[15] These often form a confluent patch that covers the entire shin, thereby resembling erysipelas. Moreover, the lesions of EN do not always evolve in an array of colors simulating a bruise; sometimes, the bright red lesions fade directly into normal skin color. Consequently, the absence of color changes does not exclude a diagnosis of EN. Finally, although the lesions usually resolve within 3 weeks, they may become chronic, persisting for months or years.

Joint Manifestations. Approximately two-thirds of patients with EN have an associated arthropathy, which usually accompanies the febrile phase but occasionally may precede it by weeks. Some patients have only arthralgias, so that although the affected joints are tender to palpation, no joint swelling is present. Early morning stiffness may also occur.

About a third of patients have objective evidence of arthritis, manifested as swelling, erythema, warmth, and effusion. The large peripheral joints (knees, ankles, wrists, and elbows) are usually involved, often symmetrically, but swelling may also occur in the small joints of the hands and feet.

The arthropathy usually resolves within a few weeks. Occasionally, it may become chronic, lasting for months, and only rarely for a year or longer. Deformity does not occur, however, even when the duration of arthritis is protracted.

Hilar Adenopathy. Unilateral or bilateral pulmonary hilar adenopathy is an integral feature of EN.[15] However, it does not occur in all cases nor is it a clue to underlying sarcoidosis, because hilar adenopathy may evolve as part of the EN syndrome irrespective of the underlying cause.

Hilar adenopathy is usually asymptomatic, being disclosed only on a chest x-ray. Consequently, the finding of pulmonary abnormalities on physical examination is a clue to underlying causes such as tuberculosis, histoplasmosis, and sarcoidosis.

DIAGNOSTIC STUDIES

Additional diagnostic clues may be provided by laboratory and x-ray studies. Although certain laboratory and radiographic abnormalities may occur with EN, all are nonspecific and none are consistently present. The basic work-up should nevertheless include a CBC, erythrocyte sedimentation rate (ESR), throat culture, antistreptolysin-O titer, tuberculin skin test, and chest x-ray.[22] Selectively, other tests to detect underlying causes, such as stool cultures for Yersinia, may be in order.

Laboratory Studies and Radiography

Elevation of the ESR and presence of other acute-phase reactants as well as a modest neutrophilic leukocytosis are laboratory abnormalities commonly observed in EN. The white blood count rarely exceeds 20,000 cells/mm^3. X-ray of the chest may disclose hilar adenopathy that is frequently but not always bilateral (Fig. 3). Laboratory abnormalities revert to normal with clinical remission of the syndrome, but roentgenographic evidence of hilar adenopathy may persist for months.

When the precipitating cause is one of the streptococcal infections, such as streptococcal pharyngitis or tonsillitis, erysipelas, or scarlet fever, throat culture may yield Group A beta-hemolytic streptococcus and the antistreptolysin-O titer may be elevated. Other tests to document other potential causes may also be obtained, but only in the proper clinical setting. Routine screening for all potential pathogens with a variety of serologic and skin tests is otherwise impractical and costly. The unavailability, as well as questions concerning the validity, of the Kveim test clearly limits its usefulness in diagnosing sarcoidosis.[22]

Biopsy

The biopsy findings in erythema nodosum are variable and depend on the depth and size of the section, the stage of the clinical lesion, and the site of biopsy. In fact, different areas of an involved site may disclose strikingly dissimilar histologic features. For this reason, excisional biopsy is preferred to punch biopsy.

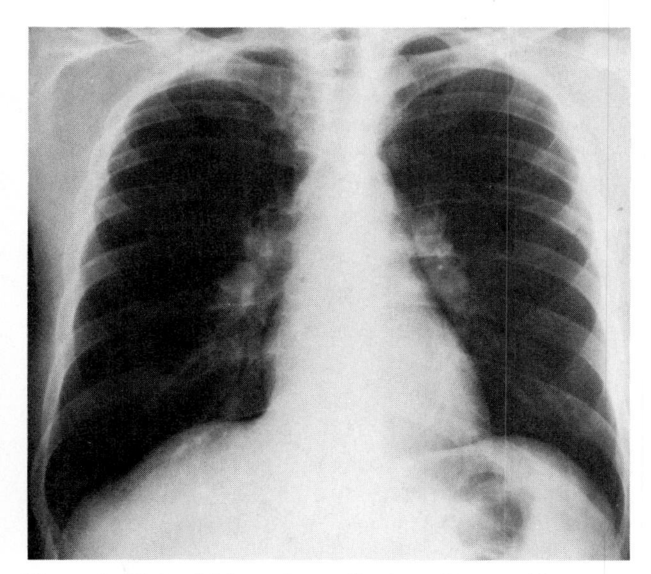

Figure 3. Bilateral hilar adenopathy in a 36-year-old woman with erythema nodosum caused by sarcoidosis.

Biopsy should be performed only when the lesions are clinically atypical and other diagnostic considerations need to be excluded. Consequently, biopsy may prove useful in differentiating other causes of inflammatory nodules of the legs, such as relapsing panniculitis (Weber-Christian disease), erythema induratum, nodular vasculitis, and superficial thrombophlebitis.[22–24] However, reliance on histologic findings alone, without correlation with clinical features, can lead to erroneous conclusions.[15]

DIFFERENTIAL DIAGNOSIS

Nodose lesions of the legs can be sorted out according to their predilection for certain sites as well as other distinguishing features (Table 2). The nodules of relapsing panniculitis, unlike those of EN, occur primarily on the thighs and trunk; they are usually painless, they may ulcerate, and the involved sites often become atrophic.[23] As in other panniculitides, fat necrosis and granulomatous inflammation distinguish relapsing panniculitis from EN.[15]

The lesions of erythema induratum usually occur on the calves and are frequently associated with ulceration.[22] Nodular vasculitis most frequently appears on the calves and ankles and is distinguished by its chronicity (the lesions persist for months). Scarring and hyperpigmentation may occur in both erythema induratum and nodular vasculitis but not in erythema nodosum.[23] On histopathologic examination, both erythema induratum and nodular vasculitis demonstrate inflammatory edema of the epidermis that is not present in EN.[23] Superficial (migratory) thrombophlebitis may be confusing initially, but its linear evolution and the cord-like consistency of the swelling on palpation serves to differentiate it readily from EN.[22]

The panniculitis secondary to pancreatic disease may occur acutely on the legs, mimicking EN. However, the clinical evidence of pancreatic abnormalities and the elevations of lipolytic enzymes in the former disorder should lead to the correct diagnosis.[22]

Intestinal bypass procedures for the treatment of morbid obesity induce rheumatic syndromes in up to one-fourth of cases.[15, 25] Arthralgias, arthritis, and cutaneous lesions of leukocytoclastic vasculitis develop. These lesions include erythematous papules, vesiculopustules, and erythema nodosum–like lesions that arise on the extremities, trunk, and face. The antigenic stimulus for this immune complex disease is believed to be bacterial, secondary to bacterial overgrowth in the excluded loop of bowel. Histologic examination of the le-

Table 2. DIFFERENTIATING FEATURES OF NODULAR DISORDERS OF THE LEGS

Entity	Most Common Sites	Other Distinguishing Features
Erythema nodosum	Shins	Hilar adenopathy; no ulceration, scarring, or hyperpigmentation
Relapsing panniculitis	Thighs, trunk	Ulceration, atrophy
Erythema induratum	Calves	Ulceration, scarring, hyperpigmentation
Nodular vasculitis	Calves, ankles	Scarring, hyperpigmentation

sions reveals minimal chronic inflammation of fatty areas without necrosis.[25]

Erythema nodosum leprosum has only recently been recognized as a different disorder both clinically and pathologically from true erythema nodosum.[15] It may be the initial manifestation of leprosy but occurs most often during the course of disease in patients receiving treatment. In contrast to lesions of the true form, the nodules of erythema nodosum leprosum rarely affect the pretibial surfaces, usually involving the arms, face, and anterior thighs.[22]

REFERENCES

1. Willan R. On cutaneous diseases. London: John Churchill, 1807.
2. Weinstein L. Erythema nodosum. DM 1969;June:1–30.
3. Blomgren SE. Erythema nodosum. Semin Arthritis Rheum 1970;4:1–24.
4. Palmer WG, Enyeart JJ. Erythema nodosum. Convergence 1981;1:75–9.
5. Salvatore MA, Lynch PJ. Erythema nodosum, estrogens, and pregnancy. Arch Dermatol 1980;116:557–8.
6. Merk H, Rusicka T. Oral contraceptives as a cause of erythema nodosum (letter). Arch Dermatol 1981;117:454.
7. Darlington LG. Erythema nodosum and oral contraceptives. Br J Dermatol 1974;90:209–12.
8. Randall OS, Abernathy WS, Berven B. Familial erythema nodosum. Mich Med 1973;72:283–9.
9. Doxiadis SA. Erythema nodosum in children. A review. Medicine 1951;30:283–334.
10. Cupps TR, Fauci AS. The Vasculitides. Philadelphia: WB Saunders, 1981;147–9; Major problems in internal medicine vol. 21.
11. Scott DG, Rowell NR. Preliminary investigations of arteritic lesions using fluorescent antibody techniques. Br J Dermatol 1965;77:211–20.
12. Parish WE. Studies on vasculitis. I. Immunoglobulins, BIC, C-reactive protein, and bacterial antigens in cutaneous vasculitis lesions. Clin Allergy 1971;1:97–109.
13. Winkelmann RK, Forstrom L. New observations in the histopathology of erythema nodosum. J Invest Dermatol 1975;65:441–6.
14. Guyatt GH, Bensen WG, Stolmon LP, Fagnilli L, Singal DP. HLA-B8 and erythema nodosum. Can Med Assoc J 1982;127:1005–6.
15. Braverman IM. Skin signs of systemic disease. 2nd ed. Philadelphia: WB Saunders, 1981:476–84.
16. Fine RM, Meltzer HD. Erythema nodosum: a form of allergic cutaneous vasculitis. South Med J 1968;61:680–6.
17. Fine RM, Meltzer HD. Chronic erythema nodosum. Arch Dermatol 1969;100:33–8.
18. Eastmond CJ, Reid TM. Campylobacter enteritis and erythema nodosum (letter). Br Med J 1982;285:1421–2.
19. Ellis ME, Pope J, Mokashi A, Dunbar E. Campylobacter colitis associated with erythema nodosum. Br Med J 1982;285:937.
20. Hicks JH. Erythema nodosum in patients with tinea pedis and onychomycosis. South Med J 1977;70:27–8.
21. Bafverstedt B. Erythema nodosum migrans. Acta Derm Venereol 1968;48:381–4.
22. Soderstrom RM, Krull EA. Erythema nodosum: a review. Cutis 1978;21:806–10.
23. Gibbs RC, Canizares O, Shapiro E, Soscia JD. Nodular lesions of the lower extremities. GP 1968;38:91–7.
24. Winkelmann RK. New inflammatory nodules of the legs. South Med J 1964;57:637–41.
25. Zapanta M, Aldo-Benson M, Biegel A, Madura J. Arthritis associated with jejunoileal bypass. Arthritis Rheum 1979;22:711–7.

ERYTHROCYTE SEDIMENTATION RATE, ELEVATED

BRIAN P. SCHMITT

☐ SYNONYMS: Sed rate, ESR (elevated)

BACKGROUND

Definition and Origins

The phenomenon of erythrocyte sedimentation has been known since the time of the ancient Greeks but was not employed clinically until the early 20th century. In 1918, Fahraeus discovered that the speed of erythrocyte sedimentation was altered in pregnancy; subsequently, he noted that many disease states accelerated sedimentation.[1] Westergren in 1926 and Wintrobe in 1935 devised the two methods commonly employed in clinical practice to measure the rate of erythrocyte sedimentation. The simplicity of these methods, their minimal expense, and the commonly held belief that they were useful in screening for the presence or absence of active disease led to the widespread popularity of ESR determination. This popularity, however, has been tempered by the difficulties that arise in interpretation of results. Is the patient with a normal ESR free of active disease? How does one interpret the elevated ESR, especially if the patient is asymptomatic? Although ESR measurement is inexpensive and simple to perform, its interpretation remains problematic.

Factors Determining Sedimentation Rate

Interpretation requires some understanding of the factors that determine erythrocyte sedimentation and how they may be altered in disease (Table 1). Sedimentation occurs because the density of red cells is greater than the density of plasma.[2] As the red cells descend they cause an upward displacement of the plasma. This displacement generates an upward inhibitory force. Normally, the upward and downward forces are nearly equal, resulting in minimal sedimentation. In disease, aggregates of red cells (rouleaux) may form. Each aggregate has an increased weight relative to its volume. Consequently, aggregate settling is enhanced and the ESR is increased. As a rule, factors that cause red cell aggregation increase the ESR and factors that inhibit aggregation or impair settling may lead to a normal ESR despite the presence of underlying disease.

Red cell aggregation does not occur under normal circumstances. Each red cell has a negative surface charge contributing to a mutually repulsive intercellular force. With disease, increased amounts of large asymmetric protein such as fibrinogen or gamma globulin can dissipate this repulsive force and enhance aggregation. A wide variety of inflammatory states, both acute and chronic, are associated with an increased fibrinogen level. Gamma globulin levels likewise may be increased in many inflammatory conditions. However, marked changes in ESR secondary to excessive plasma gamma globulin are usually the result of a lymphoproliferative disorder.[1] Red cell aggregation requires the presence not only of large asymmetric plasma proteins but also of red cells that are normal in size and shape. Alterations in size and shape can impede rouleaux formation.[1] Anisocytosis, poikilocytosis, spherocytosis, acanthocytosis, and hypochromia have been noted to inhibit aggregation. Polycythemia, increased bile salts, and the use of nonsteroidal anti-inflammatory drugs may falsely lower the ESR. Factors leading to a false or accentuated increase in ESR include anemia, azotemia, and elevated cholesterol.[1, 2]

In summary, multiple variables besides laboratory technique may influence the ESR result and make interpretation difficult.

How the Test Is Performed

Before proceeding to ESR interpretation, it is also important to know how the test is performed and how normal values for the test have been generated. As mentioned previously, the Westergren and Wintrobe methods are most commonly used. The results from one method are not interchangeable with results from the other, and the range of normal depends on the method.

In the Westergren method, 2 ml of venous blood is collected in 0.5 ml of sodium citrate solution. A cylindrical Westergren tube is filled with the blood to the 200-mm level and placed vertically in a rack. At the end of 1 hour, the distance from the top of the blood column to the top layer of red cells is measured. This distance is the sedimentation rate,

Table 1. FACTORS THAT MAY ALTER INTERPRETATION OF ESR DETERMINATIONS

Alterations in RBC size or shape
Anemia
Polycythemia
Pregnancy or oral contraceptives
Nonsteroidal anti-inflammatory drugs
Elevated blood lipids
Elevated bile salts

expressed in mm/hr.[1] With the Wintrobe method no diluent is used. Anticoagulated blood is placed in a marked, graduated tube 100 mm long and examined in 1 hour. Again, the distance from the top of the column to the top layer of red cells is measured, the rate is expressed in mm/hr.

The Westergren method has been more widely accepted and is endorsed by the International Committee for Standardization in Hematology.[3] Drawbacks of the Wintrobe method include a limitation of the magnitude of any ESR abnormality and problems with reliability. The Wintrobe tube is only 100 mm long, so an ESR higher than 60 mm/hr can rarely be measured because RBC packing impedes further settling. Also, the narrow bore of the Wintrobe tube may at times cause nonreproducible results.[1] Technical sources of error for both methods have been described elsewhere.[4] Some laboratories have attempted to correct the ESR results for anemia; however, the usefulness of these correction factors is subject to controversy.[1, 2, 5]

Normal Values

What value of ESR should be considered abnormal? Understanding the manner in which the upper limit of normal is selected is crucial for interpretation. Clinicians often approach the ESR as if the test separates diseased from nondiseased individuals. However, normal limits for the ESR are statistically derived from groups of persons presumably in good health. Specifically, a population of healthy (normal) individuals is identified and tested. The upper limit of normal is usually selected to ensure that 90 to 95 per cent of the values obtained fall below the limit.[3, 6] Although this approach separates usual (normal) from unusual (abnormal) test values, it says nothing about distinguishing diseased from nondiseased persons. In fact, by definition, 5 to 10 per cent of healthy individuals have abnormal erythrocyte sedimentation rates even though they are free of disease.

Determining the upper limit of normal is further complicated by the fact that healthy subgroups of the population have different "normal" ESR values.[6, 7, 8] Women as a group have higher rates than men, and the elderly as a group have higher rates than younger people. Furthermore, within individuals there tends to be an age-related increase in the ESR. Consequently, selecting a limit to separate normal from abnormal test values is confounded by inter- and intra-individual variability. At best, the limit selected can give information only about the usualness of the individual value. Additional study of the ESR using appropriate clinical epidemiologic methods[9] is needed if its measurement is to be used to separate diseased from nondiseased individuals within the context of a specific problem.

Clinical Application

The ESR has been used clinically for a variety of screening, diagnostic, and monitoring purposes.[1, 2] For example, some clinicians order the test routinely for every patient in an attempt to identify unsuspected or occult disease. Others reserve it for patients with nonspecific symptoms, in hopes of separating those with a functional disorder from those with organic disease. The clinician using the ESR for either purpose generally regards a normal test result as reassuring and an abnormal result as the basis for further evaluation. Unfortunately, the ESR has not been appropriately assessed for these applications. The available literature does suggest that a significant percentage of those with localized and potentially curable malignant disease may have an ESR lower than 20 mm/hr.[10] At the other extreme, some patients with a grossly elevated ESR (100 mm/hr or higher) may have no evidence of clinical disease after extensive evaluation and long-term follow-up.[5, 11] Consequently, the physician ordering an ESR evaluation must make tentative any interpretation of the results and must refrain from premature reassurance or alarm. More data regarding the test's sensitivity, specificity, and predictive value in specific clinical situations are needed.

In order to improve the diagnostic usefulness of the ESR, some investigators have studied patients with extreme elevations.[11–22] Zacharski and Kyle studied 263 patients with rates of 100 mm/hr or higher at the Mayo Clinic and found that 58 per cent had malignant disease.[11] Their findings suggested that the ESR may be helpful in identifying patients with malignant disease. However, when ambulatory and general hospital populations were surveyed, the prevalence of malignant disease ranged between 11 and 23 per cent (see Table 3).[12–20] Most patients with both malignant disease and a grossly elevated ESR had metastatic spread. In the majority of patients in these studies, an underlying infection or a connective tissue disorder was associated with an elevated ESR. A small percentage of the patients with high rates had no identifiable disease. Most patients with a grossly elevated ESR in these studies had diseases that could be identified, although a causal relationship was not clearly demonstrated. Despite these associations, the usefulness of the ESR for screening and diagnosis continues to be a source of debate.

The ESR has also been used to monitor disease activity and response to treatment. For example, serial ESR tests may be made in a patient with osteomyelitis to seek evidence of clinical response to treatment. Others have found it helpful to follow the activity of rheumatoid arthritis and other connective tissue disorders; a falling ESR may corroborate other early signs of clinical improvement, and a rising ESR may signal disease recurrence. As a monitoring device, the ESR still has a useful role.

HISTORY

An extensive list of disorders associated with an elevated sedimentation rate is provided in Table 2. Using the list to guide collection of historical data could be exhaustive. Consequently, a selective approach emphasizing common etiologies is preferable. Many patients with an elevated ESR have one or more diseases from four general categories: infections, connective tissue disease, malignancy, and renal disease (Table 3). Keeping in mind these categories and the most common disease entities within each, the clinician can select his or her patient queries in order to obtain appropriate leads.

Table 2. CONDITIONS ASSOCIATED WITH AN ELEVATED ERYTHROCYTE SEDIMENTATION RATE

Infections	Most symptomatic bacterial infections
	Pulmonary
	Genitourinary
	Osteomyelitis
	Otitis media
	Secondary syphilis
	Leptospirosis
	Viral infections
	Infectious hepatitis
	Systemic fungal infections
Malignancies	Hematologic malignancies
	Leukemia
	Lymphoma
	Myeloma
	Carcinomas
	Lung
	Breast
	Colon
	Genitourinary
	Other
Connective tissue diseases	Rheumatoid arthritis
	Systemic lupus erythematosus
	Temporal arteritis
	Rheumatic fever
	Other
Renal disorders	Nephrotic syndrome
	Acute glomerulonephritis
	Other
Miscellaneous conditions	Inflammatory bowel disease
	Cholecystitis
	Pancreatitis
	Thyroiditis
	Postsurgical condition
	Sarcoid

Subjective Data

History of Present Illness. In studies of ambulatory and general hospital populations, infections have been found to be the most common category of disease associated with an elevated ESR.[13, 18] A history of fever, chills, or rigors suggests infection. In view of the high rate of respiratory and urinary tract sources of infection, questions directed at these areas may provide a lead. Does the patient complain of cough, chest pain, hemoptysis, shortness of breath, or increased sputum production? Does the patient complain of urinary frequency, dysuria, hematuria or costovertebral angle tenderness?

Connective tissue diseases are another common disease category associated with abnormally high sedimentation rate. In adults, rheumatoid arthritis, systemic lupus erythematosus, and polymyalgia rheumatica including temporal arteritis are commonly associated diseases. A history of joint discomfort or swelling, especially if symmetric, is significant. Also, it is important to ask about skin rash, proximal muscle aches, headache, and visual disturbances. In children, rheumatic fever is frequently associated,[14] although the incidence of rheumatic fever itself is decreasing.[23] A history of migratory arthralgias, skin nodules, skin rash, and preceding sore throat is helpful.

Of the malignant diseases associated with an elevated ESR, solid tumors are more common than hematologic disorders. Lung, breast, colorectal, and urinary tract neoplasms are commonly identified solid tumors.[11, 12, 15] Leukemia, lymphoma, and myeloma are common hematologic diseases.[11, 18] Several questions may provide further leads regarding these etiologies: Does the patient complain of hemoptysis, weight loss, or shortness of breath? Was the patient a cigarette smoker? Has the patient ever had a breast lump or abnormal nipple discharge? Is there a family history of breast cancer? Has there been blood in the stools or a change in bowel habits? Has there been any hematuria or urinary difficulty? Does the patient complain of increasing fatigue (anemia), recurrent infections (neutropenia), or recurrent nosebleeds (thrombocytopenia)? Has the patient noted swollen glands? Has the patient noticed easy bruising?

Renal disease is the fourth category. Specifically, patients with azotemia, nephrotic syndrome, and acute or chronic glomerulonephritis often have an

Table 3. CATEGORIES OF DISEASE ASSOCIATED WITH A GROSSLY ELEVATED ESR*

Study	No. Patients in Series	ESR Criterion (mm/hr)	Infection No.	(%)	Connective Tissue Disease No.	(%)	Malignancy No.	(%)	Renal Disease No.	(%)	Other No.	(%)	No Cause No.	(%)
Zacharski and Kyle[11]	263	≥ 100	22	(8)	34	(13)	154	(58)	22	(8)	29	(11)	17	(6)
Payne[13]	100	> 100	53	(53)	33	(33)	14	(14)	0		0		0	
Hart et al.[18]	348	100	120	(34)	31	(9)	80	(23)	11	(3)	100	(29)	6	(2)
Cheah and Ransome[12]	360	≥ 100	159	(44)	87	(24)	42	(12)	21	(6)	50	(14)	0	
Abengowe[17]	100	—	62	(62)	27	(27)	11	(11)	—		—		—	
Wyler[16]	200	≥ 100	70	(35)	16	(8)	30	(15)	7	(3.5)	56	(28)	14	(7)
McDonald[19]	39	≥ 100	18	(46)	1	(3)	10	(26)	1	(3)	9	(23)	0	
Ford et al.[15]	100	≥ 100	60	(60)	26	(26)	28	(28)	11	(11)	41	(41)	0	
Schimmelpfennig and Chusid[14]	156	≥ 100	87	(55)	25	(16)	21	(13)	14	(9)	7	(4)	2	(1)

*In some series, the sum of percentages does not equal 100 because more than one disease was identified in some patients.

ESR elevation. Is there a history of ankle swelling (suggesting hypoalbuminemia)? Has the patient ever had renal disease or hematuria?

Family History. Is there a family history of connective tissue disease? If the patient is female, is there a history of breast cancer in her mother or sisters?

Social and Occupational History. Does the patient have functional limitations at home or work? Does he or she work in an area that may be associated with increased risk of neoplasm (exposure to asbestos or radiation)? If the patient is female and sexually active, could she be pregnant?

Drug History. Is the patient taking any nonsteroidal anti-inflammatory drugs, including aspirin, that might alter ESR interpretation? Does the patient smoke or drink (raising the possibility of lung cancer or cirrhosis)?

Previous Medical History. Has the patient had a recent operation? Is there a history of inflammatory bowel disease or skin rash? Has the patient had a previous ESR determination, which could be used for comparison? Is there a history of sickle cell disease? Does the patient have a prosthetic bone device (which might predispose to osteomyelitis)?

General Considerations. Was the elevated ESR identified as part of a diagnostic work-up for a given problem, or was it obtained through routine screening of an asymptomatic individual? The extent of evaluation may be tempered by the reason for ordering an ESR determination.

High-Payoff Queries

The following questions summarize the preceding discussion and may be helpful in directing the search for potential causes of an elevated ESR.

1. *Do you have a productive cough or a fever, or have you felt short of breath?* An affirmative answer might point to a pulmonary disease, such as pneumonitis, pulmonary embolus, lung cancer, or lung abscess.
2. *Do you have pain or discomfort on your side? Do you have difficulty urinating? Do you have a fever?* These questions explore the possibility of renal or genitourinary disease, such as a urinary tract infection (including pyelonephritis), perinephric abscess, acute glomerulonephritis, or hypernephroma.
3. *Do any of your joints ache? Have you noticed a skin rash? Have you had any muscle aches lately? Do you have a fever?* If the patient answers "Yes," the clinician should suspect a connective tissue disease, such as rheumatoid arthritis or systemic lupus erythematosus, or a systemic disease, such as subacute bacterial endocarditis.
4. *Have you lost weight lately? Do you have blood in your sputum, a lump in your breast, or bloody urine?* Any of these signs and symptoms might indicate a malignant disease with solid tumor, such as lung cancer, breast cancer, hypernephroma, or bladder cancer.
5. *Have you noticed swelling in any of your glands (lymph nodes)? Are you tired? Has your nose bled a lot lately? Do you have a fever?* An affirmative answer might signal a hematologic malignancy, such as leukemia, lymphoma, or myeloma.
6. *Have you been feeling well lately?* If so, there may be no disease associated with the high erythrocyte sedimentation rate.

PHYSICAL EXAMINATION

A physical examination directed at the suspected cause of the ESR elevation will be guided by the history. Specific physical findings often seen in the patient with a high ESR are listed in Table 4, along with possible significance or cause.

Temperature. Infection, malignant disease, and connective tissue disease may all be associated with a fever. Consequently, temperature should

Table 4. PHYSICAL FINDINGS ASSOCIATED WITH ESR ELEVATION AND THEIR POSSIBLE SIGNIFICANCE

Finding	Significance
Tender, palpable temporal artery	Temporal arteritis
Localized or generalized adenopathy	Lymphoma, leukemia, cancer
Dullness to chest percussion	Malignant effusion, empyema, pneumonia with consolidation
Bronchial breath sounds	Pneumonia, lung tissue above an effusion
Aortic or mitral regurgitation murmur with fever	Subacute bacterial endocarditis
Lump in breast	Breast cancer
Splenomegaly	Lymphoma, leukemia, infection
Costovertebral angle tenderness	Pyelonephritis
Pelvic mass	Uterine cancer
Adnexal mass	Ovarian cancer
Rectal mass, occult blood in stool	Rectal or colonic cancer
Skin rash	Systemic lupus erythematosus, rheumatic fever
Symmetric joint swellings	Rheumatoid arthritis
Bone pain	Osteomyelitis

be measured, noted, and followed. Spiking fevers, chills, and rigors would suggest infection with associated bacteremia.

DIAGNOSTIC STUDIES

The decision to employ further laboratory investigations depends upon the symptomatic status of the patient and data obtained from the history and physical examination. In symptomatic patients with important historical findings, laboratory studies will be ordered to pursue specific leads. In symptomatic patients without an obvious cause for elevated ESR, further evaluation is justifiable; however, additional evaluation need not be extensive or invasive unless specific leads are identified. Zacharski and Kyle,[11] in their study of patients with rates of 100 mm/hr or more at the Mayo Clinic, were able to make a diagnosis or find significant clues for all but 12 of 263 patients by means of a complete history, physical examination, hemoglobin determination, white blood cell and differential blood cell counts, chest x-ray, and urinalysis. In the 12 undiagnosed patients, serum protein electrophoresis was of major diagnostic importance in six patients, bone marrow examination in eight, and BUN measurement in two. It should be noted that in the highly selected population seen by these investigators, only 8 per cent had an infection and 58 per cent had malignant disease. In an ambulatory and general hospital population, Abengowe[17] reported that microbiologic investigations of urine, blood, and sputum, complete blood count, chest x-rays, and intravenous pyelography identified the cause of a grossly elevated ESR in most patients. In their study of patients hospitalized on a general medical ward with ESR values of 100 mm/hr or higher, Ford and colleagues[15] found that a careful history and physical examination led to a diagnosis in most patients. In those in whom the diagnosis remained uncertain, they recommended obtaining a complete blood count, BUN and electrolytes determinations, serum protein analysis, urinalysis, culture of urine and sputum when available, ECG, and chest x-ray. This approach established a diagnosis in 54 per cent of their patients and stimulated further investigation resulting in a diagnosis in 41 per cent. It would appear that the setting in which a physician practices may be an important determinant of the type of diagnostic evaluation needed. Consequently, the diagnostic approach to the patient with an elevated ESR remains empirical, although one should rely heavily on the historical and physical findings when choosing among the alternatives.

ASSESSMENT

Identifying the cause of an elevated ESR requires a careful history and physical examination and a limited laboratory evaluation. The data acquired are then compared and contrasted with the clinical characteristics of the diseases listed in Table 2. Rather than providing an extensive review of the characteristics of each disease in the differential list, it would seem more appropriate here to focus on the diagnostic approach. The clinical characteristics of these diseases are thoroughly presented elsewhere.[23]

One approach to evaluation of the patient with an elevated ESR is presented in the algorithm. The asymptomatic patient presents a dilemma. Should the physician subject a potentially healthy individual to the expense and anxiety of more extensive evaluation? Conversely, can the physician justify not pursuing further investigation to identify a potentially serious and treatable illness? The approach presented here utilizes regular patient observation in lieu of further testing. The use of the

DIAGNOSTIC ASSESSMENT OF ELEVATED ERYTHROCYTE SEDIMENTATION RATE

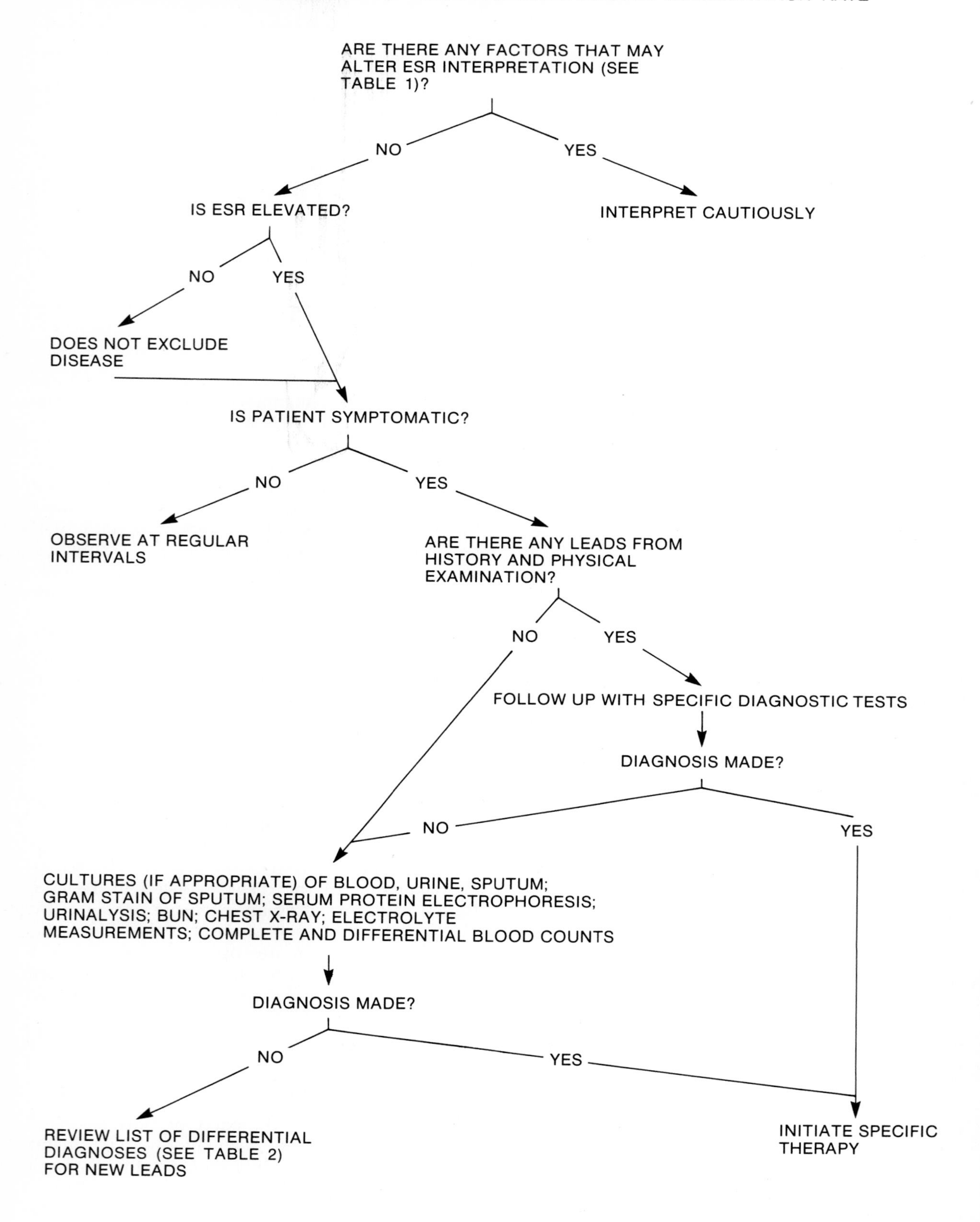

ESR in asymptomatic patients for the purpose of case finding has not been justified by the available literature and does not fulfill the accepted criteria for a screening test.[9] As mentioned previously, the presence of an abnormal ESR cannot be equated with the presence of disease (see Table 1). Even if one assumes that a disease is present, it is important to consider the implications of further testing and diagnostic labeling. If the patient has malignant disease, an elevated ESR might signal metastatic disease.[11] For an asymptomatic patient, discovery of metastatic disease would likely provide a label without a cure and more time to suffer the psychological impact of the disease. If the patient has an infection, lack of signs or symptoms would force one to seriously question its clinical significance; following the clinical course would not be unreasonable. If a connective tissue disease is present, labeling the problem would not provide a change in therapy because cure is usually not possible and the need for therapy is generally guided by the patient's symptoms.

Continuing evaluation of the asymptomatic patient does carry risks. The more the physician looks for disease the more likely one is to be identified, whether or not it truly exists and whether or not it is the cause of the elevated ESR. The process of disease labeling may have an impact of its own on the patient.[22] Evaluation of the symptomatic patient is justified, because the physician, without guarantee, is attempting to identify and ameliorate the patient's problem. However, to the asymptomatic patient the physician makes an implicit guarantee of improvement by early disease detection. If improvement is not possible, then further evaluation may have adverse effects. Consequently, the recommended approach would avoid further evaluation until the patient becomes symptomatic. For clinicians who choose further evaluation, it is important to recognize the diagnostic limits of the ESR result and to minimize the amount of additional testing. The laboratory test list in the algorithm is one guide to further evaluation.

REFERENCES

1. Kushner I. The acute phase reactants and the erythrocyte sedimentation rate. In: Kelly W, Harris E, Ruddy S, Sledge C, eds. Textbook of rheumatology. Philadelphia: WB Saunders, 1981;669–76.
2. Lascari AD. The erythrocyte sedimentation rate. Pediatr Clin North Am 1972;113–21.
3. International Committee for Standardization in Hematology: Recommendation for measurement of erythrocyte sedimentation rate of human blood. Am J Clin Pathol 1977;68:505
4. Nelson DA. Basic methodology. In: Henry JB, ed. Clinical diagnosis and management by laboratory methods. Philadelphia: WB Saunders, 1979;914–5.
5. Zacharski LR. The erythrocyte sedimentation rate. Br J Hosp Med 1976;16:53–62
6. Rafnsson V, Bengtsson C, Lennartsson J, Lindquist O, et al. Erythrocyte sedimentation rate in a population sample of women with special reference to its clinical and prognostic significance. Acta Med Scand 1979;206:207–14.
7. Sparrow D, Rowe J, Silbert J. Cross-sectional and longitudinal changes in the erythrocyte sedimentation rate in men. J Gerontol 1981;36:180–4.
8. Sharland D. Erythrocyte sedimentation rate: the normal range in the elderly. J Am Geriatr Soc 1980;28:346–8.
9. Fletcher RH, Fletcher SW, Wagner EH. Clinical epidemiology—the essentials. Baltimore: Williams & Wilkins, 1982;18–74.
10. Peyman MA. The effect of malignant disease on the erythrocyte sedimentation rate. Br J Cancer 1962;16:56–71.
11. Zacharski LR, Kyle RA. Significance of extreme elevation of erythrocyte sedimentation rate. JAMA 1967;202:264–6.
12. Cheah JS, Ransome GA. Significance of very high erythrocyte sedimentation rates (100 mm or above in one hour) in 360 cases in Singapore. J Trop Med Hyg 1971;74:28–30.
13. Payne RW. Causes of the grossly elevated erythrocyte sedimentation rate. Practitioner 1968;200:415–7.
14. Schimmelpfennig RW Jr, Chusid MJ. Illness associated with extreme elevation of the erythrocyte sedimentation rate in children. Clin Pediatr 1980;19:175–8.
15. Ford MJ, Parrish FM, Allan NC, et al. The significance of gross elevations of the erythrocyte sedimentation rate in a general medical unit. Eur J Clin Invest 1979;9:191–4.
16. Wyler DJ. Diagnostic implications of a markedly elevated erythrocyte sedimentation: a re-evaluation. South Med J 1977;70:1428–30.
17. Abengowe CV. Clinical importance of grossly increased erythrocyte sedimentation rate (letter). Can Med Assoc J 1975;113:929–30.
18. Hart GD, Soots M, Sullivan J. Significance of extreme elevation of erythrocyte sedimentation rate. Appl Therapeut 1970;12:12–13.
19. McDonald CR. Elevated ESR (letter). South Med J 1978;71:880.
20. Kirkeby AK, Leren P. Betydningenau storkt forhøyt senkningsreaksjon: 348 tilfelle med SR over 100 mm. Nord Med 1952;48:1193–5.
21. Liljestrand A, Olhagen B. Persistently high erythrocyte sedimentation rate. Acta Med Scand 1955;151:441–9.
22. Haynes RB, Sackett DL, Taylor DW, et al. Increased absenteeism from work after detection and labeling of hypertensive patients. N Engl J Med 1978;299:741–4.
23. Calin A. Acute rheumatic fever. In: Rubinstein E, Federman D, eds. Scientific American medicine. New York: Scientific American, 1979, VIII;1–5.

FACIAL PAIN

JERRY TEMPLER

☐ SYNONYMS: "Toothache," "sinus," headache, earache

BACKGROUND

Because pain in the face may arise from the paranasal sinuses, teeth, arteries, cranial nerves, nasopharynx, deep spaces, intracranial structures, or a psychogenic illness or may be referred from nearby structures, a large number of medical and dental specialists are interested in the subject. The resultant differing philosophies and approaches[1-4] bring to mind the poem "The Blind Men and the Elephant." Chronic facial pain frequently exasperates the doctor as well as the patient. In a large percentage of patients the diagnosis is presumptive, based on the clinical course, and there are no physical, x-ray, or biopsy findings to confirm it. Many of the entities are purely descriptive and their treatment is empirical. Headache and facial pains are frequently overlapping, because headache frequently occupies the forehead and temples. Facial pain might even be considered a form of headache. Measurement of pain is not possible, and even a university facial pain clinic using the most sophisticated and extravagant means will neither diagnose nor help all patients. The physician treating patients with facial pain needs to be aware of the large number of entities in order to accomplish a diagnosis and treatment. He or she first must separate serious or life-threatening disease from the chronic pain syndromes, which in turn are separated from the trivial or short-lived problems. Once progressive disease has been ruled out, a compassionate but pragmatic approach is necessary. The temptation to use narcotics must be resisted in most instances.

HISTORY

Diagnosis is essential if effective therapy is to be provided. Of the factors in diagnosis—the history, physical examination, laboratory and other diagnostic studies, response to medication, and follow-up—the history is by far the most important element in facial pain.[5] After obtaining a detailed history, one should have a pretty good idea as to the diagnosis. Other procedures rarely reveal an abnormality that is not suspected on the basis of the history and physical examination. History-taking is therefore reviewed in some detail.

Age and Circumstances of Onset. In general, pains beginning early in life are most frequently vascular in origin. Onset of pain in middle age suggests depression or emotional factors. Facial pain that begins in elderly patients must be suspected to be neuritis, temporal arteritis, or other organic disease. Trauma occurring at the onset of pain must be considered in all age groups.

Characteristics of Pain. The patient will describe the clinical course of his or her pain. The physician wants to know the frequency and duration of attacks. He or she must know the evolution of a typical attack, including precipitating factors, auras, type of onset, character of the pain, and what the patient does during the attack. Previous treatment and response to it are also important. Migraine frequently occurs in the face, and the pain is usually unilateral in the frontal or temporal area. Migraine is an episodic disorder and does not occur every day. It may recur twice a week or only once every year or so.

The nature of the pain is also important. Vascular pain is frequently pulsatile or throbbing. Cluster headache may be a constant severe, boring pain. Psychogenic pain may be described as pressure, heaviness, or fullness. The time of day when the attacks occur is helpful. Migraine may occur during the night, but a cluster headache frequently occurs at the same hour night after night. Prodromal symptoms are associated only with migraine. It is important to know whether there are associated symptoms such as nausea, vomiting, photophobia, hypersensitivity to noise, and odors. The patient should be asked whether environmental factors trigger attacks. Bright lights, weather changes, pollution, and carbon monoxide may induce migraine attacks. Cold air exposure may trigger trigeminal neuralgia. Aggravation by chewing or eating suggests dental or temporomandibular joint problems. Emotional stress, anxiety, tension, or depression may be recognized by the patient and may parallel the course of the disease. Some patients are convinced that certain foods cause their pain. The history of a head injury preceding pain may be significant. The patient should be asked whether more than one type of pain occurs, and each distinct type should be described.

Facial pain is often present in patients with allergies, but there is difficulty in proving that the allergies cause the pain. The patient should be questioned about previous response to medications. Abuse of analgesics is a very common problem in patients with chronic pain.

High-Payoff Queries

The questions asked for facial pain are the same questions asked for headache (see p. 209). The only other questions are:

1. *Do you have disease of the teeth and gums? What have you done about it?*
2. *Do you have decreased hearing, ringing of the ears, or drainage from the ears?*

PHYSICAL EXAMINATION

As with other diseases, a careful physical examination is essential, including a check of vital signs to rule out hypertension and fever. Observing the patient's behavior provides some clues. The patient with trigeminal neuralgia may protect his or her face and may not allow a trigger area to be touched.

Every square millimeter of the mucosa of the upper airways and digestive tract is examined to rule out a malignant tumor, especially in elderly men who smoke and consume large amounts of alcohol. The head and neck area should be inspected for asymmetry and swelling. The neck is palpated for abnormal masses, and the pulses are checked and bruits listened for. The cranial nerves should be examined in a systematic fashion; overlooking them might cause one to miss a clue to an organic disease.[6] The patient is questioned regarding the status of or changes in sense of smell, which is tested objectively with coffee or another common aroma. The eyes are palpated for tenderness or abnormal tension. The fields of vision are checked by gross confrontation. The eye grounds are examined, and the pupils are tested for reaction to light. The extraocular muscle function is ascertained by having the patient look in all directions. The fifth nerve should be checked by sensation to pinprick across the face. The corneal reflex is elicited with a wisp of cotton, and the nasal tickle is checked by inserting a cotton-tipped applicator in the nose. The muscles of mastication are palpated and their strength is ascertained. The seventh nerve is examined by voluntary movement of each area of the face. Taste is evaluated by rubbing the lateral aspect of the tongue with an applicator saturated with a sugar or salt solution. The patient should be able to identify these tastes without putting the tongue back in the mouth. The hearing is tested with tuning forks; however, if the patient complains of tinnitus or there is a possibility of hearing loss, formal audiometry is performed. If one does not examine the eighth cranial nerve, one might miss an acoustic neurinoma irritating the trigeminal nerve. The vestibular division is stimulated with iced water; 1 to 3 ml of iced water are placed on the tympanic membrane under direct vision with the head elevated 30 degrees from horizontal and are left in contact with the tympanic membrane for at least 20 seconds. The patient should have a lateral beating nystagmus in the opposite direction from the tested ear. The physician should wait at least 5 minutes before testing the other ear. The posterior pharynx is stimulated to elicit a gag reflex. The larynx is viewed with a mirror to determine whether both vocal cords move. The 11th cranial nerve is tested by movement of the trapezius and sternocleidomastoid muscles; lastly, the twelfth nerve is tested by having the patient protrude the tongue and move it laterally against resistance.

A headlamp or head mirror is required for illumination and visualization of the nose, mouth, hypopharynx, and larynx. The nasal mucosa is inspected; if swollen, it should be sprayed with a vasoconstrictor to permit visual inspection. Significant findings include mass lesions, pus in the nose, and sharp deviations of the nasal septum. The nasopharynx is examined with a mirror or angled lens to see above the palate. The larynx and hypopharynx are also examined with a mirror. All painful areas are carefully palpated in a search for mass lesions or inflammation.

DIAGNOSTIC STUDIES

In general, only the tests that are suggested by the history and physical findings should be ordered. A CBC, a screening chemistry profile, electrolyte determinations, and sedimentation rate measurements should be obtained routinely. X-rays of the paranasal sinuses and dental films are needed. A CT scan of the head should be done if the diagnosis has not been confirmed by the previous procedures. After excluding structural disease via the work-up, one may have to institute a therapeutic trial with various medications in order to arrive at a diagnosis; for example, cases of migraine may be difficult to diagnose but may respond to one of the ergotamine preparations.

CAUSES OF FACIAL PAIN

Paranasal Sinus Disease

Patients with chronic recurring facial pain are often convinced that pain is due to sinus disease. Inflammation of the paranasal sinuses can certainly cause pain, but the pattern of the pain should parallel the course of an acute febrile illness.[7] Occasionally, an indolent disease such as mucocele, an osteoma, or an infection such as actinomycosis may extend over several months or years.[8] Chronic allergy may cause severe edema of the turbinates, thereby stimulating pain receptors. Chronic sinus disease only infrequently causes pain but can occur in a patient with chronic facial pain. Malignant tumors of the nose or paranasal sinuses cause pain, but there is a crescendo of signs and symptoms over weeks or months rather than a protracted episodic course.

Paranasal sinus films are necessary when disease within the sinuses is expected. During an acute infection, the ostia are frequently blocked and pus cannot be seen within the nose. The thin-walled, air-filled cavities provide excellent contrast for x-ray examination. Soft tissue masses and thickening of the mucosa or air-fluid levels are readily apparent. A series of films is needed to examine all of the paranasal sinuses. The skull is a rough sphere, and the sinuses are best demonstrated by superimposing them on relatively smooth cranial bones. The head is tipped back to project the maxillary sinus above the petrous portion of the temporal bone in the Waters view. The high profile of the frontal sinuses makes them easily visible in the anteroposterior projection. The ethmoid cells and sphenoid sinuses are superimposed in the anteroposterior film. CT scans delineate soft tissue masses within the sinuses, orbits, central nervous system, and other adjacent structures (Fig. 1).

When fluid is seen within a sinus a trochar may be inserted to aspirate fluid or irrigate the sinus for diagnosis. This is easily accomplished in the maxillary sinus, but also can be done in the frontal and sphenoid sinuses. Wolff[9] has reported placing a balloon in the maxillary antrum and raising the pressure to 250 mm Hg before producing pain. High negative pressure in the sinuses is painful, and persons flying in an airplane with obstructed sinuses may experience severe pain during ascent and descent. X-ray films made shortly after a flight may show what appears to be hematomas, apparently from the mucosa being torn from the bone by the high negative pressure. Almost one atmosphere of pressure may be produced in the sinuses by a rapid descent. High pressure differentials do not occur in stationary patients; however, in some patients pain may be triggered by rather mild changes in pressure.

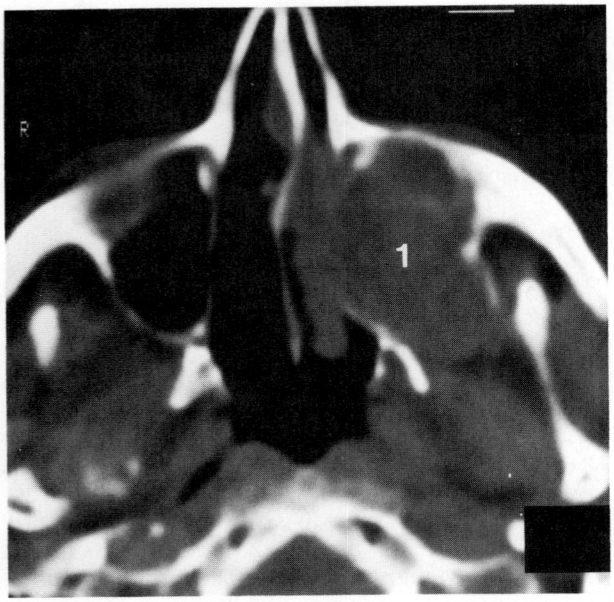

Maxillary Sinusitis. The maxillary antrum is the most frequently infected sinus, probably because of its relation to the roots of the maxillary teeth. It is frequently incriminated as the cause of cheek pain, but the diagnosis must be made objectively. It does not cause chronic or recurring pain. The pain of maxillary sinusitis is fairly well localized over the cheeks. The maxillary teeth are often sensitive on the side of the infection. A bacterial infection should respond to medical treatment and should not be a recurring problem.

Frontal Sinusitis. Pain in frontal sinusitis may be severe. Occasionally, an osteoma, mucocele, or acute exacerbations of chronic infection may cause recurring pain. Acute infection in this area is alarming because of the danger of spread to the central nervous system. Pain can be elicited by tapping the anterior wall, and the floor of the frontal sinus is exquisitely tender.

Ethmoid Sinusitis. Pain from the anterior ethmoid cells is medial to the orbit. Pain from the posterior ethmoid cells is not well localized and is described as a vertex headache. The ethmoidal sinuses are frequently involved by allergic disease and may be the source of large polyps. Polyps probably do not cause pain, which is present only with acute infection. The ethmoid sinuses are very poor containers for disease, and most processes quickly spill over into adjacent structures—the orbit, nose, or anterior cranial fossa.

Figure 1. CT scan through level of the maxillary sinus. The patient had cheek pain and hypesthesia of the infraorbital nerve. A mass *(1)* is seen filling the maxillary antrum and eroding through the medial and posterior walls.

Infratemporal Fossa Disease

The infratemporal fossa is bounded laterally by the ramus of the mandible, and medially by the posterolateral wall of the maxillary sinus. The portion of the sphenoid bone that forms the floor of the middle fossa is the roof of the infratemporal fossa. The fossa contains, among other things, the pterygoid muscles and the third division of the trigeminal nerve. Persistent preauricular and facial pain is the most common symptom of a malignant tumor in this area. Later, trismus and hypesthesia of the lower face are seen. Direct examination of this area is not easy. The best technique is computed tomography. If a mass is found, diagnosis requires biopsy through surgical exposure across the maxillary sinus.

Disorders of the Parapharyngeal Space

The parapharyngeal space extends from the base of the skull to near the hyoid bone. It is bounded laterally by the mandible and medially by the constrictors of the pharynx. Cranial nerves IX and XII and the contents of the carotid sheath traverse this area. Benign tumors in this area manifest as mass lesions without other symptoms. Malignant tumors cause facial pain or loss of motor or sensory function of the nerves in the area. Bimanual palpation is the single best method of inspecting this area. Computed tomography also gives excellent detail of this area and often shows the relationship of the mass to other structures.

Ear Pain

Otalgia is a frequently encountered complaint, and patients often equate pain with inflammation. Acute otitis media and acute otitis externa do not pose great diagnostic problems because the ear is easily accessible to examination and these diseases have a short course. However, chronic recurring ear pain without other signs or symptoms may challenge even the most experienced diagnostician. Hearing loss, tinnitus, vertigo, or otorrhea suggests organic disease. A basal cell or squamous cell carcinoma of the concha or external ear canal may invade bone or cartilage and cause severe pain. However, such tumors are visible and readily accessible to biopsy. Suspicious areas should be palpated with a cotton-tipped applicator to determine whether the pain is arising from them.

The status of the tympanic membrane is ascertained by otoscopy. The patient should be able to inflate the eustachian tube by occluding the nose and swallowing. The tympanic membrane should move perceptibly with this (Toynbee) maneuver. Failing this, the patient should try to forcibly inflate the eustachian tube by a modified Valsalva maneuver. Unilateral eustachian tube dysfunction in an adult without previous ear disease is suggestive of nasopharyngeal carcinoma. Tumors that involve the apical portion of the temporal bone cause a deep retro-orbital pain. With tumor growth, cranial nerves VI through XI may be involved, so each should be carefully tested. If the examination does not reveal local disease, the pain is assumed to be referred from some other area. Painful lesions involving nerves V, IX, and X may cause referred otalgia.

Neuritis and Neuralgias

Trigeminal Neuralgia. Trigeminal neuralgia is an episodic, recurring, very severe unilateral pain that occurs in one or more branches of the trigeminal nerve.[10] The pain is of high intensity and usually of short duration. The older name, tic douloureux, suggests the lightning speed of the pain. However, in some patients there is a slow aching component. The disease occurs almost exclusively in the elderly, and when present in younger patients suggests multiple sclerosis.[11] It is associated with a "trigger zone," i.e., an area about the face that when palpated triggers the pain. The patient attempts to avoid touching the trigger area and may avoid washing the face, shaving, or even chewing to avoid pain. In contrast, patients often massage areas that are painful from other causes. In most patients with trigeminal neuralgia, there is no sensory deficit in the distribution of the pain.

Glossopharyngeal Neuralgia. Glossopharyngeal neuralgia is probably similar to trigeminal neuralgia; however, both are of unproven etiology. In the glossopharyngeal disorder, the pain is precipitated by chewing, swallowing, or yawning and is generally in the area of the tonsil, posterior pharynx, and ear.

Atypical Facial Pain. This is simply a descriptive term for what may be a number of pain syndromes of the lower half of the face that we cannot otherwise categorize.[12] There is apt to be a steady diffuse pain not consistently associated with one pain nerve distribution. It usually has no trigger zone. If the pain is pulsatile or throbbing, it may be migraine that occurs in the face. When persistent, atypical facial pain requires a systematic approach for diagnosis. The patient should be seen by a dentist interested in facial pain, a neurologist, and an otolaryngologist as well as the primary physician. If the pain appears to be associated with stress, a psychiatrist should be consulted.

Sphenopalatine neuralgia, or Sluder's neuralgia, is one of the described syndromes in this group. It is a unilateral paroxysmal pain of the medial canthus, lateral nose, and cheek. Injection of the ganglion with lidocaine should temporarily interrupt the pain.

Post-Herpetic Neuritis. Occasionally, pain recurs after herpes zoster involvement of the trigeminal nerve. It is intense and long-lasting and may be so severe as to almost "ruin" the life of the patient. This pain is particularly difficult to handle, and if it does not resolve spontaneously, it may not respond to any known treatment.

Pain Arising in the Teeth, Mandible, or Temporomandibular Joint

Disorders Involving the Temporomandibular Joint. Perhaps no other area engenders such a wide divergence of opinions and philosophies as temporomandibular joint (TMJ) dysfunction. Some clinicians doubt that TMJ syndrome even exists. The literature on the subject is voluminous, and there is confusion within the dental profession concerning diagnosis and treatment. Recently, the disorder has been called myofascial pain dysfunction syndrome. The pain is thought to be due to spasm of the muscles of mastication, especially the masseter and temporalis. It may be caused by overstretching of these muscles.[13] Bruxism or loss of teeth resulting in malocclusion may cause the disorder. Recently, several authors have strongly suggested that a majority of cases of muscle contraction headache, and migraine, and even symptoms in distant systems may be caused by temporomandibular joint dysfunction.

Most affected patients are women in the third through the sixth decade. Earache is the most common complaint, but the pain may be poorly localized over the face and may even radiate into the neck and shoulder. It may be constant or intermittent, and is deep and dull. Generally, there is tenderness of the muscles of mastication, clicking or popping of the joint, and at times limitation of movement.

Most patients with this pain have visited several physicians or dentists. Many have had multiple expensive procedures to correct dental occlusion. The diagnosis may be reinforced by response to therapy. Very tender areas or trigger points may be injected with a mixture of lidocaine and a steroid.

Pain Arising From a Tooth. Whether or not pain arises from a tooth seems to be a trivial question, but it may be quite difficult to answer. Frequently, dental pain may mimic neuralgic pain. An obvious abscess or a tooth that is very tender to percussion is highly suggestive. A dentist is required for confirmation of the diagnosis and for treatment to relieve the pain. The mandibular x-rays made in a hospital radiology department will show large lytic lesions, but they do not have the detail of dental films.

Unusual problems, such as the "cracked tooth" syndrome, which is thought to be an incomplete tooth fracture, can cause atypical and even intermittent pain. Frequently, chewing certain types of food causes pain but chewing other foods does not. The pain is frequently made worse by cold liquids.

Patients with persistent facial or head pain, particularly unilateral, that has not been diagnosed should be seen by a dental specialist.

Vascular Headaches

Migraine. Migraine can take numerous forms and at times may be located in the forehead, temple, orbit, or cheek. Affected patients frequently assume that they have sinus disease. Migraine is usually unilateral but shifts from side to side at different times. It is a chronic recurring pain, frequently described as throbbing. It may be accompanied by nausea and vomiting. A family history of headache is usually elicited. Migraine is more common in women than in men. It usually begins before the age of 40, commonly in the second or third decade, and tends to decrease with advancing age. Migraine may be precipitated by alcohol, especially wines, and by aged cheese, chocolate, and canned figs. Some patients have an aura preceding the pain. The duration of an attack is usually from several hours up to 18 or 36 hours. The patient may feel better when lying quietly, and jarring or moving about aggravates the pain.

Cluster Headache. Cluster headache occurs mostly in middle-aged men. It is a severe boring pain around the eye, almost always unilateral, and lasts for 30 to 60 minutes in most cases.[14] As the name suggests, the pains come in clusters. They may occur several times in 24 hours or may waken the patient at the same time night after night. Accompanying the attacks may be lacrimation, injection of the conjunctiva, and nasal stuffiness on the same side. There may be remissions for months or even years. Many affected patients smoke and drink more than the average population, and they have been described as having a leonine appearance. Frequently, there is a ruddy complexion with skin that is thick, coarse, and deeply pitted.

Temporal Arteritis (Giant Cell Arteritis). This entity is a vasculitis that may occur in several medium-sized arteries. It frequently occurs in the temporal arteries of elderly people. The pain is described as an aching or burning in the temple or jaws. The artery is usually enlarged and ropelike on palpation. The diagnosis is made by excising a segment of the artery and examining it microscopically. It is important to diagnose this disease early, since it may involve the arteries to the eyes, leading to blindness.

Pain Around the Eyes

The eye and orbit may be sources of facial pain.

The symptoms of eyestrain headache are usually pain and tiredness of the eyes or the forehead above the eyes. It is always associated with sustained visual effort and seems to be due to a refractive error or problem of the oculomotor system. Examination by the primary physician will probably be unrevealing. The patient should be seen by an ophthalmologist.

Other pains about the eye may be due to conjunctivitis or diseases of the cornea. Corneal disease usually is felt as a foreign body or manifests as photophobia. Patients with glaucoma frequently have severe pain in the eye and usually distorted or decreased vision. The eyes are frequently red and the cornea appears edematous. The eye is very hard to palpation.

Inflammation of the orbit, including orbital cellulitis and dacryoadenitis, may be obvious. Orbital cellulitis is frequently secondary to inflammation within the paranasal sinuses. Orbital pseudotumor

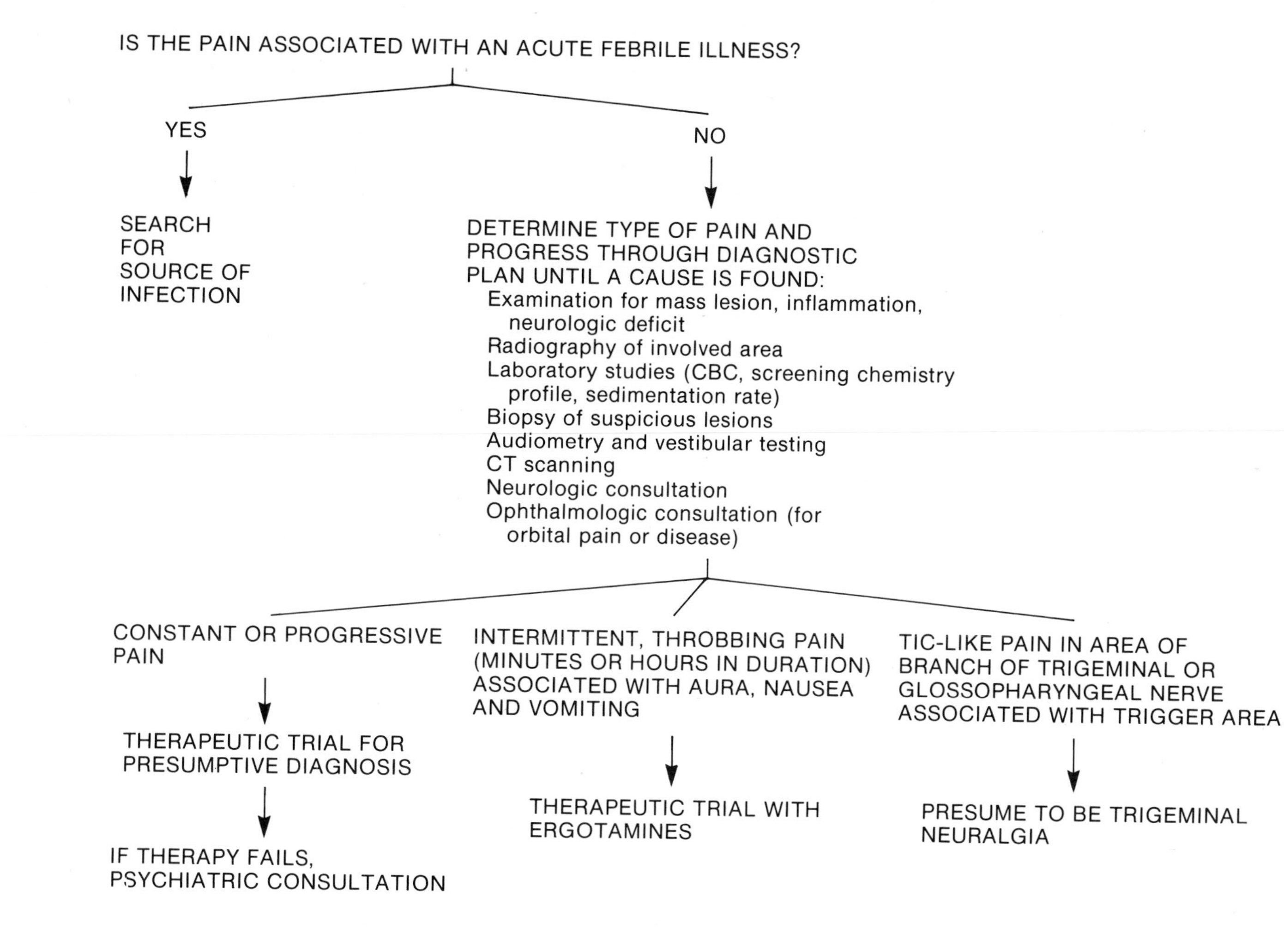
DIAGNOSTIC ASSESSMENT OF FACIAL PAIN
IS THE PAIN ASSOCIATED WITH AN ACUTE FEBRILE ILLNESS?
YES
NO
SEARCH FOR SOURCE OF INFECTION
DETERMINE TYPE OF PAIN AND PROGRESS THROUGH DIAGNOSTIC PLAN UNTIL A CAUSE IS FOUND:
Examination for mass lesion, inflammation, neurologic deficit
Radiography of involved area
Laboratory studies (CBC, screening chemistry profile, sedimentation rate)
Biopsy of suspicious lesions
Audiometry and vestibular testing
CT scanning
Neurologic consultation
Ophthalmologic consultation (for orbital pain or disease)
CONSTANT OR PROGRESSIVE PAIN
INTERMITTENT, THROBBING PAIN (MINUTES OR HOURS IN DURATION) ASSOCIATED WITH AURA, NAUSEA AND VOMITING
TIC-LIKE PAIN IN AREA OF BRANCH OF TRIGEMINAL OR GLOSSOPHARYNGEAL NERVE ASSOCIATED WITH TRIGGER AREA
THERAPEUTIC TRIAL FOR PRESUMPTIVE DIAGNOSIS
THERAPEUTIC TRIAL WITH ERGOTAMINES
PRESUME TO BE TRIGEMINAL NEURALGIA
IF THERAPY FAILS, PSYCHIATRIC CONSULTATION

manifests as severe eye pain, decreased movement of the extraocular muscles, and proptosis. It is frequently diagnosed on CT scanning, and its rapid response to steroids may be diagnostic. Pain associated with proptosis and extraocular muscle dysfunction is sometimes due to serious disease within the orbit that may be life-threatening or may cause loss of vision. The patient should be seen by an ophthalmologist immediately.

DIAGNOSTIC APPROACH

A diagnostic approach to the patient with facial pain is presented in the algorithm.

REFERENCES

1. Poser CM. Facial pain: diagnostic dilemma, therapeutic challenge. Geriatrics 1975;30:110–5.
2. Calkins RA. Facial pain: a neurological perspective. J Iowa Med Soc 1973;63:13–5.
3. Ratner EJ, Person P, Kleinman DJ, Shklar G, Socransky SS. Jawbone cavities and trigeminal and atypical facial neuralgias. Oral Surg 1979;48:3–19.
4. Dalessio DJ. Evaluation of the patient with chronic facial pain. Am Fam Physician 1977;16:84–92.
5. Schramm VL. A guide to diagnosing and treating facial pain and headache. Geriatrics 1980;35:78–90.
6. McFarland HR. Differential diagnosis of chronic facial pain. Am Fam Physician 1981;23:137–44.
7. Templer JW. Inflammatory diseases of the paranasal sinuses. In: English G. ed. Textbook of otolaryngology. Hagerstown, Maryland: Harper and Row, 1976.
8. Wyllie JW, Kern BB, Djalilian M. Isolated sphenoid sinus lesions. Laryngoscope 1973;83:252–65.
9. Wolff JG. Headache mechanisms. Intern Arch Allergy 1955;7:210–25.
10. Hart RG, Easton JD. Trigeminal neuralgia and other facial pains. Mo Med 1981;78:683–93.
11. Bayer DB, Stenger TG. Trigeminal neuralgia. Oral Surg 1979;48:393–9.
12. Paulson GW. Atypical facial pain. Oral Surg 1977;43:338–41.
13. Marbach JJ, Lipton JA. Treatment of patients with temporomandibular joint and other facial pains by otolaryngologists. Arch Otolaryngol 1982;108:102–7.
14. Kunkel RS. Cluster headache. Ohio State Med J 1977;73:131–8.

FAILURE TO THRIVE, INFANT

ELLEN F. SOEFER

☐ SYNONYMS: Growth retardation, growth failure, inadequate progression of growth before 2 years of age

BACKGROUND

Definition

Failure to thrive should be regarded not as a diagnosis but rather as a descriptive phrase requiring a systematic approach to the determination of its cause.[1] By commonly held definition, the term describes an individual who is two standard deviations below the mean for weight (below the third percentile) or is chronically below his or her own established growth curve, often including length and head circumference as well as weight.[2] This chapter deals with infants, who are by definition younger than 2 years. About 3 per cent of normal children have growth parameters that fall below the third percentile, including those with constitutional short stature.[2] The onus, however, is on the health care provider to determine whether such infants are indeed normal.

Origins

Use of the word thrive in relation to the growth of infants can be traced to Holt in 1899.[3] Chapin, as early as 1915, began alerting pediatricians to the association of growth and development failure with poverty and institutional care of infants and children.[4] In 1945, Spitz reported his observations of anaclitic (so-called dependence upon others) depression, malnutrition, and growth failure in infants under 1 year of age kept in foundling homes.[2, 4] In 1947, Talbot and Sobel suggested that caloric insufficiency might be responsible for failure of some infants to thrive in their homes as well as in institutions.[2, 4] Bakwin, 2 years later, described unhappy facial expressions, poor muscle tone, slow movements, and little interest in the environment in emotionally deprived hospitalized infants.[4] Prader contributed the idea in 1963 that catch-up growth could occur following illness or starvation.[4] Continued research and observation since that time has lead to further identification of causes of and therapeutic interventions for growth failure in infancy.

Incidence and Causes

Patients who are failing to thrive may account for 1 to 5 per cent of hospital admissions.[5, 6] Incidence, however, depends on the location of the practice or hospital. In tertiary care settings, organic causes may predominate, whereas nonorganic causes may be more common in primary care settings.[6]

Essentially, the broad categories of causes of growth failure are organic disorders (conditions associated with actual disease), nonorganic reasons (including psychosocial difficulties and environmental deprivation) and a combination of both.[7] There is also a percentage of patients for whom the etiology of growth failure is undeterminable.[6, 8] Surveys over the years indicate that organic diagnoses account for 18 to 85 per cent of the total, environmental deprivation accounts for 15 to 55 per cent, and no diagnosis can be determined in 9 to 32 per cent.[6] Possible organic causes are such entities as: chronic gastroenteritis, pyloric stenosis, gastroesophageal reflux, chalasia, celiac disease, cystic fibrosis, central nervous system disorders, recurrent pneumonia, congenital heart disease, hypothyroidism, metabolic and chromosomal abnormalities, and immune deficiency diseases. More obscure diseases are possible but much less likely causes.

HISTORY

A detailed history, along with a comprehensive physical examination and observation of family dynamics, provides the key to diagnosing the etiology of failure to thrive in an infant.[4]

Standard medical history questions will serve to elicit appropriate data. However, certain subject areas lead more quickly to helpful diagnostic information. The following mnemonic highlights these areas, which are discussed in detail.

*F*amily
*A*pgar scores and birth history
*I*ntrauterine insult
*L*earning ability
*U*nusual circumstances
*R*eview of systems
*E*conomics

*T*emperament
*H*ealth care history
*R*ecognition of problem
*I*ntake
*V*erification of growth parameters
*E*nvironment

Family. Information about the family, including medical history and growth stature of members as well as psychosocial dynamics, is crucial. Often a conversational approach is the most successful way to discuss such issues.[2]

Apgar Scores and Birth History. Birth history supplies initial growth parameters and percentiles, and information about problems encountered perinatally that could persist throughout infancy (e.g., vomiting, breathing problems, feeding difficulty). Apgar scores reflect birth trauma or anoxia, which can affect the infant's developmental progress. Neurologic damage at birth can also affect the infant's ability to feed.

Intrauterine Insult. Perinatal history gives information about an intrauterine insult that might influence the growth of the infant. Alcohol ingestion, anticonvulsant medications such as phenytoin sodium (Dilantin) and trimethadione (Tridione), smoking, gestational hypertension, gestational infections with toxoplasmosis, rubella, cytomegalovirus, and herpes simplex (TORCH diseases), syphilis, and addictive drug ingestion can produce small babies, often with anomalies and resultant growth retardation in infancy.[5, 9] Gestational age assessment labels the baby as small (SGA), appropriate (AGA), or large (LGA) for gestational age. Although the evidence is contradictory, growth patterns for SGA term and preterm infants appear to vary from those of AGA term and preterm infants. Catch-up growth during infancy appears to differ in these categories.[9]

Learning Ability. The infant's ability to learn is suggested by the developmental milestones he or she has passed. The Denver Developmental Screening Test is a useful tool for screening and following a baby's development via history as well as office testing. Deficits in all categories (gross motor, fine motor, language, and personal-social) suggest environmental deprivation or a global neurologic insult. Delays in specific categories suggest focal neurologic deficits and a need for detailed investigation.

Unusual Circumstances. A history of unusual circumstances relating to the family itself, to prior pregnancies, or to the perinatal period of the infant in question often illuminates the reason for the infant's failure to thrive. An example is neglect of an infant who reminds a parent of someone in his or her past who has caused pain, fear, or anger.[10] Abuse, neglect, or psychosocial growth failure of one of the caretakers may be repeated for the infant in question.

Review of Systems. A thorough and complete review of body systems is the key to diagnosing organic cause of failure to thrive. Gastrointestinal, cardiovascular, endocrine, renal, and nervous systems are most frequently affected. If one considers failure to thrive to be the result of an imbalance between the supply and the proper use of energy by the body, any gastrointestinal abnormality leading to one of these components (such as oral cavity anomalies interfering with intake or a malabsorption syndrome interfering with energy utilization) may be the primary culprit.[11]

Growth failure in children with congenital heart disease may have a variety of causes, but growth of those with cyanotic lesions seems to be significantly more impaired than growth of those with acyanotic lesions.[12]

Endocrinopathies are found relatively infrequently as causes of failure to thrive, although hormonal disturbances (i.e., alterations of homeostatic control of growth hormone, insulin, thyroid hormone, cortisol, aldosterone, catecholamine, and antidiuretic hormone production) may be associated with, but may not necessarily cause, growth failure.[13]

Renal causes of failure to thrive include a variety of urinary tract defects, such as obstructive uropathy. Renal failure is often, but not always, present. Speculation on the cause of the growth failure seen in these infants includes the association of acidosis, osteodystrophy, protein-calorie malnutrition, alterations in hormone production and metabolism, anorexia, electrolyte imbalances, chronic glucocorticoid administration, anemia, and hyposthenuria.[14]

Diseases of the nervous system causing growth failure may be suggested by specific deficits, as described earlier. In addition, an entity called the diencephalic syndrome is a disturbance of the neuroendocrine function of the hypothalamus, presumably from the presence of a tumor. Abnormalities in growth hormone and plasma cortisol production are detected in these patients.[13]

Economics. The economic situation of the family is vital information. The baby's growth failure may simply be the result of inadequate energy intake due to lack of food availability. Conditions of poverty at home may make it difficult for the caretakers to provide a nurturing environment for the infant.

Temperament. Learning about the temperament of the baby is quite helpful. Infants failing to thrive are often difficult feeders with disturbances in sleep patterns and elimination behavior. They may engage in rumination (self-induced regurgitation of food followed by rechewing and reswallowing) and other self-stimulatory actions. Such behavior often results from an impaired caretaker-infant relationship and leads to increasing discomfort of each with the other, making successful nurturing more difficult.

Health Care History. Information about the infant's past problems as well as the caretaker's level of responsibility in caring for the infant can be gleaned from the health care history. Missing immunizations and infrequent visits to a health care provider suggest poor compliance and probable neglect.

Recognition of Problem. Whether or not the caretakers perceive growth failure is an important issue, because frequently they do not. They may instead present the infant to the health care provider for somatic complaints. It is often difficult to convince the caretakers that the infant is growing inadequately. This issue should be addressed directly, but nonthreateningly, during the history-taking session.

Intake. Complete details of dietary intake are crucial components of the infant's history. They should include the types of solids and liquids ingested as well as quantities, methods of preparation, and caloric content. Without adequate caloric intake, appropriate growth cannot occur. Growth failure has even been demonstrated in solely breast-fed infants of mothers with inadequate milk production.[15] Improper feeding techniques as well as poor dietary content may contribute. Evidence suggests that in order for growth recovery to occur in an infant with growth failure, caloric intake must exceed the level suggested for normal growth for that infant's ideal weight for age and height.[4]

Verification of Growth Parameters. Knowledge of previous weight, length, and head circumference values will establish the actual pattern of growth. In situations of malnutrition, weight is lost first, followed by arrest in length and, lastly, arrest in head growth.[2] To obtain this information, one may need to contact previous health care providers and the hospital of birth.

Environment. Details about the infant's environment are also crucial to diagnosis and therapeutic intervention. Daily routines affect feeding schedules. Is the environment one that fosters love for the infant? Was this baby unwanted? Do older siblings require significant care, leading to competition with the infant's care? Is good hygiene practiced? Does the infant interact with people and objects in his or her environment? Answers to these questions give direction to further investigation.

PHYSICAL EXAMINATION

Clinical criteria determined during the initial assessment (i.e., history and physical examination) should allow the physician to identify more than 80 per cent of those cases in which organic disease is responsible for all or part of the failure to thrive.[7] Clues from the history should suggest areas of special focus, but a thorough physical examination is essential.

Careful measurements of height, weight, and head circumference are key elements for suggesting that the infant is failing to thrive. Skin-fold thickness demonstrates the status of stored fat and may help determine the degree and duration of malnutrition.

General appearance reveals level of hygiene, presence of obvious anomalies, bruises suggesting abuse, degree of eye contact with observer, and natural posture of the infant. Abnormal vital signs point to the organ system needing further investigation.

Abnormalities of the head and eyes suggest genetic syndromes, intrauterine insults, or neglect. Cataracts may be caused by intrauterine viral infections as well as enzyme deficiencies such as galactosemia. Breathing and swallowing functions should be observed. Abnormalities interfere with caloric intake and may cause over- or underutilization of energy. Examination of the chest, heart, and abdomen will reveal problem areas, helping to identify possible organic disorders.

Genital anomalies may suggest endocrine disease. Chromosomal aberrations may be associated with abnormal dermatoglyphics. Anomalies of the extremities may also suggest a chromosomal problem or a familial (genetic) disease.

Any neurologic abnormality may cause growth failure. Even infants with nonorganic failure to thrive may have differences in strength, muscle tone, and developmental abilities. A detailed neurologic exam along with in-depth developmental testing provides necessary information. Occupational and physical therapists are often asked to perform these evaluations.

DIAGNOSTIC STUDIES

Laboratory tests should not be ordered indiscriminately in the evaluation of an infant with failure to thrive. Clearly, a specific abnormality found through history-taking or physical examination should be appropriately investigated; examples are a barium swallow roentgenogram in a patient with a history of vomiting and aspiration to check for gastroesophageal reflux, and a sweat test in a patient with foul-smelling, fatty stools and a history of recurrent pneumonia to check for cystic fibrosis. It is reasonable to obtain a complete blood count with differential counts, urinalysis, urine culture, and serum electrolyte and CO_2, BUN, and creatinine determinations as baseline tests.

Experience has shown that only a small proportion (0.8 to 1.4 per cent) of laboratory studies are of assistance in diagnosing the cause of failure to thrive.[8, 16] Reliance on such technology can be costly in terms of time and patient discomfort as well as money.

It is beyond the scope of this chapter to describe every organic condition that causes growth failure and to suggest appropriate laboratory tests. Several of the more common and appropriate screening tests not already mentioned include: thyroid function tests for hyperthyroidism or hypothyroidism; chest x-ray for chronic infection, anomalies, or cardiac disease; ECG for cardiac disease; intravenous pyelogram for chronic urinary tract infection or renal anomalies; liver function tests when there is evidence of liver disease; calcium and phosphorus determinations for rickets or parathyroid disease; computed tomography of the head for focal neurologic abnormalities; serum immunoglobulins for immunodeficiency diseases; erythrocyte sedimentation rate for inflammatory or collagen vascular diseases; fasting blood sugar if there is glucose in the urine; determination of stool pH and presence in the stool of reducing substances or fat as evidence for disaccharide or fat malabsorption; and upper and lower (barium enema) gastrointestinal x-rays for malformations, Hirschsprung's disease, or pyloric stenosis.

Bone age x-rays are often helpful in categorizing types of linear growth delays. An infant or child who has genetically limited growth potential due to familial short stature, gonadal dysgenesis, chondrodystrophy, or primordial dwarfism will have a normal linear growth velocity and a bone age equal to his or her chronologic age. An infant or child growing slightly below but parallel to the third percentile whose linear growth velocity is within the normal range and whose bone age is equal to height age has a constitutional delay in growth. An infant or child whose growth is parallel to but far below the third percentile, with growth velocity at the lower limits of or slightly below normal and bone age behind chronologic age and equal to height age, is likely to have a systemic disease. Characteristically, an infant or child whose growth progressively deviates downward away from the third percentile or from a previous growth curve and has a markedly retarded bone age has a chronic systemic or endocrinologic disease.[17]

If abnormalities are uncovered through laboratory screening tests, it is important to keep their significance in perspective. Before definitive diagnostic labels are applied, laboratory test results must be viewed in relation to history and physical findings.

ASSESSMENT

The assessment of an infant with failure to thrive involves one more step, observation. This may be performed on an outpatient basis if the growth failure is not significant enough to be life-threatening and if the caretakers' compliance is believed to be adequate. More often, however, the situation requires inpatient observation. An intermediate care setting is ideal for observation but is frequently unavailable. The purposes of observation are to corroborate symptoms elicited from the history, to evaluate infant-caretaker interaction, to accomplish in-depth developmental assessment, and to involve the parents or guardians in specialized care of the infant, including feedings. If organic disease is suspected from the history, physical, and initial laboratory findings, hospitalization can facilitate additional testing.

Observing for 1 week or more allows one to monitor the infant's caloric intake and weight status. If weight gain is achieved under conditions of adequate nutrition and nurturing, it is likely that a component of the problem is psychosocial deprivation along with inadequate caloric intake. Lack of weight gain over a 1-week span does not rule out these possible causes, however.

Assessment of such infants, on either an inpatient or outpatient basis, is enhanced by using a multidisciplinary team approach. Team members may be a nutritionist, physician, behaviorist, occupational or physical therapist, social worker, nurse practitioner or clinical specialist, speech therapist, and play therapist. Each should focus on his or her area of expertise to assess the problem. Often when psychosocial deprivation is the cause, simple bonding by the parent or guardian to a concerned health professional not only provides clues to the diagnosis but actually becomes a first step in the infant's treatment.

The period of observation can provide evidence of new symptomatology. Frequent interactions of the observer(s) with the family may illuminate a need for intervention such as foster placement for the infant. It is clearly the responsibility of the primary health care provider to assess the situation and recommend further tests, dietary changes, follow-up developmental stimulation programs, and follow-up medical care. Parents or caretakers often require explicit directions regarding activities such as feeding techniques, structured play, and appropriate positioning after meals to prevent gastroesophageal reflux and subsequent vomiting.

SUMMARY

The approach to an infant with failure to thrive involves a thorough history, complete physical examination, minimal laboratory testing unless organic disease is strongly suspected, and subsequent assessment based on an analysis of the data obtained via these mechanisms in addition to a period of observation. During the observation period, further diagnostic testing may be accomplished, along with further data-gathering. The latter process is enhanced by involving a multidisciplinary team, if at all possible. The data should be reviewed to determine whether the growth failure is due to an organic condition, psychosocial (emotional) deprivation (which may include inadequate caloric intake), or a combination of both. Therapeutic intervention can then be instituted on the basis of the cause, or continued if the period of observation actually resulted in early amelioration of the problem. Irrespective of the diagnosis, an early, effective bond between the infant's caretakers and health care personnel will facilitate evaluation and treatment.

REFERENCES

1. English PC. Failure to thrive without organic reason. Pediatr Ann 1978; 7:774–81.
2. Cupoli JM, Hallock JA, Barness LA. Failure to thrive. Curr Prob Pediatr 1980;10:1–43.
3. Smith CA, Berenberg W. The concept of failure to thrive. Pediatrics 1970;46:661–3.
4. Goldbloom RB. Failure to thrive. Pediatr Clin North Am 1982;29:151–66.
5. Levine MI. Failure to thrive: introduction. Pediatr Ann 1978;7:737–42.
6. Berwick DM. Nonorganic failure-to-thrive. Pediatr Rev 1980;1:265–70.
7. Homer CH, Ludwig S. Categorization of etiology of failure to thrive. Am J Dis Child 1981;135:848–51.
8. Sills RH. Failure to thrive. Am J Dis Child 1978;132:967–9.
9. Fischer RH. Growth patterns of low-birth-weight infants. Pediatr Ann 1978;7:782–8.
10. Fraiberg S, Adelson E, Shapiro V. Ghosts in the nursery. J Am Acad Child Psychiatry 1975;14:387–421.
11. Lavy U, Bauer CH. Pathophysiology of failure to thrive in gastrointestinal disorders. Pediatr Ann 1978;7:743–9.
12. Ehlers KH. Growth failure in association with congenital heart disease. Pediatr Ann 1978;7:750–9.
13. Abrams CAL. Endocrinologic aspects of failure to thrive. Pediatr Ann 1978;7:760–6.
14. Friedman J, Lewy JE. Failure to thrive associated with renal disease. Pediatr Ann 1978;7:767–73.
15. O'Connor PA. Failure to thrive with breast feeding. Clin Pediatr 1978;17:833–5.
16. Berwick DM, Levy JC, Kleinerman R. Failure to thrive: diagnostic yield of hospitalization. Arch Dis Child 1982;57:347–51.
17. Fiser RH Jr, Meredith PD, Elders MJ. The child who fails to grow. Am Fam Physician 1975;11:108–15.

FEVER OF UNKNOWN ORIGIN

DANIEL M. MUSHER

☐ SYNONYM: Fever of undetermined origin, FUO

BACKGROUND

Fever of unknown origin (FUO) is a source of great concern to patient and doctor alike. The patient has a potentially serious symptom with no ready explanation and is subjected to extensive (and expensive) studies, the results of many of which are negative or, even worse, "suggestive," without conclusion. The physician has to analyze a difficult problem, often in the absence of helpful clues or in the presence of misleading ones, and daily must face the patient without an answer. The consultant, for whom FUO is still unusual no matter how much time he or she spends studying infectious diseases or related subspecialties, has to generate a diagnostic approach, knowing that even when correct principles are followed the route to a correct diagnosis is tortuous and that in some cases the goal is never achieved.

Fever occurs as a part of so many disease states that the list seems endless—every body system and every class of disease may be responsible. Because of this complexity, most discussions of FUO are personal, being influenced by the experience and interest of the discussant. Nevertheless, as we shall see, certain basic principles are common to all.[1–9] My definition of FUO, which departs slightly from the traditional one,[1] is as follows:

1. Illness of more than 3 weeks' duration.
2. Fever continuously or intermittently present.
3. Documentation.
4. No obvious diagnosis with initial complete routine examination (very flexible definition).
5. Presence of fever, usually higher than 99.4°F (37.5°C), but any temperature higher than normal for the individual.

For practical reasons, patients are not considered to have FUO unless they have a febrile illness for more than 3 weeks. The evaluation for FUO is arduous, and many trivial, self-limited diseases are excluded by this requirement, especially childhood illnesses.[7–9] Fever, defined as any temperature greater than normal for a particular individual, must be documented during most of these 3 weeks. Generally, adult males do not have a temperature higher than 99.4°F (37.5°C), whether measured orally or rectally, and I regard anything higher than that as a fever. Children often have higher temperatures, as do women in association with the menstrual cycle. In addition, there must be no obvious diagnosis at the end of an initial complete, routine evaluation. The definition of FUO offered by Petersdorf and Beeson[1] required that patients be in the hospital for 1 week without a diagnosis being reached. This requirement served two purposes, to document the fever and to eliminate readily diagnosable conditions. My reasons for not insisting on a full week in the hospital without diagnosis are that a great deal may depend on who does the initial evaluation (as in the first case report) and also that new technology now makes it possible to accomplish, during 1 week in hospital, studies that would have been inconceivable in the 1950s.

DIAGNOSTIC EVALUATION

The evaluation must begin with the epidemiologic and clinical characteristics of the patient. There are so many different causes of FUO, and therefore so many different ways of evaluating a febrile patient, that the overall direction in each case must be determined by the clinical situation. When this basic principle is followed, seemingly complicated diagnostic problems may yield simple diagnoses.

The approach to evaluating patients with FUO is shown in the algorithm. A complete history must come first, and must include medical, social, and occupational factors. Information about travel, hobbies, and animal exposure is important, as well as previous operations and ingestion of drugs, including alcohol. There is then the careful and meticulously complete physical examination followed by routine laboratory studies, such as blood counts, blood chemistries, routine x-rays, electrocardiogram, and urinalysis. Cultures of urine and blood are included as part of the routine evaluation of a febrile patient.

Out of these findings, a few possible diagnoses are likely to emerge. The physician must keep in mind that an initial diagnosis is no more than a scientific hypothesis, which may be supported or opposed by additional data. As hypotheses are developed from available data, it is still important for the physician to expand his or her horizons by referring to reviews of systems, classes of disease (Table 1), or lists of causes of FUO (Table 2). It is essential to retake the history and examine the patient again, especially as new insights emerge from physical and laboratory findings and as hy-

DIAGNOSTIC ASSESSMENT OF FEVER OF UNKNOWN ORIGIN (FUO)

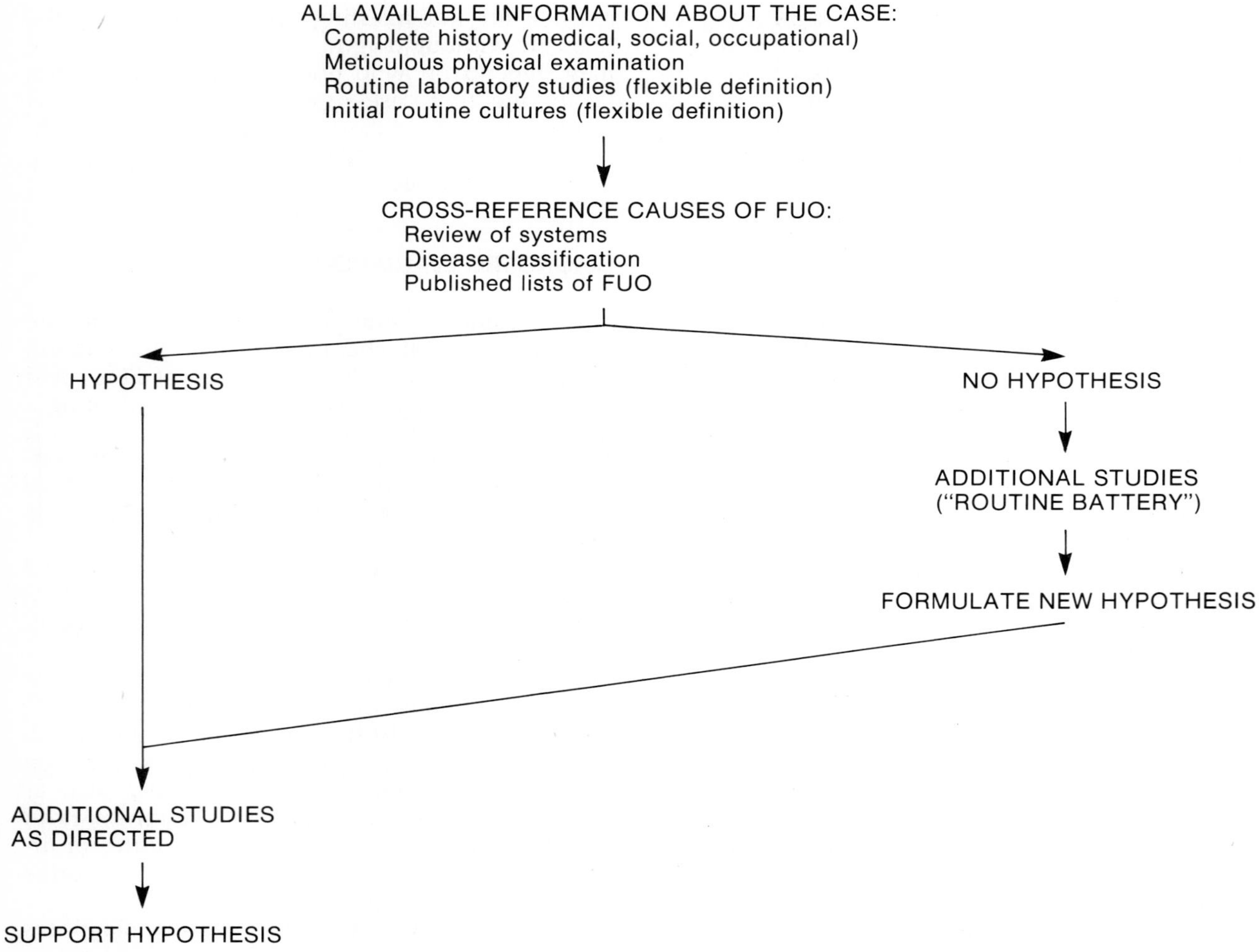

ALL AVAILABLE INFORMATION ABOUT THE CASE:
Complete history (medical, social, occupational)
Meticulous physical examination
Routine laboratory studies (flexible definition)
Initial routine cultures (flexible definition)

↓

CROSS-REFERENCE CAUSES OF FUO:
Review of systems
Disease classification
Published lists of FUO

HYPOTHESIS

NO HYPOTHESIS

↓

ADDITIONAL STUDIES
("ROUTINE BATTERY")

↓

FORMULATE NEW HYPOTHESIS

↓

ADDITIONAL STUDIES
AS DIRECTED

↓

SUPPORT HYPOTHESIS

Table 1. CLASSIFICATION OF DISEASE STATES

Infectious	Toxic
Neoplastic	Endocrine
Immunologic	Metabolic
Other collagen vascular	Congenital
Vascular	Traumatic
Degenerative	Unknown
Demyelinating	

potheses are developed. In other words, while evaluating a patient with FUO, the physician focuses on the patient's own clinical picture but continually keeps in mind a broad range of possibilities. If these factors suggest a reasonable hypothesis, the physician pursues that one first; only if they do not should the large battery of additional studies that are generally considered helpful in a so-called FUO work-up be undertaken. Within that general framework, the basic approach is first to perform noninvasive studies directed at problem areas suggested by the historical and physical findings, and then move to more invasive and less directed studies.

The following cases will illustrate these principles.

Infection by a Somewhat Uncommon Organism

Case Report. A 56-year-old man was in excellent health until 2 months before admission, when he began to notice intermittent fever (documented on many occasions up to 101.5°F), fatigue, and weight loss. He felt tired and depressed, and his back ached. Otherwise, there were no symptoms; he specifically denied respiratory, urinary, or gastrointestinal symptoms. On physical examination, he looked older than his stated age. There was no heart murmur, his liver and spleen were not enlarged, and the neurologic examination was unrevealing. He had a swollen and tender testis. Results of initial laboratory studies—hemoglobin measurement, white blood cell (WBC) count, serum creatinine and electrolyte determinations, liver function studies, serum protein measurements, urinalysis and urine culture, chest x-ray, and electrocardiogram—were all normal.

At this point, having failed to uncover an obvious diagnosis, many physicians might think it appropriate to refer to a published list of common causes of FUO, for example, the "Big Three"—infections, neoplasms, and collagen-vascular diseases.[3] They might judge that the cause in this patient has an equal chance of falling into any one of these categories and so might undertake a diagnostic evaluation for each. Thus, because in the first category (infection) tuberculosis predominates, a tuberculin skin test, acid-fast stains of sputum or gastric washings, and mycobacterial cultures would be undertaken. To cover the second category (malignancy), a search might be initiated for tumors of all kinds. A screening for connective tissue diseases, the third category, may also be done.

The problem with this approach is that it opposes the basic principle of FUO evaluation, that data about the individual patient should serve as the starting point for evaluation. In this case the initial history was not thorough enough, and some essential aspects were omitted. It is true that the patient had always been in excellent health; he worked hard as a cattle rancher in Texas, a state that has a high incidence of brucellosis. In fact, there had been some sickness among his cattle; a few weeks before the onset of illness, one of his cows had aborted, and working bare-handed, the patient had delivered the animal of the retained products of abortion. The diagnosis was brucellosis, supported by detection of antibody at 1:2,048 dilution and eventually by positive results of blood cultures.

Several instructive points arise from this case. First, this patient had a single, uncomplicated infection in its typical form.[10] History of the present illness closely followed the textbook description of brucellosis—if the physician had only known to elicit the epidemiologic information and had been able to figure out which part of the textbook to use. This diagnosis can readily be made on the basis of history alone, supported by a single laboratory test, namely, a Brucella agglutination titer. The *general* rarity of this disease did not decrease the likelihood of its occurring in this *specific* patient, on the basis of his occupational history and exposure to sick cattle. Second, it is apparent on hindsight that the patient need not have been hospitalized for 1 week without a diagnosis in order for him to be regarded as having FUO. A careful history was obtained in this case within a few days of admission, and the serologic test readily confirmed the diagnosis within a week, although the patient clearly had a febrile disease of 8 weeks' duration. Third, minor variations in the clinical setting (i.e., the historical information) may greatly alter the diagnostic approach. Let us say, for example, that the patient had been raised by his grandparents because his mother and father both contracted tuberculosis during his childhood. Moreover, let us suppose that he lived in midtown Manhattan and had never received antituberculous therapy. Although it would still have been possible for him to have acquired brucellosis, for example, by eating unpasteurized cheese imported from Mexico or Greece, this diagnosis would have been exceedingly unlikely. In other words, with exactly the same immediate history of the present illness and identical physical and laboratory findings, the diagnostic approach would take a completely different direction because of the overall epidemiologic and clinical setting. This last point reiterates the basic principle of evaluating FUO:

Table 2. CAUSES OF FEVER OF UNKNOWN ORIGIN

Infections	
Generalized	
Bacterial	Typhoid
	Brucellosis
Mycobacterial	Tuberculosis
Spirochetal	Syphilis
	Leptospirosis
Fungal	Histoplasmosis
Protozoal	Malaria
	Toxoplasmosis
Parasitic	Strongyloidiasis
	Visceral larva migrans
Viral	Cytomegalovirus
	Epstein-Barr virus
Localized	
Cardiovascular	Infective endocarditis
	Infected aneurysm or vascular graft (including entero-vascular fistula)
	Suppurative thrombophlebitis
Thoracic	Empyema
Intra-abdominal	Peritonitis (tuberculous, bacterial)
	Hepatitis (viral, bacterial, amebic)
	Cholangitis
	Abscess (splenic, subphrenic, hepatic, subhepatic, pancreatic, cholecystic, colonic including appendiceal, pelvic, tubo-ovarian)
Urinary tract	Intrarenal
	Perinephric
	Prostatic
Skin or bone	Decubitus ulcer tract infection, with or without osteomyelitis
	Osteomyelitis
	Dental infection
Neoplasms	
Hematologic	Lymphoma
	Hodgkin's disease
	Acute leukemia
	Angioblastic lymphadenopathy
	Other
Tumors	Hepatoma
	Hypernephroma
	Atrial myxoma
	Metastatic, from any primary

Table continued on opposite page

the physician must first deal with likely causes of fever in an individual case, i. e., those specifically suggested by the history and the physical and laboratory findings, before considering diagnoses that are said to be more likely in a textbook list of causes of FUO.

Other infective agents likely to cause FUO are listed in Table 2. Generalized infections may cause no localized findings that would serve as clues to the diagnosis. Disseminated histoplasmosis occurs far more commonly in the southern and southwestern than in the northeastern United States and does manifest as FUO.[11] Patients with typhoid fever have generally traveled in other countries where sanitation is poor. Infections caused by Epstein-Barr virus (infectious mononucleosis) or cytomegalovirus are readily identified through examination of the peripheral blood smear and serologic tests. They may occur in patients of any age, although cytomegalovirus infection is seen especially following transfusion or in immunocompromised hosts. It should be noted that the list of possible causes expands even more when FUO occurs in an immunocompromised host, who cannot mount an inflammatory response; these are beyond the scope of the present chapter. Leptospirosis and syphilis are said to cause FUO; although the former is likely to resolve spontaneously before 3 weeks have elapsed, fever due to the latter may persist for a month or more.[12] Amebic colitis or hepatitis (with or without an abscess) usually has symptoms relating to these systems; a diagnostic work-up is readily accomplished in most cases, and this presentation has not been a diagnostic dilemma in my experience.

Infections of individual organs usually have some manifestation to point in the appropriate direction. Endocarditis is often diagnosed in the first few days in a hospital because blood cultures are done far more frequently now than in the

Table 2. CAUSES OF FEVER OF UNKNOWN ORIGIN *(Continued)*

Drug ingestion	Antibiotics (especially penicillins) Antihypertensives Beta-lactam antibiotics Hydralazine Phenytoin Others
Presumed immune complex disorders	Systemic lupus erythematosus Rheumatoid arthritis Rheumatic fever
Vasculitides	Temporal arteritis Periarteritis nodosa Isolated angiitis Takayasu's arteritis Others
Liver disorders	Granulomatous hepatitis Alcoholic liver disease
Gastrointestinal disorders	Inflammatory bowel disease Whipple's disease
Central nervous system disorders	Infection Tumor
Uncommon disorders	Familial Mediterranean fever Weber-Christian disease Cyclic neutropenia Eosinophilic fasciitis
Miscellaneous disorders	Sarcoidosis Recurrent pulmonary emboli
Factitious fever	
Undiagnosed FUO	Disappears spontaneously Disappears spontaneously but recurs at regular or irregular intervals Disappears with empiric therapy with or without recurrence

1950s and better media are commercially available. True culture-negative endocarditis is unusual unless antibiotics have already been administered.[13–15] There may be no localized findings in endocarditis; usually, however, a heart murmur or peripheral lesions of endocarditis can be detected. If a patient has previously documented damage to a heart valve, the diagnosis is suspected more strongly. Infected vascular grafts[16] or, more rarely, infected aneurysms[17] may also cause FUO; these should certainly be suspected on the basis of the history. Infections in other organ systems such as the lung, the pleural space, the peritoneal cavity, the urinary tract, soft tissues, and bones are of great importance and are discussed in the following pages.

Malignancy

Case Report. A 50-year-old man was referred to the infectious disease service because of fever of several weeks' duration. The patient had generally been in excellent health. About 3 to 4 weeks before admission he began to have fever up to 102°F with occasional chills. His joints ached all the time, and he noticed a large lymph node in his neck. He lost 16 lb during this time. There was no history of exposure to blood products, needles, kittens, or persons with tuberculosis or infectious mononucleosis, and he had no skin rash, pruritus, or genital lesions. He was heterosexual. He had an 80 pack per year history of cigarette smoking. The patient had already received a course of intravenous antibiotics (a "knee-jerk" therapeutic response with strikingly little to defend it) without defervescence. Physical examination showed a relatively normal-appearing man with enlarged lymph nodes in the anterior and posterior cervical areas as well as in the axillary and inguinal regions. Hematocrit, WBC count, and differential counts were entirely normal, as were results of serum chemistry tests and liver function studies. The clinical diagnosis of lymphoma was proven by lymph node biopsy.

In my own practice at a Veterans Administration Hospital, malignancy is responsible for slightly more than one-half of all referrals for FUO, the same proportion reported in the recent paper by Larson and colleagues.[6] Proposed mechanisms by which tumors produce fever include production of pyrogen by tumor cells (probably responsible in this patient), necrosis, and obstruction.[18] Within the broad category of malignancy there may be a great variety of tumor types. Lymphoma and Hodgkin's disease lead the list, but many other kinds are represented. Disseminated cancer is more likely to be implicated than a solitary tumor, but either can be responsible. A few unusual primary tumors, such as hepatoma and hypernephroma, are said to have a striking propensity to cause fever, as is any tumor metastatic to the liver.[6, 19, 20] Nevertheless, when tabulating causes of FUO at my hospital, I found common tumors (e. g., of lung and prostate) to be the most commonly implicated. A particularly frequent occurrence is bronchogenic carcinoma with radiographic evidence of an infiltrate around or distal to it in a patient who has persistent fever for weeks despite therapy with a variety of antibiotics. Necrosis need not appear radiographically, obstruction is uniformly present, and often the fever may remit spontaneously. Although I do not know the mechanism(s) involved, I have seen that virtually any kind of tumor can be responsible for prolonged fever, even in the absence of obvious necrosis or infection of the tissues. The mechanisms may be obscure, but the observation is unquestionable. The special situation of fever in a patient with malignancy who is receiving chemotherapy is beyond the scope of this discussion.

The patient who presents with fever and lymphadenopathy opens up an interesting set of diagnostic possibilities. Although physicians often think of proceeding directly to biopsy of involved tissues, this procedure is not necessarily the best way to establish the diagnosis. There are many causes in which the histologic changes are nonspecific, ranging from syphilis, which is entirely treatable and potentially dangerous, to infectious mononucleosis and cytomegalovirus infection, which are essentially untreatable and self-limited. As noted, the order of diagnostic studies should be determined by the invasiveness of each proposed test. Even when a lymph node biopsy may be most likely to yield the specific answer, as in the case just presented, serologic tests for syphilis and infectious mononucleosis and perhaps those for lymphogranuloma venereum and cytomegalovirus should be done first. If the actual diagnosis is lymphoma or lung cancer, a critic might argue that a few days in the hospital have been lost to serologic testing. At the same time, if the final diagnosis is syphilis, demonstrated by a VDRL titer positive at 1:128 dilution, the performance of an unnecessary lymph node biopsy will have been embarrassing for the physician and expensive and painful for the patient.

Connective Tissue Disease

Case Report. A 72-year-old man was hospitalized for evaluation of fever of 2 years' duration. He had been in excellent health all his life, working as a laborer until he retired, and thereafter remaining entirely healthy. Two years before admission, he began to have fever up to 101°F but without shaking chills, and he began to lose weight. Except for a possible loss of sensation in his feet, there were no specific symptoms, such as cough, sputum production, abdominal pain, urinary infection, and arthralgias. He had not traveled outside urban Houston and had no pets. He was hospitalized twice during this period, and on each occasion was given some kind of "fever work-up" with negative results. Physical examination showed a wasted elderly man who walked with a broad-base gait and had loss of sensation (light touch, pinprick, and vibration) in the lower legs. Hemoglobin level was 12.5 gm/dL and WBC count was 4200 cells/mm^3; renal function and electrolyte levels were normal, as were results of liver function studies. Because the history suggested occult malignancy, an extensive evaluation for a source was begun. Although he did not really have muscle pain, the possibility of myositis as part of a paraneoplastic syndrome was raised; a muscle biopsy showed "necrotizing arteritis." The antinuclear antibody test was positive, as was the test for antibody to DNA. The final diagnosis was systemic lupus erythematosus.

This is a relatively pure example of FUO, in that the admitting physician obtained no clues from the history or physical examination that might have led to the diagnosis. As already noted, the proper diagnostic approach is to perform a general battery of screening studies beginning with simple (blood and serologic) tests and progressing to more complex ones. The order of studies should always be tempered by an estimation of the likelihood of a positive result. Certainly an antinuclear antibody test ought to have been done before screening studies for occult malignancy or blind biopsy of muscle tissue, even though the latter led to the correct diagnosis. Because of the frequency of temporal arteritis in elderly patients,[21] I would probably have performed a biopsy of the temporal artery before the muscle, but I would not have done either until the initial serologic studies, including the antinuclear antibody and anti-DNA antibody assays, were done.

Despite the designation of infection, malignancy, and collagen vascular disease as the "Big Three" causes of FUO, in my experience collagen vascular disease has been relatively rare. This rarity may be in part related to my patient population, but other series have not shown more than 10 to 15 per cent of cases to be due to this cause. In their recent paper on FUO, Larson and colleagues[6] comment that the widespread knowledge of autoimmune diseases and the availability of antinuclear antibody assays and related tests have decreased the likelihood that a patient with such a disease would present with unexplained fever. The propensity of any kind of vasculitis to cause fever[22] is reason to consider this group of diseases in evaluating any patient with FUO.

FUO With Many Potential Sources (Due to a "Miscellaneous" Cause)

Case Report. A 46-year-old quadriplegic man was referred for evaluation of FUO. Six weeks before admission he had been in an automobile accident, in which he had sustained a compound fracture of the femur that had been repaired with a plate and screws, and lacerations of the liver and bowel for which débridement, resection, and irrigation of the peritoneal cavity had been performed. Postoperatively he had pneumonia with a pleural effusion. He had been treated almost continuously since his accident with cephalothin, gentamicin, and, more recently, ampicillin. Physical examination revealed a quadriplegic male with signs of wasting already apparent. He had no skin rash. His eyes, ears, and throat were normal. His neck was not stiff. There was dullness to percussion of the chest and decreased breath sounds at the right lung base. The abdominal wall was not entirely flaccid, although it was also not rigid, and no masses were palpable. His abdominal wound did not appear to be infected. The area over the repaired femur was indurated but not inflamed. There was no obvious purulence at the site of intravenous lines. His hematocrit was 32 per cent. The WBC count was 16,000 cells/mm^3, with increased immature polymorphonuclear neutrophils. Urinalysis showed many WBCs and bacteria; urine culture yielded *Serratia* species and *Candida albicans.* Chest x-ray showed an abnormality at the right costophrenic angle, consistent with pleural reaction, fluid, or an infiltrate.

Unlike the first patient, who had a "pure" FUO that developed outside a medical setting from an uncommon cause, this patient represents a more frequently encountered situation. Certainly, he should not be evaluated in accord with a general FUO scheme. The proper approach is to begin with causes of fever that are likely in this individual and this clinical setting and to explore less likely causes only if a search for the more likely ones is unrewarding. Thus, a tuberculin skin test might perhaps have a place, because stress to the system can always activate tuberculous infection, but tests for Salmonella and Brucella antibody are simply not recommended, no matter how noninvasive, because nothing suggests the presence of salmonellosis and brucellosis and, as a basic principle, the evaluation should proceed along logical lines.

Likely sources of this patient's fever can be chosen on the basis of initial evaluation. First, he may have an *intra-abdominal abscess.* He sustained trauma to the liver and small bowel, with both blood and fecal contents in the peritoneal cavity when admitted to the hospital after the accident. An examination of the abdomen in a quadriplegic patient with intra-abdominal infection may be normal or it may show nontender guarding or rigidity of the abdominal wall due to reflex transmission of impulses through the spinal cord. The evaluation for an intra-abdominal abscess might include ultrasonography, gallium scanning, and computed tomography. If all three procedures suggest a single diagnosis, they are quite likely to be correct; however, discrepancies among them may occur and make interpretation difficult. Moreover, no single test is anywhere near as reliable as the earlier literature on the procedures might have led us to believe. A number of recent articles, including one from our own hospital, have shown a surprisingly high incidence of error. We observed an even higher rate of lack of diagnostic usefulness—a situation in which the wrong diagnosis was suggested or there was no more definitive diagnosis—afterward than there had been before the study was done.[23]

A second area for attention is the abnormality in the right lower lung field. It is often taught that a patient who does not cough or bring up sputum is not likely to have bacterial *pneumonia.* Although this is still a good general rule, it may be misleading in consideration of a quadriplegic patient, who may have mechanical deficiencies that prevent an adequate cough. Even more likely in this case, however, would be *empyema* due to a previous pneumonia or to an intra-abdominal process.

Osteomyelitis is another likely diagnosis. The broken bone was contaminated at the time of fracture, and a foreign body was placed at the time of surgery. Meticulous surgical technique and intraoperative antibiotic therapy would have reduced, but by no means eliminated, the likelihood of infection; without these appropriate precautions, the likelihood of osteomyelitis would be even greater, and a careful review of the operative record will help to determine what actually was done. Pain at the site of such an infection, usually a reliable finding, would be absent in this patient because of his lack of sensation. A bone scan would not be useful because it would yield positive results for months after trauma, but x-rays may show rapidly progressive osteomyelitis, and a strongly positive gallium scan this long after surgery would also be suggestive. Demonstration of pus by needle aspiration of the involved area would still be the most reliable way to establish the diagnosis.

A *urinary tract infection* could be responsible for persistent fever. The patient may have had a series of reinfections, most currently with *Serratia* and *Candida,* or he could even have developed a perinephric abscess with suppression of the causative organism in the urine by antibiotic therapy and recolonization with new organisms.[24]

An *infection at the site of an intravenous catheter* could be the cause of fever, especially if the catheter had been in place for several weeks, as often happens in complicated cases. There may be no physical findings at the area, although the presence of pus strongly suggests significant infection with seeding of the blood stream.[25, 26] Removing the line and culturing the end by rolling it across an agar plate is a good way of making the diagnosis.[25] Alternatively, blood drawn back through the catheter that is positive on culture, especially if peripheral blood cultures are negative, strongly implicates the catheter as a source of infection.[26]

Decubitus ulcers with or without underlying osteomyelitis are a serious problem in bedridden patients. Infection of these ulcers is caused by mixed facultative and anaerobic bacteria. The problem is that it can be extremely difficult to determine whether a decubitus ulcer is infected or whether an infection is the cause of fever. Establishing the diagnosis of osteomyelitis underlying a decubitus ulcer is even more difficult. A recent study at our hospital showed that if a histologic diagnosis is used as the definition of osteomyelitis, none of the standard techniques, including bone and gallium scanning, wound culture, and culture of bone specimens, establishes a diagnosis with certainty.[27] In the patient who has been bedridden for a long time, the ulcer may dissect into deeper tissue planes, leaving the superficial aspect with a benign appearance.

Transfusion-related infections, such as hepatitis B, non-A, non-B hepatitis, and cytomegalovirus infection, are also likely causes of fever if the patient received many transfusions, another piece of information that must be obtained by careful review of the records.

Several noninfectious sources of fever must also be considered. *Pulmonary emboli* are relatively commonly implicated as causes of FUO[28, 29] and deserve special consideration in a bedridden patient. Alcoholic hepatitis, a very common cause of FUO,[28] could be disregarded in this case. There are some unusual causes of fever that specifically affect quadriplegics. Soon after their injury they may become febrile, and fever may persist for many weeks; the diagnosis of *quadriplegia fever*[30] obviously requires exclusion of other identifiable causes. Formation of new bone around the femurs (so-called heterotopic bone formation) may cause clinical and radiologic findings of osteomyelitis, and is said to cause fever.[31]

The possibility of *drug fever* must also be raised in patients who are in the hospital and receiving a variety of medications. Our patient had been receiving beta-lactam antibiotics continuously for 5 weeks. He had no previous history of allergies or skin rash, and no eosinophilia. Nevertheless, as part of the evaluation, antibiotics were discontinued. The fever promptly defervesced, and the patient remained afebrile until he was rechallenged with ampicillin; the prompt recurrence of fever supported the diagnosis of drug fever. Thus, in spite of all the possible infections that might have been present, this particular patient's fever was due to a drug reaction.[32]

This complicated case was chosen to illustrate the basic principle that in evaluating an individual patient it is essential to deal with the case itself. The careful physician begins with known abnormalities and moves from them to areas of likely abnormalities in the specific clinical setting, rather than using a checklist of generally likely or unlikely causes of FUO.

Unexplained FUO of Many Years' Duration

Case Report. A 66-year-old man had chills and fevers lasting for 1 to 3 weeks once or twice per year for 15 years. They were not accompanied by any symptoms other than weakness and malaise. Extensive work-ups, including cultures of blood, urine, and bone marrow for bacteria, viral cultures, repeated examinations for parasites, and evaluation of every organ by every known test (including newer ones as time progressed) all were negative. Because he had done military duty in the South Pacific, blood smears for parasites were also done but results were negative.

No diagnosis has been reached in this case, and none is likely to be. Unexplained fevers in adults may be divided into three groups: those that disappear spontaneously and do not recur; those that disappear but recur (as in this case), always without explanation; and those that persist in association with debilitation but respond to empiric therapy such as aspirin or glucocorticosteroid administration. This last group probably includes fever in patients with diseases akin to temporal arteritis, sarcoidosis, or granulomatous hepatitis in which biopsy results just happen to be negative. I have seen several such cases in which no diagnosis is achieved and fever responds well to prednisone given empirically because of continued wasting, only to recrudesce when the drug is discontinued. The absence of weight loss is said to be a favorable sign when no cause is found for a fever.[28]

Fever of unknown etiology that occurs at regular intervals has been included under the rubric periodic fever; Dinarello and Wolff[34] state that only cases associated with cyclic neutropenia have been well-documented in recent studies, although Hodgkin's disease may have such a presentation.[35] A varying proportion of FUO cases go unexplained; the proportion may reach 30 to 42 per cent in pediatric cases[7–9] because of spontaneous resolution without recurrence; generally a smaller proportion of adult cases remain unexplained.

Finally, one must consider factitious fever, either a falsification of temperature recordings (now harder to achieve thanks to the electronic temperature monitoring devices in widespread use) or autoinoculation with pyrogenic substances.[35] People who work in a medical environment are more likely to express underlying disturbed personality patterns in this fashion. They are technically competent and highly manipulative; thus, this diagnosis is often overlooked and is difficult to establish once it is thought of.

ASSESSMENT

Having presented these few illustrative cases, I would like now to refer again to the algorithm and discuss the proper approach to evaluating patients with FUO. It is essential to use all the information available from a complete history. Only some of this information is medical; social and occupational data may contain clues that lead to a diagnosis. Careful clinical examination also yields diagnostic information. For example, patients with disseminated tuberculosis may be found to have choroid tubercles during funduscopic examination. Although intravenous lines are always suspect and need not be visibly abnormal to be the source of fever, the presence of a small degree of redness or, especially, any tiny amount of purulence may signal the cause of fever in a hospitalized patient with complications. Rectal examination may uncover a perirectal or prostatic abscess. Decubitus ulcers are often overlooked. These are findings that most consultants in infectious disease make; it is unusual for them to detect a meaningful heart murmur or find a palpable spleen that others have missed. In laboratory studies, it is usually his or her concern about the quality of a specimen and attention to fine details in interpreting the results of ordinary tests that make a consultant helpful, rather than recommendation of a procedure that no one else has thought of. For example, recognizing that a poorly obtained urine specimen is responsible for a large number of bacteria with a nondiagnostic urinalysis may help to direct diagnostic efforts to disease outside the urinary tract, and focusing attention on the small number of *Staphylococcus aureus* found on a urine culture may enable diagnosis of deep-seated staphylococcal infection.

These clinical and laboratory data should lead to consideration of a diagnosis or hypothesis that is formulated by induction from available data. It is useful to use, as a cross reference, three overlapping ways of categorizing information. They will stimulate the physician to derive additional data related to the working hypothesis as well as suggest alternative hypotheses:

1. The review of systems needs to be perfectly complete, with every possible area covered.

Table 3. CLASSES OF INFECTING ORGANISMS THAT MIGHT CAUSE FEVER OF UNKNOWN ORIGIN

Bacteria	Fungi
Mycobacteria	Amoeba
Actinomyces	Protozoa
Spirochaeta	Parasites
Mycoplasma	Viruses
Chlamydia	Unclassified
Rickettsia	

2. The classes of disease (see Table 1) should be examined carefully for other diagnostic possibilities. Within each of these classes, there are means of further subcategorization; for example, the 13 broad classes of infective organisms that can be identified in the category of infectious diseases (Table 3) represent a rough guide for thinking about different kinds of infectious agents rather than a formal biologic classification.

3. One should go through the published list of causes of FUO (see Table 2), but only *after* the other approaches have been tried. As has been repeatedly stressed, what appears to be a likely cause of FUO in someone else's list may have nothing whatever to do with one's own patient.

When consideration of all these factors leads to the formulation of one or more hypotheses, diagnostic studies should be undertaken to support them. The general principle is to seek support for more likely diagnoses before less likely ones, with a preference for less invasive studies. Cost-effectiveness should be considered in ordering noninvasive studies; otherwise the expense of a so-called FUO work-up can be enormously high. Newer techniques, such as CT scanning, render much of the old and not-so-old literature obsolete, e.g., treatises on lymphangiography or laparotomy in FUO. However, the newer techniques do yield false-positive and false-negative results, and no procedure can be allowed to replace good clinical judgment and a rational approach. If there are no clues at all, a diagnostic evaluation should be undertaken in accord with previously published lists of causes of FUO; once again, less invasive studies should take precedence. Therapeutic trials in the absence of a good hypothesis are best avoided because of great difficulty in interpreting the results.

SUMMARY

Despite many advances in clinical medicine, diagnostic evaluation of a patient with FUO remains a challenging and interesting problem for the thoughtful physician. A logical and disciplined approach might seem to be too slow and indirect in any individual case, but in the long run it is the best way. A definite cause of FUO can be identified in most, but by no means all, cases. In patients who have prolonged history of fever (more than two years) and no apparent source, a cause is not generally detected with currently available techniques.

REFERENCES

1. Petersdorf RG, Beeson PB. Fever of unexplained origin: report on 100 cases. Medicine 1961;40:1–30.
2. Molavi A, Weinstein L. Persistent perplexing pyrexia: some comments on etiology and diagnosis. Med Clin North Am 1970;54:379–96.
3. Jacoby GA, Swartz MN. Fever of undetermined origin. N Engl J Med 1973;289:1407–10.
4. Wolff SM, Fauci AS, Dale DC. Unusual etiologies of fever and their evaluation. Ann Rev Med 1975;26:277–81.
5. Esposito AL, Gleckman RA. A diagnostic approach to the adult with fever of unknown origin. Arch Intern Med 1979;139:575–79.
6. Larson EB, Featherstone HJ, Petersdorf RG. Fever of undetermined origin: diagnosis and follow-up of 105 cases, 1970–1980. Medicine 1982;61:269–92.
7. McClung HJ. Prolonged fever of unknown origin in children. Am J Dis Child 1972;124:544–50.
8. Pizzo PA, Lovejoy FH Jr, Smith DH. Prolonged fever in children: review of 100 cases. Pediatrics 1975;55:468–73.
9. Feigin RD, Shearer WT. Fever of unknown origin in children. Curr Probl Pediatr 1976;6(10):1–64.
10. Young EJ. Brucellosis. Rev Infect Dis 1983;5:821–42.
11. Goodwin RA Jr, Shapiro JL, Thurman GH, Thurman SS, DesPrez RM. Disseminated histoplasmosis: clinical and pathologic correlations. Medicine 1980;59:1–33.
12. Musher DM. Syphilis: an unusual cause of FUO. Hosp Pract 1978;13(Oct):134–36.
13. Roberts RB, Krieger AG, Schiller NL, Cross KC. Viridans streptococcal endocarditis: the role of various species, including pyridoxal-dependent streptococci. Rev Infect Dis 1979;1:955–66.
14. Van Scoy RE. Culture-negative endocarditis. Mayo Clin Proc 1982;57:149–54.
15. Pazin GJ, Saul S, Thompson ME. Blood culture positivity: suppression by outpatient antibiotic therapy in patients with bacterial endocarditis. Arch Intern Med 1982;142:263–8.
16. Kierman PD, Pairolero PC, Hubert JP Jr, Much P Jr, Wallace RB. Aortic graft-enteric fistula. Proc Mayo Clin 1980;55:731–8.
17. Case records of the Massachusetts General Hospital. Case 46–1981. N Engl J Med 1981;305:1205–10.
18. Dinarello CA, Wolff SM. Molecular basis of fever in humans. Am J Med 1982;72:799–819.
19. Weinstein EC, Geraci JE, Green LF. Hypernephroma presenting as fever of obscure origin. Proc Mayo Clin 1961;36:12–9.
20. Fenster LF, Klatskin G. Manifestations of metastatic tumors of the liver. Am J Med 1961;31:238–48.
21. Huston KA, Hunder GG, Lie JT, Kennedy RH, Elveback LR. Temporal arteritis: a 25-year epidemiologic, clinical and pathologic study. Ann Intern Med 1978;88:162–7.
22. Fauci AS, Haynes BF, Katz P. The spectrum of vasculitis: clinical, pathologic, immunologic, and therapeutic considerations. Ann Intern Med 1978;89:660–76.
23. Pitcher WD, Musher DM: Critical importance of early diagnosis and treatment of intra-abdominal infection. Arch Surg 1982;117:328–33.
24. Hoverman IV, Gentry LO, Jones DW, Guerriero WG: Intrarenal abscess: report of 14 cases. Arch Intern Med 1980;140:914–6.
25. Maki DG, Weise CE, Sarafin HW. A semiquantitative culture method for identifying intravenous catheter-related infection. N Engl J Med 1977;296:1305–9.
26. Moyer MA, Edwards LD, Farley L. Comparative culture methods on 101 intravenous catheters: routine, semiquantitative and blood cultures. Arch Intern Med 1983;143:66–9.
27. Sugarman B, Hawes S, Musher DM, Klima M, Young EJ, Pircher F. Osteomyelitis beneath pressure sores. Arch Intern Med. 1983;143:683–9.
28. Gleckman R, Crowley M, Esposito A. Fever of unknown origin: a view from the community hospital. Am J Med Sci 1977;274:21–5.
29. Murray HW, Ellis GC, Blumenthal DS, Sos TA. Fever and pulmonary embolism. Am J Med 1979;67:232–5.
30. Sugarman B. Fever in recently injured quadriplegic persons. Arch Phys Med Rehab 1982;63:639–40.
31. Venier LH, Ditunno JF Jr. Heterotopic ossification in the paraplegic patient. Arch Phys Med Rehab 1971;52:475–9.
32. Young EJ, Fainstein V, Musher DM. Drug-induced fever: cases seen in the evaluation of unexplained fever in a general hospital population. Rev Infect Dis 1982;4:69–77.
33. Simon HB, Wolff SM. Granulomatous hepatitis and prolonged fever of unknown origin: a study of 13 patients. Medicine 1973;52:1–21.
34. Dinarello CA, Wolff SM. Fever of unknown origin. In: Mandell GL, Douglas RG Jr, Bennett JE, eds. Principles and practice of infectious diseases. New York: John Wiley & Sons, 1979;407–28.
35. Williams TW Jr. Personal communication.
36. Aduan RP, Fauci AS, Dale DC, Herzberg JH, Wolff SM. Factitious fever and self-induced infection: a report of 32 cases and review of the literature. Ann Intern Med 1979;90:230–42.

GASTRIC STASIS SYNDROMES

RICHARD W. McCALLUM □ DOMINICK A. RICCI

BACKGROUND

Recently, there has been increased interest in delineating disorders of gastric motility. Definition and treatment of gastric stasis syndromes rely on clinical diagnosis and radionuclide and electrophysiologic studies as well as pharmacotherapeutic advances. In terms of gastric emptying, the stomach may be physiologically divided into two compartments that govern the handling of the solid and liquid components of a meal. Newer diagnostic parameters such as dual-isotope radionuclide–labeled meals, which measure both solid and liquid emptying, can elucidate gastric motility disorders. Pathophysiologic diagnostic studies are beginning to address gastric electrophysiology, presaging the next era in this field. Much of the renewed interest in gastric motor disorders stems from the advent of effective gastrointestinal prokinetic agents, namely metoclopramide and domperidone.

Physiology

Gastric emptying may be divided into liquid and solid phases, since different parts of the stomach are involved in each. The fundus and proximal corpus of the stomach are mainly concerned with liquid emptying, which is effected through a gastroduodenal pressure gradient generated by gastric contractions (Fig. 1). The reservoir or food storage function of the proximal stomach allows for large volumes to be accepted while relatively low intragastric pressures are maintained. This adjustment is known as receptive or adaptive relaxation, and truncal vagotomy as well as superselective or parietal cell vagotomy abolishes this reflex, resulting in rapid emptying of liquids.

Solid food emptying is primarily a function of the distal stomach. Circular rings of muscle contraction in the distal stomach increase in strength toward the pylorus, generating a grinding effect on solid food in conjunction with pepsin and acid from the proximal stomach. The pylorus will not accept food particles larger than 0.5 mm, and hence the initial boluses are rejected and retropelled. The repetitive grinding and mixing action of the antrum—trituration—continues until a more chymous form is produced, upon which gastric emptying proceeds.

Neural control is mediated via efferents from both vagal (stimulatory) and sympathetic (inhibitory) nerves. Dopaminergic (inhibitory) pathways have also been implicated in the control of gastric emptying.[1] A gastric pacemaker located in the midcorpus along the greater curvature is responsible for pacesetter or slow-wave activity propagated aborally at a rate of 3 to 4 per minute. Distal gastric contractions superimposed on the pacesetter potentials have a velocity and frequency determined but not initiated by these pacesetter potentials (see Fig. 1).

Interdigestive or fasting motor activity varies from the fed state, in that migrating motor complexes propagated from the stomach to the ileum have been described, comprising four phases.[2] Phase III activity, lasting 5 to 15 minutes at a rate

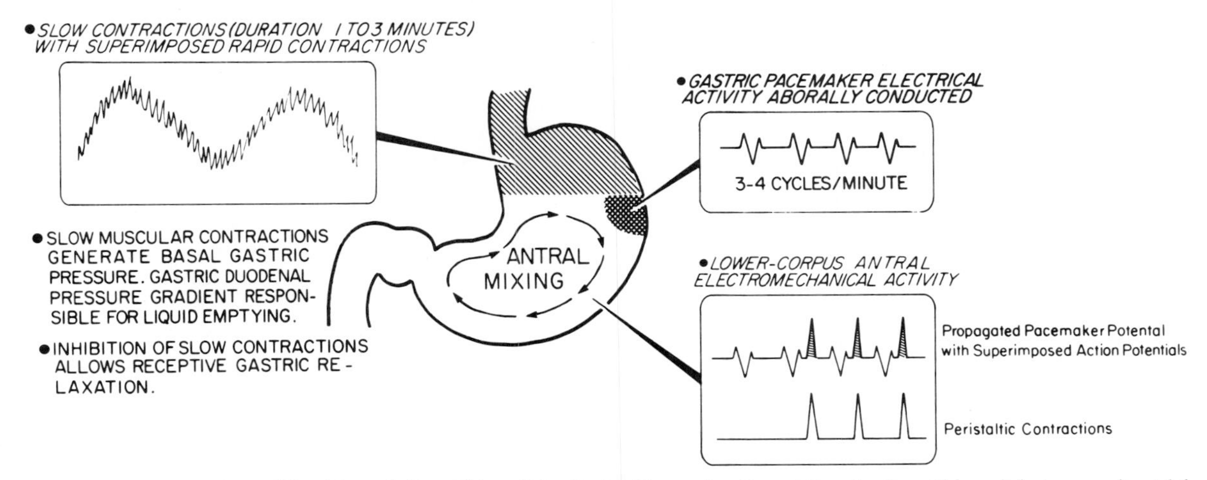

Figure 1. Gastric emptying of liquids and digestible solids. Peristaltic contractions triturate digestible solids to near-liquid form.

of 3 contractions/min., sweeps undigested particles through an open pylorus. Hence these motor complexes have been called the housekeepers of the gastrointestinal tract.

Motility disorders of the antrum result in delayed emptying of solids, although liquid emptying is largely undisturbed owing to the preserved gastroduodenal pressure gradient. In theory, proximal gastric motility disturbances could lead to solid and liquid retention, because the stomach would be unable to evacuate the chymous triturated solids secondary to the decreased gastroduodenal pressure gradient. Although isolated antral motility abnormalities and hence gastric stasis for solids are well recognized, there is no clinical entity resulting in isolated liquid retention. However, a combined impairment of solid and liquid emptying may be observed, usually in more severe or advanced cases, e.g., diabetic gastroparesis. On the other hand, liquid emptying may be rapid (dumping) and solid emptying slow, as in gastric stasis occurring after partial gastric resection with a Billroth I or II anastomosis.

Symptoms

The clinical manifestations of delayed gastric emptying usually form a constellation of symptoms. Occasionally, the patient may experience only one or two "uncomfortable" symptoms. Nausea and vomiting are the most disquieting of all the symptoms. Some patients with gastric emptying disorders may complain only of postprandial bloating or fullness, which is probably due to the accumulation of solids or liquids in a distended stomach. Anorexia and early satiety, although of possible constitutional origin, in the framework of the appropriate signs and symptoms may indicate gastric stasis. Although abdominal pain is occasionally found in gastric retention states, also probably owing to distension, its presence should arouse the suspicion of clinical entities, either anatomically independent from the stomach or mechanically related, that result in delayed gastric emptying. These would include gastric ulcer, posterior penetrating duodenal ulcer, gastric cancer, smoldering pancreatitis, biliary tract disease, "upset stomach" possibly related to gastritis or a viral insult, and pancreatic cancer.

Physical findings may be entirely normal or remarkable only for epigastric distension or fullness. A succussion splash, although characteristic of gastric outlet obstruction, may be found in gastric stasis patients, especially those with significant liquid retention. Epigastric tenderness may be elicited but is an uncommon finding. Sometimes a bezoar found on radiographic or endoscopic studies may be the first clue to delayed gastric emptying.

Causes

Obviously, any organic lesion obstructing the antropyloric or duodenal region will produce gastric retention, initially of solids and later of liquids. Pyloric stenosis due to peptic ulcer disease, hypertrophic pyloric stenosis of the infantile or adult variety, or obstruction by antral carcinoma may explain gastric stasis.

Delayed gastric emptying may be found with varied clinical situations not associated with organic gastric outlet obstruction, many of which are transient (Table 1). One common situation is the delayed gastric emptying that occurs in postoperative ileus from both intra-abdominal and extra-abdominal surgery. Retention of both solids and liquids has been seen but is rarely a prolonged clinical problem. Norepinephrine is released after surgery and is present in high concentrations in the gut and systemically. Norepinephrine may inhibit part of the gastric interdigestive cycle. Transient gastric retention is said to occur with septicemia, peritonitis, pancreatitis, and other clinical conditions of stress and/or pain, possibly through a similar mechanism.

Metabolic derangements, including hyperglycemia, hypercalcemia, hypokalemia, hypocalcemia, hypomagnesemia, hypothyroidism, hepatic encephalopathy, and uremia, have been implicated in delayed gastric emptying, but only hyperglycemia conditions have been studied.[3] Diabetic ketoacidosis and hyperosmolar states impair gastric emptying.

Viral syndromes, especially viral gastroenteritis, have been implicated in delayed gastric emptying, which usually resolves after the acute illness subsides. No chronic gastric retention state has, as yet, been definitely ascribed to a viral cause. Although the mechanism is still unclear, total parenteral nutrition has also been shown to produce significant gastric retention.[4] Delayed emptying of solids has been demonstrated to occur in association with cigarette smoking.

With the increased awareness of gastric stasis and the advent of using radionuclide-labeled meals to test gastric emptying, varied clinical situations have been studied and identified as causes of gastric stasis. We will now review each of these clinical states, of which some are generally familiar by virtue of their previous association with gastric stasis but others may be relatively unfamiliar in the context of a gastric motor abnormality.

Diabetic Gastroparesis

Gastric stasis in diabetic patients is a well-recognized phenomenon originally suspected more than 50 years ago. In 1958, the term diabetic gastroparesis was coined.[5] Some discrepancy has arisen in the incidence reports for this disorder,

Table 1. CAUSES OF DELAYED GASTRIC EMPTYING

Pharmaceutical agents and hormones	Opiates, including endorphins and narcotics (e.g., morphine) Anticholinergics Tricyclic antidepressants Beta-adrenergic agonists Levodopa Aluminum hydroxide antacids Gastrin Cholecystokinin Somatostatin
Causes of acute or transient gastric retention	Postoperative ileus Viral gastroenteritis Hyperglycemia and other metabolic abnormalities Elemental diets Total parenteral nutrition Cigarette smoking
Causes of chronic or prolonged gastric retention	Diabetes mellitus Gastric surgery (truncal, superselective, or gastric vagotomy with or without pyloroplasty; antrectomy; subtotal gastrectomy) Gastroesophageal reflux Achlorhydria and atrophic gastritis with or without pernicious anemia Anorexia nervosa Gastric ulcer disease Amyloidosis Progressive systemic sclerosis Idiopathic intestinal pseudo-obstruction Systemic lupus erythematosus Dermatomyositis Myotonia dystrophia Progressive muscular dystrophy Familial dysautonomia Idiopathic gastroparesis (gastric dysrhythmias)

mainly through variations in patient selection and the obvious limitations in quantitating gastric retention using radiologic techniques. Gastric emptying may now be accurately quantitated using radionuclide-labeled test meals.

Initial theories held that diabetic gastroparesis resulted from a vagal neuropathy; however, vagotomy usually produces rapid liquid emptying or dumping, which is not characteristic of diabetes. The neuropathy is now thought to be caused by the abnormal metabolic products that accumulate in diabetic patients. The level of myoinositol, a necessary part of the normal nerve unit, has been found to be elevated in the urine of poorly controlled diabetics and to normalize in the normoglycemic state. Also, an inverse correlation has been observed between blood glucose level and gastric emptying rate.[3]

The basic defect may be impaired neural control. The rate and duration of antral contractions are diminished in diabetic gastroparesis. Phase III interdigestive myoelectric activity, normally propagated through the upper gastrointestinal tract to the distal ileum, was found to be absent only in the stomachs of symptomatic diabetic patients,[6] suggesting that the stomach does not respond or responds poorly to existing motor stimuli. Further evidence of the neurogenic origin of the defect is substantiated by the reestablishment of Phase III activity after metoclopramide administration.[6]

Chronic gastric stasis occurs via the mechanisms discussed. However, acutely uncontrolled diabetics in ketoacidosis or nonketotic hyperosmolar states may have transitory gastric stasis. The nausea and vomiting are transient and are attributed to the metabolic imbalance.

Gastroparesis may occur in asymptomatic patients. It may be insidious in onset, disclosed only by radiographic studies. In time in some patients, the stasis progresses to a complicated downhill course with persistent vomiting and weight loss, usually in conjunction with evidence of advancing disease elsewhere and an accompanying peripheral neuropathy. It is important to recognize that gastric stasis in this clinical setting adversely affects control of the underlying diabetes. As mentioned, an inverse correlation between blood glucose levels and gastric motility has been demonstrated. Logically, to overcome this vicious cycle and to facilitate metabolic control of the diabetes, early restoration of gastrointestinal function is vital.

Gastric Surgery and Vagotomy

Sectioning of the vagus nerve at the level of the proximal stomach (proximal gastric or superselective vagotomy) would cause alteration in gastric receptive relaxation, increasing the gastroduodenal pressure gradient and causing rapid emptying of liquids. Truncal vagotomy (sectioning of both the proximal and the distal branches of the vagus) would decrease antral motility and slow solid food emptying. The consequent decrease in gastric acid production may also be involved in the delay of gastric emptying. Clinically, however, there is some degree of variability in the frequency and degree of gastric motor abnormalities, as demonstrated in an extensive study using radionuclide-labeled meals, reported by Kalbasi and associates.[7]

The effects of truncal vagotomy and pyloroplasty on gastric emptying are transient. By 3 years after operation, gastric emptying has returned to normal. After truncal vagotomy, the time to complete liquid emptying is prolonged. When pyloroplasty is also performed, liquid emptying is normal. After antrectomy there is usually a slight increase in liquid emptying rates. One month after antrectomy with truncal vagotomy, gastric emptying of solids is delayed; however, normalization of the gastric emptying rate is achieved by the sixth postoperative month. From the foregoing information, it is obvious that severely symptomatic gastric stasis after these varied surgical procedures is distinctly uncommon. Surgeons generally concur that the presence of gastric retention 1 month postoperatively without gastric outlet obstruction probably signals a chronic disorder; it occurs in 3 to 9 per cent of patients.

A more prolonged period of postoperative gastric stasis was noted by Kalbasi and associates[7] in patients with preoperative gastric outlet obstruction. However, the overall incidence of postoperative gastric retention was not affected in patients undergoing truncal vagotomy and hemigastrectomy. The probable cause for such an occurrence is a chronically distended stomach with its attendant overly stretched and poorly responsive gastric smooth muscle.

Another interesting observation has been noted in patients undergoing vagotomy and hemigastrectomy. Postoperatively, patients with symptomatic gastric stasis were found to have no Phase III interdigestive motor activity, unlike asymptomatic patients.[8] Myoelectric activity was reestablished after administration of metoclopramide, a gastrointestinal prokinetic agent. In some cases, high gastric resection may interfere with the gastric pacemaker, accounting for the slow emptying.

Achlorhydria and Atrophic Gastritis With or Without Pernicious Anemia

Experimental gastric emptying studies have been conducted in patients with achlorhydria and low acid output states, with varied results. Dual-isotope radionuclide studies in patients with pernicious anemia and others with atrophic gastritis alone have yielded interesting findings. Patients with pernicious anemia had delayed solid but normal liquid emptying, whereas those with atrophic gastritis alone had delayed emptying of both solids and liquids. The majority of both groups were not symptomatic for gastric stasis. We hypothesize that atrophic gastritis causing the achlorhydria may also impair neuromuscular function of the antrum.

Intestinal Pseudo-Obstruction

Chronic pseudo-obstruction most notably affects the small and large intestine and occasionally the esophagus.[9] The stomach may also be involved. Recently, some changes have been observed in intestinal pseudo-obstruction. A myopathic form called hereditary hollow visceral myopathy (familial visceral myopathy) has been described, in which there is degeneration of the smooth muscle. Accompanying these changes is the intramural formation of collagen. Evidence also suggests the existence of visceral myopathy without familial tendency. A neuropathic form (familial visceral neuropathy) exhibits a diffusely abnormal myenteric plexus with normal smooth muscle. Gastric retention is known to occur in secondary intestinal pseudo-obstruction, in which an identifiable cause is revealed. Examples include some of the muscular diseases, such as myotonic dystrophy and progressive muscular dystrophy.[10, 11] In familial dysautonomia, or Riley-Day syndrome, gastric stasis is known to occur along with other signs of autonomic dysfunction, namely, peripheral neuropathy, labile hypertension, and vasomotor instability. The autonomic neuropathy of acute intermittent and variegate porphyria has been implicated. Another form of secondary pseudo-obstruction, amyloidosis, has been implicated as a cause of gastric retention.

Anorexia Nervosa

Nausea, vomiting, and epigastric bloating, distension, and pain are frequent complaints in anorexia nervosa, a psychiatric disorder of still-undetermined etiology affecting predominantly young females. Delayed gastric emptying of solids has been noted in affected patients and may contribute to the production or perpetuation of the syndrome.[12] Sorting out the primary or secondary role at this point is difficult, but neuromuscular involvement of the gastric smooth muscle has been implicated by the notable reversal of the emptying delay after administration of metoclopramide. The exact role of the psychiatric component in the initiation or aggravation of anorexia, as well as the role of malnutrition, is debatable. The occurrence of delayed gastric emptying in these patients should prompt the clinician to consider a liquid diet and pharmacologic augmentation of gastric emptying as initial therapeutic approaches.

Gastric Ulcer Disease

Conflicting data have been reported about gastric emptying in patients with gastric ulcer, owing mainly to nonstandardized forms of assessment. Several studies indicate a temporary slowing of gastric emptying, particularly if the active ulcer is in the proximal stomach. There is speculation that chronic gastritis may be a cause and that the high recurrence rate in gastric ulcer disease may, in part, be explained by chronic motor dysfunction.

Progressive Systemic Sclerosis and Other Connective Tissue Diseases

Progressive systemic sclerosis is probably best noted for its disturbance of motility in the esophagus and to some degree in the small and large intestine.[13] Weakness or absence of peristalsis in the body of the esophagus and prolonged patency of the lower esophageal sphincter characterize the disease affecting the esophagus. Involvement of the stomach, at present, does not appear to be an important clinical characteristic of the disease process until it is well-advanced. In some patients with limited esophageal disease, delayed emptying of solid food from the stomach has been thought to augment the tendency for gastroesophageal reflux and severe esophagitis. When more extensive gastrointestinal involvement is noted, liquid emptying is also delayed. In spite of smooth muscle degeneration and collagen deposition, the degree of involvement is unpredictably patchy, and gastric stasis may improve with pharmacologic treatment.

Unconfirmed results have been reported with other collagen vascular diseases. A small minority of patients with systemic lupus erythematosus were found to have gastrointestinal dysmotility problems, and either a vasculitis or an autonomic neuropathy has been cited as the cause. Atony of the small and large intestine as well as the stomach has been seen in dermatomyositis. The collagen vascular diseases usually do not produce severe clinical gastric motility disorders but should be included in the differential diagnosis.

Gastroesophageal Reflux

In theory, a contributing factor in gastroesophageal reflux would be a delay in the evacuation of gastric contents, which would allow more time for a greater volume of liquids, solids, or acid to flow back into the esophagus. One study using radionuclide-labeled solid and liquid meals demonstrated that esophagitis patients, as a group, have slow emptying of a solid meal.[14] Fifty-seven per cent of those with reflux had delayed solid emptying, but all of them had normal liquid emptying. Only one-fourth of the group with delayed gastric emptying were symptomatic, having nausea and vomiting. On the basis of this information, clinicians should be alert to the fact that patients with gastroesophageal reflux may have typical subjective and objective evidence of impaired gastric emptying. In addition, signs and symptoms of slow emptying may be the first manifestations of incipient gastroesophageal reflux. The primary or secondary nature of the gastric motility disorder is yet undetermined, but recent information suggests that histologic gastritis in the antrum, possibly secondary to duodenal (bile) reflux, may result in antral motor dysfunction.[15] In addition, the information gained from gastric emptying studies provides further support for some of the treatments empirically recommended in the past. Small soft or semisolid meals make good sense, and a low-fat diet is important because fat decreases lower esophageal sphincter pressure and inhibits gastric emptying.

Among pediatric patients, infants with severe gastroesophageal reflux resulting in failure to thrive or pulmonary aspiration may display severe gastric retention of liquids with the use of radionuclide-labeled formula.

Idiopathic Gastric Stasis

Many clinical conditions not previously implicated in delayed gastric emptying are now recognized to be part of the differential diagnosis of this disorder, thanks to an increased awareness of the disorder, availability of radionuclide scintigraphic studies, and the advent of pharmacotherapeutic trials. One other advance has been responsible for delineating a recently defined contribution to the knowledge about "idiopathic gastric stasis." Electrogastrography, which utilizes intraoperative placement of serosal surface electrodes and peroral suction electrodes (available at specialized centers), has raised the question of whether gastric dysrhythmias may alter the flow of gastric contents. Employing these electrodes, researchers have described electromechanical events such as tachygastria and tachydysrhythmia. The gastric pacemaker normally emits pacesetter potentials at about 3 to 4 cycles/min. Potentials occurring at greater frequency with similar wave form morphology and intervals are known as tachygastria.[2] Abnormally rapid potentials with irregular intervals and different morphology are termed tachydysrhythmias. Such abnormal electromechanical events are believed to originate from an ectopic antral pacemaker and potentially are capable of slowing gastric emptying, resulting in regurgitation or vomiting.[16] Dyssynchrony between gastric and intestinal segments prevents passage of gastric contents beyond the pylorus or proximal small intestine, leading to a protracted course of vomiting without any obvious etiology.[17] Surgery has finally been resorted to in some cases because of refractoriness to pharmacologic agents. These situations are fortunately very infrequent but may leave the patient incapacitated by protracted vomiting and weight loss.

Pharmacologic Agents

Gastric emptying has been substantially delayed by endogenous and exogenous opiates, beta-adrenergic agents, anticholinergics, tricyclic antidepressants, and levodopa. Morphine and its derivatives, well-known causes of delayed gastrointestinal transit, may produce gastric stasis by augmented transpyloric resistance from increased pyloric or duodenal contractions. The activity of endogenous peptides, endorphins, and enkephalins is similar to that of exogenous opiates, and these agents have been shown to delay gastric emptying of a radionuclide-labeled semisolid meal. These effects may occur directly on the gastrointestinal tract or indirectly through the central nervous system.

Beta-adrenergic agents such as salbutamol and isoproterenol delay gastric emptying, as measured by scintigraphic techniques.[18] Propranolol, a beta-adrenergic blocker, when given alone at doses of 160 mg/day for at least 1 week accelerates gastric emptying.

Anticholinergic agents such as atropine and diphenhydramine have delayed liquid emptying rates in rats.[19] Tricyclic antidepressants such as imipramine have diminished intestinal absorption, probably by a delay in gastric emptying. The mechanism has been postulated either to be anticholinergic or to occur through norepinephrine enhancement.

Levodopa delays emptying of a semi-solid meal, possibly by activating gastric inhibitory dopamine receptors.[20]

Cigarette smoking delays emptying of solid food through stimulation of the nicotinic inhibitory neurons.[21] Antacids containing aluminum alone may delay gastric emptying experimentally, but the clinical relevance of this finding is questionable.[22]

Given such a formidable list of chemical agents, one must regard a thorough drug history as an absolute necessity for ruling out causes of gastric stasis, especially considering the ubiquitous use of these substances, which are not infrequently given in combination.

CLINICAL METHODS OF MEASURING GASTRIC EMPTYING

Clinically, there are currently three methods employed for assessing gastric emptying: gastric or gastroduodenal intubation, radiologic techniques, and use of radionuclide-labeled test meals. Gastric aspiration, alone or after fluid loading, was initially employed, but its efficacy was reduced by questions of gastric secretion and whether complete sampling of gastric contents was achieved. Radiologic methods essentially represent qualitative measurements, since residual barium cannot be quantitated, and the procedures involve significant radiation exposure. Modifications, which have included "barium burger" test meals and liquid barium meals alone, do not satisfy the condition of "physiologic emptying."

Radionuclide-labeled meal tests employ ^{99m}technetium (^{99m}Tc). The standard test meal is prepared as follows: ^{99m}Tc sulfur colloid is injected into the wing vein of a chicken, and 90 per cent of the dose is incorporated into the Kupffer cells. The chicken is then killed and its liver is excised and chopped into 1-cm cubes. The liver is mixed with 7½ ounces of untagged canned beef stew, heated in a microwave oven, and fed to the patient with two saltine crackers. Liquid phase emptying can be measured in the same study period by having the patient drink 100 ml of water labeled with 50 microcuries of ^{111}Indium.

With the patient in the supine position, a gamma camera is used to monitor passage of the radiolabeled meal; having a computer interfaced with the gamma camera makes precise measurement possible (Figs. 2 and 3). Abnormal gastric emptying has been determined, using this technique, as more than 70 per cent retention of the solid meal after 2 hours (mean ± 2 S.D.) with the patient in the supine position.[23] (Gastric emptying is no faster when the patient is sitting or standing.)

This technique has been modified in our laboratory to obviate destruction of an animal. Cooked cubes of commercially obtained chicken liver are injected with ^{99m}Tc sulfur colloid and then mixed with beef stew and water. Gastric emptying rates are similar to those obtained by the standard method, and this modification is more applicable in a community hospital with nuclear medicine facilities.

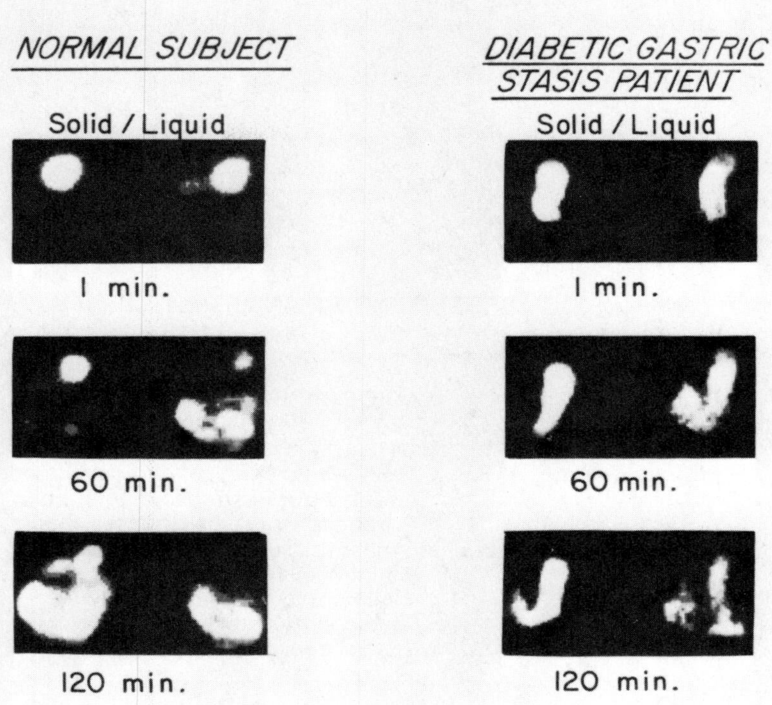

Figure 2. Gastric emptying in diabetic gastroparesis (dual isotope technique).

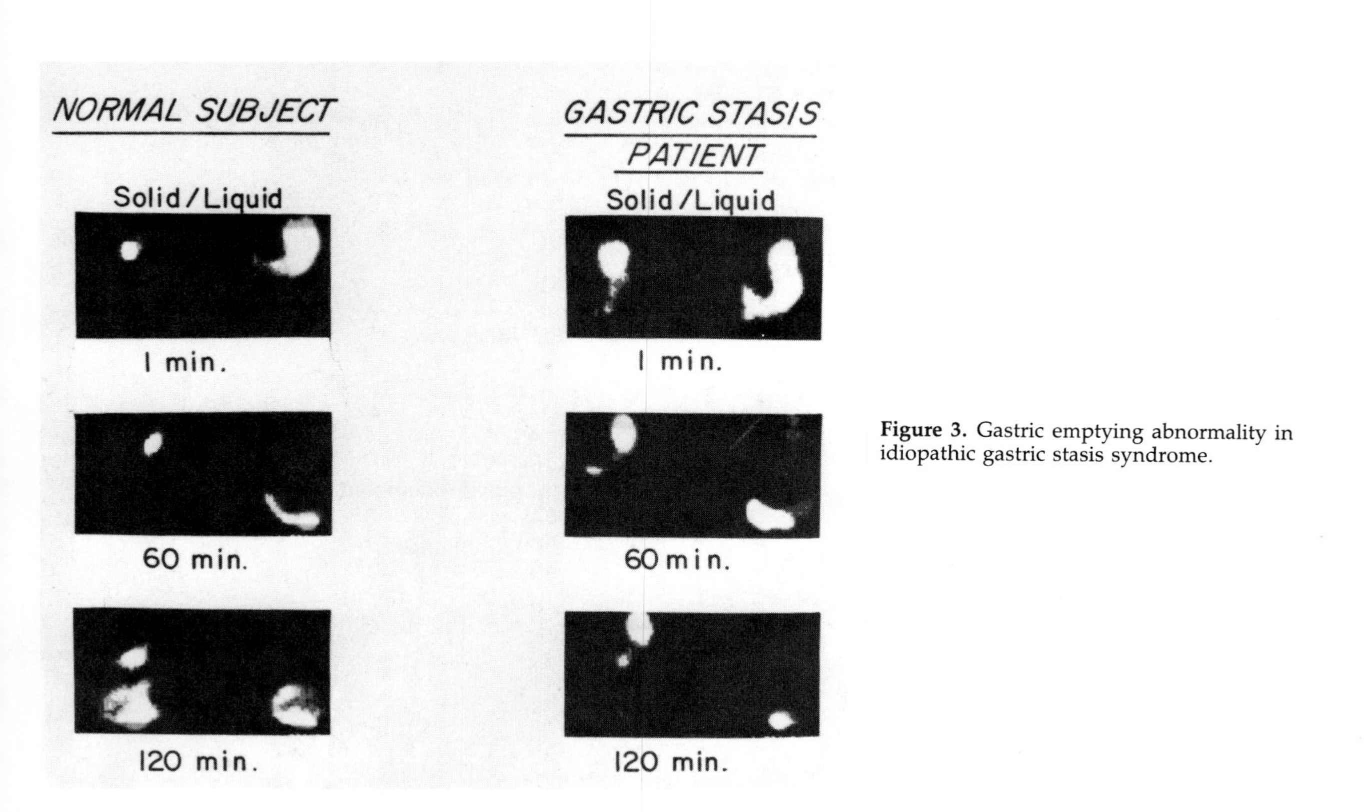

Figure 3. Gastric emptying abnormality in idiopathic gastric stasis syndrome.

DIAGNOSTIC ASSESSMENT OF AND TREATMENT APPROACH TO GASTRIC STASIS

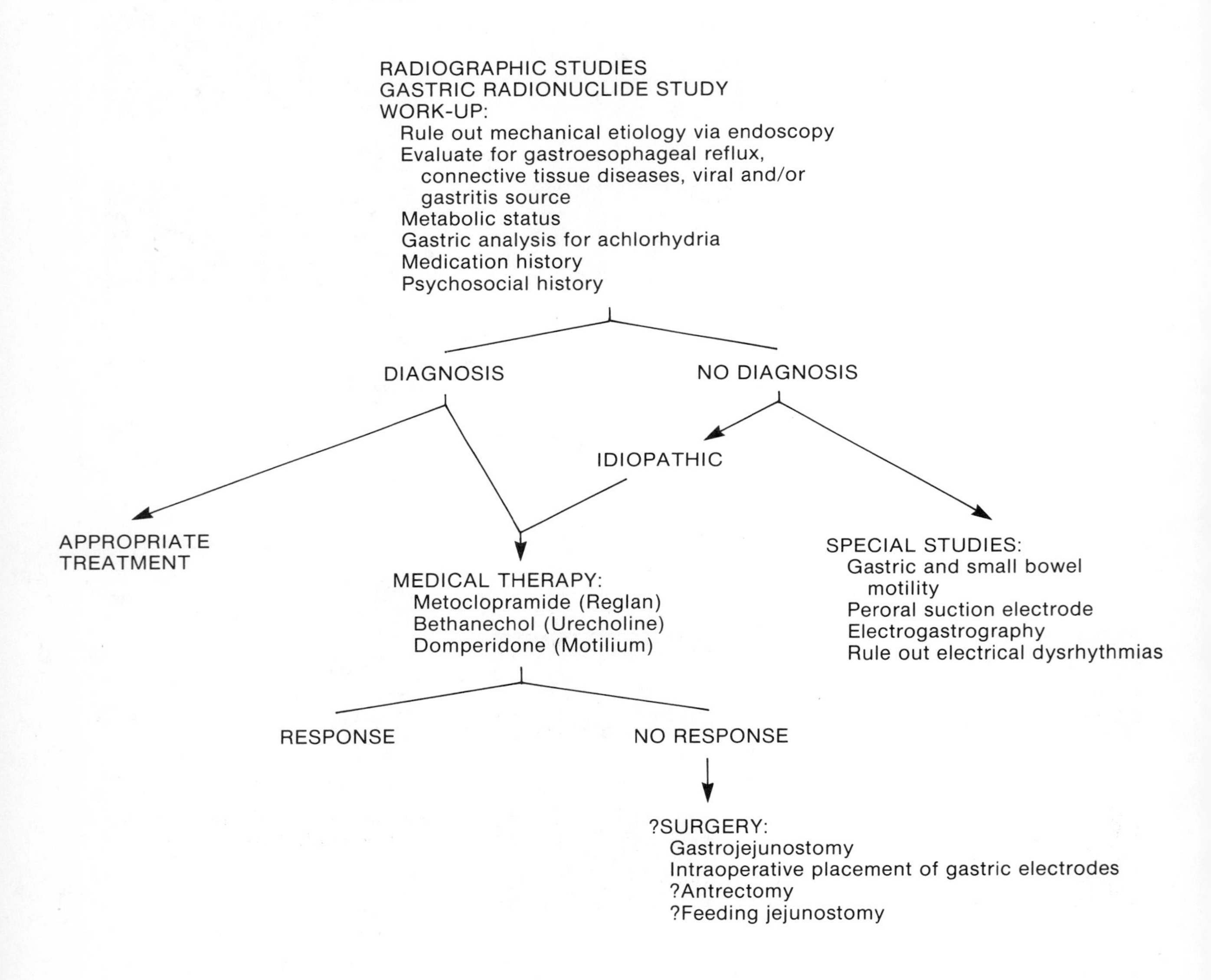

ASSESSMENT

Gastric stasis syndromes have traditionally been difficult to deal with, even prompting surgery in the most intractable cases. Evolving knowledge of the underlying pathophysiologic events and the introduction of new pharmacologic agents have aided greatly in practical therapy.

Other diagnostic studies after radionuclide testing often are relied upon. They range from upper gastrointestinal endoscopy to the intraoperative placement of serosal surface electrodes or electrogastrography using peroral mucosal electrodes. These last studies, performed in patients for whom no diagnosis has been established, may require referral to specialized centers.

The stages of the work-up and the order of diagnostic tests are summarized in the algorithm.

Roles of Medication and Surgery

Parasympathomimetic agents, such as bethanechol, have demonstrated some ability to improve gastric emptying, limited in addition by the untoward effect of cholinergic stimulation. With the introduction of a new category of agents that both stimulate cholinergic receptors and antagonize the inhibitory dopamine receptors present in the gastrointestinal tract, treatment of gastric stasis syndromes has improved. A procainamide analog known to antagonize dopaminergic receptors, metoclopramide, is an antiemetic and gastrointestinal prokinetic agent that affects gut smooth muscle, increasing the frequency and amplitude of gastric contractions and partially inhibiting gastric receptive relaxation.[1, 24] Stomach and small intestine motor activity becomes enhanced and more coordinated, resulting in movement of gut contents in the aboral direction. Dopaminergic agonists stimulate the medullary chemoreceptor trigger zone and produce emesis, whereas dopaminergic antagonists, such as metoclopramide, are effective antiemetics. At present, metoclopramide is the treatment of choice for gastric stasis syndromes. Domperidone, a benzimidazole derivative, is also a dopamine antagonist devoid of any side effects related to dopamine antagonism in the central nervous system; its use, however, is currently limited to experimental investigation.

Surgical intervention may play a role in those few patients whose gastric stasis syndrome has not responded to medical therapy and who undergo careful manometric and electrophysiologic studies using peroral or serosal electrodes. Patients with tachygastria or dysrhythmias and patients whose symptoms are due to gastrointestinal dyssynchrony may be candidates for gastrojejunostomy, antrectomy, or placement of small-bowel feeding tubes.

REFERENCES

1. Valenzuela JE. Dopamine as a possible nerve transmitter in gastric relaxation. Gastroenterology 1976;71:1019–22.
2. Code CF, Marlett JA. Canine tachygastria. Mayo Clin Proc 1974;49:325–32.
3. MacGregor IL, Deveney C, Way LW, Meyer JH. The effect of acute hyperglycemia on meal stimulated gastric, biliary pancreatic secretion and serum gastrin. Gastroenterology 1976;70:197–202.
4. MacGregor IL, Wiley ZO, Lavigne ME, et al. Total parenteral nutrition slows gastric emptying of solid foods (abstract). Gastroenterology 1978;74:1059.
5. Kassander P. Asymptomatic gastric retention in diabetes (gastroparesis diabeticorum). Ann Intern Med 1958;48:797–812.
6. Fox S, Behar J. Pathogenesis of diabetic gastroparesis: a pharmacologic study. Gastroenterology 1980;78:757–63.
7. Kalbasi H, Hudson FR, Herring A, Moss S, Glass HI, Spencer J. Gastric emptying following vagotomy and antrectomy and proximal gastric vagotomy. Gut 1975;16:509–13.
8. Malagelada JR, Rees WD, Mazzotta LJ, et al. Gastric motor abnormalities in diabetic and post vagotomy gastroparesis: effect of metoclopramide and bethanechol. Gastroenterology 1980;78:286–93.
9. Lipton AB, Knauer CM. Pseudo-obstruction of the bowel. Therapeutic trial of metoclopramide. Am J Dig Dis 1977;22:263–5.
10. Goldberg HI, Sheft OJ. Esophageal and colon changes in myotonia dystrophica. Gastroenterology 1972;63:134–9.
11. Bevans M. Changes in musculature of gastrointestinal tract and in myocardium in progressive muscular dystrophy. Arch Pathol 1945;40:225–38.
12. McCallum RW, Grill BB, Lange R. Definition of a gastric emptying abnormality in patients with anorexia nervosa. Clin Res 1981;29:667.
13. Peachy RD, Creamer B, Pierce JW. Sclerodermatous involvement of the stomach and the small and large bowel. Gut 1969;10:285–92.
14. McCallum RW, Mensh R, Lange R. Definition of gastric emptying abnormalities present in gastroesophageal reflux patients (abstract). Gastroenterology 1981;80:1226.
15. Behar J, Ramsly G. Gastric emptying and antral motility in reflux esophagitis. Gastroenterology 1978;74:253–6.
16. Telander RL, Morgan KG, Kreulen DL, et al. Human gastric atony with tachygastria and gastric retention. Gastroenterology 1978;75:497–501.
17. You CH, Chey WY, Kae YL, et al. Gastric and small intestinal myoelectric dysrhythmia associated with chronic intractable nausea and vomiting. Ann Intern Med 1981;95:449–51.
18. Rees MR, Clark RA, Holdsworth CD. The effect of beta-adrenoceptor agonists and antagonists on gastric emptying in man. Br J Clin Pharmacol 1980;10:551–4.
19. Feldman S, Putcha L. Effect of anti-Parkinsonian drugs on gastric emptying and intestinal transit in the rat. Pharmacology 1977;15:503–11.
20. Berkowitz DM, McCallum RW. Interaction of levodopa and metoclopramide on gastric emptying. Clin Pharm Ther 1980;27:414–20.
21. Harrison A, Ippoliti A. Effect of smoking on gastric emptying (abstract). Gastroenterology 1979;76:1152.
22. Hurwitz A, Robinson RG, Vats TS. Effects of antacids on gastric emptying. Gastroenterology 1976;71:268–73.
23. McCallum RW, Berkowitz DM, Lerner E. Gastric emptying in patients with gastroesophageal reflux. Gastroenterology 1981;80:285–91.
24. Shulze-Delrieu K. Metoclopramide. Gastroenterology 1979;77:768–79.

GASTROINTESTINAL BLEEDING OF UNKNOWN ORIGIN

STUART JON SPECHLER

☐ SYNONYMS: Occult gastrointestinal bleeding/hemorrhage, cryptogenic gastrointestinal bleeding/hemorrhage

BACKGROUND

Definition and Prevalence

A patient has gastrointestinal bleeding of unknown origin when the cause of such bleeding is not established by conventional diagnostic techniques. Because there are no universally accepted criteria for what constitute "conventional diagnostic techniques" in this setting, the definition of gastrointestinal bleeding of unknown origin is not standardized. Furthermore, many studies of patients with this condition predate the availability of modern techniques of arteriography, radionuclide scanning, and flexible fiberoptic endoscopy—techniques that might now be considered "conventional." Hence, there are wide variations in reports of the prevalence of gastrointestinal bleeding of unknown origin among patients seen initially for gastrointestinal hemorrhage. Prevalences ranging from 4 to 43 per cent have been reported, depending largely upon the authors' criteria for identifying the episode of gastrointestinal bleeding as one of unknown origin.[1]

For the purpose of this chapter, gastrointestinal bleeding of unknown origin is defined operationally according to the following criteria:

1. The patient has guaiac-positive stools.
2. The patient has no apparent coagulopathy.
3. The conventional techniques of sigmoidoscopy, barium contrast examination of the upper and lower gastrointestinal tracts, and panendoscopy of the upper gastrointestinal tract either have normal findings or reveal lesions that are judged not to be the source of the hemorrhage.

Using these criteria, one can estimate that gastrointestinal bleeding of unknown origin will be encountered in approximately 5 to 10 per cent of patients who present with gastrointestinal hemorrhage.

CAUSES

Gastrointestinal bleeding of unknown origin may result from common and uncommon disorders. Common causes of gastrointestinal hemorrhage that are likely to be found through the early use of conventional diagnostic techniques are listed in Table 1. These disorders may escape detection by conventional diagnostic modalities, however, and thus may cause gastrointestinal bleeding of unknown origin. Such common lesions may be missed if they are of unusual size, shape, or location or because of technical inadequacies. With the exception of colonic diverticulosis, those disorders listed in Table 1 are not discussed specifically. Only causes of gastrointestinal bleeding that frequently escape detection by conventional diagnostic techniques are dealt with here.

Vascular Abnormalities

Aortoenteric Fistula. An aortoenteric fistula is a communication between the aorta and the gut. The third portion of the duodenum, which lies just anterior to the aorta, is the site most frequently involved. Such a fistula may occur spontaneously or, more commonly, as a late complication of aortic reconstructive surgery. The incidence of aortoenteric fistulization following such surgery is be-

Table 1. COMMON CAUSES OF GASTROINTESTINAL TRACT BLOOD LOSS LIKELY TO BE FOUND THROUGH EARLY USE OF CONVENTIONAL DIAGNOSTIC TECHNIQUES

Organ	Disorder
Esophagus	Esophagitis
	Ulcer
	Varices
	Neoplasm
	Laceration (Mallory-Weiss tear)
Stomach	Gastritis
	Ulcer
	Neoplasm
Small intestine	Duodenal ulcer
	Marginal ulcer
	Regional enteritis
Large intestine	Hemorrhoids
	Stercoral ulcer
	Rectal neoplasm
	Ulcerative colitis
	Granulomatous colitis
	Ischemic colitis
	Diverticulosis

tween 0.4 and 2.4 per cent.[2] Characteristically, the patient with an aortoenteric fistula presents with brisk gastrointestinal bleeding that stops abruptly. This so-called herald hemorrhage is typically followed hours to days later by massive exsanguination. Aortoenteric fistula is fatal unless diagnosed and treated promptly. The possibility of aortoenteric fistula should be explored immediately in any patient with gastrointestinal bleeding who has undergone aortic reconstructive surgery. If the bleeding is not immediately life-threatening, such a patient should undergo upper gastrointestinal panendoscopy. This procedure infrequently demonstrates the fistula but is useful in ruling out other, more common bleeding lesions of the esophagus, stomach, and duodenum. The utility of other nonoperative diagnostic modalities such as colonoscopy, barium contrast roentgenography, and arteriography in this setting is controversial; these procedures may be helpful in ruling out other bleeding lesions, but they infrequently demonstrate the fistula, their results are often misleading, and their performance may result in fatal delays in initiating surgical therapy. Surgical exploration following an unrevealing upper gastrointestinal endoscopy may be the diagnostic and therapeutic procedure of choice.[2] The patient who has undergone aortic reconstructive surgery and develops massive, life-threatening hemorrhage should have *immediate* surgical exploration with no antecedent diagnostic procedures.

Aneurysm. Gastrointestinal bleeding of unknown origin has uncommonly resulted from leakage of aneurysms of the gastric, hepatic, splenic, superior mesenteric, pancreaticoduodenal, small pancreatic, and iliac arteries. Arteriography is the most useful diagnostic technique to demonstrate these lesions.

Arteriovenous Malformation. Arteriovenous malformation (AVM) is a non-neoplastic, localized dilatation of arterial and venous structures. AVM may be congenital or acquired and is a frequent cause of gastrointestinal bleeding of unknown origin. Arteriovenous malformation may be classified as one of three clinical types.[3]

Type I. Commonly called colonic angiodysplasias, type I AVMs appear to result from a degenerative process of aging, and hence are found predominantly in patients older than 60 years.[4] Affected patients frequently have multiple type I AVMs involving principally the right colon. The lesions are small (usually less than 5 mm in diameter) and are easily missed by the surgeon at the time of laparotomy and by the pathologist using standard histologic techniques. Type I AVM is an important cause of colonic bleeding in older patients, perhaps even more common than bleeding colonic diverticula.[4–6] Characteristically, patients present with episodes of painless, brisk lower gastrointestinal hemorrhage. Some patients have chronic low-grade blood loss, however. For unclear reasons, approximately one-fourth of patients with type I AVMs have aortic stenosis. Type I AVMs may be identified on colonoscopy, but selective mesenteric arteriography appears to be the diagnostic procedure of choice.

Type II. This type differs from type I AVM in several respects. Type II AVMs appear to be uncommon congenital lesions; they are found predominantly in patients younger than 50 years; they involve the small bowel most frequently; and they tend to be larger, often grossly visible at laparotomy. Selective mesenteric arteriography is the preferred diagnostic procedure.

Type III. These lesions are telangiectases that occur throughout the gastrointestinal tracts of affected patients. Their presence is better known as hereditary hemorrhagic telangiectasia or Osler-Weber-Rendu syndrome. Type III AVMs are inherited as an autosomal dominant trait, and thus most patients have a family history of the disorder. Patients typically present in late middle life with repeated episodes of epistaxis and gastrointestinal hemorrhage. The diagnosis of type III AVMs can usually be established by physical examination, which reveals the characteristic telangiectases of the face and the oropharyngeal and nasopharyngeal mucosa. The lesions may also be demonstrated by arteriography or endoscopy.

Diverticula

Colonic Diverticula. Colonic diverticula are intimately associated with prominent vasa recta, which can rupture into the diverticular lumen and cause substantial hemorrhage. Bleeding from colonic diverticula has been considered the most common cause of brisk lower gastrointestinal hemorrhage in the elderly. This notion has recently been challenged, however, because it now appears likely that many cases of lower gastrointestinal bleeding that had been attributed to colonic diverticula were in fact due to type I arteriovenous malformations.[4–6] Nevertheless, colonic diverticula remain an important cause of gastrointestinal bleeding of unknown origin. Diverticular hemorrhage is typically brisk and painless; such bleeding infrequently accompanies diverticulitis.[7] In the majority of documented cases, the bleeding originates from an uninflamed diverticulum in the right side of the colon.[8] Diverticulosis is extremely common in older individuals, and it may be tempting to attribute an elderly patient's gastrointestinal bleeding of unknown origin to colonic diverticula. In the absence of direct evidence, however, the clinician should be reluctant to do so, particularly if the hemorrhage is not brisk.

Meckel's Diverticulum and Enteric Duplication Cyst. Meckel's diverticulum is a relatively common congenital anomaly that arises from the antimesenteric side of the ileum as a result of incomplete obliteration of the embryonic vitelline duct. An enteric duplication, a cyst that shares a common wall and blood supply with the adjacent bowel, occurs most frequently on the mesenteric side of the ileum. Both Meckel's diverticulum and enteric duplication cyst may be lined by an acid-producing gastric type of epithelium that can cause peptic ulceration and bleeding in the adjacent gut.[9] This ectopic gastric epithelium can concentrate technetium, and thus these lesions can be identified by ^{99m}Tc sodium pertechnetate scanning.

Other Small Intestine Diverticula. Although it is not uncommon to find diverticula of the duodenum and jejunum on a barium contrast examination of the upper gastrointestinal tract, these lesions are rarely the site of hemorrhage. In the absence of direct evidence, the clinician should be reluctant to attribute bleeding to small intestine diverticula.

Neoplasms

Colonic Neoplasm. Colonic neoplasm is a common cause of occult gastrointestinal bleeding in older patients. The bleeding is usually low-grade; brisk hemorrhage from colonic neoplasms is uncommon. Two recent studies have examined the role of colonoscopy in patients with rectal bleeding who have normal barium enema findings.[10, 11] In both studies neoplasms were detected by colonoscopy in approximately one-fourth of such patients. Clearly, colonoscopy is a valuable tool for identifying tumors of the colon.

Small Intestine Neoplasm. Bleeding is a frequent complication of primary neoplasms of the small bowel, which fortunately are uncommon.[12] Small bowel tumors are often missed by conventional barium contrast examinations. They may be identified via arteriography and via fiberoptic endoscopy using extra-long instruments.

Hemangioma. A hemangioma is a vascular neoplasm that may occur anywhere in the gastrointestinal tract. The blue rubber bleb nevus syndrome is a rare disorder in which patients have both cutaneous and visceral hemangiomas; the diagnosis can be established on physical examination by the finding of multiple blue, raised, wrinkled cutaneous hemangiomas. Visceral hemangiomas can be identified by arteriography.

Hemobilia

Blunt trauma and penetrating wounds to the liver may result in bleeding into the biliary tract, called hemobilia. Other even rarer causes of hemobilia include gallstones, hepatic artery aneurysms, hepatobiliary tumors, and hepatobiliary ascariasis. Blunt trauma usually precedes the onset of symptoms of hemobilia by approximately 4 weeks. Patients characteristically present with paroxysmal abdominal pain, jaundice, and upper gastrointestinal hemorrhage. Flexible fiberoptic endoscopic demonstration of bleeding from the ampulla of Vater establishes the diagnosis of hemobilia, but not the cause. Arteriography, the most valuable diagnostic procedure, should be performed early if hemobilia is suspected.[13]

Pancreatic Disease

Pancreatitis is complicated by gastrointestinal hemorrhage from common lesions such as gastritis, peptic ulcer, esophageal varices, and Mallory-Weiss tears in up to one-fifth of cases.[14] Pancreatitis may result in gastrointestinal bleeding of unknown origin by any of several mechanisms. First, bleeding may occur within a pancreatic pseudocyst either as a result of hemorrhage from small vessels in its walls or from the erosion of a major adjacent vessel with the formation of a pseudoaneurysm. Second, rupture of a pancreatic pseudocyst into a hollow viscus may be accompanied by hemorrhage. Third, pancreatitis may result in the formation of true aneurysms of the splenic and pancreatic arteries, which may subsequently rupture. In such circumstances, arteriography is the diagnostic procedure of choice.

Vasculitis

Gastrointestinal bleeding of unknown origin may result from any vasculitis involving the visceral vessels. Such involvement is characteristic of Henoch-Schönlein purpura and polyarteritis nodosa, and it may also occur in the vasculitis that complicates connective tissue diseases like lupus erythematosus, rheumatoid arthritis, and dermatomyositis.

The diagnosis of Henoch-Schönlein purpura is made in patients who have a vasculitis of small vessels and clinical manifestations including nonthrombocytopenic purpura of the lower extremities, polyarthritis, glomerulonephritis, abdominal pain, and gastrointestinal bleeding.[15] Adults can be affected, but the disease is more common in children.

The manifestations of polyarteritis nodosa include arthritis, polyneuritis, pericarditis, pleuritis, renal failure, abdominal complaints, and gastrointestinal bleeding.[16] The vasculitis involves muscular arteries and arterioles, particularly at their bifurcations, resulting in the formation of multiple small aneurysms at the bifurcations of small and medium-sized visceral arteries, a pathognomonic pattern easily recognized on arteriography. Thus, arteriography is the preferred diagnostic procedure.

Inherited Disorders of Connective Tissue

Pseudoxanthoma Elasticum (Grönblad-Strandberg Syndrome). Pseudoxanthoma elasticum is a rare hereditary disorder in which there is an accumulation of abnormal elastic tissue throughout the body. Involvement of visceral vessels may result in spontaneous gastrointestinal bleeding. The diagnosis can often be established by physical examination, which reveals the characteristic xanthoma-like papules of the skin and angioid streaks of the ocular fundus.

Ehlers-Danlos Syndrome. Ehlers-Danlos syndrome is also a rare hereditary disorder of connective tissue. Gastrointestinal bleeding may be the result of colonic diverticula, which occur commonly in affected patients, or of visceral artery rupture. The characteristic physical findings are hyperextensibility of the skin and hypermobility of the joints.

Drugs

Gastritis and gastrointestinal bleeding have been reported in association with the ingestion of many drugs, including alcohol, aspirin, and a variety of nonsteroidal anti-inflammatory agents.[17] Drug-induced gastritis may heal quickly and thus may be missed at endoscopy if the procedure is performed too long after ingestion of the offending agent. The clinician should obtain a detailed history of any medications taken by the patient with gastrointestinal bleeding of unknown origin.

Miscellaneous Causes

Amyloidosis. Gastrointestinal bleeding is a frequent complication of systemic amyloidosis. Bleeding may be due to the fragility of the amyloid-infiltrated blood vessels, to ulceration of a markedly infiltrated region or amyloid "tumor" of the gut, or to esophageal varices caused by hepatic amyloidosis. The diagnosis may be established by the demonstration of amyloid deposits in biopsy specimens of rectum, gingiva, or small bowel.

Ulcerations of the Jejunum and Ileum. Ulcerations of the jejunum and ileum may be idiopathic or may occur in association with gastrinoma, Crohn's disease, syphilis, tuberculosis, typhoid fever, histoplasmosis, foreign bodies, arsenic poisoning, Richter's hernia, vasculitis, ectopic gastric mucosa, radiation, ischemia, nontropical sprue, and the ingestion of enteric-coated potassium chloride or mercaptopurine. These lesions often cause small bowel obstruction, but hemorrhage may be the only clinical manifestation. The lesions are easily missed on routine barium contrast examination. Fiberoptic endoscopy with extra-long instruments may be helpful.

Nasopharyngeal and Pulmonary Lesions. Blood oozing from a lesion of the nasopharynx or lung may be swallowed, resulting in guaiac-positive stools. These lesions may be detected on chest x-ray, bronchoscopy, and examination of the nasopharynx.

HISTORY

Historical data can be helpful in localizing the bleeding lesion to the upper or lower gastrointestinal tract. A history of hematemesis bespeaks a lesion proximal to the ligament of Treitz. If the patient has ingested no iron or bismuth preparations, the passage of black, tarry stools also suggests a lesion of the upper gastrointestinal tract; such stools may rarely result from a bleeding lesion of the right colon, however. The passage of bright red blood per rectum suggests bleeding from the colon but occasionally results from massive hemorrhage from an upper gastrointestinal source. The passage of small quantities of bright red blood per rectum suggests a lesion of the sigmoid colon or rectum.

The association of abdominal pain with the episode of hemorrhage may be useful in establishing a differential diagnosis. Table 2 shows the association of pain and hemorrhage in some causes of gastrointestinal bleeding of unknown origin.

High-Payoff Queries

The following questions are especially likely to elicit important historical data:

1. *Have you had any abdominal operations?* A history of aortic reconstructive surgery suggests aortoenteric fistula. A history of surgery for bleeding peptic ulcer raises the possibility of recurrent ulcer.
2. *What medications do you use? Do any of them contain aspirin?* Gastrointestinal bleeding is associated with the ingestion of aspirin and many other nonsteroidal anti-inflammatory agents. Many patients do not consider aspirin a "medication" and must be asked about its ingestion specifically.
3. *Do you drink?* If so, bleeding from alcoholic gastritis and pancreatic disease should be considered strongly.

Table 2. THE ASSOCIATION OF ABDOMINAL PAIN WITH HEMORRHAGE IN SOME CAUSES OF OCCULT GASTROINTESTINAL BLEEDING

Commonly cause pain	Aortoenteric fistula Hemobilia Pancreatic disease Vasculitis
Commonly do not cause pain	Arteriovenous malformation Diverticulum Neoplasm Drugs Amyloidosis

4. *Have you had any injuries to your abdomen in the past few months?* Blunt abdominal trauma typically precedes symptoms of hemobilia by about 4 weeks.[13]

5. *Have other members of your family had problems with internal bleeding?* A strong family history of gastrointestinal bleeding is characteristic of the patient with type III arteriovenous malformations.

PHYSICAL EXAMINATION

Some causes of gastrointestinal bleeding that have distinctive physical features are listed in Table 3.

Temperature. Fever accompanied gastrointestinal hemorrhage in 45 per cent of patients with aortoenteric fistulae in one recent series.[2] It is also frequently associated with bleeding in patients with vasculitis.

Head and Neck. More than 90 per cent of patients with type III AVM have visible telangiectases of the face and the mucosa of the oropharynx and nasopharynx. Scleral icterus is often noted in patients with hemobilia. Angioid streaks of the ocular fundus are characteristic of pseudoxanthoma elasticum. An enlarged tongue suggests amyloidosis. Finally, careful examination of the oropharynx and nasopharynx may reveal a bleeding neoplasm.

Chest. A murmur of aortic stenosis is present in about one-fourth of patients with type I AVM.

Abdomen. A careful examination of the abdomen may reveal a mass suggestive of an aneurysm, a pancreatic pseudocyst, or a neoplasm.

Rectum. The character of the stool may reflect the magnitude of the bleeding. Loose, tarry, black, or maroon stools suggest recent brisk hemorrhage. Formed brown stools without visible evidence of blood that are guaiac-positive suggest low-grade bleeding. Note that to report a patient's stools merely as "guaiac-positive" hides important data.

Joints. Ehler-Danlos syndrome is characterized by marked hypermobility of the joints. Arthritis may be a manifestation of vasculitis.

Skin. Careful examination of the skin may reveal the palpable purpura typical of Henoch-Schönlein and other vasculitides; the blue, raised, wrinkled hemangiomas of the blue rubber bleb nevus syndrome; the fragility of amyloid-laden cutaneous capillaries; the xanthoma-like papules of pseudoxanthoma elasticum; or the hyperextensibility characteristic of Ehlers-Danlos syndrome.

DIAGNOSTIC STUDIES

Nonspecific Diagnostic Techniques

Occasionally, lesions escape detection even by modern techniques such as flexible fiberoptic endoscopy, arteriography, and radionuclide scanning. Lesions that are small, located beyond the reach of the endoscope, not primarily vascular, and not bleeding rapidly are particularly likely to be missed. In such circumstances, diagnostic techniques that identify the general area from which the bleeding originates may be helpful.[18, 19] These nonspecific techniques are as follows.

Fluorescein String Test. The patient swallows a weighted string that is allowed to traverse a chosen segment of the gastrointestinal tract, after which 10 to 20 ml of fluorescein is injected intravenously. The string is removed several minutes later and examined under ultraviolet light for flu-

Table 3. CAUSES OF GASTROINTESTINAL BLEEDING THAT HAVE DISTINCTIVE PHYSICAL FINDINGS

Disorder	Distinctive Physical Findings
Type III AVM	Telangiectases of the face and of the oropharyngeal and nasopharyngeal mucosa
Blue rubber bleb nevus syndrome	Multiple blue, raised, wrinkled cutaneous hemangiomas
Henoch-Schönlein purpura	Purpuric rash of the lower extremities
Amyloidosis	Enlargement of the tongue, fragility of cutaneous capillaries
Pseudoxanthoma elasticum	Xanthoma-like papules of the skin, angioid streaks of the ocular fundus
Ehlers-Danlos syndrome	Hypermobility of the joints, hyperextensibility of the skin

orescent areas, which may correspond to sites where bleeding has occurred during the fluorescein exposure period. This test has largely been abandoned because it is very insensitive, not specific, and fraught with technical difficulties.

Stepwise Aspiration of Intestinal Contents. The patient swallows a long tube, and the intestinal contents are aspirated as the tube traverses the small bowel. The station at which the aspirate becomes bloody or changes from guaiac-negative to guaiac-positive may correspond to the site of the lesion. A modification of this approach involves the intravenous injection of red blood cells tagged with sodium chromate ^{51}Cr after passage of the long tube. Presence of radioactivity in the aspirated fluid confirms fresh bleeding and may aid in localizing the lesion.[18] This technique is time-consuming, usually not helpful, and seldom performed.

Nuclear Imaging Techniques. Nuclear imaging techniques for identifying the site of gastrointestinal bleeding use two basic approaches. In the first approach, an imaging substance that is rapidly extracted from the blood is injected intravenously (e.g., ^{99m}Tc sulfur colloid). Bleeding into the bowel lumen then appears on scintigraphy as an area of activity that persists after the rest of the marker has been cleared from the intravascular space. Although bleeding rates as low as 0.05 ml/min have been detected in animals by this technique, its limitations are that the subject must be actively bleeding at the time of injection and that the labeled liver and spleen may mask overlying foci.[19] In the second approach, a nondiffusable indicator is injected intravenously (e.g., ^{99m}Tc-labeled red blood cells); this indicator then accumulates at the bleeding site during a specified time. The indicator is not rapidly cleared from the circulating blood, so it is possible to monitor the patient for active hemorrhage over an extended period. For example, such monitoring can be performed for up to 24 hours after injection of the ^{99m}Tc-labeled red blood cells. Thus, sites that bleed only intermittently can be identified by this method.

These nuclear imaging techniques appear to be valuable diagnostic tools. Limited clinical experience with ^{99m}Tc-labeled red cell scanning suggests that it is more sensitive than arteriography in identifying the site of gastrointestinal bleeding of unknown origin.[19]

Surgical Exploration

The role of surgical exploration in the patient with submassive gastrointestinal bleeding of unknown origin remains unclear. In patients whose bleeding sites are not identified by means of conventional diagnostic modalities or modern techniques such as flexible fiberoptic endoscopy, arteriography, and nuclear imaging, the diagnostic yield of exploratory surgery is probably less than 10 per cent.[20] Some authors believe that the yield can be increased by performing endoscopic examination of the bowel at the time of laparotomy.[21] In the event of a nondiagnostic surgical exploration, some authors have advocated (1) "blind" resection of the right colon, (2) the performance of an ileostomy to differentiate colonic and small intestine bleeding, or (3) the performance of a transverse colostomy to differentiate bleeding from the right and left sides of the colon; there are little data to support or refute these approaches. However, "blind" gastric resection, a procedure once advocated for gastrointestinal bleeding of unknown origin, is ineffective and should be strongly discouraged.[1]

ASSESSMENT: DIAGNOSTIC APPROACH

Some of the disorders discussed so far are so rare that the likelihood of a given patient's having one of them may be less than the chance that a more common lesion has been missed. Therefore, in the patient with gastrointestinal bleeding of unknown origin who has a history suggestive of one of the common disorders listed in Table 1, it is wiser to repeat the appropriate conventional diagnostic studies than to pursue a more exotic diagnosis.

By the definition proposed at the beginning of this chapter, the patient with gastrointestinal bleeding of unknown origin has had unrevealing sigmoidoscopy, barium contrast examinations, and upper gastrointestinal panendoscopy. In many such patients, findings of a careful history and physical examination provide clues to direct further diagnostic efforts. The patient's age is also an important consideration in formulating a diagnostic approach. For example, colonic neoplasm, type I AVM, and colonic diverticulosis are particularly common causes of gastrointestinal bleeding of unknown origin in the elderly. Thus, early diagnostic efforts in elderly patients should be so directed. Alternatively, a ^{99m}Tc sodium pertechnetate scan to identify a bleeding Meckel's diverticulum should be an early diagnostic test in children with occult gastrointestinal bleeding; in adults, in whom this disorder is very rare, such a scan is of far lower priority.

When the history and physical examination provide few diagnostic clues, the diagnostic approach to the patient with gastrointestinal bleeding of unknown origin is determined by the rapidity of blood loss. Is the gastrointestinal hemorrhage massive, brisk, or subacute?

Massive Gastrointestinal Bleeding of Unknown Origin

Diagnostic efforts must not take precedence over resuscitative ones in patients with massive life-threatening bleeding. The first goal is to achieve hemodynamic stability with the transfusion of blood and blood products and other supportive measures. There is little joy in establishing an accurate diagnosis in a patient who has exsanguinated. Rarely, a patient may present with uncontrollable hemorrhage of such magnitude that immediate surgical exploration is both the diagnostic and therapeutic procedure of choice (especially if aortoenteric fistula is a consideration). If there is time, arteriography may be helpful in localizing the hemorrhage for the surgeon and may even be used for therapy.[22]

Brisk Gastrointestinal Bleeding of Unknown Origin

If the bleeding is brisk but not immediately life-threatening, ^{99m}Tc-labeled red blood cell scintigraphy can localize the site of hemorrhage and thus direct subsequent arteriography or surgical exploration. If the nuclear imaging findings are unrevealing and brisk bleeding persists, arteriography should be the next step. The diagnostic yield of arteriography in patients with active gastrointestinal bleeding is about 50 per cent.[23] Surgical exploration must be considered for the patient with persistent brisk bleeding in whom no lesion is demonstrable by arteriography.

Subacute Gastrointestinal Bleeding of Unknown Origin

^{99m}Tc-labeled red blood cell scintigraphy should be performed early in the evaluation of the patient with subacute or chronic bleeding; a positive result can be used to direct further diagnostic studies. If the scan is not helpful, colonoscopy is a reasonable next step, having demonstrated utility in this setting. If no lesion is found on colonoscopy, a rectal biopsy to detect amyloidosis or ^{99m}Tc sodium pertechnetate scintigraphy to detect a Meckel's diverticulum may be performed. If these studies are unrevealing, arteriography should be done to seek an AVM, aneurysm, or neoplasm. If after all of these studies are completed the cause of bleeding is still not apparent, the chance that surgical exploration will reveal the diagnosis is likely to be small. In such a patient, the chance of surgical morbidity and mortality may be greater than the chance of establishing a diagnosis. It may be preferable to support the patient with oral iron therapy or even intermittent blood transfusion and to plan to repeat some of the investigations in the future. Surgical exploration may be indicated for the patient with persistent subacute bleeding in whom these less invasive diagnostic techniques have repeatedly failed to determine the cause.

REFERENCES

1. Douvres PA, Jerzy-Glass GB. Cryptogenic gastrointestinal bleeding. In: Jerzy-Glass GB, ed. Progress in gastroenterology. Vol. II. New York: Grune & Stratton, 1970;466–93.
2. Kiernan PD, Pairolero PC, Hubert JP, Mucha P, Wallace RB. Aortic graft-enteric fistula. Mayo Clin Proc 1980;55:731–8.
3. Moore JD, Thompson NW, Appelman HD, Foley D. Arteriovenous malformations of the gastrointestinal tract. Arch Surg 1976;111:381–8.
4. Boley SJ, Sammartano R, Adams A, DiBiase A, Kleinhaus S, Sprayregen S. On the nature and etiology of vascular ectasias of the colon. Degenerative lesions of aging. Gastroenterology 1977;72:650–60.
5. Welch CE, Athanasoulis CA, Galdabini JJ. Hemorrhage from the large bowel with special reference to angiodysplasia and diverticular disease. World J Surg 1978;2:73–83.
6. Broor SL, Parker HW, Ganeshappa KP, Komaki S, Dodds WJ. Vascular dysplasia of the right colon. An important cause of unexplained gastrointestinal bleeding. Dig Dis 1978;23:89–92.
7. Meyers MA, Alonso DR, Gray GF, Baer JW. Pathogenesis of bleeding colonic diverticulosis. Gastroenterology 1976;71:577–83.
8. Casarella WJ, Kanter IE, Seaman WB. Right sided colonic diverticula as a cause of acute rectal hemorrhage. N Engl J Med 1972;286:450–3.
9. Case Records of the Massachusetts General Hospital (Case 16-1980). N Engl J Med 1980;302:958–62.
10. Tedesco FJ, Waye JD, Raskin JB, Morris SJ, Greenwald RA. Colonoscopic evaluation of rectal bleeding. A study of 304 patients. Ann Intern Med 1978;89:907–9.
11. Teague RH, Thornton JR, Manning AP, Salmon PR, Read AE. Colonoscopy for investigation of unexplained rectal bleeding. Lancet 1978;1:1350–2.
12. Miles RM, Crawford D, Duras S. The small bowel tumor problem: an assessment based on a 20 year experience with 116 cases. Ann Surg 1979;189:732–8.
13. Bismuth H. Hemobilia. N Engl J Med 1973;288:617–9.
14. Marks IR, Bank S, Louw JH, Farman J. Peptic ulceration and gastrointestinal bleeding in pancreatitis. Gut 1967;8:253–9.
15. Cream JJ, Gumpel JM, Peachey RDG. Schönlein-Henoch purpura in the adult. A study of 77 patients with anaphylactioid or Schönlein-Henoch purpura. Q J Med 1970;39:461–84.
16. Cabal E, Holtz S. Polyarteritis as a cause of intestinal hemorrhage. Gastroenterology 1971;61:99–105.
17. Simon LS, Mills JA. Nonsteroidal antiinflammatory drugs. N Engl J Med 1980;302:1179–85, 1237–43.
18. Pillow RP, Hill LD, Ragen PA, Siemsen JS, Walker LA. Newer methods for localization of obscure small-bowel bleeding. JAMA 1962;179:23–6.
19. Markisz JA, Front D, Royal HD, Sacks B, Parker JA,

Kolodny GM. An evaluation of ^{99m}Tc-labelled red blood cell scintigraphy for the detection and localization of gastrointestinal bleeding sites. Gastroenterology 1982;83:394–8.
20. Spechler SJ, Schimmel EM. Gastrointestinal tract bleeding of unknown origin. Arch Intern Med 1982;142:236–40.
21. Myers RT. Diagnosis and management of occult gastrointestinal bleeding: visualization of the small bowel lumen by fiberoptic colonoscope. Am Surg 1976;42:92–5.
22. Athanasoulis CA. Therapeutic applications of angiography. (Parts I and II). N Engl J Med 1980;302:1117–24, 1174–8.
23. Shiff AD, Grnja V, Osborn DJ, Spiro HM. Angiography in the diagnosis of gastrointestinal diseases. Ann Intern Med 1972;77:731–40.

GYNECOMASTIA

HOWARD D. GROVEMAN

□ SYNONYM: Male breast enlargement

BACKGROUND

Definition and Origins

Gynecomastia is the presence of palpable breast tissue in one or both breasts in the male. It is a condition whose earliest description dates back to Greek mythology, in which male breast enlargement was described as a punishment by the gods for human misdeeds. Pronounced gynecomastia is depicted in the statues of Tutankhamen and in other hereditary pharaohs of his time, suggesting that a familial form of the condition may have been present.[1] It has only been in recent years that the pathophysiologic mechanisms of gynecomastia have been elucidated.

Clinical Presentation

The male breast is a rudimentary organ composed of a nipple with a small underlying duct system and a fatty stroma. These underlying structures are not palpable during the physical examination unless they have become enlarged owing to one of a variety of hormonal or other influences. The patient may present with a history of painful or painless breast enlargement, or the enlargement may be found during a routine examination in an asymptomatic patient. Clinically, gynecomastia most commonly takes the form of a unilateral or bilateral subareolar plate of tissue, 2 to 5 cm in diameter, that is easily distinguished from surrounding subcutaneous fat. Histologic examination shows intraductal epithelial hyperplasia in a loose cellular stroma, which may after several months or years progress to a dense, hyalinized stroma without prominent ductal structures.[2] Occasionally gynecomastia may manifest as a more diffuse enlargement of the breast and may at times be difficult to distinguish from subcutaneous fat. In these instances, mammography and ultrasonography are useful diagnostic tools.[3] The histologic features of gynecomastia lend no clues to its particular etiology, and biopsy for this purpose will be unrewarding.

As in any patient presenting with a breast mass or breast enlargement, the possibility of cancer, albeit exceedingly small in the male, must be considered. Features of male breast tumors that help distinguish them from gynecomastia are: a nonsubareolar location, bloody nipple discharge, fixation, axillary adenopathy, overlying skin changes, and ulceration.[4] Any patient with suspicious findings should have a biopsy. The high prevalence of gynecomastia in the general population makes routine biopsy an otherwise costly and unnecessary procedure.

Importance

In 1963, Williams[5] showed that gynecomastia might be a more common entity than previously described; his study revealed histologic findings consistent with gynecomastia in 40 per cent of 447 autopsied males. In recent separate clinical studies, Nuttal[6] and Carlson[7] have confirmed this high incidence (36 and 32 per cent, respectively) in routine examinations of asymptomatic adult males. Considering how common the condition is, it is quite appropriate to ask if any systematic approach to the patient with gynecomastia is necessary. The answer to this question is "Yes," because gynecomastia (1) may be a normal physiologic feature of infancy, adolescence, and aging; (2) may be of major clinical significance in the early diagnosis of certain systemic illnesses and endocrine disorders; (3) may be a side effect of various drugs; and (4) may have profound psychologic significance for the patient and his family.

HISTORY

In all cases of gynecomastia a careful history should be obtained.

History of the Present Illness. The age of onset, the presence or absence of pain, and the duration of breast enlargement should be determined. A careful drug history is most important, especially in regard to those medications listed in Table 1. A history of weight loss or gain, testicular pain or enlargement, or change in libido would be most significant. The history should also address symptoms related to a systemic illness or endocrinologic abnormality. Of importance would be any historical features of hyperthyroidism, uremia, alcoholism, and nutritional deficiency.

Previous Medical History. An early childhood history should be taken to determine the presence or absence of congenital or developmental abnormalities. Anorchia, undescended testes, and other genital anomalies would be significant. Information about pubertal development should also be recorded.

Family History. Familial disorders of which gynecomastia is a feature are exceedingly rare.[8] A family history of a genetic disturbance such as Klinefelter's syndrome, however, would be quite important to ascertain.

PHYSICAL EXAMINATION

Patients with gynecomastia should have a careful breast examination to exclude the possibility of concomitant malignancy. The features of breast carcinoma have previously been discussed.

During the physical examination it is important to assess overall growth and development. The testes should be examined for masses, unilateral enlargement, lack of descent, atrophy and absence. The finding of small, firm testes should also be noted. The abdominal examination should focus on liver size and the presence or absence of a mass lesion, which might indicate an adrenal or other neoplasm. During the remainder of the examination, particular search should be made for stigmata of systemic or endocrinologic disorders.

PATHOPHYSIOLOGIC CONSIDERATIONS

The many and various causes of gynecomastia are listed in Table 1.

In the normal adult male, estrogens and androgens are produced in a ratio of approximately 1:100; this ratio is in contradistinction to that in the adult female, which approaches 1:10.[9] It is now clear that this balance of estrogens and androgens is responsible for breast development or lack thereof. Any condition in the male that actually raises the estrogen-androgen ratio (as in disorders causing decreased testosterone synthesis, elevated estrogen production, or both) or effectively raises it (as in conditions that cause increased plasma binding of testosterone or decreased end-organ receptivity to testosterone) may cause gynecomastia. This physiologic relationship is a most important one, being the etiologic factor in most cases of gynecomastia. Surprisingly, prolactin has been shown to play little if any direct role in the development of male breast enlargement.[10]

Physiologic Gynecomastia

Gynecomastia is a frequent finding during three periods of normal physiologic change: the newborn period, adolescence, and old age.

Palpable breast tissue, a common finding of the newborn examination, represents the stimulatory effect of placental estrogens on the infant breast. Regression usually occurs within a few weeks. It is always a good idea to include this fact in the anticipatory guidance given new parents.

In a series of 2,369 normal male adolescent examinations, Nydick and associates[11] found gynecomastia in 38.7 per cent, with a peak incidence of 64.6 per cent in 14-year-olds. Breast enlargement in the adolescent can be unilateral or bilateral and is occasionally painful. Regression usually takes place within 2 years of onset.[12] This phenomenon is generally believed to be due to the fact that testicular estrogen production reaches adult levels in advance of testosterone production, thereby creating a temporary elevation in the estrogen-androgen ratio.[13]

Gynecomastia is also a frequent physiologic concomitant of old age. Although more serious causes must be considered, the decrease in testosterone production by the testes in many elderly males creates a setting of relative estrogen excess.[14] Increasing adiposity with age may also cause higher peripheral production of estrogen from androgenic precursors, by way of the aromatase system.

Prepubertal Gynecomastia

Although premature thelarche in the female can have a physiologic basis, prepubertal gynecomastia may have graver implications. Fortunately this condition is exceedingly rare.

Table 1. CAUSES OF GYNECOMASTIA

Physiologic gynecomastia	Newborn period Adolescence Old age
Systemic disorders	Recovery from malnourished state Hyperthyroidism Renal failure Cirrhosis Paraplegia
Disorders of testosterone synthesis or action	Klinefelter's syndrome Mumps orchitis Congenital anorchia Lepromatous leprosy Undescended testes Testicular feminization syndrome
Disorders manifested by increased estrogen production	Feminizing adrenal tumors Germinal cell tumors Interstitial cell testicular tumors Lung cancer or other malignancy with hCG elevation True hermaphroditism
Drugs	Androgens Busulfan Cimetidine Diazepam Digitalis Estrogens Heroin Isoniazid Ketoconazole Marijuana Methyldopa Nitrosoureas Penicillamine Phenothiazines Reserpine Spironolactone Tricyclic antidepressants Vincristine

Exposure to exogenous estrogens must be the first diagnostic consideration. Accidental ingestion of estrogen or exposure to estrogenic creams may produce gynecomastia. An epidemic of breast enlargement has been reported at an Italian school in which estrogen-contaminated meat was implicated.[15] A variety of other drugs can also affect this age group (see Table 1).

Gynecomastia can also be secondary to a variety of tumors in prepubertal males.[16] Interstitial cell tumors of the testes may cause overproduction of testosterone or estradiol. Testosterone overproduction causes gynecomastia by a mechanism of increased peripheral conversion to estrogens. Another tumor, the gonadotropin-secreting germinal cell tumor—either of the testes or in an ectopic location—produces excessive amounts of human chorionic gonadotropin (hCG), which in turn stimulates the normal Leydig cells of the testes to overproduce estradiol. A much rarer neoplasm is the feminizing adrenal tumor, which causes oversecretion of estrogenic precursors and a marked elevation in the estrogen-androgen ratio; a palpable abdominal mass can frequently be found in patients with feminizing adrenal tumors.[17] Adrenal hyperplasia without tumor has also been reported in prepubertal patients with gynecomastia.[18]

Finally, certain types of local breast disease may mimic gynecomastia in this age group. So-called pseudogynecomastia has been reported with breast tumors, hemangiomas, and neurofibromatosis.[19]

Systemic Illnesses and Gynecomastia

Gynecomastia is frequently seen as a manifestation of hyperthyroidism, renal failure, and cirrhosis. It can also be found in patients recovering from a malnourished state and in paraplegics.

Hyperthyroidism. Elevations in sex hormone–binding globulin (SHBG) in patients with hyperthyroidism lead to increases in serum levels of

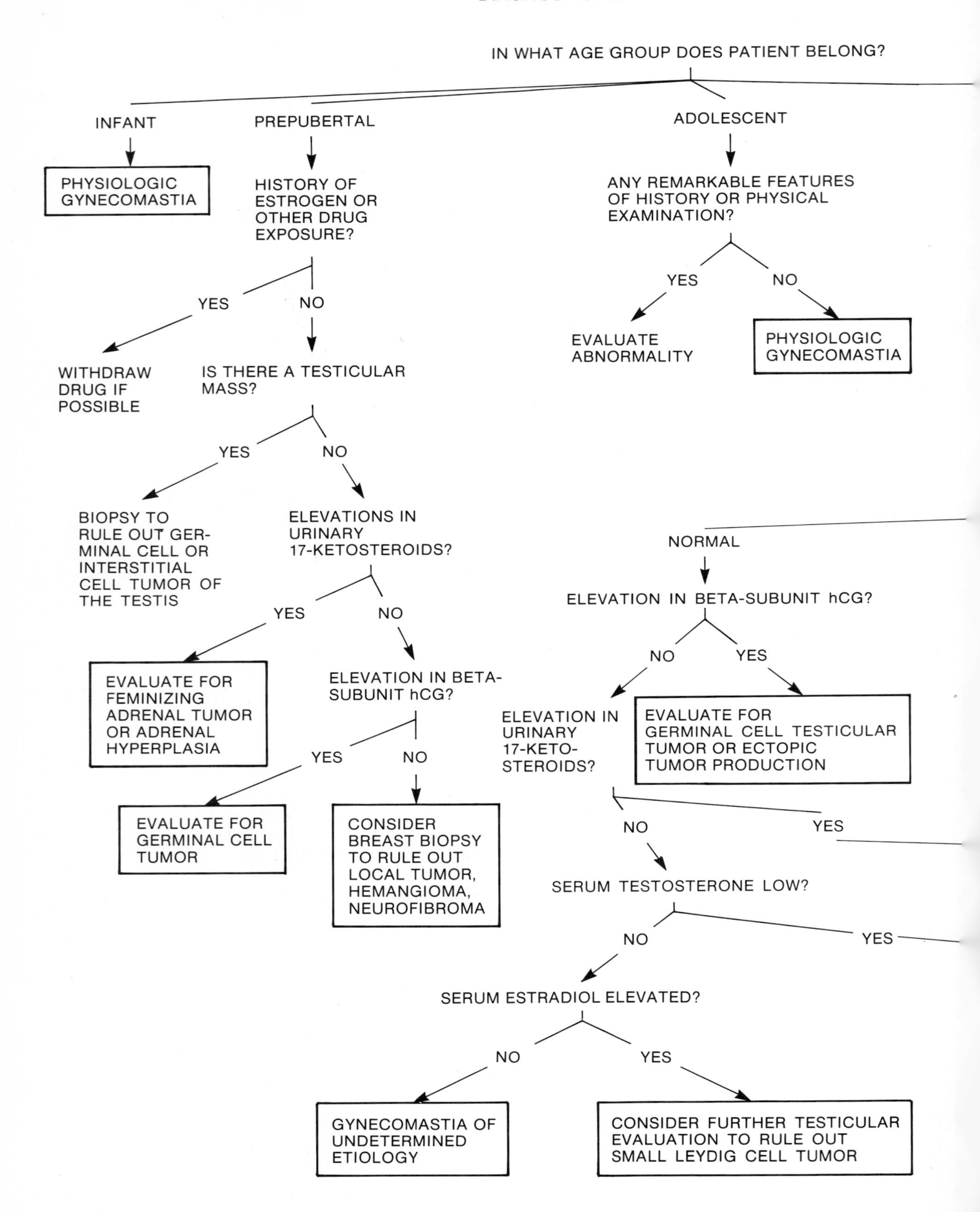
DIAGNOSTIC ASSESSMENT OF GYNECOMASTIA
IN WHAT AGE GROUP DOES PATIENT BELONG?
INFANT
PREPUBERTAL
ADOLESCENT
PHYSIOLOGIC GYNECOMASTIA
HISTORY OF ESTROGEN OR OTHER DRUG EXPOSURE?
ANY REMARKABLE FEATURES OF HISTORY OR PHYSICAL EXAMINATION?
YES
NO
YES
NO
WITHDRAW DRUG IF POSSIBLE
IS THERE A TESTICULAR MASS?
EVALUATE ABNORMALITY
PHYSIOLOGIC GYNECOMASTIA
YES
NO
BIOPSY TO RULE OUT GERMINAL CELL OR INTERSTITIAL CELL TUMOR OF THE TESTIS
ELEVATIONS IN URINARY 17-KETOSTEROIDS?
NORMAL
ELEVATION IN BETA-SUBUNIT hCG?
YES
NO
NO
YES
EVALUATE FOR FEMINIZING ADRENAL TUMOR OR ADRENAL HYPERPLASIA
ELEVATION IN BETA-SUBUNIT hCG?
ELEVATION IN URINARY 17-KETO-STEROIDS?
EVALUATE FOR GERMINAL CELL TESTICULAR TUMOR OR ECTOPIC TUMOR PRODUCTION
YES
NO
EVALUATE FOR GERMINAL CELL TUMOR
CONSIDER BREAST BIOPSY TO RULE OUT LOCAL TUMOR, HEMANGIOMA, NEUROFIBROMA
NO
YES
SERUM TESTOSTERONE LOW?
NO
YES
SERUM ESTRADIOL ELEVATED?
NO
YES
GYNECOMASTIA OF UNDETERMINED ETIOLOGY
CONSIDER FURTHER TESTICULAR EVALUATION TO RULE OUT SMALL LEYDIG CELL TUMOR

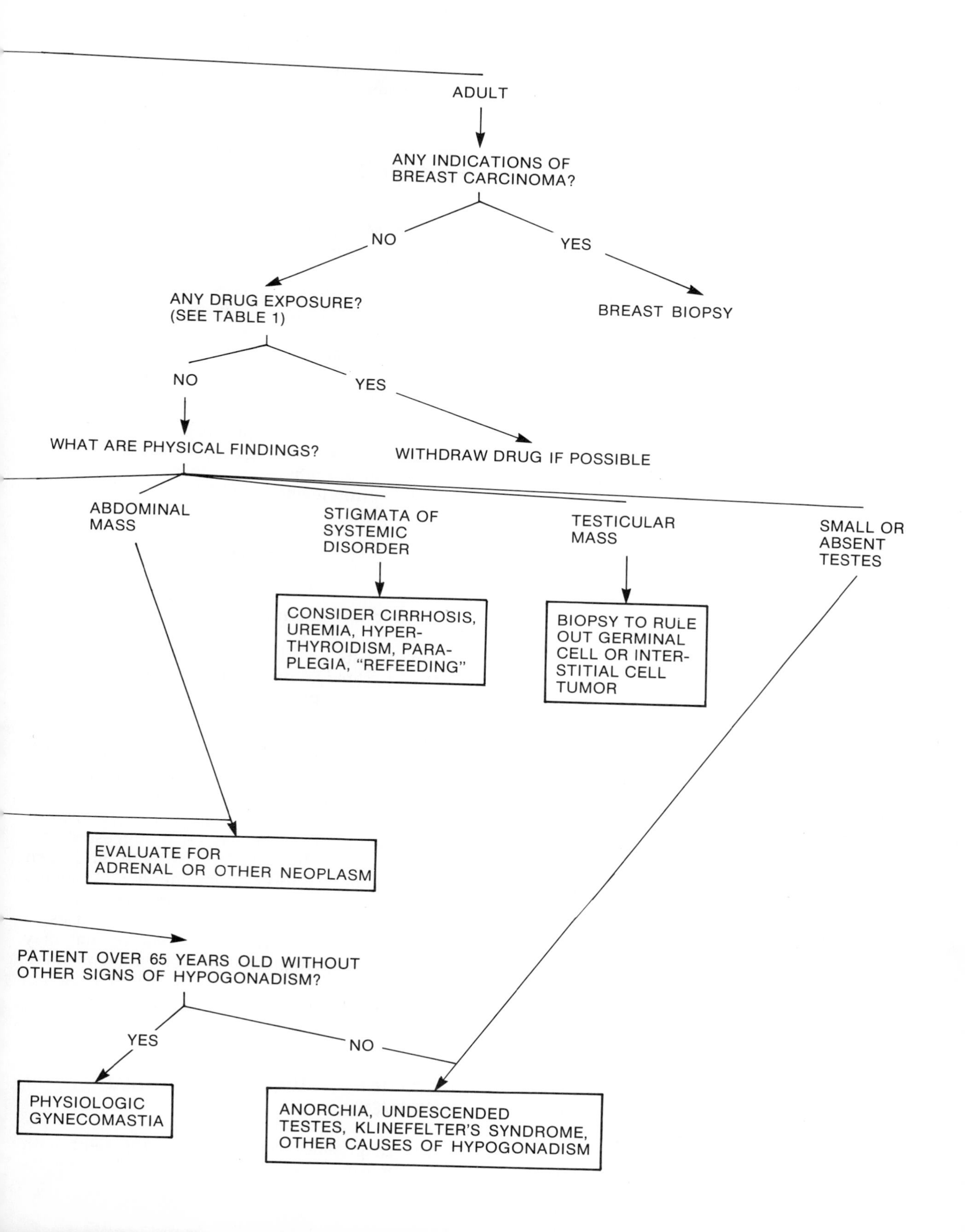
ADULT
ANY INDICATIONS OF BREAST CARCINOMA?
NO
YES
BREAST BIOPSY
ANY DRUG EXPOSURE? (SEE TABLE 1)
NO
YES
WITHDRAW DRUG IF POSSIBLE
WHAT ARE PHYSICAL FINDINGS?
ABDOMINAL MASS
STIGMATA OF SYSTEMIC DISORDER
TESTICULAR MASS
SMALL OR ABSENT TESTES
CONSIDER CIRRHOSIS, UREMIA, HYPER-THYROIDISM, PARA-PLEGIA, "REFEEDING"
BIOPSY TO RULE OUT GERMINAL CELL OR INTER-STITIAL CELL TUMOR
EVALUATE FOR ADRENAL OR OTHER NEOPLASM
PATIENT OVER 65 YEARS OLD WITHOUT OTHER SIGNS OF HYPOGONADISM?
YES
NO
PHYSIOLOGIC GYNECOMASTIA
ANORCHIA, UNDESCENDED TESTES, KLINEFELTER'S SYNDROME, OTHER CAUSES OF HYPOGONADISM

estradiol as well as testosterone.[20] Preferential binding of testosterone by SHBG may be the mechanism by which the free estradiol level is elevated in hyperthyroidism. The free testosterone level, however, is normal, leading to an elevation in the estrogen-androgen ratio at the cellular level. Additionally, increased peripheral conversion of androgens to estrogens may play a role.

Renal Failure. Testicular dysfunction in uremia leads to both impaired spermatogenesis and decreased testosterone production.[21] This hypogonadal state is the most likely cause of gynecomastia in renal failure. Elevation in pituitary gonadotropins is also common, secondary to decreased renal clearance as well as the lack of feedback inhibition by testosterone. Elevations in luteinizing hormone (LH) may stimulate the remaining Leydig cells of the testes to overproduce estradiol, thereby causing a further increase in the estrogen-androgen ratio.

Cirrhosis. As in renal failure, the development of a hypogonadal state may be the primary etiology of the gynecomastia seen in alcohol-related liver disease. This mechanism has been postulated to be due either to the direct toxic effects of alcohol on the testes or to an alteration in the hypothalmic-pituitary axis.[21] In addition, liver dysfunction can lead to a diminished extraction of estrogenic precursors such as androstenedione, and hence to an excessive peripheral production of estrogen. Elevations of SHBG in liver disease (possibly due to the direct effect of elevated estrogens) may cause a further reduction in free testosterone.

Malnutrition and the Refeeding Phenomenon. Although the mechanisms are probably quite complex, malnutrition can lead to abnormalities in the hypothalmic-pituitary axis, simulating the prepubertal state.[22] Refeeding, then, can normalize this axis, producing gynecomastia through mechanisms similar to those in adolescence. This situation has been likened to a "second puberty" and may occur on recovery from any prolonged illness.

Paraplegia. The mechanism for gynecomastia in paraplegia is unclear. A refeeding mechanism may be involved in the recovery period following spinal cord trauma. Decreased testicular function has also been demonstrated, resulting from an elevation in gonadal temperature caused by interruption of the lumbar sympathetic nerve supply.[21]

Disorders of Testosterone Synthesis or Action

As discussed previously, any disorder that produces a hypogonadal state can cause gynecomastia. Conditions of testicular dysfunction can lead to decrease or absence of testosterone synthesis. These conditions include mumps orchitis, congenital anorchia, undescended testes, and lepromatous leprosy. Of particular importance is Klinefelter's syndrome, which is not uncommon in the general male population and of which gynecomastia is a prominent feature. Other features of this syndrome include small, firm testes, azoospermia, and a characteristic 47,XXY karyotype.[23]

Gynecomastia can also develop as the consequence of a defect in testosterone action. Absence of or decrease in androgen receptors, as in the testicular feminization syndrome, leads to unopposed estrogen action at the cellular level.[9]

Disorders Manifested by Increased Estrogen Production

Feminizing adrenal tumors, although rare, are frequently malignant. They produce excessive amounts of estrogenic precursors and can be detected by elevations in urinary 17-ketosteroids.[17] Gynecomastia can also result from germinal cell tumors, which liberate hCG, thereby stimulating excessive estradiol secretion by the testes. Other sources of ectopic hCG production, such as lung tumors, can also cause gynecomastia and can be detected by elevations in urinary or, more frequently, serum levels of hCG.[9]

Finally, true hermaphroditism can cause gynecomastia if functioning ovarian tissue secretes feminizing amounts of estrogen.[24]

Drugs and Gynecomastia

Table 1 lists a variety of medications that have been implicated in gynecomastia. In a recent study by Carlson,[7] 62 per cent of patients with gynecomastia were found to be taking one or more medications thought to cause breast enlargement.

A hormonal mechanism may be responsible for certain drug-induced cases. Spironolactone, for example, which has long been associated with gynecomastia, acts primarily by blocking androgen receptors.[25] Similarly, it has been suggested that cimetidine acts by interference with androgen binding sites.[26] Cancer chemotherapeutic agents (e.g., busulfan) can cause gynecomastia secondary to testicular damage with resultant decreases in testosterone levels. Another substance that may have a hormonal mechanism of action is marijuana; it is postulated that similarities exist between the drug's active ingredient, tetrahydrocannabinol (THC), and estradiol.[27]

LABORATORY EVALUATION AND GENERAL ASSESSMENT

The diagnostic approach to any patient with gynecomastia must be tailored to the clinical presentation. The algorithm suggests a systematic approach to patient evaluation. The physiologic nature of breast enlargement in early infancy and adolescence, for example, obviates the need for extensive evaluation, unless physical findings or a prolonged duration suggests otherwise. In prepubertal gynecomastia, however, serious disorders may be present, such as feminizing adrenal tumor, germinal cell tumor, or interstitial cell testicular tumor; an extensive evaluation is therefore warranted.

It is in the adult or elderly patient with gynecomastia in whom a balance must be found between diagnostic fervor and cost-effectiveness. There have been no studies evaluating the cost-benefit ratio of any particular "screening panel" for gynecomastia. Considering the high incidence of gynecomastia in normal men, Carlson[7] has suggested that no further evaluation be undertaken in an otherwise healthy patient whose gynecomastia is asymptomatic and of long or uncertain duration; he also quite appropriately points out that the etiology of such gynecomastia may remain uncertain, even after extensive laboratory evaluation.

In most cases of drug-induced gynecomastia, withdrawal from medication will be both diagnostic and curative—especially if the enlargement is of recent onset. The benefits and risks of drug withdrawal must therefore be considered. Gynecomastia itself does not seem to predispose to breast cancer, except in the clinical setting of Klinefelter's syndrome, in which yearly breast examinations are justified.[28]

The psychologic implications of breast enlargement must also be assessed in each patient. Surgery may sometimes be justified if altered self-image or family dysfunction is pronounced. In mild cases of gynecomastia, counseling and patient education are of utmost importance.

REFERENCES

1. Paulshock BZ. Tutankhamun and his brothers: familial gynecomastia in the Eighteenth Dynasty. JAMA 1980;244:160–4.
2. Nocolis GL, Modlinger RS, Gabrilove JL. A study of the histopathology of human gynecomastia. J Clin Endocrinol Metab 1971;32:173–8.
3. Wigley KD, Thomas JL, Bernardino ME, Rosenbaum JL. Sonography of gynecomastia. AJR 1981;136:927–30.
4. Crichlow RW. Breast cancer in men. Semin Oncol 1974;1:145–52.
5. Williams MJ. Gynecomastia: its incidence, recognition and host characterization in 447 autopsy cases. Am J Med 1963;34:103–12.
6. Nuttall FQ. Gynecomastia as a physical finding in normal men. J Clin Endocrinol Metab 1979;48:338–40.
7. Carlson HE. Gynecomastia. N Engl J Med 1981;303:795–9.
8. Edwards JA, Bannerman RM. Familial gynecomastia. Birth Defects 1971;7:193–5.
9. Emerson K Jr. The mammary gland: a mirror of the endocrine system. Med Times 1980;108:35–45.
10. Turkington RW. Serum prolactin levels in patients with gynecomastia. J Clin Endocrinol Metab 1972;34:62–6.
11. Nydick M, Bustos J, Dale JH Jr, Rawson RW. Gynecomastia in adolescent boys. JAMA 1961;178:449–54.
12. Groveman HD, Norcross WA. Adolescent breast masses. Hosp Med 1982;18:65–84.
13. Large DM, Anderson DC. Twenty-four hour profiles of circulating androgens and oestrogens in male puberty with or without gynecomastia. Clin Endocrinol 1979;11:505–21.
14. Rubens R, Dhont M, Vermeulen A. Further studies on Leydig cell function in old age. J Clin Endocrinol Metab 1974;39:40–5.
15. Fara GM, Del Corvo G, Bernuzzi S, et al. Epidemic of breast enlargement in an Italian school. Lancet 1979;8137:295–7.
16. August GP, Chandra R, Hung W. Prepubertal male gynecomastia. J Pediatr 1972;80:259–63.
17. Gabrilove JL, Sharma DC, Wotiz HH, Dorman RI. Feminizing adrenocortical tumors in the male: a review of 52 cases including a case report. Medicine (Baltimore) 1965;44:37–79.
18. Gabrilove JL, Nicholis GL, Sohval AR. Non-tumorous feminizing adrenogenital syndrome in the male subject. J Urol 1973;110:710–3.
19. Lipper S, Willson CF, Copeland KC. Pseudogynecomastia due to neurofibromatosis—a light microscopic and ultrastructural study. Hum Pathol 1981;12:755–9.
20. Chopra IJ, Tulchinsky D. Status of estrogen-androgen balance in hyperthyroid men with Graves disease. J Clin Endocrinol Metab 1974;38:269–77.
21. Morley JE, Melmed S. Gonadal dysfunction in systemic disorders. Metabolism 1979;28:1051–73.
22. Smith SR, Chhetri MK, Johanson AJ, Radfar N, Migeon CJ. The pituitary-gonadal axis in men with protein-calorie malnutrition. J Clin Endocrinol Metab 1975;41:60–9.
23. Paulsen CA, Gordon DL, Carpenter RW, Gandy HM, Drucker WD. Klinefelter's syndrome and its variants: a hormonal and chromosomal study. Recent Prog Horm Res 1968;24:321–63.
24. Wilson JD, Aiman J, MacDonald PC. The pathogenesis of gynecomastia. Adv Intern Med 1980;25:1–32.
25. Greenblatt DJ, Koch-Weser J. Gynecomastia and impotence: complications of spironolactone therapy. JAMA 1973;223:82.
26. Winters SJ, Bank JL, Loriaux DL. Cimetidine is an antiandrogen in the rat. Gastroenterology 1979;76:504–8.
27. Harmon J, Aliapoulios MA. Gynecomastia in marihuana users. N Engl J Med 1972;287:936.
28. Cuena CR, Becker KL. Klinefelter's syndrome and cancer of the breast. Arch Intern Med 1968;121:159–62.

HEADACHE, ACUTE

ROBERT B. TAYLOR

☐ SYNONYMS: Cephalgia, head pain

BACKGROUND

Definition and Origins

Headache describes a sensation of pain or other discomfort related to structures of the head and neck. Although the bony structures and brain parenchyma are insensitive to pain, virtually all other tissues have pain-sensitive fibers that may respond to a variety of stimuli. The arteries are especially sensitive, and vascular changes characteristically cause a deep, aching pain. Pain may arrive via the cranial nerves, especially the trigeminal (fifth cranial) nerve. Also sensitive to pain on direct stimulation are the glossopharyngeal (ninth cranial), the vagus (tenth cranial), the spinal accessory (11th cranial), and the hypoglossal (12th cranial) nerves. The superior sagittal and other venous sinuses are sensitive to painful stimuli, although the response is not as intense as that arising in the arteries. Pain may occur when there is traction on the small tributary veins of the venous sinuses. Head pain may also be caused by stimulation of the first, second, or third cervical nerves, generally manifested as pain near the vertex and the back of the head and neck.

This chapter discusses *acute* headache, i.e., headache having a recent onset and relatively severe course. Recent onset is defined as within 1 week and is likely to be measured in hours. Although chronic and recurrent headaches are among the most common ailments of mankind, this chapter focuses on the diagnostic approach to the "new" headache; the recurrent headache syndromes—notably migraine and muscle contraction–tension headaches—are discussed only as they relate to the differential diagnosis of acute headache.

Incidence and Causes

Headache was the seventh most frequent symptomatic reason for visits given by patients in the National Ambulatory Medical Care Survey taken in the United States in 1977–1978, constituting an estimated 18,341,923 visits to office-based physicians.[1] Of those reported visits in which the headache constituted a new problem, the time since onset of the complaint was less than one week in 43.9 per cent of females and 49.3 per cent of males.

Headache is, of course, a symptom and not a diagnosis. Table 1 presents the principal diagnoses in patients presenting in an emergency department with headache as the chief complaint.[2] In these patients, there were high incidences of headache caused by extracranial infection (39.3 per cent) or trauma (9.3 per cent). These patients had one-half the incidence of migraine headache and a much lower incidence of hypertension-related headache than the patients in the National Ambulatory Medical Care Survey. In a similar study by Leicht, muscle contraction–tension headache and migraine headache were the most common diagnoses, accounting for 54 per cent of 485 emergency department patients evaluated for nontraumatic headaches.[3] In another study of 124 patients with nontraumatic headache seen at a university hospital emergency room, Dickman and Masten found that 50 per cent had headaches described as "benign, tension, undefined, associated with virus or fever," 20 per cent had headaches from upper respiratory infection, 10 per cent from hypertension, 3 per cent from migraine, and 17 per cent from miscellaneous causes.[4] Headache patterns of children differ from those of adults; in one study 15 per cent of children referred to a pediatric neurology clinic because of headache were found to have a seizure equivalent.[5]

Possible causes of acute headache are listed in Table 3 and discussed later in the chapter. Many of the problems listed here are encountered infrequently but must be considered in the differential diagnosis of the patient presenting with severe cephalgia of recent onset. Several of these causes merit special mention. With the current interest in

Table 1. DIAGNOSES IN EMERGENCY DEPARTMENT PATIENTS PRESENTING WITH HEADACHE AS THE CHIEF COMPLAINT

Final Diagnosis in Emergency Department	Number	Percentage
Tension headache	168	19.3
Vascular (migraine type)	39	4.5
Post-traumatic	81	9.3
Infection other than intracranial	343	39.3
Hypertension-related	42	4.8
Migraine and tension	4	0.5
Subarachnoid hemorrhage	8	0.9
Meningitis	5	0.6
Miscellaneous	130	14.9
No Diagnosis	52	6.0
Total	872	100

(From Dhopesh V, Anwar R, Herring C: A retrospective assessment of emergency department patients with complaint of headache. Headache 19:37–42, 1979. Reprinted by permission.)

physical exercise, more patients have experienced headaches related to exertion, including some who develop major hemorrhage from previously unsuspected intracranial neoplasms while running.[6] Exercise-related headache has also been reported in a patient with pheochromocytoma.[7] Because of the relatively long headache-free intervals, patients with cyclical migraine may present with symptoms of acute headache; these headaches occur in cycles that last an average of 6 weeks recurring about five times per year.[8]

Psychogenic disorders that may cause headache include anxiety, depressive reactions, and conversion reactions.[9] Packard has defined *conversion headache* as one in which a peripheral pain mechanism is not present and the prevailing clinical disorder is a conversion reaction.[10] In affected patients the pain may begin as a local process, prolonged as an hysterical symptom after the physical problem (such as trauma) has healed.

Temporomandibular joint (TMJ) dysfunction may cause headache, especially in young women.[11] Headache is also common in women during the first postpartum week, particularly between days 3 and 6.[12] A rare cause of headache in young women is pseudotumor cerebri, characterized by headache, diplopia, and papilledema.

HISTORY

In most patients, acute headache can be diagnosed by means of a carefully taken history.[3]

Subjective Data

History of the Present Illness. The medical history should record the headache's onset, location, and frequency as well as the quality and intensity of pain and any associated symptoms.[4] Is the pain constant or intermittent? If the headache is intermittent, how long does an episode last? Are there associated symptoms such as visual phenomena, nausea, vomiting, and vertigo? Has there been a head injury? Has the patient fainted or had a convulsion? Has there been nasal congestion or discharge? Does the pain seem to be increasing or decreasing in severity? What has been done to relieve the pain?

Information regarding the patient's mental status, including mood change, alterations in habits, and presence of delusions or hallucinations, may be obtained from both patient and family.

Other questions might be prompted by circumstances: Has there been pain in peripheral joints (temporal arteritis associated with polymyalgia rheumatica)? Has there been a recent infection involving the middle ear or midfacial structures (brain abscess)? Might the patient have been hunting (tularemia), have eaten undercooked pork (trichinosis), or have traveled in a tropical area (malaria)? Has he or she been using cleaning fluid (carbon tetrachloride), spraying for insects (insecticides), or repairing an automobile in a closed garage (carbon monoxide)? Has the patient recently begun taking a new medication (indomethacin, vasodilators, oral contraceptives)? Has there been generalized flushing (carcinoid tumor), eye pain (glaucoma), blurred vision (benign intracranial hypertension), or jaw pain (TMJ dysfunction)?

Family History. A family history of migraine headaches is found in approximately half of all migraineurs. Other important components of family history of patients with headache include: hypertension, stroke, mental disorder, recent febrile illness in the household, drug abuse, and glaucoma.

Social and Occupational History. What is the patient's job and what potential headache causes are involved? Is the patient under stress at home or on the job? What are the patient's habits regarding sleep, exercise, and nutrition?

Drug History. A history of drug use can provide important clues, including an index of the severity of the headache. The drug history should include the patient's habits regarding tobacco, alcohol, and caffeine.

Previous Medical History. Is there a history of headaches of any kind? Has the patient suffered any injuries, notably trauma to the head or neck? Has the patient ever had an acute infection of the brain such as meningitis or encephalitis? Is there a history of convulsions, or has the patient ever taken anticonvulsant medication? Has the patient had tuberculosis, venereal disease, or cancer? Has the patient ever had a surgical operation or been hospitalized for other reasons?

General Considerations. Early assessment of an acute headache should include determining the patient's expectations for the visit. Is the patient's objective the alleviation of pain, relief of concern regarding the cause, legitimization of sick-role behavior, or some other purpose?[13] How does the headache interfere with usual activities? Is the patient receiving secondary gain from the headache symptom?

High-Payoff Queries

The following ten questions are especially likely to elicit noteworthy information:

1. *Where is your headache located?* Tension headache is generally worst at the back of the neck (62 per cent of respondents), whereas migraine headache is more common around the eye (60.2 per cent).[14] Hypertension headache is often described as localized to the back or top of the head.

2. *Does your headache occur at a particular time of*

day? A migraine headache often awakens the patient from sleep, a hypertensive headache is generally worse in the morning, and a tension headache may become worse as the day progresses.[14] Headaches related to brain tumors often occur in the morning and subside during the day.[15]

3. *Do you see spots before your eyes, blind spots, or flashing lights?* Such symptoms occur in 40.8 per cent of migraine patients.[14]

4. *Is your headache associated with trauma or exertion?* An affirmative answer suggests the presence of subarachnoid hemorrhage, concussion, neoplasm, or hypertension.

5. *Have you been sick with a fever recently?* If so, an intracranial or extracranial infectious disease may be the cause of the acute headache.

6. *Have you ever had cancer of the lung, breast, or other area?* If so, a metastatic lesion must be ruled out.

7. *Do you have weakness in your legs or arms?* An affirmative answer is a red flag strongly suggesting an intracranial lesion.

8. *What sort of special stress is present in your life at this time?* This open-ended question forces the patient to consider emotional causes of headache.

9. *What drugs—over-the-counter, prescribed, or "recreational"—do you use?* The examiner should consider both drug side effects and withdrawal symptoms.

10. *Have you ever taken an ergot preparation?* One-fourth of migraine patients give an affirmative answer to this question.[14]

PHYSICAL EXAMINATION

Although the extent of the physical examination will be determined by the patient's age, the history of the present illness, and other circumstances of the chief complaint, certain basic data should always be recorded.

In their study of 124 consecutive emergency department records of adults presenting with a chief complaint of headache, Dickman and Masten found the following information to be fundamental to an accurate diagnosis.[4]

Temperature Determination. Only 4.8 per cent of patients in their study had a temperature in excess of 38.2° C (100.6° F).

Blood Pressure Measurements. A diastolic blood pressure of greater than 100 mm Hg was recorded in 6.5 per cent of patients.

Head and Neck Examination. This includes thorough assessment of the head, eyes, ears, nose, throat, sinuses, and related structures. Changes that may be noted include ptosis, pupillary abnormalities, discharge from the nose or ear, pharyngitis, tenderness or opacification of the paranasal sinuses, and enlarged cervical lymph nodes.

Neurologic Examination. The focus and extent of the neurologic examination depends on the history, vital signs, and findings of head and neck examination. Important data include the patient's emotional state, intellectual function, affect, speech, and mental status. There should be an assessment of the function of all cranial nerves. The motor system should be tested for tone, strength, and function. Sensory function examination includes tests for deep and superficial pain perception, vibratory sense, perception of hot and cold, proprioception, and balance sense. The examination of the reflexes should include the corneal and pupillary responses, deep tendon and abdominal reflexes, and specialized signs (e.g., Babinski, Kernig, Brudzinski).

Physical Findings and Their Significance: Key Findings

Because an elevated temperature is uncommon with acute headaches, the detection of fever is a sign that the cause may be an intracranial or extracranial infection.

In a study by Dhopesh and colleagues, 13 (31 per cent) of 42 patients thought to have headaches related to hypertension had diastolic blood pressures of less than 99 mm Hg, and the remainder had blood pressures above 99 mm Hg; almost all were known hypertensives.[2] Another study, however, found no correlation between headache and hypertension unless the diastolic blood pressure was more than 130 mm Hg.[16]

Examination of the head and neck may reveal evidence of papilledema, pupillary abnormalities, or nuchal rigidity, all signs suggesting severe central nervous system (CNS) disease.

Significant findings on neurologic examination are listed in Table 2.

Louis has proposed a simple bedside test using the Valsalva maneuver and superficial temporal artery compression to discriminate between extracranial and intracranial vascular dilatation headache.[17] The patient performs Valsalva's maneuver for approximately 5 seconds and relaxes, and then repeats the maneuver while the physician obstructs both superficial temporal arteries with pressure anterior to the tragus. During both phases of the maneuver the patient is asked to comment on the state of the headache. In all vascular dilatation headaches the pain improves during straining and increases following the end of straining in a crescendo, gradually settling thereafter. In the second part of the test the pain returns only when the vessel pressure is released, if the headache is due to dilatation of the external carotid system. Patients with intracranial or both types of dilatation note that pain is improved during Valsalva's ma-

Table 2. NEUROLOGIC FINDINGS IN ACUTE HEADACHE

Finding	Significance and Possible Causes
Visual field defects	Hysteria Tumor Optic neuritis Multiple sclerosis
Blindness	Methanol, ethanol, or other drug poisoning Hysteria
Ptosis	Aneurysm of the basilar arteries Brain tumor
Oculomotor palsy	Brain tumor Cerebral thrombosis or hemorrhage Complicated migraine
Facial weakness	Stroke Bell's palsy
Hearing impairment	Ear infection Acoustic neuroma
Soft palate immobility, dysphagia, or slowing of heart rate due to vagus nerve lesions	Tumor Cerebral hemorrhage Intracranial infection
Torticollis	Trauma or infection of the cervical vertebra Tumor Enlargement of cervical lymph nodes
Tongue deviation	Cerebral hemorrhage Tumor
Change in muscle tone	CNS bleeding or tumor
Tremor	Stress Alcoholism Hysteria
Gait disturbance	Alcoholism Cerebellar lesion
Hyperactive deep tendon reflexes	CNS tumor Stroke
Hypoactive deep tendon reflexes	Severe infectious disease Status post convulsion or stroke
Upgoing Babinski's reflex	Recent epileptic seizure Upper motor neuron lesion
Kernig's or Brudzinski's sign	Meningitis
Sensory deficit	Meningitis Stroke Tumor

neuver and is only partially helped or is not helped at all by obstruction of both superficial temporal arteries. Straining produces no change in the headache of patients with encephalitis or meningitis.[17]

Other examinations that may be useful include: general physical examination to detect evidence of primary or metastatic cancer, joint examination for evidence of rheumatic disease, skin examination for signs of herpes zoster, transillumination of the maxillary and frontal sinuses, determination of ocular tension to detect evidence of glaucoma, and examination of the bite to detect TMJ dysfunction.

DIAGNOSTIC STUDIES

Although history and physical examination constitute the basis upon which most acute headaches are assessed and diagnosed, laboratory tests are necessary in a small but significant group of patients. Of the 18 million headache patients reported in the National Ambulatory Medical Care Survey for 1977–1978, 16.2 per cent required clinical laboratory tests and 9.0 per cent received x-rays; other tests utilized included electrocardiogram (ECG), vision test, and blood pressure check.[1]

Laboratory Tests

Useful laboratory determinations in acute headache include complete blood count, erythrocyte sedimentation rate, blood chemistry tests, serologic test for syphilis, thyroid function tests, and cultures and other clinical laboratory tests performed on blood, urine, exudates, or other material. In the group of emergency department patients described by Dickman and Masten, 18 per cent had complete blood counts, 22.2 per cent had blood chemistry tests, 2.4 per cent had erythrocyte sedimentation rate determinations, and 0.8 per cent had urinalyses. Specialized tests that might be performed on blood or urine include a slide test for infectious mononucleosis, complement fixation or hemagglutination tests for various infectious diseases, thick blood smear for malaria, assays for toxic chemicals, carboxyhemoglobin determination, urinary determinations of 5-hydroxyindoleacetic acid and catecholamines, and assays for various prescription and illicit drugs.

Diagnostic Imaging

Routine radiographs of the skull continue to be useful, particularly when localized bony tenderness is noted, metastatic bone disease of the skull is suspected, or a pituitary abnormality is considered.[3] Other abnormalities that might be detected are widening of suture lines (or fontanelles in the infant) owing to increased intracranial pressure and shifting of the pineal gland, suggestive of an intracranial mass. Certain brain tumors, such as craniopharyngioma and meningioma, contain calcium and can be seen on routine skull x-rays,[15] although use of the CT scan is preferred in such instances.[3]

The radionuclide brain scan, useful in detecting isodense subdural hematomas or primary and metastatic brain tumors, is used less often than in the past, owing to the popularity of CT scanning. Angiography, ventriculography, and pneumoencephalography are seldom used in the assessment of acute headaches.

Sinus x-rays that reveal opacification may help to confirm a diagnosis of headache owing to referred pain from nasal and sinus structures.

The chest x-ray may reveal pneumonia or tuberculosis as a cause of systemic symptoms or a lung tumor as the origin of cerebral metastasis.

Computed tomography remains the "gold standard" in the assessment of complicated headache syndromes. The CT scan, with and without contrast enhancement, was found to be the most accurate and most informative neurodiagnostic method in evaluating 2,928 patients, 1,071 of whom had intracranial tumors.[18] A CT scan was ordered in 18 (4 per cent) of 485 emergency department patients in the series reported by Leicht, eight of whom had abnormal findings.[3] Leicht concluded, "The CT scan has become the emergency procedure of choice, when available, for any stable patient with suspected intracranial tumor, intracranial bleed, including subarachnoid hemorrhage, brain abscess, and obstruction to CSF flow."[3] There is controversy regarding the use of CT scans in evaluation of headache problems, however.[19] In a study of 161 selected patients with headache who were reviewed to determine the cost effectiveness of neurodiagnostic evaluations, Larson and associates concluded that a carefully taken history and thorough physical and neurologic examinations were adequate to detect intracranial mass lesions or systemic disease associated with headache, and that in patients with normal neurologic findings, no clinically significant abnormalities were detected by CT scan, skull roentgenogram, angiography, or radionuclide brain scan.[20]

Other Tests

The electroencephalogram (EEG) may be important, particularly when a seizure equivalent is suspected in a pediatric patient. Jay and Tomasi found the EEG to be significant in differentiating between migraine headaches and recurrent seizures.[5] The electroencephalogram may aid in localization of a cortical tumor with enlarged delta waves that correspond to the site of a neoplasm.

Audiometry may help detect an acoustic neuroma.

An electrocardiogram was ordered in 9.7 per cent of emergency department patients reviewed by Dickman and Masten, whose final diagnostic impression was hypertension in 10 per cent of these patients.[4]

Lumbar puncture is mandatory when meningitis or encephalitis is suspected and a mass lesion is unlikely. Opening and closing pressures and fluid color should be carefully noted, and a specimen should be sent for cell count, and glucose, protein, chloride, and urea determinations. When intracranial bleeding is suspected, lumbar puncture should be deferred until a CT scan has been obtained, because in the presence of intracranial bleeding a lumbar puncture examination either can be hazardous or can yield a false-negative result.

Thermography has limited utility in diagnosis of acute headache and is chiefly used in demonstrating vascular changes during acute migraine attacks.

ASSESSMENT

The physician solves complicated diagnostic problems by following a sequence of steps: aggregation of groups of findings into patterns, selection of a "pivot" or key finding, generation of a cause list, pruning of the cause list, selection of a diagnosis, and validation of the diagnosis.[21] The physician assessing the patient with an acute headache must keep in mind that there are a few potentially serious and life-threatening causes that must be accorded due regard in diagnosis.

Constellations of Findings

The following are constellations of findings that characterize the various types of acute headaches listed in Table 3. Key findings are printed in italics.

Extracranial Infections. The most common causes of headaches, extracranial infections include a wide variety of diseases likely to be manifested as *fever*, malaise, lethargy, and loss of appetite in the absence of nuchal rigidity or mental change. There may also be nausea, vomiting, diarrhea, cough, or sore throat. Other persons in the patient's household may have similar symptoms.

Psychogenic Causes. Within this group is the tension (muscle contraction) headache, which the patient generally describes as "tightness" or "pressure." Patients with psychogenic headache may have anxiety, depression, or conversion reaction. There may accordingly be signs of autonomic hyperactivity (anxiety), vegetative signs such as anorexia or insomnia (depression), or symbolization and secondary gain (conversion headache).[10] A *history of personal or family stress* and a lack of significant physical findings are likely.

Post-Traumatic Headache. These patients have in common a *history of trauma to the head or neck,* although careful questioning of family and friends may be necessary to elicit this important bit of data. There may or may not be focal neurologic signs. Fever is generally absent. A skull x-ray or CT scan will detect any evidence of fracture or intracranial bleeding.

Hypertensive Headache. Patients with this diagnosis are likely to have a history of *high blood pressure,* whether treated or untreated. Physical examination reveals elevated diastolic blood pressure in most but not all.[2] The headache is often described as an occipital pain present upon awakening, becoming less intense during the day, and sometimes aggravated by physical activity. The detection of elevated blood pressure is not sufficient evidence that an acute headache is being caused by hypertension.

Vascular Headache of the Migraine Type. This group of headaches, which includes migraine and cluster headaches, has in common *episodic* cephalgia that is generally *one-sided,* and an absence of permanent structural changes. The recurrent nature of these headaches is generally sufficient to distinguish them from other types of acute headache.

Intracranial Bleeding or Thrombosis. Patients with intracranial bleeding or thrombosis generally complain of very severe headaches of *rather sudden onset.* The patient may have a stiff neck or hemiparesis. Focal *neurologic signs* may be noted. A *CT scan* generally reveals the lesion.

Intracranial Infection. Encephalitis, meningitis, or brain abscess is likely to be associated with fever, systemic signs of toxicity, and *nuchal rigidity.* There may be impairment of mental function. The *lumbar puncture* examination shows CSF leukocytosis and other changes.

Vascular Headache of the Nonmigraine Type. There may be a *history of drug (including alcohol) use or exposure to toxic chemicals.* Hypoglycemia is a rare cause of acute headache.

Traction Headache. The pain is often described as deep, dull, steady, and oppressive. Throbbing is uncommon. Coughing or bending may abruptly increase the headache, and assuming an upright posture may bring relief. There may be nausea, vomiting, and dizziness—all concomitants of migraine that can complicate the diagnosis. If the cause is a tumor, the *CT findings* will be diagnostic.

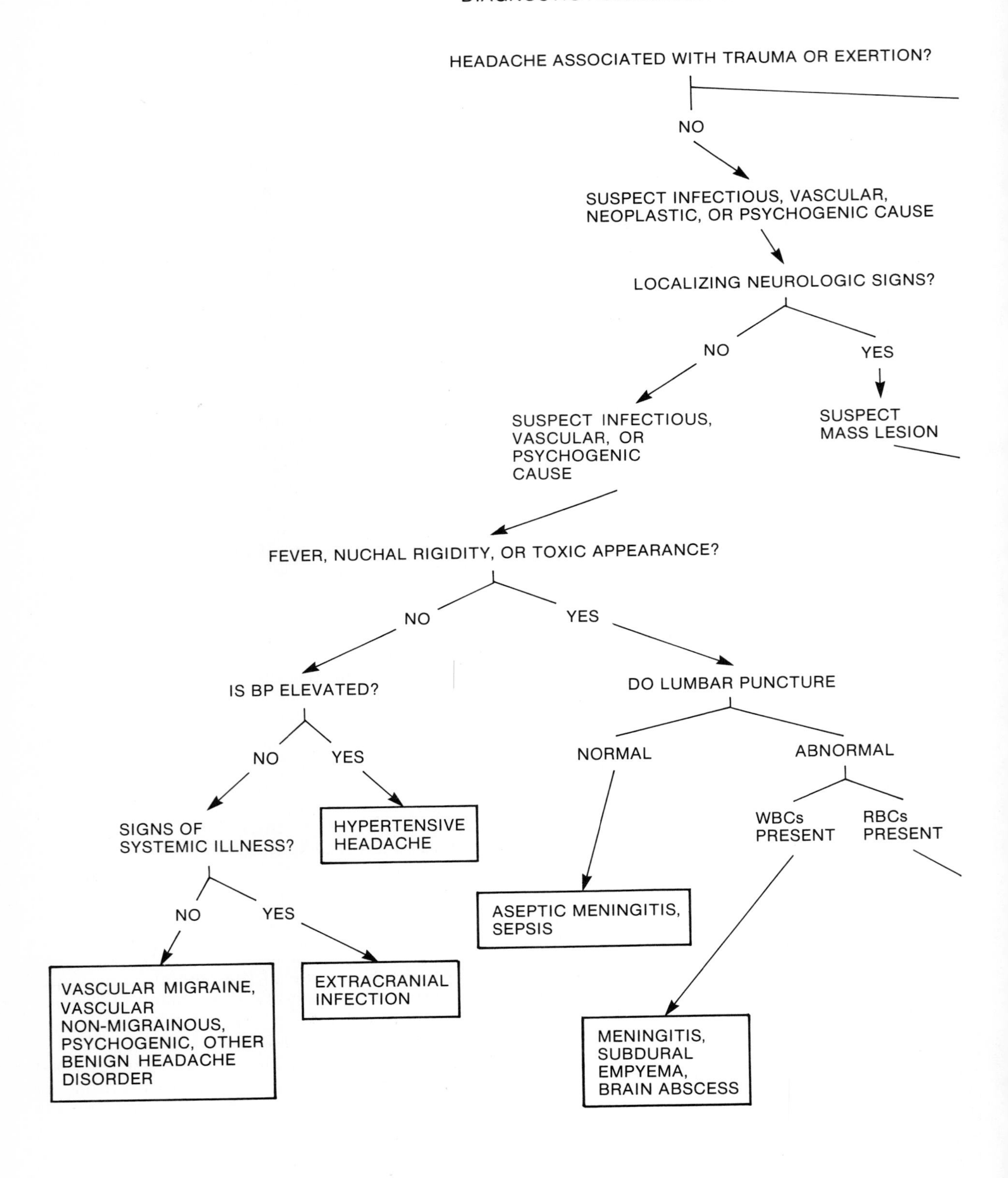
DIAGNOSTIC ASSESSMENT OF ACUTE HEADACHE
HEADACHE ASSOCIATED WITH TRAUMA OR EXERTION?
NO
SUSPECT INFECTIOUS, VASCULAR, NEOPLASTIC, OR PSYCHOGENIC CAUSE
LOCALIZING NEUROLOGIC SIGNS?
NO
YES
SUSPECT INFECTIOUS, VASCULAR, OR PSYCHOGENIC CAUSE
SUSPECT MASS LESION
FEVER, NUCHAL RIGIDITY, OR TOXIC APPEARANCE?
NO
YES
IS BP ELEVATED?
DO LUMBAR PUNCTURE
NO
YES
NORMAL
ABNORMAL
SIGNS OF SYSTEMIC ILLNESS?
HYPERTENSIVE HEADACHE
WBCs PRESENT
RBCs PRESENT
NO
YES
ASEPTIC MENINGITIS, SEPSIS
VASCULAR MIGRAINE, VASCULAR NON-MIGRAINOUS, PSYCHOGENIC, OTHER BENIGN HEADACHE DISORDER
EXTRACRANIAL INFECTION
MENINGITIS, SUBDURAL EMPYEMA, BRAIN ABSCESS

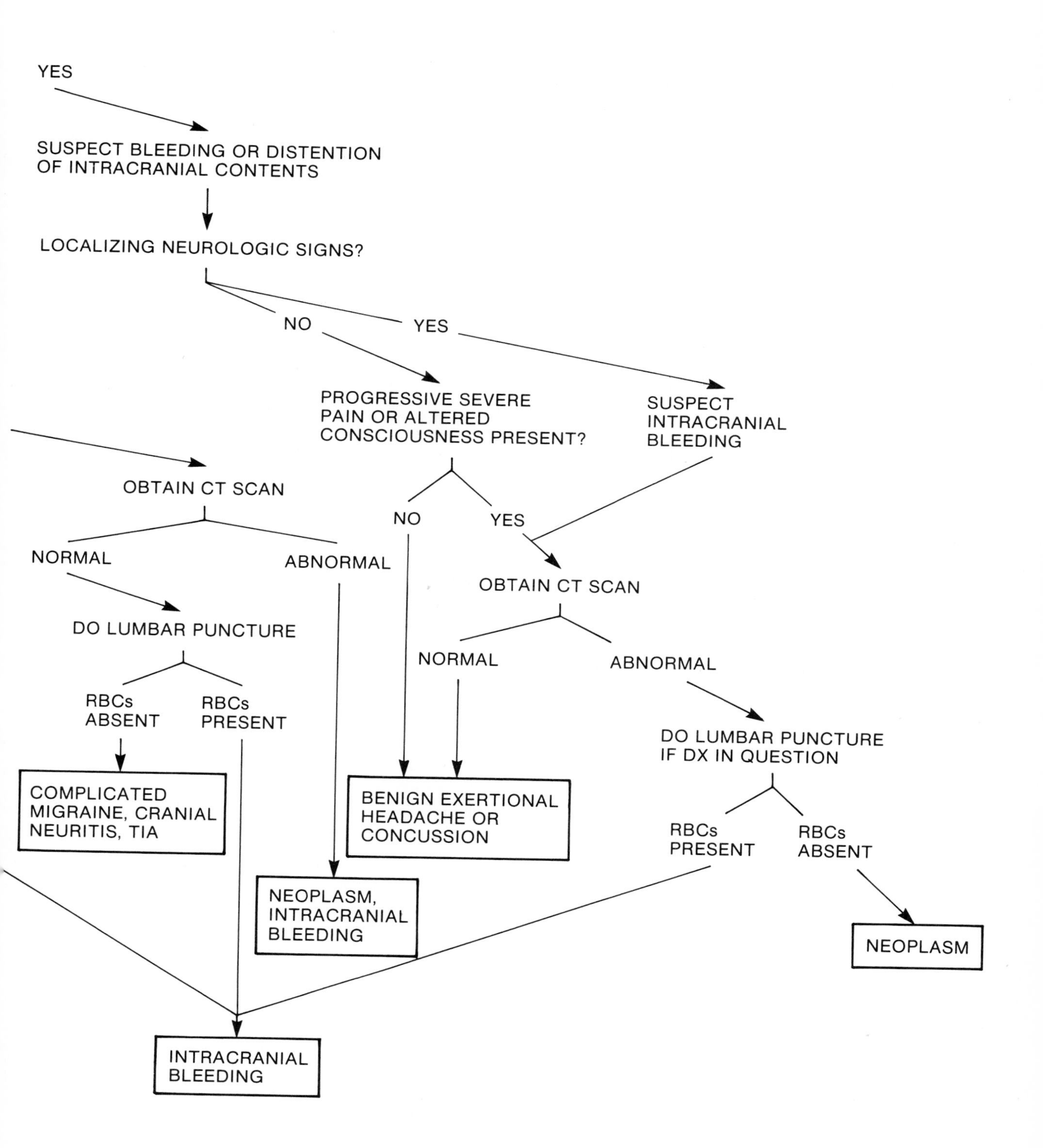
YES
SUSPECT BLEEDING OR DISTENTION OF INTRACRANIAL CONTENTS
LOCALIZING NEUROLOGIC SIGNS?
NO
YES
PROGRESSIVE SEVERE PAIN OR ALTERED CONSCIOUSNESS PRESENT?
SUSPECT INTRACRANIAL BLEEDING
OBTAIN CT SCAN
NO
YES
NORMAL
ABNORMAL
OBTAIN CT SCAN
DO LUMBAR PUNCTURE
NORMAL
ABNORMAL
RBCs ABSENT
RBCs PRESENT
DO LUMBAR PUNCTURE IF DX IN QUESTION
COMPLICATED MIGRAINE, CRANIAL NEURITIS, TIA
BENIGN EXERTIONAL HEADACHE OR CONCUSSION
RBCs PRESENT
RBCs ABSENT
NEOPLASM, INTRACRANIAL BLEEDING
NEOPLASM
INTRACRANIAL BLEEDING

Table 3. CAUSES OF ACUTE HEADACHE

Extracranial infection	Febrile illness of childhood
	  Measles
	  Mumps
	  Tonsillitis
	Infectious mononucleosis
	Influenza
	Malaria
	Otitis media or externa
	Salmonellosis
	Sinusitis
	Trichinosis
	Tularemia

Psychogenic	Tension (muscle contraction) headache
	Headache related to specific psychiatric syndromes
	  Anxiety
	  Depression
	  Conversion reaction

Post-traumatic	Concussion Contusion of brain Traumatic dysautonomic cephalgia
Hypertension	Essential hypertension Pheochromocytoma

Migraine-type vascular	Migraine headache
	  Classic
	  Common
	  Complicated
	  Cyclical
	Cluster headache
	Migraine variants (e.g. orgasmic headache)

Intracranial bleeding or related cause	Aneurysm Arteriovenous malformation Intracerebral bleeding Subarachnoid bleeding Subdural bleeding Vascular insufficiency (transient ischemic attack)
Intracranial infection	Brain abscess Encephalitis Meningitis Subdural empyema

Nonmigraine vascular	Drug effects
	  Vasodilators
	  Oral contraceptives
	  Indomethacin
	Drug withdrawal
	  Amphetamines
	  Ergot preparations
	  Caffeine
	Toxic chemicals
	  Benzene
	  Nitrates
	  Tyramine
	  Phenylethylamine
	  Monosodium glutamate
	  Carbon monoxide
	  Carbon tetrachloride
	  Insecticides
	  Lead
	Alcohol (hangover)
	Fever
	Hypoxia
	Hypoglycemia

Traction	Brain swelling
	Brain tumor
	  Primary
	  Metastatic
	Obstruction of CSF flow
	Post–lumbar puncture

Miscellaneous	Benign exertional headache
	Eye/visual causes
	  Glaucoma
	  Refractive error, e.g., astigmatism, hyperopia
	  Iritis
	Cranial neuritis or neuralgia
	Benign intracranial hypertension
	TMJ pain-dysfunction syndrome
	Temporal arteritis

Miscellaneous Causes. This extremely diverse group of causes (see Table 3 for a list) can be responsible for a variety of clinical syndromes, which *differ according to the cause of the headache.* The onset of headache in the person over age 60 should suggest temporal arteritis.

Diagnostic Approach

The algorithm illustrates a logical diagnostic approach to the patient with an acute headache, one that aims to identify first those causes of headache that necessitate prompt intervention. The algorithm stops short of differentiating among the many benign chronic headache syndromes.

Implications of Acute Headache

Acute headache syndromes do not always fall neatly into diagnostic categories. For example, sinus headache may be associated with stress.[22] The patient with a conversion headache may have suffered severe trauma.[10] There may be significant overlap between migraine and tension headaches.[2] Therefore, while striving for diagnostic specificity, the physician must first exclude the possibility of serious or life-threatening causes.

Fortunately, life-threatening causes of acute headache are uncommon. Dhopesh and colleagues have reported that only 11 (1.2 per cent) of 872 patients in their study of emergency department headache complaints had serious neurologic conditions.[2] Only two (1.6 per cent) of the 124 patients studied by Dickman and Masten had neurologic disease.[4] Leicht reported a 5 per cent incidence of serious neurologic conditions in his group of 485 ED patients.[3] Using the diagnostic approach described in this chapter, the clinician should be able to identify such serious neurologic disorders early, thus allowing prompt treatment of illnesses that may cause disability or death and permitting subsequent evaluation of the more common but less serious acute headache syndromes.

REFERENCES

1. Headache as the reason for office visit. National Ambulatory Medical Care Survey: United States, 1977–78. Advanced data from vital and health statistics of the National Center for Health Statistics. U.S. Department of Health and Human Services, Public Health Service, Office of Health Research, Statistics, and Technology, 1981;67:1–7.
2. Dhopesh V, Anwar R, Herring C. A retrospective assessment of emergency department patients with complaint of headache. Headache 1979;19:37–42.
3. Leicht MJ. Nontraumatic headache in the emergency department. Ann Emerg Med 1980;9:404–9.
4. Dickman RL, Masten T. The management of nontraumatic headache in a university hospital emergency room. Headache 1979;19:391–6.
5. Jay GW, Tomasi LG. Pediatric headaches: a one year retrospective analysis. Headache 1981;21:5–9.
6. Downey R, Antunes JL, Michelsen WJ. Hemorrhage within brain tumors during jogging. Ann Neurol 1980;7:496.
7. Paulson GW, Zipf RE, Beekman JF. Pheochromocytoma causing exercise-related headache and pulmonary edema. Ann Neurol 1979;5:96–8.
8. Medina JL, Diamond S. Cyclical migraine. Arch Neurol 1981;38:343–4.
9. Weatherhead AD. Psychogenic headache. Headache 1980;20:47–54.
10. Packard RC. Conversion headache. Headache 1980;20:266–8.
11. Reik L Jr, Hale M. The temporomandibular joint pain-dysfunction syndrome: a frequent cause of headache. Headache 1981;21:151–6.
12. Stein GS. Headaches in the first post partum week and their relationship to migraine. Headache 1981;21:201–5.
13. Taylor RB, Burdette JA, Camp L, Edwards J. Purpose of the medical encounter: Identification and influence on process and outcome in 200 encounters. J Fam Pract 1980;10:495–500.
14. Diehr P, Wood RW, Barr V, Wolcott B, Slay L, Tompkins RK. Acute headaches: presenting symptoms and diagnostic rules to identify patients with tension and migraine headaches. J Chronic Dis 1981;34:147–58.
15. Ebersold MJ. The early diagnosis of brain tumors. Cont Educ Fam Phys 1981;15(2):15–20.
16. Badran RH, Weir RG, McGuiness JB. Hypertension and headache. Scot Med J 1970;15:48–51.
17. Louis S. A bedside test for determining the sub-types of vascular headache. Headache 1981;21:87–8.
18. Baker HL, Houser OW, Campbell K. Evaluation of computed tomography in the diagnosis of intracranial neoplasms. Radiology 1980;136:91–6.
19. Sargent JD, Lawson RC, Solbach P, Coyne L. Use of CT scans in an out-patient headache population: an evaluation. Headache 1979;19:388–90.
20. Larson EB, Omenn GS, Lewis H. Diagnostic evaluation of headache: impact of computerized tomography and cost-effectiveness. JAMA 1980;243:359–62.
21. Eddy DM, Clanton CH. The art of diagnosis. N Engl J Med 1982;306:1263–8.
22. Hamilton JG Jr, Haynes SN, Gannon L, Safranek RA. Sinus headache: a psychophysiological study. Headache 1980;20:258–60.

HEMATURIA

GEORGE S. BENSON □ EILEEN D. BREWER

□ SYNONYM: Blood in the urine

BACKGROUND

Every patient who presents with hematuria, either gross or microscopic, requires evaluation. Although multiple factors merit consideration, the patient's age and sex and the relationship of the hematuria to trauma are of primary importance in governing the direction and extent of the evaluation. For example, glomerulonephritis is responsible for 40 to 50 per cent of cases of hematuria in children referred for evaluation of nontraumatic gross or microscopic hematuria.[1, 2] Neoplasia, primarily Wilms' tumor and bladder and prostatic rhabdomyosarcoma, is an uncommon cause of hematuria in this age group. On the contrary, neoplasia, both benign and malignant, is the most common cause of hematuria in the hospitalized adult, and glomerulonephritis is uncommonly diagnosed in adults.[3] Accordingly, each discussion in this chapter is further subdivided into consideration of the symptom in the adult, in the child, and secondary to trauma.

No one will argue that gross hematuria is an important symptom that requires evaluation. The definition of significant microscopic hematuria is, however, controversial. In children, microscopic hematuria has been defined as more than five red blood cells per high-powered field in a centrifuged sediment in at least two of three successive urinalyses.[4] In the adult, however, such a definition may lead to diagnostic error, because bladder and renal cancers may bleed intermittently. When in doubt, the physician should personally examine the urine under the microscope. If doubt persists, a reasonable screening laboratory and radiologic evaluation is preferable to possibly overlooking significant urinary tract disease.

HISTORY

Hematuria in the Adult

In general, the presence of hematuria in the adult requires laboratory and radiographic evaluation, and the history is of paramount importance in determining the extent and direction of this investigation. The primary goal of history-taking is to distinguish between lower urinary tract (urethra, prostate, and bladder) and upper urinary tract (kidneys and ureters) symptoms and to determine a reasonable differential diagnosis on the basis of patient's age and sex.

Hematuria associated with urinary frequency, urgency, dysuria, and suprapubic pain in the young female is most commonly the result of cystitis secondary to a gram-negative bacterial infection. Similar symptoms in a young male are commonly associated with prostatitis or urethral stricture disease. In the older male one must consider infection associated with bladder outlet obstruction caused by benign prostatic hyperplasia, prostatic cancer, or urethral stricture. Therefore, the presence of obstructive symptoms—hesitancy, straining to void, and decreased force and caliber of the urinary stream—should be ascertained in male patients with hematuria.

The presence of flank or upper abdominal pain is usually indicative of hematuria originating in the upper urinary tract. Pain that radiates from the flank or abdomen to the testis or labia is commonly seen with an obstructing ureteral stone. Similar pain may also occur with ureteral obstruction caused by blood clots, which may be secondary to a bleeding renal cell carcinoma or sickle cell disease, or a sloughed renal papillus, which may be associated with diabetes mellitus, sickle cell disease, tuberculosis, or phenacetin abuse. Therefore, detailed patient history and family history relating to these disease entities should be obtained. In the older patient, flank pain and hematuria may be caused by a renal artery embolus. A history of heart disease and cardiac medications is mandatory for proper evaluation.

Hematuria associated with fever, particularly in the female, is also usually associated with upper urinary tract infection. Significant fever is rarely, if ever, present in patients with uncomplicated cystitis. In the female, hematuria associated with fever may be secondary to nonobstructive pyelonephritis or a "closed-space" infection with ureteral obstruction caused by any of the disease states discussed in the preceding paragraph. In the male, hematuria and fever (particularly in the presence of lower urinary tract symptoms) may indicate the presence of prostatitis or prostatic abscess. Fever, usually chronic and low-grade, is occasionally associated with renal cell carcinoma.

Otherwise-asymptomatic hematuria, particularly in patients over the age of 40, should alert the examining physician to the possibility of urinary tract cancer. Occupational exposure in the aniline dye, rubber, and petroleum industries and cigarette smoking have been linked to bladder cancer.[5, 6] Subtle and relatively nonspecific bone pain may be secondary to metastatic prostatic carcinoma. Otherwise-asymptomatic hematuria is a common presentation of renal as well as bladder carcinoma. Flank and nonspecific abdominal pain may also occur in the patient with a renal cancer; in addition, symptoms secondary to paraneoplastic syndromes are occasionally associated with this tumor.[7] The presence of diarrhea, symptoms of peripheral neuropathy, and confusion or lethargy secondary to hypercalcemia should be noted. Other significant disease entities, such as adult polycystic kidney disease, may also be present in the patient with hematuria who is otherwise asymptomatic.

Cyclical hematuria occurring at the time of the menstrual cycle strongly suggests the presence of a bladder endometrioma. Drugs such as cyclophosphamide and anticoagulants may be directly responsible for urinary blood. Hematuria has been reported after exercise (in joggers, marathon runners, etc.), but a history of jogging does not preclude further urologic evaluation.[8] In addition, symptoms compatible with a glomerular lesion—edema, hypertension, arthralgias, and antecedent pharyngitis—should be sought in the young adult as well as in the child.

Hematuria in the Child

Hematuria is one of the most important early markers of significant renal or urologic disease in childhood. The diagnostic evaluation will vary depending on whether the hematuria is associated with an acute illness or trauma, or whether it is discovered in an asymptomatic child during a routine well-child, school, or pre-camp physical examination. A careful history is important at the outset to establish whether the hematuria is associated with symptoms.

Pain in the abdomen or flank, fever, frequency, urgency, or dysuria suggests a urinary tract infection. In the infant or younger child, only fever or lower abdominal pain may be the presenting symptom. Severe abdominal pain may occur with renal or ureteral stones in a child who has recurrent infections and a congenital anomaly of the urinary tract or a metabolic disorder (hypercalciuria, renal tubular acidosis, cystinuria, primary hyperoxaluria) predisposing to stone formation.

Swelling suggests that glomerulonephritis is the cause of hematuria. In the child, swelling may first be noted by parents when the child's clothes are too tight at the waist or when the eyes are swollen on awakening in the morning. Specific inquiries about these symptoms are often necessary to determine how long swelling has been present. If the onset of swelling and hematuria is acute, postinfectious glomerulonephritis should be suspected, and a history of a sore throat or impetiginous skin infection preceding the symptoms by 7 to 10 days should be sought. According to one study of children presenting with edema and nephrotic syndrome, hematuria may be present in as many as 25 per cent of cases of minimal change nephrotic syndrome and 50 per cent of cases of focal segmental glomerulosclerosis or membranoproliferative glomerulonephritis.[9]

Other forms of glomerulonephritis may also be suggested by specific symptoms associated with hematuria. A purpuric rash of the lower extremities, joint pains, abdominal pain, and hematuria are characteristic of Henoch-Schönlein purpura. A transient malar flush or butterfly rash on the face and arthritis or arthralgias can occur in systemic lupus erythematosus in children. Gross hematuria at the time of an upper respiratory febrile illness in older children and adolescents is suggestive of IgA nephropathy,[10] although many types of glomerulonephritis may result in gross hematuria during a febrile illness. Bloody diarrhea may herald the onset of hemolytic uremic syndrome or Henoch-Schönlein purpura. Severe diarrhea and dehydration in an infant may be followed by hematuria and palpably enlarged kidneys resulting from renal venous thrombosis.

One should always ask about recent trauma or vigorous exercise as a potential explanation for gross or microscopic hematuria. However, for an active, playful young child, a history of mild abdominal or flank trauma that may have nothing to do with the etiology of the hematuria is often quite easily elicited. On occasion it may be necessary to ask the child quite directly whether or not he or she has inserted a foreign body into the urethra or vagina to cause apparent hematuria. Vigorous masturbation in boys occasionally may be a cause of transient microscopic hematuria.

The asymptomatic child with hematuria often presents the most difficult diagnostic dilemma. If the child is asymptomatic, establishing whether the hematuria is gross or microscopic may be helpful. Gross hematuria can be either bright red or brown or tea-colored. Bright red urine suggests trauma to the urinary tract, bladder infection, a kidney stone, or possibly an arteriovenous malformation or hemangioma in the kidney or bladder. Reddish-brown or tea-colored urine, on the other hand, suggests some form of glomerulonephritis. Gross hematuria is often episodic. If so, one should determine whether microscopic hematuria remains when the gross hematuria abates. Such is often the case in IgA nephropathy.[11] Microscopic hematuria can also be episodic or persistent. Asymptomatic episodic microscopic hematuria is often the most difficult type for which to determine the cause.

A few other specific inquiries may be quite useful in the history of a child with hematuria. Does the child have a known bleeding disorder (hemophilia, von Willebrand's disease, idiopathic thrombocytopenic purpura)? Has the child been taking a hematuria-causing drug (methicillin or other penicillin-related drugs, cyclophosphamide, anticoagulants)? Is there a close contact (family member, babysitter) with known tuberculosis? Does the child have a hearing loss, which would suggest Alport's hereditary nephritis?

A careful family history is also essential in the evaluation of hematuria in the child. One should specifically inquire about nephritis or death from kidney or Bright's disease, especially in adult males. A positive response plus a history of the early onset of deafness in family members is highly suggestive of Alport's hereditary nephritis. A history of asymptomatic hematuria in adult family members may suggest the more benign condition, familial hematuria. In black families, a history of sickle disease, sickle trait, and sickle–hemoglobin C disease should be sought. All these conditions may be associated with gross or microscopic hematuria. Polycystic kidney disease of either the infantile or adult form is hereditary and may manifest as hematuria in childhood. In the southeastern and southwestern United States, hematuria associated with hypercalciuria without definite stones has been reported.[12, 13] A family history of renal stone disease may guide the physician to a more careful evaluation for hypercalciuria in the child.

Hematuria Secondary to Trauma

Hematuria, either gross or microscopic, associated with a history of trauma demands immediate evaluation. The history often will localize the source of hematuria to the lower or upper urinary tract. If a patient has sustained significant abdominal or pelvic trauma and has not voided since the injury, trauma to the urinary tract must be presumed until proven otherwise. A "straddle" type injury to the perineum is commonly associated with a bulbus urethral tear. Suprapubic or diffuse abdominal pain with vomiting may be seen with an intraperitoneal bladder rupture. Flank or upper abdominal pain may signify renal injury. It is important to ascertain whether the injury is secondary to blunt or penetrating trauma. Most blunt renal injuries can be managed conservatively, whereas all penetrating renal injuries require surgical intervention. A history outlining prior urologic disease or urologic operative procedures should be obtained. As all of these patients require radiographic evaluation, previous allergic reactions to contrast media should be noted. With penetrating trauma, the patient's tetanus immunization status is important.

PHYSICAL EXAMINATION

Hematuria in the Adult

An elevated temperature (> 101° F) in a patient with hematuria is usually associated with infection (pyelonephritis, prostatitis); minimal temperature elevations (< 101° F) may be associated with a ureteral stone in the absence of associated infection. Tachycardia and hypotension may signify either sepsis or significant blood loss from the urinary tract. Pain associated with ureteral calculi may be responsible for a tachycardia. The heart should be examined for rhythm and murmurs. An irregularly irregular heart rate in the older adult with flank pain and hematuria should raise the possibility of a renal artery embolus from a mural thrombus in association with atrial fibrillation. A cardiac murmur in the patient with hematuria and fever may signify subacute bacterial endocarditis. A pleural effusion is sometimes seen with renal and perirenal infections. Costovertebral angle tenderness is often indicative of pyelonephritis or ureteral obstruction.

Palpation of the upper abdomen may reveal tenderness or guarding secondary to underlying renal disease (infection, hydronephrosis, or intrarenal or perinephric hematoma secondary to bleeding renal tumor). In the adult, normal kidneys are only rarely palpated. Palpable renal masses direct one's attention to renal neoplasms, polycystic kidney disease, and xanthogranulomatous pyelonephritis. A palpable bladder usually signifies bladder outlet obstruction or urinary retention secondary to neurogenic bladder disease.

All females with hematuria should undergo a careful pelvic examination. Suprapubic, urethral, and bladder tenderness are common findings in the female with cystitis. A urethral caruncle or urethral diverticulum should be carefully excluded. The adnexae should be evaluated for masses that may be related to the hematuria (ovarian carcinoma or endometriosis with bladder invasion).

In the male, the genitalia should be specifically examined for evidence of trauma and for meatal condyloma acuminatum. The urethra should be palpated for evidence of carcinoma. Rectal examination to look for rectal and prostate cancer must always be performed as part of the routine examination in the male. A soft, tender prostate usually signifies prostatitis; discrete prostatic nodules or diffuse hardness may indicate carcinoma. A large but otherwise normal-feeling prostate may indicate benign prostatic hyperplasia. Although this disorder is a common cause of hematuria in the older male, the evaluation of the patient's hematuria should not stop before other more serious coexistent conditions are excluded.

Hematuria in the Child

Physical examination in the child should always include comparisons of height and weight measurements with the standards for age. If the height and weight are below the third percentile for age, renal disease and compromised renal function may have been present for a significant period. A blood pressure measurement should also be obtained in any child with hematuria, no matter what the size or age. Normal blood pressure is lower for children than for adults.[14] A reading of 70/40 is normal for a term infant.[15] Blood pressure rises slowly with age, to reach adult normal in the teen years. Thus, a blood pressure of 120/80, which would be normal for an adult, would be hypertensive for a 3-year-old. If hypertension is present, funduscopic examination may reveal the arteriolar narrowing of long-standing hypertension or, occasionally, hemorrhages associated with acute hypertension. The child's temperature should also be recorded. Fever may or may not be associated with urinary tract infections. Many types of glomerulonephritis may lead to gross hematuria at the time of a febrile illness.

The skin should be carefully examined for evidence of a rash, skin infection, or petechiae. A purpuric rash on the lower extremities is characteristic of Henoch-Schönlein purpura. Impetigo caused by a nephritogenic strain of streptococcus may be the forerunner of poststreptococcal glomerulonephritis. A malar flush or butterfly rash on the face suggests systemic lupus erythematosus. The presence of scattered petechiae or ecchymoses may indicate a bleeding disorder that can also account for the hematuria.

The child should be carefully examined for the presence of edema. If he or she has been at bedrest during the day or asleep overnight, no ankle edema may be present; however, significant periorbital edema, sacral edema, ascites, or edema of the genitalia may be seen. If the child has been up and active, little periorbital edema may be evident, although there may be ankle edema. In the child with anasarca, pleural effusions may be present. Tachycardia and an enlarged heart may be found on physical examination of the child with acute glomerulonephritis and edema from volume overload.

Examination of the abdomen may reveal suprapubic or flank tenderness in a child with urinary tract infection. Point tenderness along the course of the ureter may be indicative of a ureteral stone. In the infant, hydronephrosis and hydroureter may be appreciated as an abdominal mass. Hematuria occurs transiently in about 15 per cent of patients with hydronephrosis.[16] Infantile polycystic disease or renal venous thrombosis may cause palpably enlarged kidneys and hematuria. In general, kidneys are not normally palpable after the newborn period. Hematuria, especially gross hematuria, can occur with Wilms' tumor, usually at a time when the mass can be palpated. Abdominal tenderness and intussusception may occur with Henoch-Schönlein purpura.

Careful examination of the genitalia may reveal an external abrasion, wound, sore, or diaper rash, which might account for apparent hematuria.

Arthritis and arthralgias accompany some forms of glomerulonephritis, notably Henoch-Schönlein purpura and lupus nephritis. The joints should be evaluated carefully for any signs of swelling, tenderness, increased warmth, or erythema.

In an asymptomatic patient with hematuria, a screening test for hearing loss may be helpful in determining whether Alport's hereditary nephritis is present. Often there are few or no physical findings in a child who may have a significant renal abnormality as the cause for hematuria.

Hematuria Secondary to Trauma

The pulse and blood pressure should be monitored and their values used as a guide for intravenous fluids or blood replacement. A complete physical examination should be performed, with special attention paid to the thorax. Renal trauma is often associated with rib fractures and pulmonary trauma.

Blood is often found at the urethral meatus in patients who have sustained a urethral injury. A palpable bladder usually signifies urinary retention. A urethral injury should also be suspected in patients with a perineal hematoma, a "high-riding" prostate, or a pelvic fracture.

Hematuria is present in the majority of patients with bladder injury. Suprapubic and abdominal tenderness and guarding are usually present, and abdominal distention and ileus often accompany an intraperitoneal rupture. The diagnosis of renal trauma should be entertained if a flank mass, flank tenderness, or abdominal distention is present. In addition, abdominal or flank ecchymoses or evidence of penetrating trauma requires urologic investigation. Because many patients with renal trauma also have trauma to other abdominal organs, a careful physical examination with attention directed toward the spleen and gastrointestinal tract should be undertaken.

DIAGNOSTIC STUDIES AND ASSESSMENT

Hematuria in the Adult

Although the history and physical examination are important in the initial assessment of the adult with hematuria, most patients require further laboratory evaluation (Fig. 1). The exception to this is the young woman with hematuria, signs and symptoms of uncomplicated cystitis, and a positive urine culture result. Such a patient should be treated for cystitis. If a follow-up urinalysis is normal and the culture results are negative, no further investigation is needed.[17] If, however, the hematuria persists after antibiotic therapy, evaluation of hematuria should continue. Hemogloblin electrophoresis should be performed for blacks with hematuria to rule out sickle cell disease or trait. Except in the young woman with cystitis, intravenous pyelography (IVP) is mandatory and usually provides direction for further investigation. If there is clinical doubt concerning the patient's renal function, a serum creatinine measurement should be determined before IVP. A radiolucent filling defect in the renal pelvis or ureter usually represents a transitional cell tumor, blood clot, sloughed renal papillus, or non-opaque stone. A retrograde ureteropyelogram is often helpful in delineating the nature of the filling defect. If a renal pelvic or ureteral tumor is suspected, cystoscopy should be performed to rule out a coexistent bladder tumor.

The finding of a renal parenchymal mass on IVP necessitates determining whether the mass is a tumor or a benign renal cyst. The radiologic evaluation of a renal mass is controversial. In general, we prefer ultrasonography as the initial study in the evaluation of a renal mass. If all criteria for a benign cyst are met, the lesion is aspirated. If clear fluid is obtained and the cytologic findings are negative, no further evaluation is necessary.[18] A mixed or solid ultrasonographic pattern, bloody fluid aspirate, positive cytologic findings, or calcification of the mass requires surgical exploration for diagnosis and therapy. An arteriogram is often helpful before surgery to determine the renal vascular anatomy, to determine renal vein involvement by tumor, or to make an angiographic diagnosis of renal cell carcinoma to allow radical nephrectomy without first inspecting and performing a biopsy of the lesion. Alternatively, computed tomography (CT) scanning may be used to differentiate benign cysts from renal tumors.[19]

Further diagnostic studies are necessary in the evaluation of hematuria in the adult even if the IVP findings are normal. A bladder tumor must be ruled out via cystoscopy. If no bladder tumor is visualized and the IVP findings and serum creatinine level are normal, further evaluation depends primarily on the age of the patient and the degree of hematuria. The evaluation of hematuria in an elderly patient with microscopic hematuria can reasonably stop at this point. A patient who is young or has persistent gross hematuria should have further evaluation. Gross efflux of blood from a ureteral orifice can be evaluated by arteriography (to rule out arteriovenous malformation or fistula), CT scan (to rule out anterior or posterior mass lesions that may not be seen on the IVP), or retrograde ureteropyelography (if the ureter is not completely visualized on the IVP).

Glomerular lesions should be considered in younger patients with persistent microscopic hematuria. Creatinine clearance and quantitative urine protein values should be obtained. With reduced creatinine clearance or significant proteinuria, renal biopsy is usually warranted. Rarer causes of hematuria in the adult (coagulopathies and tuberculosis) should also be considered.

Hematuria in the Child

Hematuria in any child warrants laboratory investigation. The extent of the laboratory investigation depends upon the presence or absence of urinary tract infection, as documented by a urine culture, and the presence or absence of proteinuria or red blood cell casts, as documented by a urinalysis of a fresh urine specimen. A reasonable sequence of laboratory investigation is outlined in Figure 2. If the child has hematuria as well as a positive culture result and symptoms of urinary tract infection, the infection should be treated and follow-up urinalysis and urine culture obtained (Fig. 2*a*). If these test results are negative, no further investigation may be needed, unless the patient is an infant girl, a boy with a first urinary tract infection, a girl with a second urinary tract infection, or a child whose stature is less than the third percentile for standards for age; such children should have an intravenous pyelogram and voiding cystourethrogram. A negative urine culture result should be obtained before a voiding cystourethrogram is performed. Radiographic studies may reveal the presence of congenital anomalies of the urinary tract, stones, or a foreign body in the bladder or urethra that predisposes the child to infection. If the findings on the intravenous pyelogram and the voiding cystourethrogram are normal, evaluation may stop, but if the hematuria persists even after treatment of the infection, the evaluation should continue.

Hematuria alone, without other abnormalities on urinalysis, may require extensive laboratory and radiologic evaluation (Fig. 2*b*). If a lesion of the external genitalia has been identified as a potential cause, urinalysis should be repeated after the lesion heals. Only if hematuria persists on this follow-up urinalysis should further evaluation proceed. If a child is receiving a hematuria-causing drug and the drug can be stopped or changed, a follow-up urinalysis should be performed after the change in therapy; if hematuria persists, further evaluation should proceed. A history of a recent upper respiratory or skin infection always raises

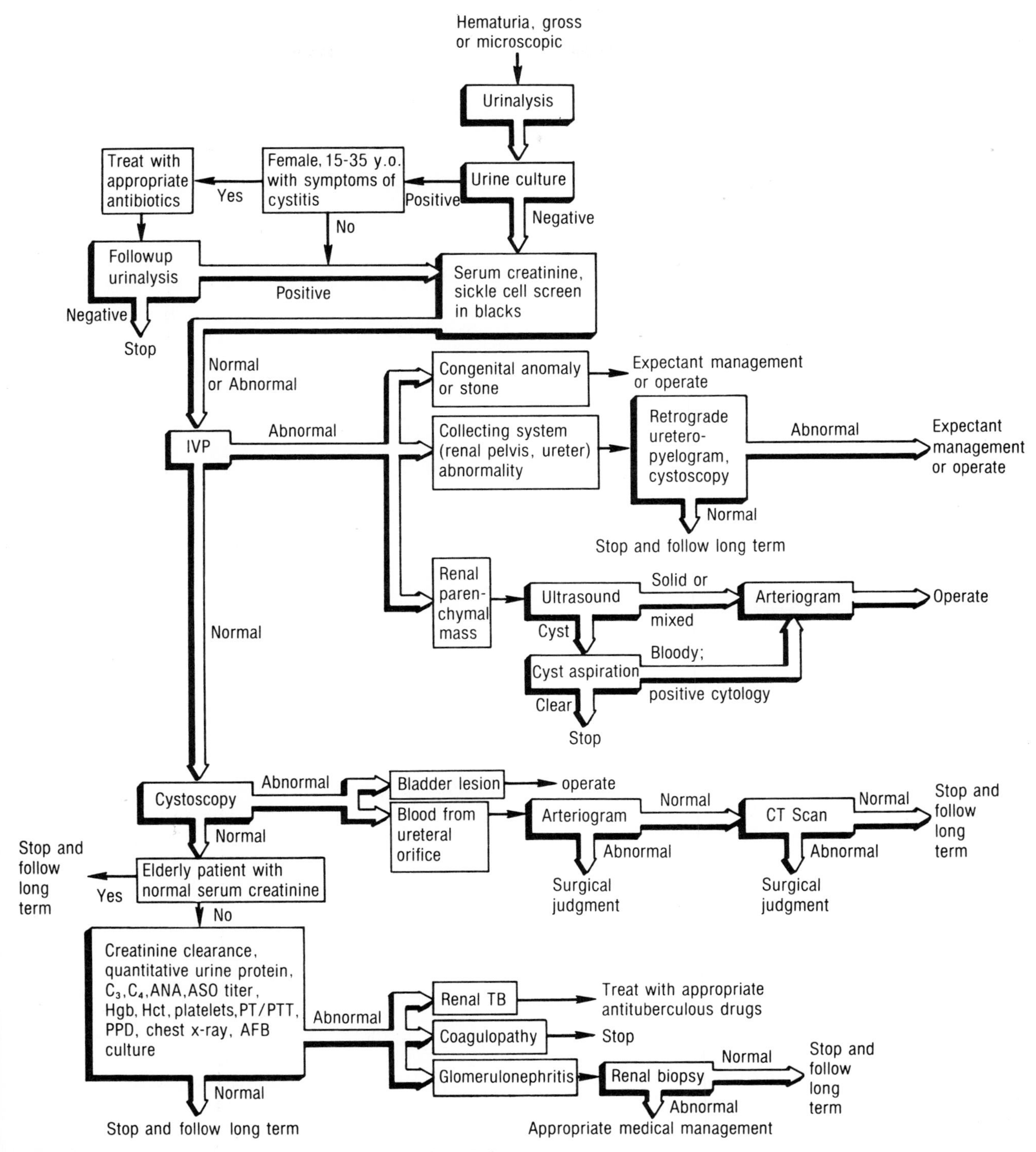

Figure 1. Diagnostic evaluation of hematuria in the adult. *IVP*, intravenous pyelogram; *ANA*, antinuclear antibody; *ASO*, antistreptolysin-O; *Hgb*, hemoglobin; *Hct*, hematocrit; *PT*, prothrombin time; *PTT*, partial thromboplastin time; *AFB*, acid-fast bacillus. (From Benson GS, Brewer ED. Hematuria: algorithms for diagnosis. II. Hematuria in the adult and hematuria secondary to trauma. JAMA 1981; 246:993–6. Copyright 1981, American Medical Association. Reprinted with permission).

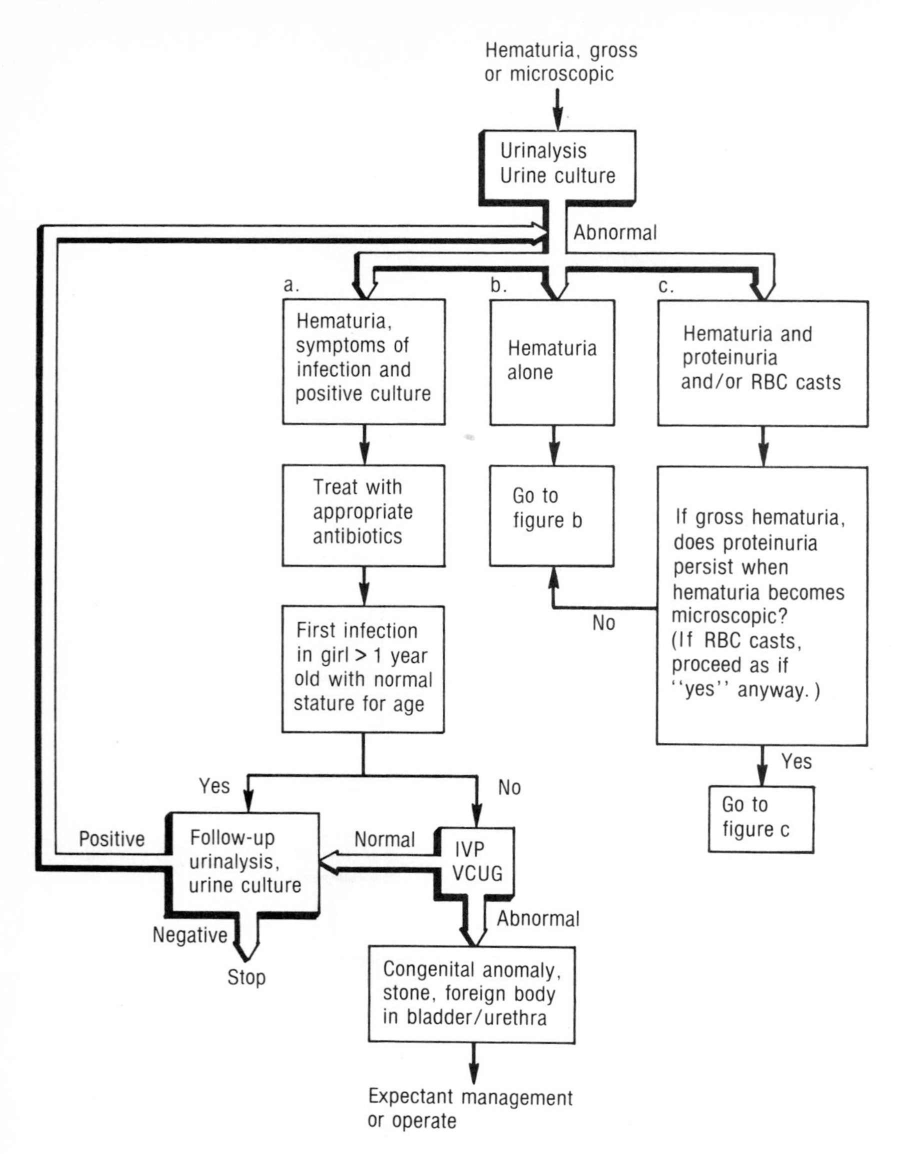

Figure 2. Approach to evaluation of child with hematuria alone, with symptoms of infection and positive culture, and with proteinuria or RBC casts on urinalysis. *VCUG,* voiding cystourethrogram. See Fig. 1 for other abbreviations. (From Brewer ED, Benson GS. Hematuria: algorithms for diagnosis. I. Hematuria in the child. JAMA 1981; 246:877–80. Copyright 1981, American Medical Association. Reprinted with permission).

Illustration continued on opposite page

the possibility of postinfectious glomerulonephritis even in a relatively asymptomatic child. Evidence of a recent streptococcal infection can be either a positive culture result or a rising antistreptolysin O, antihyaluronidase, or antideoxyribonuclease B titer. If there is evidence of a recent streptococcal infection and if the serum C_3 level is low, a presumptive diagnosis can be made and renal function should be assessed. The child may then be followed expectantly with appropriate medical management and no further laboratory investigation. If, however, the serum C_3 level remains low after 1 or 2 months, another form of glomerulonephritis, such as membranoproliferative glomerulonephritis, must be considered and further laboratory evaluation pursued.

In the asymptomatic child with persistent hematuria (present on three urinalyses performed on three different days) or episodic hematuria without other abnormalities on urinalysis, renal function should be tested by determination of the serum creatinine concentration. Normal values for serum creatinine concentrations are lower in children than in adults and will vary with age, sex, and muscle mass.[20] A number of other blood tests may also provide useful information at this stage of the work-up. Early membranoproliferative glomerulonephritis or lupus nephritis may be suspected if the serum concentration of C_3 or C_4 is low. A positive antinuclear antibody titer will help make the diagnosis of lupus nephritis. In black children, a sickle cell screening test is necessary to determine whether the hematuria is associated with sickle cell trait, sickle cell–hemogloblin C disease or sickle cell crisis. Hematuria can be associated with a coagulopathy (hemophilia,

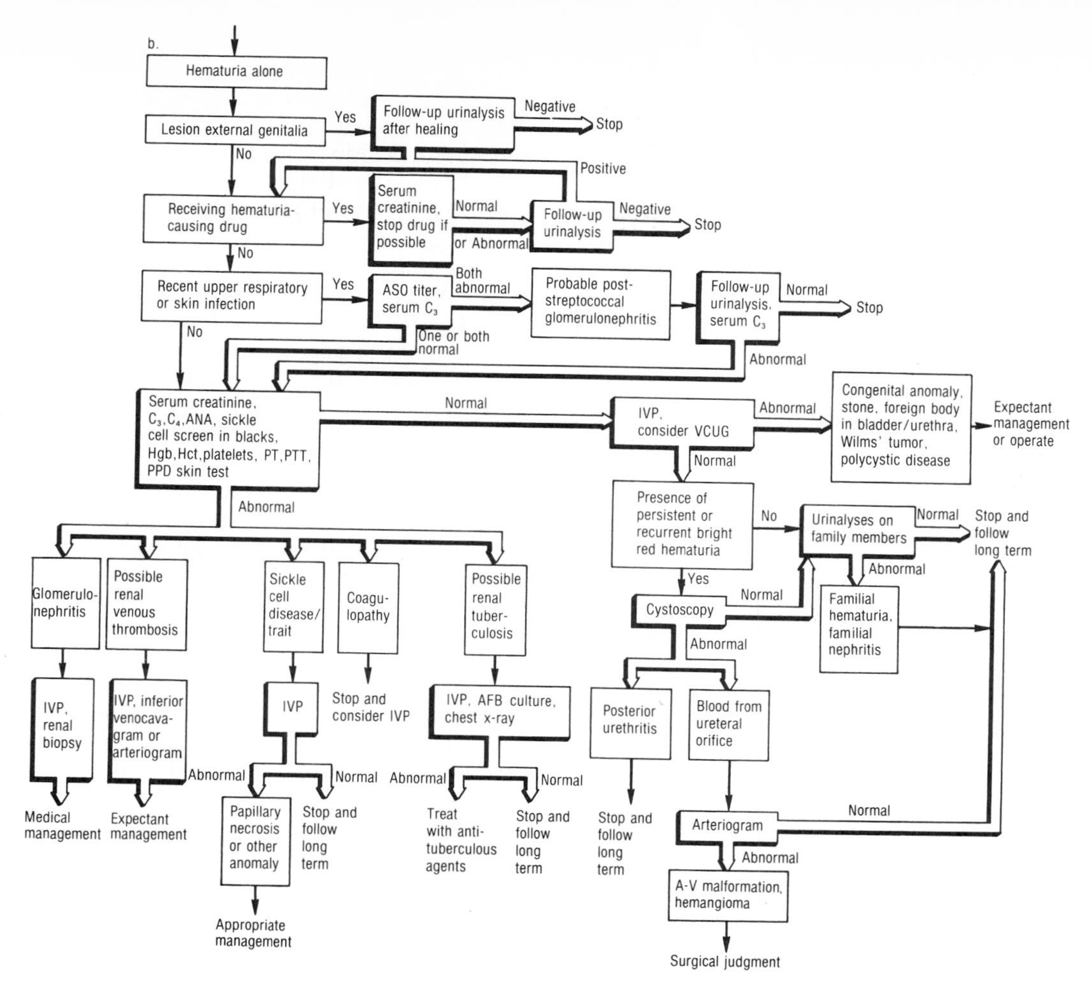

Figure 2*b* *Continued*

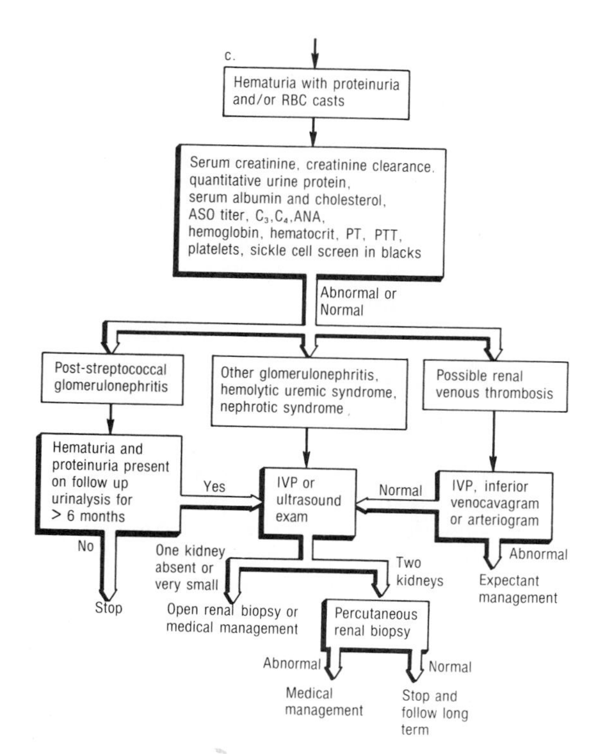

Figure 2*c* *Continued*

thrombocytopenia, disseminated intravascular coagulopathy) and thus warrants appropriate laboratory investigation, including hemoglobin, hematocrit, and platelet values, and measurements of prothrombin and partial thromboplastin times. Specific clotting factor determinations should be assessed as indicated by the type of bleeding disorder. Rarely, a child with asymptomatic hematuria has renal tuberculosis, which can be verified by a PPD skin test.

Hypercalciuria may be a cause for asymptomatic microscopic or gross hematuria in children.[12, 13] Screening for this abnormality can be performed with a fasting spot urine calcium-creatinine ratio determination (normal <0.20) or a 24-hour urine calcium excretion measurement (normal <4 mg/kg/24 hrs).[12, 13]

After blood and urine screening tests are performed, radiologic evaluation should be made. An intravenous pyelogram is almost always indicated in the evaluation of hematuria alone. This study may show hydronephrosis, Wilms' tumor, bladder rhabdomyosarcoma, hemangioma, polycystic kidney disease, renal venous thrombosis, stones, or a foreign body in the bladder or urethra. A voiding cystourethrogram may provide additional information and should be considered in each case.

In general, cystoscopy is rarely necessary in the evaluation of hematuria in the child.[21, 22] Bladder tumors are quite rare in childhood and are not likely to be missed on radiologic studies. Posterior urethritis is usually symptomatic, and cystoscopy does not change the therapy. In the child with bright red urine, however, cystoscopy may be helpful at the time of active bleeding to localize blood to one or both ureteral orifices. An arteriogram may be necessary to diagnose a renal arteriovenous malformation or a small hemangioma.

If the results of blood and urine tests and radiologic studies are negative, urinalyses of family members may help make the diagnosis of familial hematuria or Alport's hereditary nephritis, even when no family history of the disorder has been obtained. When the results of the entire evaluation are normal, hematuria may represent an early stage of glomerulonephritis or benign hematuria. Benign hematuria is a diagnosis of exclusion, and long-term follow-up is necessary to affirm it. If over years of follow-up the child grows normally, maintains a normal blood pressure, has normal renal function, and does not develop proteinuria or red blood cell casts, he or she probably has benign hematuria, with a good long-term outlook. If the persistence of hematuria for several years without other symptoms is source of anxiety for parents and the child, a renal biopsy to look for glomerulonephritis may be worth the small risk of the procedure.[16]

The symptomatic or asymptomatic child with proteinuria, either in the presence of microscopic hematuria or persisting after gross hematuria becomes microscopic, is likely to have a renal parenchymal lesion. The presence of red blood cell casts is usually diagnostic of a glomerular lesion. Laboratory evaluation in this child should always include an assessment of renal filtration function, determination of serum albumin and cholesterol levels, and quantitative measurement of urine protein (Fig. 2*c*). Evidence of a recent streptococcal infection in the presence of a low C_3 value suggests poststreptococcal glomerulonephritis. A renal biopsy is usually not necessary to confirm the diagnosis if the child follows the usual clinical course for this disease. If no biopsy is done, the child should be followed carefully, and if the serum C_3 concentration does not return to normal after 1 to 2 months, or if hematuria and proteinuria persist for 6 to 12 months, further evaluation, including a renal biopsy, is indicated. Other types of glomerulonephritis, including membranoproliferative glomerulonephritis, lupus nephritis, rapidly progressive glomerulonephritis, Alport's hereditary nephritis, IgA nephropathy, mesangial proliferative glomerulonephritis, focal segmental glomerulosclerosis, and other focal nephritides require a renal biopsy for diagnosis. A percutaneous renal biopsy, which can be performed even in a small child by an experienced pediatric nephrologist, should be attempted only after IVP or ultrasonography has confirmed the presence of two kidneys. If one kidney is absent or small, an open renal biopsy is preferred. If a renal biopsy is performed, tissues should be submitted for evaluation by light, electron, and immunofluorescence microscopy to allow accurate pathologic diagnosis. Renal biopsy may be useful for determining long-term prognosis in the child with hematuria and proteinuria attributable to Henoch-Schönlein purpura nephritis or in treatment of the child with hemolytic uremic syndrome. Focal nephritis or early focal segmental glomerulosclerosis may be missed on examination of a percutaneous needle biopsy specimen taken in the early stages of the disease, so the child with a normal biopsy result should receive long-term medical follow-up.

Neonatal Hematuria. Hematuria in the neonate is a special problem. Red urine in this age group can be caused by hemogloblin, bile pigments, porphyrins, or urates. Betadine, which may be used to clean an infant's perineum before obtaining a bagged urine specimen, can also give a false-positive result on dipstick test for blood.[23] Thus, a urinalysis on a fresh specimen is mandatory to detect red blood cells. When hematuria is present, one must consider the diagnostic possibilities of infection, obstructive uropathy, Wilms' tumor, congenital nephrosis, infantile polycystic kidney disease, renal venous thrombosis (especially in an infant of a diabetic mother, an infant with preceding severe diarrhea, or an infant who has received a large dose of contrast material for cardiac angiography), renal artery thrombosis (especially in the ill neonate with an umbilical artery catheter), cortical or medullary necrosis, and antibiotic-induced nephritis. Glomerulonephritis is exceedingly rare in infants. The laboratory evaluation for these diagnostic possibilities often requires radiologic studies. Newborn infants do not concentrate their urine well and may have much bowel gas overlying the kidneys, rendering interpretation of an intravenous pyelogram difficult until at least a week or two after birth. Renal ultrasonography may be useful in the meantime to detect a congenital anomaly, cystic structures, or enlarged kidneys.

Hematuria Secondary to Trauma

Hematuria secondary to trauma (either blunt or penetrating) requires immediate radiologic investigation (Fig. 3). The entire urinary tract can, in general, be visualized using three studies: retrograde urethrogram (urethra), cystogram (bladder), and IVP (kidneys and ureters). If a urethral injury is suspected in a man on the basis of previously described historical and physical findings, a retrograde urethrogram to rule out injury should be performed before urethral catheterization is attempted. Urethral injuries are rare in women and for the most part can be discounted. If the urethrogram result is normal, a urethral catheter should be inserted and a cystogram performed. If the cystogram or urethrogram demonstrates a urethral or bladder injury, operative intervention is generally indicated only after IVP has ruled out significant renal and ureteral injury.[24]

If results of retrograde urethrography and cystography are normal, or if these studies are not performed because there is no clinical suspicion of lower urinary tract trauma, IVP is the initial

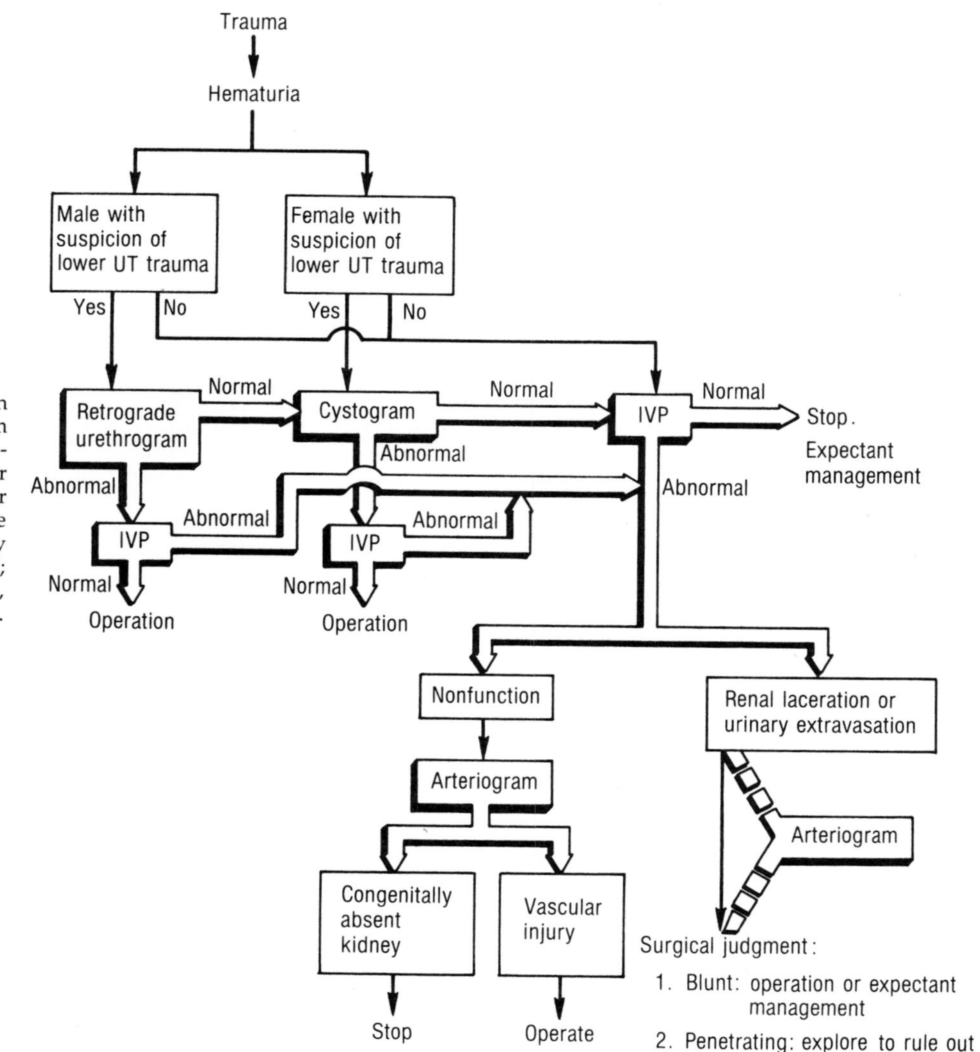

Figure 3. Diagnostic evaluation of hematuria resulting from trauma. *IVP*, intravenous pyelogram. (From Benson GS, Brewer ED. Hematuria: algorithms for diagnosis. II. Hematuria in the adult and hematuria secondary to trauma. JAMA 1981; 246:993–6. Copyright 1981, American Medical Association. Reprinted with permission.)

study of choice to assess renal or ureteral injury. The patient with suspected renal injury and a normal IVP result should be treated expectantly. Unilateral nonfunction suggests either a major vascular injury or renal agenesis; the study of choice to differentiate these two entities is a renal arteriogram. The further assessment of renal lacerations or urinary extravasation seen on IVP is controversial.[25, 26] An arteriogram is usually extremely helpful in assessing the degree of injury and determining whether immediate surgical exploration is necessary. In general, however, all patients with penetrating renal trauma should undergo surgical exploration to rule out other associated injuries (to pancreas, spleen, liver, or bowel).

REFERENCES

1. Harrison WE, Habib HN, Smith EI, McCarthy RP. Nontraumatic hematuria in children. J Urol 1966;96:95–100.
2. Wyatt RJ, McRoberts JW, Holland NH. Hematuria in childhood: significance and management. J Urol 1977;117:366–8.
3. Carter WC, Rous SN. Gross hematuria in 110 adult urologic hospital patients. Urology 1981;18:342–4.
4. Dodge WF, West EF, Smith EH, Bunce H. Proteinuria and hematuria in school children: epidemiology and early natural history. J Pediatr 1976;88:327–47.
5. Miller AB. The etiology of bladder cancer from the epidemiological viewpoint. Cancer Res 1977;37:2939–42.
6. Morgan RW, Jain MG. Bladder cancer: smoking, beverages, and artificial sweeteners. Can Med Assoc J 1974; 111:1067–70.
7. Gibbons RP, Montie JE, Correa RJ Jr, Mason JT. Manifestations of renal cell carcinoma. Urology 1976;8:201–6.
8. Boileau M, Fuchs E, Barry JM, Hodges CV. Stress hematuria: athletic pseudonephritis in marathoners. Urology 1980;15:471–4.
9. International Study of Kidney Disease in Children. Nephrotic syndrome in children: prediction of histopathology from clinical and laboratory characteristics at time of diagnosis. Kidney Int 1978;13:159–65.
10. McCoy RC, Abramowsky CR, Tisher CC. IgA nephropathy. Am J Pathol 1974;76:123–40.
11. Southwest Pediatric Nephrology Study Group. A multicenter study of IgA nephropathy in children. Kidney Int 1982;22:643–52.
12. Kalia A, Tavis LB, Brouhard BH. The association of idiopathic hypercalciuria and asymptomatic gross hematuria in children. J Pediatr 1981;99:716–9.
13. Roy S, Stapleton FB, Noe HN, Jerkins G. Hematuria preceding renal calculus formation in children with hypercalciuria. J Pediatr 1981;99:712–5.
14. National Heart, Lung and Blood Institute's Task Force on Blood Pressure Control in Children. Report of the task force on blood pressure control in children. Pediatrics 1977;59(Supp):797–820.
15. DeSwiet M, Fayers P, Shinebourne EA. Systolic blood pressure in a population of infants in the first year of life: the Brompton study. Pediatrics 1980;65:1028–35.
16. West CD. Asymptomatic hematuria and proteinuria in children: causes and appropriate diagnostic studies. J Pediatr 1976;89:173–82.
17. Fair WR, McClennan BL, Jost RG. Are excretory urograms necessary in evaluating women with urinary tract infection? J Urol 1979;121:313–5.
18. Pollack HM, Goldberg BB, Bogash M. Changing concepts in the diagnosis and management of renal cysts. J Urol 1974;111:326–9.
19. McClennan BL, Stanley RJ, Melson GL, et al. CT of the renal cysts: is cyst aspiration necessary? AJR 1979; 133:671–5.
20. Schwartz GJ, Haycock GB, Spitzer A. Plasma creatinine and urea concentration in children: normal values for age and sex. J Pediatr 1976;88:828–30.
21. Walther PC, Kaplan GW. Cystoscopy in children: indications for its use in common urologic problems. J Urol 1979;122:717–20.
22. Johnson DK, Kroovand RL, Perlmutter AD. The changing role of cystoscopy in the pediatric patient. J Urol 1980;123:232–3.
23. Rasoulpour M, McLean RH, Raye J, Shah BL. Pseudohematuria in neonates. J Pediatr 1978;92:852–3.
24. Morehouse DD, MacKinnon KJ. Posterior urethral injury: etiology, diagnosis and initial management. Urol Clin North Am 1977;4:69–73.
25. Wein AJ, Murphy JJ, Mulholland SG, et al. A conservative approach to the management of blunt renal trauma. J Urol 1977;117:425–7.
26. Carlton CE. Surgery in renal trauma (editorial). Urology 1974;3:671.

HEMOPTYSIS

JUDD SHELLITO

☐ SYNONYM: Coughing up blood

BACKGROUND

Incidence and Age Distribution

Hemoptysis is the coughing up of blood. The amount of blood expectorated may vary, from blood tinging the sputum to frank blood. Hemoptysis is a common symptom of cardiopulmonary disease and is the presenting complaint of approximately 15 per cent of patients seen in an urban chest clinic.[1] Hemoptysis is more common in older patients, the median age in most series being 50 to 55 years.

Source of Bleeding

Blood coming from the patient's mouth is not an infallible sign of hemoptysis, because its origin may be the nose, mouth, larynx, or stomach rather than the tracheobronchial tree. The first step in the evaluation of any patient with hemoptysis is to localize the bleeding to the respiratory tract.

Bleeding from lesions in the nose, mouth, or throat may be misinterpreted as hemoptysis, particularly in children. With questioning, however, most patients can localize the source of bleeding. Epistaxis may not be recognized as such by some patients, because nasal blood may be aspirated and then expectorated. For this reason, a nasal examination is important in every patient with suspected hemoptysis. The mouth and throat should be carefully examined for bleeding lacerations or tumors. Bleeding sites beneath dentures are easily overlooked. Laryngeal sources of bleeding, usually tumors, are often not considered because they are not visualized on physical examination. A mirror examination of the larynx should therefore be a part of any hemoptysis work-up.

Hematemesis—the vomiting of blood—may also be mistaken for hemoptysis by both patient and physician. Again, with questioning, most patients can distinguish hematemesis from hemoptysis, but in some cases, the sudden welling up of blood from the esophagus into the pharynx stimulates coughing, making the distinction difficult. Some features help to distinguish hematemesis from hemoptysis. Coughed-up blood is usually mixed with air and has a foamy appearance; vomited blood is rarely foamy. Coughed-up blood is usually bright red; vomited blood, owing to the action of gastric acid, is dark red to black. Patients with hematemesis may give a history of gastrointestinal bleeding, ulcer disease, liver disease, or alcoholism. Testing expectorated blood with pH paper usually shows alkaline values in hemoptysis and acid values in hematemesis. Once an initial episode of hemoptysis subsides, the patient often expectorates blood-tinged sputum for several days; this sequela is unusual with hematemesis. Rarely, it is necessary to pass a nasogastric tube to separate hematemesis from hemoptysis. However, only the aspiration of bright red blood from the tube localizes the bleeding to the stomach, because coughed-up blood is commonly swallowed.

On rare occasions, patients may expectorate reddish material that is not blood ("pseudohemoptysis"). Pulmonary infections with reddish-pigmented strains of *Serratia marcescens* may be associated with sputum that looks like blood. Similarly, the coughing up of "anchovy paste" sputum from a bronchial rupture of an amoebic abscess may be mistaken for hemoptysis.

Causes of Hemoptysis

Bleeding from the respiratory tract is associated with a wide variety of disorders. The source of bleeding may be the pulmonary arterial or the bronchial circulation. For centuries, tuberculosis was the most common cause of hemoptysis.[2] With the control of tuberculosis, other causes of hemoptysis were recognized, and the incidence rates for the various disorders associated with hemoptysis changed accordingly. Two recent patient series reported in the United States indicate that bronchitis and bronchiectasis together account for 40 to 46 per cent of cases of hemoptysis.[3, 4] Lung neoplasms, both benign and malignant, are found in 23 to 24 per cent, and tuberculosis is now the cause of hemoptysis in only 3 to 6 per cent of cases. These figures apply only to the United States; tuberculosis undoubtedly remains a more common cause of hemoptysis in other parts of the world.

The potential causes of hemoptysis are legion. A complete listing of disorders associated with hemoptysis is presented in Table 1. It is helpful to consider the possible causes of hemoptysis by disease mechanism (infectious, neoplastic, etc.) Only the more common causes of hemoptysis are discussed in this chapter.

Infectious Diseases

Hemoptysis due to bronchitis usually is minimal in quantity and presumably is due to mucosal inflammation. Bronchiectasis is almost invariably

Table 1. CAUSES OF HEMOPTYSIS

Category	Causes

Infectious diseases	Bronchitis
	  Acute
	  Chronic
	Bronchiectasis
	Tuberculosis
	Pneumonia
	  Viral
	  Bacterial (pneumococcal, staphylococcal, klebsiella, pseudomonas)
	Lung abscess
	Fungal infections, including mycetoma

Neoplasms	Bronchogenic carcinoma Benign lung tumors (bronchial adenomas) Metastatic tumors, particularly choriocarcinoma, osteogenic sarcoma Tracheal tumors
Cardiovascular disorders	Mitral stenosis Pulmonary infarction Pulmonary arteriovenous fistula Aortic aneurysm Pulmonic stenosis Eisenmenger's reaction in left-to-right shunt
Traumatic causes	Puncture of lung in rib fracture or bullet or stab wound Pulmonary contusion Inhalation of smoke or toxic fumes Aspiration of gastric contents Mucosal tear from prolonged coughing Bronchial fracture
Parasitic disorders	Paragonimiasis Strongyloidiasis Ancylostomiasis Trichinosis Schistosomiasis Echinococcosis Ascariasis
Congenital abnormalities	Cystic fibrosis Pulmonary sequestration Pulmonary artery atresia Bronchogenic cyst Hereditary hemorrhagic telangiectasia
Immunologic disorders	Goodpasture's syndrome Wegener's granulomatosis Acute lupus pneumonitis Periarteritis nodosa Sarcoidosis Behçet's syndrome
Iatrogenic conditions	Bronchoscopy Transtracheal aspiration Transthoracic needle aspiration Swan-Ganz catheterization Bronchial stump blowout after pneumonectomy Suture granuloma Anticoagulant therapy

Miscellaneous causes	Foreign body aspiration
	Idiopathic pulmonary hemosiderosis
	Primary pulmonary hypertension
	Endometriosis with pulmonary implants
	Broncholithiasis
	Blood dyscrasias
	  Hemophilia
	  Leukemia
	  Thrombocytopenia
	Uremic pneumonitis
	Lymphangioleiomyomatosis
	Isolated bronchial wall telangiectasia
	Pulmonary amyloidosis
	Emphysematous bullae
	Factitious hemoptysis

Idiopathic hemoptysis	

associated with hemoptysis at some point in the progression of the disorder. In most cases, hemoptysis is accompanied by a typical history of chronic cough with copious sputum production. However, in upper lobe bronchiectasis related to tuberculous or fungal infection, there may be no history of productive cough. In about half the cases of such "dry bronchiectasis," hemoptysis may be the presenting symptom.[5]

Tuberculosis remains an important cause of hemoptysis. More often than coming from a ruptured Rasmussen's aneurysm in a cavity wall, bleeding in tuberculosis is related to the development of anastomoses between the bronchial and pulmonary arterial circulations, with capillary leakage due to the entrance of high-pressure bronchial blood into the low-pressure pulmonary circuit.[6] It is important to recall that hemoptysis in tuberculosis bears no relationship to activity of infection. Adequately treated residual tubercular cavities may be associated with massive hemoptysis, and hemoptysis may also occur when no cavities are visible on x-ray.[7]

Hemoptysis may be seen with a wide variety of bacterial pulmonary infections. Definite hemoptysis is actually not very common in pneumococcal pneumonia, although the sputum is often dark brown. Bleeding is more common with pneumonia due to staphylococcus, *Klebsiella* ("currant jelly" sputum), and *Pseudomonas*. Hemoptysis occurs in 11 per cent of patients with lung abscess, massively in a little more than 5 per cent.[8] Surgical resection may be required to control hemoptysis associated with a lung abscess.

Any of the pulmonary fungal infections (coccidioidomycosis, histoplasmosis, etc.) can cause hemoptysis, but the pulmonary fungal infection most commonly associated with bleeding is the mycetoma, or fungus ball. This lesion usually represents *Aspergillus fumigatus* growing within an old tuberculous cavity. Most patients with mycetoma experience hemoptysis at some time during their lives. The cause of mycetoma-associated bleeding may relate to friction caused by the freely moving fungal mass, proteolytic enzymes released by the fungi, or local invasion.[9]

Neoplasms

Hemoptysis occurs in approximately 50 per cent of cases of bronchogenic carcinoma at some time in the course of disease.[10] The bleeding is usually not profuse and is presumably due to bronchial neovascularization associated with the growing tumor. Benign lung tumors, including bronchial adenomas, are even more likely to manifest as hemoptysis. Metastatic tumors to the lung rarely cause hemoptysis, because they originate as microemboli far from the airways; exceptions to this rule include metastatic choriocarcinoma and osteogenic sarcoma.

Cardiovascular Disorders

Hemoptysis is seen in 10 to 20 per cent of patients with mitral stenosis, which should be particularly suspected in a younger patient whose hemoptysis occurs after exertion. Bleeding is due to rupture of pulmonary veins or capillaries that have been distended by increased intravascular pressure. Thirty-six per cent of patients with pulmonary embolism and infarction experience hemoptysis, usually along with dyspnea and pleuritic chest pain.[11] The possibility of pulmonary infarction should be considered in every patient with hemoptysis.

Traumatic Causes

Hemoptysis is common after penetrating chest injuries or rib fractures, usually coupled with pneumothorax. Pulmonary contusion after blunt chest trauma, as from a steering wheel injury, may result in expectoration of blood. Mucosal damage from the inhalation of smoke or toxic fumes or following the aspiration of gastric contents may also cause hemoptysis. Rarely, protracted coughing causes a mucosal tear, with resultant bleeding.

Parasitic Disorders

Parasitic lung disease, particularly paragonimiasis (lung fluke), is a common cause of hemoptysis in many geographic areas.

Congenital Abnormalities

Hemoptysis is common in cystic fibrosis owing to the underlying bronchiectasis and demands aggressive, usually nonsurgical, management. Pulmonary sequestration and bronchogenic cysts may also cause bleeding in association with superimposed infection.

Immunologic Disorders

Bleeding in Goodpasture's syndrome follows damage to the alveolar capillary basement membrane by membrane-directed antibody. Hemoptysis may also be seen in Wegener's granulomatosis, acute lupus pneumonitis, periarteritis nodosa, sarcoidosis, and Behçet's syndrome.

Iatrogenic Conditions

Hemoptysis due to medical or surgical procedures is becoming increasingly common. Blood-streaked sputum is often noted after bronchoscopy, particularly with a transbronchial biopsy, or following transtracheal aspiration, transthoracic needle aspiration, or Swan-Ganz catheterization. The Swan-Ganz catheter can produce hemoptysis by causing pulmonary infarction or rupture of pulmonary vessels by an overinflated balloon.

Miscellaneous Causes

An aspirated foreign body may present as hemoptysis. This fact is important to consider with hemoptysis in children. Radiolucent aspirated foreign bodies causing scanty hemoptysis have been mistakenly treated as childhood asthma because of the associated wheezing. In endometriosis with pulmonary implants of endometrial tissue, hemoptysis may occur, sometimes only during menses. Broncholithiasis causes bleeding as calcified lymph nodes erode into a bronchus. Often, blood mixed with gritty white material is expectorated.

Idiopathic Hemoptysis

Even after thorough evaluation, 5 to 15 per cent of cases of hemoptysis are unexplained.[12]

HISTORY

History of the Present Illness. As with most diagnostic problems, the evaluation of hemoptysis starts with a well-taken history. The initial part of the patient interview should be devoted to questions designed to distinguish hemoptysis from nonpulmonary bleeding. The patient should be questioned carefully regarding possible epistaxis, bleeding oral lesions, and hematemesis. The age of the patient is important, because bronchiectasis and mitral stenosis are more common causes of hemoptysis before the age of 40.[13] The elicited information should include the amount of blood, its appearance, whether the blood was mixed with sputum, the duration of bleeding, and whether a cough was present before the patient began to bring up blood. Defining the rate of bleeding is particularly important, because it has a direct bearing on prognosis (see "Assessment").

Other symptoms associated with hemoptysis may suggest a diagnosis. Is there a history of fever, shaking chills, or purulent sputum mixed with blood (pneumonia, lung abscess)? Does the patient have a history of chronic productive cough (chronic bronchitis or bronchiectasis)? Has the patient noticed weight loss, anorexia, or hoarseness (lung carcinoma)? Is there a history of pleuritic chest pain or paroxysmal dyspnea (pulmonary embolism with infarction)? Is there a history of hemoptysis associated with exertion (mitral stenosis)? Has the patient experienced recent chest trauma or inhaled smoke or toxic fumes? Is there a history of nasal or sinus pain (Wegener's granulomatosis) or hematuria (Goodpasture's syndrome)? Rarely, patients may notice subjective chest sensations that localize the bleeding site within the chest.

Previous Medical History. The previous history should focus on prior lung disease, tuberculosis, abnormal chest x-ray findings, or a known heart murmur. Approximately 30 per cent of patients presenting with hemoptysis have had a prior episode of hemoptysis. A history of peptic ulcer disease or gastrointestinal bleeding may suggest that hematemesis rather than hemoptysis is occurring. A history of a bleeding disorder or the use of anticoagulant drugs is of obvious importance.

Social History. A history of smoking is important in defining a risk factor for both chronic bronchitis and lung carcinoma. Excess alcohol intake may indicate bleeding from esophageal varices, whereas a history of illicit drug use may suggest septic pulmonary emboli. Careful inquiry should be made into the patient's occupation and hobbies for possible exposure to toxic inhalants.

PHYSICAL EXAMINATION

In the physical examination, the nose should be checked carefully for bleeding sites and for ulceration of the nasal septum. Buccal telangiectasia may indicate hereditary hemorrhagic telangiectasia. The larynx should be visualized for a possible bleeding site. In the chest, a localized wheeze or signs of pleural effusion may indicate malignant disease. Bilateral basilar rales may point to mitral stenosis. Physical signs of consolidation (egophony, increased fremitus) may indicate either pneumonia or pulmonary infarction. Unfortunately, blood spreads rapidly throughout the lungs, often causing harsh airway sounds far from the source of bleeding. Therefore, abnormal physical findings may not correlate with the actual bleeding site. The heart should be carefully auscultated for the opening snap and diastolic rumble of mitral stenosis. Abdominal masses may suggest metastatic disease to the chest. Digital clubbing is most often associated with bronchogenic carcinoma, bronchiectasis, or lung abscess. Lymphadenopathy may indicate lymphoma or bronchogenic carcinoma.

DIAGNOSTIC STUDIES

Laboratory Studies

All patients with hemoptysis should have a complete blood count and tests for coagulation such as a platelet count, prothrombin time, and partial thromboplastin time. Hemoptysis is an uncommon cause of anemia; few patients expectorate enough blood to become hypovolemic or iron-deficient. Anemia is a more likely indication of an underlying malignancy or immunologic disorder such as Wegener's granulomatosis.

Sputum smears and cultures are of obvious importance in the diagnosis of bacterial pulmonary infections. Most patients with hemoptysis should also have at least three sputum examinations for acid-fast bacilli (both smear and culture). Cytologic examination of sputum is helpful in patients more than 40 years of age.

Diagnostic Imaging

Standard posteroanterior and lateral chest x-rays are of primary importance in the evaluation of hemoptysis. The chest x-rays may indicate changes typical of a disease process responsible for the bleeding, such as lobar pneumonia, cardiomegaly with Kerley B lines (mitral stenosis), lung abscess, cavitary tuberculosis, diffuse nodular densities (Wegener's granulomatosis), and intracavitary mycetoma. However, the physician should be cautious about interpreting an abnormality on chest x-ray as the cause of the bleeding reported by the patient. The presence of a lesion on chest x-rays does not necessarily confirm it as a source of bleeding. For example, chronic postinflammatory changes, such as from old fungal infection, may coexist with a subradiographic bleeding lung tumor. In addition, blood spreads rapidly throughout the tracheobronchial tree and may produce infiltrates on chest x-rays far from the origin of bleeding. A normal chest x-ray appearance is not uncommon in patients with hemoptysis, being seen in up to 50 per cent of patients in some series. Normal radiographic findings are particularly common in cases of bleeding associated with bronchiectasis and chronic bronchitis.

If appearance on chest x-ray is abnormal, additional radiographic studies may be of value. Tomography may be helpful in better defining mass lesions seen on chest x-rays or in detecting additional lesions. Computed tomography (CT) of the chest is also helpful in this regard. Neither standard tomography nor CT scanning should be employed, however, if the standard chest x-ray findings are normal. Ventilation-perfusion radionuclide lung scanning may help in the diagnosis of suspected pulmonary embolism. Surprisingly, arteriography is rarely of much value in diagnosing either the cause or the location of nonmassive hemoptysis, for two reasons: First, hemoptysis can arise from either the pulmonary arterial or bronchial circulation. Arteriographic visualization of both circulations is impractical. Second, arteriography is of benefit only for active bleeding and gives the physician little or no information once the bleeding has stopped. Radiographic visualization of the bronchial tree (bronchography) is no longer routinely performed in patients with hemoptysis, probably because of both a decline in the incidence of bronchiectasis and the development of fiberoptic bronchoscopy. At present, bronchography is usually reserved for patients in whom bronchiectasis is suspected and bronchoscopic findings are normal. Bronchography should be delayed until after bleeding ceases, because blood clots in the bronchi may produce misleading irregularities of contour.

Bronchoscopy

After chest radiography, bronchoscopy is probably the most widely used investigative technique in patients with hemoptysis. In the past, there was much debate about when bronchoscopy should be performed (during or after an episode of hemoptysis) and whether bronchoscopy might precipitate additional bleeding. Recent patient series, however, have established that bronchoscopy can be safely performed and highly informative during an episode of active bleeding.[1, 3] Fiberoptic bronchoscopy is most commonly performed in patients with hemoptysis, because the small size and the flexibility of the instrument allow for better penetration into the tracheobronchial tree. Utilizing fiberoptic bronchoscopy, Smiddy and Elliott[3] localized the bleeding site in 93 per cent of their patients with active hemoptysis. Performing the procedure during active bleeding had no adverse effects. For patients expectorating large amounts of blood (massive hemoptysis), most pulmonary physicians prefer to evaluate the respiratory tract with a rigid bronchoscope. The rigid scope is larger than the fiberoptic scope, can clear much larger amounts of blood from the trachea and large airways, and can serve as an airway for ventilation if necessary.

ASSESSMENT

Establishing the Rate of Bleeding

The first step in evaluating a patient with hemoptysis is to establish the rate of bleeding, which has a direct relationship to prognosis and determines the assessment approach. Patients should be carefully questioned in an effort to quantitate the amount of hemoptysis that has occurred before seeking medical attention. Most authorities agree that patients who cough up 600 ml of blood or more within a 24-hour period are in a high-risk group. A standard hospital emesis basin holds about 600 ml, as do three styrofoam coffee cups. Once a bleeding patient has been hospitalized, all coughed-up sputum and blood should be collected and measured. By establishing the rate of bleeding, the physician can assign the patients to one of two categories: those with massive hemoptysis and those with nonmassive hemoptysis. The diagnostic approaches differ for the two categories.

Assessment in Massive Hemoptysis

As mentioned, *massive hemoptysis* may be arbitrarily defined as the loss of greater than 600 ml of blood within a 24-hour period. The cause of massive hemoptysis is more likely to be inflammatory (tuberculosis, lung abscess, or bronchiectasis) than neoplastic. Massive pulmonary bleeding is also more likely to arise from the bronchial than the pulmonary arterial circulation. Patients with massive hemoptysis have a mortality rate of 50 to 100 per cent.[14, 15] Treatment of these patients with surgical resection of bleeding pulmonary tissue decreases the mortality rate to between 17 and 23 per cent.[14, 15] The work-up for the patient with massive hemoptysis involves maintaining the airway, determining whether the patient is a candidate for surgical resection, locating the bleeding site, and performing the operation. Making a specific diagnosis in such patients is considered secondary to identification of the side that is bleeding and surgical intervention.

All patients with massive hemoptysis should be cared for in a facility where thoracic surgery can be performed if necessary, and surgical consultation should be obtained early in the evaluation. The patient with massive hemoptysis should be given supplemental oxygen, and intubation should be done if he or she is unable to maintain the airway. The patient should lie with the bleeding side down, if it is known; a Trendelenberg position may be necessary to keep the airway clear. All such patients should be given intravenous fluids and blood should be cross-matched for 6 units. A brief history should be obtained, along with a chest x-ray, and simple spirometric evaluation, if possible. The managing physician should try to establish whether the patient is a candidate for surgery. Patients who would not be considered surgical candidates include those with widely metastatic tumors or severe underlying pulmonary disease that would prevent removal of any lung tissue. After the initial evaluation and consultation with a thoracic surgeon, these patients should be examined with a rigid bronchoscope. The purpose of bronchoscopy in these patients is to determine which side the blood is coming from rather than what the specific cause of bleeding is. Once the bleeding lung is identified, it can be isolated from the airway necessary for ventilation, and the bleeding lobe or lung can be resected. In patients who are not surgical candidates, control of bleeding may be attempted using endobronchial balloon tamponade or bronchial artery embolization.[16, 17]

Assessment in Nonmassive Hemoptysis

Most patients with nonmassive hemoptysis should be hospitalized for diagnostic evaluation. This is not an inflexible rule, but the work-up proceeds more smoothly in the hospital, and most patients ultimately require bronchoscopy, which is also best performed in the hospital. The approach to these patients concentrates much more on establishing a specific diagnosis than the approach to patients with massive hemoptysis. It should be emphasized that there can be no treatment of nonmassive hemoptysis until a diagnosis is made. "Conservative management" of undiagnosed hemoptysis is no treatment at all. After the initial history taking and physical examination, most patients should be given supplemental oxygen and a mild sedative, i.e., not enough to depress the cough reflex. A suction machine with suction catheters should be at the bedside, along with a laryngoscope and endotracheal tubes for possible intubation. For all patients, an initial blood count, coagulation profile, and chest x-ray, and for most patients, sputum studies for bacterial and mycobacterial pathogens and cytologic examination, should be performed. It is often wise to wait for the results of these initial evaluations before proceeding further. If no obvious diagnosis can be achieved on the basis of the history, physical examination, chest x-ray, and sputum smear findings, most patients should be examined with the fiberoptic bronchoscope. As already mentioned, this procedure is best performed when the bleeding is active, although recent evidence suggests that bronchoscopy may be delayed without sacrificing the chance of a diagnosis.[4] Certainly, there is no need to schedule emergency bronchoscopy at night or during weekend hours to evaluate a patient with nonmassive hemoptysis.

Additional diagnostic studies depend upon the results of the initial evaluation. A radionuclide lung scan may be necessary for suspected pulmonary embolism with infarction, or a pulmonary arteriogram may be necessary for suspected pulmonary arteriovenous fistula. In most patients, the diagnosis will be obvious after the history taking, physical examination, initial laboratory work, chest x-ray, and bronchoscopic examination have been done.

Special Considerations

A question often raised regarding the evaluation of hemoptysis is whether all bleeding patients require bronchoscopy. In some patients, the diagnosis is obvious, and bronchoscopy is not necessary; examples are active unilateral tuberculosis, unilateral pneumonia, and unilateral lung carcinoma with a diagnostic sputum cytology result. Bronchoscopy is required for persistent or recurrent bleeding, however. Chronic bronchitis is one of the most common causes of hemoptysis. Many patients with this disease contact their physician to report purulent sputum associated with a single episode of blood streaking. They should be evaluated with caution, because most patients with chronic bronchitis are also at risk for lung carcinoma. At a minimum, chronic bronchitis patients reporting blood-streaked sputum in association with a clear-cut exacerbation of bronchitis should undergo chest radiography and three cytologic examinations of the sputum. If the results of these studies are negative and hemoptysis does not continue, bronchoscopy may be deferred. It has been shown, however, that most such patients bleed again, and an aggressive initial evaluation, including bronchoscopy, simplifies management of additional bleeding episodes. Weaver and associates[18] examined 110 hospitalized patients with nonmassive hemoptysis with regard to the need for bronchoscopy. Their study indicated that bronchoscopy can be deferred if the following three factors are present: age less than 40 years, a normal chest x-ray appearance, and hemoptysis lasting less than 1 week. If any one of these factors is not present, bronchoscopy should be performed. All patients with recurrent hemoptysis require bronchoscopy.

The evaluation of nonmassive hemoptysis in extremely elderly or demented patients requires a good deal of clinical judgment. Usually, the controversy revolves around whether to perform bronchoscopy to rule out a pulmonary malignancy. In such patients, as full a history as possible should be taken, and physical examination, complete blood count, coagulation profile, chest x-ray, and sputum studies should be performed. Additional evaluation should take into consideration what treatment will be instituted in the individual patient. Specifically, bronchoscopy need not be performed to rule out a pulmonary malignancy, if no therapy would be directed at that malignancy once detected.

Idiopathic Hemoptysis

In 5 to 15 per cent of patients with hemoptysis, no explanation is found for bleeding, even after a thorough evaluation including bronchoscopy and bronchography. Fortunately, several clinical studies have indicated that these patients have a good prognosis.[12, 19] Douglass and Carr,[12] reporting on 55 such patients followed for longer than 5 years, found that less than half bled again, and in only one case was the second episode associated with more bleeding than the first episode. Only one patient was found to have a bronchogenic carcinoma on follow-up. The cause of bleeding in such patients is believed to be either bronchitis beyond the view of the bronchoscope or bronchiectasis not detected on bronchography.

REFERENCES

1. Purcel JE, Lindskog GE. Hemoptysis: a clinical evaluation of 105 patients examined consecutively on a thoracic surgical service. Am Rev Respir Dis 1961;84:329–36.
2. Abbot OA. The clinical significance of pulmonary hemorrhage: a study of 1,316 patients with chest disease. Dis Chest 1948;4:824–42.
3. Smiddy JF, Elliott RC. The evaluation of hemoptysis with fiberoptic bronchoscopy. Chest 1973;64:158–62.
4. Gong H Jr, Salvatierra C. Clinical efficacy of early and delayed fiberoptic bronchoscopy in patients with hemoptysis. Am Rev Respir Dis 1981;124:221–5.
5. Gillis DA, Miller RD. Dry bronchiectasis. JAMA 1958;167:1714–9.
6. Ishihara T, Inove H, Kohayashi K, et al: Selective bronchial arteriography and hemoptysis in non-malignant lung disease. Chest 1974;66:663–8.
7. Middleton JR, Sen P, Lange M, et al: Death producing hemoptysis in tuberculosis. Chest 1977;74:601–4.
8. Thoms NW, Pura HE, Arbulu A. The significance of hemoptysis in lung abscess. J Thorac Cardiovasc Surg 1970;59:617–29.
9. Varkey B, Rose HD. Pulmonary aspergilloma: a rational approach to treatment. Am J Med 1976;61:626–31.
10. Cohen S, Hossain M. Primary carcinoma of the lung—a review of 417 histologically proven cases. Dis Chest 1966;49:67–74.
11. Sasahara A, Hyers T, eds. The urokinase pulmonary embolism trial. New York: American Heart Association, 1973;II–61.
12. Douglass BE, Carr DT. Prognosis in idiopathic hemoptysis. JAMA 1972;150:764–5.
13. Moersch MJ. Clinical significance of hemoptysis. JAMA 1952;148:1461–5.
14. Crocco J, Rooney J, Frankushen D, et al. Massive hemoptysis. Arch Intern Med 1968;121:495–8.
15. Courin A, Garzon A. Operative treatment of massive hemoptysis. Ann Thorac Surg 1974;18:52–69.
16. Gottlieb L, Hillberg R. Endobronchial tamponade therapy for intractable hemoptysis. Chest 1975;67:482–3.
17. Magilligan D Jr, Ravipati S, Zayat P, et al: Massive hemoptysis: control by transcatheter bronchial artery embolization. Ann Thorac Surg 1981;32:392–400.
18. Weaver L, Solliday N, Cugell D. Selection of patients with hemoptysis for fiberoptic bronchoscopy. Chest 1979; 76:7–10.
19. Barrett R, Tuttle W. A study of essential hemoptysis. J Thorac Cardiovasc Surg 1960;40:468–74.

HIRSUTISM AND HYPERTRICHOSIS

LAWRENCE T. CHOY □ RICHARD F. WAGNER, JR.

□ SYNONYM: Excessive hair growth

BACKGROUND

Definition and Origins

The evaluation of excessive hair growth should begin with the distinction that is drawn between hirsutism and hypertrichosis. Hirsutism involves increased androgen-dependent male-pattern hair growth in a child or a woman, and may be an early sign of virilization; by definition, hirsutism cannot occur in a man. Hypertrichosis involves hair growth that is not dependent on androgen and is not associated with virilization; hypertrichosis can occur in children, women, and men.

An embryologic perspective aids in understanding abnormal hair growth. Hair development begins in the third gestational month, with very fine, lightly pigmented lanugo hair on the entire fetus. By the time of birth, soft, fine, nonpigmented vellus hair has replaced lanugo hair. At puberty, vellus hair changes to thick, coarse, pigmented terminal hair, which can be either dependent on or independent of sex steroids. Eyelashes and eyebrows do not depend on sex hormones for growth, but other facial hairs as well as body, axillary, and pubic hairs depend on hormonal stimulation for full development.[1] Hirsutism involves excessive sex steroid–dependent terminal hair growth over androgen-sensitive areas of a patient's body. Hypertrichosis involves increased nonsexual vellus hair; such hair growth does not reflect an imbalance of sex hormones. This chapter discusses the recognition of hirsutism, its differentiation from hypertrichosis, and the diagnostic evaluation required to determine the etiology of the hirsute state.

Causes

Most commonly, hirsutism is primary (idiopathic), i.e., there is no detectable underlying disease process.[2] Hirsutism also has familial and genetic causes. Hirsutism may coexist with various physiologic states, such as normal puberty, precocious puberty, pregnancy, and menopause.[3]

Drugs are well-known causes of hirsutism. Steroid drugs include androgens such as danazol (Danocrine) as well as glucocorticoids, birth control pills, and ACTH.[4] Other drugs that cause hirsutism include phenytoin (Dilantin), diazoxide (Proglycem), minoxidil (Loniten), cobalt, hexachlorobenzene, streptomycin, and cyclosporin A.[2, 5]

There are various ovarian causes of excess androgen production resulting in hirsutism. The ovaries can be a major source of excess androgen in patients with idiopathic hirsutism. The most common ovarian cause of excess androgens is the polycystic ovary syndrome (Stein-Leventhal syndrome).[5] Others are hilar cell hyperplasia and stromal hyperthecosis. Both primary ovarian tumors (arrhenoblastoma, hilar cell tumor, adrenal rest tumor, and granulosa-theca cell tumor) and metastatic tumors to the ovaries can result in hirsutism.[3]

Adrenal diseases with excess androgen production include congenital and noncongenital adrenal hyperplasia, adrenal adenoma, and adrenal carcinoma.

There is an entity of mixed adrenal-ovarian hyperandrogenemia; in this condition the excess androgen is produced by both the ovaries and the adrenals. Four mechanisms are described: (1) the deficient activity of $\Delta 5,3\beta$-hydroxysteroid dehydrogenase, an enzyme that is normally found in both the adrenal glands and the ovaries; (2) blockade of adrenal steroidogenic enzymes by androgens that are synthesized by the ovary; (3) adrenal androgens causing polycystic changes in the ovaries; and (4) adrenal enzymes ectopically present in the ovaries, perhaps owing to the presence of adrenal rests.[5]

Endocrine causes of hirsutism include hypothyroidism, hyperthyroidism, and acromegaly. Hyperprolactinemia is associated with adrenal androgen overproduction.[5] Nonendocrine malignancies that produce ACTH-like substances and anorexia nervosa can also result in hirsutism. (The causes of precocious puberty are listed in the chapter on that subject.)

The causes of hypertrichosis are also numerous but should be divided according to whether they result in localized or generalized hypertrichosis. Localized hypertrichosis is caused by local chronic chemical or mechanical trauma or is associated with physical conditions such as spina bifida, hamartoma, and nevi.[6]

Generalized hypertrichosis may be seen in a large number of conditions. The congenital or hereditary forms are reported more frequently than the acquired forms.[7] Congenital anomalies include hypertrichosis lanuginosa, also known as hypertrichosis universalis congenita, a rare condition that involves the entire hair-bearing surface of the body. Fewer than 30 unrelated families with this disorder are known.[6] Other congenital anomalies include Cornelia de Lange's syndrome, bird-headed dwarfism of Seckel, trisomy E syndrome, and Hurler's syndrome.[3]

Noncongenital forms of generalized hypertrichosis result from ingestion of various medications, such as diphenylhydantoin (Dilantin), penicillamine (Cuprimine, Depen), diazoxide (Proglycem), and hexachlorobenzene.[4, 8] Hypertrichosis lanuginosa, which can occur in adult life in the absence of a family history, is also known as "malignant down" because it is associated with internal malignancies. Various nervous system disorders, such as postencephalitis, multiple sclerosis, concussion of the brain, and hyperostotic internal craniopathy (Morgagni's syndrome), may be associated with generalized hypertrichosis. The psychiatric disorders schizophrenia and anorexia nervosa can also cause hypertrichosis. Other causes include erythropoietic porphyria, porphyria cutanea tarda, dermatomyositis, hypothyroidism, starvation, acrodynia, epidermolysis bullosa, and malnutrition due to infection or malabsorption.[3, 4, 9]

HISTORY

A thorough history is necessary in the evaluation of excess hair growth. The essential points of the history-taking in hirsutism are described.

History of the Present Illness. The age and the menstrual history of the patient with hirsutism are crucial in the diagnosis. The onset of hirsutism before puberty may indicate precocious puberty, which is defined as sexual development occurring in a boy less than 10 years old or in a girl less than 8 years old. Precocious puberty is either complete or incomplete. In complete precocious puberty, isosexual maturation is due to a hypothalamic-pituitary mechanism, and the condition may be associated with fertility. In incomplete precocious puberty, sexual maturation may be either isosexual or heterosexual, and although secondary sexual characteristics develop, the gonads fail to mature and the patient is infertile.

Hirsutism at puberty is seen in the combined adrenal-ovarian abnormalities. Affected patients may demonstrate no other signs of virilization, and as a group they have slightly elevated plasma testosterone levels associated with an increased testosterone production rate.

Typically, the polycystic ovary syndrome begins to manifest itself in the teenage years.[5] In a review of over 1,000 patients with the syndrome, hirsutism was found in 69 per cent, dysfunctional uterine bleeding in 29 per cent, relative infertility in 74 per cent, obesity in 41 per cent, and hyperandrogenemia in most of these patients.[10] Hirsutism and virilization during pregnancy are usually due to ovarian overstimulation by human chorionic gonadotropic hormone.[5]

Hirsutism may occur along with menopause, when estrogen levels generally fall.[5]

Family History. A family history of hirsutism should always be identified.

Drug History. A complete drug history is always essential.

General Considerations. At all ages, the presence of hirsutism should arouse the suspicion of underlying tumor, especially if there is a rapid onset of hirsutism, virilization, and menstrual irregularities.

High-Payoff Queries

The following questions are helpful in evaluating hirsutism and hypertrichosis.

1. *Is there a family history of hirsutism?* Although hirsutism is most likely familial and idiopathic, without an identifiable underlying disease, a family history of hirsutism may be seen in congenital adrenogenital syndrome and polycystic ovary syndrome.[5]

2. *What drugs have you been taking? How long have you been taking them?* A woman may be on chronic steroid treatment for malignancy, rheumatologic disease, or pulmonary disease, or as post–kidney transplantation therapy. She may be taking a birth control pill, minoxidil for hypertension, or phenytoin for epilepsy.

3. *How long has the excess hair been present?* A diagnostic work-up may be avoided in a fertile woman with a long history of mild hirsutism and normal menstrual periods. An investigation is needed, however, when the onset of hirsutism is recent or when there is moderate to severe hirsutism of any duration.

4. *Please describe your menstrual periods.* Hirsutism may be found in association with various benign physiologic states, such as puberty, pregnancy, and menopause. A history of either abnormal menstruation or infertility should arouse suspicion of a pathologic state that requires evaluation. One should always be aware that a patient may not realize that she is pregnant.

5. *Have you noticed any change in your voice or skin, or the size of your clothes?* The history may reveal virilization, signified by the new onset of voice deepening, acne, or a decrease in breast size. Virilization should be identified in the history-taking, and its finding necessitates a thorough physical examination. Increasing libido is also a symptom of virilization.

6. *Have you lost weight or your appetite?* An affirmative answer to this query should prompt an

investigation for neoplastic disease and anorexia nervosa.

7. *Have you had a psychiatric disorder?* Excess hair growth has been reported in several psychiatric diseases, such as schizophrenia and anorexia nervosa.

PHYSICAL EXAMINATION

The physical examination should differentiate hypertrichosis from hirsutism. Chronic physical or chemical exposure may be identified as the cause of localized hypertrichosis. Bruises, nerve injuries, exposure to chemicals, local skin irritation by plasters, and hormonal stimulation have been implicated. Localized hypertrichosis has been found in mental patients who practice self-mutilation, and in sackbearers of India secondary to chronic irritative stimuli.[7] Localized hypertrichosis that appears as tufts of hair in the cervical and lumbar regions may be congenital.[6] Hypertrichosis may occur in hamartomas or nevi, such as pigmented nevi with hair, nevus pilosus, and pigmented hairy epidermal nevi. Although a pigmented nevus may be noticed at birth, excess hair may grow later. Hypertrichosis may also be associated with spina bifida.[6]

Acquired hypertrichosis lanuginosa requires a thorough evaluation for an underlying carcinoma. One review included nine patients with ages ranging from 34 to 78 years old who developed generalized lanugo hair; 56 per cent of the tumors were of gastrointestinal origin and 22 per cent were pulmonary.[9]

In the classification of hirsutism proposed by Ferriman and Gallwey,[11] the body is divided into nine regions of androgen-sensitive hair growth: upper lip, chin, chest, abdomen, pubic area, upper arms, thighs, and back. In a normal female it is not unusual to find a few hairs growing on several androgen-sensitive regions. Each of the nine body regions is given a grade, from *one,* which indicates minimal terminal androgen-sensitive hair, to *four,* which identifies frank virilization. The grades for all nine regions are added; a total score of eight or more suggests hirsutism. About 5 per cent of all premenopausal women have a score of eight or more.[1]

Signs of virilization should be identified. The voice may have a deep pitch, and the patient may appear to have a male body habitus. The skin examination may reveal temporal balding, oiliness, malodorous perspiration, and acne. The breasts and uterus may appear atrophic, and there may be clitoromegaly.

The clinical finding of obesity may be associated with various causes of hirsutism. Ettinger and associates[12] reported obesity in 75 per cent of patients evaluated for hirsutism. Truncal obesity, hypertension, hyperpigmentation, and purple striae are found in Cushing's syndrome. The etiology of Cushing's syndrome may be due to the use of exogenous steroids, adrenal hyperplasia, an adrenal adenoma, or a carcinoma. Hirsutism is seen in 80 per cent of patients with Cushing's syndrome.[13] Nonendocrine ACTH-producing tumors include oat-cell carcinoma, bronchial adenoma of the lung, tumors of the thymus, pancreas, and thyroid, and pheochromocytoma. In ectopic ACTH production due to tumor, weight gain, central obesity, and striae are rare, but hypokalemic alkalosis, edema, hyperpigmentation, and hypertension are more common.[13] Obesity may also be noted in a large percentage of patients with polycystic ovary syndrome and in hypothyroidism. Very thin young women with hirsutism may have anorexia nervosa, although hypertrichosis with lanugo hair is more common.[14]

A breast examination should be performed. Galactorrhea may be secondary to enhanced prolactin release from pituitary tumors such as prolactin secreting tumors, mixed growth hormone and prolactin secreting tumors, and chromophobe adenomas.[15]

In the girl with precocious puberty, periodic abdominal and rectal examinations are necessary for 2 years after the onset of virilization in order to exclude ovarian disease.

In a woman, an abdominal examination may reveal an abdominal mass due to an ovarian or an adrenal tumor. A pelvic bimanual examination is also indicated.

Virilization at puberty with variable breast development is seen in patients with a congenital 17β-hydroxysteroid dehydrogenase deficiency. These patients are 46,XY males, mostly with female phenotype, who have a blind-ending vagina and inguinal or abdominal testes. No uterus or fallopian tubes are found. This enzyme deficiency is probably the most common defect in testosterone production causing male pseudohermaphroditism.[16]

The adrenogenital syndrome (congenital adrenal hyperplasia) in females includes a variety of other hormonal defects in testosterone synthesis that cause hirsutism. The most common form is a deficiency of the 21-hydroxylase enzyme. Such defects are congenital and usually manifest at birth or in adolescence, but hirsutism and virilization may be of late onset, occurring in an adult female. Late-onset hirsutism has been described for 21-hydroxylase, 11β-hydroxylase, and 3-β-ol-dehydrogenase enzyme deficiency syndromes.[5] Hypertension and hypokalemia develop in the 11β-hydroxylase deficiency owing to the accumulation of 11-deoxycorticosterone, which has mineralocorticoid activity.[13]

The discovery of virilization should always lead the physician to search for an adrenal or ovarian tumor. Carcinoma is the most common virilizing adrenal tumor.[13] Some adrenal tumors are massive enough to be palpable on abdominal examination.[17] An ovarian tumor may be felt as an adnexal mass, but often it is not palpable because such a tumor cannot be palpated abdominally until it reaches 15 cm in diameter.[18]

A patient who has the symptoms of polycystic ovary syndrome should have an internal examination, because endometrial carcinoma is associated with the condition.[4]

Pituitary tumors may cause other physical findings. Visual field deficits should be identified. Coarse facial features and enlarged extremities are found in acromegaly.

A psychiatric examination may reveal the poor self-esteem, fear of obesity, or depression common to patients with anorexia nervosa.[14]

DIAGNOSTIC STUDIES

Hormone Determinations

Blood tests are more direct measurements of body hormonal levels than urinary tests and are therefore preferable. Androgen levels are elevated in most hirsute patients, but certain guidelines are useful to identify specific diagnoses.[4]

Initially, serum testosterone, serum dihydrotestosterone (DHT), and serum dehydroepiandrosterone sulfate (DHEA-S) should be measured. A serum testosterone level greater than 2.0 ng/ml or a serum DHEA-S level greater than 7,000 ng/ml suggests a virilizing tumor.

Several points should be noted concerning the serum testosterone level. This hormone has been found to be increased in 30 to 82 per cent of hirsute patients.[4] In some laboratories, the reported value may actually be a total value that includes androgenic compounds besides testosterone. Excess testosterone may come from either the ovaries or the adrenals. The free testosterone level should be measured, because a portion of serum testosterone is bound to a testosterone-binding globulin, TeBG (testosterone estradiol–binding globulin), and to albumin. Exogenous progesterone, androgens, and steroids decrease TeBG and increase free testosterone but the total testosterone value remains normal. Estrogen ingestion, pregnancy, and hyperthyroidism increase TeBG and reduce the free testosterone level. This level correlates better with the amount of hirsutism, and therefore may be a better index of androgenicity.[4] Because the release of testosterone is pulsatile during the menstrual cycle, a mean value should be obtained from three pooled blood samples.

Dihydrotestosterone (DHT) is secreted by both the ovaries and the adrenals and is the most potent androgen.[4] The DHT level does not fluctuate during the menstrual cycle. An elevated DHT level suggests either a mixed ovarian-adrenal problem or excess adrenal secretion of androgen.[4]

DHEA-S production is largely confined to the adrenals, so high levels of this substance usually indicate an adrenal source of excess androgens.

Dexamethasone Suppression Test

The dexamethasone suppression test is an important part of the laboratory investigation. The test is used to screen for Cushing's syndrome and to distinguish adrenal hyperplasia from adrenal tumor. It is also used, with modifications, to help identify the cause of an elevated androgen level.

The 1-mg overnight dexamethasone suppression test is the best screening test for Cushing's syndrome.[13] After 1 mg is administered to a patient at midnight, blood is taken at 8:00 A.M. for a cortisol measurement; a value above 5 μg/dl is abnormally high, and prompts the further use of 0.5 mg of dexamethasone every 6 hours for 2 days, followed by a measurement of a 24-hour urinary 17-hydroxysteroid level on the second day. If this level is higher than 3 mg, the patient has Cushing's syndrome. Further testing with a 2-mg dose of dexamethasone every 6 hours for 2 days with measurement of blood ACTH and cortisol levels (high-dose dexamethasone test) helps to differentiate adrenal hyperplasia from adrenal adenomas and carcinomas. The metyrapone test, in which 750 mg of metyrapone is given every 4 hours for six doses with subsequent measurement of the urinary 17-hydroxysteroid excretion, may be used as an alternative to the high-dose dexamethasone test.

A modified dexamethasone suppression test has been proposed by Abraham and associates[19] for identifying the cause of hirsutism.[19] This test should not be performed when the patient is suffering a severe depression, because the cortisol levels in such a patient may not be suppressed. This test should also not be done if a tumor is suspected; when the serum testosterone value is greater than 2 ng/ml or the DHEA-S level is greater than 7,000 ng/ml, a tumor should first be ruled out. If the testosterone level is more than 2 ng/ml, there is probably an ovarian tumor, but an adrenal tumor is also possible.[4] A DHEA-S level greater than 7,000 ng/ml strongly suggests an adrenal tumor. A predetermined dose of dexamethasone given daily for at least 2 weeks is needed in most patients for adequate adrenal suppression. Most evidence shows that dexamethasone does not suppress ovarian function. The dose of dexamethasone varies with body weight. Prior to the test, three consecutive morning blood samples are drawn for serum cortisol, testosterone, androstenedione, DHT, and DHEA-S determinations. The mean values are used as the pretest values. These blood tests are repeated on the last 3 days of the test. Tables of control values are available for pretest and postsuppression hormone levels in normal patients. At the end of the 2-week period, if the serum cortisol value is above 40 ng/ml and the DHEA-S level is above 400 ng/ml, adrenal suppression is inadequate. In such a case, a 1-mg overnight dexamethasone suppression test is done. If cortisol is still inadequately suppressed, Cushing's syndrome needs to be excluded. If cortisol is adequately suppressed but DHEA-S is not, a 1-month dexamethasone suppression test is needed.

When there is adequate suppression of cortisol and DHEA-S, further steps are needed to evaluate the data. If an androgen level is initially elevated during the pretest period and is subsequently suppressed to normal in the postsuppression period, then the excess androgen is likely to be of adrenal origin. If androgen is not suppressed, and the difference between the pretest and the postsuppression levels is equal to the normal adrenal component, the source of the excess androgen is considered to be the ovaries. When the androgen is partially suppressed, with elevated postsuppression levels, and if the difference between the pretest and the postsuppression levels is greater than the normal adrenal component, the excess androgen is considered to be of mixed adrenal-ovarian origin. If the pretest levels of all of the androgens are normal, the patient may have hypersensitivity of the pilosebaceous unit.[20]

Other Studies

The diagnosis of a tumor may be supported by ultrasonography and computed tomography. Computed tomography (CT) scanning of the adrenal glands has been shown to be more sensitive, specific, and accurate than ultrasonography, although the latter procedure remains valuable in the patient who is very thin or has a large mass in the upper abdomen.[21, 22] Ultrasonography is better for evaluating an adnexal mass, although computed tomography is excellent for assessing associated lymphadenopathy, extension of tumor into osseous structures, and tumor invasion into paravaginal, parametrial, and retroperitoneal fat and muscle.[23] In a girl with precocious puberty, serial ultrasonographic examinations of the ovaries should be performed for 2 years after the onset of hirsutism, in order to exclude an ovarian neoplasm. In a boy with precocious puberty, periodic CT scanning of the brain is indicated to rule out intracranial disease. Occasionally, laparotomy is necessary when a tumor is strongly suspected and is impossible to exclude by other means. Arteriography may be needed to visualize an adrenal tumor. Difficult cases may require adrenal and ovarian vein catheterization.

Evaluating Diagnostic Findings

In one study, measurements of serum DHEA-S, DHT, testosterone, and cortisol have detected hyperandrogenemia in 100 per cent of hirsute patients.[19] It should be noted that in postmenopausal women, hirsutism may be seen with normal androgen levels, probably owing to a relatively high androgen-estrogen ratio.[4]

Patients with polycystic ovary syndrome may show a lack of suppression on the dexamethasone suppression test. These patients may have minimally to markedly elevated plasma androgen levels and normal to extremely high luteinizing hormone (LH) levels. Some investigators have found elevated LH levels in half of all their patients with polycystic ovary syndrome.[24]

Adrenal virilization secondary to a mild acquired or congenital enzyme defect should always be considered in adult women, because it may mimic polycystic ovary syndrome. A specific diagnosis of enzyme deficiency depends on the measurement of the specific steroid precursor in question. In the 21-hydroxylase deficiency, the plasma 17-hydroxyprogesterone level and the progesterone level should be elevated. In the 11-hydroxylase deficiency, blood levels of 11-deoxycortisol and deoxycorticosterone are elevated. In the 3-β-ol-dehydrogenase deficiency, an isolated elevation of DHEA-S is found. In patients with a 17-β-hydroxysteroid dehydrogenase deficiency, plasma androstenedione is elevated, and obtaining a karyotype is necessary in some of these patients.[25]

ASSESSMENT

In the diagnostic evaluation of the hirsute patient, one must be alert for the life-threatening diseases that manifest as hirsutism.

Constellations of Findings

The following clinical descriptions represent common presentations in hirsutism.

Benign Hirsutism. A family history of hirsutism along with currently normal menstruation and fertility suggest a benign cause.

Polycystic Ovary Syndrome. There is a broad

clinical spectrum ranging from relatively normal menstruation and absence of hirsutism to abnormal menstruation and frank hirsutism. A family history of hirsutism may also be found.

Ovarian Carcinoma. A description of ovarian dysfunction, such as unusually heavy menstruation, dysmenorrhea, or miscarriages in a woman more than 40 years of age may be obtained via the history. There also may be gastrointestinal symptoms such as vague abdominal discomfort, dyspepsia, increasing flatulence, and gas with abdominal distension.

Anorexia Nervosa. Extreme thinness with amenorrhea, episodes of bulimia, low blood pressure, and bradycardia are consistent with this illness. Anorexic patients often engage in vigorous exercise.

Cushing's Syndrome. Truncal obesity with associated hypokalemia, hypertension, hyperpigmentation, purple striae, and a plethoric "moon" facies are common features of this syndrome.

REFERENCES

1. Ackerman AB. Structure and function of the skin. Development, morphology, and physiology. In; Moschella SL, Pillsbury DM, Hurley HJ, eds. Dermatology. Philadelphia: WB Saunders, 1975; 1–60.
2. Wagner RF Jr. Hirsutism. J Dermatol Allergy 1982;5:17–23.
3. Maguire HC. Diseases of the hair. In: Moschella SL, Pillsbury DM, Hurley HJ, eds. Dermatology. Philadelphia: WB Saunders, 1975;1197–1221.
4. Maroulis GB. Evaluation of hirsutism and hyperandrogenemia. Fertil Steril 1981:36:273–305.
5. Hatch R, Rosenfield RL, Kim MH, et al. Hirsutism: implications, etiology, and management. Am J Obstet Gynecol 1981;140:815–830.
6. Danforth CH. Studies on hair with special reference to hypertrichosis. Arch Dermatol Syph 1925;12:380–401.
7. Fretzin DF. Malignant down. Arch Dermatol 1967;95: 294–7.
8. Hensley GT, Glynn KP. Hypertrichosis lanuginosa as a sign of internal malignancy. Cancer 1969;24:1051–6.
9. Hegedus SI, Schorr WF. Acquired hypertrichosis lanuginosa and malignancy; a clinical review and histopathologic evaluation with special attention to the "mantle" hair of Pinkus. Arch Dermatol 1972;106:84–8.
10. Goldzieher JW, Green JA. The polycystic ovary. I. Clinical and histologic features. J Clin Endocrinol Metab 1962;22:235–8.
11. Ferriman D, Gallwey JD. Clinical assessment of body hair growth in women. J Clin Endocrinol Metab 1961;21: 1440–7.
12. Ettinger B, von Werder K, Thenaers GC, et al. Plasma testosterone stimulation-suppression dynamics in hirsute women. Am J Med 1971;51:170–5.
13. Williams GH, Dluhy RG, Thorn GW. Diseases of the adrenal cortex. In: Isselbacher KJ, Adams RD, Braunwald E, et al, eds. Harrison's principles of internal medicine. New York: McGraw-Hill, 1980;1711–94.
14. Boyar RM. Anorexia nervosa. In: Isselbacher KJ, Adams RD, Braunwald E, et al, eds. Harrison's principles of internal medicine. New York: McGraw-Hill, 1980;416–8
15. Emerson K Jr, Wilson JD. Diseases of the breast and of milk formation. In: Isselbacher KJ, Adams RD, Braunwald E, et al, eds. Harrison's principles of internal medicine. New York; McGraw-Hill, 1980;1787–94.
16. Wilson JD, Griffin JE: Disorders of sexual differentiation. In: Isselbacher KJ, Adams RD, Braunwald E, et al, eds. Harrison's principles of internal medicine. New York: McGraw-Hill, 1980;1794–1808.
17. Liddle GW. The adrenals. In: Williams RH, ed. Textbook of Endocrinology. 6th ed. Philadelphia: WB Saunders, 1974;233–322. 1981;249–290.
18. Barber HRK. Ovarian carcinoma. Etiology, diagnosis, and treatment. New York: Masson, 1978;99.
19. Abraham GE, Maroulis GB, Boyers SP, et al. Dexamethasone suppression test in the management of hyperandrogenized patients. Obstet Gynecol 1981;57:158–65.
20. Abraham GE, Maroulis GB, Buster JE, et al. Effect of dexamethasone on serum cortisol and androgen levels in hirsute patients. Obstet Gynecol 1976;47:390–402.
21. Sample WF, Sarti DA. Computed tomography and gray scale ultrasonography of the adrenal gland: a comparative study. Radiology 1978;128:377–83.
22. Abrams HL, Siegelman SS, Adams DF, et al. Computed tomography versus ultrasound of the adrenal gland: a prospective study. Radiology 1982;143:121–8.
23. Fleischer AC, Walsh JW, Jones HW III, et al. Sonographic evaluation of pelvic masses. Method of examination and role of sonography relative to other imaging modalities. Radiol Clin North Am 1982;20:297–412.
24. Givens JR, Andersen RN, Umstot BS. Clinical findings and hormonal responses in patients with polycystic ovarian disease with normal versus elevated LH levels. Obstet Gynecol 1976;47:388–94.
25. Silver HK, Gotlin RW, Klingensmith GW. Endocrine disorders. In: Kemp CH, Silver HK, O'Brien D, eds. Current pediatric diagnosis and treatment. Los Altos, Cal.: Lange, 1982;706.

HYPERCALCEMIA

MICHAEL R. WILLS □ B. LEWIS BARNETT, JR.

□ SYNONYM: Elevated serum calcium level

BACKGROUND

Definition

Hypercalcemia may be simply defined as an increase in serum calcium concentration to a value above the upper limit of the reference range. The reference range values for serum calcium vary slightly from laboratory to laboratory, the most commonly quoted values being between 8.5 and 10.5 mg/100 ml (2.15 to 2.60 mmol/liter). The interlaboratory variations are a reflection of different analytical techniques. In any consideration of an individual result it is important to make sure that the sample has been carefully collected and that venous stasis has not been induced during collection. Venous stasis during blood collection is an important artifactual cause of hypercalcemia; it results in an increase in calcium concentration by in vivo ultrafiltration and its effect on serum protein concentrations. Similarly, fluid shifts and protein variations associated with changes in posture (from the horizontal to vertical position) can cause false elevations in the estimated total calcium concentration. The major protein species that binds calcium is the albumin fraction. In the clinical interpretation of a serum calcium value it is important to know the simultaneously estimated albumin concentration. The simultaneous estimation of total protein and albumin concentrations is of particular importance when one is monitoring and interpreting serial calcium values in any one patient over a long period.

Incidence

There are many possible and probable causes of hypercalcemia. The incidence of hypercalcemia and the relative importance of its various causes are uncertain.[1] It is recognized that hypercalcemia, and particularly hyperparathyroidism, is common and that many patients either are asymptomatic or only have vague symptoms. Fisken and colleagues[1] reported that there appears to be a distinct difference in both the incidence and causes of hypercalcemia between the general population or unselected series of outpatients and hospital inpatients. From a review of the literature, these researchers concluded that the incidence of hypercalcemia in the general population or unselected outpatients ranges from 0.1 to 1.6 per cent, and in general hospital inpatients from 0.5 to 3.6 per cent. Hyperparathyroidism appeared to be the most common cause in some of the reported series of general population or unselected outpatients, but not in others; other causes reported to occur with relatively high incidences in this classification include the administration of thiazide diuretics, thyroid disease, milk-alkali or milk-drinker's syndrome, and immobilization. Malignancy is more common in general hospital inpatients than in the general population, and in most of the reported series it is the most common cause of hypercalcemia.

In either classification of patients, the evaluation and differential diagnosis of hypercalcemia essentially depend on the clinical evaluation of the patient and the correct interpretation of the associated biochemical findings. The diagnostic approach must be based on a full understanding of the mechanisms involved in normal calcium homeostasis and the disturbances in these mechanisms that are associated with disease states.

Calcium Homeostasis

The normal steady-state regulation of calcium involves dietary intake and, more important, physiochemical factors and hormonal control. Disturbances in any of these systems due to disease are associated with disorders of calcium homeostasis, which are manifested as either hypercalcemia or hypocalcemia.

All of the calcium in the body tissues and fluids is derived from the diet. The dietary intake and the various digestive mechanisms ultimately control the amount of calcium that is available for intestinal absorption. In a child, calcium is absorbed and retained for skeletal growth, whereas in the adult, only enough is absorbed and retained to offset obligatory losses, which normally occur in urine and feces. A woman who is pregnant or lactating needs more calcium, for fetal skeletal formation or milk production. In the kidney, calcium excretion is controlled by the processes involved in renal tubular reabsorption. Both children and adults need to adapt intestinal calcium absorption to meet the requirements for maintenance of the skeleton and to ensure calcium balance in the face of variations in dietary intake and excretion. The adaptive mechanisms involved in the maintenance of steady-state balance involve variations in hormone secretion rates. In addition to skeletal maintenance, there is the overriding need to maintain the constant concentration of ionized calcium essential for normal neuromuscular function and probably for other cell functions such as secretion and transport.

The major physiochemical factors of calcium homeostasis are those involved in the maintenance of the skeleton and include weight bearing and muscle activity. Any disease that affects the rate of either bone deposition or resorption can cause a disturbance of steady-state calcium regulation, with consequent changes in serum concentration.

In the blood compartment, calcium exists in three forms: ionized, protein-bound, and complexed. The complexed fraction constitutes approximately 10 per cent of the total; the calcium is in complex with phosphate, bicarbonate, citrate, and similar ions. The protein-bound fraction constitutes approximately 40 per cent of the total and is mainly bound to albumin. The ionized fraction constitutes approximately 50 per cent of the total serum concentration. It is considered to be the physiologically active portion, which is both the controlled and controlling mechanism in hormone secretion. A fall in the serum concentration of ionized calcium is the major stimulus to parathyroid hormone (PTH) production and secretion. A negative feedback mechanism between serum calcium concentration and PTH secretion is responsible for the relative constancy of the serum concentration. The calcium-sensitive receptors in the parathyroid gland respond immediately to changes in ionized calcium concentration by increasing production and secretion.

The hormones that are essential in the steady-state regulation of calcium are parathyroid hormone (PTH), 1,25-dihydrocycholecalciferol (1,25-DHCC), and calcitonin. The precise physiologic role of calcitonin in humans, if any, is not well-defined and awaits further clarification. It has, however, been recently proposed that calcitonin is important in the maintenance of steady state.[2] In this model, calcitonin aids in the routing of calcium obtained from intestinal absorption into bone fluid, where it is temporarily stored and from which it is returned to the extracellular fluid compartment as required during intervals between oral intakes of calcium. A number of other hormones also involved in overall calcium and skeletal homeostasis include: growth hormone, prolactin, the sex steroids, thyroxine, and cortisol, all of which have only subsidiary roles. The essential hormones exert their control over calcium homeostasis by their actions on the rate of calcium deposition in or mobilization from bone, the urinary excretion of calcium, and the rate of absorption of calcium from the intestinal tract.

The biologic actions of PTH involve target tissues in the kidney, bone, and gastrointestinal tract. In the target tissues, PTH acts on specific cell membrane receptors that are linked to adenyl cyclase; there is a consequent intracellular release of cyclic adenosine monophosphate, which transmits the stimulus within the cell. The action of PTH on the kidney is accompanied by an increased excretion of cyclic adenosine monophosphate (cyclic AMP) in the urine, and this action is of differential diagnostic value. In the kidney, the biologic actions of PTH involve the handling of calcium, phosphate, and other ions together with an effect on the production of 1,25-DHCC. In the absence of PTH, 97 per cent of the filtered load of calcium is reabsorbed by the renal tubules. PTH increases the tubular reabsorption of calcium and raises the renal calcium threshold and hence the serum concentration. PTH decreases the tubular reabsorption of phosphate, lowers the renal phosphate threshold, and allows the same excretion of phosphate at a lower serum concentration; the overall effect is to cause a reduction in serum phosphate concentration. PTH also has an effect on cholecalciferol metabolism; it stimulates the renal production of 1,25-DHCC from its precursor 25-hydroxycholecalciferol (25-HCC). The biologic action of PTH on bone is to cause an increase in resorption in which both the mineral and collagen phases are broken down and released into the circulation.

Cholecalciferol is formed in the skin photochemically from 7-dehydrocholesterol. The first step in the conversion of cholecalciferol to its ultimate biologically active form occurs in the liver with hydroxylation at the C-25 position and the formation of 25-HCC. The latter is further hydroxylated in the kidney at the C-1 position with the formation of 1,25-DHCC, which is the major biologically active metabolite and the hormonal form of cholecalciferol. The kidney is the production site of another dihydroxymetabolite, 24,25-dihydroxycholecalciferol (24,25-DHCC); although it may have a role in calcium and phosphate metabolism, such a role remains to be defined, as does the role of other di- and tri-hydroxy metabolites. In hypocalcemic situations renal synthesis is oriented to 1-hydroxylation and 1,25-DHCC production with a transition to 24,25-DHCC production as the serum calcium concentration increases to the normal range. The production of 1,25-DHCC is controlled by two systems. The first consists of calcium, phosphate, PTH, and 1,25-DHCC itself; this system regulates 1,25-DHCC production to suit the short-term needs for calcium and phosphate and is under negative feedback control. The second system, which is probably designed for long-term homeostasis, consists of growth hormone, prolactin, and the sex steroids; which of these has the major control in any particular situation is as yet ill-defined.

The major biologic sites of action of 1,25-DHCC are bone and the gastrointestinal tract, where it acts on specific nuclear cellular receptors. There is virtually no active transport of calcium across the gut wall in the absence of 1,25-DHCC, although calcium can diffuse across passively if the dietary intake is high enough. 1,25-DHCC dramatically increases such active transport and causes an increase in serum concentration. The uncalcified osteoid present in patients with rickets and osteomalacia is remineralized following treatment with 1,25-DHCC. Mineralization may involve extracellular calcium and phosphate concentrations and the factors that regulate the coupling process in bone between resorption and mineralization. The increase in bone resorption is clearly seen following overtreatment with either vitamin D or its biologically active metabolites. Other tissues on which 1,25-DHCC has a biologic action include the parathyroid glands, kidneys, and muscle. Specific receptors for vitamin D are present in the cells of the parathyroid glands, the secretion rate of which can be altered by vitamin D metabolites in experimental animals. When 1,25-DHCC is given therapeutically to hypoparathyroid patients, there is an eventual increase in renal tubular reabsorption of phosphate, with consequent corresponding changes in their serum concentrations. Proximal muscle weakness, a striking feature of vitamin D deficiency, is relieved by treatment with 1,25-DHCC.

HISTORY

Hypercalcemia may manifest clinically in many ways or it may be discovered on routine biochemical screening of an asymptomatic patient. In recent years, with the widespread use of automated biochemical profile instrumentation, there has been a dramatic increase in the "accidental" discovery of hypercalcemia. Even when hypercalcemia is symptomatic, the patient may have only vague symptoms such as tiredness, weakness, lassitude, and depression. These general symptoms may take on a more neuropsychological nature, such as hallucinations, paranoia, and neurotic behavior. In addition to neuropsychiatric presentation, the patient with hypercalcemia may present with other symptoms that may be confined to specific systems such as the gastrointestinal or genitourinary tract. The gastrointestinal symptoms include constipation, anorexia, nausea, vomiting, and upper abdominal pain; the latter may be due either to peptic ulceration or to acute pancreatitis. Genitourinary symptoms, including polydipsia and polyuria are common. Patients may also present with loin pain or other symptoms attributable to renal stones.

The cardiovascular system may be affected, giving rise to hypertension. Electrocardiographic changes may occur with either an extreme elevation or a depression in serum calcium concentration. In severe hypercalcemia there may be shortening of the QT interval and an increase in the amplitude of the T wave, which appears to begin immediately after the end of the QRS complex, such that the ST segment appears to be absent.

Some patients with hypercalcemia have metastatic calcification, which may prompt them to seek medical care. A relatively common site for calcification is in the cornea; it should be looked for at the limbus of the cornea and is unlike arcus senilis, which is continuous with the scleral margin. Patients with hypercalcemia may develop a symptomatic acute "red eye" owing to conjunctival calcification.

The multiple clinical modes of presentation of hypercalcemia mean that it must be considered *frequently* in differential diagnosis. A request for the estimation of serum calcium concentration is justified as a part of an initial work-up in many patients. A major problem of hypercalcemia is the risk that irreversible renal damage may occur if it is allowed to continue undiagnosed and untreated. There is also the risk that the hypercalcemia may, for a variety of reasons, undergo a sudden increase and give rise to a hypercalcemic crisis, which has a high mortality rate and must be treated as a medical emergency. In this situation death may occur from dehydration, coma, and anuria.

The severity of the clinical symptoms in general correlates well with the degree of hypercalcemia, regardless of the underlying cause. It is important to recognize the fact that the finding of hypercalcemia is not a final diagnosis but only the start of an investigation of its cause.

PHYSICAL EXAMINATION

In the patient who has hypercalcemia, there may be absolutely normal physical findings. Indeed, 2.5 per cent of persons tested will have elevated calcium levels, but some will be healthy individuals whose value falls at the upper end of the distribution curve.[3] The making of the clinical diagnosis then involves the physical examination, which must be thorough, but does not depend totally upon it. The combined evaluation of all historical, physical, and chemical data is imperative. The diagnostic difficulty arises from the vague nature of symptoms and the lack of physical signs. In general, findings may relate to urologic problems, gastrointestinal syndromes, psychiatric syndromes, or skeletal problems.[4]

In some cases of hypercalcemia, proximal muscle weakness can be demonstrated. Late in the disease, examination of the eyes may reveal corneal band keratopathy, which appears as grayish white calcium deposits in the superficial layers of the cornea at the medial and lateral borders. Mental clarity can be affected adversely in some older patients. Hypertension may be one of the physical findings. Weight loss is noted with associated neoplasms. Pancreatitis manifests as epigastric tenderness. Gross hematuria may be seen with renal stones. Frequent fractures and joint tenderness may also give clues.

If there are no abnormal physical findings on repeated examinations, and the hypercalcemia persists, one must be aware of the possibility of occult malignancy.

DIAGNOSTIC STUDIES

Serum Calcium — Total and Ionized

As already stated, particular attention should be paid to the technique used for venipuncture when collecting blood for serum calcium estimation to avoid the problems of artifactual hypercalcemia. Ideally, the patient should be fasting prior to collection of blood for calcium estimation. Fasting is, however, not essential, because during a normal working day, increments in serum calcium concentration of only about 0.5 to 0.8 mg/100 ml (0.13 to 0.20 mmol/liter) occur, after either the intake of a normal meal or a large load of oral calcium. The simultaneous estimation of total protein and, particularly, albumin concentrations is of value when comparing the calcium results in any one patient over time, because variations in total serum calcium concentration may reflect alterations in total serum protein and albumin concentrations.

The diagnostic value of the routine measurement of ionized calcium concentration in the evaluation of patients with hypercalcemia is controversial. In our own observations, the ionized calcium level in the majority of patients bears a constant percentage relationship to the total serum concentration. We therefore consider the measurement of ionized calcium to be of value only in the assessment of hypercalcemic patients with either significant alterations in albumin concentration or multiple myelomatosis.

Serum Phosphate

Because of the action of parathyroid hormone in blocking the net tubular reabsorption of phosphate, hypophosphatemia has in the past been considered the hallmark of hypercalcemia due to primary hyperparathyroidism. In primary hyperparathyroidism, however, consistently low serum phosphate concentrations are usually the exception rather than the rule, even in the presence of normal renal function. A consistently low serum phosphate concentration is highly suggestive of primary hyperparathyroidism, but the diagnosis is not excluded in the presence of a normal or high concentration. Hypophosphatemia is also a biochemical feature of pseudohyperparathyroidism, owing to the renal tubule actions of the PTH-like peptide secreted by the nonendocrine tumor.

Phosphate Excretion Tests

A variety of phosphate excretion tests have been described. They are all based on the action of parathyroid hormone at the renal tubular level in blocking net phosphate reabsorption. The tests were devised prior to the availability of parathyroid hormone assays; they were developed in an attempt to improve the diagnostic accuracy in borderline primary hyperparathyroidism and to differentiate hypercalcemia due to primary hyperparathyroidism from hypercalcemia due to other causes. The phosphate excretion tests have employed a variety of clearance equations and can be divided according to whether they involve simple or more complex procedures. If the patient is on a metabolic unit with a controlled phosphate intake, has normal or nearly normal renal function, and does not have glycosuria, these tests may be useful in the diagnosis of borderline primary hyperparathyroidism. Abnormalities in the renal handling of phosphate, however, also occur in a variety of other conditions that may themselves cause hypercalcemia. Because of the control requirements and the technical difficulties in performing these tests, some of which require constant phosphate infusion and a rigidly controlled dietary phosphate intake, phosphate excretion tests are of limited differential diagnostic value.

Serum Proteins and Albumin

In patients with hypercalcemia, routinely estimating total serum protein and albumin concentrations simultaneously with the total calcium concentration is of diagnostic value in the interpretation of the calcium value, particularly of intermittent values measured over a long period. Serum protein electrophoresis is helpful in the differential diagnosis of hypercalcemia, especially for the identification of those patients with either sarcoidosis or myelomatosis.

Alkaline Phosphatase

For the differential diagnosis of hypercalcemia, the estimation of serum alkaline phosphatase activity is by itself of little aid. In primary hyperparathyroidism, the plasma alkaline phosphatase level correlates with the specific radiologic findings of hyperparathyroidism (osteitis fibrosa). In hypercalcemia due to malignant disease, an elevation in alkaline phosphatase activity may indicate metastatic deposits in bone or other organs.

Parathyroid Hormone (PTH)

The phenomenon of immunoheterogeneity of circulating PTH is probably the major determinant of the results of serum immunoreactive-PTH (i-PTH) measurement with a given radioimmunoassay procedure. Knowledge of the immunospecificity of the assay being used is crucial to the interpretation of test results as well as of the simultaneous serum calcium determination. The routine assay of i-PTH in an individual blood sample using a procedure that employs an antisera with specificity for the carboxyterminal region of PTH is of value in the diagnosis of primary hyperparathyroidism and the differential diagnosis of hypercalcemia. In making these interpretations, Broadus and Rasmussen emphasize, the individual physician "must know and understand the characteristics and track record of the PTH method from which his assay results are derived."[5] They also state that extreme caution should be used "in accepting as diagnostic values within the normal range which are judged nomographically or by computer as 'inappropriate.' In the latter context, "laboratories which report predominantly inappropriate results in patients with primary and secondary hyperparathyroidism are using assays which are clearly insensitive and of little value in differentiating primary hyperparathyroidism from other causes of hypercalcemia."[5]

Assays that employ antisera with specificity for the amino-terminal region of PTH should be used for multiple venous sampling; these assays reflect acute changes in the secretion rate of PTH. Multiple venous sampling of the neck region in an attempt to localize a parathyroid adenoma by i-PTH assay should be reserved for patients who have undergone neck surgery and have either persistent or recurrent hypercalcemia; the procedure is not a part of the routine differential diagnostic evaluation of hypercalcemia.

25-Hydroxyvitamin D and 1,25-Dihydroxycholecalciferol

Assays of 25-hydroxyvitamin D (25-OHD) and 1,25-dihydroxycholecalciferol (1,25-DHCC) should be performed for the differential diagnosis of hypercalcemic states that are either known or considered to be caused by disorders in vitamin D metabolism. Serum 1,25-DHCC may be elevated in primary hyperparathyroidism.

Calcitonin

An increase in serum immunoreactive calcitonin level can occur in many disease states, particularly cancer. It is of no differential diagnostic value in hypercalcemia.

Urine Calcium

The total 24-hour urine calcium excretion rate should be estimated in all patients with hypercalcemia, in order to confirm the blood findings and also to exclude those very rare patients with familial hypocalciuric hypercalcemia.

Urine Hydroxyproline

Hydroxyproline is a nonessential amino acid that occurs almost exclusively in collagen, where it accounts for some 14 per cent of total amino acids. In primary hyperparathyroidism, the urinary excretion of hydroxyproline is increased, probably because of accelerated bone turnover and collagen degradation. In these patients the increase in urine hydroxyproline excretion appears to be a more sensitive index of bone involvement than the serum alkaline phosphatase activity. Because urine hydroxyproline excretion is of itself directly correlated with the rate of bone destruction, however, its estimation is of no value in the differential diagnosis of patients with hypercalcemia, in whom bone destruction due to a variety of causes may account for the hypercalcemia.

Urine Cyclic AMP

An increase in urine cyclic AMP (cAMP) excretion represents the target tissue (renal tubule) response to the action of PTH and has been reported to be slightly superior to the i-PTH assay in the differential diagnosis of hypercalcemia. Relatively poor correlations of urine total cAMP excretion with i-PTH concentration have been reported because of renal impairment. This problem can be overcome by reporting the results as nephrogenous cAMP, which takes into account both the glomerular filtration rate and the plasma cAMP concentration.[5] In view of the difficulties in measuring the latter, an alternative approach has been used, in which the total urine cAMP excretion is expressed as a function of the glomerular filtration rate, and has been termed "nephrogenous" cAMP. The urine cAMP excretion appears to be of considerable diagnostic value in the differential diagnosis of hypercalcemia when used in conjunction with the serum i-PTH assay.

Cortisone Suppression Test

Although it is not strictly a laboratory investigation, the cortisone suppression test is included here for the sake of completeness.

It was originally reported that following the administration of cortisone there was a significant reduction in the hypercalcemia associated with sarcoidosis, myelomatosis, thyrotoxicosis, vitamin D intoxication, and malignant disease, and that such a reduction did not occur in the hypercalcemia associated with primary hyperparathyroidism. Since the original description of this test, there have been many reports of patients with proven primary hyperparathyroidism in whom hypercalcemia has been suppressed, as well as of patients with hypercalcemia due to various other causes who have failed to show suppression. In the majority of these conflicting reports the workers have not used the method as originally described and have used other various steroid substitutes. It is recognized that even when correctly performed, this test is not completely reliable, as both suppression of hypercalcemia due to primary hyperparathyroidism and nonsuppression of hypercalcemia due to other causes may occur. Despite this limitation, the test is of value in the differential diagnosis of hypercalcemia when other tests have failed to show definitive diagnostic patterns. The test as originally described involves the oral administration of a standard 10-day load of cortisone given orally in a dose of 50 mg three times a day; recently hydrocortisone (40 mg three times a day) has been used instead with comparable results.[6] This test has been reported to have a high degree of diagnostic accuracy; false-positive results may occur in patients with osteitis fibrosa.[7]

ASSESSMENT

In the assessment of a patient with hypercalcemia it is important to recognize that the symptoms due to the hypercalcemia per se are vague and nonspecific and are the same irrespective of the causative mechanism. The symptoms, and many of the clinical signs, are generally proportional to the degree of elevation in the serum calcium concentration and offer no clue to the etiologic mechanism. The accurate differential diagnosis of hypercalcemia is important if rational treatment is to be instituted for the underlying disorder. In many situations a particular diagnosis can be made or excluded by either a carefully taken clinical history or a detailed physical examination. Frequently, however, the underlying disease is not obvious and there are equivocal clinical and even radiologic findings; in such cases the differential diagnosis of hypercalcemia has to be based on an evaluation of the associated biochemical findings. Such an evaluation must be related to the potential causes of an increase in serum calcium concentration.

It has already been stated that the incidences of hypercalcemia differ in outpatient and inpatient hospital populations. In the diagnostic approach these variations in incidence should be considered.

Carcinoma

The most common cause of hypercalcemia in a general hospital population is carcinoma, and approximately 10 per cent of patients with neoplasia have hypercalcemia at some time in their illness. In the outpatient situation, hypercalcemia of recent onset in a patient who is apparently otherwise well is often associated with malignant disease and justifies the search for a primary neoplasm. The search should be oriented toward the types of tumor known to be associated with metastatic bone disease and hypercalcemia. In carcinoma, a variety of mechanisms can cause bone dissolution and consequent hypercalcemia, the most common being osteolytic bone metastases. The most common sources of such metastases are primary neoplasms located in the breast, bronchus, kidney, and thyroid. In patients with bone dissolution due to metastases there is a simultaneous increase in both the serum calcium and phosphate concentrations.

Hypercalcemia may occur in patients with carcinoma in whom there are no demonstrable metastatic bone lesions either on radiologic bone survey during life or on careful histologic examination of the bones at autopsy. In this group of patients a variety of mechanisms can account for the hypercalcemia, including the secretion of parathyroid hormone–like polypeptides, prostaglandins, osteoclast activity factor, and osteolytic sterols.

The secretion by a primary tumor of a polypeptide that has actions similar to those of a naturally occurring hormone allows the tumor to be classified as a nonendocrine hormone-secreting tumor. Some primary carcinomas may synthesize a parathyroid hormone–like polypeptide that causes both hypercalcemia and an associated hypophosphatemia; this syndrome has been termed pseudohyperparathyroidism. It is the most common endocrine syndrome associated with bronchial carcinoma and occurs most frequently with tumors of squamous cell origin. The i-PTH–like material secreted by these nonendocrine tumors may be immunologically different from the hormone present in the serum of the patient with primary hyperparathyroidism but it may cross-react in some assay systems. In this situation, i-PTH concentration may be reported as either elevated or inappropriate for the simultaneous calcium concentration. The differentiation of pseudohyperparathyroidism from primary hyperparathyroidism is of considerable importance, because in the patient with pseudohyperparathyroidism there may be a small, relatively symptomless primary neoplasm. In some patients, pseudohyperparathyroidism can be distinguished from primary hyperparathyroidism on the basis of acid-base balance. Patients with hypercalcemia in primary hyperparathyroidism tend to have a metabolic acidosis (low plasma bicarbonate and high plasma chloride), whereas those with hypercalcemia due to all other causes, including pseudohyperparathyroidism, tend to have a metabolic alkalosis (high plasma bicarbonate, low plasma chloride).[8]

Primary Hyperparathyroidism

Primary hyperparathyroidism is a common cause of hypercalcemia; its accurate diagnosis is important because it is amenable to surgical treatment. Primary hyperparathyroidism is usually due to an adenoma of one of the parathyroid glands, rarely to hyperplasia of all four glands, and very rarely to carcinoma.

The classic clinical presentation of primary hyperparathyroidism was as "bones, stones, or abdominal groans," but in recent years its incidence has increased with the advent of health screening programs and the discovery of asymptomatic hypercalcemia. A recent study reported that more than 75 per cent of the patients with primary hyperparathyroidism appeared to have asymptomatic disease.[9] The reported incidence of subsequently proven primary hyperparathyroidism in health screening programs has varied from 1 to 4 per 1,000 individuals screened. Hypertension has been reported to be twice as common in hyperparathyroid patients as in the general population.[9]

The presentation of primary hyperparathyroidism with symptoms attributable to the development of either renal stones or metabolic bone disease has been attributed to the type of the tumor. According to this concept, a slow-growing tumor causes renal stones, whereas a more active, faster-growing tumor gives rise to overt bone disease. The metabolic bone disease seen in patients with hyperparathyroidism is osteitis fibrosa. It may cause pain but may be asymptomatic and found accidentally during a radiologic examination. Radiologic bone disease is most often seen in the hands as subperiosteal erosions in the phalanges; it may also involve the skull or long bones. In long bones it can be seen as bone cysts, which appear either as asymptomatic swellings or with pathologic fractures. The incidence of primary hyperparathyroidism is higher in women than in men, with a peak between 40 and 70 years of age in both groups. Primary hyperparathyroidism may also be a feature of the pluriglandular syndrome associated with acromegaly.

In a recent study, Lafferty[10] reported that the most useful discriminant laboratory tests, in descending order of value, are serum chloride, calcium, hematocrit, phosphorus, and i-PTH determinations. Multivariate discriminant analysis of serum calcium, phosphorus, chloride, and hematocrit tests provided 98 per cent accuracy in separating primary hyperparathyroidism from other causes of hypercalcemia.

Thiazides

The occurrence of a mild degree of hypercalcemia has been reported in a large proportion of patients receiving diuretics of the thiadiazine group. Thiazides are unique among diuretic agents in that they stimulate the renal tubular reabsorption of calcium. The effect of thiazides on the intestinal absorption of calcium in normal humans is not clearly defined; it appears to be either unaltered or slightly increased during treatment. Some of the increase in total calcium concentration in patients receiving thiazides may reflect an increase in the protein-bound fraction; a consequence of a diuretic-induced reduction in extracellular fluid volume with an associated increase in total protein concentration. The occurrence of a significant degree of hypercalcemia (> 11.0 mg/100 ml or 2.75 mmol/liter) in a patient on thiazide diuretic therapy justifies immediate cessation of such therapy.

Hematologic Malignancy (Myeloma, Leukemia, Hodgkin's Disease)

Hypercalcemia is a recognized complication of a variety of hematologic malignancies. Hypercalcemia may occur in approximately 50 per cent of patients with myelomatosis at some time during the course of their disease. In patients with myelomatosis, the hypercalcemia is in excess of the increase that can be accounted for either by changes in serum protein levels or by the extent of the bone lesions. In lymphoid cell lines derived from patients with myeloma, a soluble factor capable of stimulating osteoclastic bone resorption in vitro has been isolated; this factor is not PTH, prostaglandins, or a vitamin D–like sterol. The factor, which has been termed osteoclast-activating factor (OAF), is capable of stimulating bone resorption in organ culture. OAF has also been obtained from lymphoid cell lines from patients with Burkitt's lymphoma and malignant lymphoma. The effect of OAF is probably confined to bone, where it is formed locally during invasion by tumor, and accounts for the local bone destruction. OAF and its production by neoplastic cells can be regarded as a part of the cellular immune response to neoplasia. In other hematologic malignancies, including lymphosarcoma and Hodgkin's disease, there is evidence that the tumors are capable of the ectopic production of a PTH-like peptide and prostaglandins.

Vitamin D Intoxication

Hypercalcemia is an important complication of the long-term treatment with either vitamin D or its various mono- and di-hydroxy analogs. The importance of this complication is that it can be avoided by awareness and surveillance. Vitamin D and its various metabolites are cumulative toxic compounds. The hypercalcemia of vitamin D intoxication is caused by an increased absorption of calcium from the gastrointestinal tract. In patients receiving treatment with vitamin D or its metabolites, changes in 24-hour urine calcium excretion may be of predictive value.

Sarcoidosis

Hypercalcemia is a rare complication in patients with sarcoidosis and, when present, is usually associated with severe and disseminated disease; the latter is, however, by no means a constant feature. There is a wide variation in the reported incidence of hypercalcemia in sarcoidosis both within any one country and from country to country. The hypercalcemia was in the past attributed to hypersensitivity to all of the actions of cholecalciferol; there is now evidence that it is due to an abnormality in the regulation and excessive production of 1,25-DHCC.[11] Production of the excess 1,25-DHCC appears to involve extrarenal sites and may be from the macrophages involved in the disease process.

A number of patients have been reported in whom primary hyperparathyroidism and sarcoidosis coexist; it would seem unlikely, however, that there is any direct etiologic relationship between these two conditions.

Thyrotoxicosis

Hypercalcemia may occur in association with hyperthyroidism either as a direct complication or as a manifestation of associated primary hyperparathyroidism. The mechanism of the hypercalcemia that occurs as a direct complication of hyperthyroidism is not clear. It is, however, recognized that thyroxine has a direct effect on the mobilization of calcium in bone.

An association has been reported between hyperthyroidism and primary hyperparathyroidism, although it is probably not a variant of the syndrome of multiple endocrine adenomatosis or hyperplasia.

Milk-Alkali Syndrome (Milk-Drinker's Syndrome)

The features of this syndrome, which occurred with a relatively high frequency in the past, are hypercalcemia with a metabolic alkalosis. The syndrome occurred in patients with peptic ulcer pain who classically had an excessive intake of both milk and an absorbable alkali; they usually also had evidence of previous renal disease. The hypercalcemia usually resolved with stopping of the excessive intake of milk and alkali. The milk-alkali syndrome has become relatively rare with changes in peptic ulcer therapy, particularly with the use of nonabsorbable alkalis. The syndrome does, however, still occur with the self-administration, by peptic ulcer patients, of proprietary "anti-acid" preparations that contain calcium carbonate. These patients are liable to present with hypercalcemia and/or renal failure.

The mechanism for the hypercalcemia in this syndrome is complex.[12] Among the factors involved is an increase in calcium absorption from the intestinal tract together with a diminution in urine calcium and bicarbonate excretion. The ingestion of an absorbable alkali, such as calcium carbonate, can of itself cause renal damage. The diagnostic criteria for this syndrome include a history of alkali intake and the characteristic laboratory findings of hypercalcemia and a metabolic alkalosis in the presence of some degree of renal impairment.

Multiple Endocrine Adenomatosis

Hypercalcemia associated with either hyperplasia or an adenoma of the parathyroid glands is a recognized, but rare, occurrence in patients with pituitary adenomas. The relationship between these two glands, and the occasional associated finding of pancreatic islet cell adenomas, is not clearly defined. The generally held view is that the relationship between acromegaly and hyperparathyroidism is a manifestation of the syndrome of "multiple endocrine adenomas" or "polyendocrine adenomatosis." The syndrome is inherited as an autosomal dominant with a high degree of penetrance and appears as manifestations of hyperactivity of multiple endocrine organs. The most common abnormalities found in one study of five families with this syndrome, in decreasing order of frequency, were hypercalcemia, pancreatic tumors, peptic ulcer, and pituitary tumors. The rarity of this syndrome is such that an endocrinologic investigation of the pituitary-adrenal axis is not justified in a patient with primary hyperparathyroidism unless there are some specific clinical indications.

Paget's Disease of Bone

In patients with Paget's disease of bone (osteitis deformans), hypercalcemia is a very rare complication and occurs virtually only when the patients are immobilized and confined to bed. The hypercalcemia is related to the markedly increased bone turnover rate and the disturbance in the balance between the normally equal rates of bone resorption and deposition as the result of immobilization. The frequency of hypercalcemia in patients with Paget's disease is sufficient to justify the regular assay of serum calcium concentration in any patient with this disease process who is immobilized for any reason (e.g., stroke, pneumonia, myocardial infarction).

Tertiary Hyperparathyroidism

Tertiary hyperparathyroidism is, by definition, hypercalcemia due to an excess secretion of parathyroid hormone that has developed in a patient with long-standing hypocalcemia, which is itself usually due to chronic gastrointestinal or renal disease. All four of the parathyroid glands in this situation are hyperplastic and may be regarded as autonomous, with no response to changes in circulating calcium concentration. In the group of patients with chronic renal failure, the serum immunoreactive parathyroid hormone (i-PTH) values are "dramatically" increased, much higher than in patients with primary hyperparathyroidism. Such extremely high values are accounted for, in part, by the failure of the functionally impaired kidneys to clear biologically inactive peptide fragments from the circulation. There is also in these patients an increase in the PTH secretion rate.

Familial Hypocalciuric Hypercalcemia

This rare benign familial disorder, which does not affect life span, has been recognized only in the past decade.[13] It is inherited as an autosomal dominant trait with complete penetrance. Symptoms, when present, are usually mild and nonspecific; they include fatigue, muscle weakness, nervous and emotional difficulties, and impairment of memory. The incidence of fractures, renal stones, and peptic ulcers in patients with this disorder is similar to that in the general population. Serum i-PTH concentrations are usually not suppressed and may even be increased; these findings may be associated with an increase in "nephrogenous" cyclic AMP excretion. A diagnostic feature is that urinary calcium excretion is low in relation to the degree of hypercalcemia, in contrast to all other forms of hypercalcemia. Another pointer to this rare diagnosis is the finding of hypermagnesemia; serum magnesium concentration is not increased in primary hyperparathyroidism. The importance of recognizing patients with this rare familial syndrome is that they need not undergo either neck exploration for a parathyroid adenoma or treatment for hypercalcemia.

Idiopathic Hypercalcemia of Infancy

Hypercalcemia in infancy occurs in a mild form and a severe form, representing two different disease processes. The mild form has been attributed to either an excessive dietary intake of vitamin D or an increased sensitivity to the actions of this vitamin; it is, however, possible that variations in endogenous fecal calcium excretion may play a role. The severe form is rare and constitutes a syndrome characterized by "elfin-like" facies, mental retardation, osteosclerosis, hypercalcemia, hypercalciuria, nephrocalcinosis, and uremia; the mechanism of the hypercalcemia is unknown.

Adrenocortical Insufficiency

Hypercalcemia may occur in patients with adrenocortical insufficiency and has been reported to have an incidence comparable to that of hyponatremia; it may, however, be the only electrolyte abnormality. The mechanism for hypercalcemia in this disorder is not clearly defined.

Immobilization

An increase in serum calcium concentration may occur with long-term immobilization, although it is extremely rare.

DIAGNOSTIC DECISIONS AND VALIDATION

Before undertaking an extensive differential diagnostic evaluation of hypercalcemia, one must confirm that the serum calcium concentration is increased. This should be done using at least two blood specimens collected with meticulous attention to technique. If two subsequent calcium determinations are both normal, then it is likely that the initial high value was either a collection or contamination artifact or was due to laboratory error and can be ignored. Prior to final dismissal of the problem, it is probably of value to collect a further specimen for calcium estimation after an interval of 1 month.

The objective of the differential diagnostic evaluation is to determine the etiology of the hypercalcemia so that appropriate treatment can be instituted for the primary causative condition. In some patients the degree of elevation in the serum calcium concentration is of itself life-threatening and necessitates urgent treatment. In this latter situation it is essential to identify the underlying cause as rapidly as possible as well as to institute treatment for hypercalcemia.

The first step in the differential diagnostic evaluation is to collect a full and detailed history with particular attention to the known symptomatology associated with hypercalcemia. The history must include full details of drug therapy, physician-prescribed as well as self-administered, and nutritional history, including vitamin intake in foodstuff as well as in supplemental tablet form.

The most common causes of asymptomatic hypercalcemia are primary hyperparathyroidism and therapy with a variety of drugs. Among the latter are thiazide diuretics, vitamin D compounds, and antacids. It is possible that asymptomatic hypercalcemia may be the presenting or accidentally discovered feature in patients with "silent" neoplasms or sarcoidosis. The latter is, however, more usually symptomatic. A rare cause of asymptomatic hypercalcemia that is usually discovered accidentally is familial hypocalciuric hypercalcemia.

The initial investigational protocol should include the following:

1. Determinations of serum total calcium and phosphate.*
2. Serum electrolyte (sodium, potassium, chloride, and bicarbonate) together with blood urea nitrogen and creatinine measurements.*
3. Determinations of serum total proteins and albumin, and electrophoresis.
4. Full blood count, including a differential white count and examination of blood film.
5. 24-Hour urine collection for calcium excretion and creatinine clearance measurements.
6. Clean urine specimen collection for total protein measurement and electrophoresis.
7. *If* the history is compatible with vitamin D intoxication, initial work-up should also include serum 25-hydroxyvitamin-D assay.
8. After confirmation of the presence of hypercalcemia with hypercalciuria, the next steps in the diagnostic strategy should include a serum i-PTH assay.

If the i-PTH value is elevated, further evaluation would require estimation of "nephrogenous" cyclic AMP and possibly of 1,25-dihydroxycholecalciferol, which is increased in primary hyperparathyroidism.

If the i-PTH level is either low or undetectable, further evaluation should be directed to a search for malignancy. The extent of such a search is controversial but should include radiologic examination of the chest and, in the presence of symptoms, the gastrointestinal and renal tracts. The use of algorithms or "decision trees" may be of some value in the evaluation of hypercalcemia. In one recent study, however, the use of algorithms assigned the correct diagnostic categories in only 66 per cent of a group of 80 patients with hypercalcemia.[14]

*In many laboratories these tests are available in a cost-efficient metabolic profile.

REFERENCES

1. Fisken RA, Heath DA, Bold AM. Hypercalcemia—a hospital survey. Q J Med 1980;64:405–18.
2. Talmage RV, Grubb SA, Norimatsu H, VanderWiel CJ. Evidence for an important physiological role for calcitonin. Proc Natl Acad Sci 1980;77:609–13.
3. Branch WT Jr. Office practice of medicine. Philadelphia: WB Saunders, 1982:900–910.
4. Tretbar HA. The diagnosis of hypercalcemia. Continuing Education. Vol. 17, October, 1981;43. New York: LeJacq Publishing Co.
5. Broadus AE, Rasmussen H. Clinical evaluation of parathyroid function. Am J Med 1981;70:475–8.
6. Dent CE, Watson L. The hydrocortisone test in primary and tertiary hyperparathyroidism. Lancet 1968;2:662–4.
7. Watson L, Moxham J, Fraser P. Hydrocortisone suppression test and discriminant analysis in differential diagnosis of hypercalcemia. Lancet 1980;1:1320–5.
8. Wills MR. Value of plasma chloride concentration and acid-base status in the differential diagnosis of hyperparathyroidism from other causes of hypercalcemia. J. Clin Pathol 1971;24:219–27.
9. Harrop JS, Bailey JE, Woodhead JS. Incidence of hypercalcemia and primary hyperparathyroidism in relation to the biochemical profile. J Clin Pathol 1982;35:395–400.
10. Lafferty FW. Primary hyperparathyroidism. Changing clinical spectrum, prevalence of hypertension, and discriminant analysis of laboratory tests. Arch Intern Med 1981;141:1761–6.
11. Stern PH, De Olazabal J, Bell NH. Evidence for abnormal regulation of circulating 1α,25-dihydroxyvitamin D in patients with sarcoidosis and normal calcium metabolism. J Clin Invest 1980;66:852–5.
12. Orwoll ES. The milk-alkali syndrome: Current concepts. Ann Intern Med 1982;97:242–8.
13. Anonymous. Familial hypocalciuric hypercalcemia [Editorial]. Lancet 1982;1:488–9.
14. Lum G, Deshotels SJ. The clinical usefulness of an algorithm for the interpretation of biochemical profiles with hypercalcemia. Am J Clin Pathol 1982;78:479–84.

HYPERHIDROSIS

D. MELESSA PHILLIPS

☐ SYNONYMS: Excessive sweating or perspiration, diaphoresis

BACKGROUND

Description and Significance

Hyperhidrosis represents a dysfunction of the eccrine sweat system in which noticeably excessive amounts of sweat are produced. Inordinate sweating may occur in response to normal stimuli or as a manifestation of an underlying disease. Clinically, hyperhidrosis is classified as *localized* (when confined to the axillae, palms, soles, or face) or *generalized* (when it occurs throughout the distribution of the eccrine system).

The patient with hyperhidrosis "sweats too much." This is usually a subjective impression rather than a clinical observation. Grice,[1] however, describes hyperhidrosis of the feet so marked that "squelching sounds" are heard when "walking in shoes filled with pools of sweat." Some teenagers and young adults actually experience a visible "drip" of perspiration from the palms. These extreme cases of idiopathic hyperhidrosis are usually triggered by anxiety or stressful situations but can occur after minimal heat exposure. Persistent generalized hyperhidrosis deserves careful clinical investigation. This type of sweating is a symptom common to many endocrine, neurologic, and even neoplastic disorders (Table 1) and must be accounted for in the context of its clinical presentation.

Anatomy and Physiology of Sweating

Two types of sweat glands are found in the body, eccrine and apocrine. These secretory structures differ in their anatomic distribution as well as in the chemical composition and site of discharge of the fluids they produce.

Eccrine sweat glands are scattered throughout the surface of the skin, especially the palms, soles, axillae, face, chest, and back. Eccrine sweat is the end-product of "precursor secretion," which is itself a substance actively manufactured by epithelial cells lining the eccrine coil.[2] Selective components of precursor secretion are reabsorbed as the fluid passes through the duct portion of the gland (Fig. 1). The drops appearing on the skin are a hypotonic solution of sodium, chloride, and water. Potassium, urea, and ammonia are found in small quantities in sweat; trace amounts of calcium, phosphorus, copper, and magnesium can also be identified.[3]

Apocrine sweat glands are located in the axillae, intertriginous areas, and areolae of the breast. Originating from the pilosebaceous system, their cloudy, thick secretion is emptied into the hair follicle shaft (see Fig. 1). While structurally similar to eccrine glands, the apocrine system has little, if any, role in hyperhidrotic conditions, and therefore is not discussed in detail.

The skin, eccrine sweat glands, and hypothalamus constitute the body's thermoregulatory control system. When necessary, body heat is removed by changes in skin blood flow (vasodilatation) mediated through the sympathetic nervous system. According to Guyton,[2] sweating begins with the reception of appropriate stimuli in the preoptic area of the anterior hypothalamus. Impulses from this area are transmitted through autonomic pathways to the spinal cord and discharged to the eccrine glands via sympathetic outflow tracts. Eccrine sweating represents an interesting and paradoxic cooperation between the two divisions of the autonomic system. Sympathetic nerve fibers terminate near the secretory "coil portion" of the dermal gland (see Fig. 1). Almost all other sympathetic fibers in the body are adrenergic, but those supplying the eccrine glands are cholinergic. The eccrine system is also capable of stimulation by circulating levels of epinephrine and norepinephrine, even though there is no direct adrenergic innervation. Profuse sweating from the palmar and plantar surfaces in response to stress, fear, or anxiety may indicate that glands in these regions have dual adrenergic and cholinergic nerve supplies.

Normal sweating is a protective physiologic response to heat (external or internal) that provides evaporative cooling of the skin surface. In conditions in which the core body temperature exceeds 98.6° F, the "hypothalamic thermostat" initiates sweating to ensure dissipation of excessive body heat production.[2] The cooling effect of moisture on the skin surface lowers body temperature, and the hypothalamic thermostat resets itself to maintain normal thermoregulation.

Eight mechanisms are responsible for the pathogenesis of generalized hyperhidrosis that is symptomatic of some systemic diseases. These mechanisms and their related disorders are summarized in Table 2.

HISTORY

What does the physician need to know about the patient who complains of sweating too much?

Table 1. CLASSIFICATION AND CAUSES OF HYPERHIDROSIS

Classification	Causes
Localized hyperhidrosis	
"Idiopathic" hyperhidrosis (palmar, plantar, axillary)	
Gustatory hyperhidrosis	Food ingestion Von Frey's syndrome
Generalized hyperhidrosis	Endocrine/metabolic disorders Thyrotoxicosis Diabetes mellitus Hypoglycemia Menopause Pheochromocytoma Carcinoid syndrome Acromegaly
	Infectious disorders Septicemias Brucellosis Tuberculosis Malaria
	Neurologic disorders Parkinsonism Tabes dorsalis Stroke Diencephalic syndrome of infancy
	Neoplastic disorders Hodgkin's disease Non-Hodgkin's lymphomas Complete cord compression by metastatic tumor
	Genetic disorders Riley-Day syndrome Cystic fibrosis
	Psychogenic causes Fear Pain Anxiety Stress
	Drugs Aspirin Emetics Insulin Meperidine Pilocarpine Physostigmine Cholinergics, anticholinesterases
	Miscellaneous conditions Alcoholism Alcohol withdrawal Drug withdrawal (opiates) Mushroom poisoning Organophosphate poisoning

Table 2. MECHANISM OF GENERALIZED HYPERHIDROSIS IN SYSTEMIC DISEASE

Mechanism	Related Conditions
Increased metabolic rate	Thyrotoxicosis Fever Pheochromocytoma Exercise
Hypothalamic dysfunction	Parkinsonism Diencephalic syndrome of infancy
Endogenous pyrogen production	Septicemia Lymphoma Brucellosis
Peripheral tissue effects of hormones	Acromegaly Pheochromocytoma
Central nervous system degeneration	Tumors (metastatic) Tabes dorsalis
Autonomic nervous system degeneration	Diabetes mellitus Riley-Day syndrome
Autonomic nervous system stimulation	Drug ingestion Toxin ingestion Cholinesterase inhibitor use
Vasodilation and increased skin blood flow	Menopause Carcinoid syndrome

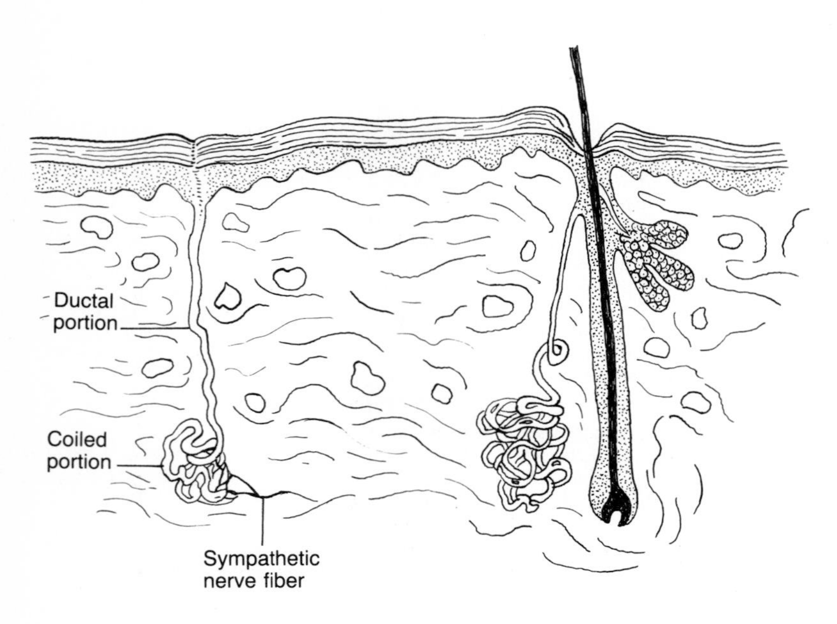

Figure 1. Eccrine and apocrine sweat glands.

Basically, the goal is to distinguish localized hyperhidrosis (a clinical diagnosis) from generalized hyperhidrosis (a symptom of underlying disease). Perfunctory questions about the onset, frequency, location, and severity of the sweating puts the condition into perspective.

History of the Present Illness. How and when did the patient first become aware of the sweating? Does he or she change clothes frequently or shower several times a day? Are clothes continually stained or decaying from sweat? Are socks always disagreeably wet, or are the feet stained after wearing dyed shoes? Does the patient wipe his or her hands constantly or even wear gloves to hide the moisture? Have family, friends, or coworkers noticed or remarked that the patient seems to sweat a lot? Is tension or stress related?

Has the hyperhidrosis interfered with patient's ability to do his or her job (typist, tailor, factory worker)? Has there been a recent change at work (promotion, more responsibility, new boss)? Has the patient been transferred from a dry climate to a hot, humid one? Has the patient been out of the country on business or vacation? Has the sweating affected recreational activities (grip on a tennis racquet or golf club)?

Are any other symptoms (headache, nervousness, flushing) present before or during the periods of sweating? Does it occur only at night? Has there been a recent change in body weight or appetite? Has there been any fatigue or insomnia?

Although gustatory hyperhidrosis is virtually self-diagnosed, clarification is helpful—does the sweating occur only on the face after eating certain foods?

Previous History and Review of Systems. A comprehensive history and systems review can eliminate or confirm suspicions of primary systemic disease. Pertinent findings and their association with known causes of hyperhidrosis are listed in Table 3.

Family History. Disorders characterized by hyperhidrosis that are known to have a familial occurrence include thyrotoxicosis, diabetes mellitus, hypertension, tuberculosis, and Hodgkin's disease. Both localized and generalized hyperhidrosis have been reported in cases of familial dysautonomia, or Riley-Day syndrome.[5] Idiopathic (localized) hyperhidrosis itself is often familial.

High-Payoff Queries

Significant conditions to be identified via the history can be summarized in the 10 following patient inquiries:

1. *Is the sweating generalized or confined to the face, underarms, palms, or soles?*
2. *Is the sweating persistent or episodic? Is it worse under stress?*
3. *Do you feel hot when others around you are comfortable or cool?*
4. *Does anyone in your family experience this type of sweating?*
5. *Is the sweating worse during the day or night?*
6. *How has the excess sweating affected your personal life, social life, and job?*
7. *Have you noticed any numbness, lack of coordination, tremor, or fatigue?*
8. *Is there a history of recurrent fever, cough or swollen glands?*
9. *Has there been a noticeable change in your weight or appetite?*
10. *Are you taking medication for hypertension, pain, or glaucoma?*

PHYSICAL EXAMINATION

The physician who actually observes an episode of hyperhidrosis is indeed fortunate. Unless the case is extreme, the paucity of physical findings in localized hyperhidrosis is disappointing, and the diagnosis is ultimately made on the basis of the history and exclusion of concurrent conditions.

The palms and soles should be inspected for scaling, maceration, or vesiculation indicative of dyshidrosis (a condition often superimposed on hyperhidrosis). The axillae should be examined for evidence of apocrine sweat gland disease (Fox-Fordyce disease, hidradenitis suppurativa). These conditions are almost always anhidrotic, but patients may credit their itching and chafing discomfort to excessive sweating. Examine the clothes (especially the underarms) and socks for evidence of discoloration or staining. If the patient describes gustatory hyperhidrosis, a provocative test with a pungent food may demonstrate the sweating.

The remainder of the physical examination should concentrate on exclusion of findings suggestive of any of the systemic diseases listed in Table 1: fever, increased blood pressure, neck mass, lymphadenopathy, visual field defects, cranial and peripheral nerve deficits, and neuromuscular motor and sensory abnormalities. Special features of these diseases are described under Assessment.

DIAGNOSTIC STUDIES

No known laboratory studies are of value in confirming localized hyperhidrosis. A basic screening panel for metabolic, infectious, and neoplastic causes of generalized hyperhidrosis includes CBC, T3, T4, and fasting blood glucose measurements, VDRL test, urinalysis, and chest x-ray.

If specific etiologies are suggested by historical and physical findings, the following special tests

Table 3. PERTINENT FEATURES OF MEDICAL HISTORY

Feature	Possible Significance
Dermatologic	
Facial flushing	Pheochromocytoma Carcinoid syndrome
Generalized pruritus	Hodgkin's disease
HEENT	
Headaches (paroxysmal)	Pheochromocytoma
Diplopia, failing eyesight	Pituitary tumor
History or symptoms of glaucoma	Pilocarpine use
Endocrinologic	
Enlarging neck	Toxic goiter
Heat intolerance	Diabetes mellitus Graves' disease
Cardiopulmonary	
Pain	Severe angina
Dyspnea, cough, night sweats	Tuberculosis Brucellosis Lymphoma
Hypertension, palpitations	Pheochromocytoma
Syncope	Hypoglycemia
Hematologic	
Easy bruisability or bleeding	Alcoholism Neoplastic marrow invasion
Lymphadenopathy	Infections Lymphoma
Gastrointestinal	
Nausea, vomiting, diarrhea, tenesmus	Carcinoid syndrome
Jaundice	Cirrhosis Hemolysis
Genitourinary	
Nocturia, polyuria	Diabetes mellitus
Loss of bladder control	Stroke Tabes dorsalis Cord lesions
Gynecologic	
Cessation of menses	Menopausal syndrome
Neuromuscular	
Tremors	Parkinsonism Hyperthyroidism
Neuralgias, paresthesias	Diabetes mellitus Tabes dorsalis
Orthopedic	
Increasing shoe or glove size	Acromegaly
Infectious diseases	
Mumps, severe parotitis	Von Frey's syndrome
Syphilis	Tabes dorsalis
Recent foreign travel	Malaria
Drug history	
Drug dependency	Withdrawal states
Use or abuse of known cholinergics, alcohol, analgesics, or insulin	

can be diagnostic: for hypoglycemia, 5-hour glucose tolerance test; for pheochromocytoma, 24-hour urine collection for determination of VMA, metanephrines, and catecholamines (results invalidated by use of methyldopa, L-dopa, MAO inhibitors, clofibrate, or nalidixic acid); for carcinoid syndrome, 24-hour urine collection for 5-HIAA test (results invalidated by use of phenothiazines, glyceryl guaiacolate, or serotonin-containing foods); for acromegaly, skull films, head CAT scan, and plasma assay for growth hormone; for tuberculosis, demonstration of acid-fast bacilli or sputum smear; for brucellosis, specific febrile agglutination titer; and for malaria, peripheral smear for plasmodia.

DIAGNOSTIC APPROACH

Clinical evaluation of the patient with hyperhidrosis is facilitated if one understands the mechanisms responsible for the excessive sweating. The known mechanisms are presented for recognized causes of both localized and generalized hyperhidrosis.

Causes of Localized Hyperhidrosis

Idiopathic Hyperhidrosis. Idiopathic hyperhidrosis is not difficult to identify. Patients present with symptoms of intense paroxysmal sweating from the palms, soles, or axillae. Any or all of these three areas may be involved, but the combination of palmar and plantar hyperhidrosis is more common than isolated axillary hyperhidrosis. Idiopathic hyperhidrosis affects both sexes equally, but studies indicate that women are seen more often than men. Most patients experience their first symptoms between the ages of 15 and 30. Spontaneous resolution is not uncommon, but without treatment the condition usually becomes chronic.

Controversy exists over the exact etiology of idiopathic hyperhidrosis. Some investigators believe there is an increase in the actual number of regional eccrine sweat glands in affected individuals. Others maintain that the glands are present in normal concentrations but are overresponsive to customary stimuli. Emotion, exercise, or heat exposure in hyperhidrotics can precipitate up to ten times the amount of sweat normally secreted. This intense regionalized sweating can usually be traced to times of unusual stress or tension. Possible mechanisms for idiopathic localized hyperhidrosis include the theory of dual autonomic innervation of eccrine glands in the palms, soles, and axillae and an enhanced reactivity of the eccrine system to the high circulating levels of epinephrine or norepinephrine adrenergically produced in emotional circumstances. The clinician should look for other symptoms that might suggest a fixed underlying anxiety or depression (insomnia, restlessness, decreased libido, etc.). A family history of localized hyperhidrosis can help confirm the diagnosis.

Gustatory Hyperhidrosis. People who experience gustatory hyperhidrosis present with a clear-cut history of facial sweating after eating. This localized form of sweating usually occurs only after ingestion of certain foods, particularly caffeine, chocolate, tea, hot liquids, and very highly seasoned dishes (e.g., curry, tomato sauce, peppers). The sweating occurs within minutes of ingestion and is most obvious on the forehead and upper lip. The exact mechanism here is not known, but the condition is probably due to an idiosyncratic response of the eccrine system.

Gustatory sweating is also a feature of von Frey's syndrome, an interesting condition that can occur after surgery or severe infections (viral or bacterial) of the parotid gland.[6] Injury to the part of the facial nerve as it passes through the gland's tissue damages both sympathetic and parasympathetic nerve fibers. As the fibers regenerate, the cholinergic fibers of the parotid become entangled and grow into the cholinergic fibers of the facial eccrine glands. Both sets of fibers are stimulated during a meal, and sweat appears on the affected area of the face. Von Frey's syndrome can also occur in infants after trauma to the facial nerve during forceps delivery.

Miscellaneous Causes. Localized hyperhidrosis has been reported in cases of pachyonychia congenita (nail bed hypertrophy) and in areas of vitiligo. It has also been observed as a phenomenon occurring around lesions of psoriasis. No specific mechanism is known.

Causes of Generalized Hyperhidrosis

Endocrine Disorders

Thyrotoxicosis. Hyperhidrosis is but one of the symptoms of hyperthyroidism shared by many of the other systemic disorders listed in Table 1. Nervousness, weight loss, palpitations, heat intolerance, weakness, increased appetite, emotional lability, and menstrual irregularities are also found in diabetes, hypoglycemia, anxiety disorders, and the menopausal syndrome. Characteristic physical findings, such as tachycardia, hypertension, widened pulse pressure, and warm moist skin, are seen with pheochromocytoma. The fine rapid tremor of thyrotoxicosis must be differentiated from the coarse resting tremor of Parkinson's disease.

The basic pathologic effects of hyperthyroidism involve excessive amounts of circulating thyroid hormone, usually caused by Graves' disease, nodular goiter, or subacute thyroiditis. The consequent hypermetabolic state is responsible for production of all of the major signs and symptoms of the disease. Physiologically, the generalized hyperhidrosis that accompanies thyrotoxicosis represents an attempt to reduce an abnormally high production of body heat that is triggered by an overall increase in tissue metabolism. Rapid utilization of oxygen in body tissues results from the increased metabolic rate, and subsequent vasodilatation increases blood flow to all body tissues, including the skin.[2] The more thyrotoxic the patient, the higher the metabolic rate and the more intense the hyperhidrosis. Enhanced eccrine sensitivity to endogenous catecholamines produced by hypermetabolism may also be a mechanism.

Guyton[2] has also made an interesting observation about hyperthyroidism: The incidence of toxic goiter is much higher in people exposed to very cold climates (Eskimos and Arctic dwellers). He proposes that continual cooling of the preoptic area of the hypothalamus initiates an increase of thyrotropin-releasing hormone, leading to greater secretion of TSH and thyroxine by the thyroid and ultimately resulting in glandular hypertrophy.

Diabetes Mellitus. Peripheral neuropathy is a well-known complication of long-standing, poorly controlled diabetes. The basic pathologic effect involves segmental demyelinization of peripheral nerves, shown in animal studies to be related to accumulations of sorbitol and fructose.[7] Concurrently, the sympathetic and parasympathetic nerve fibers can also be involved in neurologic sequelae of the disease. Heat intolerance is frequently described in the symptomatology of diabetes, and generalized hyperhidrosis, although rare, probably occurs in relation to it.

Most cases of diabetic hyperhidrosis occur in a condition called "compensatory diabetic anhidrosis," described by Goodman.[8] Diabetics with retinopathy and peripheral neuropathy were found to have marked heat intolerance and to experience profound hyperhidrosis of the head, neck, and trunk. Conversely, no sweating at all occurred below the waist. The anhidrosis was attributed to sympathetic nerve degeneration. The upper trunk hyperhidrosis is believed to represent an overcompensation of the eccrine system to dissipate body heat from the skin surface when the patient is in an overheated environment.

Hypoglycemia. Generalized sweating is a symptom commonly mentioned by patients who experience hypoglycemic episodes. This and other well-known symptoms (shakiness, palpitations, and near syncope) probably occur secondary to an excessive release of epinephrine triggered by central nervous system glucose deprivation. Several important causes of induced hypoglycemia should be kept in mind, including salicylism, ethanol ingestion, sulfonylurea use, and inappropriate administration of insulin.

Menopause. Hot flushes and intense sweats associated with cessation of menstrual activity are virtually diagnostic of the menopausal syndrome. The exact etiology of these vasomotor symptoms remains unclear, but they are likely caused by a combination of decreasing estrogen levels, increasing gonadotropin concentrations (especially FSH), and release of the circulating vasodilators, bradykinin and histamine.[9]

Pheochromocytoma. Excessive sweating experienced by a hypertensive patient offers a unique diagnostic opportunity to the astute primary care physician. The combination of hypertension and hyperhidrosis may well be the only clinical manifestation of a pheochromocytoma. Classic catecholamine attacks (palpitations, tachycardia, apprehension, and sweating) are so similar to the symptoms of hyperthyroidism, diabetes, hypoglycemia, and functional disorders that the possibility of pheochromocytoma is often overlooked. The key to accurate diagnosis is the association of these symptoms with persistent hypertension. Other clues are evidence of hypermetabolism and weight loss (in the absence of thyrotoxicosis) and orthostatic hypotension in an untreated hypertensive.[10]

These norepinephrine- and epinephrine-secreting tumors may arise from any tissue in the sympathetic nervous system. The majority are located in either the adrenal glands or the paravertebral sympathetic chains. Bursts of the adrenergic hormones released by these highly vascular tumors are transmitted throughout postganglionic sympathetic pathways and released directly into the circulation. The characteristic generalized hyperhidrosis is due to the peripheral tissue effects of these two hormones as well as to overstimulation of the sympathetic system.

Carcinoid Syndrome. Hyperhidrosis can accompany the intense vasomotor flushing pathognomonic of the carcinoid syndrome. Dermatologic expressions of this phenomenon are not infrequently distinctive for the primary location of these argentaffin cell tumors.[11] Ileal carcinoids produce facial and neck flushing of a few minutes' duration. Bronchial tree tumors cause facial flushing that may persist for hours or days. The flushing associated with gastric tumors is characterized by wheals that may occur anywhere on the body; interestingly, the palms and soles are commonly affected.

Carcinoid tumors are known to elaborate several humoral substances, particularly serotonin, histamine, prostaglandins, and the potent vasodilator, bradykinin. The flushing is thought to be indirectly mediated by sympathetic stimulation: Catecholamines normally control concentrations of bradykinin by activation of enzyme kallikrein. When excessive amounts of bradykinin are produced by a carcinoid tumor, the vasoactive substance is released into the arterial circulation, and flushing occurs. The marked vasodilatation increases blood flow to the skin, and the thermoregulatory effect of the sweating mechanism is activated, causing hyperhidrosis.

Carcinoid syndrome has fairly unique symptoms uncommon to other endocrine disorders—severe diarrhea, tenesmus, nausea and vomiting, heart failure, and hypotension. Marked weight loss may also occur, and its presence warrants exclusion of carcinoid syndrome as an etiology.

Acromegaly. Sixty per cent of patients with acromegaly experience generalized hyperhidrosis.[12] Diaphoresis is apparently a direct peripheral tissue effect of growth hormone excess produced by pituitary acidophil cell overactivity. Acidophil adenomas of the anterior pituitary are present in the majority of cases. Although the adenohypophysis and the preoptic area of the hypothalamus are anatomically close and functionally interdependent, dysfunction of the sweating control center by direct tumor extension is not reported. Visual and neurologic defects are common, however, resulting from tumor encroachment on the optic chiasm.

Acromegalic patients typically seek attention for headaches, decreasing visual acuity, and diplopia. Bitemporal hemianopsia is a common finding on ocular field testing. Other characteristics of growth hormone hypersecretion are facial chondrogenesis and marked connective tissue hypertrophy of the hands and feet. The skin becomes thick and coarse; there is exaggeration of normal skin pores (eccrine and apocrine), giving the sweat a damp, oily consistency. Hyperhidrosis in association with insidious bony, cartilaginous, and visceral enlargement should suggest acromegaly in the middle-aged patient whose body size is changing. Curiously, bromocriptine, a new long-acting dopamine antagonist, has been shown to markedly improve the hyperhidrosis of acromegaly.

Infectious Disorders

Every physician has dealt with the familiar triad of fever, chills, and sweating. Hyperpyrexia-induced hyperhidrosis can be characteristic of almost any acute or chronic infection. Interaction of fever-producing exogenous pyrogens with the body's immune system (primarily phagocytes) results in production of "endogenous pyrogen," a substance that has a potent thermal effect on the heat-sensitive neurons of the preoptic hypothalamus.[13] The hypothalamic thermostat is set to a higher level as fever rises. Chills occur during this resetting period and usually cease when a body temperature of 103° F is reached. Heating of the preoptic thermoregulatory center by endogenous pyrogen causes sudden generalized vasodilation and intense sweating, a phenomenon welcomed in the preantibiotic era ("flush" or "crisis"). Evaporative cooling of the skin surface afforded by sweating helps lower the body temperature as the thermostatic setting is reduced.

Septicemias. Bacteremia is most frequently encountered in infections caused by pyrogen-secreting organisms. These pyrogens may be endotoxins, toxins, or exotoxins; respective microbial agents include gram-negative enteric bacteria (*E. coli, Bacteroides, Proteus*), gram-positive bacteria (Group A streptococci, Group II staphylococci, *Corynebacterium diphtheriae* and the *Clostridium* species. Shaking chills, high fever, and intense sweating are well-known early clinical manifestations of these potentially life-threatening infections. Clinical diagnosis in the appropriate circumstances must be prompt, and therapy decisive.

Tuberculosis. Night sweats remain a classic symptom of pulmonary tuberculosis. Insidious constitutional symptoms, such as anorexia, fatigue, chills, and weight loss, can simulate multiple disorders, including Hodgkin's disease, lymphomas, and systemic fungal infections. Night sweats, however, occur more frequently in pulmonary tuberculosis than in any other single disease.[14] The exact cause of sweating in tuberculosis is not known. Various theories include the presence of fever, debilitation from rapid weight loss, and possible elaboration of a virulent toxic factor in the host-cellular immune response that may stimulate the hypothalamic thermoregulatory center.

Brucellosis. Brucellosis has many symptoms in common with tuberculosis, including fever-induced hyperhidrosis. Veterinarians and slaughterhouse workers are at particularly high risk for inoculation by Brucella organisms, which are known to release an exotoxin. Polymorphonuclear phagocytosis of the exotoxin induces formation of endogenous pyrogen and its effects on the thermoregulatory center. Lymphadenopathy, hepatosplenomegaly, and arthralgias are other typical manifestations of the disease.

Malaria. Relapsing fever, drenching sweats, and shaking chills are generic symptoms of infection with plasmodia. This mosquito-borne disease is still endemic in Africa, Asia, and Central and South America. Paroxysmal chills, temperature spikes to 104 to 105.8°F, headaches, and myalgias precede generalized sweating and fever reduction. Depending on the plasmodium species involved, these episodes occur predictably every 48 (*P. vivax, P. ovale*) or 72 (*P. malariae*) hours. Characteristic erythrocyte alteration and vascular endothelial damage occurs during circulatory parasitization; evidence of marked hemolytic anemia is common. A careful travel history should be taken from any patient with suggestive symptoms; identification of plasmodia in peripheral blood smears confirms the diagnosis.

Neoplastic Disorders

Hodgkin's Disease. Patients older than 40 years with widespread mixed-cellularity or lymphocyte-depletion Hodgkin's disease rarely present with the mediastinal and peripheral lymphadenopathy that characterizes the disease in younger patients.[15] Instead, severe and progressive constitutional symptoms, such as fever, night sweats, fatigue, and weight loss, predominate, often obscuring diagnosis. The Pel-Ebstein type of fever is distinctive, with late afternoon or evening temperature rises and intense sweats alternating with afebrile periods. No particular mechanism for this unusual fever pattern is known.

Non-Hodgkin's Lymphomas. This group of malignancies includes lymphocytic, histiocytic, mixed, stem-cell, lymphoblastic, and Burkitt's lymphomas. Constitutional symptoms occur but are not as prominent as in Hodgkin's disease. Human lymphoma cell lines appear to be capable of in vitro production of endogenous pyrogen.[13] Thus, the fever and sweats that occur with non-Hodgkin's lymphoma may be due to direct hypothalamic stimulation of the thermoregulatory sweating mechanism.

Metastatic Cord Transection or Compression. Although complete cord transection may occur in any metastatic carcinoma, extradural cord compression by Hodgkin's and non-Hodgkin's tumors is not uncommon. Epidural, cauda equina, and transverse spinal cord lesions may produce cord transection and, with paresthesias, paralysis or loss of bladder and bowel control. Cord interruption produces anhidrosis to heat below the level of the transection via disruption of sympathetic efferent pathways. Compensatory localized hyperhidrosis of contralateral surfaces can occur and is mediated by spinal reflexes.

Neurologic Disorders

Although sweating is autonomically mediated, both localized and generalized hyperhidrosis have been reported in some central nervous system disorders. Acetylcholine is the neurotransmitter that stimulates eccrine sweat production; eccrine glands are innervated by sympathetic efferents originating in the thoracic segments of the autonomic nervous system. Damage to the cord or peripheral fibers normally results in localized anhidrosis. However, hyperhidrosis has been reported in central pathway disruption from stroke or cerebral tumor.[6]

Parkinsonism. Facial hyperhidrosis may occur in Parkinson's disease to compensate for the anhidrosis produced by central autonomic damage.[16] It is interesting that the dopamine depletion in the caudate nucleus and putamen that results from the pathognomonic substantia nigra degeneration allows oversecretion of acetycholine by neurons in this area.[2] Presumably, it is this cholenergic excess that is responsible for the distinctive motor symptoms of Parkinsonism: rigidity, bradykinesia, resting tremor, and loss of postural reflexes.

Tabes Dorsalis. Degeneration of the posterior roots and columns of the spinal cord in tabes dorsalis results in loss of peripheral reflexes and vibratory sensation and ultimately progresses to ataxia.

Syphilis. Disruption of the dorsal nerve root fibers may cause the localized hyperhidrosis that has been reported in neurosyphilis.[17]

Stroke. Ischemic or hemorrhagic strokes of the major cerebral arteries can result in hypothalamic damage and dysfunction of the thermoregulatory control center. The middle and posterior cerebral arteries and the vertebrobasilar system are usually involved. Compensatory hyperhidrosis is usually localized, and may be ipsilateral or contralateral to the site of embolism or ischemia.

Diencephalic Syndrome of Infancy. This disorder is another pediatric syndrome characterized by excessive sweating.[18] Glioma of the anterior hypothalamus is usually responsible for the autonomic overactivity, optic atrophy, and extreme emaciation present in this definable cause of failure to thrive.

Genetic Disorders

Riley-Day Syndrome. Generalized hyperhidrosis is reported to be a cardinal symptom of familial dysautonomia.[4] This autosomal recessive disease occurs in children of Ashkenazi Jewish extraction and is characterized by a congenital decrease in the number of small unmyelinated autonomic and peripheral fibers that carry pain, temperature, and taste sensations. The syndrome manifests in early childhood as feeding difficulties (gagging, vomiting) and poor motor coordination. Autonomic dysfunction includes defects or absence of tearing, hyperhidrosis, increased salivation, and vasomotor instability (skin blotching during excitement, labile hypertension). Indifference to pain, absence of taste sensation, and developmental retardation support the diagnosis. Genetic counseling for the families of affected children is imperative.

Cystic Fibrosis. Cystic fibrosis deserves mention in any discussion of sweat gland disorders. Although hyperhidrosis is not a usual component of the disease, it is important to remember that the first observations of the abnormal sodium and chloride contents of sweat now considered diagnostic were made in children admitted to a New York hospital during a heat wave in 1949.[4] The tendency of children with cystic fibrosis to develop salt depletion, heat prostration, or shock with sweating in response to increased environmental heat may provide a clue to early diagnosis of the disorder.

Psychogenic Causes

Generalized diaphoresis is a well-known manifestation of tension, apprehension, and pain. Autonomic sympathetic activity may be the cause or the result of the symptoms frequently found in states of anxiety or depression. Hyperactivity of the sympathetic nervous system results in generalized autonomic discharge in various parts of the body simultaneously. Psychosomatic disorders may result from sympathetic hyperactivity; the autonomic system itself can be strongly stimulated by intensified reaction to fear, anger, or stress (rage, "fight or flight" reactions).

Every physician has heard the familiar phrase "broke out in a cold sweat" from patients describing the intensity of an unexpected pain. Pain can result from exogenous stimuli or come internally from tissue ischemia, chemical irritation, and spasm or overdistension of a hollow viscus.[2] Thermal signals are transmitted in the same autonomic pathways as pain, so it is understandable that profuse sweating may follow pain perception.

Drugs

Excessive sweating is listed as a potential side effect of a number of commonly used drugs, including aspirin, insulin, antiemetics, and the analgesics morphine and meperidine. Hyperhidrosis usually occurs with accidental or intentional overdoses of these agents, in which hypoglycemia, hypoperistalsis, and hypotension predominate.

Any drug capable of cholinergic stimulation can cause hyperhidrosis. Therapeutic cholinergic drugs fall into two categories, the parasympathomimetics and the acetylcholine inhibitors. Pilocarpine and bethanechol (Urecholine) are parasympathomimetics used in the treatment of glaucoma and urinary retention. Prolonged use of either may result in excessive sweating. The only current indication for long-term use of the anticholinesterases physostigmine and neostigmine is in the therapy of myasthenia gravis; hyperhidrosis during treatment of this condition is not uncommon.

Miscellaneous Disorders

Hyperhidrosis may occur as one of the most obvious manifestations of several dangerous and potentially life-threatening conditions. Substance abuse withdrawal states are frequently characterized by vasomotor disturbances, cortical irritability, and temperature instability. Tremor, agitation, and excessive sweating are common symptoms of acute alcohol and opiate abstinence reactions.

Two other emergency situations in which hyperhidrosis is a predominant symptom are organophosphate poisoning and toxic ingestion of the mushroom *Amanita muscaria.* Signs of excessive cholinergic stimulation occur in both conditions, including marked lacrimation, increased salivation, miosis, watery diarrhea, and abdominal pain. Patients presenting with hyperhidrosis who exhibit signs of generalized cholinergic discharge may require immediate intervention with atropine to reverse the effects of cholinesterase inhibition or specific mushroom toxins.

REFERENCES

1. Grice K. Hyperhidrosis and its treatment by iontophoresis. Physiotherapy 1980;66:43–4.
2. Guyton AC. Textbook of medical physiology. 6th ed. Philadelphia: WB Saunders, 1981:617–8, 650–1, 889–96, 934–7.
3. Robinson S, Robinson AH. Chemical composition of sweat. Physiol Rev 1954;34:202–16.
4. Cage GW. Diseases of eccrine sweat glands. In: Fitzpatrick TB, Arndt KA, Clark WH, Eisen AZ, Van Scott EJ, Vaughn JH, eds. Dermatology in general medicine. New York: McGraw-Hill, 1971:375–86.
5. Riley CM, Moore RH. Familial dysautonomia differentiated from related disorders. Pediatrics 1966;37:435–45.
6. Cunliffe WJ, Tan SG. Hyperhidrosis and hypohidrosis. Practitioner 1976;216:149–53.
7. Cahill GF, Jr. Diabetes mellitus. In: Wyngaarden JB, Smith LH, Jr., eds. Textbook of medicine. 16th ed. Philadelphia: WB Saunders, 1982:1053–71.
8. Goodman JI. Diabetic anhidrosis. Am J Med 1966;41:831–35.
9. Studd J, Chavracarti S, Oram D. The climacteric. Clin Obstet Gynaecol 1977;4:3–29.
10. Engleman K. Pheochromocytoma. In: Wyngaarden JB, Smith LH Jr, eds. Textbook of medicine. 16th ed. Philadelphia: WB Saunders, 1982:1306–12.
11. Engleman K. The carcinoid syndrome. In: Wyngaarden JB, Smith LH Jr, eds. Textbook of medicine. 16th ed. Philadelphia: WB Saunders, 1982:1312–17.
12. Daughaday WH. The adenohypophysis. In: Williams RH, ed. Textbook of endocrinology. 6th ed. Philadelphia: WB Saunders, 1981:73–114.
13. Dinarello CA. Pathogenesis of fever. In: Wyngaarden JB, Smith LH Jr, eds. Textbook of medicine. 16th ed. Philadelphia: WB Saunders, 1982:1393–5.
14. Bonney SG. Pulmonary tuberculosis. 2nd ed. Philadelphia: WB Saunders, 1910:158–9.
15. Rosenberg SA. Hodgkin's disease. In: Wyngaarden JB, Smith JH Jr, eds. Textbook of medicine. 16th ed. Philadelphia: WB Saunders, 1982:1053–71.
16. Grice K. Treatment of hyperhidrosis. Clin Exp Dermatol 1982;7:183–8.
17. Hatzis J, Papaioannou C, Tosca A, Varelzidis A, Capetanakis J. Local hyperhidrosis. Dermatologica 1980;161:45–50.
18. Huttenlochner PR. Diseases of the nervous system. In: Vaughn VC, McKay RJ, Behrman RE, eds. Textbook of pediatrics 11th ed. Philadelphia: WB Saunders, 1979:1793.

HYPERKALEMIA AND HYPOKALEMIA

LUIZ NASCIMENTO

☐ SYNONYMS: Hyperpotassemia and hypopotassemia

BACKGROUND

Potassium Metabolism

The regulation of potassium balance is of extraordinary importance to the maintenance of homeostasis. Relatively small changes in the concentration of extracellular potassium may be associated with extensive morbidity or death. The kidney plays a major role in the regulation of potassium balance. Under normal circumstances an individual ingests a diet containing 60 to 100 mEq of potassium per day; 5 to 10 mEq of this amount is excreted in the stool, less than 5 mEq appears in the sweat, and the remainder is excreted in the urine.[1]

Total body potassium stores are approximately 40 to 45 mEq/kg of body weight. Of this amount, 90 per cent is intracellular and is readily exchangeable with the 2 per cent found in extracellular fluid; the remaining 8 per cent of potassium is found within bone and is not readily exchangeable. The normal concentration of potassium in extracellular fluid ranges between 3.6 and 5 mEq/liter. The intracellular concentration of the ion is 140 to 160 mEq/liter. Although there is a correlation between the concentrations of extracellular fluid potassium and of total body potassium, the correlation is crude and sometimes extremely poor. It is possible for a significant deficit of total body potassium to coexist with an extracellular potassium concentration level within the normal range. Under unusual clinical circumstances, potassium in plasma serves as a useful guide to total body potassium.[2, 3]

Renal Handling of Potassium

For practical purposes, potassium can be considered to be completely filterable. Thus, concentration of potassium in glomerular filtrate will exactly match that of plasma. About 50 per cent of the potassium filtered is reabsorbed in the proximal tubule; another 40 per cent is reabsorbed in the ascending limb of the loop of Henle. There is further reabsorption of potassium in the distal tubule and collecting ducts. Most of the potassium that appears in urine, however, represents what was secreted in the distal tubule and collecting duct. The collecting duct is the final regulator of potassium secretion. It is of great importance to be aware of the factors that influence the secretion of potassium, and thus the excretion of the ion, by this segment of the nephron.[4]

Factors Influencing Distal Potassium Secretion

Perhaps the single most important factor influencing the rate of potassium secretion is the amount of sodium delivered to the collecting duct. Under circumstances in which effective arterial blood volume is contracted (glomerular filtration rate falls and proximal reabsorption rises), the absolute amount of sodium reaching the collecting duct decreases. Thus, a smaller amount of sodium is available to be exchanged for potassium, and therefore potassium secretion is diminished. The second major regulator of the rate of potassium secretion by the collecting duct is aldosterone. If the rate of distal delivery is constant, the presence of aldosterone will accelerate the exchange of sodium for potassium, whereas in the absence of aldosterone either increasing or decreasing the amount of sodium delivered to the collecting duct tends to obscure the effects of aldosterone; nevertheless, aldosterone is the major regulator of potassium secretion.[2]

Sodium can be reabsorbed as sodium chloride. If the delivery of sodium to the collecting duct is accelerated by the administration of sodium with an anion that, unlike chloride, cannot be reabsorbed (for example, sodium sulfate or sodium carbenicillin), then the only way that sodium can be reabsorbed is in exchange for either potassium or hydrogen. If aldosterone is available in abundant amounts, this exchange is enhanced. The mechanism favoring the exchange is the reabsorption of sodium, which results in a negative potential difference across the luminal epithelium in the collecting duct. With a negative potential difference at the lumen of the collecting duct, the movement of a positively charged ion is favored. Thus, the administration of sodium with a nonreabsorbable anion under appropriate circumstances can result in the development of hypokalemic metabolic alkalosis (Table 1).

Another important factor influencing the secretion of potassium by the collecting duct is the state of body adaptation to potassium, which is discussed in further detail in the following pages.

Table 1. RENAL FACTORS IN POTASSIUM HOMEOSTASIS

Factor	Effect on K Excretion	Effect on Serum K
Aldosterone deficiency	↓	↑
Change in sodium delivery to collecting duct due to:		
Volume expansion	↑	↓
CHF	↓	↑
Change in lumen potential difference of collecting duct:		
Increase	↑	↓
Decrease (due to amiloride or aldactone)	↓	↑
Therapy with:		
Nonreabsorbable anions	↑	↓
Carbenicillin or $NaSO_4$	↑	↓
Decrease in nephron mass due to chronic renal failure	Adaptive ↑	None (normal level)

(Adapted from Nascimento L, Arruda JAL. Hyperkalemia: various causes and how they influence management. Consultant 1982;22(5):55–76.)

The Role of Potassium as a Regulator of Extrarenal Metabolism

Aldosterone is a major factor influencing the excretion of potassium, and the level of potassium within the body is an important regulator of aldosterone synthesis. There is a positive feedback relationship between aldosterone and potassium. When potassium accumulates in the body through a direct effect on the cells of the zona glomerulosa of the adrenal gland, aldosterone synthesis is enhanced. The resulting increase in circulating levels of aldosterone favors the excretion of potassium, which in turn lowers body potassium. This lowering results in inhibition of further aldosterone synthesis.

An important relationship exists between potassium and insulin. An increase in the secretion of insulin favors the movement of potassium from extracellular fluid into intracellular water. Furthermore, potassium regulates the release of insulin. Hypokalemia retards release of insulin by the pancreas; it is this characteristic that is responsible for the glucose intolerance commonly seen in patients receiving long-term diuretic therapy. Thus, two hormones play a crucial role in the regulation of potassium in the extracellular fluid. Aldosterone controls the secretion of potassium by the kidney, whereas insulin controls the distribution of potassium across cell membranes. Should a patient develop a disease associated with deficiency of both hormones, hyperkalemia would most certainly be a prominent feature. As we will see subsequently, isolated hypoaldosteronism, which occurs most commonly in diabetics, is a clinical expression of the deficiency of both hormones (Table 2).[5, 6]

Potassium Adaptation

By mechanisms that are not clear, the kidney, and indeed the whole body, has the ability to adapt to changing potassium intake. If the amount of potassium in the diet is gradually increased, adaptation may occur, so that the administration of large amounts of potassium in a rapid fashion, which under usual circumstances might have proved lethal, may be accomplished with no untoward sequelae. The kidney adapts to an increase in potassium intake by increasing the amount of potassium that it may excrete per unit of time. Furthermore, extrarenal mechanisms are involved that increase the facility with which potassium may be transported into cells. The most prominent example of extrarenal potassium adaptation occurs in the lower GI tract.[2, 7]

HYPERKALEMIA

Hyperkalemia is defined by the presence of a serum potassium level above 5.5 mEq/liter. As summarized in Table 3, the syndrome may result

Table 2. FACTORS REGULATING POTASSIUM HOMEOSTASIS VIA TRANSCELLULAR FLUX

Factor	Consequence	Effect on K Level
Insulin deficiency (diabetes)	Moves K into cells	↑
Therapy with beta-adrenergic agonists	Moves K into cells	↑
Acidosis, acute	Moves K out of cells	↑
Alkalosis, metabolic or respiratory	Moves K into cells	↓

(Adapted from Nascimento K, Arruda JAL. Hyperkalemia: various causes and how they influence management. Consultant 1982;22(5):55–76.)

Table 3. CAUSES OF HYPERKALEMIA

Cause	Predisposing Factor	Recommended Evaluation(s)
Excessive intake (salt substitute or KCl therapy)	Renal disease	History
Hyperosmolality or insulin deficiency	Diabetes	History; clinical signs; serum osmolality, blood glucose level
Catecholamine deficiency	Diabetes	Evidence of blockage or sympathetic dysfunction
Hemolysis	Drugs, sickle cell disease	History; sickle cell preparation
Tissue breakdown	Rhabdomyolysis	Muscle tenderness, CPK, urinalysis
Aldosterone deficiency	Addison's disease	History; sodium, cortisol, and aldosterone levels
Selective aldosterone deficiency	Diabetes, interstitial nephritis	History; mild renal insufficiency, metabolic acidosis; K, renin, and aldosterone levels
Potassium-sparing diuretics	Renal disease	History; BUN and creatinine levels
Decreased distal delivery of sodium to the collecting duct	Volume contraction, sodium-retaining states (CHF)	History; clinical evidence; urinary sodium level
Renal tubular acidosis	Obstructive uropathy	History; clinical evidence; mild renal insufficiency; urine pH, serum and urine K, and aldosterone levels

(Adapted from Nascimento L, Arruda JAL. Hyperkalemia: various causes and how they influence management. Consultant 1982;22(5):55–76.)

from changes in total body stores of potassium or from the relative distribution of potassium between intracellular and extracellular spaces. Catabolic states and cellular damage (e.g., rhabdomyolysis) are usually associated with hyperkalemia owing to release of tissue stores of potassium into extracellular space.

History

Hyperkalemia can result in abnormalities of the neuromuscular, gastrointestinal, and cardiovascular systems. Weakness and paresthesias, ascending paralysis, and flaccid quadriplegia are the neuromuscular manifestations commonly reported. Gastrointestinal symptoms include nausea and vomiting. The most immediate danger of hyperkalemia, however, is its effect on cardiac conduction.[2]

The history may be helpful in differentiating the major syndromes in which hyperkalemia is clinically prominent. Renal failure, diabetes mellitus, ingestion of salt substitutes, use of potassium-sparing diuretics, prostate hypertrophy, renal stones, sickle cell anemia, and ureteral obstruction may be associated with hyperkalemia. The symptomatology, however, may be dominated by the underlying disease.

Physical Examination

The major clinical disorders associated with hyperkalemia may be distinguished by the initial evaluation and physical findings. Acute renal failure may manifest as fluid retention, as evidenced by edema and hypertension. In surgical cases, trauma, or rhabdomyolysis, hyperkalemia may be severe and life-threatening. Chronic renal failure of any cause usually is not associated with hyperkalemia. Hypertension, abnormal eye ground findings (hypertensive or diabetic retinopathy), and edema are usually present. Aldosterone deficiency is typically associated with diabetes mellitus and mild renal insufficiency. Weakness, paresthesias, and paralysis are the findings reported in relation to the neuromuscular system.[8]

Diagnostic Studies

It is of utmost importance for the clinician to correctly interpret the results of basic laboratory evaluation. Hyperkalemia is usually documented by a routine SMA-6 evaluation. Elevation of blood urea nitrogen (BUN) may suggest renal failure or a prerenal component (excessive volume contraction). Diabetes may be accompanied by hyperkalemia (transcellular flux, acidosis). Therapy with insulin and correction of acidosis usually control the serum potassium levels.

Most commonly, hyperchloremia and low bicarbonate levels are present in combination with hyperkalemia. Three conditions may account for hyperchloremia: dehydration, nonanion gap metabolic acidosis, and respiratory alkalosis. A normal or decreased serum sodium level eliminates the possibility of dehydration. Arterial blood gas measurements in combination with the analysis of the sequence of the clinical events allow us to separate the two acid-base disturbances. The most common causes of uncomplicated respiratory alkalosis have been reviewed recently. This acid-base alteration may be associated with processes such as congestive heart failure, liver cirrhosis, and pneumonias.[9] Alkalosis per se tends to lower serum potassium (see Table 2); however, severe volume contraction may be present (low distal delivery), favoring an increase in potassium levels in the serum (see Table 1). Determinations of urinary pH, aldosterone levels, and fractional excretion of sodium and potassium will help in the further evaluation of the renal tubular defect (see "Renal Tubular Acidosis" and Table 4).

It is imperative that the clinician be familiar with the electrocardiographic manifestations of hyperkalemia. These include peaked T waves, prolongation of P-R intervals, atrioventricular dissociation or atrial arrest, widening of the QRS complex, and shortening of the Q-T interval.[10]

Diagnostic Approach in Hyperkalemia

The clinical manifestations of hyperkalemia depend upon the ratio of intracellular to extracellular potassium. Acute hyperkalemia is more likely to be associated with an altered ratio and has important clinical manifestations. Patients in whom hyperkalemia has developed over a protracted period may have no clinical symptomatology. The role of the clinician is to critically assess the clinical background against which hyperkalemia appears. By studying the history and physical findings together with the laboratory results, the physician should be able to identify the major syndromes in which hyperkalemia is an important feature: (1) decreased renal excretion; (2) aldosterone deficiency; (3) use of diuretics that decrease potassium secretion; (4) shift of potassium from intracellular fluid; (5) renal tubular acidosis; and (6) hyperkalemic familial periodic paralysis. Each is discussed individually.

Decreased Renal Excretion

The kidney, under ordinary circumstances, is the organ that regulates potassium excretion. Marked impairment of renal function results in potassium retention. Potassium retention due to renal disease will be much more pronounced if the onset of renal insufficiency is sudden rather than gradual. It is for this reason that hyperkalemia is a much more common feature of acute renal failure than of chronic renal failure. Indeed, recent evidence suggests that many patients with chronic renal insufficiency are potassium-depleted. Potassium retention may occur in the background of chronic renal failure, especially if increased amounts of potassium are ingested in the diet or potassium is administered therapeutically, either orally or parenterally. It must be emphasized that hyperkalemia is a feature of chronic renal failure only in very severe renal insufficiency. A finding of hyperkalemia in a patient with moderate chronic renal failure should suggest another etiology for the hyperkalemia, for example, aldosterone deficiency and renal tubular acidosis.

Aldosterone Deficiency

Aldosterone is responsible for the regulation of potassium balance. Deficiency of this hormone will result in retention of potassium. Aldosterone deficiency may be the consequence of diffuse adrenal disease (Addison's disease), in which both mineralocorticoid and glucocorticoid deficiencies coexist.

Recently, a specialized form of adrenal insufficiency has been recognized and has received much attention. It has been termed isolated hyporeninemic hypoaldosteronism. As its name implies, it is a syndrome in which mineralocorticoid deficiency is not accompanied by deficiency of glucocorticoid and plasma renin activity is low.[11–13]

Regardless of its etiology or pathophysiology, aldosterone deficiency is much more common than has been supposed. It occurs in middle-aged or elderly individuals, almost all of whom have some degree of mild to moderate renal insufficiency. About 50 per cent of affected patients have diabetes mellitus. The most common type of associated renal disease is an interstitial nephritis. Hyperkalemia is the most prominent clinical feature. Metabolic acidosis is a common, although not invariable feature, and seems to be related to the degree of renal insufficiency present. A typical patient with aldosterone deficiency is a 55-year-old subject with diabetes mellitus whose laboratory profile includes hyperglycemia, hyperkalemia, a low serum bicarbonate level, and a moderately elevated creatinine concentration. Because there is a defect in mineralocorticoid hormone synthesis and release, one might suppose that the disease can be completely reversed by the administration of mineralocorticoid. This is not always the case (see "Renal Tubular Acidosis").

Aldosterone deficiency may result from two forms of the adrenogenital syndrome. Deficiency of either C-21-hydroxylase or 2-B-dehydrogenase causes impairment not only of aldosterone biosynthesis but also of steroid synthesis at a point prior to the formation of any mineralocorticoid hormone. Thus, mineralocorticoid deficiency and hyperkalemia are prominent features of both forms of adrenogenital syndrome.[12]

Use of Diuretics That Decrease Potassium Secretion

Hyperkalemia may result from the administration of a potassium-sparing diuretic such as spironolactone or triamterene. Another agent, amiloride, was recently marketed in the United States. Spironolactone exerts its potassium-retaining effect solely by blocking the action of aldosterone or other mineralocorticoid hormones. Triamterene and amiloride, on the other hand, directly affect the pump involved in the secretion of potassium by the collecting duct; these two agents exert a potassium-retaining effect in adrenalectomized animals (and humans) but spironolactone does not. With ordinary use, these agents should not result in hyperkalemia. Hyperkalemia will occur following their administration to patients with renal insufficiency or to patients given both potassium-retaining diuretics and potassium supplementation. There are instances in which it may be necessary to give potassium supplementation to the patient receiving one of these agents. One cannot overemphasize, however, that this must be done cautiously and with constant surveillance.

Shift of Potassium from Intracellular Fluid

Hyperkalemia may result from the movement of potassium from cells into extracellular fluid. In this event, total body potassium is unchanged, but the distribution of the ion is markedly altered. Transcellular shifts of potassium may occur with acidemia, digitalis intoxication, or extensive tissue damage such as muscle necrosis or hemolysis.

When evaluating a patient with hyperkalemia, one must remember that a hyperkalemic reading may be the result of hemolysis of a blood sample after it has been drawn or of poor venipuncture technique. Patients with thrombocytosis or extreme leukocytosis may also have pseudohyperkalemia.

Renal Tubular Acidosis Associated with Hyperkalemia and Hypokalemia

Renal tubular acidosis is classically described in association with hypokalemia. By definition, it is characterized by hyperchloremia (thus, nonanion gap) and an abnormally high urine pH during acidemia, implicating an intrinsic renal inability to secrete acid. Recently, several studies have shown that renal tubular acidosis may be associated with hyperkalemia and that the secretion of potassium in this syndrome is impaired, despite normal or appropriate levels of plasma aldosterone.[14]

The kidney regulates acid-base homeostasis by virtue of its capacity to secrete hydrogen ions into the tubular urine. This process is limited mainly to the proximal tubule, the distal nephron, and, most important, the collecting duct. Net acid excretion can be defined as the sum of urinary buffers minus the amount of bicarbonate in the urine; put more simply, net acid excretion = (titratable acid + ammonium) − bicarbonate. There is overlap, but the urinary buffers are titrated mainly in the distal nephron, and bicarbonate is reabsorbed mainly in the proximal segments. A defect in regulation of acid-base homeostasis, due to a derangement in this process (renal tubular acidosis), can result from a disorder in either the proximal or distal nephron. There are a number of ways that the acidification of urine in the distal nephron can become deranged, as follows.[15, 16]

Impaired Hydrogen Ion Secretion. This type of renal tubular acidosis, which results from the failure of the hydrogen ion pump to transport protons against an unfavorable hydrogen ion concentration gradient, is the mechanism responsible for the acquired type of renal tubular acidosis seen in adult patients. It is characterized by an inability to lower the urine pH below 5.5 regardless of the severity of acidemia. Affected patients titrate buffer from bone; the buffer is accompanied by calcium, and they develop hypercalciuria. Typically, both nephrocalcinosis and nephrolithiasis eventually result. The acidosis is also associated with marked hyperchloremia and failure to grow normally. Recently, it was demonstrated that normal growth in children with this disease may be restored by the administration of large amounts of bicarbonate. For reasons that are unclear, such children may excrete as much as 15 per cent of the filtered bicarbonate. The large bicarbonate excretion diminishes as the children mature, even though the renal tubular acidosis remains. Another diagnostic feature of this type of distal renal tubular acidosis is an inability to raise the urine pCO_2 with either bicarbonate administration or bicarbonate plus buffer (phosphate) administration. Because the defect is limited to the hydrogen ion pump, there is no defect in potassium secretion; indeed, affected patients typically are hypokalemic.[17]

Acid Back-Diffusion Renal Tubular Acidosis. This type of renal tubular acidosis occurs not from the failure of the proton pump to secrete hydrogen ion, but from the failure of the distal nephron membrane to maintain a steep hydrogen concentration gradient between tubular urine and blood. Once a gradient of about 100:1, or 2 pH units, has been established between blood and urine, the further secretion of protons results in back-diffusion of acid from the tubular urine to the blood. The only known cause is the chronic administration of the antifungal antibiotic amphotericin. Patients with this disease cannot lower urine pH to less than 5.5 during systemic acidosis or raise urine pCO_2 during bicarbonate loading. Administration of sodium sulfate results in a low urine pH when accompanied by an endogenous mineralocorticoid release or exogenous mineralocorticoid administration, because sodium can be reabsorbed and sulfate cannot. The reabsorption of sodium unaccompanied by sulfate yields a more negative electrical gradient in the lumen of the tubule, favoring the secretion of positively charged protons. It is believed that this negative gradient retards back-diffusion of acid in such patients, accounting for the normal response to administration of sodium sulfate.[15]

Voltage-Dependent Renal Tubular Acidosis. This syndrome, recently described by Arruda and co-workers,[18] results from the inability of a diseased kidney to reabsorb sodium normally in the distal nephron. Under normal circumstances, the reabsorption of sodium in this nephron segment generates a negative potential in the lumen. As mentioned previously, such a negative potential favors the secretion of positively charged hydrogen and also of positively charged potassium. In a patient with impaired sodium reabsorption in this segment of the nephron, the ability to secrete both hydrogen and potassium is also impaired. In other words, the patient should develop hyperkalemic hyperchloremic metabolic acidosis. During sodium restriction, the patient does not conserve sodium normally, owing to the defect in sodium transport. Since there is no defect in the renin-angiotensin-aldosterone axis, plasma aldosterone concentration is normal or even elevated owing to the hyperkalemia. The urine pH is inappropriately alkaline during acidosis, and the urine pCO_2 does not rise to expected levels in response to bicarbonate loading. The response to sodium sulfate or buffer administration is abnormal, as is the potassium excretion in response to sulfate loading. A voltage-dependent defect can be distinguished from a hydrogen ion secretory defect by the potassium excretion response to sulfate administration. Voltage-dependent renal tubular acidosis is seen in patients with interstitial nephritis and, most important, in patients with urinary tract obstruction. Consequently, the patient who presents with hyperkalemic renal tubular acidosis should be investigated for urinary tract obstruction.[14]

Aldosterone Deficiency. The deficiency of aldosterone commonly results in hyperkalemic hyperchloremic metabolic acidosis. This form of hyperkalemic acidosis can be distinguished from that seen in voltage-dependent renal tubular acidosis, because patients afflicted with aldosterone deficiency retain the ability to lower urine pH in response to systemic acidosis. Finding hyperkalemic acidosis in a patient with appropriately low urine pH suggests a diagnosis of aldosterone deficiency, which can be confirmed by the measurement of the aldosterone level in plasma.[15]

Diagnostic Evaluation. A simplified diagnostic approach to the various forms of renal tubular acidosis is outlined in Table 4. Used for this purpose are measurements of the sodium balance, the serum and urine potassium concentrations, the ability to acidify the urine during acidosis, and the ability to respond normally to bicarbonate, sulfate, or buffer administration. In addition, the plasma aldosterone concentration may be utilized to pinpoint the defect observed, particularly in the presence of hyperkalemia. With this approach, the mechanism responsible for impairment of distal urinary acidification can be readily identified.

Although part of this approach may be the domain of the specialist, the identification and initial evaluation of the syndrome are in the hands of the family practitioner and internist. It is evident, from examination of the information in Table 4, that the step following the initial clinical evaluation (history and physical exam) is a rather simple one. The measurement of serum potassium, chloride, arterial blood gases, and urinary pH should identify part of the syndrome. The bedside calculation of the fractional excretion of sodium or potassium can be achieved by spot sample measurements of serum and urinary Na, K, and creatinine. The result can be obtained by using the following formula:

$$\text{FE Na} = \frac{\text{U Na}}{\text{P Na}} \times \frac{\text{P creat.}}{\text{U creat.}}$$

where FE Na is fractional sodium or potassium excretion, U Na is urinary sodium, P Na is serum sodium, P creat. is plasma creatinine, and U creat. is urinary creatinine.

Hyperkalemic Familial Periodic Paralysis

A rare disease with an autosomal dominant mode of inheritance. When patients with this disease are resting after strenuous exercise, a significant hyperkalemia develops, leading to a flaccid paralysis that may last from minutes to several hours. Other factors that may precipitate the attacks include exposure to cold, hunger, and potassium ingestion. The capacity to accumulate potassium intracellularly seems to be deficient, because muscle stores of potassium have been shown to fall during attacks. Catecholamines reportedly ameliorate the hyperkalemic attacks, possibly because the hormones enhance the cellular uptake of potassium.[2, 19]

HYPOKALEMIA

Hypokalemia is present when the serum potassium level is below 3.0 mEq/liter. The decrease in potassium may reflect a deficit in total body potassium or may simply represent an intracellular shift. The major factors and syndromes associated with hypokalemia are outlined in Tables 2 and 5.

Table 4. CLASSIFICATION OF DISTAL ACIDIFICATION DEFECTS*

Types	Urine pH During Acidosis	Urinary-Blood pCO_2 Gradient			Serum K	Fractional Excretion of K	Aldosterone Levels	Sodium Balance	Example of Cause
		HCO_3 Loading	*PO_4 Loading*	*$NaSO_4$ Infusion*					
Proton secretory defect	>5.5	<10	<10	>5.5	N or ↓	N or ↑	N or ↑	N or impaired	Classic distal renal tubular acidosis
Back-diffusion or gradient	>5.5	<10	>30	<5.5	N or ↓	↑	N or ↓	Impaired	Amphotericin therapy
Voltage-dependent	>5.5	<10	<10	>5.5	↑	↓	↑	Impaired	Urinary tract obstruction
Aldosterone deficiency	>5.5	>30	>30	<5.5	↑	↓	↓	Impaired	Selective hyporeninism-hypoaldosteronism

*N = normal.

(From Nascimento L, Kurtzman NA: Defects in urinary acidification. Dialogues Pediatr Nephrol 1981;4:5–7. Reprinted by permission.)

Table 5. CLINICAL CONDITIONS MOST COMMONLY ASSOCIATED WITH HYPOKALEMIA

Syndrome	Clinical and Laboratory Findings	Focus of Evaluation
Diuretic therapy	Dizziness, headaches; orthostatic changes (pulse rate and blood pressure)	History; BP, pulse, hematocrit, serum uric acid, BUN, and serum bicarbonate
Primary aldosteronism	Hypertension, metabolic alkalosis	History; funduscopy (usually not associated with malignant changes); serum and urinary K, renin, serum and urinary aldosterone
Renin-secreting tumor	Hypertension, metabolic alkalosis	History; signs and symptoms; urinary K, renin, serum aldosterone, renal veins renins; renal arteriogram
Renal tubular acidosis	Failure to thrive in children, polyuria (concentration defect), kidney stones, nephrocalcinosis, acidosis	History; serum and urinary K, blood gases, urinary pH (during acidosis), aldosterone levels
Bartter's syndrome	In children; abnormal mentation and growth, muscle weakness, paresthesias, and polyuria; normal blood pressure	History (surreptitious use of diuretic?); BP, renin, aldosterone, blood gases, urinary electrolytes
Liddle's syndrome	Hypertension	History (family); serum K, arterial blood gases, renin, serum and urinary aldosterone
Vomiting or gastric suction	Metabolic alkalosis	History; arterial blood gases, serum K, urinary Na, Cl, K, and pH.

History

Clinically, hypokalemia is usually manifested by muscular weakness and easy fatigability, loss of renal concentrating ability with polyuria, decrease in carbohydrate tolerance, and postural falls in blood pressure without compensatory tachycardia.[13] In severe potassium deficiency, total muscle paralysis and rhabdomyolysis may occur. The development of such symptoms is usually associated with potassium levels below 2 mEq/liter. It is of utmost importance to collect as much information as possible about the clinical setting in which the hypokalemia occurs.

Physical Examination

The major syndromes outlined in Table 5 may manifest specific and characteristic clinical features on physical examination. Hypertension is common in the majority of the cases, except in Bartter's syndrome. It may or may not be present in association with diuretic therapy or vomiting. Hypokalemic periodic paralysis, a rare disease, is unmistakably indicated by the findings of muscle weakness and flaccid paralysis.[13] A concentration defect manifested by polyuria is the hallmark of the nephropathy of potassium depletion; this clinical setting usually implies severe potassium deficiency.

Diagnostic Approach in Hypokalemia

The major syndromes associated with hypokalemia are listed in Table 5 and discussed individually on the following pages.

Diuretic Therapy

Continuous diuretic therapy may result in hypokalemia and chronic volume contraction. The wide use of diuretics in the treatment of hypertension makes the syndrome rather common. This clinical setting is usually associated with high serum bicarbonate and uric acid levels and also with very high urinary potassium excretion, which is a consequence of increased distal delivery of sodium in the presence of secondary hyperaldosteronism. Patients may complain of dizziness, lightheadedness, and other orthostatic changes. Physical examination may reveal a significant drop in blood pressure and an increase in pulse rate when the patient moves from a supine to a standing position. The clinical consequences usually depend upon the severity of the case. Chronic hyponatremia is an associated electrolyte disturbance of diuretic therapy and usually responds to discontinuation of medication.[13]

Primary Aldosteronism

The syndrome of mineralocorticoid excess due to a tumor or adrenal hyperplasia is characterized by hypertension, hypokalemia, low renin levels, and metabolic alkalosis. Proximal tubular reabsorption is not enhanced in this type of alkalosis. The diagnosis should be suspected in any hypertensive patient presenting with hypokalemia prior to diuretic therapy. Urinary excretion of 17-ketosteroids and 17-hydroxycorticosteroids is normal. The original description by Conn[20] involved a patient with adrenal adenoma. Bilateral adrenal hyperplasia has been described, and it was demonstrated that the clinical syndrome may be suppressed with deoxycorticosterone acetate (DOCA) or aldosterone antagonist diuretic therapy. In doubtful cases the suppression test with spironolactone will help to identify hyperplasia, because adenomas do not respond to the test. Malignant tumors are rare. Of 138 patients reviewed by Conn and associates,[21] 91 per cent had single adenomas. Further steps in the work-up of patients with this clinical entity require one or a combination of the following tests: arteriogram, adrenal venography with selective blood sampling, adrenal imaging with ^{125}I-labeled 19-iodocholesterol, and computerized tomography.[13]

Renin-Secreting Tumors

Since the early description by Robertson and colleagues[22] and Kihara and associates[23] of a syndrome believed to have been induced by a juxtaglomerular cell tumor, several cases have been identified in the medical literature. The clinical picture, as further studied by Conn and co-workers,[24] includes hypertension, hypokalemia, persistently high renin and aldosterone levels, and metabolic alkalosis. The hypokalemia is a consequence of the secondary aldosteronism. The differential diagnosis consists of eliminating the possibility of renal vascular hypertension. Bilateral renal vein renin determinations and arteriography are the most useful evaluations. It should be emphasized that patients with malignant hypertension have a high incidence of hypokalemia. It is believed that this finding is due to a secondary over-secretion of aldosterone.[13]

Renal Tubular Acidosis

This syndrome is discussed under "Hyperkalemia" (p. 266).

Bartter's Syndrome

Severe potassium deficiency, metabolic alkalosis, hyperaldosteronism, and hyperplasia of juxtaglomerular cells characterize Bartter's syndrome. Usually mental and physical development is delayed in affected children. The patients initially described by Bartter and colleagues[25] were normotensive and showed a decreased vascular responsiveness to angiotensin infusion. The etiology remains unknown. More recently, several hypotheses have been advanced to explain this syndrome. Kurtzman and Gutierrez[26] postulated a defect in chloride transport at the loop of Henle; this possibility is supported by studies in which a defect in water clearance was demonstrated in affected patients.

A proximal tubular defect was excluded by the demonstration of a normal bicarbonate reabsorption in two patients. More recently, evidence was advanced for a major role for renal prostaglandin in this syndrome.[27] In support of this hypothesis, it has been demonstrated that inhibition of prostaglandin synthesis is of therapeutic value.[28, 29] Further studies are in order, however, to evaluate the long-term therapeutic consequences in this syndrome. Results of one study have suggested that patients with Bartter's syndrome tolerated this form of therapy well, with only one serious complication and an improvement in growth in all treated cases.[29] It is of interest that the hypokalemia is never completely corrected by indomethacin in these patients, despite a positive balance of sodium and potassium.

Liddle's Syndrome

This rare clinical condition, first described in two siblings, is characterized by hypertension and hypokalemic metabolic alkalosis.[30] Urinary and serum aldosterone levels are very low. Administration of spironolactone does not alter the handling of sodium and potassium by the kidney. Liddle and colleagues[30] postulated an inherited defect in renal tubular transport. The etiology is, however, not clear at present.

Excessive Ingestion of Licorice

The cause of this disorder has been shown to be glycyrrhizic acid, an ingredient in licorice that has mineralocorticoid property. Hypokalemia dominates the clinical picture of excessive licorice ingestion. Acute and rapid progressive myopathy with myoglobinuria, tetany, and convulsions has been documented.[31] When one is evaluating hypokalemia, licorice ingestion is clearly a possibility that needs to be eliminated. Careful history-taking usually suffices.

Vomiting or Gastric Suction

The loss of acid by the stomach was extensively studied by Kassirer and Schwartz.[32] Experimentally, two phases were defined in this type of metabolic alkalosis, generation and maintenance. Continuous vomiting or gastric drainage leads to a rise in plasma bicarbonate level and a decrease in plasma chloride level. Sodium bicarbonate increases in the urine, with concomitant increase in aldosterone. Characteristically, urine chloride in this phase is markedly low. The maintenance phase is characterized by a high level of plasma bicarbonate and low levels of urinary sodium and chloride. The effective arterial blood volume is contracted, as measured by proximal tubular function, and is the determinant factor in maintaining the metabolic alkalosis. Hypokalemia is present even if the potassium loss in the drainage is replaced. Thus, hypokalemia due to acid loss is a consequence of an increase in potassium excretion by the distal tubule. Saline infusion resulting in expansion of the effective arterial volume leads to correction of this type of alkalosis.

Diarrhea

In addition to diarrhea, laxative abuse, barium poisoning, and geophagia may result in hypokalemia and metabolic alkalosis. The pathophysiology involves a high rate of potassium excretion by the bowels.[2]

Villous Adenoma of the Colon

The incidence of hypokalemia in association with this tumor is variable. Jahadi and Baldwin[33] found a rate of less than 1 per cent in their retrospective study, although others have reported a higher incidence.

Burns

Patients suffering from severe burns may develop important potassium disturbances. Postburn kaliuresis may be severe and probably is a consequence of secondary aldosteronism and persistent respiratory alkalosis.[2]

REFERENCES

1. Aikawa JK, Harrell GT, Eisenberg B. The exchangeable potassium content of normal women. J Clin Invest 1952;31:367–72.
2. Kliger AS, Hayslett JP. Disorders of potassium balance. In: Brenner BM, Stein JH, eds. Acid base and potassium homeostasis. (Contemporary issues in nephrology; vol 2). New York: Churchill Livingstone, 1978:168–204.
3. Berliner RW. Outline of renal physiology (edited by Straus, M.B. and Welt, L.G.), 1977:33–86.
4. O'Connor G, Kunau RT. Renal transport of hydrogen and potassium. In: Brenner BM, Stein JH, eds. Acid base potassium homeostasis. (Contemporary issues in nephrology; vol 2). New York: Churchill Livingstone, 1978:1–29.
5. Schambelan M, Stockigt JR, Biglieri EG. Isolated hypoaldosteronism in adults. N Engl J Med 1972;287:573.
6. Nascimento L, Arruda JAL. Hyperkalemia: various causes and how they influence management. Consultant 1982;22(5):55–76.
7. Cronin RE, Knochel JP. The consequences of potassium deficiency. In: Brenner BM, Stein JH, eds. Acid base and potassium homeostasis. (Contemporary issues in nephrology; vol 2). New York: Churchill Livingstone, 1978:168–204.
8. Bull AM, Carter AB, Lowe KG. Hyperpotassaemic paralysis. Lancet 1953;2:60–64.
9. Westenfelder C, Nascimento L. Respiratory acidosis and alkalosis. Semin Nephrol 1981;1(3):220–38.
10. Marriot HJL. Practical electrocardiography. Baltimore: Williams & Wilkins, 1972:194–211.
11. Perez CO, Oster JR, Vaamonde CA. Renal acidosis and renal potassium handling in selective hypoaldosteronism. Am J Med 1974;57:809–15.
12. Perez CO, Lespier LE, Oster JR, Vaamonde CA. Effect of alterations of sodium intake in patients with hyporeninemic hypoaldosteronism. Nephron 1977;18:259–65.
13. Kaplan NW. Clinical hypertension. New York: Medcom Press, 1973.
14. Battle DC, Arruda JAL, Kurtzman NA. Hyperkalemic distal renal tubular acidosis associated with obstructive uropathy. N Engl J Med 1981;304:373–80.
15. Arruda JAL, Kurtzman NA. Mechanism and classification of deranged distal urinary acidification. Am J Physiol 1980;239:515–24.
16. Nascimento L, Kurtzman NA. Defects in urinary acidification. Dialogues Pediatr Nephrol 1981;4:5–7.
17. Narins RG. The renal acidosis. In: Brenner BM, Stein JH, eds. Acid base and potassium homeostasis. (Contemporary issues in nephrology; vol 2). New York: Churchill Livingstone, 1978:168–204.
18. Arruda JAL, Subbarayudu K, Dytka G, Mola R, Kurtzman NA. Voltage-dependent distal acidification defect induced by amiloride. J Lab Clin Med 1980;95:407–15.
19. Wang P, Clausen T. Treatment of attacks in hyperkalemic familial periodic paralysis by inhalation of salbutamol. Lancet 1976;1:221–5.
20. Conn JW. Primary aldosteronism: a new clinical syndrome. J Lab Clin Med 1955;45:6–13.
21. Conn JW, Knopf RF, Nesbit RM. Clinical characteristics of primary aldosteronism from an analysis of 145 cases. Am J Surg 1964;107:159.
22. Robertson PW, Klidjian A, Harding LK, et al. Hypertension due to a renin-secreting renal tumor. Am J Med 1967;43:963–76.
23. Kihara I, Kitamura S, Hoshino T, et al. A hitherto unreported vascular tumor of the kidney: a proposal of juxtaglomerular cell tumor. Acta Path Jap 1968;18:197–206.
24. Conn JW, Cohen EL, Lucas CP, et al. Primary reninism. Arch Intern Med 1972;129:682–96.
25. Bartter FC, Pronove P, Gill JR Jr, et al. Hyperplasia of the juxtaglomerular complex with hyperaldosteronism and hypokalemic alkalosis; a new syndrome. Am J Med 1962;33:811–20.
26. Kurtzman NA, Gutierrez LF. The pathophysiology of Bartter's syndrome. JAMA 1975;234:758–9.
27. Gill JR Jr, Frolich JC, Bowden RE, et al. Bartter's syndrome: a disorder characterized by high urinary prostaglandins and a dependence of hyperreninemia on prostaglandin synthesis. Am J Med 1976;61:43–50.
28. Verberckmoes R, Van Damme B, Clement J, Amery A, Michielsen P. Bartter's syndrome with hyperplasia of renomedullary cells: successful treatment with indomethacin. Kidney Int 1976;9:302–7.
29. Dillon MJ, Shah V, Mitchell MD. Bartter's syndrome: 10 cases in childhood. Q J Med 1979;48:429–46.
30. Liddle GW, Bledsoe T, Cappage WJ Jr. A familial renal disorder simulating primary aldosteronism but with negligible aldosterone secretion. Trans Assoc Am Phys 1963; 79:199–205.
31. Gross EG, Dexter JD, Roth RG. Hypokalemic myopathy with myoglobinuria associated with licorice ingestion. N Engl J Med 1966;274:602–6.
32. Kassirer JP, Schwartz WB: The response of normal man to selective depletion of hydrochloric acid. Factors in the genesis of persistent gastric alkalosis. Am J Med 1966; 40:10–8.
33. Jahadi MR, Baldwin A. Villous adenomas of the colon and rectum. Am J Surg 1975;130:729–32.

HYPERPROLACTINEMIA

JAMES R. JONES □ EKKEHARD KEMMANN

□ SYNONYMS: Amenorrhea-galactorrhea syndrome, elevated serum prolactin

BACKGROUND

Although prolactin has long been recognized as a distinct hormone, its significance in human clinical conditions remained a matter of conjecture until 1971, when prolactin was isolated and a specific radioimmunoassay was developed.[1] The past decade has been most fruitful in unravelling pituitary prolactin physiology and pathophysiology.

Prolactin

Human pituitary prolactin (PRL) is a polypeptide of about 200 amino acids that is biologically distinct from, but structurally related to, growth hormone (hGH) and human placental lactogen (hPL).[2] It is secreted from the lactotropic cells of the anterior pituitary gland. The regulation of PRL secretion is under hypothalamic inhibitory control, and the agent of this hypothalamic control has been termed prolactin-inhibiting factor (PIF). PIF is primarily dopaminergic and, in fact, may be dopamine itself. Thus, in normal circumstances, PIF gains access to the anterior pituitary, and therefore the lactotropic cells, via the portal circulation and suppresses the release of prolactin.[3] The dopaminergic inhibition of PRL secretion appears to be the preeminent control, even though it is known that hypothalamic thyrotropin-regulating hormone (TRH) and gonadotropin-regulating hormone (GnRH) are fairly potent stimulants for the anterior pituitary secretion of PRL.[3, 4]

Prolactin may be produced by tissue other than the pituitary. Specifically, it is secreted locally from decidual endometrium, and large quantities may be synthesized by the decidua during pregnancy and thereby enter the amniotic fluid.[5] In the nonpregnant woman, the endometrial contribution of PRL is minimal and is not an issue in the consideration of hyperprolactinemia. Prolactin has also been described as being secreted by a malignant tumor (i.e., oat cell carcinoma of the lung), but the propensity of malignancies to secrete prolactin is not high and prolactin is not considered a reliable or useful tumor marker.[6]

The functions of PRL in the animal kingdom are wide and variable. In the human, its only clear and unequivocal physiologic effect is the initiation of lactation. Thus, during pregnancy, in conjunction with other hormones (estrogens, progesterone, cortisol, insulin, thyroxine, etc.), PRL prepares the breast for lactation; in the puerperium it is critical for initiation of lactation.[7] During pregnancy, serum PRL increases markedly (to as high as 200 ng/ml, from a nonpregnancy level of less than 30 ng/ml). This increase is secondary to the direct stimulatory effect of the very high levels of estrogens secreted by the placenta. In spite of these high PRL levels, lactation itself does not occur during pregnancy. Lactation is probably inhibited by estrogens (and possibly progesterone), which block the effect of prolactin directly at the breast level.[7] At delivery the placenta is amputated, and thus the source of the high levels of steroids is removed, and within 24 hours the postpartum patient is hypoestrogenic. Although the stimulus for the increase in pituitary secretion of PRL has now been discontinued, the serum levels of PRL do not decrease to non-pregnancy levels until about 3 to 4 weeks postpartum. It is during this brief period of hypoestrogenism and hyperprolactinemia that active lactation is initiated. Lactation can be continued almost indefinitely by continued suckling or breast stimulation, which leads to pulses of increased output of PRL.[8]

Other effects of PRL in the human are less clearly defined. It is thought that PRL also takes part in pubertal breast development (mammotrophic effect).[7] Although PRL receptors have been found in the ovary, identification of the fundamental effect(s) of PRL upon gonadal function awaits further elucidation.[9]

Hyperprolactinemia

Serum levels of prolactin are measurable by radioimmunoassay (RIA). The samples are usually obtained in the morning. Normal levels range between 5 and 25 ng/ml in both males and females. Although levels of less than 5 ng/ml are occasionally found in such syndromes as hypopituitarism, hypothalamic hypogonadotropic amenorrhea (HHA), anorexia nervosa, and the climacteric, a specific syndrome associated with hypoprolactinemia has not been identified. Levels greater than 30 ng/ml are considered hyperprolactinemic.

A number of hyperprolactinemic conditions had been recognized by astute clinicians even before prolactin was reliably measured. These syndromes, generally characterized by galactorrhea and amenorrhea, include the Forbes-Albright syndrome (galactorrhea, amenorrhea, and a pituitary tumor), the Chiari-Frommel syndrome (persistent postpartum galactorrhea and amenorrhea), and the Ahumada–Del Castillo (Argonz–Del Castillo) syndrome (galactorrhea and amenorrhea not associated with a pregnancy).[10] Today the galactorrhea-amenorrhea conditions are usually classified according to the cause of the hyperprolactinemia, and the eponymic syndromes are primarily of historical interest.

In general, hyperprolactinemia states are found in association with hypogonadotropism (decreased pituitary output of FSH and LH). The exact mechanism of this association of elevated PRL levels and decreased FSH and LH release has been a subject of much conjecture. Theoretically, high circulating amounts of PRL could interfere with gonadotropin action at the ovarian level; however, the clinical significance of such peripheral PRL interference remains debatable. Exogenous gonadotropin (human FSH and LH, Perganol) therapy is effective in gonadal stimulation and in ovulation induction in patients with high prolactin levels.[11] Another possible explanation for the associated hypogonadotropism is that high PRL levels may inhibit gonadotropic secretion at the pituitary level; the evidence for this is scant. A third alternative, namely interference with GnRH at the hypothalamic level, is the most attractive.[3] It could be explained by a common defect causing deficiencies of both GnRH and PIF and resulting in hyperprolactinemia and hypogonadotropism. Alternatively, an ultrashort feedback of PRL upon the hypothalamus may cause a GnRH deficiency. Generally, the reduction of PRL to normal or near-normal levels allows gonadotropin function to resume.

Causes of Hyperprolactinemia

The various causes of serum prolactin elevation are listed in Table 1.

Physiologic Hyperprolactinemia

The increase in serum PRL found during pregnancy, the puerperium, and suckling have been discussed. Prolactin levels are also normally high in the fetus and neonate and then fall to extremely low levels during childhood. At pubescence, PRL levels rise to adult concentrations (5–25 ng/ml). A circadian rhythm of serum PRL has been described, with the highest levels found nocturnally, during non-REM sleep.[12] PRL levels also may transiently rise (much like hGH and ACTH levels) in response to stress such as surgery, vigorous exercise, or hypoglycemia.[13, 14]

Pathologic Hyperprolactinemia

Most significant among the pathologic causes of hyperprolactinemia are the structural disorders of the pituitary and the parapituitary areas. Thus, the identification of pituitary adenomas has become a most important exercise in the investigation of the hyperprolactinemic patient. Prolactin-secreting pituitary tumors are divided into microadenomas and macroadenomas.[15] The microadenomas, defined as less than 1 cm in diameter, are small pituitary adenomas (or nodules) of lactotrophic cells that seem to specifically secrete prolactin; they do not extend beyond the sella turcica and are not associated with significant alternations of the bony sella (although a "double floor" is a common radiographic finding), and other pituitary hormones are rarely affected. Prolactin-secreting macroadenomas may be associated with a significantly distorted sella turcica and may show sellar extension. Intrapituitary and extrapituitary lesions that do not secrete PRL themselves may disrupt PRL regulation and must be considered in the differential diagnosis (see Table 1).

Other causes of pathologic hyperprolactinemia include primary hypothyroidism, drugs that specifically interfere with the regulating dopaminergic transmitter process, uremia, an abnormally sensitive neurogenic reflex, and ectopic prolactin secretion. Somewhat elevated PRL levels have been found in some patients with the polycystic ovary syndrome,[16] for reasons that are not clear.

The most common cause of hyperprolactinemia is, of course, "idiopathic." This type is diagnosed after the previously listed entities have been excluded. It probably represents a hypothalamic-pituitary dysregulation of prolactin secretion. However, this category of patients may also include those with small, as yet unrecognizable prolactinomas.

HISTORY

Elevated serum PRL levels are normal in the neonate, in the adult female during pregnancy and lactation, and in response to severe stress (i.e. hypoglycemia, surgery). The clinical question before us is, What are the symptoms and signs most frequently associated with pathologic hyperprolactinemia? Because the vast majority of hyperprolactinemic states affect the female, our discussion focuses primarily upon the effects of hyperprolactinemia in the reproductive-age female, with only occasional references to the male.

Amenorrhea. Amenorrhea is defined as the absence of spontaneous menstrual bleeding for 90 or more days. Because hyperprolactinemia is usually associated with hypogonadotropic hypogonadism, amenorrhea is a leading symptom. Although

Table 1. CAUSES OF HYPERPROLACTINEMIA

Physiologic hyperprolactinemia	Pregnancy Puerperium (3–4 weeks) Suckling Fetal existence Neonatal period Nocturnal rise (non-REM sleep) Stress, i.e., anesthesia, surgery, hypoglycemia, exercise

Pathologic hyperprolactinemia	Idiopathic
	Central organic lesion
	  Pituitary
	    Pituitary adenomas
	      Microadenoma
	      Macroadenoma
	    Empty sella syndrome
	    Pituitary trauma (surgery, stalk section, etc.)
	  Parapituitary
	    Craniopharyngioma
	    Sarcoidosis
	    Glioma
	    Aneurysm
	Metabolic causes
	  Hypothyroidism
	  Uremia
	  Cirrhosis
	  Polycystic ovary syndrome
	Neurogenic stimulation
	  Chest wall lesion
	  Spinal cord lesion
	  Breast stimulation
	Ectopic PRL production
	  Neoplasm

Drug-induced hyperprolactinemia	Hormones
	  Estrogens
	  TRH
	  GnRH
	Tranquilizers
	  Thioxanthenes
	  Butyrophenones
	Narcotics
	  Morphine
	  Heroin
	Antidepressants
	  MAO inhibitors
	Antihypertensives
	  Alpha-methyldopa
	  Guanethidine
	  Reserpine
	Others
	  Sulpiride
	  Cimetidine
	  Verapamil

amenorrhea can be a symptom of a number of other entities (Table 2), hyperprolactinemia is estimated to account for about 15 per cent of cases of amenorrhea in young patients. The amenorrhea associated with hyperprolactinemia is often of long standing, and the patient may be significantly hypoestrogenic. Characteristically, affected patients do not have withdrawal bleeding when given a progestin alone (progesterone, Provera, etc.). Occasionally, patients are seen with somewhat elevated prolactin levels and irregular, infrequent menses rather than amenorrhea. This finding is usually observed in patients in whom the serum prolactin level is less than 100 ng/ml, most commonly between 30 and 50 ng/ml. This constellation of findings may be an aspect of the polycystic ovary syndrome.

Primary amenorrhea (no spontaneous menses before age 18) is a rare but possible complaint in the female with hyperprolactinemia.[17] In the woman with primary amenorrhea and hyperprolactinemia, thelarche (breast development) and

Table 2. CAUSES OF AMENORRHEA

Causes	Percentage of Cases*
Polycystic ovary (PCO) syndrome	45–50
Hypogonadotropic hypothalamic amenorrhea (HHA)	15–20
Hyperprolactinemia	10–15
Chromosome disorders	1–5
Other (ovarian failure [idiopathic], adrenal disorders, thyroid disorders)	10–15

*Percentages based upon experience of about 2,000 patients seen in reproductive-endocrine practice of the authors.

pubarche (pubic and axillary hair development) have occurred normally. Thus, it appears that puberty was initiated but not completed.

Hyperprolactinemia in women beyond the reproductive years is quite unusual. In fact, we have not seen a patient with both elevated serum prolactin levels and the markedly elevated serum gonadotropin levels seen in ovarian failure.

Galactorrhea. Galactorrhea is defined as inappropriate lactation, that is, the presence of milk at any time other than after gestation.[7] Although often of small quantity and therefore unrecognized by the patient, galactorrhea may be found by the patient during examination of the breast, during sexual foreplay, or simply because of wetting of a bra. Frequently, however, the patient is completely unaware of the presence of galactorrhea. On occasion, a postpartum patient may be unable to stop milk production after weaning (persistent lactation); this latter condition, if associated with continued postpartum amenorrhea, is referred to as Chiari-Frommel syndrome.[10]

A cardinal point about galactorrhea is that it must be looked for (see "Physical Examination"). Absence of a history of breast discharge is not sufficient to rule out galactorrhea.

Infertility. Disturbance of ovulation with resultant infertility may be the primary reason the hyperprolactinemic patient consults the physician. In general, infertility (nonovulation) associated with hyperprolactinemia tends to respond quite well to therapy.

Headaches. We have often noted that patients with hyperprolactinemia complain of frequent headaches.[18] These headaches are found in those both with and without pituitary lesions. In character, the headaches appear to be similar to "tension headaches" rather than to migraine types, and the complaints are of long duration. The cause of such headaches remains unclear.

Other Pituitary-Hypothalamic Disorders. Because pituitary PRL secretion is regulated primarily by hypothalamic inhibition, any condition that disrupts the pituitary-hypothalamic axis may result in hyperprolactinemia. Thus, any history of pituitary or hypothalamic disease, injury, surgery, or trauma is extremely relevant.

Medications. A number of drugs are known to elevate serum PRL levels (see Table 1). The eliciting of information about drug ingestion can be quite easy or surprisingly difficult. Obviously, the patient who is currently taking medications (i.e., hypertensive agents) is generally open and straightforward, but patients who may have taken medication weeks ago (perhaps for psychiatric reasons) may not remember having done so or may not be willing to discuss the matter. The nonmedical intake of medications (such as heroin ingestion) is even more difficult to detect. Once it is determined that the patient is taking a prolactin-elevating drug, whether or not to continue the therapy, and therefore whether to accept its hyperprolactinemic side effect, must be weighed in relation to its efficacy. In the patient who is medicated for psychiatric indications, we carry out testing to rule out a pituitary tumor; if test results are negative, we generally advise continuing treatment.

Estrogens and therefore estrogen-containing oral contraceptive preparations may slightly raise PRL levels. In reviews of the histories of patients with prolactinomas, it was often observed that these patients had a high degree of exposure to oral contraceptives. Concern has been voiced that there may be a possible relationship between exogenous estrogen use and the development or stimulation of such a pituitary lesion. However, it appears from retrospective studies that the risk is minimal or nonexistent.[19]

Hirsutism. Occasionally, patients with hyperprolactinemia complain of increased (and increasing) facial hair growth. This hair tends to be rather fine and soft (lanugo-like) and differs from the coarse, dark hair found in virilizing states. In addition, the patients may also note an increase in the rate of growth of arm and leg hair (hypertrichosis). The cause of these alterations in hair growth in association with hyperprolactinemia is unknown. The association of mild hyperprolactinemia with the polycystic ovary syndrome and the possibility that PRL alters adrenal androgen production are considerations.[16] The phenomenon is fundamentally unexplained.

Other Disorders. Hyperprolactinemia may also be associated with metabolic disorders such as hypothyroidism, cirrhosis, uremia, chest injury, and neoplastic production.[6, 20–23]

Male Hyperprolactinemia. Hyperprolactinemia is much less common in the male than in the female but when found is also associated with hypogonadism. In the male, advanced hypogonadism frequently manifests as impotence.[24] Galactorrhea is always pathologic in the male, and gynecomastia is another complaint that should be evaluated for hyperprolactinemia.

Family History. Currently there is no well-described syndrome of familial hyperprolactinemia. A special note on breast cancer is relevant, because of its well-described familial tendency and because its development in certain rodents is apparently prolactin-dependent. At this point, however, there are no data indicating that women with high PRL levels are at any greater risk of breast cancer.[25] In addition, studies of patients with breast cancer do not suggest present or past abnormalities of serum PRL.

PHYSICAL EXAMINATION

In the female with hyperprolactinemia, a complete examination includes specific considerations of the neurologic status, a thyroid evaluation, and thorough breast and pelvic examinations.

The general evaluation would, of course, include vital signs, height and weight, evidence of hirsutism (hypertrichosis), and needle tracks in veins. The neurologic status, specifically exclusion of optic problems (bitemporal hemianopsia), and scars of previous head trauma or surgery should be noted. The size and consistency of the thyroid gland should be checked. One should exclude chest wall injury and herpes zoster.

Typically, breast development is good. Evaluation for galactorrhea consists in "milking" the breasts by applying pressure from the edge of the areola toward the nipple. *Galactorrhea* is the finding of milk. In our experience, when the secretion looks like milk, it always is milk; it is quite unnecessary to send a specimen for cytology, fat studies, or any other laboratory testing. The galactorrhea is bilateral, and the amount of milk found is not important. Even very small amounts can be associated with very high levels of PRL.

Not all nipple secretions are galactorrhea, however. Other secretions are: blood (indicative of a possible ductal papilloma or carcinoma), pus (suggesting an intraductal infection), and fairly commonly, a clear, translucent fluid (apparently of no significance and frequently found in parous women).

Pelvic findings are usually normal, but the uterus may be found to be rather small; adnexal masses and tenderness are not expected. An enlarged uterus indicates the possibility of pregnancy, which, of course, can be associated with a rise in PRL.

In most patients the physical findings are quite normal except for the galactorrhea, which is found in about three-fourths of hyperprolactinemic patients.

DIAGNOSTIC STUDIES

Laboratory Studies

Serum Prolactin Level. Pituitary PRL is measured directly in the serum by a quite sensitive radioimmunoassay. As noted previously, the normal values in both females and males are about the same and usually do not exceed 20 to 25 ng/ml; a level of 30 ng/ml or greater is considered hyperprolactinemic. With a borderline concentration (between 20 and 29 ng/ml), the determination is repeated before the patient is definitely described as hyperprolactinemic. Attempting to assign the cause of the hyperprolactinemia on the basis of the PRL level is indeed a troublesome and dangerous exercise; nonetheless, certain very general observations seem to be helpful. Hyperprolactinemia associated with conditions such as drug ingestion, stress, polycystic ovaries, hypothyroidism, and nonsecreting pituitary or extrapituitary tumors tends to be in the lower ranges, that is, most often less than 100 ng/ml. The prolactin level associated with pituitary prolactinomas tends to be high, well over 100 ng/ml, and frequently 1000s of ng/ml or more. In the follow-up of patients with hyperprolactinemia, the frequency of the measurement of PRL is dictated by the therapy that may or may not be in progress. If simple nonintervention ("wait and see") is decided on, every 6 months seems a useful interval.

Dynamic PRL Testing. A number of prolactin stimulation and suppression tests have been developed in an attempt to discriminate between PRL-secreting pituitary adenomas and other nontumor causes of hyperprolactinemia. Unfortunately, none of the tests has survived the challenge of time, and all are less accurate in the diagnosis of pituitary microadenomas than radiography. The dynamic PRL tests that have been described include:

1. TRH stimulation test: Serum PRL increases in response to intravenously administered TRH. This response is said to be "blunted" in patients with microadenomas.[26]

2. Chlorpromazine test: Response to this stimulatory test of anterior pituitary PRL has also been described as "blunted" in the presence of a microadenoma.[26]

3. Nomifensine test: Nomifensine causes selective enhancement of hypothalamic dopaminergic activity by inhibiting uptake of dopamine by receptors in the CNS. It has been proposed that administration of the drug reduces PRL levels in patients with hyperprolactinemia secondary to functional causes but not in patients with microadenomas.[26]

4. L-Dopa and Carbidopa test: Carbidopa inhib-

its peripheral decarboxylase and thus increases dopamine activity. It is suggested that this test will effect a PRL decrease in dysfunctional but not in tumor-produced hyperprolactinemia.[26]

These tests are generally not used for routine clinical testing because of their lack of specificity. Nevertheless, the search for dynamic PRL tests to discriminate between pituitary tumor and nontumor causes of hyperprolactinemia will undoubtedly continue.

Serum FSH and LH Determinations. Serum levels of gonadotropins can be obtained in amenorrheic women at any time, but in patients with menstrual bleeding (regular or irregular) the measurements should be carried out on days 1 to 3 of a cycle. These determinations are also radioimmunoassay testings. Generally, in hyperprolactinemic patients with amenorrhea, the FSH and LH levels are low (<5 mIU/ml) to normal (5–20 mIU/ml). On occasion in the patient with the polycystic ovary syndrome, one may find slightly elevated prolactin (30–40 ng/ml), normal or low serum FSH, and elevated LH (>20 mIU/ml). Such a patient is usually managed as a polycystic ovary patient rather than as a hyperprolactinemic.

In general, obtaining serum gonadotropin concentrations serves only to distinguish among the typical hypogonadotropism of hyperprolactinemia, the slightly elevated LH level occasionally found in the polycystic ovary syndrome, and ovarian failure (in which there are castrate concentrations of FSH and LH).

Pregnancy Test. Because early pregnancy is characterized by a somewhat elevated PRL level and amenorrhea, it is obvious that on occasion a pregnancy test (urinary or serum hCG or beta-subunit hCG determination) is indicated, especially if the hyperprolactinemia is associated with an enlarged uterus.

Serum Androgen Measurements. As noted previously, an occasional hyperprolactinemic patient presents with increasing facial or body hair. In these patients serum testosterone, DHEA-S, and cortisol measurements are usually carried out. In our experience the only androgen occasionally elevated is the DHEA-S. As previously discussed, the nature of the relationship of the excessive hair growth and the hyperprolactinemia is unknown.

Growth Hormone Determination. In general, pituitary growth hormones should be measured in all patients with hyperprolactinemia, because a small number of patients with PRL-secreting pituitary tumors also have elevated growth hormone levels. The nature of the relationship between the elevated levels is difficult to define and probably varies. In some cases there is probably a coincident secretion of both PRL and growth hormone by a pituitary adenoma, in others there may be an immunologic crossover in the RIA, and in still others the PRL elevation may not reflect specific prolactin secretion by a growth hormone–secreting tumor but rather a dissociation of the anterior pituitary from hypothalamic control caused by the adenoma (essentially a stalk section).

Adrenal Studies. Serum ACTH, cortisol, and DHEA-S measurements are indicated in patients with signs of hypercortisolism or a macroadenoma.

Thyroid Studies. Since primary thyroid failure is occasionally associated with hyperprolactinemia, serum TSH and T_3 and T_4 determinations are indicated. In our experience, primary thyroid failure is a rare cause of hyperprolactinemia.

Renal Function Studies. A BUN or serum creatinine determination should be obtained to rule out severe renal disease. Uremia is rarely, if ever, diagnosed via hyperprolactinemia.

Diagnostic Imaging

Critical in patients with hyperprolactinemia is the radiographic assessment of the pituitary area. Although a number of techniques of sella turcica evaluation have evolved, the choice of one over another depends completely on the locally available method, how strongly one suspects a pituitary or parapituitary lesion, and the size of the lesion.

Computed Tomography. Early computed tomography (CT) methodologies were inadequate to detect very small pituitary lesions, but further refinements have made CT scanning the most sensitive of radiographic techniques.[27] Besides its remarkable resolution of small lesions (Fig. 1), advantages of CT scanning include: ability to define the extent of pituitary lesions beyond the sella (Fig. 2) and demonstration of certain conditions (i.e., the "empty sella") without additional neuroradiographic procedures. The disadvantages of CT scanning are cost and radiation exposure.

Polytomography. During the 1970s polytomography evolved as the method of choice for high-resolution pituitary radiographic evaluation.[28] Recently, this method has been supplanted by the better CT methods. Polytomograms are less costly than CT scans and usually are able to show significant extrasellar lesions. The disadvantages of polytomography are errors in interpretation and difficulty in detecting quite small pituitary lesions.[29]

Sellar X-Ray. The value of anteroposterior and lateral sellar x-ray views remains controversial. Massive lesions generally can be detected, yet smaller lesions or extrasellar lesions can be easily missed. Sellar x-rays have their major use in fol-

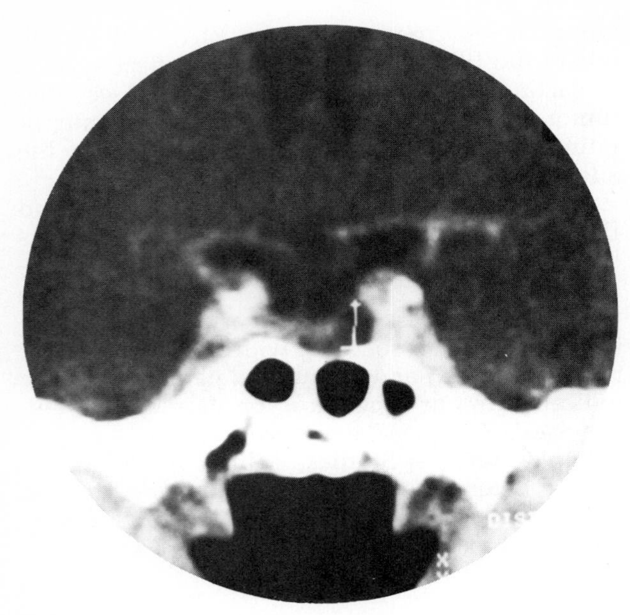

Figure 1. CT scan showing a small (0.6-cm) microadenoma within the right portion of the pituitary.

lowing a previously well-evaluated pituitary. Costs and radiation exposure are relatively low.

Other Radiographic Techniques. Further specific radiographic testing may become necessary once a sellar lesion has been identified; thus, angiography may be helpful to delineate a tumor and its extension and to rule out an aneurysm. Pneumoencephalography was important in the diagnosis of the "empty sella" syndrome but has largely been replaced by CT scanning.

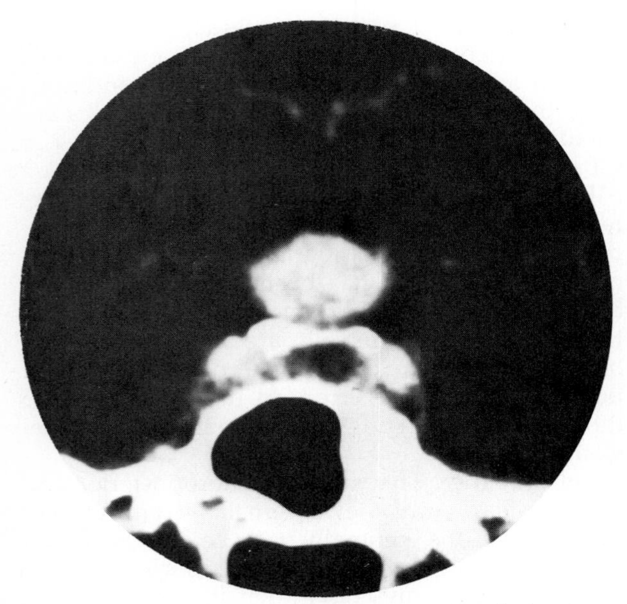

Figure 2. CT scan showing a large extrapituitary lesion (craniopharyngioma) anterior to the sella turcica.

Choice of Procedure. Controversy continues to exist as to the most accurate and appropriate radiographic methods to evaluate lesions in the sella turcica. In general, simple sellar films are probably too insensitive, the polytomogram has a significant number of false-positive and false-negative results, and in our experience, the CT scan is frequently "over-read." It seems wise to be skeptical about reports of very small (less than 0.5-cm) intrapituitary lesions. Our current choice is CT scanning for the initial evaluation and either simple sellar films or polytomography for follow-up. The specific methods used are clearly dependent on the individual circumstances. The frequency of radiographic follow-up evaluations is also individualized. In the patient whose pituitary has been adequately assessed initially, follow-up films are generally made about every 18 months.

ASSESSMENT

Hyperprolactinemia is most often found in concert with hypogonadotropic hypogonadism. In the female this disorder is most commonly displayed as galactorrhea, amenorrhea, and hypoestrogenism. Our discussion is mainly concerned with hyperprolactinemia in the female. Once hyperprolactinemia has been determined, a series of diagnostic steps must be carried out in order to arrive at the specific cause, as illustrated in the algorithm. Although flow sheets are occasionally useful and certainly concise, we strongly urge the reader not to depend on them but rather to attempt to understand the very fundamental underpinnings of assessment. By necessity, a number of factors have been deleted in the construction of this "decision tree":

1. The initial premise is that we are dealing only with females. In this instance the most common entrance of the hyperprolactinemic patient into the diagnostic system is via the complaint of amenorrhea or irregular periods with or without infertility. With the exception of this initial entry point, males are evaluated in essentially the same manner.

2. We are assuming the amenorrhea is secondary and that other reasons for amenorrhea, such as uterine synechiae (Asherman's syndrome) and hysterectomy have been ruled out. Generally these possibilities can be assessed by means of physical examination, pelvic ultrasonography, or the administration of estrogen-progestin preparations to induce uterine bleeding.

3. Dynamic PRL testing is rarely used in clinical investigations and is therefore not included.

4. A major aspect in the decision-making is the distinction between a microadenoma and a macroadenoma. Once a macroadenoma, either functional (i.e., growth hormone secretion) or non-

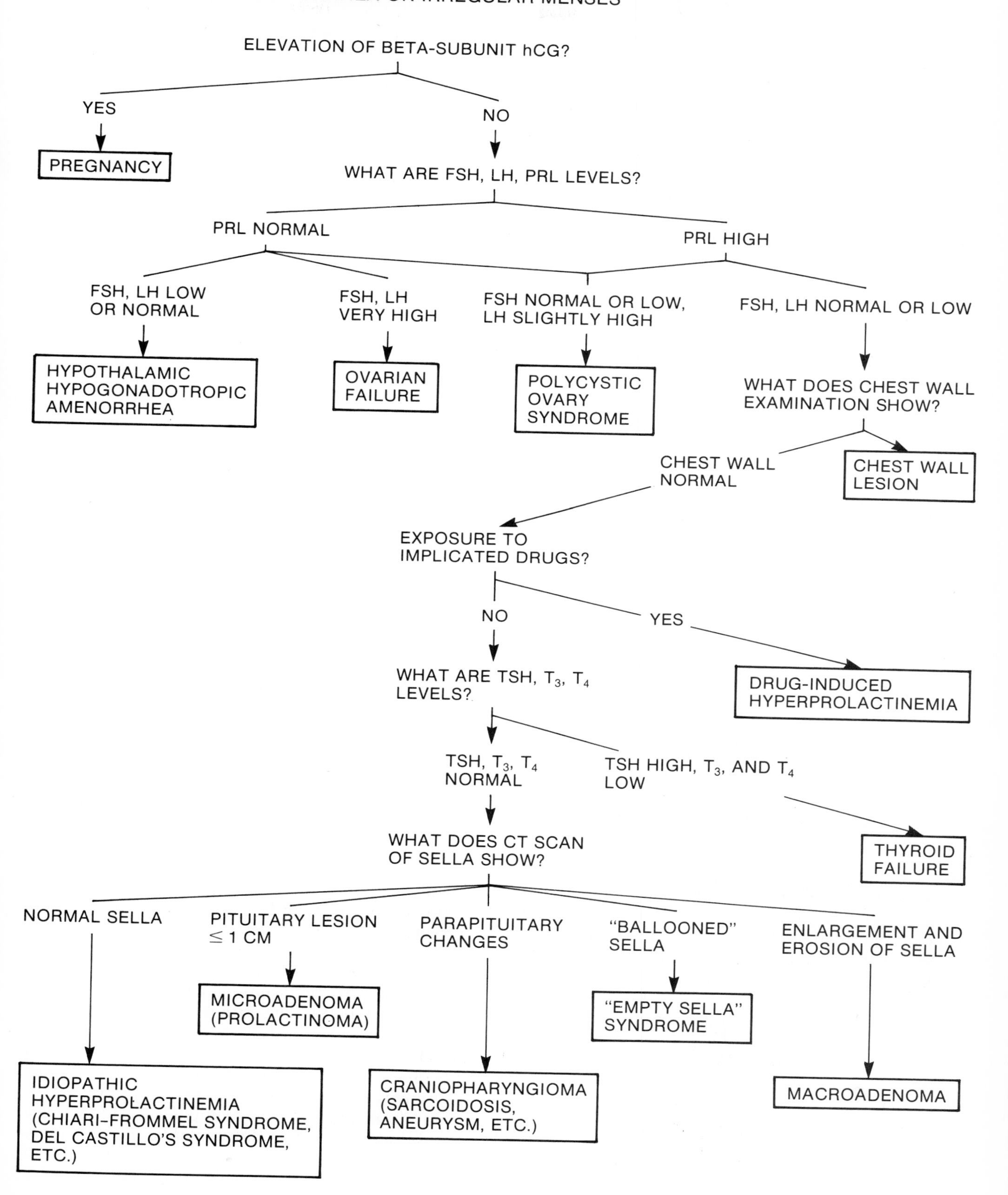
DIAGNOSTIC ASSESSMENT OF PROLACTINEMIA IN PATIENT PRESENTING WITH AMENORRHEA OR IRREGULAR MENSES
ELEVATION OF BETA-SUBUNIT hCG?
YES
PREGNANCY
NO
WHAT ARE FSH, LH, PRL LEVELS?
PRL NORMAL
PRL HIGH
FSH, LH LOW OR NORMAL
HYPOTHALAMIC HYPOGONADOTROPIC AMENORRHEA
FSH, LH VERY HIGH
OVARIAN FAILURE
FSH NORMAL OR LOW, LH SLIGHTLY HIGH
POLYCYSTIC OVARY SYNDROME
FSH, LH NORMAL OR LOW
WHAT DOES CHEST WALL EXAMINATION SHOW?
CHEST WALL NORMAL
CHEST WALL LESION
EXPOSURE TO IMPLICATED DRUGS?
NO
YES
DRUG-INDUCED HYPERPROLACTINEMIA
WHAT ARE TSH, T_3, T_4 LEVELS?
TSH, T_3, T_4 NORMAL
TSH HIGH, T_3, AND T_4 LOW
THYROID FAILURE
WHAT DOES CT SCAN OF SELLA SHOW?
NORMAL SELLA
IDIOPATHIC HYPERPROLACTINEMIA (CHIARI-FROMMEL SYNDROME, DEL CASTILLO'S SYNDROME, ETC.)
PITUITARY LESION ≤ 1 CM
MICROADENOMA (PROLACTINOMA)
PARAPITUITARY CHANGES
CRANIOPHARYNGIOMA (SARCOIDOSIS, ANEURYSM, ETC.)
"BALLOONED" SELLA
"EMPTY SELLA" SYNDROME
ENLARGEMENT AND EROSION OF SELLA
MACROADENOMA

Table 3. SUMMARY OF FINDINGS IN HYPERPROLACTINEMIC STATES

Disorder	History and Physical Findings	PRL Elevation*	FSH and LH Levels†	Sella Turcica	Other Findings
Physiologic States					
Pregnancy	Amenorrhea Enlarging uterus	Low to medium	FSH low LH high (actually hCG)	Normal	Positive pregnancy test result
Lactation	Amenorrhea Enlarged uterus but decreasing lactation	Medium	Low	Normal	—
Stress	Normal or irregular periods Normal uterus Frequently, galactorrhea	Low	Low or normal	Normal	—
Pathologic states					
Functional					
Extension of postpartum hyperprolactinemia (Chiari-Frommel syndrome)	Year or more since pregnancy Amenorrhea Small uterus Galactorrhea	Low to medium	Low or normal	Normal	—
Unassociated with pregnancy (Ahumada–Del Castillo syndrome)	Amenorrhea No recent pregnancy Small uterus Galactorrhea	Low to medium	Low or normal	Normal	—
Associated with drug ingestion	Amenorrhea or irregular periods (or infrequent but regular periods) Normal uterus Usually, galactorrhea	Low	Usually normal	Normal	—
Associated with pituitary lesion					
Microadenoma (prolactinoma)	Amenorrhea (infrequently irregular periods) Small uterus Galactorrhea	Medium to high	Low or normal	Usually not enlarged, but may show "double floor" or small (1-cm) lesion	Other pituitary functions normal No visual field problems

functional, has been diagnosed, a number of additional pituitary tests must be carried out. For example, insulin tolerance testing, water deprivation tests, and metapirone studies may be indicated. These also are not included in the algorithim.

5. Visual field assessment is not included. Generally, no harm comes by performing visual field studies on all patients. We do not assess the visual fields, however, unless the CT scan indicates something other than a microadenoma (i.e., macroadenoma, "empty sella," parapituitary lesion). Of course, such assessments are indicated if the patient's intention is pregnancy (see following paragraph).

Table 3 summarizes the characteristics of the more common disorders associated with hyperprolactinemia. This table is a general guide only. Levels of PRL are very general estimates and can be quite different in individual patients. It is our experience that determining whether one is dealing with a pathologic rather than a physiologic cause of hyperprolactinemia is relatively simple. Most of the effort and concern of the physician devolves upon whether pathologic hyperprolactinemia is related to the presence of a pituitary (or parapituitary) lesion or is simply a dysfunction of the pituitary. Frequently obtaining the answer is easy, but occasionally it is quite difficult, and sometimes nearly impossible. The justification for

Table 3. SUMMARY OF FINDINGS IN HYPERPROLACTINEMIC STATES *(Continued)*

Disorder	History and Physical Findings	PRL Elevation*	FSH and LH Levels†	Sella Turcica	Other Findings
Macroadenoma Hormone-producing	Amenorrhea (irregular periods or normal periods) Signs of acromegaly possible Uterus normal Galactorrhea	Medium to high	Usually normal	Enlarged with bony erosion	Frequently, other pituitary problems Growth hormone or ACTH may be abnormal
Non–hormone-producing	Amenorrhea (irregular periods or normal periods) Uterus normal Occasional galactorrhea	Low to medium	Usually normal	Enlarged with bony erosion	Frequently other pituitary deficiencies
Empty sella	Amenorrhea (or irregular periods) Normal uterus Occasionally, galactorrhea	Low to medium	Usually normal	Usually symmetrically enlarged, "ballooned"	Mild pituitary disruption
Parapituitary lesions	Very variable (usually irregular) periods Normal uterus Occasionally, galactorrhea	Low to medium	Usually normal	Sella normal but may show signs external pressure	Variable
Ectopic prolactin secretion	Cough	Low to medium	Variable	Normal	Abnormal chest x-ray
Polycystic ovary syndrome	Irregular periods (occasionally, amenorrhea) Uterus normal Occasionally "cystic" ovary Infrequent galactorrhea	Low	FSH usually low LH frequently > 20 mIU/ml	Normal	Hirsutism Obesity
Primary hypothyroidism	Profound hypothyroid problem	Low to medium	Normal	Normal	TSH level denotes thyroid function absent

*Low = 30–50 ng/ml; Medium = 51–200 ng/ml; High = 200+ ng/ml.
†FSH and LH levels tend to vary among laboratories.

the search for the pituitary lesion is obvious; pituitary macroadenomas or parapituitary lesions can be life-threatening, and their therapy is usually extirpative. Microadenomas, on the other hand, are generally treated conservatively, that is; without surgical or radiation extirpation. But there is still another, perhaps more remote but equally compelling, reason for the investigation. The treatment of infertility associated with hyperprolactinemia is very frequently successful, and pituitary microadenomas can and do enlarge during pregnancy and can cause minor to major problems.[30] The most effective and appropriate method of handling this clinical problem is, of course, to be aware of the possibility. In our experience, about 25 per cent of microadenoma patients who become pregnant experience significant headaches through pregnancy and rarely develop bilateral visual field defects. Obviously, such patients must be followed carefully, but in general, these neurologic manifestations do not progress extensively and the headaches and the visual field defects resolve at the termination of the pregnancy.

Hyperprolactinemia, although related to disorders that have existed for many years, is in reality a new entity. Serum prolactin measurement is a very sophisticated and rather specific method of examining the hypothalamic-pituitary axis and assessing its "wellness."

REFERENCES

1. Hwang P, Guyda H, Friesen H: A radioimmunoassay for human prolactin. Proc Nat Acad Sci USA 1971;68:1902–6.
2. Showe B, Parlow AF. Human pituitary prolactin (hPRL): the entire linear amino acid sequence. J Clin Endocrinol Metab 1977;45:1112–5.
3. Frantz AG. Prolactin. N Engl J Med 1978;298:201–7.
4. Barbarino A, DeMarinis L, Mancini A, Farabegoei C. Estrogen-dependent plasma prolactin response to gonadotropin releasing hormones in intact and castrated men. J Clin Endocrinol Metab 1982;55:1212–6.
5. Golander A, Hurley T, Barrett J, Hizi A, Handwerger S. Prolactin synthesis by human chorion-decidual tissue: a possible source of prolactin in the amniotic fluid. Science 1978;202:311–3.
6. Molitch ME, Schwartz S, Mukherji B. Is prolactin secreted ectopically? Am J Med 1981;70:803–7.
7. Kleinberg DL, Noel GL, Frantz AG. Galactorrhea: a study of 235 cases, including 48 with pituitary tumors. N Engl J Med 1977;296:589–600.
8. Noel GL, Suh HK, Frantz AG. Prolactin release during nursing and breast stimulation in post partum and non–post partum subjects. J Clin Endocrinol Metab 1974;38:413–23.
9. McNatty KP: Relationship between plasma prolactin and the endocrine microenvironment of the developing human control follicle. Fertil Steril 1979;32:433–8.
10. Forbes AP. The amenorrhea-galactorrhea syndrome: clinical features. In: Givens JR (ed), Hormone-secreting pituitary tumors. Chicago: Year Book Medical Publishers, 1982; 237–54.
11. Kemmann E, Gemzell CA, Beinert WC, Beling CB, Jones JR. Plasma prolactin changes during the administration of human menopausal gonadotropins in non-ovulating woman. Am J Obstet Gynecol 1977;129:145–9.
12. Parker DC, Rossman LG, Vanderlaan EF. Relation of sleep-entrained human prolactin release to REM-nonREM cycles. J Clin Endocrinol Metab 1974;38:646–51.
13. Konincxs P: Stress hyperprolactinemia in clinical practice. Lancet 1978;1:273.
14. May PB, Burrow GN, Kayne RD, Donabedian RK: Hypoglycemia-induced prolactin release. Arch Intern Med 1978;138:918–20.
15. Keye WR, Chang RJ, Jaffe RB. Prolactin secreting pituitary adenomas in woman with amenorrhea or galactorrhea. Obstet Gynecol Surv 1977;32:727–38.
16. Burat J, Siame-Mourot C, Fuorlinnie JC, Lemaire A, Buvat-Herbaut M, Hermand E. Androgens and prolactin levels in hirsute woman with either polycystic ovaries or "borderline ovaries." Fertil Steril 1982; 38:695–700.
17. Kemmann E, Jones JR. Hyperprolactinemia and primary amenorrhea. Obstet Gynecol 1979;54:692–94.
18. Kemmann E, Jones JR. Hyperprolactinemia and headaches. Am J Obstet Gynecol 1983;145:668–71.
19. Wingrave SJ, Kay CR, Vessey MP. Oral contraception and pituitary adenomas. Br. Med J 1980;1:685–6.
20. Honbo KS, van Herle AJ, Kettet KA. Serum prolactin levels in untreated primary hypothyroidism. Am J Med 1978; 64:782–7.
21. Nunziata V, Ceparano G, Massacca G, Budillon G. Prolactin secretion in nonalcoholic liver cirrhosis. Digestion 1978;18:157–61.
22. Lim FS, Kathpalia SC, Frohman LA. Hyperprolactinemia and impaired pituitary response to suppression and stimulation in chronic renal failure: reversal after transplantation. J Clin Endocrinol Metab 1979;48:101–7.
23. Morley JE, Dawson M, Hodgkinson H, Kalk WJ. Galactorrhea and hyperprolactinemia associated with chest wall injury. J Clin Endocrinol Metab 1977;45:931–5.
24. Spark RF, White RA, Connelly PB. Impotence is not always psychogenic. JAMA 1980;243:750–5.
25. Smithline F, Sherman L, Kolodny HD. Prolactin and breast carcinoma. N Engl J Med 1975;292:784–92.
26. Wiebe RH. Endocrine evaluation of hyperprolactinemia. Clin Obstet Gynecol 1980;23:349–65.
27. Cusick JF, Haughton VM, Hagen TC. Radiologic assessment of intrasellar prolactin-secreting tumors. Neurosurgery 1980;6:376–9.
28. Vezina JC, Sutton TJ: Prolactin-secreting pituitary microadenomas: roentgenologic diagnosis. Am J Roentgenol 1974;120:46–54.
29. Burrow GN, Wortzman G, Rewcastle NB, Holgate RC, Kovacs K: Microadenomas of the pituitary and abnormal sellar tomograms in an unselected autopsy series. N Engl J Med 1981;304:156–8.
30. Magyar DM, Marchall JR: Pituitary tumors and pregnancy. Am J Obstet Gynecol 1978;132:739–51.

HYPOCALCEMIA

L. RAYMOND REYNOLDS

☐ SYNONYMS: Tetany, hypoparathyroidism, vitamin D deficiency

BACKGROUND

The practice of routine biochemical screening has improved the recognition of disorders of calcium metabolism, particularly of asymptomatic hypercalcemia. Although hypocalcemia is found less commonly in ambulatory patients, it may be more frequent than hypercalcemia in patients with malignancy or renal disease.[1]

The serum calcium concentration is normally maintained in the range of 8.8 to 10.4 mg/100 ml, but slightly less than half the total is ionized or free of protein binding. Ionized calcium, the physiologically active portion, participates in a number of diverse metabolic processes. The total serum calcium level is therefore altered by significant changes in levels of serum proteins, especially albumin. A simple means of correcting a calcium determination for protein alterations is to increase the calcium reading by 1 mg/100 ml for each 1 gm/100 ml reduction in serum albumin below normal. Protein binding of calcium is profoundly affected by alterations in pH; an increase in pH leads to greater binding and, therefore, a decrease in ionized calcium. This principle explains the induction of hypocalcemic symptoms by the respiratory alkalosis of hyperventilation.

Calcium homeostasis depends on the interaction of parathyroid hormone (PTH) and vitamin D with specific target organs: the intestine, bone, and kidney. PTH acts primarily to increase renal reabsorption and bone resorption of calcium but also increases the conversion of 25-hydroxyvitamin D_3 to 1,25-dihydroxyvitamin D_3 (calcitriol). Calcitriol acts on the intestine to increase active calcium absorption and may also be necessary for the full expression of PTH action on bone. Symptomatic hypocalcemia, therefore, is usually the result of decreased activity of parathyroid hormone or vitamin D.

Causes

Table 1 summarizes the major causes of hypocalcemia.

Table 1. CAUSES OF HYPOCALCEMIA

Hypoalbuminemia
Hypoparathyroidism
Postsurgical
Idiopathic
Radioactive iodine
Hemochromatosis
Metastatic carcinoma
DiGeorge's syndrome
Pseudohypoparathyroidism
Hypomagnesemia
Vitamin D deficiency
Nutritional
Malabsorption
Liver disease
Anticonvulsant therapy
Chronic renal failure
Hereditary vitamin D dependency
End-organ resistance
Acute pancreatitis
Hyperphosphatemia
Blood transfusion
Cancer (osteoblastic metastases)
Neonatal hypocalcemia

Hypoparathyroidism

Hypoparathyroidism is defined as a state of decreased secretion or peripheral action of parathyroid hormone. A decrease in PTH reduces renal calcium reabsorption directly and intestinal calcium absorption indirectly through decreased production of 1,25-dihydroxyvitamin D_3. Neck surgery is the most common cause of PTH deficiency.[2] Parathyroid gland removal or injury may occur during thyroidectomy, parathyroidectomy, and radical neck surgery. Postoperative hypocalcemia commonly occurs even without significant removal of parathyroid tissue, perhaps as a result of ischemia induced by the dissection of adjacent tissues. Surgical hypoparathyroidism is commonly transient, lasting days to weeks. The "hungry bone" syndrome is a form of temporary hypoparathyroidism that often occurs after removal of a parathyroid adenoma or following thyroidectomy for hyperthyroidism.

PTH deficiency without apparent cause is called idiopathic hypoparathyroidism and embraces a heterogeneous group of disorders that occur on a familial or sporadic basis. An autoimmune mechanism is postulated in some patients because of the finding of anti-parathyroid gland antibodies and concurrent autoimmune glandular disorders, including Addison's disease, primary hypothyroidism, primary hypogonadism, diabetes mellitus, and pernicious anemia. Chronic mucocutaneous candidiasis, vitiligo, and alopecia areata may also occur in these patients. Another form of idiopathic hypoparathyroidism occurs as a sporadic, adult-onset condition without autoimmune features; the etiology is unknown, but fatty or fibrous replacement of the parathyroid glands is demonstrated pathologically.

Parathyroid gland destruction may occur in other circumstances, resulting in PTH deficiency. Irradiation injury following radioactive iodine treatment of hyperthyroidism has been rarely reported to cause overt hypoparathyroidism. Iron infiltration with subsequent hypoparathyroidism has been reported in primary or secondary forms of hemochromatosis. Neoplastic infiltration of the parathyroid glands by metastatic tumor is not unusual, particularly with breast carcinoma, but glandular destruction must be nearly total to result in hypocalcemia.[3] Defective embryologic development may result in thymic and parathyroid agenesis, or DiGeorge's syndrome.

Pseudohypoparathyroidism

As originally described by Albright in 1942, pseudohypoparathyroidism is a rare hereditary disorder characterized by hypoparathyroidism and typical somatic abnormalities. The concept of pseudohypoparathyroidism has been extended to include a group of disorders characterized by unresponsiveness of a target organ to parathyroid hormone.

In classic pseudohypoparathyroidism (type I), there is a defect in hormone receptor coupling to intercellular cyclic AMP (cAMP) or in cAMP generation, resulting in resistance to PTH in the bones and kidneys with a diminished calcemic response and a blunted rise in the phosphaturic and urinary cAMP response to exogenous PTH administration. Characteristic somatic features, including brachydactyly, short stature, round facies, and "pseudowebbing" of the neck, occur in the majority of affected patients.[4] The term pseudo-pseudohypoparathyroidism has been used to describe patients who have these somatic features but lack the biochemical abnormalities of pseudohypoparathyroidism. Other defects described in type I include hypothyroidism, prolactin deficiency, diabetes mellitus, and resistance to arginine vasopressin and glucagon, suggesting that cAMP metabolism may be altered in a generalized fashion.

A very rare form of pseudohypoparathyroidism (type II) has recently been described. These patients demonstrate hypocalcemia with a normal rise in urinary cAMP to exogenous PTH, but have a blunted phosphaturic response.[5] There are no characteristic somatic abnormalities. So few patients have been available for study that it is not clear whether this disorder is metabolically distinct from type I. Patients have also been described who appear to produce parathyroid hormone that is structurally different from normal and, therefore, they resemble patients with pseudohypoparathyroidism. These individuals, however, respond normally to exogenous PTH. This syndrome has been called pseudoidiopathic hypoparathyroidism.[6]

Magnesium Deficiency

Hypocalcemia frequently occurs in the setting of hypomagnesemia, which may be caused by chronic alcoholism, malabsorption, or magnesium-wasting nephropathy. Other causes of hypomagnesemia include treatment with magnesiuric drugs such as diuretics and aminoglycosides, prolonged intravenous feedings, and a congenital defect of intestinal magnesium absorption. Hypomagnesemia appears to cause a block in PTH secretion and a peripheral resistance to the action of parathyroid hormone on the kidney and bone. Administration of parenteral magnesium sulfate results in an immediate release of PTH and a later rise in serum calcium level.

Vitamin D Deficiency

To understand alterations in vitamin D metabolism that result in hypocalcemia requires a brief review of vitamin D biosynthesis (Fig. 1). Vitamin D is produced in the epidermis from ultraviolet sunlight exposure or absorbed in the intestine from dietary sources, primarily fortified dairy products and animal and fish oils. The vitamin then undergoes conversion in the liver to 25-hydroxyvitamin D_3 (25-OHD_3). This is the major circulating form of vitamin D, but it has little metabolic activity. 25-OHD_3 must be further hydroxylated in the kidney to 1,25-dihydroxyvitamin D_3 (1,25$(OH)_2D_3$) or calcitriol, the most potent or most metabolically active form of vitamin D. Calcitriol stimulates intestinal calcium transport and mobilizes calcium from bone.

Therefore, hypocalcemia can occur because of a deficiency in intake or absorption of vitamin D, a defect in conversion of vitamin D to 1,25$(OH)_2$ D_3, or a decrease in responsiveness of target organs to the vitamin. Nutritional deficiency of vitamin D is now rare in this country. Gastrectomy and gastric bypass cause malabsorption and may lead to vitamin D deficiency. Chronic pancreatitis, intestinal disease, and intestinal bypass surgery may decrease absorption of vitamin D and increase intestinal loss of 25-OHD_3. Severe hepatic and biliary disease may cause malabsorption of vitamin D and decreased production of 25-OHD_3.

Long-term anticonvulsant therapy can significantly alter vitamin D and calcium homeostasis. These drugs increase hepatic microsomal enzyme activity, leading to a reduction in 25-OHD_3 levels and production of less active vitamin D metabolites. Anticonvulsants may also antagonize the effects of vitamin D on intestine and bone. The resulting clinical picture includes hypocalcemia, hypophosphatemia, serum alkaline phosphatase elevation, and rickets or osteomalacia.

Chronic renal failure frequently results in hypocalcemia, also through alterations of vitamin D synthesis and action. The reduction in functioning renal tissue results in a decrease in 1,25$(OH)_2D_3$ synthesis. Production of less active vitamin D metabolites also increases, and these substances may compete at receptor sites with 1,25$(OH)_2D_3$. Reduction of 25-OHD_3 levels also occurs in uremic patients owing to poor nutrition, decreased sun-

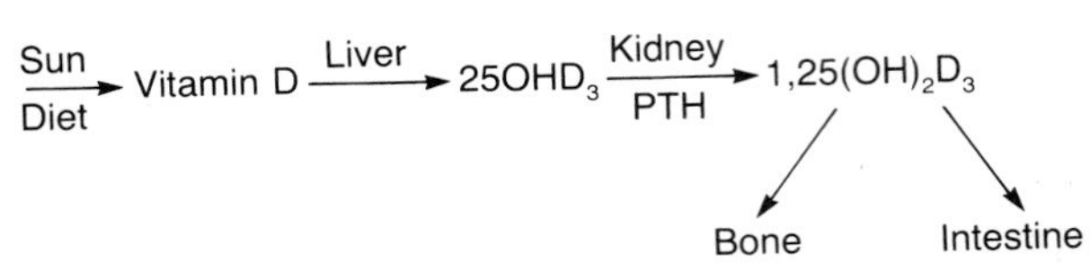

Figure 1. Vitamin D biosynthesis.

light exposure, and impaired hepatic microsomal enzyme activity. Hyperphosphatemia is common in chronic renal failure and causes hypocalcemia through a decrease in production of $1,25(OH)_2D_3$ and formation of calcium phosphate complexes in soft tissue.

A hereditary deficiency of the renal hydroxylase enzyme necessary for production of $1,25(OH)_2D_3$ results in the syndrome of hereditary vitamin D dependency. This condition manifests in infancy as hypocalcemic tetany, hypophosphatemia, serum alkaline phosphatase elevation, and rickets. Because successful treatment requires massive doses of vitamin D, the pathogenesis was believed to be peripheral resistance to vitamin D. However, resolution of this condition by physiologic doses of $1,25(OH)_2D_3$ strongly suggests that a deficiency of renal hydroxylase enzyme activity is the causal mechanism. In recent years there have also been reports of familial and sporadic forms of target-organ resistance to $1,25(OH)_2D_3$.

Miscellaneous Causes

Hyperphosphatemia. An acute rise in serum phosphate level can lead to hypocalcemia through development of extraskeletal calcification or inhibition of bone resorption. Such a rise can occur with administration of intravenous phosphate or phosphate enemas or with massive cell lysis induced by chemotherapy, burns, or rhabdomyolysis.

Acute Pancreatitis. This is a well-known cause of hypocalcemia. The calcium depletion has been attributed to precipitation of calcium with fatty acids to form "soaps" in the pancreatic bed and other areas of fat necrosis. Some investigators, however, have judged that this concept could not explain the magnitude of net calcium loss. Other postulated mechanisms include hypersecretion of glucagon, hypercalcitoninemia, and peripheral resistance to PTH. A recent study suggests that a relative parathyroid insufficiency may account for the persistent hypocalcemia of acute pancreatitis.[7]

Drugs. Many drugs can cause hypocalcemia. Phosphates, anticonvulsants, diuretics, aminoglycoside antibiotics, and antineoplastic drugs have been mentioned previously. Administration of alkali reduces ionized calcium and can cause hypocalcemic symptoms. Other implicated drugs include EDTA, calcitonin, mithramycin, and diphosphonates. Transfusion with large amounts of citrated blood can cause formation of calcium complexes and resultant hypocalcemia. Transient neonatal hypocalcemia often occurs with prematurity, with respiratory distress syndrome, and in association with maternal diabetes. Somewhat low PTH levels may be seen in these conditions. Transient hypocalcemia may also occur in a neonate given cow's milk or a formula high in phosphate during the first week of life.

Osteoblastic Metatases. Hypocalcemia in the cancer patient usually occurs in association with osteoblastic metastases. Disseminated cancers of the prostate, breast, and lung are the most common types. Osteoblastic metastases appear to have an avidity for calcium, producing a negative calcium balance. Other possible mechanisms include hypoparathyroidism, hyperphosphatemia, hypomagnesemia, and alterations in vitamin D homeostasis.[8] Hypocalcemia may be as common as hypercalcemia in the cancer patient and can result in a life-threatening crisis if not recognized early.

HISTORY

History of the Present Illness. The symptoms of hypocalcemia are not specific for the underlying disorder but are related primarily to enhanced neuromuscular excitability. Tetany, the classic manifestation of hypocalcemia, is the result of involuntary tonic muscle contractions. The earliest symptoms may be tingling of the fingertips and perioral region. The paresthesias may spread to involve larger areas of the face and extremities before overt muscle contractions of these areas begin and intensify. The patient may describe carpopedal spasm or diffuse muscle contractions in the extremities, using the term "drawing pains." Other complaints may include wheezing, dysphagia, and abdominal cramping and difficulty with urination. Less commonly, patients may experience syncope or seizures. Tetany is directly related to the rate of fall in serum calcium level and not necessarily to the absolute serum calcium level.[2]

The patient who describes episodes of tetany should be questioned regarding precipitating factors that may unmask tetany. Such factors include hyperventilation, exercise, prolonged use of an extremity, pregnancy, lactation, infection, and diuretic use. A history of such circumstances would support the diagnostic impression of tetany.

Other nonspecific symptoms may occur with chronic hypocalcemia. Subtle symptoms include voice changes, muscle stiffness, clumsiness, and difficulty with gait. Patients may also complain of fatigue, apathy, memory loss, depression, and irritability.

Previous Medical History. The previous medical history may provide the most specific information for determining the cause of hypocalcemia. Any of the following historical factors offer an immediate diagnosis and may direct the physician toward the appropriate laboratory studies. Previous thyroidectomy, parathyroidectomy, or other type of neck surgery should strongly suggest surgical hypoparathyroidism. A history of gastric surgery or ileal bypass surgery should suggest malabsorption as the cause of hypocalcemia. Previous radioactive iodine treatment, malignancy, multiple transfusions, chronic diarrhea, alcoholism, or anticonvulsant drug use could provide a specific etiology. A history of chronic fungal infections, adrenal insufficiency, premature menopause, or pernicious anemia should suggest idiopathic hypoparathyroidism.

Family History. If any of the patient's relatives have short stature or other somatic features of pseudohypoparathyroidism, the same diagnosis should be suspected in the patient, even without obvious somatic features. Since idiopathic hypoparathyroidism with its associated autoimmune disorders may be inherited with a variable expression, the patient should be asked about family members with other endocrine deficiences. If several infants in a family have tetany or bone disease, hereditary vitamin D dependency should be suspected.

PHYSICAL EXAMINATION

The effects of hypocalcemia are diverse, requiring a complete examination in each case. Special attention should be given to the skin, eyes, and neuromuscular system because of the frequency of abnormalities in these areas.

General Appearance. Direct observation of hyperventilation in a patient with tetany may provide an immediate clue. The general appearance may be diagnostic of pseudohypoparathyroidism if the patient has a short, stocky body, round facies, and short neck producing "pseudo-webbing." The unkempt malnourished derelict with alcohol on the breath should be immediately suspected of having hypomagnesemia or chronic liver disease. Evidence of previous neck surgery favors the diagnosis of surgical hypoparathyroidism. Signs of extensive weight loss or previous gastrointestinal surgery suggest malabsorption.

Skin and Appendages. The skin, appendages, and soft tissue should be examined for certain features of long-standing hypocalcemia. Dry scaly skin, brittle nails with transverse ridges, and coarse hair with areas of alopecia are nonspecific findings. Candidiasis of the nails, skin, and mucous membranes may be seen with chronic hypocalcemia of any cause but is certainly more typical of idiopathic hypoparathyroidism. The periarticular soft tissues should be palpated for ectopic calcifications, which are especially common in pseudohypoparathyroidism.[4] The teeth should be examined for excessive dental caries and delay or absence of tooth eruption, which results in fewer teeth with gaps between them; these dental abnormalities occur only with hypocalcemic states of childhood, when the teeth are developing.

Eyes. Examination of the eyes may reveal the presence of cataracts, the most common complication of chronic hypocalcemia.[2] They begin as small discrete opacities that occur in layers and eventually coalesce to form a dense opacity. Cataract development is related to the duration and severity of hypocalcemia but may occur within a year in untreated surgical hypoparathyroidism. Appropriate treatment of the hypocalcemic state arrests but does not reverse lens opacification. The presence of retinal hemorrhages or visual field loss suggests another process, because these findings have not been associated with hypocalcemia.

Cardiovascular System. The patient should be examined for signs of congestive heart failure, including elevated jugular venous pressure, pulmonary rales, cardiomegaly, and peripheral edema. Hypocalcemia may cause a reversible cardiomyopathy or precipitate congestive heart failure in patients with underlying heart disease.[9] These patients may not respond to usual therapeutic measures such as digitalization, but the correction of hypocalcemia usually restores cardiac function.

Extremities. The extremities should be examined for skeletal deformities. Shortening of the metacarpals and metatarsals may be seen with pseudohypoparathyroidism. Observation of the patient's closed fist may demonstrate absence of a knuckle or dimple over the affected metacarpal; the fourth digit is most commonly involved. Children should be examined for shortened long bones, bow legs, knock knees, and evidences of multiple fractures as seen with rickets.

Neuromuscular System. The neuromuscular system deserves special attention because of its frequent involvement in hypocalcemia. Overt tetany may be the most dramatic finding, with tonic muscle contractions of the extremities and face, carpopedal spasm, and laryngeal stridor. Subclinical tetany, however, may go unrecognized unless specific maneuvers are performed by the examiner. Chvostek's sign is elicited by tapping the facial nerve 1 inch anterior to the ear and observing for facial muscle contraction. One may observe twitching at the corner of the mouth, the nasolabial fold, and the eye. Twitching of the mouth only may be observed in 25 per cent of normal adults and is therefore of limited significance. Trousseau's sign is typical carpal spasm induced within 2 minutes of inflation of a blood pressure cuff to above systolic pressure.

Seizures may also be observed, more commonly in children. Hypocalcemia may unmask a subclinical seizure disorder of any type and lead to typical grand mal, petit mal, focal, or Jacksonian seizures. Generalized prolonged tetany may occur without loss of consciousness or other features of a generalized seizure. Extrapyramidal disorders may be observed, including a Parkinsonian syndrome, dystonic spasms, and choreoathetosis.[2] These disorders are more likely to occur in patients given major tranquilizers. Mental status evaluation may demonstrate impairment of memory or intellect, psychosis, or depression. All these findings may be reversed with correction of hypocalcemia. Mental retardation may be observed with childhood hypocalcemia. Examination of the motor system may demonstrate general hypotonia or a proximal myopathy with vitamin D deficiency states.

DIAGNOSTIC STUDIES

Appropriate laboratory investigation of the hypocalcemic patient is absolutely essential to confirm the diagnosis and to exclude other causes of tetany. In each case the laboratory must be utilized to establish a specific cause, so that appropriate treatment can be initiated.

In every patient, serum calcium, phosphorus, potassium, magnesium, albumin, alkaline phosphatase, and creatinine and arterial pH should be measured. The measurement of total serum calcium, albumin, and arterial pH is sufficient to give an accurate assessment of the calcium status in most patients. The correction formula for assessing calcium level in the presence of serum albumin alteration is discussed earlier in this chapter. Direct measurements of ionized calcium are now available in some laboratories, but technical difficulties have limited widespread application. Normal serum potassium and magnesium levels and arterial pH would exclude hyperkalemia, hypomagnesemia, and metabolic alkalosis as causes of tetany.[2] Renal function measurements are critical because of the frequency of calcium and phosphorus abnormalities in renal insufficiency. A serum alkaline phosphatase elevation indicates the presence of excessive bone formation and is useful in classification of hypocalcemic states.

If the patient has a history of weight loss or diarrhea, an evaluation for malabsorption is indicated, including studies of serum carotene, stool fat, prothrombin time, and urinary d-xylose. The patient with abdominal pain and hypocalcemia should be evaluated for acute pancreatitis by means of serum and urinary amylase determinations.

The electrocardiogram may demonstrate characteristic changes in hypocalcemia. The most typical finding is prolongation of the ST segment and QT interval. T wave changes such as peaking and inversion have also been reported, but arrhythmias are unusual. Distinct but nonspecific electroencephalographic changes have also been described, including bursts of high-voltage slow waves and irregular sharp spike and wave patterns.

Imaging

Skull x-rays to look for basal ganglia calcification are appropriate if one suspects a chronic form of hypocalcemia. Fifty per cent of patients with early-onset idiopathic hypoparathyroidism or pseudohypoparathyroidism may have such calcification.[2] Computed tomography may detect basal ganglia calcification in the patient with a radiographically normal skull. It is important to recognize these calcifications because affected patients may be more prone to develop extrapyramidal disorders.

Skeletal surveys should be completed in patients with malignancy to look for osteoblastic metastases. X-rays of the hands and feet may demonstrate metacarpal or metatarsal shortening in a patient suspected of having pseudohypoparathyroidism. Long bone and spine x-rays in vitamin D–deficient patients may demonstrate typical changes of osteomalacia or rickets, such as decreased bone density, pseudofractures, bowing of the extremities, and increased biconcavity of vertebral bodies.

Laboratory Studies

Parathyroid Hormone Measurements. Serum immunoreactive parathyroid hormone (iPTH) measurements are now widely available and are invaluable in categorizing the hypocalcemic patient. Serum iPTH levels correlate with the functioning parathyroid mass.[10] The only exception is in renal failure, which is associated with an impaired clearance of PTH and inappropriately increased serum iPTH level. Parathyroid hormone deficiency states such as surgical and idiopathic hypoparathyroidism are associated with low to low-normal iPTH levels, depending upon the severity of the deficiency. Pseudohypoparathyroidism, which is characterized by PTH resistance, is associated with increased iPTH levels. The serum iPTH level also tends to be high early in vitamin D deficiency, calcium malabsorption, and vitamin D dependency, even though the serum calcium level may still be in the low-normal range.

Vitamin D Measurements. Determinations of 25-OHD_3 have been available now for several years and are quite sensitive in detecting vitamin D deficiency. Low 25-OHD_3 levels are also found in severe chronic liver disease and neonatal hypocalcemia associated with hepatic immaturity. The recent development of a practical assay of $1,25(OH)_2D_3$ has contributed greatly to our understanding of hypocalcemic conditions.[11] Low levels of $1,25(OH)_2D_3$ in conjunction with characteristic iPTH levels can confirm the diagnosis of hypoparathyroidism, pseudohypoparathyroidism, or vitamin D dependency rickets. $25\text{-}OHD_3$ should therefore be measured when vitamin D deficiency is suspected. $1,25(OH)_2D_3$ should be measured to confirm the diagnosis in suspected parathyroid disorders or vitamin D dependency rickets.

Other Tests. Urinary cAMP of nephrogenous origin reflects the biologic effect of PTH on the kidney and therefore complements the measurement of iPTH in the evaluation of hypocalcemia.[12] Nephrogenous cAMP cannot be measured directly but must be calculated on the basis of plasma and urinary cAMP determinations in conjunction with renal function measurements. In previous years cAMP measurements were most useful when made before and after PTH infusion. The patient was then classified according to the observed phosphaturic and cAMP responses. Exogenous PTH is no longer available, requiring an increased reliance on the measurement of iPTH levels in the evaluation of hypocalcemia. In general, however, PTH deficiency and resistance are associated with low urinary cAMP levels.

ASSESSMENT

Evaluation of the hypocalcemic patient requires a logical stepwise approach utilizing specific information obtained from the history, physical examination, and laboratory tests. A basic understanding of calcium, PTH, and vitamin D homeostasis is necessary to the selection and interpretation of laboratory studies. Any alteration in serum calcium level must be interpreted in conjunction with serum albumin measurements. The symptomatic patient with tetany should be observed for hyperventilation, and other causes, including hyperkalemia, hypomagnesimia, and alkalosis, should be excluded. Table 2 summarizes the biochemical parameters of various hypocalcemic states.

Constellations of Findings

The hypocalcemic patient who has undergone neck surgery should be immediately suspected of hypoparathyroidism. This diagnosis is confirmed by the constellation of hyperphosphatemia and low iPTH urinary cAMP and $1,25(OH)_2D_3$ levels. The same biochemical pattern is seen with idiopathic hypoparathyroidism, but the patient may have onychomycosis, vitiligo, and no obvious cause of the parathyroid dysfunction.

The somatic features of short stature, brachydactyly, round facies, and "pseudo-webbing" of the neck suggest pseudohypoparathyroidism. The biochemical parameters include normal or high serum phosphorus level, increased iPTH level, decreased urinary cAMP level, and low $1,25(OH)_2D_3$ level.

Vitamin D deficiency is suggested by a history of marked weight loss, diarrhea, or poor nutritional intake. The clinical settings of long-term anticonvulsant drug use, chronic hepatic or biliary tract disease, and previous gastric surgery should also suggest a vitamin D–deficient state. The usual biochemical findings in these settings include hy-

Table 2. BIOCHEMICAL PARAMETERS IN HYPOCALCEMIA

Disorder or Condition	PO_4	Alkaline Phosphatase	Mg	iPTH	Urinary cAMP	$25\text{-}OHD_3$	$1,25(OH)_2D_3$
Hypoparathyroidism	↑	N	N	↓	↓	N	↓
Pseudohypoparathyroidism	↑,N	N	N	↑	↓	N	↓
Hypomagnesemia	N	N	↓	↓	↓	N	↓
Vitamin D deficiency	↓	↑	N	↑	↑	↓	↓,N
Anticonvulsant therapy	↓	↑	N	↑	↑	↓	↓,N
Chronic renal failure	↑	↑,N	N	↑	↑	N, ↓	↓
Hereditary Vitamin D dependency	↓	↑	N	↑	↑	N	↓
Hyperphosphatemia	↑	N	N	↑,N	N, ↑	N	↓,N
Osteoblastic metastases	↓,N	↑	N	↑,N	N, ↑	N	↑,N

DIAGNOSTIC ASSESSMENT OF HYPOCALCEMIA

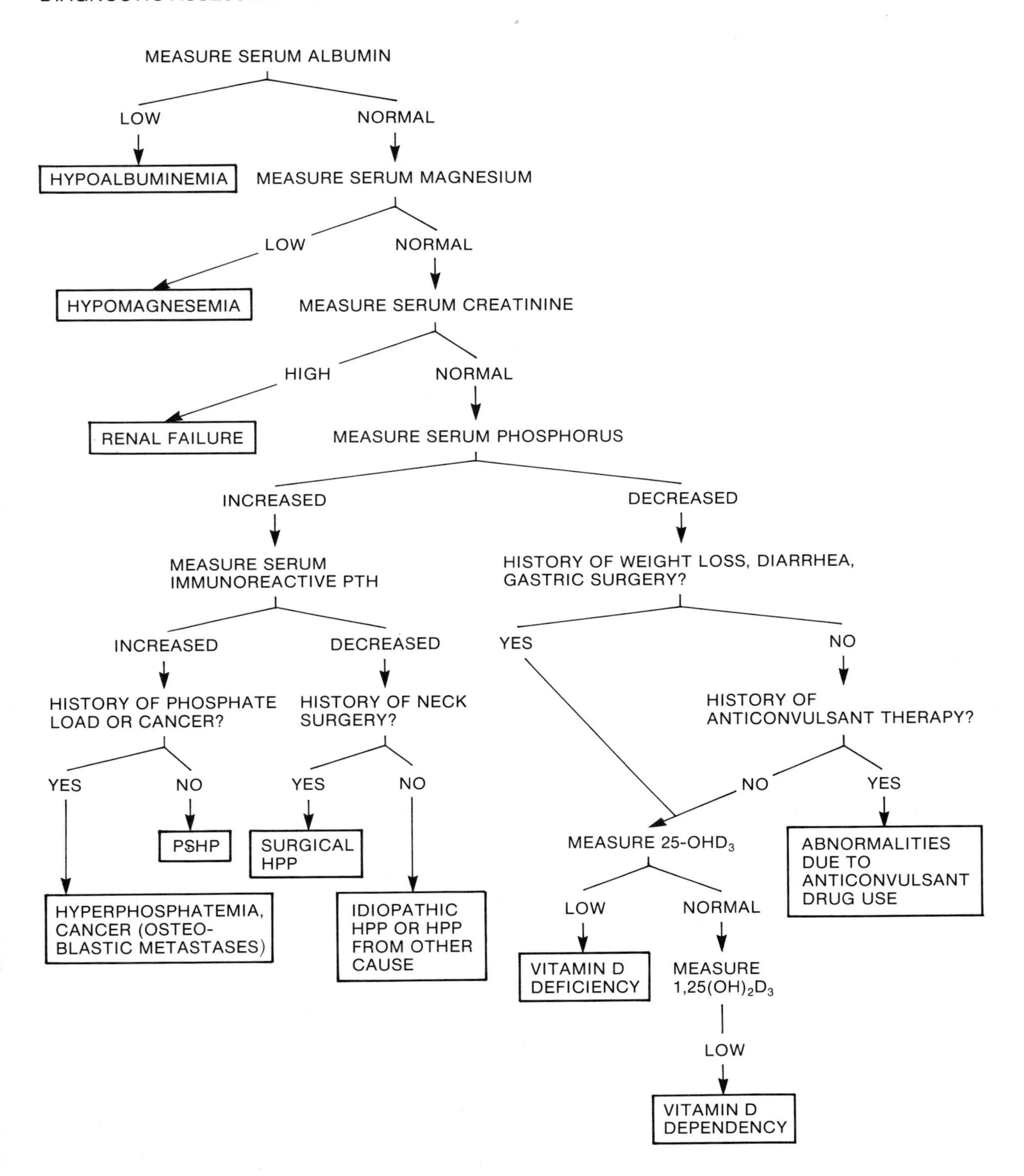

pophosphatemia, increased serum alkaline phosphatase and iPTH levels, and a decreased 25-OHD_3 level.

Patients with chronic renal failure and hypocalcemia usually demonstrate hyperphosphatemia, normal to high serum alkaline phosphatase level, increased iPTH level, and decreased levels of 25-OHD_3 and 1,25$(OH)_2D_3$.

Hereditary vitamin D dependency manifests as childhood rickets with hypophosphatemia, increased iPTH level, normal 25-OHD_3 level, and decreased 1,25$(OH)D_3$ level. A family history may be apparent, and affected individuals do not respond to usual vitamin D supplementation. The key finding is the disparity in 25-OHD_3 and 1,25$(OH)_2D_3$ levels.

The miscellaneous causes of hypocalcemia are usually apparent when one analyzes the clinical setting. The algorithm summarizes a systematic approach to the diagnosis of the hypocalcemic patient.

REFERENCES

1. Juan D. Hypocalcemia: differential diagnosis and mechanisms. Arch Intern Med 1979; 139:1167–71.
2. Parfitt MA. Surgical, idiopathic, and other varieties of parathyroid hormone-deficient hypoparathyroidism. In: DeGroot LJ, ed. Endocrinology. New York: Grune & Stratton, 1979;755–68.
3. Horwitz CA, Myers WP, Foote FW. Secondary malignant tumors of the parathyroid glands. Am J Med 1972;52:797–808.
4. Potts JT. Pseudohypoparathyroidism. In: DeGroot LJ, ed. Endocrinology. New York: Grune & Stratton, 1979;769–76.
5. Drezner M, Neelon FA, Lebovitz HE. Pseudohypoparathyroidism type II: a possible defect in the receptor of the cyclic AMP signal. N Engl J Med 1973;289:1056–60.
6. Nusynowitz ML, Klein MH. Pseudoidiopathic hypoparathyroidism: hypoparathyroidism with ineffective parathyroid hormone. Am J Med 1973;55:677–81.
7. Robertson GM, Moore EW, Switz DM, Sizemore GW, Estep HL. Inadequate parathyroid response in acute pancreatitis. N Engl J Med 1976;294:512–6.
8. Luqman WA, McCowen KD, Przasnyski EJ, Reed JW. Hypocalcemia in patients with cancer: a review. Milit Med 1980;145:96–8.
9. Bashour T, Basha HS, Cheng TO. Hypocalcemic cardiomyopathy. Chest 1980;78:663–5.
10. Ausbach GD, Marx SJ, Spiegel AM. Parathyroid hormone, calcitonin, and the calciferols. In: Williams RH, ed. Textbook of endocrinology. Philadelphia: WB Saunders, 1981;922–1031.
11. Eisman JA, Hamstra AJ, Kream BE, DeLuca HF. A sensitive, precise and convenient method for determination of 1,25-dihydroxyvitamin D in human plasma. Arch Biochem Biophys 1976;186:235–43.
12. Broadus AE. Nephrogenous cyclic AMP as a parathyroid function test. Nephron 1979;23:136–41.

HYPONATREMIA AND HYPERNATREMIA

D. M. KAJI

□ SYNONYMS: Hypo-osmolar state, water intoxication; hyper-osmolar state, dehydration

BACKGROUND

Definitions and Origins

Hyponatremia refers to a decrease in plasma (or serum) sodium concentration below 135 mEq/liter and *hypernatremia* to an increase in plasma sodium concentration above 145 mEq/liter. These terms reflect the ratio of sodium to water in the plasma and do not refer to an increase or decrease in total body sodium. Hyponatremia and hypernatremia are primarily disorders of water balance arising from a derangement in the osmoregulatory system, which is charged with the responsibility of keeping plasma osmolality within a narrow range (280–295 mOsm/kg water) primarily by variations in water excretion or intake.

Plasma osmolality (P_{osm}) refers to the total number of particles in plasma water, expressed as mOsm/kg water. Because sodium is the most abundant cation in the plasma, sodium concentration is closely paralleled by P_{osm}, as expressed in the following equation:

$$P_{osm} = 2\,(\text{Na} + \text{K mEq/liter}) + \frac{\text{glucose (mg/100 ml)}}{18} + \frac{\text{BUN (mg/100 ml)}}{2.8}$$

Effective osmolality or tonicity is given by the concentrations of those solutes that exert an osmotic gradient across cell membranes and cause water movement. Urea diffuses freely across cell membranes, is present in equal concentration in extracellular fluid (ECF) and in cells, and does not affect tonicity.

When glucose concentration is normal, plasma tonicity can be estimated as 2 × (Na + K) mEq/liter.

Acute hyponatremia and *acute hypernatremia* are conditions in which changes in the plasma sodium concentration are rapid (less than 48 hours). As discussed later, the rate of change in plasma sodium has diagnostic and prognostic implications.

Pseudohyponatremia is a spuriously low estimate of plasma sodium. Plasma normally contains more than 90 per cent water and less than 10 per cent solids. An increase in plasma solids, as in hyperlipidemia or hyperproteinemia, causes a relative decrease in plasma water. Even though the biologically relevant measurement, sodium in plasma water, is normal, the sodium concentration when expressed as mEq/liter of plasma is low.

Hyponatremia with hypertonicity refers to clinical states in which an increase in concentration of osmotically active particles other than sodium (i.e., hyperglycemia) causes a shift of water from cells to the plasma and dilutes plasma sodium.

Incidence and Causes

Hyponatremia

Hyponatremia is one of the most common electrolyte abnormalities encountered in clinical practice. Its causes are listed in Table 1. Acute hyponatremia is seen most often in hospitalized patients who are given hypotonic fluids in excess of their capacity to excrete free water. Administration of massive amounts of hypotonic fluid is most often iatrogenic, as with giving intravenous dextrose. Rarely, patients with schizophrenia and psychogenic polydipsia present with acute hyponatremia.[1] Because normal individuals possess the capacity to clear as much as 15 to 20 liters of water per day, severe hyponatremia is seen only when there is massive administration of hypotonic fluids (more than 15 liters/day) or a concomitant impairment of the capacity to excrete free water, as in cardiac or renal failure, cirrhosis of the liver, or persistent antidiuretic hormone secretion due to drugs or hypovolemia.

Chronic hyponatremia is more common than acute hyponatremia and often occurs in edematous states. The observation of hyponatremia in cirrhosis or heart failure with modest water intake (1.5 liters/day or less) suggests an advanced state of sodium and water retention and a poor prognosis.[2]

Drugs are among the most common causes of hyponatremia.[3] Diuretics, oral hypoglycemic agents, opiates, and barbiturates are most often incriminated in the pathogenesis of hyponatremia.

Although the secretion of antidiuretic hormone (ADH) is normally triggered by a rise in plasma sodium (and osmolality), several physiologic, nonosmolar stimuli are capable of triggering ADH release. When osmolar and nonosmolar stimuli for the release of ADH coincide and conflict, as in hyponatremia leading to ADH suppression and the nonosmolar stimuli causing ADH release, the nonosmolar stimuli predominate, causing persistent ADH release in the face of hyponatremia. Pain, nausea, vomiting, hypotension, hypovolemia, and emotional distress are all potent stimuli for ADH release.[4]

Advanced, untreated hypothyroidism bordering on myxedema coma may, at times, cause hyponatremia.[5] "Reset osmostat," another rare cause of hyponatremia, is a state in which the threshold for ADH suppression is below the mean value of 275 mOsm/kg found in normal subjects.[6] Adrenal insufficiency may cause hyponatremia not only by virtue of volume contraction secondary to mineralocorticoid deficiency, but also through persistent ADH release secondary to pure glucocorticoid insufficiency, as with hypopituitarism or following the abrupt withdrawal of pharmacologic doses of glucocorticoids.[7]

The syndrome of inappropriate ADH (SIADH) is described with a growing list of conditions mainly affecting the central nervous system and the lungs (see Table 1). Oat cell bronchogenic carcinoma remains the most common cause of this clinical syndrome. Acute intermittent porphyria, alcohol withdrawal, and delirium tremens are noteworthy metabolic causes of SIADH.

Hypernatremia

The causes of hypernatremia are given in Table 2. Acute hypernatremia has been described in infants given formula feedings of hypertonic solutions.[8] Chronic hypernatremia in children is most often seen in gastroenteritis with diarrhea or in infections causing fever and increased respiratory losses of water.[9]

In adults, hypernatremia is more often chronic than acute. An inability to ingest water, as with debilitated states or depressed sensorium, is a common denominator of almost all the causes of chronic hypernatremia in adults (see Table 2). Sometimes, an impairment of the thirst mechanism may be responsible for hypernatremia. Elderly patients given high-protein tube feedings without adequate provision for water intake develop hypernatremia rapidly because of large fluid losses secondary to osmotic diuresis from urea.[10]

Acute hypernatremia in adults is uncommon.

Table 1. CAUSES OF HYPONATREMIA

Pseudohyponatremia	Hyperlipidemia
	Hyperproteinemia
	  Multiple myeloma
	  Waldenström's macroglobulinemia

Hyponatremia with hypertonicity	Hyperglycemia
	Mannitol infusion
	Ingestion of toxins
	  Ethylene glycol
	  Ethyl alcohol
	  Methanol

"True" hyponatremia (hyponatremia with hypo-osmolality)	
With volume overload	Nephrotic syndrome Cirrhosis Congestive heart failure Acute or chronic renal failure

With volume contraction	Extrarenal losses
	  Gastrointestinal
	    Vomiting
	    Diarrhea
	  Third spacing
	    Peritonitis
	    Pancreatitis
	    Burns
	Renal losses
	  Diuretic administration
	    Thiazides
	    Amiloride
	  Mineralocorticoid deficiency
	  Osmotic diuresis
	  Salt-losing states
	    Renal tubular acidosis
	    Medullary cystic disease
	    Postobstructive states

Table 1. CAUSES OF HYPONATREMIA *(Continued)*

With clinically euvolemic states	Syndrome of inappropriate ADH release
	Central nervous system diseases
	Trauma
	Meningitis
	Encephalitis
	Brain abscess
	Brain tumor
	Guillain-Barré syndrome
	Acute psychosis
	Epilepsy
	Pulmonary diseases
	Oat cell bronchogenic carcinoma
	Bacterial pneumonia
	Tuberculosis
	Aspergillosis
	Acute respiratory failure
	Other neoplasms
	Pancreatic
	Duodenal
	Thymic
	Lymphoma
	Leukemia
	Metabolic states
	Acute intermittent porphyria
	Alcohol withdrawal state, including delirium tremens
	Ingestion of drugs causing water retention
	Diuretics
	Oral hypoglycemic agents
	Chlorpropamide
	Tolbutamide
	Sedative-hypnotics
	Opiates
	Barbiturates
	Antineoplastic agents
	Vincristine
	Cyclophosphamide
	Anti-inflammatory drugs
	Indomethacin
	Aspirin
	Acetaminophen
	Clofibrate
	Carbamazepine
	Isoproterenol
	Pure glucorticoid insufficiency
	Hypopituitarism
	Abrupt withdrawal from large doses of glucorticoids
	Hypothyroidism
	Severe potassium depletion with/without diuretics
	"Reset osmostat"

Table 2. CAUSES OF HYPERNATREMIA

Acute hypernatremia	Intravenous sodium bicarbonate administration
	After cardiac arrest
	For lactic acidosis
	Dialysis with hypernatremic solution (accidental)
	Accidental introduction of hypertonic saline into mother's blood during induced abortion
	Near-drowning in sea water
	Accidental feeding of hypernatremic formula to infants
Chronic hypernatremia	Impaired thirst mechanism
	Inability to ingest water
	Debilitation
	Depressed sensorium
	Large losses of hypertonic fluids
	Fever with tachypnea
	Osmotic diuresis
	Mannitol infusion
	High-protein tube feedings
	Diabetes mellitus
	Recovery from obstructive uropathy or renal failure
	Central diabetes insipidus
	Head injury
	Surgical ablation near the hypophysis
	Metastatic tumors
	Craniopharyngioma
	Pinealoma
	Lymphoma
	Leukemia
	Granulomatous disease
	Tuberculosis
	Sarcoidosis
	Infection
	Meningitis
	Encephalitis
	Vascular accidents
	Hemorrhage
	Thrombosis
	Ligation of internal carotid or anterior communicating artery
	Idiopathic
	Nephrogenous diabetes insipidus
	Drug ingestion
	Lithium
	Demeclocycline
	Methoxyflurane
	Amphotericin
	Vinblastine
	Colchicine
	Chronic renal disease, especially tubulo-interstitial
	Hypokalemia
	Hypercalcemia
	Sickle cell disease
	Multiple myeloma, amyloid
	Sjögren's disease
	Sarcoidosis
	Idiopathic, familial

Accidental use of hypernatremic solutions in dialysis and accidental administration of hypertonic saline to the mother during attempts to induce abortion have been reported to cause severe hypernatremia.[11, 12] Patients given large amounts of sodium bicarbonate after cardiac arrest or for lactic acidosis may also present with acute hypernatremia.

Central diabetes insipidus is secondary to partial or complete cessation of ADH release. Although in the past idiopathic diabetes insipidus and brain tumors were considered to be the most common causes of central diabetes insipidus, trauma and hypophysectomy are currently recognized to be responsible for the majority of cases.

Nephrogenous diabetes insipidus refers to a renal resistance to the action of ADH. Drugs (lithium, demeclocycline, methoxyflurane) and electrolyte disorders (hypercalcemia, hypokalemia) are among the most common causes of acquired renal resistance to ADH.

HISTORY

Hyponatremia

A careful review of the patient's chart, including the nurses' and physicians' progress notes, order sheets, intake and output sheets, records of weight and of intravenous fluids administered just prior to the change in plasma sodium, is of great value and should supplement data obtained from the patient, relatives, and other physicians.

History of the Present Illness. The history should record the onset of hyponatremia or hypernatremia and note the presence or absence of mental changes temporally associated with the change in plasma sodium level.

A history of vomiting, diarrhea, dizziness, recent weight loss or gain, ascites, edema, and puffiness of face may provide clues to the status of ECF volume.

The history of pain is important, because pain may cause ADH release and because anti-inflammatory agents used to relieve pain may cause water retention.

Family History. A family history of renal disease may be obtained from some patients with salt-losing states, such as polycystic kidneys and medullary cystic disease.

Social History. Is there a history of heavy beer-drinking (beer-drinker's hyponatremia)? Heavy chain-smoking may contribute to the persistence of ADH in the blood.

Drug History. The list of drugs causing hyponatremia can be found in Table 1. A careful drug history is essential for the evaluation of hyponatremia.

Previous Medical History. A history of thyroid or pituitary surgery may lead to the diagnosis of hypothyroidism or glucocorticoid insufficiency.

Hypernatremia

The following questions are most likely to reveal the source of hypernatremia:

1. *What is the urine output?* Polyuria with hypernatremia signifies an impairment of ADH secretion (central diabetes insipidus) or ADH action on the tubules (nephrogenous diabetes insipidus).
2. *Is the patient thirsty?* Absence of thirst is abnormal with hypernatremia and may be responsible for hypernatremia.
3. *Is the patient able to respond to thirst by drinking water?* Debilitation or impaired sensorium may lead to hypernatremia through failure to replace water losses.
4. *Is the insensible fluid loss greater than normal?* Fever with tachypnea or gastroenteritis with diarrhea may lead to large losses of hypotonic fluids that may be difficult to replace.
5. *Is the patient being given a high-solute load?* Administration of high-protein tube feeding or intravenous sodium bicarbonate may lead to hypernatremia.

PHYSICAL EXAMINATION

The most important aspect of the physical examination is a careful assessment of the extracellular fluid (ECF) volume status, which allows a rational approach to both hyponatremic and hypernatremic states. The findings listed in Table 3 deserve special emphasis.

DIAGNOSTIC STUDIES

Hyponatremia

Determinations of blood urea nitrogen, creatinine, glucose, and electrolytes are helpful in all but the most obvious cases. Pseudohyponatremia may be suspected when the total protein level exceeds 10 gm/100 ml or the total lipid level exceeds 1000 mg/100 ml.

Hyperglycemia lowers plasma sodium in a predictable fashion (1.6 mEq/liter fall in sodium for every 100 mg/100 ml rise in glucose).[13]

Generally, it is not necessary to measure plasma osmolality (P_{osm}), which can be estimated from plasma sodium, potassium, glucose, and BUN values, as discussed under "Background." An abnormally large gap ($>$10mOsm/kg) between measured and calculated P_{osm} may be a clue to the

Table 3. PHYSICAL FINDINGS OF SIGNIFICANCE IN HYPONATREMIA OR HYPERNATREMIA

Finding	Possible Significance
Orthostatic rise in pulse	ECF volume contraction
Orthostatic fall in blood pressure	ECF volume contraction
Head and neck	
Puffy face	Nephrotic syndrome, hypothyroidism
Abnormal pupils, papilledema, neck rigidity	Central nervous system lesion associated with SIADH
Engorged neck veins	Fluid overload
Chest	
Unilateral wheezing	Bronchogenic carcinoma with SIADH
Cardiac	
S_3 gallop, tachycardia	Congestive heart failure
Abdominal	
Ascites	Cirrhosis of liver
Edema	Congestive heart failure, cirrhosis, nephrotic syndrome
Neurologic	
Apathy, lethargy, Cheyne-Stokes respirations, depressed tendon reflexes	Severe hyponatremia
Increased muscle tone, increased muscle twitching, increased tendon reflexes, convulsions	Severe hypernatremia

presence of a poison such as ethyl alcohol, methanol, or ethylene glycol.

The measurement of "spot" urinary sodium concentration is of great help in differentiating among the various causes of hyponatremia (see algorithm).

A low urinary potassium level (<20 mEq/liter) may be seen with acute renal failure, adrenal hormone deficiency, administration of potassium-sparing diuretics or cation-exchange resins (i.e., Kayexelate). High urinary potassium excretion may be seen with diuretic administration, salt-losing nephropathy, renal tubular acidosis, and metabolic alkalosis. The presence of a low urinary chloride value with a high urine sodium value suggests bicarbonaturia and is seen in metabolic alkalosis with sodium and volume depletion.

The presence of urine osmolality above 750 mOsm/kg water, strongly suggests SIADH or adrenal insufficiency, but such a high value is not required for the diagnosis of SIADH. Thus, urine osmolality of 240 mOsm/kg water is inappropriately high in the presence of severe hypo-osmolar syndrome.

The calculation of free water clearance (C_{H_2O}) may help in the diagnosis of hyponatremia; it is obtained with the following formula:

$$C_{H_2O} = V - \frac{U_{osm} \times V}{P_{osm}}$$

where V is urine volume and U_{osm} is urine osmolality. The effective free water clearance ($e - C_{H_2O}$) may be more useful in hyponatremia than C_{H_2O}.[14] Effective water clearance is obtained with the following formula:

$$eC_{H_2O} = V\left(1 - \frac{U_{Na} + U_K}{P_{Na}}\right)$$

where U_{Na} and U_K are the urinary Na and K, respectively, and P_{Na} is the plasma sodium, all expressed in mEq/liter. Calculation of free water clearance may help to clarify the relative contribution of excess water intake and reduced free water excretion capacity to the cause of hyponatremia. Under the stimulus of hypo-osmolality, C_{H_2O} in normal subjects may reach as much as 10 ml/min, or up to 15 liters/day. Thus, in a paraplegic man with progressive hyponatremia, P_{Na} of 124 mEq/liter, U_{Na} of 20 mEq/liter, and U_K of 11 mEq/liter, and urine volume of 6000 ml/24 hr, both a reduced effective free water clearance (4500 ml/day) and a water intake in excess of 4.5 liters/day are responsible for the hyponatremia.

The ability to excrete a water load may be tested by measurement of U_{osm} for up to 4 hours after rapid oral water intake of 20 ml/kg body weight (about 1200 ml over 10 to 15 min). Normal subjects may achieve U_{osm} values as low as 50 to 150 mOsm/kg. Patients with a diluting defect are unable to achieve this degree of dilution of urine. This test does not differentiate among the various causes of diluting defect.

Ancillary tests such as chest x-ray and tomograms, brain scan, electroencephalogram, and CT scan of the brain may all be useful in localizing the lesion responsible for SIADH.

Hypernatremia

Many of the laboratory measurements employed in hyponatremic patients (blood chemistry, urine electrolytes, and urine osmolality) are useful in evaluating hypernatremic patients as well.

The response of urine specific gravity (or, preferably, U_{osm}) to dehydration and exogenous ADH is of great help in making a diagnosis of diabetes insipidus. Normal subjects are able to raise U_{osm} to about 1,000 mOsm/kg with 12 to 15 hours of fluid deprivation. Hospitalized patients with nonrenal diseases may be able to achieve U_{osm} of up to 750 mOsm/kg.[15] Both normal subjects and patients with nonrenal diseases show no further elevation in U_{osm} when ADH is given after fluid deprivation. In contrast, patients with complete central diabetes insipidus are unable to make a hypertonic urine with dehydration (maximum U_{osm} 150–200 mOsm/kg) and show a marked rise in U_{osm} (to 450 mOsm/kg) with exogenous ADH.[15] Those with partial central diabetes insipidus may be able to elaborate a slightly hypertonic urine (U_{osm} 400–500 mOsm/kg) and show a further increase in U_{osm} with exogenous ADH. Patients with nephrogenous diabetes insipidus are unable to raise U_{osm} above 150 or 200 mOsm/kg with either dehydration or ADH administration.[15]

Water deprivation may be hazardous to a patient with diabetes insipidus and should be stopped when the body weight falls by 3 per cent or more during the test.

Other tests, such as hypertonic saline infusion, are occasionally employed in hyponatremia, but they may be difficult to interpret and pose the danger of precipitating heart failure in susceptible subjects.

ASSESSMENT

Hyponatremia

The diagnostic approach to hyponatremia is illustrated in the algorithm. The assessment of extracellular fluid volume is the key to the differential diagnosis of hyponatremia, once the clinician is able to exclude both pseudohyponatremia and hyponatremia with hypertonicity.

Hyponatremia with Volume Contraction. Affected patients present with tachycardia, postural hypotension, decreased axillary sweating, oliguria, a rise in urea nitrogen, and, at times, a smaller rise in serum creatinine. The presence of increased BUN, hyponatremia, hyperkalemia, and mild metabolic acidosis with normal anion gap constitutes a pattern strongly suggestive of adrenal insufficiency.

Hyponatremia and Volume Overload. These patients have either renal failure or an edema-forming state. Hyponatremia occurs late in the history of the edema-forming states and is associated with oliguria and low urine sodium (< 20–30 mEq/liter).

Hyponatremia with Clinically Euvolemic States. Patients in this category are often the hardest to diagnose and treat. The syndrome of inappropriate ADH (SIADH) is largely a diagnosis of exclusion. The criteria for diagnosis include:

1. Normal renal, adrenal and pituitary function.
2. Hyponatremia with hypotonicity.
3. Urine osmolality higher than expected for the degree of hyponatremia. Normally, a 1–3 per cent fall in plasma sodium and osmolality should give rise to urine specific gravity of 1,003 or less (urine osmolality of 100 mOsm/kg water or less).
4. High urine sodium (> 20 mEq/liter).
5. Absence of clinical signs of volume contraction or overload.
6. Correction of plasma sodium with water restriction.[16]

Patients with "reset osmostat" have chronic hyponatremia, a debilitating disease such as tuberculosis, persistence of ADH in blood at P_{osm} of 275 mOsm/kg below, and normal response to water loading (urine osmolality less than 100 mOsm/kg).

Pure glucocorticoid deficiency is not the same as Addison's disease, the former being associated normal mineralocorticoid secretion and absence of volume contraction. Such a deficiency cannot be easily distinguished from SIADH. Goldberg[14] has recommended a therapeutic trial of 50 mg of IV hydrocortisone as a way to distinguish glucocorticoid-deficient patients from SIADH patients. He suggests that a large rise in urine volume and a fall in urine specific gravity within 3 to 6 hours of glucocorticoid administration may be specific for glucocorticoid deficiency.

Hypernatremia

The assessment of a hypernatremic patient is also aided by an evaluation of ECF volume.

Hypernatremia with Volume Overload. Patients in this group are uncommon, and their clinical condition suggests the administration of hypernatremic solutions. They may present with pulmonary congestion or engorged neck veins rather than peripheral edema because the volume overload is sudden in onset.

Hypernatremia with Hypovolemia. Patients with volume depletion due to extrarenal losses present with urinary sodium concentrations below 20 mEq/liter and high urine osmolality. Patients

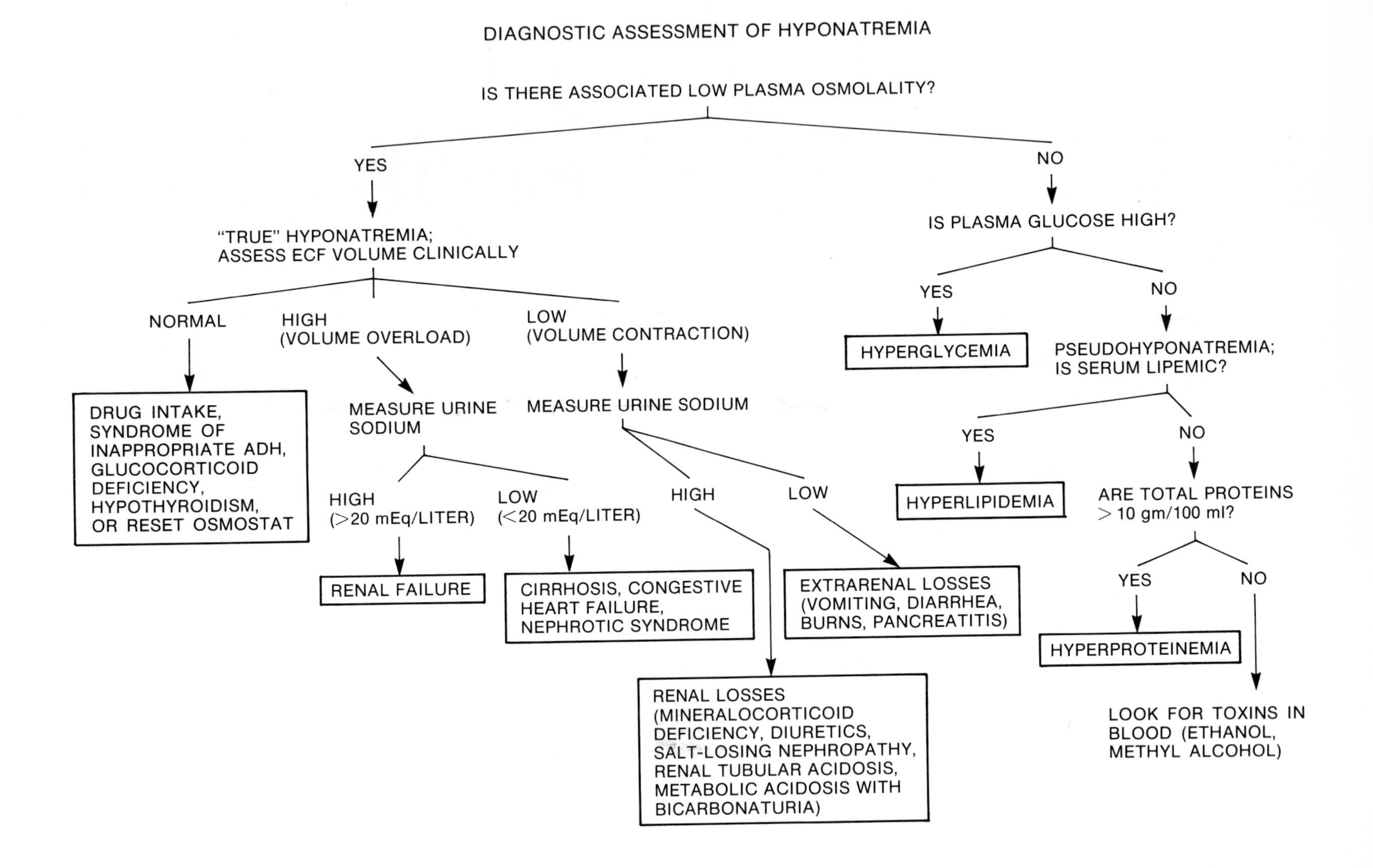
DIAGNOSTIC ASSESSMENT OF HYPONATREMIA
IS THERE ASSOCIATED LOW PLASMA OSMOLALITY?
YES
NO
"TRUE" HYPONATREMIA; ASSESS ECF VOLUME CLINICALLY
IS PLASMA GLUCOSE HIGH?
NORMAL
HIGH (VOLUME OVERLOAD)
LOW (VOLUME CONTRACTION)
YES
NO
HYPERGLYCEMIA
PSEUDOHYPONATREMIA; IS SERUM LIPEMIC?
DRUG INTAKE, SYNDROME OF INAPPROPRIATE ADH, GLUCOCORTICOID DEFICIENCY, HYPOTHYROIDISM, OR RESET OSMOSTAT
MEASURE URINE SODIUM
MEASURE URINE SODIUM
YES
NO
HIGH (>20 mEq/LITER)
LOW (<20 mEq/LITER)
HIGH
LOW
HYPERLIPIDEMIA
ARE TOTAL PROTEINS > 10 gm/100 ml?
RENAL FAILURE
CIRRHOSIS, CONGESTIVE HEART FAILURE, NEPHROTIC SYNDROME
EXTRARENAL LOSSES (VOMITING, DIARRHEA, BURNS, PANCREATITIS)
YES
NO
HYPERPROTEINEMIA
RENAL LOSSES (MINERALOCORTICOID DEFICIENCY, DIURETICS, SALT-LOSING NEPHROPATHY, RENAL TUBULAR ACIDOSIS, METABOLIC ACIDOSIS WITH BICARBONATURIA)
LOOK FOR TOXINS IN BLOOD (ETHANOL, METHYL ALCOHOL)

with renal losses present with urine sodium concentrations above 20 mEq/liter and variable urine osmolality. Signs of ECF volume depletion (described earlier) are common to both these groups of patients.

Euvolemic Hypernatremia. Patients with euvolemic hypernatremia lack signs of ECF volume contraction or volume overload. They have primarily water losses without loss of sodium. Those with extrarenal water losses present with hypertonic urine.

The patient with complete central diabetes insipidus typically presents with a history of brain tumor or surgery for brain tumor, sudden onset of polyuria (> 5 liters/day), and hypotonic urine (specific gravity < 1003, urine osmolality < 150–200 mOsm/kg) with low urine sodium (< 20 mEq/liter). Patients with partial central diabetes insipidus who are dehydrated may present with mildly hypertonic urine but are unable to achieve maximal urine osmolality unless they are given exogenous vasopressin (ADH). The method of differentiating between complete central, partial central, and nephrogenous diabetes insipidus is described under "Diagnostic Studies."

Implications of Sodium Abnormality

Neurologic manifestions have been reported in about 60 per cent of patients with plasma sodium levels below 128 mEq/liter.[17] Acute hyponatremia (onset less than 12 hours) generally results in stupor, coma, or seizures.[17] Chronic hyponatremia may be associated with lethargy, apathy, weakness, gastrointestinal symptoms, cramps, altered mental state with depressed or abnormal tendon reflexes, Cheyne-Stokes breathing, and hypothermia.[17] Mortality rates over 50 per cent are reported in patients with acute hyponatremia, in contrast to 12 per cent with chronic symptomatic hyponatremia. No deaths have been reported in chronic asymptomatic hyponatremia.[18]

In children with plasma sodium levels above 150 mEq/liter, neurologic signs have been reported in 16 to 90 per cent in different series.[18] The signs include irritability, hyperactive tendon reflexes, increased muscle tone, twitching, convulsions, and focal paresis.[18] Adults have been reported to show chorea, convulsions, muscular irritability, and depressed sensorium.[18] Data compiled by Covey and Arieff[18] from several series reveal that the mortality rate exceeds 40 per cent in children with acute hypernatremia and is less than 10 per cent in children with chronic hypernatremia.

Two-thirds of children have neurologic sequelae after recovery from acute hypernatremia. In adults, the mortality rate with acute hypernatremia is in excess of 65 to 70 per cent and with chronic hypernatremia, as high as 60 per cent, but the high rates may be consequences of serious underlying conditions such as lactic acidosis, diabetic hyperosmolar coma, and recovery from cardiac arrest.[18]

These findings illustrate the need for an aggressive and swift approach to the diagnosis and treatment of acute changes in plasma sodium level. Even chronic asymptomatic hyponatremia or hypernatremia should initiate a diagnostic search because it may be the only clue to the presence of a serious and potentially treatable disease, such as adrenal insufficiency or lung cancer.

REFERENCES

1. Hariprasad MK, Eisinger RD, Nadler IM. Hyponatremia in psychogenic polydipsia. Arch Intern Med 1980;140:1639–42.
2. Schwartz TB. Disorders of fluid electrolyte and acid-base balance. In: Beeson PB, McDermott W, Wyngaarden JB, eds. Cecil textbook of medicine. 15th ed. Philadelphia: WB Saunders, 1979;1950–69.
3. Miller M, Moses AM. Drug-induced states of impaired water excretion. Kidney Int 1976;10:96–103.
4. Robertson GL, Aycinena P, Zerbe RL. Neurogenic disorders of osmoregulation. Am J Med 1982;72:339–53.
5. Goldberg M, Reivich M. Studies on the mechanism of hyponatremia and impaired water excretion in myxedema. Ann Intern Med 1962;56:120–30.
6. DeFronzo RA, Goldberg M, Agus ZS. Normal diluting capacity in hyponatremic patients. Ann Intern Med 1976;84:538–42.
7. Linas SL, Berl T, Robertson GL, Aisenbrey GA, Schrier RW, Anderson SL. Role of vasopressin in the impaired water excretion of glucocorticoid deficiency. Kidney Int 1980;18:58–67.
8. Finberg L. Hypernatremic (hypertonic) dehydration in infants. N Engl J Med 1973;289:196–98.
9. Banister A, Siddiqi SAM, Thatcher GW. Treatment of hypernatremic dehydration in infancy. Arch Dis Child 1975;50:179–86.
10. Gault MH, Dixon EE, Doyle M, Cohen WM. Hypernatremia, azotemia and dehydration due to high-protein tube feeding. Ann Intern Med 1968;68:778–82.
11. Bleumle LW. Current status of hemodialysis. Am J Med 1968;44:749–66.
12. Cameron JM, Dagan AD. Association of brain damage with therapeutic abortion induced by amniotic-fluid replacement: report of two cases. Br Med J 1966;1:1010–3.
13. Katz MA. Hyperglycemia-induced hyponatremia—calculation of expected serum sodium depression. N Engl J Med 1973;289:843–4.
14. Goldberg M. Hyponatremia. In: Beck LH, ed. Symposium on body fluid and electrolyte disorders. Med Clin North Am 1981;65:251–70.
15. Miller M, Dalakos T, Moses AM, Fellerman H, Streeten DHP. Recognition of partial defects in antidiuretic hormone secretion. Ann Intern Med 1970;73:721–9.
16. Schwartz WB, Bennett W, Curelop S, Bartter FC. Syndrome of renal sodium loss and hyponatremia probably resulting from inappropriate secretion of antidiuretic hormone. Am J Med 1957;23:529–42.
17. Arieff AI. Kidney, water and electrolytes in diabetes mellitus. In: Brenner BM, Rector FC, eds. The kidney. Philadelphia: WB Saunders, 1976;1257–96.
18. Covey CM, Arieff AI. Disorders of sodium and water metabolism and their effects on the central nervous system. In: Brenner BM, Stein JH, eds.: Contemporary issues in nephrology. Sodium and water homeostasis. New York: Churchill Livingstone, 1978;212–41.

IMPOTENCE

IRWIN GOLDSTEIN

☐ SYNONYMS: Erectile impotence, erectile insufficiency, erectile failure, erectile incompetence

BACKGROUND

Erectile impotence may be defined as the inability to generate sufficient corporal body pressure within the penis to achieve vaginal penetration, or the inability to maintain this corporal body pressure until ejaculation (barring any ejaculatory disturbances).[1] This form of male sexual dysfunction is distinct from other forms involving abnormal libido, orgasm, emission, or ejaculation. Penile rigidity, the major determinant of erectile potency, is directly related to the amount of corporal body pressure. A corporal body pressure of approximately 90 mm Hg exists when the penis, undergoing erection, elevates to a 90-degree angle from the abdomen. This degree of pressure is usually adequate for vaginal penetration.

Several classifications are in clinical use. *Primary impotence* exists if the individual has never been able to achieve potency. *Secondary impotence* exists if the potency has once been established and at some point becomes impaired. Another classification utilizes suspected pathophysiology. Impotence in this way may be defined as either primarily psychological or primarily organic, with the latter subdivided into vascular, neurologic, hormonal, mechanical, and some combination thereof.

This discussion of erectile impotence focuses on the diagnostic approach used to gain an understanding of the pathophysiology of the disorder. Correct differential diagnosis in this regard ultimately allows for appropriate therapy such as hormonal replacement, sex therapy, prosthetic surgery, or vascular or microvascular surgical reconstruction.

Incidence and Causes

In a study of more than 14,000 men, Kinsey[2] observed that the incidence of erectile dysfunction is age-dependent. He found that until the age of 45, impotence occurred rarely; however, from age 50 to age 80, the incidence increased exponentially. Approximately 10 per cent of the male study population in the sixth decade was found to be impotent, whereas approximately 80 per cent was in the ninth decade. Similar studies by Masters and Johnson,[3] Finkle and associates,[4] and others have noted similar age dependence. If a conservative estimate of the male population is assumed (approximately 35 to 50 per cent of all males are over age 50), the problem of impotence can be seen as rather extensive, afflicting millions of American men.

The causes of impotence are listed in Table 1. This is a clinical classification and is based on the suspected pathophysiologic cause of the disorder. This latter information is more readily available now that testing for impotent patients has become more objective.

In 1959, Wershub[5] stated that impotence was psychological in more than 90 per cent of cases. Although this statement may or may not still be true, recent observations support a greater appreciation for the role of abnormal physical factors. In fact, some studies (including my own) of patients with impotence report abnormal physical factors existing in well over 50 per cent of patients evaluated.[6]

Organic Impotence

Impotence is organic when abnormal physical factors affect the patient's ability to generate and maintain penile erections.

Vasculogenic Impotence. This may be the most common abnormal physical factor. The hypogastric-cavernous arterial bed, which supplies blood to the penis, consists of the internal iliac (hypogastric), internal pudendal, penile, and cavernosal arteries. This bed is unique in its ability to supply rapidly increasing blood flow at the time of pelvic nerve (sexual) stimulation. In normal individuals, blood flows have been recorded ranging from approximately 10 ml/min at rest to approximately 60 ml/min during stimulation.[1] It is this rapid rise in blood flow along with the neurologic redistribution of the flow into the corporal spaces that results in penile erection.

Insufficient blood pressure in the small vessels of the arterial bed at the time of sexual stimulation results in delivery of an inadequate volume into the corporal bodies and a "partial erection." This

Table 1. CAUSES OF IMPOTENCE

Organic	Vasculogenic Neurologic Endocrinologic "Mechanical"
Psychological	Primary Secondary*

*This may become apparent after reversal of an organic cause.

is most likely the major explanation for the strong association between impotence and aging found by Kinsey and others.

The degree of disease within this arterial bed may vary, resulting in a spectrum of corporal body pressures due to varying degrees of restriction of the increase in blood flow. For example, a complete absence of erection may represent severe vascular disease, whereas a relatively firm erection at rest that disappears during coital movement may represent less severe vascular disease. In this latter situation, there may be a vascular steal syndrome within the pelvic circulation. When arterial inflow into the hypogastric arteries is restricted and occlusive disease occurs within the internal pudendal artery, blood flow within the hypogastric-cavernous arterial pathway may be redirected into lower-resistance exercise muscle beds. One such bed is the gluteal muscle bed, a parallel vascular bed fed by the large superior and inferior gluteal arteries, which are branches of the hypogastric and internal pudendal arteries. Clinically, the redistribution of blood flow during exercise has been labeled the pelvic steal syndrome. It may manifest as the loss of erections during active coital movement.[7]

Neurologic Impotence. Abnormal neurologic factors may impair the ability to generate and sustain a penile erection. Three neurologic pathways may be considered important to the generation of an erection. The major efferent pathway involves the *parasympathetic pelvic nerve.* It originates in the intermediolateral aspect of the sacral cord segments S2, S3, and S4 and terminates on the blood vessels within the corporal body. There appears to be a preganglionic neuron whose neurotransmitter is probably acetylcholine, as well as a short postganglionic neuron whose neurotransmitter is as yet unknown. Research into this area is still ongoing, and it is very possible that vasoactive intestinal polypeptide plays a major role in redirecting the pelvic nerve–stimulated blood into the corporal spaces. A disorder of the pelvic nerve (due to surgical trauma, diabetic autonomic neuropathy) or, in addition, of the cauda equina or sacral cord may result in impaired redistribution of this corporal blood flow and inadequate generation of corporal body pressure.

The second major pathway is afferent and involves the *somatic pudendal nerve.* It begins in the somesthetic skin receptors of the penile and genital skin, passes to the sacral cord segments S2, S3, and S4 and travels through ascending spinal cord pathways to synapse in the corticomedullary junction and thalamus. It then terminates in the contralateral primary sensory area deep in the interhemispheric fissure. The importance of this pathway in normal sexuality has been established in animal and clinical studies.[8] Abnormalities in the pudendal pathway may cause inability to sustain an erection during coitus.

The third pathway involves the numerous tracts that combine to form the *cortical-sacral efferent pathway.* Experimental studies in this area have established the following locations as important in the cerebral control of penile erections: the anteromedial portion of the hypothalamus, the paraventricular nucleus, the medial forebrain bundle, the gyrus rectus, the septum pellucidum, the mamillothalamic tracts, the cingulate gyrus, and the hippocampus. Cerebral outflow from these and other pathways appears to follow a course through the substantia nigra in the midbrain to the ventrolateral portion of the pons.[9] Information is then passed through descending tracts to the sacral parasympathetic nuclei. This pathway allows for the cerebral control of penile erections. Abnormalities in the cortical-sacral efferent pathway (multiple sclerosis, syringomyelia, transverse myelitis, head injuries) may ultimately affect the modulation of the parasympathetic pelvic nerve pathway and result in impaired erectile capacity.

Several authors have proposed that the thoracolumbar sympathetics participate in the generation of an erection. Recent clinical observations and experimental studies, however, have shown that these long tract sympathetics play a role in ejaculation only, and not in generating penile erection.[9] Patients with testicular cancer who undergo removal of the thoracolumbar sympathetic ganglia during radical retroperitoneal lymphadenectomy usually have full erectile capacity.

Endocrinologic Impotence. Abnormalities within the hypothalamic-pituitary-gonadal axis or other endocrine system can affect the ability to generate or sustain penile erection. The pathophysiologic mechanisms for this form of impotence are as yet unknown. It is not clear, at present, how endocrinopathy has the ability to affect either the delivery of blood flow or the local neurologic redistribution of blood flow into the corporal spaces. On the other hand, a central mechanism for control of libido is a better-established role for endocrinologic parameters. A central feature of both hypogonadism and hyperprolactinemia is depressed libido.[10] Other suspected causes of endocrine impotence include hyperthyroidism and elevated endogenous estrogen levels.

Psychological Impotence

Inability to obtain a sufficiently rigid penile erection can result primarily from abnormal psychological factors. In males with erectile dysfunction, abnormal psychological factors can be found frequently. The important question is not whether these factors exist but whether they are *causing,* or are the *result* of, the impotence. Often, careful psychological testing is necessary to distinguish between primary and secondary psychological factors in erectile dysfunction.

A physical basis for primary psychological impotence may be postulated as failure to adequately stimulate the cortical-sacral efferent pathway. Reasons for this may be multiple, including the effects of sympathetic overstimulation, which may result from anxiety, depression, anger, or guilt occurring at the time of sexual stimulation.

Other Causes of Impotence

Those causes that are not discussed here include: mechanical factors such as Peyronie's disease, post–partial penectomy, and congenital deformities of the penis such as severe epispadias and microphallus.

Many pharmacologic agents, mostly antihypertensives, have been reported to cause impotence. The mechanisms of drug-associated impotence are poorly understood and may involve a combination of central and peripheral effects. Likely peripheral effects include direct blocking of the neurotransmitter action during pelvic nerve stimulation and overall reduction in the systemic arterial perfusion pressure, which may be the major peripheral effect. A minimally stenotic vascular bed may allow for the adequate delivery of corporal blood only when the systemic perfusion pressure is elevated. This possibility may explain why some patients may achieve "normal" erections when not taking medication (hypertension uncontrolled) and have poor erections when taking medication (hypertension controlled). More commonly, however, occlusive vascular disease is more severe, and changing antihypertensive medication does not usually restore erectile function completely. In addition, this latter hypothesis also may explain why hydrochlorothiazide alone can cause changes in erectile function.

HISTORY

A carefully taken history can often provide a very accurate assessment of the pathophysiology of erectile impotence. It may be divided into the sexual history (identifying the sexual dysfunction) and the medical history (identifying etiologic factors).

Sexual History

The physician must determine what the patient means by the term impotence. Other disorders commonly confused with erectile impotence are decreased libido and ejaculatory disturbances.

Loss of libido is characterized by the lack of sexual interest in the postpubertal male and, strictly speaking, is not impotence. Patients often have no problem with erections and are occasionally referred for medical attention at the insistence of the spouse or partner. The causes of libido loss include clinical depression and endocrinologic abnormalities such as hypogonadism and hyperprolactinemia.

Ejaculatory disturbances, i.e., premature and retarded ejaculation, are often associated with a normal ability to achieve erection. In some cases, ejaculation may be so premature as to occur prior to vaginal penetration. There are few organic causes that would explain the occurrence of premature ejaculation. In retarded or delayed ejaculation, the patient may be unable to achieve intravaginal ejaculation. In the absence of alpha-adrenergic blocker therapy or previous retroperitoneal surgery, delayed ejaculation is most commonly a psychological problem.

The sexual history should include: (1) the approximate period of the patient's complaint and the time course of the change; (2) the frequency of coitus at present and prior to onset of the problem; (3) the ability to ejaculate; (4) the desire to have sexual intercourse; and (5) the quality of the erection with masturbation, upon awaking in the morning, with sexual stimulation, with other partners, during vaginal penetration, and during subsequent coital movement.

Using these sexual characteristics, several patterns of erectile impotence become obvious. Patients with organic impotence (usually vascular) generally report a gradual decline in erectile function over a period of years, from several coital episodes per week to rare coital episodes in a month. The libido is usually preserved, ejaculation is either unaffected or slightly premature, and the quality of the erection is poor regardless of the sexual stimulation. In contrast, patients with primary psychological impotence may have a sudden change in potency over several days to weeks, with the ability to achieve good erections in some situations but not in others, and they often have both libido and ejaculatory complaints.

Medical History

Vascular History. In 1923, Leriche[11] described a syndrome caused by atherosclerotic occlusion of the distal aorta and common iliac arteries. The findings consisted of lower extremity claudication, leg atrophy and pallor, and inability to achieve an erection. The majority of patients with vasculogenic impotence, however, do not have such severe disease in the major vessels. They appear to have stenoses and occlusions acting in a more confined and selected location within the hypo-

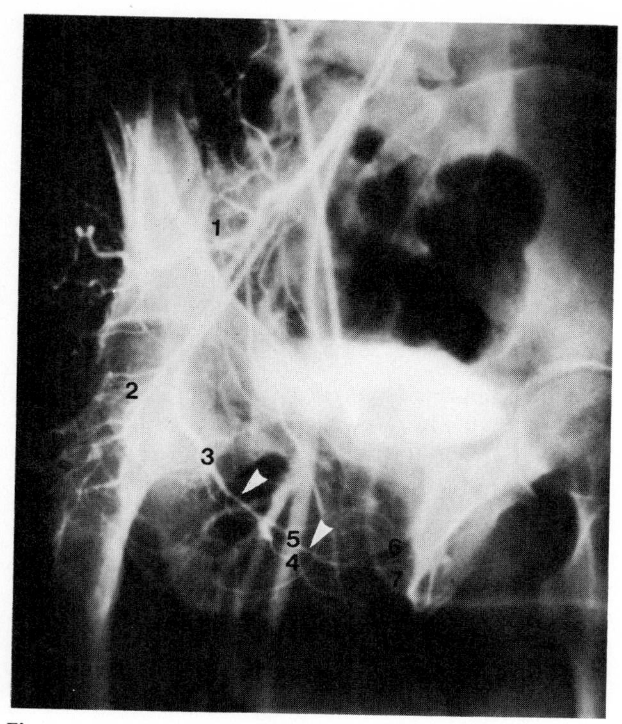

Figure 1. A selective internal pudendal arteriogram in a patient with vasculogenic impotence. *1*, superior gluteal artery; *2*, inferior gluteal artery; *3*, internal pudendal artery; *4*, perineal/scrotal artery; *5*, penile artery; *6*, dorsal artery; *7*, corporal artery. There are stenotic lesions *(white arrows)* in the internal pudendal and penile arteries.

gastric-cavernous arterial bed. Vascular disease in this bed, which interferes with arterial pressure in the corporal artery and with blood volume delivery to the corporal bodies, is similar in vascular effects to the Leriche syndrome (Fig. 1).

Vasculogenic impotence may be suspected in the patient with vascular risk factors such as family history of vascular disease, cigarette smoking, hypercholesterolemia, hypertension, diabetes, blunt pelvic trauma, and pelvic radiation therapy. The quality and length of smoking habit as well as the duration and severity of both systemic hypertension and diabetes should be estimated in all cases. In addition, complications of vascular risk factors should be looked for, such as bronchitis, emphysema, coronary artery disease, and peripheral vascular disease (associated with smoking), cerebrovascular accidents and headaches (associated with hypertension), and nephropathy, neuropathy, and retinopathy (associated with diabetes). A thorough drug history should be obtained, especially concerning agents that lower systemic arterial perfusion pressure, such as diuretics, antihypertensive agents, tranquilizers, sympatholytics, and antidepressants.

Neurologic History. Normal sexual function depends on an intact nervous system, so lesions affecting the nervous system may result in erectile impotence.

Patients with known neurologic disease, especially spinal cord injury, should be questioned about the level and completeness of the lesion. What is the temporal relationship between the development of the neurologic lesion and the development of impotence? All impotent patients should be assessed for the development of decreased sensation, especially in the penis or external genitalia (associated with diabetes, alcoholism, or uremic pudendal neuropathy), upper and lower extremity weakness or visual disturbances (associated with multiple sclerosis, spinal cord trauma, neoplasms, or infections), and back pain and bowel or urinary dysfunction (associated with sacral cord or cauda equina syndrome). Rarely, a neurologic disorder may first manifest as erectile impotence. For the most part, in an unselected population of impotent patients, approximately 10 per cent will have impotence secondary to neurologic factors. Some will complain of total inability to obtain an erection (complete sacral cord lesion), and others of an inability to adequately sustain and maintain the erection (pudendal neuropathy, incomplete suprasacral cord or cerebral lesion).

Endocrinologic History. Impotence secondary to a direct endocrine dysfunction is uncommon and, in descending order of frequency, may be related to hypogonadism, hyperprolactinemia, and hyperthyroidism. Classic historical features are subtle and consist of loss of libido, decreased beard growth, gynecomastia, sweating, and hand tremor. Some medical disorders, such as hepatic cirrhosis, may result in the abnormal metabolism of estrogens. Information concerning alcohol intake, hepatitis, and jaundice may also be useful. Exogenous estrogens such as those given for treatment of prostate cancer may result in depressed libido.

Psychological History. Impotent men commonly have at least some psychological problems, as identified by history-taking, because self-esteem, self-worth, and ego are often closely allied to "adequate" sexual performance. Therefore, one should attempt to elicit information about performance anxiety, anger, depression, guilt, or feelings of impaired worth. These factors, however, are often difficult to identify as primary or secondary causes of impotence.

High-Payoff Queries

The following eight questions are likely to provide valuable insight into the pathophysiology of the impotence:

1. *How long have you had problems with impotence? How quickly did the impotence develop?* Primary impotence is lifelong and, in the presence of abnormal nocturnal penile tumescence, may have an underlying *organic* etiology. Secondary impotence

is variable in onset and classically may be the result of either an acute problem (weeks to months) or a gradual, progressive one (months to years). An acute onset may imply a situational psychological etiology; a gradual onset may be consistent with a physical factor, usually vascular.

2. *How often do you have intercourse now compared with before you started having impotence problems?* This question will establish a "baseline" coital frequency and will help the physician understand the patient's interpretation of his erectile problem. Often an individual may complain of "impotence" for several years but may still be able to perform intercourse several times per week. His impotence may be more of a problem with performance under different situations or with different partners. It may also be related to partner satisfaction or to libido or ejaculation problems. This question may help clarify a patient's interpretation of his problem.

3. *Do you have difficulty with ejaculation?* Ejaculatory problems, especially premature ejaculation, often interfere with self-confidence and partner satisfaction and are harbingers of the fear of failure and anxiety.

4. *What is the quality of your erections during masturbation, when you awaken in the morning, after sexual stimulation, and with different partners?* Erections can be graded on a scale by assuming the patient is standing in an upright position. The flaccid penis rests at 6 o'clock; a good erection sufficient for vaginal penetration may be 90 degrees from the abdomen at 9 o'clock; a more rigid erection can be at 10 o'clock or even 11 o'clock. Most partial erections are described as being at 7 or 8 o'clock. Classically, an organic problem involves an erection that is consistently partial and lower than 9 o'clock under most circumstances.

5. *Is it difficult to achieve vaginal penetration?* A partial erection will usually require mechanical assistance to achieve penetration.

6. *During coital activity, do you lose the erection or does it increase in rigidity?* The former condition may imply a vascular steal phenomenon, the latter insufficient stimulation during foreplay prior to coitus.

7. *Do you smoke? Do you have high blood pressure, diabetes, or exercise-related chest or leg pain?* It is essential to identify all vascular risk factors in patients undergoing impotence evaluation.

8. *Have you had any neurologic injuries, back operations, a stroke, numbness or weakness, or bladder or bowel dysfunction?* It is essential to identify any antecedent neurologic history in patients undergoing impotence evaluation.

PHYSICAL EXAMINATION

A careful physical examination often reveals some clues that substantiate the pathophysiologic possibilities gleaned from the history. It is more common, however, for the history to offer a more accurate assessment as to the genesis of the dysfunction.

Vascular Findings. An arterial pulse can usually be palpated on the dorsum of the penis at the level of the suspensory ligament. This is the dorsal artery pulse, and its presence can be classified on a zero to 3 scale. Palpation of other arteries, such as the femoral, may give an estimation of the degree of proximal aortoiliac or external iliac artery disease. The presence of an active femoral pulse, however, does not rule out small-vessel disease in the hypogastric-cavernous arterial bed. Other signs of peripheral vascular disease such as leg atrophy and pallor and loss of leg hair growth may be supportive of an overall vasculogenic impairment.

Neurologic Findings. The neurologic examination should be concentrated in the perineal and lower extremity area. One should assess the sensation (light touch, pinprick) in the external genitalia and the lower extremities. In addition, the deep tendon reflexes should be assessed including the quadriceps (L3, L4) and Achilles tendon (L5, S1, S2) reflexes. The bulbocavernosus reflex is evoked by palpating the glans penis. The response is determined by palpating the resultant muscle contraction of either the bulbocavernosus muscle or the external anal sphincter muscle. The reflex subserving the sacral cord segments S2, S3, S4 is clinically present in most normal males.

Endocrinologic Findings. The level of androgen stimulation can be assessed by observing the secondary sex characteristics such as body and facial hair pattern, muscular development, and size and consistency of the prostate and testes. The degree of estrogenic stimulation can be judged according to the presence or absence of gynecomastia.

Miscellaneous Findings. A thorough physical examination should include palpation of the corpora cavernosa to assess their bulk and detect the presence of plaque formation. This latter problem (so-called Peyronie's plaques) is significant in that the presence of plaques may herald a mechanical inability to achieve a straight erection. In addition, such problems as phimotic foreskin and scrotal mass, which affect penile size, should be identified.

DIAGNOSTIC STUDIES

A clinical suspicion of the etiology of impotence is usually established during the history and physical examination. In the majority of cases, however, objective erectile function testing is necessary to confirm the pathophysiology. For example, a patient with underlying psychological impotence may deny the presence of morning erections and may observe his erectile capacity changing gradually instead of abruptly. On the other hand, patients with underlying organic impotence may have relatively normal morning erections and may also experience sudden rather than gradual change in erectile function, especially if the change is temporally related to radical pelvic surgery. Moreover, organic impotence may have psychological factors, making affected patients indistinguishable from those with primary psychological impotence.

The purpose of erectile function testing is to objectively assess with a battery of examinations certain aspects of the erectile physiology. Erectile function testing usually consists of nocturnal penile tumescence studies and various vascular, neurologic, endocrinologic, and psychological evaluations.

Evaluation of Nocturnal Penile Tumescence (NPT)

This procedure is broadly indicated for every patient complaining of erectile dysfunction. Using strain-gauge plethysmography, it attempts to document the involuntary unconscious erections normally obtained during sleep. The test is useful in distinguishing patients with primary psychological impotence and normal nighttime erections from those with organic impotence and impaired nighttime erections.[12] Normal nighttime erections may be described as three to four tumescence periods lasting 30 to 45 minutes each with circumferential changes greater than 2 cm. Abnormal nighttime erections, in contrast, last 7.5 to 15 minutes each with circumferential changes less than 2 cm. The NPT tracing records penile circumferential changes instead of penile rigidity and thus has a potential diagnostic pitfall, especially in recording those episodes of tumescence with sufficient penile rigidity but only minimal circumferential change. Nevertheless, the NPT test is a useful diagnostic procedure in impotence screening.

Vascular Evaluation

All patients with erectile insufficiency should undergo evaluation of the hypogastric-cavernous arterial bed. The method most commonly used to assess adequacy of pelvic blood flow noninvasively is penile Doppler ultrasonography. A standard 9.5-kilohertz Doppler probe is positioned over each cavernosal artery. A 2.5-cm cuff is placed at the base of the penis, and penile systolic occlusion pressures are noted; when these are compared with the systemic systolic occlusion pressures (brachial), a penile-brachial index (PBI) is established.[13] Knowledge of the resting index provides insight into the degree of drop in arterial pressure that occurs from stenotic arterial lesions along the hypogastric-cavernous arterial bed.

Since resting PBI values appear somewhat insensitive, dynamic or exercise PBI testing is also performed. In this latter evaluation, the pelvic steal test, the patient performs a gluteal exercise for 3 to 5 minutes. A positive result consists of a significant fall in PBI during exercise. The most appropriate explanation for this drop is an exercise-associated pelvic blood flow redistribution phenomenon, in which inflow to the restricted, high-resistance hypogastric-cavernous arterial bed is diverted to the low-resistance gluteal arterial bed. Documentation of a redistribution phenomenon may help identify patients with vasculogenic impotence, who may otherwise have normal resting PBI values.[14]

Redistribution phenomenon may be further identified by recording penile (intraurethral) temperature during exercise. Urethral temperatures closely reflect cavernous temperatures, especially when a rigid intraurethral temperature probe is positioned against the larger-volume corporal body. A drop in penile temperature during exercise implies a pelvic blood flow redistribution pattern.

Other noninvasive techniques used to identify adequacy of pelvic blood flow consist of plethysmography and radioisotopic procedures. Selective pudendal arteriography is performed principally in those patients who have abnormal results on noninvasive studies and desire treatment by invasive vascular procedures, such as balloon angiodilation, vascular reconstruction, and microsurgical revascularization. Pudendal arteriography should not be performed to confirm a suspected vascular disorder if no vascular therapy is planned.

Neurologic Evaluation

Neurologic testing should be performed in patients complaining of erectile dysfunction, especially if there exists an antecedent neurologic disorder or a history indicative of neurologic impairment.

The first neurologic evaluation may be penile vibration perception threshold (VPT) testing. This procedure, performed with a biothesiometer, is inexpensive and painless, and its results quantitative and reproducible. Abnormalities in vibration sensitivity have been shown to be early features of peripheral neuropathy. A tactor is placed on the glans and on the right and left midshaft surfaces of the penis. The amplitude of vibration is increased while the patient is asked to note the first vibration stimulus he perceives. This test is repeated several times until a reproducible value is obtained. Unlike evoked response testing, this evaluation is performed with minimum nerve stimulation and thus may be a more sensitive index of pudendal peripheral sensory neuropathy.

Other neurologic evaluations include perineal electromyography, sacral latency testing, and genital-cerebral evoked response testing. These evaluations are more invasive and are generally not used as screening procedures in unselected impotent patients.

Perineal electromyography involves placing a fine sterile concentric needle electrode within the bulbocavernosus muscle. An analysis is then made of the resting as well as contracting perineal electromyograms to look for potentials characteristic of pudendal nerve denervation.

In a sacral latency test, the glans or shaft of the penis is electrically stimulated, and subsequent reflex perineal contractions are recorded with perineal electromyography. An average of 16 to 32 stimulations are made for each recording. The result is a neurophysiologic representation of the bulbocavernosus reflex and may be used to objectively evaluate the sacral cord segments S2, S3, and S4 in suspected cases of sacral spinal cord disease.[15]

Upper motor neuron impotence may be evaluated by dorsal nerve somatosensory evoked response testing. In this procedure, the right or left penile shaft is repetitively stimulated. The subsequent evoked response waveform is recorded over the sacral spinal cord as well as the cerebral cortex. Reproducible latency values consistent with the spinal cord synapse and the primary cortical sensory area synapses have been identified. In addition, a possible thalamocortical synapse may occasionally be seen preceding the cortical latency. Thus the dorsal nerve somatosensory evoked response can be divided into peripheral and central conduction times. Abnormalities of latency values between synapse locations may imply a localized upper motor neuron lesion affecting the pudendal suprasacral afferent pathway. Abnormalities within this pathway do not define neurologic impotence per se but rather imply its existence.

Correlating the objective indications of neurologic function with other erectile function test results allows for identification of neurologic impotence.[16]

Endocrine Evaluation

The minimal endocrine evaluation should consist of serum testosterone, luteinizing hormone, and prolactin measurements. All impotent patients should undergo a minimal endocrine evaluation, especially those who have described a decrease in libido. More complete evaluation for possible endocrinologic dysfunction may include assessments of the alternative pathways of testosterone such as estrone and the metabolic products of testosterone such as dihydrotestosterone, estradiol, and the unbound portion of testosterone (free testosterone). If abnormal screening results are identified, admission to a metabolic unit for more specialized testing may be considered. This specialized testing may consist of determinations of tripooled gonadotropins, testosterone, and estradiol; a 24-hour urine collection for 17-ketosteroids, free cortisol, and creatinine measurements; polytomography of the sella turcica; CT scanning and visual field analysis; and human chorionic gonadotropin stimulation testing and luteinizing hormone–releasing factor evaluation for gonadotropin assessment.

Psychological Evaluation

Formal psychological evaluation may be necessary in patients who complain of erectile dysfunction, especially if: the baseline history is strongly suggestive of a causal, psychological association such as situational impotence; there are previous psychological problems; there is an obvious psychological disorder such as depression, anxiety, hostility, guilt, or shame; or the patient desires such an interview. Whenever possible, the presence of the patient's partner for at least a portion of the interview helps provide a more adequate sexual history. In addition, the partner's presence has been found to make any subsequent psychological treatment easier. Psychological evaluation may play an important role in the ultimate success and sexual rehabilitation of patients treated even for organic impotence, particularly those who receive nonprosthetic surgical or endocrine treatment.

Overview of Diagnostic Studies

An organized multidisciplinary approach, involving vascular, neurologic, endocrine and psychological evaluations as well as nocturnal penile tumescence testing, is utilized. This battery of evaluations, which constitute erectile function testing, is used to assess the specific physiologic mechanisms that play a role in the erectile process. The aim of erectile function testing is to provide the clinician with objective data about the erectile dysfunction. In this manner, a diagnosis can be confirmed and an appropriate treatment plan may be developed.

A typically structured evaluation may consist of the following: The initial evaluation comprises a thorough history and physical examination. Following judgment as to the sexual problem, several screening procedures are performed. The first of these examinations may consist of nocturnal penile tumescence testing, penile Doppler ultrasonography, penile temperature measurement, vibration perception threshold testing, and endocrine screening of the hypothalamic-pituitary-gonadal axis. If abnormalities within each group are identified, more specific specialized testing may be performed to document them. For instance, if vascular abnormalities are identified, the nocturnal penile tumescence test result is abnormal, and the patient is considered to be as a candidate for microsurgical revascularization, a selective pudendal arteriogram should be performed. If results of both vibration perception threshold and nocturnal penile tumescence testing are abnormal, the patient should undergo appropriate further neurologic testing as previously described. Lesions identified on testing that were not suspected clinically may be evaluated further via CT scanning, electroencephalography, or myelography. If the endocrine screening values and nocturnal penile tumescence test results are abnormal, a more complete endocrine evaluation as previously described may be considered.

ASSESSMENT

Impotence can be a relatively frustrating diagnostic problem for both patient and physician. From the patient's point of view the problem may be private, emotional, and difficult to discuss. From the physician's point of view the problem may be one of "role frustration," e.g., difficulty understanding the time investment, the pathophysiology, and the potential for both medical and surgical (prosthetic and nonprosthetic) rehabilitation.

The physician assessing the patient with erectile impotence must keep in mind that much research and information have been generated in the last decade and that previous teachings and concepts have been re-evaluated. The diagnostic evaluation of male impotence is no longer limited solely to history-taking and physical examination, and the dysfunction is no longer exclusively a psychological problem.

Constellations of Findings

The following are constellations of findings that characterize the various types of erectile impotence. Key findings are in italics.

Vasculogenic Impotence. The most common type of organic impotence, vasculogenic impotence, is especially common in the patient with a history of *cigarette smoking, hypertension, diabetes, peripheral vascular disease, coronary artery disease,* or *cerebrovascular insufficiency.* The change in erectile insufficiency is gradual, usually occurring in the sixth or seventh decade. It is associated with a decrease in the frequency of intercourse, normal or premature ejaculation, partial erection with sexual stimulation, partial morning erection, failure to achieve vaginal penetration, and inability to maintain erection. Patients are often receiving antihypertensive medication, which commonly appears to aggravate the erectile dysfunction. Two subgroups of patients with vasculogenic impotence include those in their 20s and 30s who have suffered blunt perineal trauma, especially in motor vehicle accidents,[17] and those who have undergone pelvic irradiation, especially for prostate cancer.[18] Dysfunction in the former subgroup can be completely reversed with microsurgical revascularization.

Neurologic Impotence. The next most common type of organic impotence occurs in patients with neurologic lesions affecting the *parasympathetic pelvic pathway,* the *pudendal sensory afferent pathway,* or the *cortical-sacral efferent pathway.* The patient may complain of either gradual or acute onset of erectile dysfunction, depending on the etiology of the neurologic lesion. Erections may be totally absent or partial, with an inability to maintain adequate rigidity. Neurologic conditions affecting potency include alcoholism, diabetes, post–radical pelvic surgery; spinal cord infection, tumor, or trauma, syringomyelia, degenerative disc disease, transverse myelitis, multiple sclerosis; brain tumors or trauma, and cerebral insufficiency. Drug-related impotence may possibly act by adversely affecting the neurotransmitter released during pelvic nerve stimulation, although a vascular mechanism is more likely.

Simultaneous neurologic and vasculogenic impotence may exist, especially in patients with diabetes mellitus. The accurate determination of abnormal neurologic factors is particularly important in assessing patients with possible combined causes. Unrecognized neurologic factors could possibly result in continued erectile dysfunction despite technically satisfactory vascular reconstructive procedures.

Endocrinologic Impotence. The classic symptom of endocrinologic impotence is decreased libido. Subtle physical findings such as small testes and decreased body hair may indicate hypogonadism; depression and loss of visual acuity may accompany hyperprolactinemia; sweating and hand tremors may signify hyperthyroidism. A low testosterone level is not, in and of itself, pathognomonic for endocrinologic impotence. Clinical observations have shown that normal erections can occur with testosterone levels well below normal and even in patients who have been castrated. Nevertheless, in the patient with decreased libido and abnormally low testosterone level, androgen replacement has had therapeutic benefit.

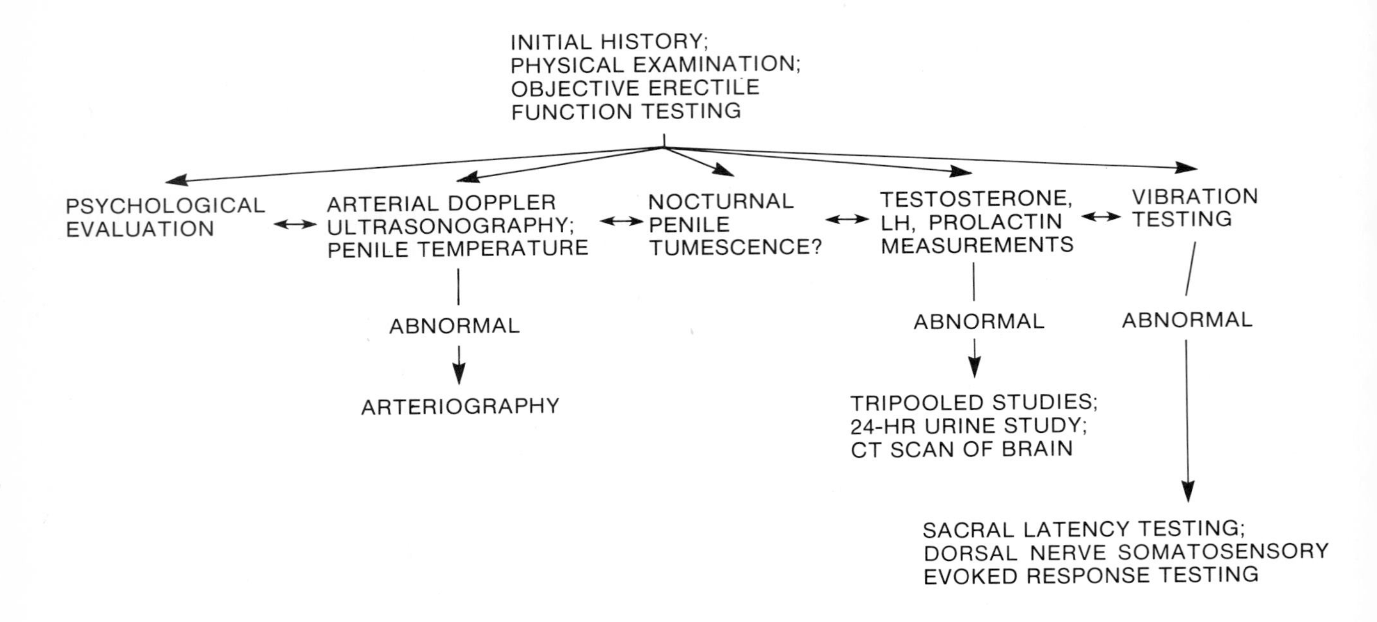

Psychological Impotence. The identification of psychological factors in patients with erectile insufficiency is common but may not in most instances imply a primary etiologic role. Feelings such as anxiety, depression, anger, guilt, loss of self-esteem, and loss of self-worth may be identified in both the presence and absence of organic disease. The patient with primary psychological impotence is usually younger (age 40 or less) and has an abrupt onset of impotence related to a recognizable, usually social event. He may also have situational impotence, i.e., the inability to perform coitus in certain situations.

Diagnostic Approach

The algorithm illustrates a typical structured approach designed to organize the evaluation of patients with erectile impotence.

Implications of Impotence

Erectile impotence is rarely a life-threatening disorder, and so generally does not command widespread physician interest or attention. The usual response is that its evaluation takes too much time, the problem is usually psychological, and only occasionally is successful treatment possible.

The last several years, however, have seen a dramatic alteration in the way physicians view the problem of male impotence. It is being appreciated that the disorder afflicts, by conservative estimates, many millions of American men. Numerous centers for treating male reproductive disorders around the country have recently been established to attempt to deal with the diagnostic problems. An organized, rational, multidisciplinary approach to understanding erectile physiology is now becoming available. Such an approach has enabled, in many situations, the precise pathophysiology to be determined. Treatment plans can now be tailored to the individual patient's problem and clinical results can now be maximized. New treatment forms, especially microvascular surgical reconstruction, can reverse the impotence in some cases without the use of prosthetic material. The ultimate aim is to develop a better awareness of the nature of the problem of male impotence, its etiology, treatment, and, it is to be hoped, subsequent prophylaxis.

REFERENCES

1. Metz P, Wagner G. Penile circumference and erection. Urology 1981;18:268–70.
2. Kinsey A, Poneroy W, Martin C. Sexual behavior in the human male. Philadelphia: WB Saunders, 1948;7:218–62.
3. Masters WH, Johnson VE. Human sexual response. Boston: Little, Brown, 1966:248–70.

4. Finkle AL, Moyers TG, Tobenkin MI, Karg SJ. Sexual potency in aging males. I. Frequency of coitus among clinic patients. JAMA 1959;170:1391–3.
5. Wershub LP. Sexual impotence in the male. Springfield, Ill. Charles C Thomas, 1959:29.
6. Karacan I, Moore CA. Nocturnal penile tumescence: an objective diagnostic aid for erectile dysfunction. In: Bennett AH, ed. Management of male impotence. Baltimore: Williams & Wilkins, 1982;62–72.
7. Michal V, Kramar R, Pospichal J. External iliac steal syndrome. J Card Surg 1978;19:355–7.
8. DeGroat WE, Booth AM. Physiology of male sexual function. Ann Intern Med 1980;92(2 Pt2);329–31.
9. Siroky MB, Krane RJ. Physiology of male sexual dysfunction. In: Krane RJ, Siroky MB, eds. Clinical Neuro-Urology. Boston: Little, Brown, 1979;45–62.
10. Weideman CL, Northcutt RC. Endocrine aspects of impotence. In: Furlow WL, ed. Male sexual dysfunction. Philadelphia: WB Saunders, 1981;8:143–51.
11. Leriche R. Des oblitérations artérielles hautes (oblitération de la terminaison de l'aorte) comme cause d'insuffisance circulatoire des membres inférieures. Bull Soc Chir (Paris) 1923;49:1404–8.
12. Karacan I, Ilaria RL. Diagnostic advances in impotence. Encephale 1978;4:81–92.
13. Queral LA, Whitehouse WM Jr, Flinn WR, Zarins CK, Bergan JJ, Yao JST. Pelvic hemodynamics after aorto-iliac reconstitution. Surgery 1979;86:799–809.
14. Goldstein I, Siroky MB, Nath RL, Menzoian JL, Krane RJ. Vasculogenic impotence: role of the pelvic steal test. J Urol 1983;128:300–6.
15. Krane RJ, Siroky MB. Studies on sacral evoked potentials. J Urol 1980;124:872–6.
16. Goldstein I. Neurologic impotence. In: Krane RJ, Siroky MB, Goldstein I, eds. Male sexual dysfunction. Boston: Little, Brown, 1983; 193–201.
17. MacGregor RJ, Konnak JW: Treatment of vasculogenic erectile dysfunction by direct anastomosis of the inferior epigastric artery to the central artery to the corpus cavernosum. J Urol 1982;127:136–9.
18. Goldstein I, Feldman MI, Babayan RK, Siroky MB, Krane RJ. The mechanism of radiation-associated impotence: a clinical study. JAMA 1984: in press.

INFERTILITY

JAMES R. DINGFELDER

□ SYNONYMS: Primary infertility, secondary infertility, female infertility, male infertility, sterility, unexplained infertility, habitual abortion, reproductive failure

BACKGROUND

Definitions

Infertility is the inability of a couple to conceive or to maintain a pregnancy until fetal viability. *Primary infertility* exists when a couple has not achieved conception after 1 year of regular intercourse. *Secondary infertility* exists when a couple who have previously conceived are unsuccessful in achieving another conception.

In *male infertility*, male factors are at least partly responsible for a couple's inability to conceive. Such factors include azospermia (total absence of sperm in the semen), oligospermia (sperm density less than 20 million/ml), abnormal sperm motility and morphology, and sperm antibodies.

Female infertility refers to adverse factors in the female reproductive system, including fallopian tube obstruction, ovulation failure, and cervical mucus problems.

In some instances, the problem is said to be a *couple factor* or *combined factor*. Examples include poor or ill-timed coital techniques, infections in both individuals (mycoplasma, Chlamydia), and use of spermicidal lubricants. It is useful to approach every case of infertility as a couple problem, even when the infertility factor is limited to one individual, because the resultant infertility affects both partners, and infertility treatments often require the cooperation and understanding of the unaffected partner.

Incidence and Outcomes

Infertility should be recognized as a major medical problem because it affects up to 15 per cent of married couples. Although in 90 per cent of such couples the specific cause of infertility is identified, in only 50 per cent can it be treated successfully.[1, 2] The remaining couples are forced to resort to artificial insemination with donor semen, when appropriate, or to adoption, a less available alternative in recent years.

Up to 10 per cent of all couples who seek evaluation are found to have no identifiable problem, and have so-called *unexplained infertility*. The percentage of unexplained infertility cases has declined in recent years as more sophisticated evaluation methods have evolved through the renewed interest in basic research that has been stimulated by the marked reduction in numbers of infants offered for adoption. Contemporary therapeutic abortion policies, and the fact that 95 per cent of single mothers now keep their infants, have contributed to this situation.

Causes of Infertility

The causes of infertility can be subdivided into several categories (Table 1). It is evident that male factors and factors in which the male is partially involved (coital problems, sperm antibodies, timing of intercourse) constitute a major portion of infertility problems. The relatively large contribution of male factors to the overall problem has been little appreciated until recently. A decline in sperm counts in the general population has been noted in the last 20 to 30 years. This observation is of serious concern to specialists in the field because it raises the possibility that environmental factors, particularly the toxic by-products of our industrialized society, may be contributing to the decline.

Tubal factors in the female compose the other major category of infertility. Although congenital defects and endometriosis are occasionally responsible for tubal obstruction, gonorrheal and chlamydial infections and infectious complications of the use of intrauterine contraceptive devices are responsible for most tubal disease. Surgical repair of the infectious sequelae is an important therapeutic skill frequently demanded of infertility specialists. The increase in venereal disease in recent decades undoubtedly has been the principal cause of tubal disease and was a major impetus to the development of in vitro fertilization technology.

Evaluation Resources

Most infertile couples first seek advice from the wife's physician, usually an obstetrician-gynecologist. In recent years many gynecologists have concentrated solely on infertility problems and have become skilled in the evaluation of male factors as well. Reproductive endocrinology and infertility is now a recognized and certifiable subspeciality requiring fellowship training beyond the standard residency in obstetrics and gynecology.

Many family physicians have acquired expertise in the initial evaluation of the infertile couple. They are often in the unique position of knowing both partners' medical histories and are able to appreciate the impact of infertility on the couple's interpersonal dynamics. The family physician usually has no hesitation or reluctance about performing a complete physical examination of both partners, whereas the gynecologist by tradition has been reluctant to examine, or even discouraged from examining, the husband.

The urologist, in the same tradition, has been restricted to evaluation and treatment of male infertility. Unfortunately, until recently many urologists had meager interest or training in this area.

Table 1. CAUSES OF INFERTILITY

Infertility Factor	Percentage
Ovulatory factors	10–15
Numbers and quality of ova	
Follicle rupture mechanics	
Endocrine factors	
Timing	
Ovulatory failure (congenital, acquired)	
Male factors	40
Sperm quantity and quality	
Semen-mucus interaction	
Endocrine factors	
Sperm antibodies	
Tubal and uterine factors	20–30
Uterine anomalies and adhesions	
Tubal obstruction	
Tubo-ovarian adhesions	
Cervical factors	5
Deficient mucus	
Sperm antibodies	
Infections	
Combined factors	5
Sperm antibodies	
Adverse coital techniques	
Infections	
Unexplained infertility	10–15

Their infertility treatment skills are often limited to surgical repair of varicoceles, vasectomy reversal, and testicular biopsy. Like their counterparts in obstetrics and gynecology, only a minority of urologists are truly qualified by experience as infertility specialists. The American Fertility Society, through its official journal *Fertility and Sterility* and by sponsorship of annual meetings and regional seminars, has brought gynecologists, urologists, and basic medical scientists into an organization that promotes interdisciplinary study and understanding. It is unlikely that the traditional training of urologists and gynecologist will ever be modified to allow the emergence of a specialist skilled in the medical and surgical aspects of both male and female infertility. Ideally, the infertile couple is best served by a urologist-gynecologist team whose members devote a major share of their practices to infertility problems and are supported by a competent endocrinology-andrology laboratory.

HISTORY

The husband should be encouraged to accompany his wife to the initial evaluation interview. His perspective on common problems, his contributions to the taking of a complete history, and facilitation of his understanding about the relative importance of male factors are good reasons for this recommendation. He should be informed that a semen analysis is the first diagnostic step in an evaluation and ought to be done before other more expensive and invasive tests and procedures are considered. Including the husband from the outset promotes his continued involvement in what sometimes is a prolonged, frustrating, and expensive course of treatment.

Careful and detailed history-taking is essential in every infertility evaluation. Important clues may be elicited that quickly direct the course of evaluation toward specific factors of obvious importance.

Family History. The history of relative infertility in parents or other close relatives on rare occasions yields clues about the existence of an abnormal chromosome. One example is the syndrome of male infertility due to incomplete androgen expression, a partial androgen insensitivity in the testicular tissues that results in severe oligospermia or azospermia.[3] Polycystic ovarian disease with anovulation has also been reported to have a familial tendency, transmitted as an autosomal dominant, but it is responsive to ovulation-inducing agents.

More important is maternal history of infertility, recurrent abortion, reproductive difficulty, or a disease associated with decreased reproductive efficiency, especially diabetes mellitus. Infertile couples whose mothers have such a history may have been exposed to diethylstilbestrol (DES) in utero. DES exposure has now been reported as a cause of both male and female infertility.[4, 5] The female exposed in utero to DES may have cervical abnormalities and defective mucus, an increased rate of ectopic pregnancy, or a T-shaped uterus (demonstrated by hysterosalpingography). Male infertility due to DES exposure is reflected in epididymal cysts, hypotrophic testes, and severe sperm abnormalities.[4]

Social History. Infertility of either partner in a previous marriage naturally directs attention toward the involved partner but should not forestall the complete basic evaluation of both individuals, which should include the following information.

1. *Occupations.* Both partners should be queried regarding their exposure to environmental and industrial toxins, particularly chemicals, pesticides, herbicides, heavy metals, gases, anesthetic agents, and radiation sources. Prolonged exposure of the scrotal area to extremes of heat and cold may have deleterious effects on spermatogenesis.
2. *Social habits.* The adverse effects of alcohol, tobacco, marijuana, and other recreational drugs and their association with impaired fertility should be reviewed with the couple. Both partners should be urged to abstain from the use of these agents, permanently if possible, because all have been shown to be deleterious.
3. *Coital habits and technique.* The coital frequency and routines of the couple should be reviewed. The use of coital lubricants should be discouraged because they are generally spermicidal. Infrequent intercourse impairs fertility by reducing the opportunities for fertilization at the time of ovulation and by permitting a relative increase in the numbers of aging and less motile sperm. Too frequent intercourse is rarely an impediment. Daily ejaculation may diminish total sperm numbers but the percentage of motile sperm will be correspondingly increased. Alternate-day intercourse from the tenth to 18th days of the menstrual cycle will usually result in pregnancy if mistimed coitus is the only problem. Problems with premature ejaculation and ejaculatory failure may not be volunteered, but specific questions should be asked about such matters if the postcoital test shows absence of sperm in spite of a normal sperm count
4. *Previously undisclosed fertility.* The existence of previous proof of fertility in either partner, which may have been concealed from the other partner for obvious reasons, should be elicited by discreet questioning of each partner in the absence of the other. Positive information in this regard is invaluable but must remain confidential and unwritten lest it threaten the relationship of a couple whose ties may already be somewhat strained by their infertility problem.

Table 2 is a summary of the remaining sections

Table 2. ASSESSMENT OF INFERTILITY ACCORDING TO FACTOR

	History	Physical Examination	Diagnostic Studies
Ovulatory factors	Menstrual interval Age at menarche Mittelschmerz Weight change Dysmenorrhea Lactation Amenorrhea	Estrogen effects Cervical mucus Breast mass Vagina Androgen excess Hair pattern Clitoromegaly Acne Ovarian size Galactorrhea	Basal temperature chart Prolactin level Progesterone level LH and FSH levels Androgen profile Endometrial biopsy
Tubal and uterine factors	Menstrual pattern Previous surgery Infections IUD use Dysmenorrhea Habitual abortion Postpartum fever Pelvic pain	Uterus: Size Shape Position Tenderness Adnexa: Tenderness Masses Nodularity	Hysterosalpingography Laparoscopy Hysteroscopy Cultures
Male factors	Infections: Mumps Venereal disease Prostatitis Tuberculosis Cystic fibrosis Occupation Undescended testis Drug intake Surgery Recent febrile illness	Testes: Size Consistency Cryptorchidism Presence of epididymis and vas deferens Gynecomastia Hair pattern Hypospadias Varicocele	Semen analysis Zona-free hamster ova penetration test Postcoital test Antibody tests Endocrine tests: LH level FSH level Prolactin level Testosterone level Testicular biopsy
Cervical factors	Surgery: Conization Cauterization Induced abortion Habitual abortion Ovulation mucus DES exposure Venereal disease	Mucus: Amount Color Stenosis Lacerations Eversion-erosion Vaginitis	Mucus evaluation: Cellularity Fern pattern Spinnbarkeit Postcoital test Sperm penetration test Culture

of this discussion, in which the important aspects of medical history, physical examination, and diagnostic studies are detailed for each of the more difficult or controversial infertility factors enumerated in Table 1.

OVULATORY FACTORS

History

In women who report having predictably regular menstrual cycles at intervals of 25 to 32 days, one can usually assume that regular ovulation is occurring without resorting to clinical or laboratory assays for confirmation. Only a rare woman would have regular (monthly) anovulatory withdrawal bleeding episodes. Despite this fact, ovulation is generally confirmed by hormonal assays because it cannot be thought of as an all-or-none phenomenon. The hormonal quality of ovulation is an important concept. Similarly, a history of amenorrhea, infrequent menses, or irregular cycles suggests that infrequency or absence of ovulation needs to be considered. The clinician must obtain a precise previous and current menstrual history. When did menarche occur? When, if ever, were there regular monthly cycles? Have there been prolonged periods of secondary amenorrhea? Have there been occasional episodes of heavier bleeding, occurring 1 or 2 weeks after the period was expected, which suggest recurrent early spontaneous abortions? Has the patient experienced gradually worsening acne, hair growth, irregular cycles, and weight gain, suggesting polycystic ovary disease? Does the patient experience menstrual cramps (which frequently accompany ovulatory cycles)? Does she experience midcycle ovulation discomfort (mittelschmertz)? Has she charted her basal body temperature (BBT) throughout one or more cycles? Does the patient experience 2 or more days of premenstrual spotting, which would suggest an inadequate luteal phase due to diminished progesterone production after ovulation?

Physical Examination

A complete physical examination should be performed at the beginning of every infertility evaluation in which ovulatory dysfunction is suspected. The examiner looks for signs of increased circulating androgens—classically manifested by a male-pattern hair distribution (facial hair, coarse hair on the chest, inner thighs, and abdomen), acne lesions on the face and upper back, and clitoral enlargement. Increased circulating androgens can arise from the adrenals, ovaries, or exogenous sources.

A palpably enlarged or nodular thyroid gland may suggest thyroid dysfunction, which when extreme can lead to anovulation. Characteristic changes in skin, gastrointestinal function, and deep tendon reflexes may also point to this diagnosis.

The pelvic examination may disclose enlarged, firm ovaries typical of polycystic ovary disease. Cervical mucus may be abundant and clear, reflecting increased amounts of circulating estrogen derived from excessive luteinization of multiple immature follicles. Evaluation of pelvic organs is essential in cases of primary amenorrhea, because congenital absence of the vagina, cervix, and/or uterus may be associated with rare congenital disorders such as testicular feminization (androgen insensitivity syndrome), wherein XY individuals with insensitivity to normal circulating testosterone levels develop a typical female phenotype with large breasts, absence of pubic and axillary hair, absence of internal female pelvic organs, and presence of gonads (usually located inguinally) that must be removed because of their high malignant potential.

Extremes of body weight should also be noted. Anovulation is common in the very obese and in the woman whose body fat percentage has fallen below 20 per cent (commonly owing to deliberate weight loss, anorexia, or vigorous exercise habits). The breasts should be examined for inappropriate lactation (galactorrhea), which is seen when prolactin levels are increased. Table 3 lists a variety of causes for prolactin elevation.

Table 3. SOURCES OF ELEVATED PROLACTIN AND AMENORRHEA-GALACTORRHEA SYNDROME

Primary hypothyroidism
Adrenocortical insufficiency
Thoracotomy scars, chest burns
Pelvic surgery
Cervical spine lesions
Herpes zoster
Excessive nipple stimulation and suckling
Pituitary and hypothalamic tumors or lesions
Stress
Medications
Phenothiazines and derivatives
Opiates
Oral contraceptives
Methyldopa
Amphetamines
Diazepines
Butyrophenones
Reserpine and derivatives
Thioxanthenes

Diagnostic Studies

Ovulation, the physical release of the ovum from the ovarian follicle, is an event rarely witnessed and generally assumed only from indirect evidence or from a subsequent successful pregnancy. Indirect assessment of ovulation includes a biphasic basal body temperature chart (see Fig. 1), a properly timed midluteal serum progesterone determination, ultrasonographic demonstration of the formation and disappearance of an ovarian follicle (Fig. 2), and premenstrual endometrial biopsy.

A serum progesterone value greater than 10 ng/ml is an excellent indicator of adequate function of the corpus luteum, the postovulatory involuting follicle site on the overy that secretes progesterone. As shown in Figure 3, progesterone levels reach a peak about 1 week after ovulation. Samples obtained 1 to 2 days before or after this peak are generally greater than 10 ng/ml in successful conception cycles.[6] An endometrial biopsy specimen obtained 1 to 2 days before expected menstruation is a human bioassay for progesterone. An experienced pathologist can diagnose inadequate progesterone effect from the delay in expected maturation seen in the endometrial sample.

Inadequate luteal phase is diagnosed when the endometrial biopsy or progesterone determination demonstrates an abnormal progesterone level, which is presumed to be a cause of absolute infertility or habitual abortion. This diagnosis has been questioned by many experts. Most criticism points to the failure to demonstrate that the disorder occurs repetitively. No study has been published showing the defect to occur in large numbers of patients over several consecutive cycles. Controversy also extends to treatment of alleged progesterone insufficiency. One approach advocates postovulatory replacement with progesterone suppositories,[7] and another uses clomiphene-hCG preventive treatment in the follicular phase of the cycle.[6]

Luteinized unruptured follicle (LUF) syndrome, also a controversial new entity, is the diagnosis when

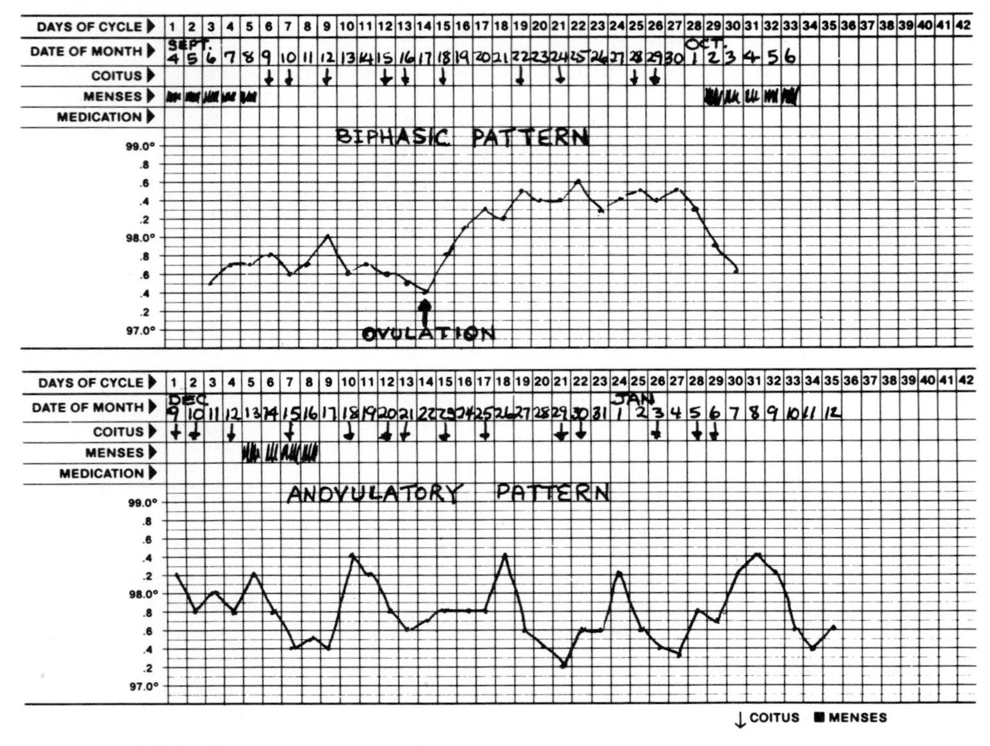

Figure 1. Basal body temperature charts illustrating biphasic ovulation cycle and monophasic anovulatory pattern.

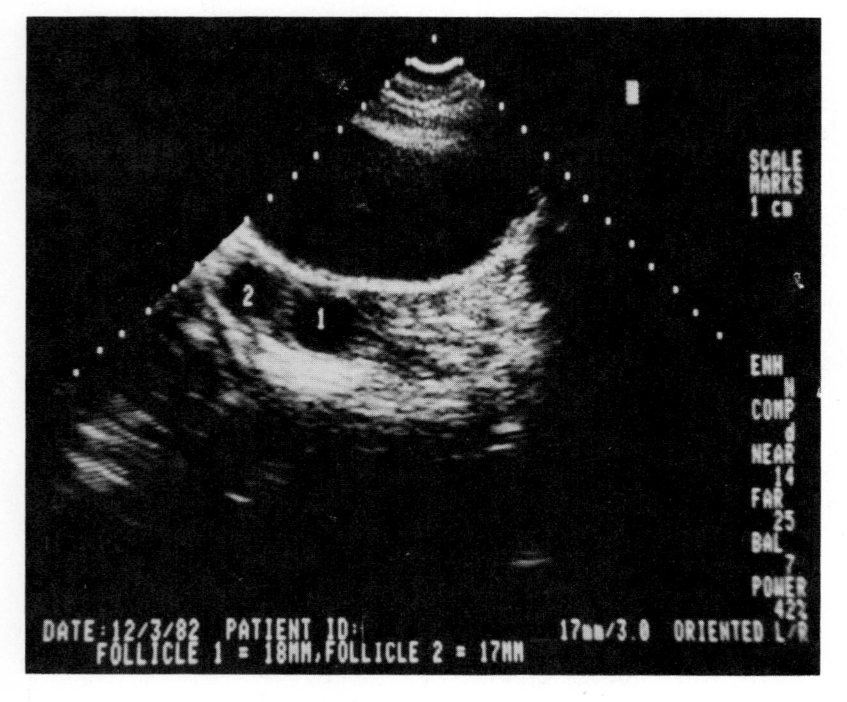

Figure 2. Ultrasound sector scan of pelvis showing mature ovarian follicle.

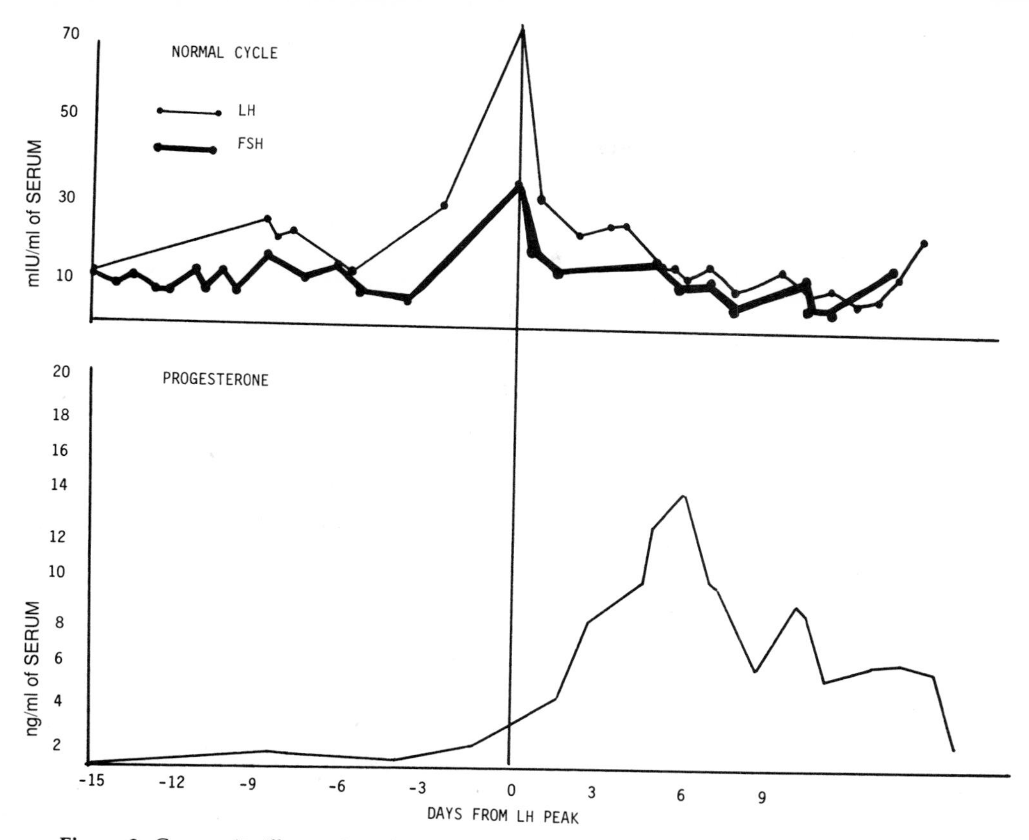

Figure 3. Composite illustration of changing endocrine values throughout the ovulatory cycle.

laparoscopy performed 1 to 2 days after apparent ovulation fails to show a typical ovulation stigma (the follicle opening seen after physical extrusion of the ovum) on the follicle surface. Although its etiology is obscure, LUF syndrome is associated with an increased incidence of simultaneous endometriosis. Some investigators believe that decreased peritoneal fluid levels of estrogen and progesterone, presumably due to failure of these steroids to be excreted directly by the unruptured follicle, favor the growth of intraperitoneal endometriosis implants that would normally be suppressed.[8] Critics of this concept cite failure to show that the phenomenon occurs in repetitive cycles, a finding that would require repeated laparoscopy, which no patient would tolerate. An hCG injection at the time of presumed ovulation is claimed to prevent this syndrome, possibly by promoting the factors necessary for follicular rupture (prostaglandins, enzymatic activity, increased follicular pressure) and may explain the higher pregnancy rates seen with a clomiphene-hCG regimen for ovulation induction than with clomiphene alone.

Hyperprolactinemia may impair or prevent normal ovulation and conception. Mild prolactin elevations in the luteal phase have been associated with infertility in patients who otherwise appear to have a normal ovulation cycle. There is normally a slight increase in the prolactin level during the luteal phase, so it is appropriate to measure both progesterone and prolactin levels in the midluteal phase, about 1 week after ovulation. Mild increases in prolactin may diminish the response of the endometrium to progesterone or, more likely, may impair the production of progesterone by the corpus luteum. More substantial elevations of prolactin (greater than 50 ng/ml) have a direct effect on production of gonadotropins from the pituitary and are often associated with absolute absence of ovulation. Prolactin elevation may be due to any of the causes listed in Table 3, which should be eliminated by appropriate investigation. Levels greater than 100 ng/ml, when not otherwise explained, may be caused by functioning pituitary tumor, particularly microadenoma, which should be ruled out by obtaining polytomogram x-rays of the pituitary sella. Trans-sphenoidal resection of prolactin-secreting adenomas is an accepted surgical remedy that has restored fertility to many anovulatory patients. Bromoergocryptine, an effective prolactin-suppressing agent, has been used with success in many hyperprolactinemic states, including some small pituitary adenomas.

Anovulation or infrequent ovulation, as distinguished from deficiencies in the otherwise normal ovulatory cycle, may be categorized as having one

Table 4. CATEGORIES OF OVARIAN FAILURE

Category	Laboratory Values	Clinical States
Primary ovarian failure	FSH >40 mIU/ml	Normal menopause Premature menopause Gonadal dysgenesis (Turner's syndrome, mosaic forms) Resistant ovary syndrome Gonadal agenesis Gonadotropin-secreting tumors
Hypothalamic-pituitary disorders	FSH <5 mIU/ml LH <5 mIU/ml	Pituitary tumors Pituitary insufficiency Anorexia nervosa Malnutrition Stress Postpill amenorrhea
Gonadotropin asynchrony	LH >25 mIU/ml FSH low or normal	Polycystic ovary disease Adrenal hyperplasia Obesity Androgen-producing ovarian tumor

of three distinct causes: primary ovarian failure, hypothalamic-pituitary disorders, or gonadotropin asynchrony (Table 4).

Anovulation or infrequent ovulation may be suspected on the basis of a history of amenorrhea or infrequent menstrual bleeding. Preliminary confirmation is offered by absence of a biphasic temperature pattern on the BBT chart (see Fig. 1). A luteal phase temperature elevation above 98.0°F is a direct biologic effect of progesterone but may be seen with a progesterone level as low as 2 ng/ml, which may not be compatible with sustained pregnancy. The premenstrual endometrial biopsy shows (1) "proliferative endometrium," the absence of a progesterone effect, (2) "atrophic" changes in cases of low estrogen activity, or (3) "hyperplasia" when estrogen levels are sustained or elevated (as in the polycystic ovary syndrome).

The best screening laboratory test is a measurement of gonadotropins—luteinizing hormone (LH) and follicle-stimulating hormone (FSH). Table 4 shows how LH and FSH levels determine the category of anovulatory disorder and direct the clinician toward a more precise diagnosis.

Ovarian Failure

Primary ovarian failure (hypergonadotropic hypogonadism) is diagnosed when FSH levels are greater than 40 mIU/ml. It implies gonadal failure with exhaustion or congenital absence of primordial oocytes. Since ovulation is impossible in such cases, infertility is absolute and the use of ovulation-inducing agents would be futile. This process is the normal course of events seen at the menopause, which may occur as early as age 35 (premature menopause). In younger patients, primary or secondary amenorrhea due to primary ovarian failure is most often due to congenital sex chromosome disorders such as Turner's syndrome (XO) or the other mosaic forms of gonadal dysgenesis such as XO/XX, XO/XY, and XX/XY. The importance of these disorders is two-fold. First, although most patients with a typical clinical appearance of Turner's syndrome (short stature, shield chest, webbed neck, increased carrying angle) will be karyotyped as XO, a few are XO/XX mosaics with XX gonads. Such women have a limited ovulation potential that may soon be exhausted. More important are mosaic individuals with Y chromosomes in their gonads (usually streak gonads). Such Y-bearing gonads have a high malignant potential and should be removed upon detection, to prevent both malignant change and virilization of the phenotypic female. Karyotyping of peripheral blood may not detect all mosaics with Y chromosomes. The use of H-Y antigen assays is increasingly used to detect Y chromosome–bearing tissues in such individuals.

The *resistant ovary syndrome* is a rare disorder in which an anovulatory patient with elevated gonadotropins has a normal XX karyotype. Ovarian biopsy reveals the presence of normal ovarian follicles. These rare individuals, as well as a few normal patients with apparent premature ovarian failure, may ovulate after receiving very high doses of human menopausal gonadotropins (hMG), an equal mixture of FSH and LH. It is presumed that their ovarian tissue has gonadotropin receptors deficient in numbers or sensitivity. *Gonadal agenesis* is total absence of gonadal tissue, either congenital or acquired through prepubertal viral, metabolic, or immunologic injury.

Hypothalamic-Pituitary Disorders

Hypothalamic-pituitary disorders (hypogonadotropic hypogonadism) are those conditions that result in inadequate gonadotropin (LH, FSH) stimulation of otherwise normal ovaries. The clinical presentation may be identical to that of primary ovarian failure, but the prognosis is infinitely better. The challenge lies in detecting the etiologic conditions that are treatable or potentially dangerous, and in separating pituitary disorders from those of higher origin in the hypothalamus. Clinically, affected women are usually normal except for signs of estrogen deficiency (vaginal mucosal atrophy, breast atrophy, scanty cervical mucus, amenorrhea, failure to have withdrawal menses after progestin challenge). A few may show systemic manifestations of pituitary diseases, including acromegaly, Cushing's syndrome, Addison's disease, galactorrhea, and hypothyroidism. Routine evaluation for evidence of pituitary malfunction when the gonadotropins (LH, FSH) are abnormally low includes determination of serum prolactin, ACTH, thyroid-stimulating hormone (TSH), and growth hormone levels. Abnormal elevations or subnormal levels of these pituitary hormones compel the clinician to search for a pituitary tumor via sellar polytomograms and, if necessary, pneumoencephalograms. After appropriate treatment of the pituitary disorder, if pregnancy is permitted by the patient's general condition, ovulation can usually be induced with human menopausal gonadotropins (hMG), an equal mixture of FSH and LH.

Hypothalamic disorders, generally diagnosed by the exclusion of pituitary disease, are the most common conditions in this category. Most are related to temporary stress, such as the transient anovulation and amenorrhea seen in young women entering college or professional school. In most cases the condition is temporary, and ovulation returns a few months after abatement of the stressful situation. A more troublesome example is *anorexia nervosa,* a psychiatric disorder manifested by severe weight loss that can eventuate in cachexia and death. Ovulation should not be induced with gonadotropins until the underlying psychiatric disorder has been remedied. Successful therapy and weight gain usually lead to spontaneous ovulation.

Gonadotropin Asynchrony

The remaining disorders, of which *polycystic ovarian disease* (PCO) is the most common example, involve disordered ovulation in previously normal ovaries. The precise etiology of polycystic ovary disease (Stein-Levinthal syndrome) is unknown. Many believe that it involves a gradual and progressive deterioration in the complex feedback system between the ovarian steroids, especially estradiol, and the centers of gonadotropin regulation and stimulation in the hypothalamus. The estrogen (estradiol) feedback regulation involves both "tonic" and "cyclic" gonadotropin responses in the hypothalamic-pituitary axis. Thus, either an abnormally sustained estrogen feedback or a failure of the "cyclic" gonadotropin response could result in a "steady state" of pituitary gonadotropin secretion rather than the "surges" that appear to trigger ovulation.

Whatever the primary defect, the result is a constant overproduction of luteinizing hormone (LH) in the face of a normal or low level of follicle-stimulating hormone (FSH). This situation causes a large number of follicles to undergo minimal enlargement (from FSH) while being excessively luteinized (from increased LH). Such polycystic ovaries secrete abundant levels of estrogen as well as excessive levels of androgens, particularly androstenedione and testosterone, owing to chronic LH stimulation of the ovarian stroma. Peripheral conversion of adrenal or ovarian androgens to estrogens adds further to the persistent estrogen elevation. The lack of variability or cyclicity in estrogen levels reinforces the gonadotropin "steady state" secretion and perpetuates the chronic anovulation. Excessive androgen output, if sustained, may gradually result in signs of virilization (acne, weight gain, excessive hair growth).

Successful therapy depends on interruption of the steady state and restoration of cyclic estrogen and gonadotropin production. Removal of functioning ovarian tissue with a wedge resection causes an abrupt decline in ovarian estrogen and androgen sources and restores cyclicity and ovulation in a majority of patients. Clomiphene citrate, a rather weak estrogen, restores cyclicity and ovulation by occupying and inducing a reduction in estrogen receptors in the hypothalamus, causing it to "sense" a lowered estrogen level. The hypothalamus responds with a gonadotropin-releasing hormone surge, which then triggers pituitary FSH production, normal follicle maturation, and ovulation. Any physiologic or pathologic disease process that contributes added estrogen and dampens the normal cyclic variation in estrogen levels could compound or even initiate the problem. Conversion of the androgens originating from mild adrenal hyperplasia, and more efficient conversion in the adipose tissues of an obese woman, are both possible contributions to the problem. The end result is identical: a steady state of chronic anovulation with estrogen and androgen excess.

When the LH and FSH values are consistent with this diagnosis (LH elevated, FSH low or low normal), serum testosterone and dehydroepiandrosterone sulfate (DHEA-S) levels should be measured. Abnormally elevated testosterone levels (>2.0 ng/ml) indicate a need to search for an ovarian or adrenal tumor. An elevated DHEA-S level implicates the adrenal as the source of the increased androgens. Adrenal hyperactivity should be verified by a dexamethasone suppression test, which will temporarily reduce the androgens to normal levels.

TUBAL AND UTERINE FACTORS

Blockage or damage to the fallopian tubes and intrauterine disease are factors that must be sought and excluded early in the course of an infertility evaluation. Important elements of their assessment are outlined in Table 2.

History

The amount of menstrual flow should be assessed. Scanty menstruation, or secondary amenorrhea occurring in women who have regular monthly premenstrual symptoms, is seen with *Asherman's syndrome* (intrauterine synechiae). Intrauterine adhesions occur when the endometrium has been denuded by a vigorous dilatation and curettage procedure after an incomplete abortion or postpartum hemorrage, accompanied by an intrauterine infection or endometritis. Heavy or prolonged periods may result from intrauterine endometrial polyps or submucous leiomyomata (fibroids). *Habitual abortion*, the occurrence of three consecutive early pregnancy losses in the absence of a preceding viable pregnancy, increases suspicion of a congenital uterine duplication anomaly such as a bicornuate or septate uterus (Fig. 4).

A history of pelvic inflammatory disease or previous use of an intrauterine contraceptive device (IUD) is associated with increased rates of damage and blockage of the fallopian tubes. Postpartum endometritis and salpingitis occasionally are misdiagnosed as urinary tract infections but may result in identical tubal damage. Atypical dysmenorrhea of relatively late onset, with symptoms predominating after the first day of flow, suggests endometriosis.

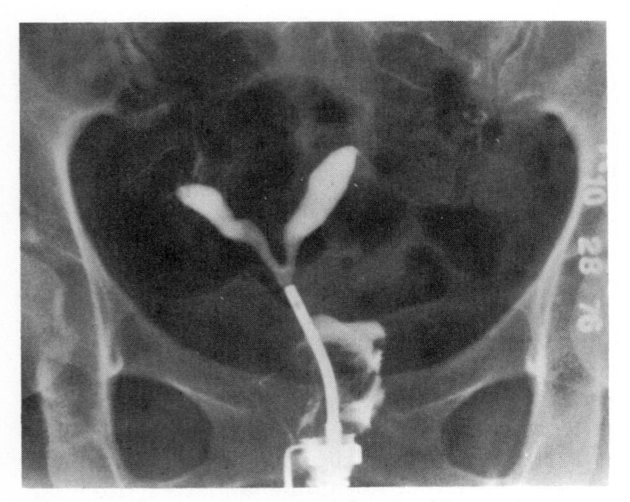

Figure 4. Hysterosalpingogram showing bicornuate uterus.

Previous pelvic surgery, especially with infectious complications, has a high potential for subsequent tubal damage. A ruptured appendix may spread infection to the tubes. Manipulation of the tubes or ovaries during surgery for tubal ectopic pregnancy or during an ovarian wedge resection for polycystic ovarian disease carries a high probability of subsequent tubal or tubo-ovarian adhesions, which are thought to be due to abrasions or drying of serosal or peritoneal surfaces with subsequent fibrin deposition and scarring. Ectopic pregnancy is often caused by intrinsic or congenital tubal disease and is likely to recur.

Physical Examination

The uterus should be of normal size, with a symmetric contour and smooth surface. Passive movement of the organ should not be uncomfortable. Uterine retroversion is not in itself abnormal, although a fixed retroverted uterus may be the result of a previous cul-de-sac abscess or endometriosis. Uterine enlargement suggests possible adenomyosis (myometrial endometriosis), whereas asymmetry or palpable external nodularity points to concomitant intrauterine fibroids.

Unusual tenderness on uterine or adnexal motion or palpation may occur with endometriosis and tubo-ovarian adhesions secondary to infectious processes. Cervicitis or purulent cervical mucus is seen with infections by gonococcus or Chlamydia, the two organisms that appear to be responsible for the majority of cases of salpingitis and pelvic infection.[9]

Tender uterosacral nodularity is the hallmark of endometriosis and is best appreciated when palpation is performed during menstruation.

Diagnostic Assessment

The contemporary assessment of tubal and uterine factors depends on an extension of physical inspection made possible by recent improvements in technical instrumentation. Hysterosalpingography is an indispensible diagnostic tool that should be used early in the evaluation, especially when the history suggests a tubal factor (Fig. 5). A water-soluble x-ray contrast medium is injected transcervically into the uterus, and the filling of the uterus and fallopian tubes is monitored fluoroscopically. The test is done in the week between the end of menstruation and ovulation. Optimally,

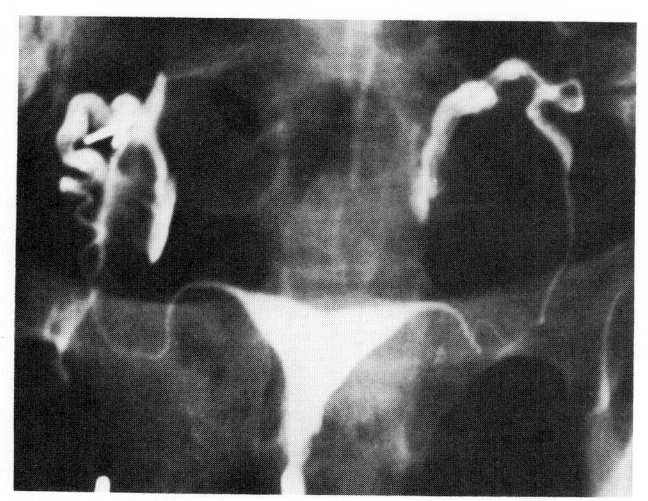

Figure 5. Hysterosalpingogram showing normal uterine cavity, normal Fallopian tubes, and bilateral spill of contrast medium into peritoneal cavity.

it is a combined effort of radiologist and gynecologist.

The normally triangular intrauterine contour is assessed. Bicornuate shapes and midline septa are obvious, but even minimal "subseptate" indentations of the superior fundal contour have been reported to cause infertility.[10] The DES infertility syndrome may be diagnosed after discovery of a "T-shaped" uterine cavity. Polyps should be suspected when an area of decreased radiographic density is seen. Intrauterine adhesions present a grossly distorted, moth-eaten appearance.

After filling of the uterine cavity, there should be prompt bilateral filling of both fallopian tubes and rapid intraperitoneal spill within a few minutes. Residual contrast medium should outline the rugal folds of the lateral ampullary portion of the tubes. Fimbrial occlusion presents a typical dilated distal tubal appearance characteristic of hydrosalpinx (Fig. 6). Modern microsurgical techniques make possible tubal patency and subsequent pregnancy in a high percentage of such cases. It is therefore important to accurately identify the precise point of obstruction, so that the infertility surgeon can resect a small portion of obstructed tube and anastomose the remaining patent segments.

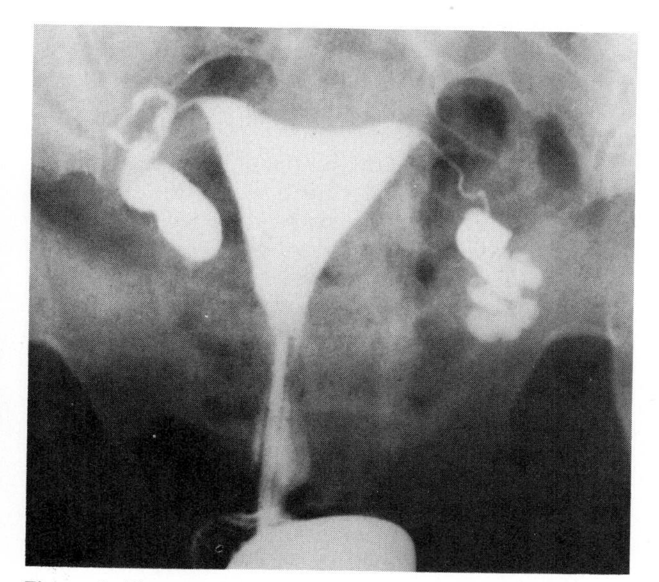

Figure 6. Hysterosalpingogram showing bilateral fimbrial occlusion with resultant hydrosalpinx.

Laparoscopy has become the most valuable tool in the assessment and treatment of tubal and tubo-ovarian disease. Insertion of the 10-mm diameter fiberoptic instrument through a periumbilical incision enables an unobstructed direct view of the pelvic viscera. The diagnostic and prognostic value of this technique is remarkable. Tubal patency can be confirmed by introducing dilute methylene blue dye solution through the cervix. Endometriosis is easily identified, and small implants can be coagulated with instruments introduced through the laparoscopy incision or through second-puncture sites in the suprapubic area. Avascular adhesions involving the tubes, ovaries, or uterus can be cut with operating scissors. Ova contained in mature ovarian follicles can be aspirated through special needles, an important step in the in vitro fertilization procedure. "Second look" laparoscopy is frequently used for prognosis after tubal surgery or medical therapy of endometriosis.

A similar instrument of smaller diameter, the hysteroscope, is introduced through the cervix to visualize the endometrial cavity, permitting diagnosis and treatment of intrauterine adhesions, polyps, fibroids, and septa. Although the hysteroscope has only recently been introduced, most infertility specialists expect it to be in routine use in the near future.

The recent introduction of in vitro fertilization procedures offers new hope to women with irreparable tubal damage and may soon be utilized for a wide variety of infertility problems. It is potentially useful in situations of oligospermia, antisperm antibodies, hostile cervical mucus, and "unexplained" infertility, although the procedure is still in the developmental stage and its ultimate success rate and utility are yet to be determined.

MALE FACTORS

History

Too often, the male partner's complete history is taken only after a semen analysis has revealed an abnormality of sperm morphology, motility, or count (sperm density). Table 2 outlines several historical elements that may explain an adverse male factor.

Mumps orchitis, if bilateral, may produce azospermia through destruction of the sperm-producing germinal epithelium that lines the seminiferous tubules. Tuberculosis and gonorrhea may involve and obstruct the vas deferens. Gonorrhea and other bacterial infections of the genital tract often depress sperm count and motility. Cystic fibrosis is sometimes associated with congenital absence of the vas deferens. If an undescended testicle (cryptorchidism) is corrected before age 6 fertility is seldom compromised.

Any acute febrile illness can cause a moderate temporary depression of sperm production. Since the entire spermatogenic cycle takes 64 days, it is wise to repeat the sperm count after 3 months before diagnosing an adverse male factor solely on the basis of semen analysis. Obviously, azospermia or severe oligospermia should be investigated whenever the condition becomes known.

Occupational history is important in determining exposure to extremes of heat and cold as well as to industrial chemicals, toxins, and pesticides. Extreme cold and heat, which depress spermatogenesis, have been reported to cause infertility in truck drivers, steel workers, and devotees of the sauna and hot tub. A wide variety of industrial solvents, chemicals, heavy metals, pesticides, radiation sources, radar emanations, and other agents encountered in our industrialized society have the potential to adversely affect male fertility. Limitation of exposure to these agents may lead to an improvement in seminal parameters, although a direct causal relationship remains speculative or unproven in most cases.

The medical history is often more rewarding. An inguinal hernia repair may compromise the testicular blood supply or accidentally obstruct the vas deferens. Perineal or pelvic surgery may affect sympathetic innervation and lead to retrograde ejaculation, a condition also associated with diabetes mellitus and the ingestion of certain antihypertensive medications (guanethidine, barbiturates, phenothiazines). Chemotherapy for leukemia and Hodgkin's disease, especially the use of busulfan (Myleran) and cyclophosphamide (Cytoxan), usually results in permanent sterility. The nitrofurantoins, antibiotics frequently used for urinary tract infections, may arrest spermatogenesis temporarily. Monamine oxidase inhibitors frequently cause severe depression of the sperm count. Amebicides and antimalarials have been associated with temporary oligospermia, recovery from which may take 6 to 12 months. Excessive use of alcohol, heroin, and marijuana has been reported to impair fertility. Spironolactone and cimetidine may impair spermatogenesis by occupying testosterone receptors.

Physical Examination

The general examination may yield clues about systemic and endocrine disease. Gynecomastia and aberrations of height, weight, and hair pattern direct attention toward rare chromosomal disorders such as Klinefelter's syndrome (XXY). More often, direct inspection and palpation of the external genitalia yield the most information. Hypospadias and penile lesions should be obvious. Presence of the vas deferens should be confirmed. Nodularity or beading of the vas deferens or epididymis indicates possible obstruction or chronic infection of the structure. A varicocele—a dilated internal spermatic vein—may impair sperm production, producing the so-called stress pattern (increased immature forms with decreased motility) on semen analysis. Surgical repair of varicoceles improves the sperm count in more than 75 per cent of cases and will lead to pregnancy in at least 50 per cent.

The size and consistency of the testicles should be ascertained. Decreased size and softening are frequently seen with hypogonadism and lack of androgen stimulation or as infection sequelae. Rectal examination should be performed to confirm prostatic size, consistency, and tenderness. Prostatic fluid, if obtained, should be examined for leukocytes, the presence of which suggests infection.

Diagnostic Assessment

The specimen for a semen analysis, the single most important test of male fertility, is customarily obtained at the couple's first or second visit. The female should never be subjected to costly, invasive, or time-consuming tests and procedures until the results of the semen analysis are known. The essential elements of an optimal semen analysis are shown in Figure 7. Fertility is generally impaired when a sperm count is below 20 million/ml, and fertility is unusual if it is less than 10 million/ml. Subnormal counts and motility often occur together, indicating a basic problem of spermatogenesis at the testicular level.

The presence of more than 4 white blood cells per high-power microscopic field is highly suggestive of infection. Tetracycline therapy may be rewarding in such cases, because recent evidence indicates that T mycoplasma *(Ureaplasma urealyticum)* and chlamydial infections may be associated with infertility in both partners.

Complexes of agglutinated spermatozoa may be seen on microscopic examination of a drop of semen. Hundreds of sperm may be involved in these complexes, which form when sperm react with antibodies in the seminal plasma. Antibodies

SEMEN ANALYSIS

Name: ______	Viscosity: ____
Physician: ______	1. normal
Type of Specimen: ____	2. slightly viscous
1. fresh	3. very viscous
2. diluted	Count: ____ × 10⁶/ml
3. post-thaw	Total Count: ____ × 10⁶
Date of Specimen: ______	Progressively Motile: ____ %
Time of Collection: ______	Mean Progressive Motility: ____
Complete Sample: ____	0. none
1. yes	1. poor
2. no	2. good
Days of Abstinence: ____	3. excellent
Method of Collection: ____	Agglutination: ____
1. masturbation	0. none
2. intercourse interrupt	1. small clumps
3. other (specify): ______	2. large clumps
Time Since Collection: ____ hrs	Agglutination Type: ____
Liquefaction Time: ____ min	1. head-to-head
Volume: ____ ml	2. head-to-tail
pH: ____	3. tail-to-tail
Color: ____	Normal Spermatozoa: ____ %
1. normal	Abnormal Spermatozoa: ____ %
2. white	Abnormal Forms, Predominant Type(s): ______
3. yellow	Leukocyte Concentration: ____

Figure 7. Sample of a semen analysis record.

are frequently seen after vasectomy and may reduce fertility rates after vasectomy reversal. It is presumed that vasectomy promotes extravasation of sperm antigens into the general circulation, with resultant antibody formation. Shulman and colleagues[12] have reported successful treatment of male sperm antibodies with short-term high-dose steroid therapy. Most often, the individual with sperm antibodies has no history of vasectomy, infection, or testicular trauma.

When the semen analysis shows moderate or marked diminution in sperm density, motility, and morphology, an endocrinologic basis is often suspected. Testosterone, LH, FSH, and prolactin levels are generally measured. In most cases the results are normal, although the FSH level may be elevated in some cases of azospermia or extreme oligospermia.

The evaluation of impaired male fertility is often quite frustrating. In less than 10 per cent of infertile men can any definite cause be found, and successful treatment is equally rare. Many "empirical" regimens have evolved, using thyroid, androgens, clomiphene, human chorionic gonadotropins, and prolactin inhibitors, to name only a few. It is doubtful that any will be shown to result in significant improvement in male fertility. Artificial insemination with donor semen (AID) has enjoyed increasing popularity in recent decades as a solution to the still largely unexplained state of male infertility.[13]

One new test offers additional prognostic information. The zona-free hamster ova penetration test (Fig. 8) calculates the percentage of hamster ova, freed of zona pellucida covering by enzymatic treatment, that are penetrated by human spermatozoa.The resultant percentages correlate well with clinical male fertility potential.[14] In a small proportion of cases, a man with a normal semen analysis result has a very low hamster ova penetration score, indicating a qualitative defect of the spermatozoa. Low scores may also be seen in the presence of sperm antibodies and increased leukocytes.

CERVICAL FACTORS

Adverse cervical factors are a diagnostic and therapeutic challenge to infertility specialists, because the cervix is subject to a wide variety of immune, infectious, congenital, endocrine, and traumatic disorders.

History

Previous medical-surgical events are primary items of importance in the evaluation of adverse cervical factors (see Table 2). Destruction of mucus-producing endocervical glands by conization or cauterization procedures can reduce the amount of cervical mucus available for reception and transport, and perhaps storage, of spermatozoa in and through the cervix. Repeated spontaneous abortions, especially after one or more induced abortions, suggest a structural weakness in the cervix itself, a condition amenable to surgical repair. The patient with predictable monthly cycles is often aware of a midcycle mucus secretion. Prenatal exposure to diethylstilbestrol (DES syndrome) can produce characteristic genital tract changes, including cervical hoods, "cock's-comb" deformities, a T-shaped uterine cavity, adenosis (deposits of ectopic cervical-type glands in the vagina), and deficient cervical mucus.[5] The presence of T mycoplasmas and Chlamydia in cervical mucus have been associated with abnormal postcoital test results and poor sperm survival.

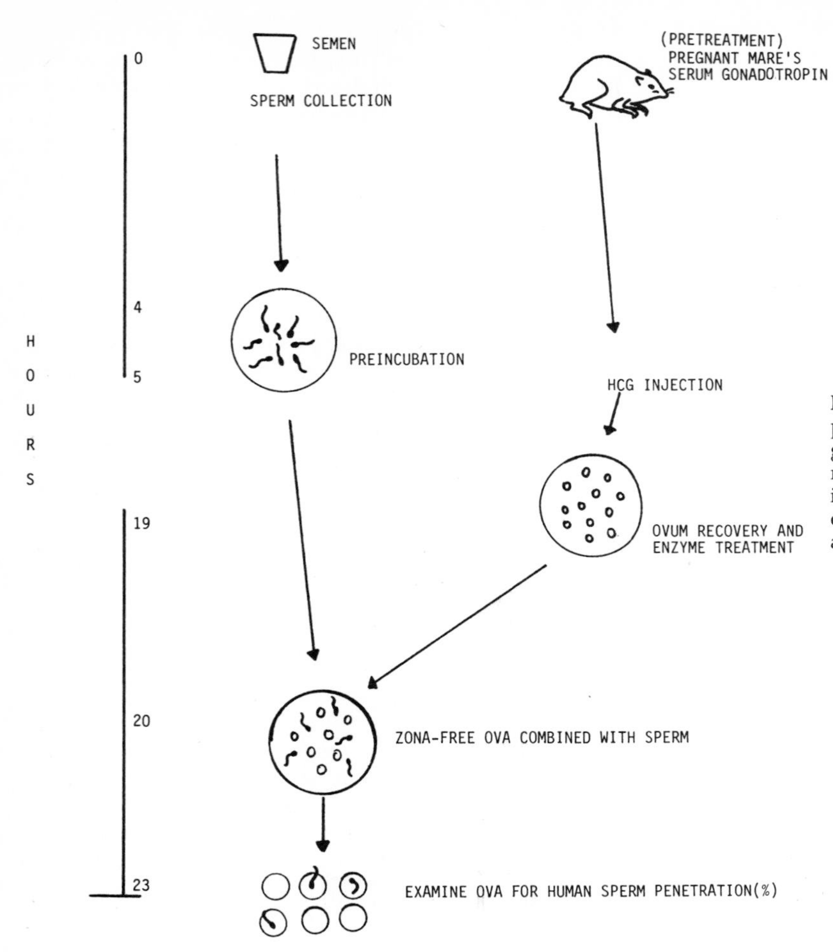

Figure 8. The zona-free hamster ova sperm penetration test. The ova of super-ovulated golden hamsters are treated with enzymes to remove the zona pellucida covering. After incubation with human sperm, the percentage of eggs penetrated is compared with results of a test using a fertile control.

Physical Examination

Deviations from the normal appearance of the cervix should be noted, with the cyclic variation of mucus production taken into account. Mucus production peaks in the days preceding ovulation and parallels the estrogen surge resulting from rapid growth of ovulation follicles. A severe "fish-mouth" cervical laceration from previous childbirth can expose the endocervical glandular epithelium to vaginal pathogens and reduce normal mucus production. Previous surgery or a congenital condition can result in a narrowed, stenotic cervical os. It is doubtful that stenosis per se is a cause of infertility. Associated damage to endocervical epithelium and mucus glands is the more probable cause. At times other than midcycle, cervical mucus may be thick and reduced in quantity, but it should not be purulent at any time. A visible yellowish cast, with heavy leukocytic infiltration on microscopic examination, strongly suggests an infectious process. Concurrent vaginitis and infections of the endocervix and mucus glands are relative rather than absolute impairments to fertility, but they may assume greater importance when combined with other adverse factors, especially diminished sperm count and presence of sperm antibodies.

Diagnostic Assessment

The *postcoital test* is invaluable in assessing the cervical factor.[15] It should be scheduled to coincide with the presumed day of ovulation or the day preceding, and proper timing should be confirmed with concurrent BBT recordings or ultrasonographic demonstration of mature ovarian follicle development (>20 mm diameter). Intercourse should be performed from 8 to 16 hours before the test; if it is done much earlier than this, the delayed adverse effects of infection or mucus antibodies might not be apparent. Specimens of mucus are collected at the external cervical os and from a point higher up in the endocervical canal. The higher specimen should show at least 10 motile spermatazoa per high-power microscopic field. Gross inspection of the cervix should reveal abundant, crystal-clear mucus that can be drawn out in 15- to 20-cm threads (spinnbarkeit), a reflection of increased estrogen effect resulting in increased sodium chloride and water content. This same biochemical phenomenon is responsible for the crystalized "fern pattern" seen when periovulatory mucus is viewed microscopically after being air-dried.

The sperm penetration test is a recent innovation that serves as an in vitro assay of sperm progression in mucus.[16] A 6-inch column of bovine cervical mucus is placed in a semen sample, and the depth of sperm penetration into the mucus column is assessed after 2 hours. Failure to penetrate a minimal length of the mucus column indicates that the sperm have an inherent defect in motility or are being affected by seminal sperm antibodies or infection. The use of standardized bovine mucus eliminates variables associated with individual patient mucus samples.

Sperm antibodies may be produced by either partner against antigens from several distinct parts of the spermatozoon.[17] It is necessary to utilize a number of tests in a complete antibody survey of the couple. Ordinarily, each partner's serum is tested against both the husband's sperm and antibody-free donor sperm. Treatment of antibody problems is difficult and may be approached in two ways. The first involves lowering the female antibody titer by avoiding sperm contact through prolonged (6 to 12 months) use of condoms. Alternatively, either or both partners can receive large-dose short-term suppressive steroid therapy.[12]

UNEXPLAINED INFERTILITY

Despite a decade of intensive investigation into the causes of infertility, no abnormality can be detected in at least 10 per cent of couples. Many such couples are presumed to be affected with subtle enzymatic deficiencies, immunologic problems (perhaps to surface antigens of the ovum), sperm metabolic deficits, and other conditions. It is a serious error to tell these couples that there is "nothing wrong." Their chances of achieving a pregnancy are extremely low. Donor insemination and in vitro fertilization may be offered as a last resort, but a favorable outcome could not be expected. Although it is tempting to offer "empirical" therapy, such treatment is usually fruitless and expensive and offers false hope. A more realistic approach is to tell the couple that present diagnostic tests are unable to detect the cause of their problem but the physician believes a problem exists, and that their present chances for pregnancy are low. They should be offered periodic reassessment, in the event that new discoveries may be applicable to them, and advised that adoption may be the only current alternative.

REFERENCES

1. Speroff L. Investigation of the infertile couple. In: Speroff L, Glass RH, Kase NG, eds. Clinical gynecologic endocrinology and infertility. Baltimore, Williams & Wilkins, 1978;315–41.
2. Hammond MG, Talbert LM. Infertility—a practical guide for the physician. Chapel Hill, NC, Health Services Consortium, Inc, 1981.
3. Morris J. Gonadal anomalies and dysgenesis. In: Gehrman SJ, Kistner RW, eds. Progress in infertility. Boston, Little, Brown, 1975;265–79.
4. Gill WB, Schumacher GFB, Bibbo, M. Pathological semen and anatomical abnormalities of the genital tract in human male subjects exposed to diethylstilbestrol in utero. J Urol 1977;117:477–80.
5. Herbst AL, Poskanzer DC, Robboy SJ, Friedlander L, Scully RE. Prenatal exposure to stilbestrol. A prospective comparison of exposed female offspring with unexposed controls. N Engl J Med 1975;292:334–9.
6. Shepard MK, Senturia YD. Comparison of serum progesterone and endometrial biopsy for confirmation of ovulation and evaluation of luteal function. Fertil Steril 1977;28:541–8.
7. Jones GS, Aksel S, Wentz AC. Serum progesterone values in the luteal phase defects. Effect of chorionic gonadotropin. Obstet Gynecol 1974;44:26–34.
8. Koninckx PR, Ide P, Vandenbroucke W, Brosens IA. New aspects of the pathophysiology of endometriosis and associated infertility. J Reprod Med 1980;24:257–60.
9. Westrom L. Effect of acute pelvic inflammatory disease on fertility. Am J Obstet Gynecol 1975;121:707–13.
10. Nickerson, CW. Infertility and uterine contour. Am J Obstet Gynecol 1977;129:268–73.
11. Toth A, Martin LL, Brooks B, Labroila A. Subsequent pregnancies among 161 couples treated for T-mycoplasma genital tract infection. N Engl J Med 1983;308:505–7.
12. Shulman S, Harlin B, Davis P, Reyniak JV. Immune infertility and new approaches to treatment. Fertil Steril 1978;29:309–13.
13. Steinberger E, Smith KD. Artificial insemination with fresh or frozen semen. JAMA 1973;233:778–83.
14. Stenchever MA, Spadoni LR, Smith WD, Karp LE, Shy KK, Moore DE, Berger R. Benefits of the sperm (hamster ova) penetration assay in the evaluation of the infertile couple. Am J Obstet Gynecol 1982;143:91–6.
15. Gibor Y, Garcia CJ, Cohen MR, Scommegna A. The cyclical changes in physical properties of the cervical mucus and the results of the postcoital test. Fertil Steril 1970;21:20–7.
16. Moghissi KS, Segal S, Meinhold D, Agronow SJ. *In vitro* sperm cervical mucus penetration: studies in human and bovine cervical mucus. Fertil Steril 1982;37:823–7.
17. Menge AC, Medley NE, Mangione CM, Dietrich JW. The incidence and influence of antisperm antibodies in infertile human couples on sperm–cervical mucus interactions and subsequent fertility. Fertil Steril 1982; 38:439–46.

JAUNDICE

ROBERT T. MANNING

☐ SYNONYM: Icterus

BACKGROUND

Definitions

Jaundice, a yellow discoloration of the skin or sclera, is produced by accumulation of bilirubin in the serum with subsequent deposition in subcutaneous tissues. The word jaundice is derived from the French *jaune* meaning yellow and the word *icterus* from the Greek word meaning a yellow discoloration.

Total serum bilirubin, routinely determined by clinical laboratories, may be fractionated by chemical methods into unconjugated and conjugated portions. Synonyms for unconjugated bilirubin include: indirect and delayed serum bilirubin; and for conjugated bilirubin: direct, immediate, prompt, or "1-minute" serum bilirubin. Most hospital laboratories continue to use *indirect bilirubin* for the unconjugated form and *direct bilirubin* for the conjugated fraction.

Normal range for total serum bilirubin is 0.2 to 1.2 mg/100 ml. Ordinarily, the conjugated fraction is less than 15 per cent of the total, or 0 to 0.2 mg/100 ml with an upper limit of 1.0 mg/100 ml for unconjugated bilirubin. Visual detection of jaundice is usually not possible until the total serum bilirubin is more than 3 mg/100 ml. Jaundice with higher levels of bilirubin may be missed if the patient is viewed in dim light, under incandescent lighting, or in a room with yellow or brownish walls. It is best to observe the patient in daylight, wherever possible, in order to detect early jaundice.

Physiology

Bilirubin arises from degradation of the porphyrin ring of heme as senescent red cells are destroyed in the reticuloendothelial system, destruction of 1 gm of hemoglobin producing approximately 36 mg of bilirubin. Additionally, bilirubin is a by-product of intramarrow hemolysis (so-called "ineffective" erythropoiesis) and of the porphyrin component of the cytochrome oxidase system within the liver cell. The latter is frequently termed the "early labeled peak" and may account for between 15 and 25 per cent of the bilirubin produced under physiologic conditions. Bilirubin turnover is approximately 40 mg/kg/day.[1, 2]

The initial product of heme degradation is biliverdin, a green water-soluble pigment. The initial step removes one carbon of the porphyrin ring as carbon monoxide, the only endogenous reaction in humans that produces carbon monoxide.[3] Subsequently, biliverdin is reduced to bilirubin, which is not water-soluble and requires conjugation for excretion. Because bilirubin is nonpolar it is transported in the blood attached to albumin, and delivery depends, in part, on hepatic blood flow. Specific binding proteins for bilirubin are present in the liver cell (ligandins) that promote "trapping" of bilirubin inside the hepatocyte. Subsequent to the entry of bilirubin into the cell, one mole of glucuronic acid is attached to bilirubin at one of the propionic acid side chains (catalyzed by uridine diphosphate glucuronyl transferase). The resultant product, bilirubin monoglucuronide, then undergoes transglucuronidation with another molecule of bilirubin monoglucuronide, producing bilirubin diglucuronide and free bilirubin.[4, 5] Bilirubin diglucuronide is excreted by an active process across the canalicular membrane into the bile. Under physiologic conditions, 95 per cent or more of the bilirubin in bile is bilirubin diglucuronide.

Within the intestinal tract, bilirubin is hydrogenated through a series of steps, ultimately producing the pigments that give the stool its ordinary brown color, the various urobilinogens. Urobilinogen is water-soluble and can be reabsorbed from the bowel and re-excreted by the liver, producing a so-called enterohepatic circulation of urobilinogen. These steps are illustrated in Figure 1.

Pathogenesis

The presence of jaundice should be confirmed by estimation of the total serum bilirubin level and its fractionation. The causes of jaundice may be classified as unconjugated, mixed, or conjugated. Unconjugated jaundice may be due to increased production of bilirubin, as with hemolysis, or to problems in delivery of bilirubin to the liver or its uptake or conjugation (Table 1). Problems associated with the delivery to or uptake of bilirubin by the liver cell do not, ordinarily, produce unconjugated bilirubin levels above 4 mg/100 ml; therefore, levels exceeding this amount suggest overproduction or problems with conjugation or excretion of bilirubin by the hepatocyte.[1]

Mixed hyperbilirubinemia is characteristically associated with abnormalities of both uptake and excretion and indicates generalized liver cell injury and dysfunction. Increased conjugated bilirubin, in the presence of normal total or normal uncon-

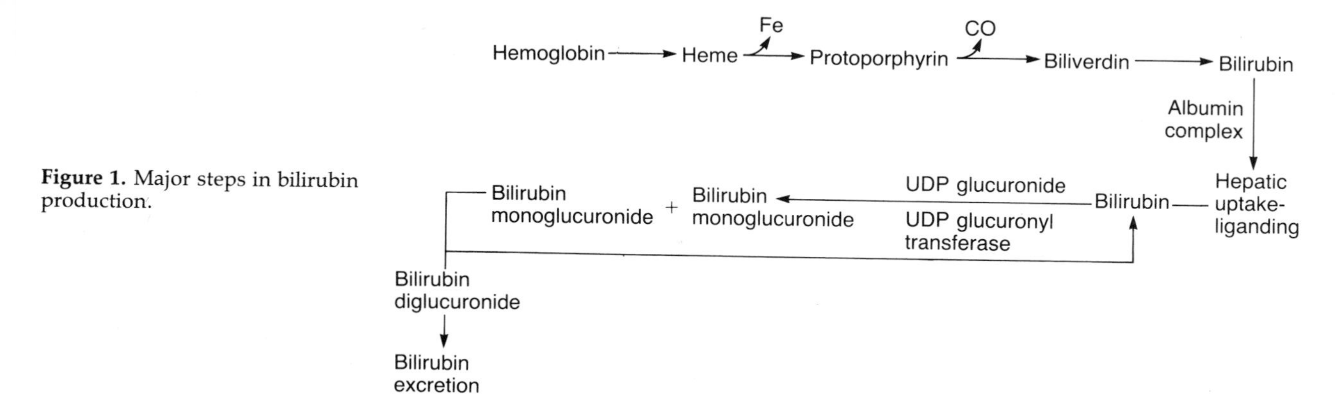

Figure 1. Major steps in bilirubin production.

jugated bilirubin, is associated with congenital abnormalities (Table 2).

The clinical setting in which the jaundiced patient is seen is an important factor in differential diagnosis, as well as the age of the patient, whether the patient is well or sick, and associated findings. A pathogenetic classification of jaundice is presented in Table 3.

CLINICAL EVALUATION

The Neonate

Jaundice in the neonatal period may be "physiologic" jaundice of the newborn, which is thought to be due to a delay in maturation of the enzyme system necessary for conjugation of bilirubin, resulting in unconjugated hyperbilirubinemia. More striking examples may occur if there has been an ABO-Rh incompatibility or if there are intrinsic hemoglobin or red cell abnormalities that lead to hemolysis during the neonatal period. Unconjugated bilirubin can cross the blood-brain barrier in the neonate, producing the threat of kernicterus. Exchange transfusions for this disorder are usually undertaken when the indirect serum bilirubin reaches 20 mg/100 ml.[6] In addition, the "bili-light" may decrease the levels of unconjugated bilirubin by conversion of unconjugated bilirubin to a water-soluble "photobilirubin" incident to molecular rearrangement caused by the absorption of ultraviolet light by the bilirubin molecule.[7] Other causes of neonatal jaundice include breastfeeding[8]—some women excrete a pregnanediol derivative that impairs bilirubin uptake or conjugation—and familial neonatal jaundice, the Lucey-Driscoll syndrome. A rare congenital disorder, the Crigler-Najjar syndrome, may become evident in the neonatal period with marked elevations of the unconjugated fraction. Crigler-Najjar syndrome may be present as types I or II, depending upon the response to phenobarbital enzyme induction therapy.[9-11]

Neonatal hepatitis usually produces a mixed hyperbilirubinemia and is most commonly due to the transmission of the hepatitis B virus from an infected mother to the offspring at the time of delivery. Women at high-risk should be screened for hepatitis B surface antigen and e antigen close to term, and if results of either test are positive, the infant should receive hyperimmune B globulin shortly after delivery. High-risk patients include immigrants from the Asian subcontinent, health professionals who handle blood, individuals who work in institutions for the mentally retarded, those who have been refused as blood donors, and any woman who develops jaundice or hepatitis syndrome during the course of pregnancy.[12]

Table 1. FACTORS ALTERING BILIRUBIN LEVELS

Bilirubin Fraction	Factors Causing an Increase	Factors Causing a Decrease
Unconjugated	Fasting Exercise Infection Drugs (oral cholecystographic dyes) Alcohol Pregnancy Estrogen	Ultraviolet light Glucocorticoids Drugs
Conjugated	Drugs (anabolic steroids) Pregnancy Renal failure	Glucocorticoids

Table 2. CONGENITAL CAUSES OF HYPERBILIRUBINEMIA

Unconjugated hyperbilirubinemia	Gilbert's disease
	Criger-Najjar syndrome
	Lucey-Driscoll syndrome
Conjugated hyperbilirubinemia	Dubin-Johnson-Sprinz syndrome
	Rotor's syndrome

Table 3. PATHOGENETIC CLASSIFICATION OF JAUNDICE

Cause	Examples
Increased production of bilirubin	
Intrinsic	
Hemoglobinopathies	Sickle cell disease
Enzyme abnormalities	Glucose-6-phosphate dehydrogenase deficiency
Cell structure abnormalities	Spherocytosis
Ineffective erythropoiesis	Thalassemia
	Sideroblastic anemias
Extrinsic	
Drugs	Alpha-methyldopa
	Alcohol
Infection	Mycoplasma
	Viruses
Immunologic	
ABO-Rh incompatibility	
Autoimmune	Systemic lupus erythematosus
Malignancy	Leukemia
Trauma	Prosthetic valves
Hepatic dysfunction	
Intrinsic	
Defective hepatic uptake	Gilbert's disease
Defective conjugation	Crigler-Najjar syndrome
Defective excretion	Dubin-Johnson-Sprinz syndrome
Cytoplasmic injury	Hemochromatosis
	Alpha$_1$-antitrypsin deficiency
	Wilson's disease
Extrinsic	
Defective conjugation	Familial neonatal jaundice (Lucey-Driscoll syndrome)
	Breast milk jaundice
Drugs	Isonicotinic acid hydrazide
	Alpha-methyldopa
	Erythromycin estolate
	Cholecystographic agents
Infections	Viral hepatitis
	Cytomegalovirus
	Epstein-Barr virus
	Amebiasis
	Leptospirosis
Immunologic	Chronic active hepatitis
	Primary biliary cirrhosis
Focal lesion	Granulomatous disease (sarcoid, tuberculosis)
Malignancy	Hepatoma
	Metastatic disease
Biliary drainage	
Intrahepatic	
Drugs	Chlorpromazine
Infection	Schistosomiasis
Immunologic	Primary biliary cirrhosis
	Sclerosing cholangitis
Extrahepatic	
Infection	"Ascending cholangitis"
Calculous disease	Choledocholithiasis
Trauma	Bile duct stricture
Malignancy	Bile duct carcinoma
	Carcinoma of head of pancreas

The Adolescent

Type A, type B, and non-A, non-B hepatitis may occur during the adolescent period and produce a mixed hyperbilirubinemia. Infectious mononucleosis and cytomegalovirus also may produce a hepatitis syndrome with a similar combined elevation of unconjugated and conjugated fractions.

Any adolescent who presents with jaundice and a hepatitis-like syndrome should be screened for Wilson's disease, which may be clinically indistinguishable from viral hepatitis. Appropriate screening tests include serum ceruloplasmin and urinary copper measurements, followed when indicated by tissue copper estimation via liver biopsy. Wilson's disease, although rare, should be considered because it is treatable and life-threatening. Choledochal cysts may produce extrahepatic obstruction and jaundice in the adolescent period, more commonly in males than females.

The Well Adult

Otherwise healthy persons may discover or may be told by friends that their eyes have a yellow discoloration. Such asymptomatic jaundice is usually due either to a compensated hemolytic disorder or to Gilbert's disease, a hereditary abnormality of uptake and conjugation of bilirubin. When one is presented with an otherwise well adult, particularly aged 15 to 25 years, who is jaundiced and has an unconjugated hyperbilirubinemia, initial evaluation should include a reticulocyte count and erythrocyte studies in order to detect a compensated hemolytic disorder producing an "overproduction" unconjugated hyperbilirubinemia. If the reticulocyte count and hemologic studies reveal no evidence of hemolysis, one should consider Gilbert's disease, the most common inheritable disorder producing unconjugated jaundice.[13] The exact mechanism of the hyperbilirubinemia in Gilbert's disease is not clear but probably relates to a defect in ligandins and uptake of bilirubin by the liver and, perhaps in some, to a depressed glucuronide-conjugating capacity. Because it is characteristic for patients with this disorder to experience jaundice during periods of fasting or intercurrent illness, the diagnosis may be confused with other causes of jaundice such as hepatitis. Characteristically, the unconjugated fraction is between 1.5 and 4.0 mg/100 ml. Presumptive confirmation of Gilbert's disease may be obtained by measuring unconjugated bilirubin before and after a fast of 24 to 48 hours. If the jaundice is due to Gilbert's disease there should be a doubling of the unconjugated fraction following such a fasting period.[14] Gilbert's disease is important to recognize because the patient will experience episodes of jaundice throughout life, but there is no evidence that it produces morbidity, mortality, or liver injury. Liver biopsies and other studies in such patients yield normal results and so are not indicated. Less common are the Dubin-Johnson-Sprinz syndrome and Rotor's syndrome, both of which produce a conjugated hyperbilirubinemia and are associated with diminished excretion of organic ions such as cholecystographic dyes.[15–17]

The Sick Adult

Jaundice associated with other manifestations of illness direct the clinician's attention to the hematologic system and to primary or secondary liver dysfunction. The various hemolytic syndromes may produce jaundice with characteristic elevation of unconjugated bilirubin. With a mixed hyperbilirubinemia, attention should be directed to liver dysfunction caused by acute or chronic hepatic injury and to intrahepatic or extrahepatic bile duct obstruction.

Acute Liver Cell Injury

The hepatitis syndrome consists of clinical manifestations of lassitude, easy fatigability, nausea, occasional vomiting, myalgia, and jaundice. However, only about one-third of patients with viral hepatitis develop clinically detectable jaundice. Liver cell injury is best detected by measuring serum transaminase levels. When one encounters a patient with the clinical syndrome and elevated serum aminotransferase level, a detailed epidemiologic history of contact with jaundiced persons and information about sexual contacts, receiving or handling blood or blood products, and details about drug ingestion[18] and occupation are essential.

Type A viral hepatitis, transmitted by the fecal-oral route, frequently occurs in epidemics when food or water supplies are contaminated by untreated sewage and, more recently, has been described in individuals working in day care centers for toddlers. Type B hepatitis is transmitted horizontally by intimate mucous membrane contact, notably in sexual contact, and vertically from mother to offspring during the period of delivery (vita supra).[19] Post-transfusion hepatitis is now most commonly due to non-A, non-B virus, because donor blood is screened for the B antigen and type A hepatitis is not an agent of post-transfusion hepatitis.[20] The diagnosis of non-A, non-B hepatitis is made in the appropriate setting following exclusion of types A and B by serologic testing. The Epstein-Barr virus and cytomegalovirus, which may also produce a hepatitis syndrome, are detected by Monospot slide test and studies for cytomegalovirus infection, respectively.

As noted, Wilson's disease should always be considered, particularly in an adolescent who presents with a hepatitis-like syndrome. Additional unusual causes include alpha$_1$-antitrypsin deficiency (commonly associated with lower lobe emphysematous changes) and hemochromatosis. Other transmissible causes include amebiasis and bacteria-associated liver abscess. Amebiasis should be suspected in anyone who has traveled to an endemic area and presents with fever, chills, and a hepatitis syndrome.[21] Pyogenic liver abscess may occur without associated causes but is more common in individuals who have had intra-abdominal sepsis or are immunosuppressed.[22] Bacterial hepatitis is very unusual.

Chronic Liver Cell Injury

In the United States, the most common etiologic and pathogenic factor in chronic liver cell injury producing jaundice is excessive ingestion of alcohol. A careful history of alcohol intake should be taken in any patient with jaundice or with biochemical manifestations of liver cell injury. Although a variety of factors are important in the development of alcoholic liver injury, the consumption of more than 70 gm (100 ml) of alcohol per day usually leads to detectable liver cell injury. Because patients tend to be circumspect regarding their alcoholic intake, careful, nonjudgmental questioning is essential. Criteria for diagnosis of alcoholism have been published in a joint statement by the American College of Physicians and the American College of Psychiatry.[23] Chronic alcoholic liver injury is characteristically associated with a variety of clinical markers, including spider nevi, gynecomastia, "liver palms," white nails, parotid enlargement, and the biochemical manifestations of liver cell injury. The aspartic transaminase level is characteristically greater than the alanine transaminase level in alcoholic liver injury; this finding may be helpful in distinguishing alcoholism from other nonalcoholic causes of liver injury, in which the reverse is true.

Chronic persistent or chronic active hepatitis may be due to type B virus, non-A, non-B virus, or drugs.[24] Appropriate serologic studies for hepatitis B antigens and antibodies (hepatitis B surface antigen, anti-core antibody) and the clinical history usually reveal the cause. Differentiation of chronic persistent hepatitis from chronic active hepatitis is based on clinical grounds and the appearance of the liver biopsy specimen. Patients will be periodically jaundiced, but jaundice may be absent in the presence of surprising elevations of serum transaminase levels. Both alcoholic liver injury and persistence of B virus or non-A, non-B virus infection may lead, ultimately, to necrosis, fibrosis, and regenerative nodules or cirrhosis.

Primary biliary cirrhosis may manifest as jaundice and should be suspected in a woman between the ages of 30 and 50 who presents with jaundice and pruritus as initial manifestations.[25] The disorder, of unknown cause, is associated with immunologic injury to the ducts within the liver and, characteristically, marked elevation of alkaline phosphatase, lesser elevations of the transaminases, and the presence of antimitochondrial antibody. The disease is progressive and relentless, and to date, no clearly effective therapy is available. The female-to-male incidence ratio is between 8:1 and 10:1.

A variety of disorders may be associated with granulomas within the liver that produce a hepatitis syndrome and jaundice. Tuberculosis, histoplasmosis and other fungi, and sarcoid may produce granulomatous infiltration of the liver and are usually associated with fever, lymphadenopathy, hepatosplenomegaly, and pulmonary manifestations.[26] Histoplasmosis may, in addition, be associated with oral mucosal ulcerations. Some drugs may also produce a granulomatous involvement of the liver.[18] Characteristic biochemical findings include a disproportionate increase in alkaline phosphatase level in comparison with the transaminase elevations, and mixed hyperbilirubinemia.

Obstructive Disease

Impairment of flow of bile from the liver may have an intrahepatic or extrahepatic cause. The obstructive syndrome, characterized by a mixed hyperbilirubinemia, may be associated with so-called painless jaundice. Itching is more commonly associated with bile duct obstruction than with intrahepatic disease. Mechanical obstruction of the extrahepatic biliary system occurs with choledocholithiasis and with tumors either within or surrounding the extrahepatic biliary system, notably carcinoma of the head of the pancreas. Jaundice may be an early manifestation of such extrahepatic obstruction, although careful history-taking usually indicates associated manifestations of malaise, fatigue, unexplained weight loss, nausea, and, occasionally, vomiting. Common duct obstruction by a stone is usually associated with clinical evidence of calculous disease of the gallbladder, although some patients have "silent gallstones" and do not develop symptoms until a stone gains access to the extrahepatic biliary system, lodging at the ampullary area.[27] Colicky right upper quadrant pain associated with increasing levels of bilirubin and elevations of transaminase and alkaline phosphatase) calls for further studies of the extrahepatic biliary system. Stenosis of the extrahepatic biliary system may occur because of pre-existing common duct injury incident to prior gallbladder surgery. Sclerosing cholangitis, an unusual disorder more common in males than females, commonly occurs in the setting of ulcerative colitis and may produce jaundice as a prominent manifestation. The effects of some drugs, notably chlorpromazine (Thorazine), mimic the clinical and biochemical manifestations of obstructive disease.[18]

In the past, differentiating between so-called medical jaundice and surgical jaundice was a major clinical problem. At present, newer techniques, such as ultrasonography followed by thin-needle transhepatic cholangiography or endoscopic retrograde cholangiopancreatography, allow anatomic visualization of the extrahepatic biliary system and make the differential diagnosis much more straightforward. Any patient presenting with the clinical and biochemical manifestations of obstruction of the extrahepatic biliary system should undergo one or both of these procedures for delineation of the system. Hepatic radioisotope scintigraphy and upper abdominal CT scanning may be helpful in selected patients.[28]

Tumor Involvement of the Liver

Tumor involvement of the liver may be benign,[29] or primary hepatocellular or metastatic. Primary hepatocellular carcinoma occurs predominantly in the setting of pre-existing hepatitis B infection as the oncogenic agent.[30] Clinical manifestations are varied but include unexplained fever, erythrocytosis or anemia, weight loss, elevated serum transaminase and alkaline phosphatase levels, and one or more markers of pre-existing hepatitis B virus infection.[31] Primary hepatocellular carcinoma characteristically invades the hepatic tributaries, and metastases to the lungs are frequently present by the time the malignancy becomes otherwise manifest.

Metastatic disease to the liver most commonly occurs with intra-abdominal malignancies and produces a disproportionate elevation of alkaline phosphatase level compared with the transaminase levels. Any patient presenting with an isolated elevation of alkaline phosphatase, with or without jaundice, in the absence of osteoblastic disease should be surveyed for malignant invasion of the liver. Isotope scanning and upper abdominal CT scanning are useful in detecting focal defects in the substance of the liver.[32] Definitive diagnosis depends on liver biopsy or exploratory laparotomy. Occasionally, a disease of the Hodgkin's-lymphoma group can invade the liver, producing a hepatitis-like syndrome. Malignant involvement of the liver does not usually produce jaundice until late in the course of the disorder, unless it is associated with a hemolytic phenomenon.

Important Features of the History

The medical history should include the following items:

1. A careful, detailed history of consumption of alcoholic beverages.
2. Drug ingestion data.
3. Information about associated disease, particularly inflammatory bowel disease or evidence of malignancy.
4. Careful epidemiologic history of the patient's environment, including exposure to industrial toxins, jaundiced individuals, and the presence of an epidemic in the community. Health care workers in dialysis units and oncology units and those who frequently handle blood are at risk for hepatitis B.
5. Family history of disorders associated with hemolysis or liver disease, suggesting hereditary disorders such as alpha$_1$-antitrypsin deficiency, Wilson's disease, and hemochromatosis.
6. Information about travel to areas where amebiasis is endemic or hepatitis infection is prevalent in the community.
7. Data on sexual practices, particularly homosexuality in males.
8. History of the receipt of blood transfusions or blood products or of having been refused as a blood donor.

DIAGNOSTIC STUDIES

Initial laboratory studies in the jaundiced patient should include an estimation of total bilirubin and its fractionation into conjugated and unconjugated portions, serum transaminases, and alkaline phosphatase. With clinical manifestations of hepatitis, anti-HAV, IgM, hepatitis B surface antigen, and anti-core antibody tests are essential. Subsequent evaluation will depend upon the clinical setting and the laboratory variations, as discussed. A total serum bilirubin level greater than 25 mg/100 ml suggests that more than one pathogenetic factor is producing the elevation of serum bilirubin, such as hemolysis plus liver cell injury.

Choice of special studies depends on the clinical situation. In patients suspected of having malignant disease involving the liver, ultrasonography or radioisotope or upper abdominal CT scanning may be helpful. Oral cholecystography is useful in detecting the presence of gallstones, but visualization is usually not adequate if the patient's total serum bilirubin is above 4 to 5 mg/100 ml. Radioisotope studies using labeled materials excreted by the liver may allow visualization of the extrahepatic biliary system and nonvisualization of the gallbladder, suggesting intrinsic gallbladder disease.[33] In patients in whom bile duct obstruction is suggested by the clinical picture, transhepatic cholangiography or endoscopic retrograde cholangiopancreatography is essential for anatomic visualization.[34]

Liver biopsy may be useful to detect malignant involvement of the liver and assist in identifying causes of the hepatitis syndrome. The procedure is also of value in differentiating chronic persistent from chronic active hepatitis and alcoholic hepatitis from fatty infiltration of the liver. Liver biopsy provides useful information regarding prognosis as well as an etiologic diagnosis.

If the patient presents with an unconjugated hyperbilirubinemia, appropriate hematologic studies, including red cell indices and reticulocyte count, should be carried out to detect the presence of a hemolytic disorder.

REFERENCES

1. Berlin NI, Berk PD. Quantitative aspects of bilirubin metabolism for hematologists. Blood 1981;57:983–99.
2. Berk PD. Total body handling of bilirubin. In: Goresky CA, Fisher MM, eds. Jaundice. New York; Plenum, 1975:135–57.
3. Berk PD, Rodkey FL, Blaschke TF, Collison HA, Waggoner JG. Comparison of plasma bilirubin turnover and carbon monoxide production in man. J Lab Clin Med 1974;83:29–37.
4. Schmid R. Bilirubin metabolism: state of the art. Gastroenterology 1978;74:1307–12.
5. Chowdhury JR, Jansen PLM, Fischberg EB, Daniller A, Arias IM. Hepatic conversion of bilirubin monoglucuronide to diglucuronide in uridine disphosphate-glucuronyl transferase-deficient man and rat by bilirubin glucuronoside glucuronosyltransferase. J Clin Invest 1978;62:191–6.
6. Cashore WJ, Stern L. Neonatal hyperbilirubinemia. Pediatr Clin North Am 1982;29:1191–1203.
7. McDonagh AF, Palma LA, Lightner DA. Blue light and bilirubin excretion. Science 1980;208–145–51.
8. Hargreaves T, Piper RF. Breast milk jaundice: effect of inhibitory breast milk and 3α,20β-pregnanediol on glucuronyl transferase. Arch Dis Child 1971;46:195–8.
9. Israel JB, Arias IM. Inheritable disorders of bilirubin metabolism. Adv Intern Med 1975;21:34–40.
10. Crigler JF Jr, Najjar VA. Congenital familial nonhemolytic jaundice with kernicterus. Pediatrics 1952;10:169–80.
11. Arias IM, Gartner LM, Cohen M, Ezzer JB, Levi AJ. Chronic nonhemolytic unconjugated hyperbilirubinemia with glucuronyl transferase deficiency. Am J Med 1969; 47:395–409.
12. Centers for Disease Control. Hepatitis Surveillance Report No. 47. December 1981.
13. Powell LW, Hemingway E, Billing BH, Sherlock S. Idiopathic unconjugated hyperbilirubinemia (Gilbert's syndrome): a study of 42 families. N Engl J Med 1967; 277:1108–12.
14. Felsher BF, Rickard D, Redeker AG. The reciprocal relation between caloric intake and the degree of hyperbilirubinemia in Gilbert's syndrome. N Engl J Med 1970;283:170–2.
15. Dubin IN, Johnson FB. Chronic idiopathic jaundice with unidentified pigment in liver cells: a new clinicopathologic entity with a report of 12 cases. Medicine 1954;33:155–97.
16. Sprinz H, Nelson RS. Persistent nonhemolytic hyperbilirubinemia associated with lipochrome-like pigment in liver cells: report of four cases. Ann Intern Med 1954;41:952–62.
17. Wolkoff AW, Wolpert E, Pascasio FN, Arias IM. Rotor's syndrome: a distinct inheritable pathophysiologic entity. Am J Med 1976;60:173–9.
18. Zimmerman HJ. Drug-induced liver disease. Drugs 1978;16:25–44.
19. King JW. A clinical approach to hepatitis B. Arch Intern Med 1982;142:925–8.
20. Czaja AJ, Davis GL. Hepatitis non A, non B: manifestations and implications of acute and chronic disease. Mayo Clin Proc 1982;57:639–52.
21. Katzenstein D, Rickerson V, Braude A. New concepts of amebic liver abscess derived from hepatic imaging, serodiagnosis, and hepatic enzymes in 67 consecutive cases in San Diego. Medicine 1982;61:237–46.
22. Butler TJ, McCarthy CF. Pyogenic liver abscess. Gut 1969;10:389–99.
23. National Council on Alcoholism, Criteria Committee. Criteria for the diagnosis of alcoholism. Ann Intern Med 1972;77:249–58.
24. Hodges JR, Millward-Sadler GH, Wright R. Chronic active hepatitis: the spectrum of disease. Lancet 1982;1:550–2.
25. Sherlock S, Scheuer PJ, The presentation and diagnosis of 100 patients with primary biliary cirrhosis. N Engl J Med 1973;289:674–8.
26. Simon HB, Wolff SM. Granulomatous hepatitis and prolonged fever of unknown origin: a study of 13 patients. Medicine 1973;52:1–21.
27. Wenckert A, Robertson B. The natural course of gallstone disease: eleven-year review of 781 nonoperated cases. Gastroenterology 1966;50:376–81.
28. Whalen JP. Caldwell Lecture. Radiology of the abdomen: impact of new imaging methods. Am J Radiol 1979;133:587–618.
29. Knowles DM II, Casarella WJ, Johnson PM, Wolff M. The clinical, radiologic, and pathologic characterization of benign hepatic neoplasms: alleged association with oral contraceptives. Medicine 1978;57:223–37.
30. Beasley RP, Lin CC, Hwang LY, Chien CS. Hepatocellular carcinoma and hepatitis B virus: a prospective study of 22,707 men in Taiwan. Lancet 1981;2:1129–32.
31. Margolis S, Homcy C. Systemic manifestations of hepatoma. Medicine 1972;51:381–91.
32. Tempero MA, Petersen RJ, Zetterman RK, Lemon HM, Gurney J. Detection of metastatic liver disease: use of liver scans and biochemical liver tests. JAMA 1982;248:1329–32.
33. Pelot D, Berk JE, Wistow BW, Morton ME. PIPIDA excretory scintigraphy in the diagnosis of hepatobiliary disorders. Am J Gastroenterol 1981;75:22–6.
34. Matzen P, Haubek A, Holst-Christensen J, Lejerstofte J, Juhl E. Accuracy of direct cholangiography by endoscopic or transhepatic route in jaundice—a prospective study. Gastroenterology 1981;81:237–41.

LYTIC LESIONS IN BONE

THOMAS LEE POPE, JR. □ THEODORE E. KEATS

□ SYNONYMS: Bony lysis, bony destruction, osteolysis, bone loss, bony erosion, osteoclasia

BACKGROUND

Normal Bony Development, Anatomy, and Physiology

A brief review of the normal development of bone as well as its pertinent anatomic and physiologic features is necessary to any approach to lytic lesions in bone. As all connective tissue, bone develops from primitive mesenchymal cells, which are pluripotential. These cells develop into chondrocytes (which produce and maintain cartilage) and osteoblasts (which lay down bone), and eventually become osteocytes (which maintain bony integrity) and osteoclasts (which destroy bone).

In the developing embryo, there are two mechanisms of bone formation, intramembranous and enchondral development. Intramembranous bone is formed directly from mesenchyme without an intervening cartilaginous phase and is thought to be derived phylogenetically from the dermis of the skin. These bones, which become ossified earlier than bone developed from enchondral formation, are listed in Table 1.

Enchondral formation is the major mechanism of most bony growth. In this process, mesenchymal cells produce a rough structure in cartilage. When the cartilage matures, it is invaded and destroyed by vessels and cells. The dead cartilage is then replaced by bone produced by osteocytes. Such activity takes place mainly at the ends of bones, the epiphyseal centers of ossification. This continual process—laying-down of cartilage, cartilage death, and subsequent replacement by bone—is the method of bony maturation. Because of this mechanism of formation, bone can be divided into three separate anatomic regions, the epiphysis, metaphysis, and diaphysis. The difference between immature and mature bone is the presence or absence of the growth plate, which intervenes between the metaphysis and epiphysis during growth (Fig. 1).

There are two radiographically distinct types of bone, cancellous (spongy or trabecular) and cortical (compact) (Fig. 2). Cancellous bone makes up the marrow space and is primarily concentrated in the subarticular region (i.e., the metaphyseal area). In long bones, its main function is to support the endplate and to transmit forces to the cortex on the articular surface. Cortical bone, on the other hand, is most prevalent in the diaphysis, where there is a paucity of trabecular bone. It functions mainly as a supporting structure. Thus, there is a reciprocal relationship between cancellous and cortical bone.[1]

Maintenance of normal bone is a dynamic process of continual breakdown by osteoclasts and buildup by osteoblasts. On the inner surface of the cortex is a theoretical layer of connective tissue fibroblasts termed the endosteum. When cancellous bone is resorbed or lysed, the fibroblasts transform into osteoclasts, which break down bone, and osteoblasts simultaneously repair this process. Inside cortical bone, there are individual cylindrical units called haversian canals or osteones, interconnected by perpendicular passages termed Volkmann's canals. Cortical bone is lysed by cooperative osteoclasts lining up, and the space is then refilled by layers of lamellar bone.[2]

Normal control of this process is accomplished through a complex interaction of parathormone and calcitonin. This subject is not particularly relevant to our discussion but can be reviewed if desired.[3]

Definition of Bony Lysis

Bony lysis, as perceived radiographically, is an imbalance of bony destruction and production. In this situation, osteoclasts destroy cancellous and cortical bone faster than osteoblasts can rebuild it. The net result is bone loss, a two-fold process. First, the mineral component of the bony matrix is removed, and second, the matrix is enzymatically digested. It is important to remember that *only osteoclasts can destroy bone.*[4]

Generally, cancellous bone can be destroyed faster than cortical bone. However, large amounts

Table 1. STRUCTURES DERIVED FROM INTRAMEMBRANOUS BONE FORMATION

Parietal bone
Squamous and tympanic portions of temporal bone
Occipital squamosa
Frontal bone
Vomer
Medial pterygoid plate
Facial bones
Mandible
Clavicles (although secondary ossification centers do develop)

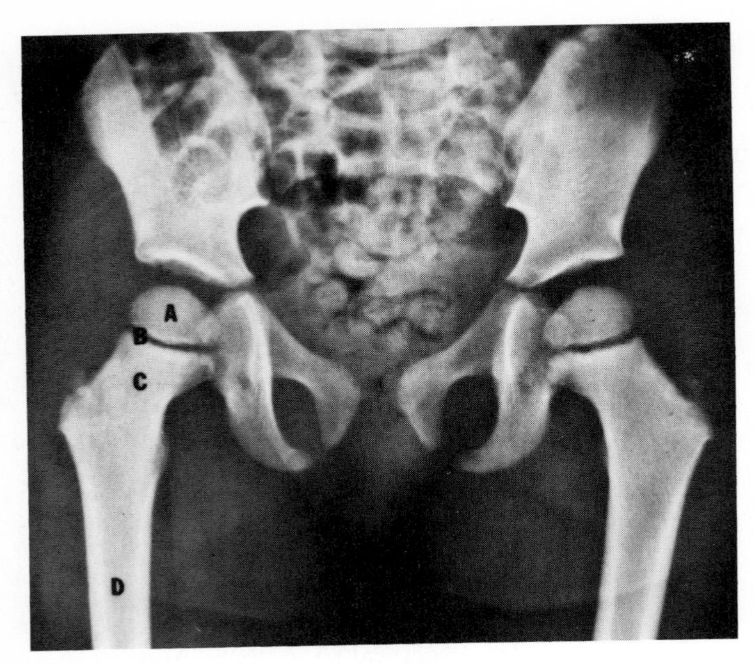

Figure 1. AP view of pelvis in a 3 year old. *A*, femoral capital epiphysis; *B*, epiphyseal plate; *C*, metaphysis of right femur; *D*, diaphysis of right femur.

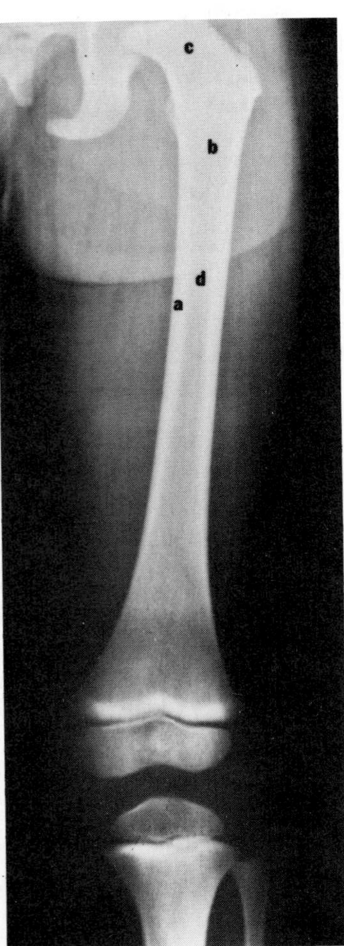

Figure 2. AP view of left femur in a 3 year old. *A*, diaphyseal cortical bone; *B*, metadiaphyseal spongy bone; *C*, metaphysis of left femur; *D*, diaphyseal spongy (cancellous) bone. Note that cortical bone is most prominent in regions where spongy bone is least prominent, and vice versa.

(up to 50 per cent) of cancellous bone must be lost before the destruction is perceived radiographically.[5] Cortical bone is destroyed more slowly, yet because of its density, its loss is more easily seen on x-ray. In either case, however, radiographic perception of destruction is usually not evident until 10 days after the initial bony insult.[6]

Categories of Bone Lesions

In general, bone lesions may be divided into categories as outlined in Table 2. In approaching any lytic lesion of bone, one should review mentally each of these potential etiologies and correlate them with the individual radiographic pattern and clinical symptomatology. This approach usually allows one to generate a differential diagnosis for a particular lesion.

HISTORY

Generally, age of the patient is an important consideration in bone disease. Certain benign con-

Table 2. CATEGORIES OF BONE DISEASE

Congenital
Acquired
Inflammatory
Traumatic
Neoplastic
Benign
Malignant
Primary
Secondary
Metabolic or ischemic

ditions, such as a fibrous cortical defect, occur only in young patients, but lytic metastatic disease to bone is the most common lytic lesion in patients older than 40 years.

A family history of a congenital bone disease may be important, although most such diseases are quite uncommon. For example, neurofibromatosis, a congenital disease of mesodermal and neuroectodermal elements first described by Smith in 1849, can cause bony erosion and lysis, and it is important to know whether this disease exists in the family when analyzing such lesions.[7] Likewise, the very rare cystic angiomatosis of bone may cause lytic lesions of bone.

Of course, fever and systemic symptoms are important in inflammatory diseases of bone. Any infecting agent can cause bony lysis, and the location of bony lysis in infection is usually characteristic and important to diagnosis.

Pain can sometimes be a presenting symptom in lytic lesions of bone. In such cases, infection, ischemia, and malignancy should be considered. Rarely do benign neoplasms present with pain. They are usually diagnosed fortuitously when the bone is radiographed for another reason.

A pre-existing disease known to spread to bone, such as lymphoma or cancer, can be a helpful historic finding in the assessment of certain lytic lesions of bone. Known metabolic diseases such as gout and hyperparathyroidism can also be pertinent. Finally a previous history of infection, especially tuberculosis, can be helpful in certain lytic bone diseases.

PHYSICAL EXAMINATION

Rarely is physical examination helpful in diagnosing lytic lesions of bone. If the patient has pain, the general anatomic region may be localized, but referred pain can complicate this procedure.

In direct spread of inflammation to bone, the skin over the affected bone will usually be indurated and quite tender, a potentially helpful diagnostic finding.

In some primary tumors, the soft tissue mass representing the extension of the neoplasm may be palpated. This is a late finding, however, and the patient usually presents with pain before this time.

DIAGNOSTIC STUDIES

Elevated white blood cell counts with a high percentage of polymorphonuclear leukocytes and an elevated serum erythrocyte sedimentation rate may be supportive evidence in lytic lesions thought to be secondary to infection.[8]

Certain metabolic diseases that cause lytic lesions have characteristic laboratory findings. Patients with hyperparathyroidism usually have elevated serum calcium and decreased phosphorus levels, although both may be normal in patients with low serum protein levels.[9, 10] The patient with gout may have an elevated serum uric acid level because of its overproduction from purine or its retention due to decreased renal excretion.[11]

ASSESSMENT

Before describing the most common specific entities under the general categories of bone disease, we should discuss a few more fundamental considerations in lytic bone disease: the margins of the lesion, the matrix of the lesion, and whether the patient has single or multiple lesions.

The Margins of the Lesion

In general, the radiographic appearance of all lytic lesions of bone is really a measure of the lesion's biologic activity. A well-demarcated, dense, sclerotic border or margin around an area of bony lysis usually indicates a "nonaggressive" lesion that has given the bone time to respond to it (Fig. 3). "Aggressive" lesions tend to have wider

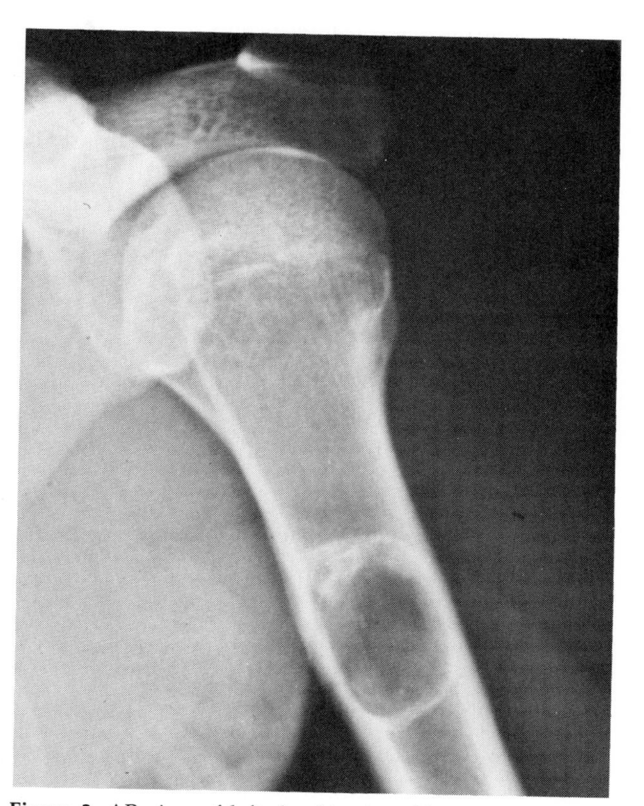

Figure 3. AP view of left shoulder in a 20 year old showing the characteristic appearance of a simple bone cyst in the humerus. Note various sclerotic "nonaggressive" margins.

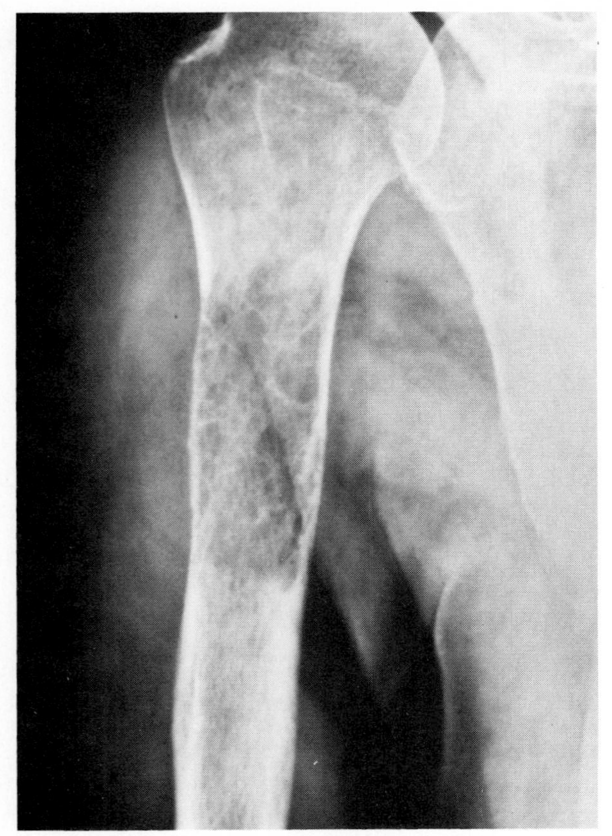

Figure 4. AP view of shoulder in a 65-year-old patient with known renal carcinoma shows a very aggressive lytic process in the proximal humerus with ill-defined margins. This was metastatic renal carcinoma.

zones of transition and poorly demarcated borders or margins, thus indicating that the bone has not had time to properly surround the insult (Fig. 4).[1]

In all lytic lesions, therefore, the margin should be assessed in relation to the anatomic location of the lesion and the clinical picture.

The Matrix of the Lesion

Radiographic matrix is defined as the substance within lytic lesions of bone produced by certain interior cells.[12] The matrix of a lesion is usually an indication of the predominant cells within the lytic area and may be cartilaginous calcification (chondroid matrix), osseous calcification (osteoid matrix), and fibrous density (fibromyxoid matrix).

Many bone lesions are entirely lytic on radiograph, signifying that there is no perceptible interior matrix mineralization. Such lesions may contain collagen, normal marrow cells, blood, fat, fluid, or vascular spaces, none of which normally shows up on radiographic examination unless it contains some mineralization.

Cartilaginous or chondroid matrix is produced primarily by chondroblasts and is usually visualized radiographically as irregular rings and arcs or flocculations of calcium (Fig. 5). Osseous matrix produced mainly by osteoblasts that mineralize (or calcify) is usually more regular and more uniformly dense than cartilage (Fig. 6). Fibrous matrix may or may not partially mineralize. If it does not, the radiograph shows no definable matrix. If it does mineralize, the lesion has a cloudy, slightly dense matrix pattern, as seen in fibrous dysplasia (Fig. 7).

Therefore, the matrix may be very helpful in predicting the most likely diagnosis of a lytic bone lesion.

Single vs. Multiple Lesions

Single lytic lesions may occur in the entire range of possible etiologies of bone disease. Each solitary lesion, therefore, must be assessed using the previously described criteria.

Multiple areas of osteolysis generally have a narrower range of diagnostic possibilities, however. In the young patient, congenital disorders and infection are the most common causes of multiple lesions and should be sought first. In patients over 40, bony metastases, myeloma, and metabolic causes are more common.

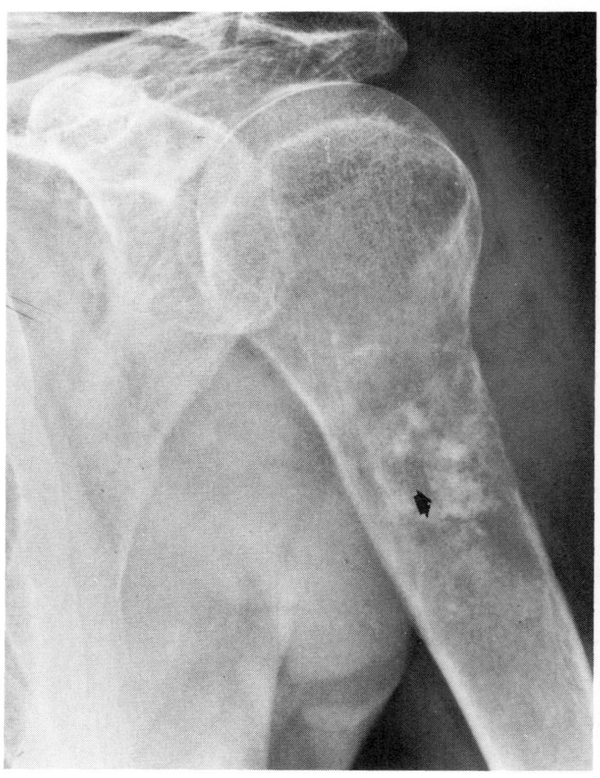

Figure 5. AP view of shoulder in a 73-year-old man shows an aggressive lesion involving the proximal portion of the bone. Bony lysis and cartilaginous calcification *(arrowhead)* can be seen.

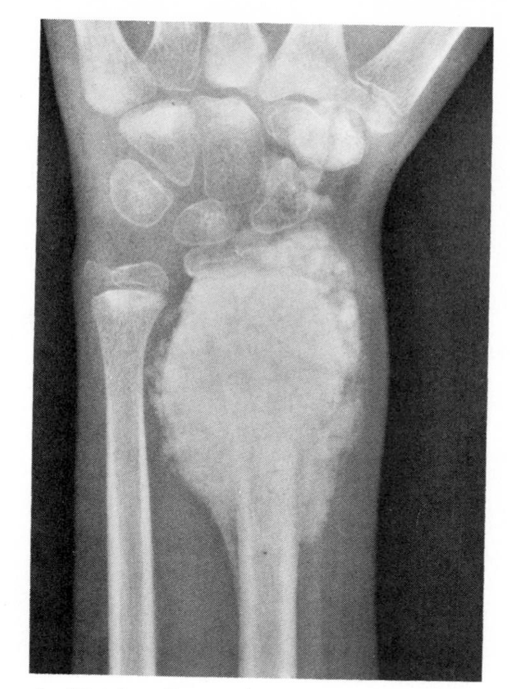

Figure 6. Distal radius and ulna in a 9-year-old patient with disseminated osteosarcomatosis. Note the characteristic cloudy, osteoid matrix in the radius.

In the assessment of any lytic bone lesion, the following data should then be considered: the age of the patient, the bone involved and the anatomic location of the lytic area, the margins and matrix of the lesion, and whether the lesion is solitary or one of many.

SPECIFIC LYTIC LESIONS OF BONE

We now discuss characteristic lytic lesions in each category of bone disease. The examples presented are "typical" and are intended mainly as guides. As discussed previously, diagnosing bone disease is mainly a process of generating a differential list of possible diagnoses on the basis of the radiographic appearance and narrowing this list by considering the age of the patient, the historical and physical findings, and the laboratory data. The major features of each entity are discussed and references are provided for further reading and research. However, the radiographic appearance is the primary focus in each discussion.

Congenital Lesions

Overall, congenital diseases are an uncommon cause of lytic lesions of bone. Often the disease is known before the lytic lesion develops. In some of the less common diseases, however, bony lysis may be the initial presentation, and biopsy is usually required for diagnosis. Cystic lymphangiomatosis of bone has been chosen as the typical example of congenital lytic bone disease.

Cystic Angiomatosis of Bone (Fig. 8). First described by Jacobs and Kimmelstiel[13] in 1953, cystic angiomatosis of bone is a rare disease causing lytic lesions of bone. The etiology is unknown, and the diagnosis is usually made when the patient is young (10 to 15 years old). Males are affected twice as often as females, and over half the patients have a history of fracture. The angiomatous bone lesions may also be associated with similar changes throughout the body, particularly in the spleen.[14]

Generally, the diagnosis is difficult to make. Any bone may be involved, but there is a predilection for the axial skeleton. The lesions are usually central cystic lucent regions 1 or 2 mm to several centimeters in diameter with well-defined sclerotic margins. They are typically round to oval

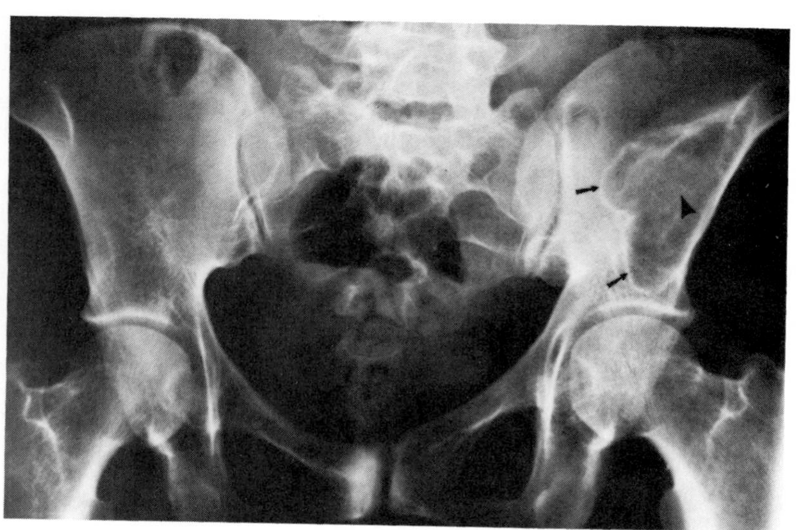

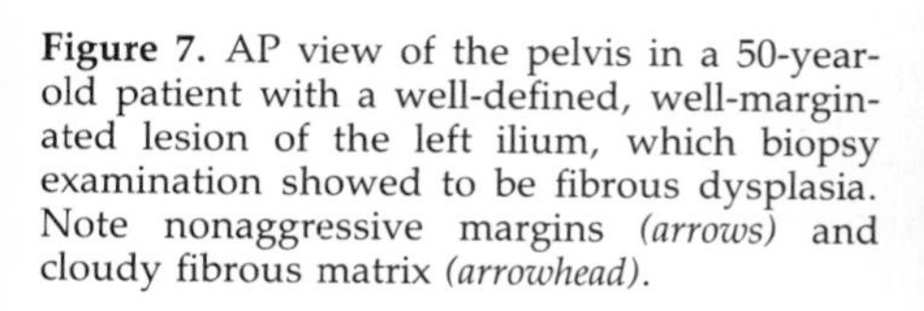

Figure 7. AP view of the pelvis in a 50-year-old patient with a well-defined, well-marginated lesion of the left ilium, which biopsy examination showed to be fibrous dysplasia. Note nonaggressive margins *(arrows)* and cloudy fibrous matrix *(arrowhead)*.

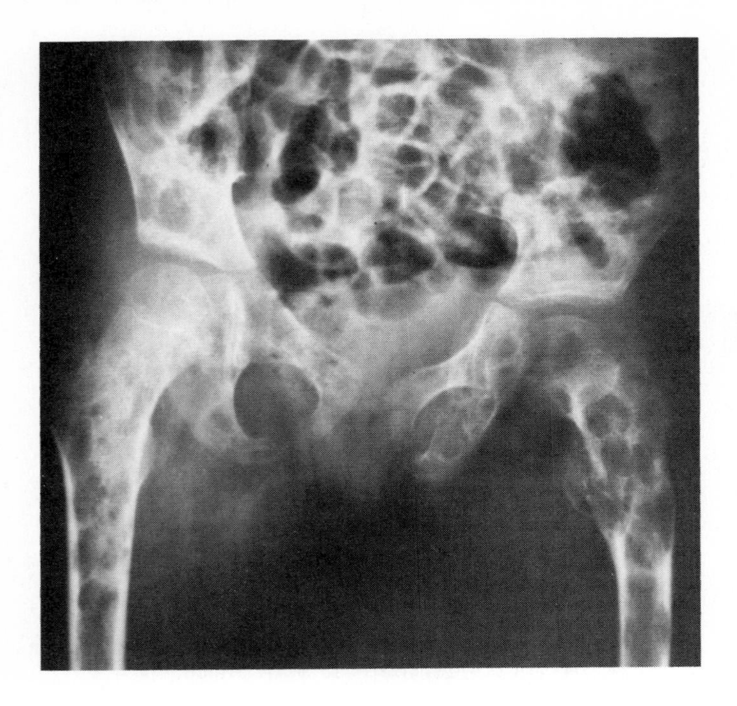

Figure 8. AP view of pelvis and both femurs of a 10-year-old child with known cystic angiomatosis of bone. Note multiple lytic lesions throughout the bones.

and situated in the medullary cavity, and they can reach any size. They have no matrix.

The differential diagnosis in such cases includes eosinophilic granuloma, polyostotic fibrous dysplasia, metastases, and multiple myeloma. Diagnosis requires biopsy.

Acquired Lesions

As discussed previously, this category of bone lesions can be divided into subcategories: inflammation, trauma, benign or malignant neoplasm, and metabolic or ischemic disease. We discuss each category briefly and choose classic examples of the bone lesions seen in each.

Inflammatory

Osteomyelitis

Osteomyelitis causing lytic lesions of bone can be further divided into acute hematogenous osteomyelitis and secondary or contiguous, soft-tissue extension osteomyelitis.

Acute Hematogenous Osteomyelitis (Fig. 9).[15] This disease is more common in infants and children and has become more widespread with the heightened use of intravenous catheters. The infecting organism is most commonly *Staphylococcus aureus,* followed in order of decreasing frequency by tuberculosis, syphilis, and streptococcus. The most common sites are the spine, sacroiliac joints, symphysis pubis, and sternoclavicular joints, although the long bones are also commonly involved.

The lesion usually occurs in the distal metaphysis or metaphyseal-equivalent areas of bone. Blood normally sludges in this region because of its small arterial and venous interconnections. Embolic bacteria occlude these small branches and begin the infective process.

No radiographically detectable bony changes occur for at least 3 days. In suspected cases, bone or gallium scanning may be helpful in this early period.[16] The earliest finding in adults is deep soft-tissue swelling adjacent to the affected bone. However, in children and infants the earliest manifestation may be a metaphyseal lytic lesion. The margins are usually ill-defined and "aggressive-looking." Periosteal reaction, a later finding, is usually exuberant if the infection is not treated. In children, the epiphyseal plate often acts as a barrier to spread into the adjacent joint, but adults commonly have an associated septic arthritis. Of course, as mentioned in the introductory paragraphs, the clinical picture may be very helpful in the diagnosis of acute hematogenous osteomyelitis.

Occasionally, a chronic cavity of Brodie's abscess may develop without an antecedent acute phase. In this case, the patient presents with pain in the involved region and the x-ray may show a wide variety of findings. The lesion is virtually always lucent and may be of varying size. It is located in either the diaphysis or the metaphysis and may have no margin or a dense rim of sclerosis around its periphery (Fig. 10). It may also show thick periosteal reaction and be mistaken radiographically for an osteoid osteoma.[17]

Secondary Osteomyelitis (Fig. 11).[18] This form

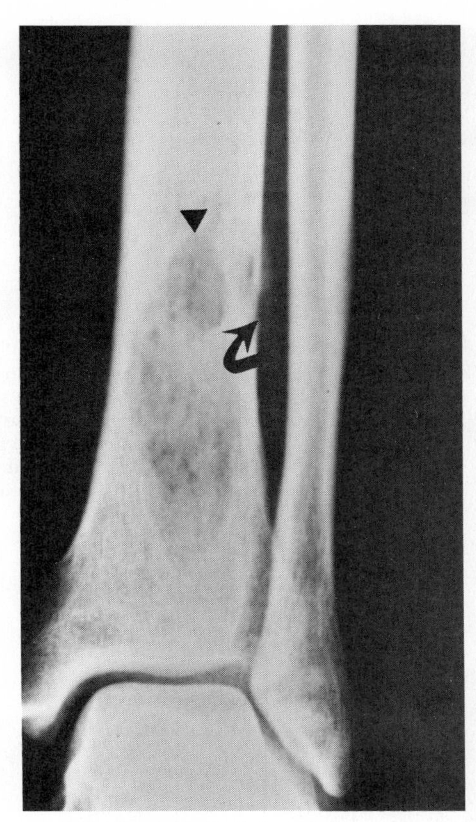

Figure 9. AP view of distal tibia and fibula in a 36-year-old man with sepsis. Note areas of bony lysis *(arrowhead)* and periosteal reaction *(curved arrow)*, which are characteristic of acute hematogenous osteomyelitis.

of bone infection occurs most commonly in patients with diabetes mellitus or vascular insufficiency. The bone adjacent to the soft tissue infection is invaded by the organism and destroyed or lysed. Radiographically, the involvement may manifest as bony cortical destruction (radiolucency), osteosclerosis, periosteal new bone formation, or any combination of these findings.

Traumatic

In this category, there are few true lytic lesions of bone. Of course, in any fracture there is lysis of some bone as the reorganization toward healing occurs. The history of trauma is most commonly known. Repeated trauma, however, can cause marked bony resorption and lysis, most frequently seen in acute neuropathic arthropathy.

Acute Neuropathic Arthropathy (Fig. 12).[18] The first description of neuropathic joint was made by Charcot in 1868. The disease is primarily secondary to two main processes: disruption of sensory nerves and repeated trauma. At one time, syphilis was the most common predisposing disease. In recent years diabetes mellitus has become more common, and neuropathic changes occur in about 6 per cent of diabetic patients.[19] The changes of neuropathic arthropathy usually take years to develop.

Acute neuropathic arthropathy, a variant of the Charcot joint, is characterized by fragmentation of the articular ends of bone and subluxation in less than 2 months. This rapidity of development often leads to misdiagnoses such as trauma and infection.

Radiographic changes include bony destruction, fragmentation, and loss of articular cartilage. Calcific debris may be seen in the surrounding soft tissues and may dissect along muscle planes. The hip, knee, and shoulder are most prone to acute neuropathic arthropathy.

The diagnosis should be suspected in patients with known predisposing conditions who develop the typical radiographic manifestations.

Neoplastic

By far the most common causes of lytic lesions of bone belong in this category. Benign lesions of bone are quite common and usually are diagnosed incidentally when the involved bone is radiographed for trauma. Such lesions are typically asymptomatic, and certain lesions occur in characteristic locations. Malignant bone lesions may be primary or secondary. Secondary involvement of bone by a primary tumor is exceedingly more common than primary tumor of bone. The most typical manifestations of a few of these lesions are described.

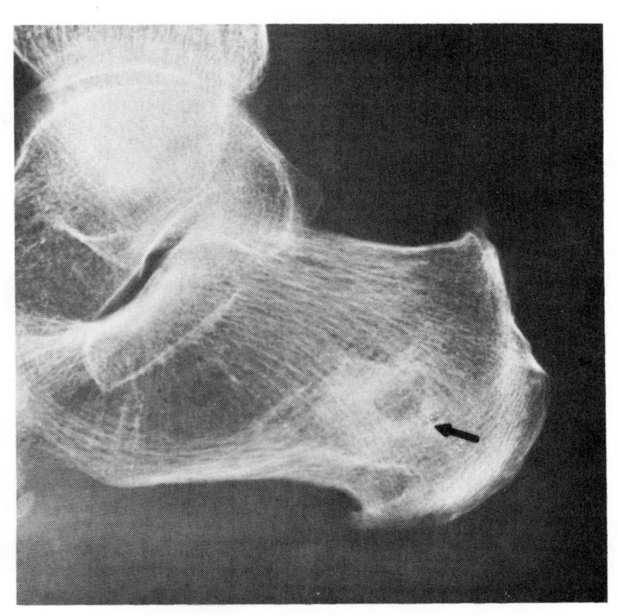

Figure 10. Lateral view of calcaneus in a 25-year-old woman with positive blood culture results. Note well-circumscribed lucency within the calcaneus surrounded by a wide zone of sclerosis *(arrow)*. This picture is characteristic of a Brodie's abscess.

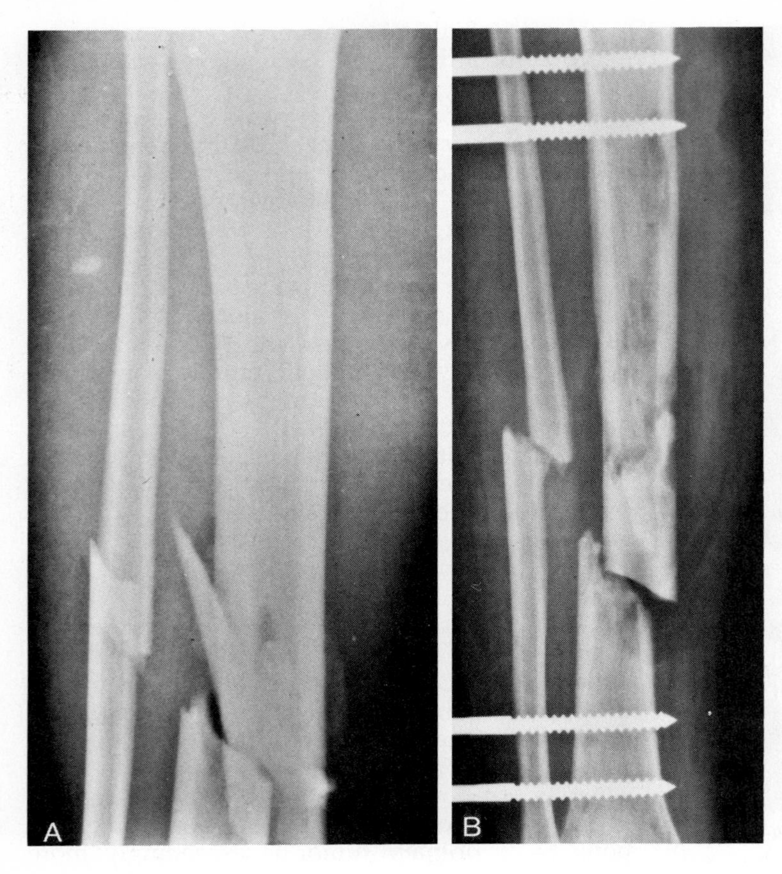

Figure 11. *A,* AP view of tibia and fibula in a 25-year-old man following automobile accident shows comminuted fractures of both bones. These were open fractures. *B,* AP view of tibia and fibula in same patient 5 months later. Note marked bony lysis, particularly in the tibia, which is characteristic of secondary osteomyelitis.

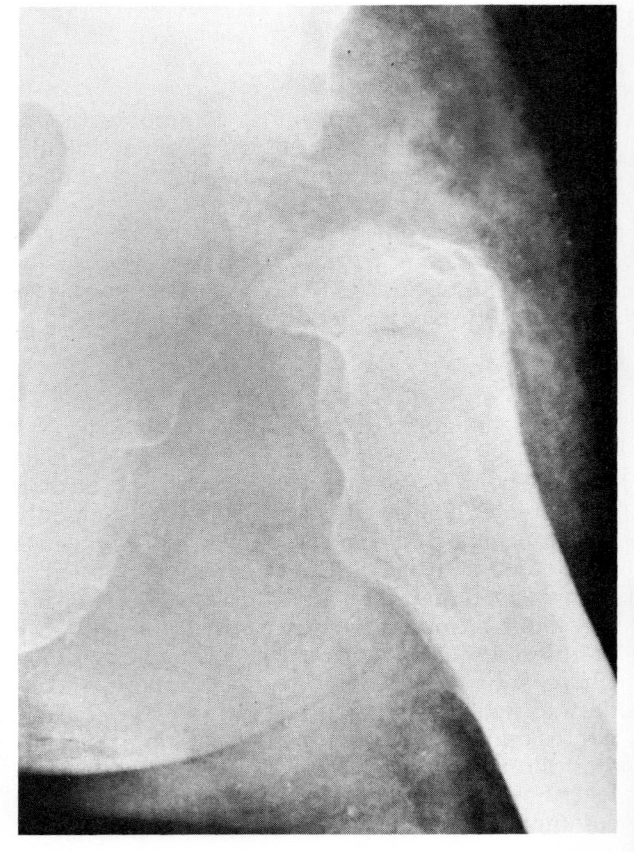

Figure 12. Left hip of a 25 year old shows marked bony destruction, fragmentation, and loss of articular cartilage. This appearance is characteristic of acute neuropathic arthropathy.

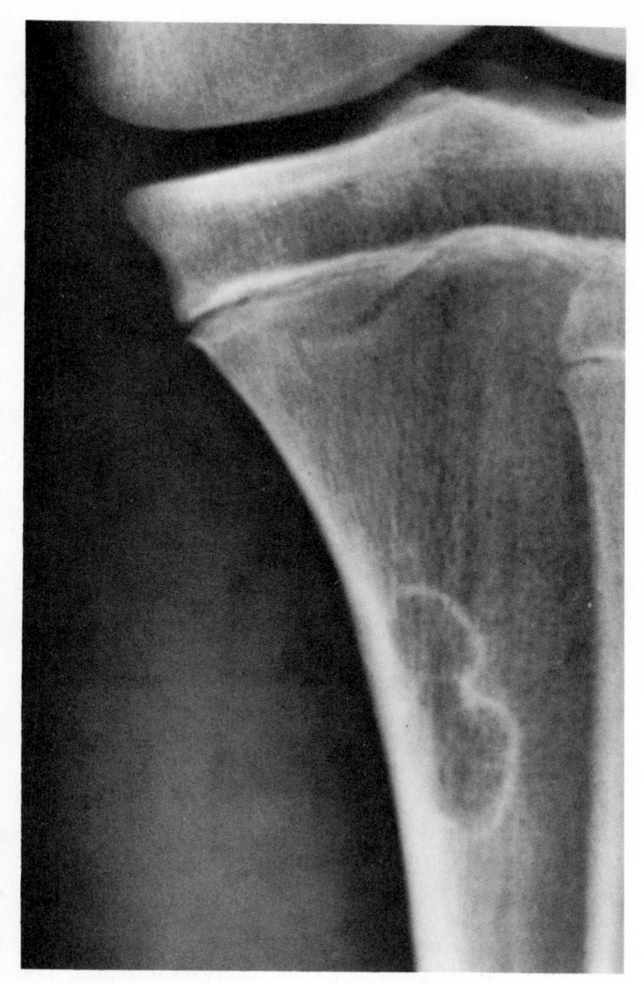

Figure 13. Coned-down view of proximal tibia in a 9-year-old boy shows typical appearance of a fibrous cortical defect.

Benign Neoplasms

Fibrous Cortical Defect (Fig. 13).[19] This normal variant is a lytic lesion of bone whose radiographic appearance is so characteristic that no other diagnostic workup is needed when it is encountered.[19] Children aged 4 to 8 most often have this lesion, and spontaneous regression is the rule. Males exhibit the finding more often than females, and the lesions are asymptomatic.

The most common site is the posteromedial distal femur, although fibrous cortical defect can occur in the tibia or fibula. Radiographically, there is a small round, ovoid, or irregular lucency adjacent to the cortex. The margins are densely sclerotic and well-demarcated and never erode through the cortex.

Benign Chondroblastoma (Fig. 14).[20, 21] Presumed to be derived from chondroblasts, this primary bone tumor is relatively rare. The peak age range is 10 to 25 years, and approximately 50 per cent of these lesions involve the knee joint. Benign chondroblastoma has been reported in unusual sites such as the patella and can occur in any flat bone that was preformed in cartilage.[22]

The chief presenting complaint is joint pain. Tenderness, swelling, limitation of motion, weakness, numbness, local heat, and muscle atrophy have also been reported.

The lesion is almost always confined to the epiphysis. In fact, this diagnosis should be the first consideration in any lytic lesion of the epiphysis in a patient of the right age. The margins of the tumor are usually thin and sclerotic and therefore "nonaggressive" in appearance. The size of the lesion ranges from 3 to 19 cm, and eccentric ovoid expansion of the cortex can occur; yet periosteal reaction should not be a feature of the disease. The matrix in approximately 50 per cent of the tumors has an amorphous "fluffy cotton-wool" appearance.

The differential diagnosis includes the rare Brodie's abscess, which affects only the epiphysis, the even rarer eosinophilic granuloma of the epiphysis, and giant cell tumor. However, giant cell tumor should have a more "aggressive" appearance.

Unicameral (Simple) Bone Cyst (see Fig. 3).[23] This benign bony lesion of unknown origin is a true fluid-filled cyst. Approximately 80 per cent of such lesions occur in children aged 3 to 14, males being more commonly affected. The most common locations in patients under 17 are the proximal

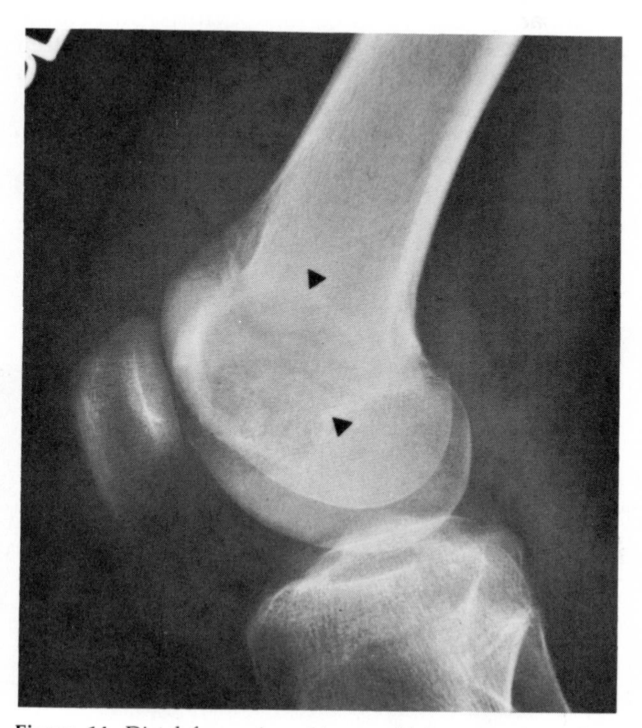

Figure 14. Distal femur in a 14-year-old boy contains a lytic lesion with well-defined margins *(arrowheads)* in the distal femoral epiphysis. Biopsy examination of this lesion revealed chondroblastoma.

humerus and proximal femur, and in patients over 17, the pelvis and calcaneus.

The radiologic features of unicameral bone cyst are very characteristic. It is most commonly a central metaphyseal lytic lesion with nonaggressive margins located either adjacent to or a small distance from the epiphyseal plate. The lesion is usually broader at the metaphyseal end and narrower at the diaphyseal end, and its long axis is greater than its diameter. The width is hardly ever broader than the epiphyseal plate, and the cyst never erupts into the soft tissues.

Interestingly, however, a common mode of presentation is pathologic fracture. In such cases, a fragment of bone may fall into the most dependent portion of the radiolucent tumor—the "fallen fragment sign."[24] The differential diagnosis includes giant cell tumor, aneurysmal bone cyst, enchondroma, and chondromyxoid fibroma. However, chondromyxoid fibroma and aneurysmal bone cyst are usually more eccentric and have predilection for different locations. Enchondromas usually have stippled cartilaginous calcification, and giant cell tumors look like much more aggressive lesions.

The treatment is surgical curettage, although recurrence is not uncommon.

Eosinophilic Granuloma of Bone (Fig. 15).[25, 26] Eosinophilic granuloma of bone is included in the benign neoplasm category as part of the spectrum of entities including Letterer-Siwe disease (acute or subacute disseminated histiocytosis) and Hand-Schüller-Christian disease (chronic disseminated histiocytosis). The clinical syndrome and age of presentation in these diseases are dissimilar; the cited references can be consulted for specifics. Bone is not necessarily involved. Generally, however, when bone is involved there is associated pain and limitation of motion. Local inflammatory signs may also be present. Skull, ribs, mandible, spine, pelvis, and extremities are the most common sites of involvement.

Radiologically, the bone lesions are punched-out osteolytic areas. The margins may be sharp and somewhat sclerotic or ill-defined. Often the margin seems to have an undulating contour, giving it a "hole-within-a-hole" configuration. Periosteal reaction in varying degrees of severity may be seen with this lesion. Skull involvement typically demonstrates both inner and outer table erosion, and a double contour may be seen if each is unevenly involved. One characteristic of mandibular involvement is resorption around the roots of teeth, creating the appearance of "floating teeth." One other typical lesion is the flattened, almost totally collapsed vertebra plana occasionally seen with spine involvement in this disease.

Histologically, these lytic lesions of bone contain reticular cells with varying degrees of lipid or granulomas with histiocytes and eosinophils. Diagnosis is usually made via biopsy.

Malignant Neoplasms

Osteosarcoma (Fig. 16).[27, 28] Osteosarcoma is the second most common sarcoma of bone, surpassed in frequency only by multiple myeloma. The predominant cellular element consists of osteocytes that have undergone malignant degeneration. The tumor can be classified according to its site in bone as central medullary osteosarcoma, parosteal (juxtacortical) osteosarcoma, multiple osteosarcomatosis, and soft-tissue osteosarcoma. We limit our brief discussion to the central medullary osteosarcoma.

Males are affected twice as often as females. The peak age range of incidence for this neoplasm is the second and third decades. The most common presenting complaint is pain at the site of involvement, although pathologic fracture can be the inciting factor in the diagnosis. Early metastases and poor prognosis are characteristic of osteosarcoma. Amputation followed by adjuvant chemotherapy is the preferred treatment regimen.

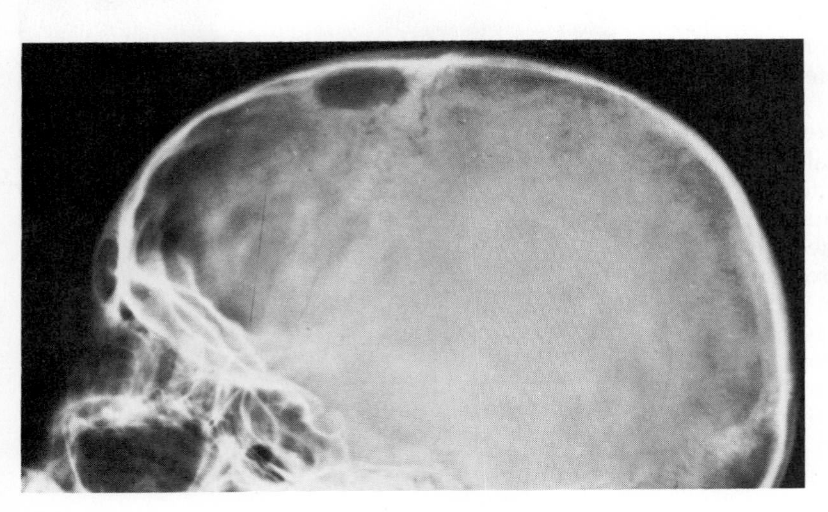

Figure 15. Lateral view of the skull of an 11 year old with known eosinophilic granuloma shows lytic calvarial lesions characteristic of this disease.

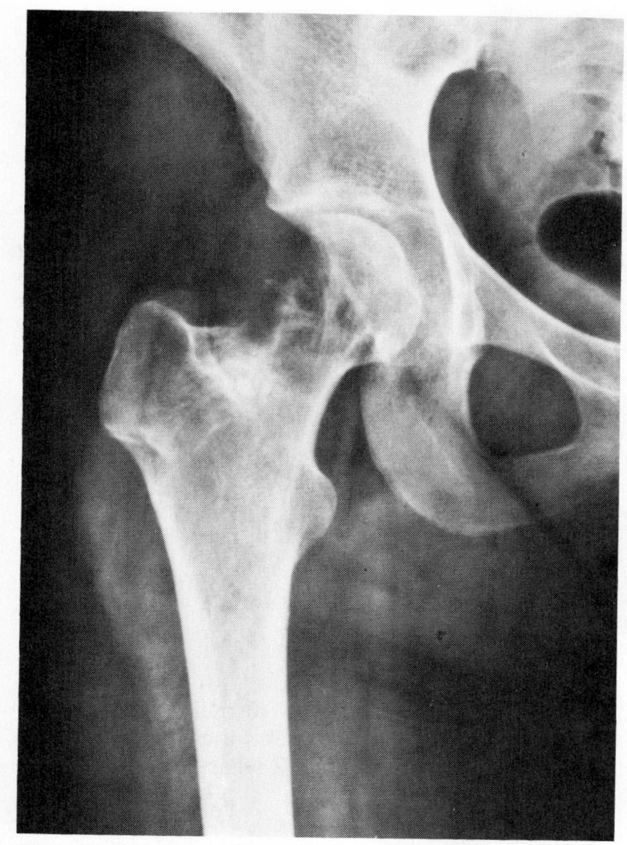

Figure 16. AP view of right hip in a 17-year-old woman shows osteolytic destruction of the femoral neck and proximal portion of the femoral head. On biopsy, this lesion proved to be osteolytic osteosarcoma.

The most common site of involvement is the distal femur and proximal tibia (about three-fourths of cases), although any bone can be affected. The metaphysis is most commonly involved but diaphyseal osteosarcoma is not uncommon. If the tumor begins prior to epiphyseal closure, the epiphyseal cartilage usually functions as a barrier to extension into the epiphysis.

Radiologically, the tumor may appear as a densely sclerotic lesion, moderately ossified tumor, purely lytic area, or combination of any of these. Pure lysis without mineralized matrix is rare. Any variation in density is due to the degree of mineralization within the tumor cells themselves.

The classic osteosarcoma is a sclerotic, ill-defined lesion in the metaphysis of a long bone that has broken through the cortex and extended into the soft tissues. There is commonly a spiculated periosteal reaction that extends perpendicular to the shaft of the bone, the so-called sunburst appearance. This soft-tissue extension may be quite large, and computed tomography can be helpful in determining its extent.[29]

In osteolytic osteosarcoma there are spotty areas of bony lysis interspersed with more sclerotic areas, a radiographic picture that may cause diagnostic confusion with osteomyelitis. Biopsy will clarify the diagnosis.

Ewing's Sarcoma (Fig. 17).[30, 31] Ewing's sarcoma was first described in 1866; in 1921, Ewing renewed interest in the tumor, which he called diffuse endothelioma or endothelial myeloma. This relatively rare disease has a predilection for young patients, being very unusual in a patient over the age of 30. There is an approximately equal male-to-female ratio, with the long bones of the lower extremity and the pelvis being the most common sites of involvement.

Patients with Ewing's sarcoma usually present with fever, leukocytosis, and increased sedimentation rates and are often thought to have infections. There may be pain and swelling in the involved area, which also may be taken for signs of osteomyelitis.[32]

Radiographically, the most common appearance is a diaphyseal lesion with a very aggressive, permeative pattern and poorly defined margins. There is often a parallel, multilayered, so-called onion-skin

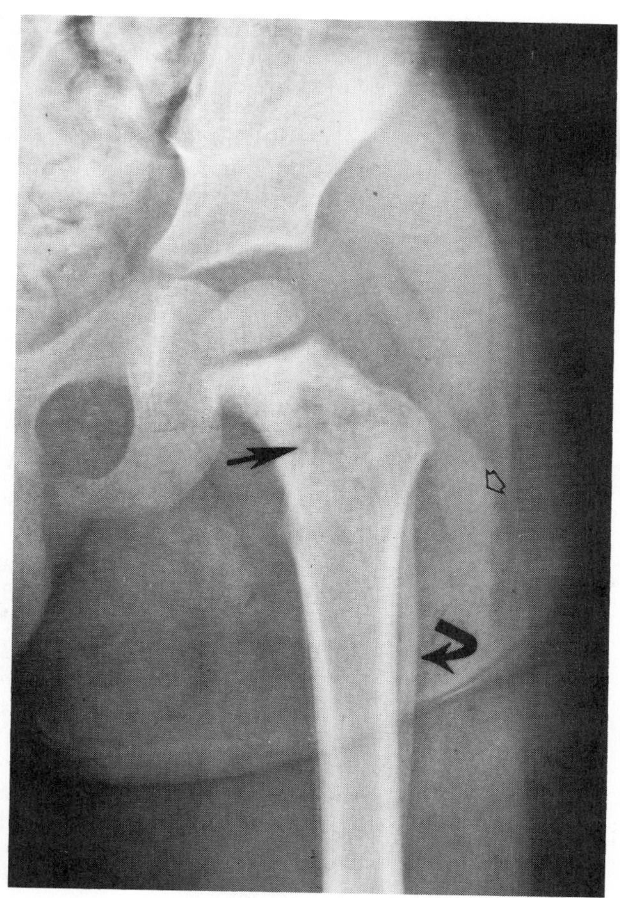

Figure 17. Ewing's sarcoma. AP view of left femur in a 4-year-old girl with hip pain shows marked osteolytic destruction of the proximal femur *(arrow)* with "onion-skin" periosteal reaction associated with the shaft of the femur *(curved arrow)*. Note also large soft tissue mass *(open arrowhead)*.

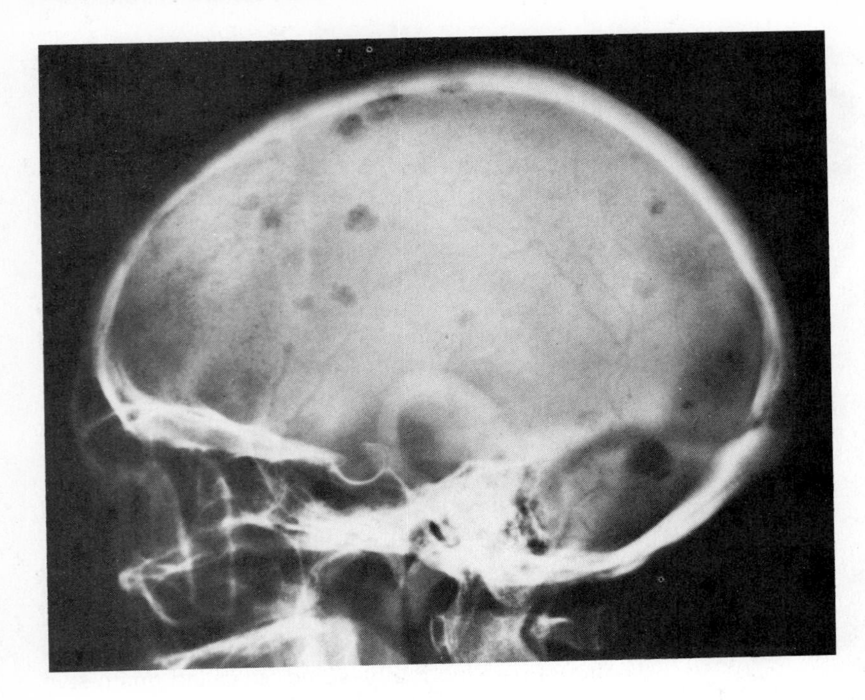

Figure 18. Lateral skull view in a 57-year-old woman with known multiple myeloma shows multiple lytic defects throughout the calvarium, characteristic of this disease. The differential diagnosis would also include metastatic disease.

periosteal reaction. Cortical destruction may also be present in a permeative pattern. Commonly, a large soft tissue mass surrounds the bone lesion.

The differential diagnosis includes osteomyelitis, osteosarcoma, and malignant lymphoma in this age group. The prognosis in this disease is poor regardless of therapy, the 5-year survival rate ranging from 4.8 to 12.6 per cent.

Multiple Myeloma (Fig. 18).[33, 34] This lesion represents more than one half of all malignant bone tumors. Multiple myeloma is the most common neoplasm of bone in adults. The incidence approaches three cases per 100,000 population in the United States. There is a slight predilection for males, and the average age of discovery is 60 years. Any bone with hematopoietic elements may harbor myeloma, but interestingly, the mandibles and maxillae are involved in over 30 per cent of cases.[33] There is also a distinct preference for larger bones.

Clinically, pain suggesting neuralgia or arthralgia is the presenting symptom. Soft-tissue swelling and palpable masses may be seen in some patients. The advanced stages of the disease produce widespread bony deformities, and hypercalcemia from bone breakdown is common. Azotemia may also be a prominent feature.

Characteristic radiographic patterns of diffuse, lytic "punched-out" areas are most commonly seen in this disease. Such areas are often irregular and do not usually have sclerotic borders. They do not contain any definable matrix, and the margins are often ill-defined and very "aggressive."

The differential diagnosis includes osteolytic metastases, although some authors point out that soft-tissue masses and generalized osteoporosis favor myeloma.[36] Prognosis, once dismal, has been improved by a variety of chemotherapeutic agents, and remissions of almost 2 years have been reported.

Metastatic Carcinoma (Fig. 19).[37] Metastases, together with myeloma, are probably the most common cause of lytic lesions in bone. In fact, a lytic

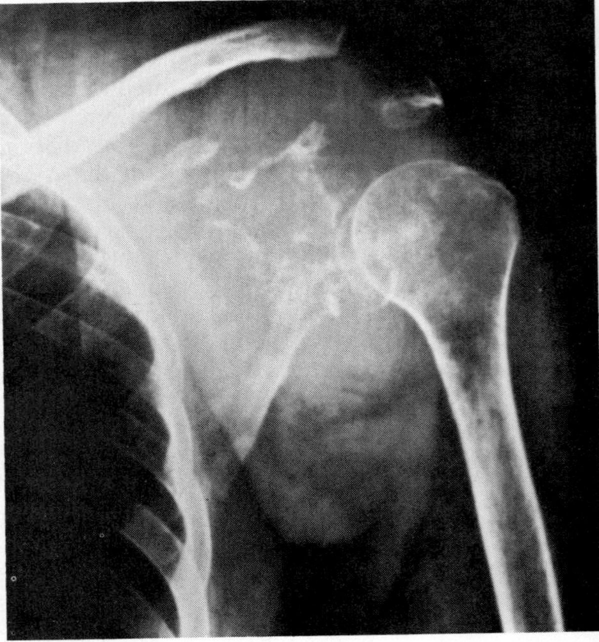

Figure 19. AP view of left shoulder in a 65-year-old woman with known breast cancer shows marked destruction and osteolysis of the scapula, which biopsy examination proved to be a metastatic deposit.

lesion in a patient older than 60 years is considered a metastasis or myeloma until proven otherwise. Spread to bone may occur in any bone via direct extension, lymphatics, or blood stream.

The primary tumors most often responsible for lytic lesions are those of breast, lung, thyroid, kidney, and, rarely, prostate and gastrointestinal tract. Of course, any of these tumors may also produce bony reaction or sclerosis, causing osteoblastic metastases. Commonly there is a mixed pattern.

The radiographic changes in metastases are varied. Usually, bone is destroyed in a random manner and the lesion is typically "aggressive," with ill-defined margins. There commonly are multiple areas of involvement, a characteristic that helps to exclude a malignant primary tumor of bone.

Plain x-rays do not often show the full extent of bony involvement in metastatic disease and are therefore very insensitive tools for monitoring progression or regression of disease. Bone scanning with any of a variety of radioactive nuclides is the preferred method of surveying bony involvement today. Often, however, correlation of the bone scan findings with plain x-rays is important, particularly when degenerative arthritis, a common plain film finding in this age group, is encountered.[38, 39]

Metabolic

In the metabolic category, a variety of disorders may cause bony lysis. Bony erosions may be seen with gout, pseudogout, and other arthritides. However, the typical example of a metabolic lytic lesion of bone is one caused by hyperparathyroidism. (Refer to references 40–43 for discussion of other metabolic diseases.)

Hyperparathyroidism (Fig. 20).[44, 45] Hyperparathyroidism may be divided into primary and secondary forms. Primary hyperparathyroidism is most commonly due to parathyroid adenomas or hyperplasia of the gland, and secondary hyperparathyroidism is a compensatory effect of rickets, osteomalacia, pregnancy, renal insufficiency, calcium deprivation, or maternal hypoparathyroidism. The disease is most common in the third through fifth decades and affects females approximately three times as often as males. Laboratory data usually show elevated calcium levels with lower phosphorus levels, although in the patient with a low serum protein concentration, the calcium level may be normal.

The skeletal lesions of primary and secondary hyperparathyroidism are identical, and about half of all patients have recognizable roentgen signs. Classic radiologic features include subperiosteal cortical bone erosions, especially on the radial side of the middle phalanges of the hand; generalized deossification; articular, tendinous, and ligamentous calcification; and localized lytic lesions of bone, so-called brown tumors.

These lytic areas are common and may affect any bone. Characteristically, they are large, eccentric, expanding destructive regions in the metaphyses of long bones. The margins may be either well-demarcated or ill-defined, and there is no demonstrable matrix. Histologically the "tumors" of hyperparathyroidism are filled with giant cells (osteoclasts) and may be difficult to distinguish radiographically from true giant cell tumors of bone. Usually, however, there is other roentgen evidence of hyperparathyroidism.[9]

Therapy is oriented toward treating the underlying cause of hyperparathyroidism. Rapid regression of the bone lesions with treatment is the rule.

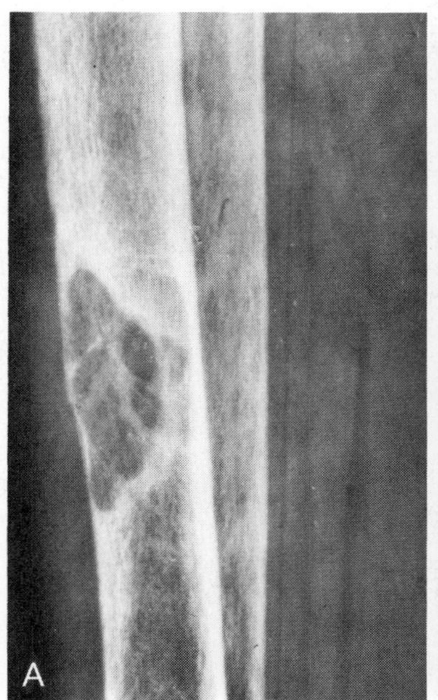

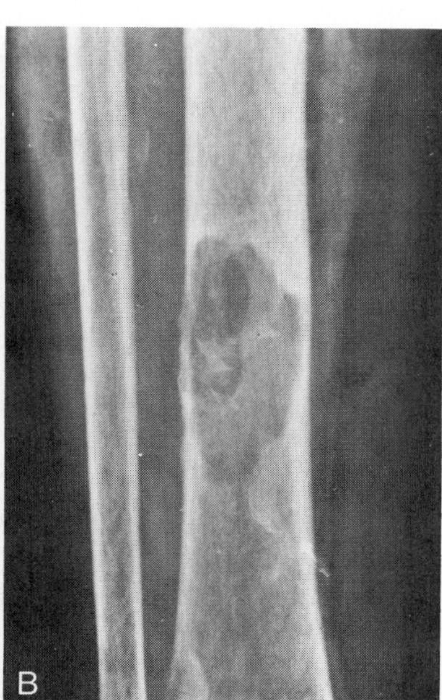

Figure 20. AP *(A)* and lateral *(B)* views of tibia in a patient with marked elevation of serum calcium level and marked depression of serum phosphorus level. This lytic lesion was a "brown tumor" of hyperparathyroidism.

REFERENCES

1. Madewell JE, Ragsdale BD, Sweet DE. Radiologic and pathologic analysis of solitary bone lesions. Part I: internal margins. Radiol Clin North Am 1981;19:715–48.
2. Johnson LC. The kinetics of skeletal remodeling. In: structural organization of the skeleton. Birth Defects 1966;2:21–36.
3. Chambers TJ. The cellular basis of bone resorption. Clin Orthop Rel Res 1980;151:283–93.
4. Lodwick GS. Reactive response to local injury in bone. Radiol Clin North Am 1964;2:209–19.
5. Ardran GM. Bone destruction not demonstrable by radiography. Br J Radiol 1951;24:107–9.
6. Edeiken J. Roentgen diagnosis of diseases of bone. 3rd ed. Baltimore: Williams & Wilkins, 1981:9.
7. Smith R. Treatise on the pathology, diagnosis, and treatment of neuroma. Dublin: Hodge Smith, 1849.
8. Staab EV, McCartney WH. Role of gallium 67 in inflammatory disease. Semin Nucl Med 1978;8:219–33.
9. Steinbach HL, Gordan GS, Eisenberg E, Crane JT, Silverman S, Goldman I. Primary hyperparathyroidism: a correlation of roentgen, clinical, and pathologic features. Am J Roentgenol 1961;86:329–43.
10. McClean FC, Hastings AB: Clinical estimation and significance of calcium-iron concentration in the blood. Am J Med Sci 1935;189:601–9.
11. Steinberg VL, Wenley WG, Mason RM. Gout. Br J Clin Pract 1962;16:173–82.
12. Sweet DE, Madewell JE, Ragsdale BD. Radiologic and pathologic analysis of solitary bone lesions. Part III: Matrix patterns. Radiol Clin North Am 1981;19:785–814.
13. Jacobs JE, Kimmelstiel P. Cystic angiomatosis of skeletal system. J Bone Joint Surg [Am] 1953;35:407–20.
14. Boyle WJ: Cystic angiomatosis of bone. J Bone Joint Surg [Br] 1972;54:626–36.
15. Capitano MA, Kirkpatrick JA. Early roentgen observations in acute osteomyelitis. Am J Roentgenol 1970;108:488–96.
16. Lisbona R, Rosenthall L. Observations on the sequential use of ^{99m}Tc-phosphate complex and ^{67}Ga imaging on osteomyelitis, cellulitis, and septic arthritis. Radiology 1977;123:123–9.
17. Miller WB, Murphy WA, Gilula LA: Brodie abscess: reappraisal. Radiology 1979;132:15–23.
18. Norman A, Robbins H, Milgram JE. The acute neuropathic arthropathy—a rapid, severely disorganizing form of arthritis. Radiology 1968;90:1159–64.
19. Greenfield GB. Radiology of bone diseases. Philadelphia: JB Lippincott, 1975:596–7.
20. McLeod RA, Beabout JW. The roentgenographic features of chondroblastoma. Am J Roentgenol Radium Ther Nucl Med 1973;118:464–71.
21. Nolan DJ, Middlemiss H. Chondroblastoma of bone. Clin Radiol 1975;26:343–50.
22. Cohen J, Cahen I. Benign chondroblastoma of the patella. A case report. J Bone Joint Surg [Am] 1963;45:824–6.
23. Cohen J. Etiology of simple bone cyst. J Bone Joint Surg [Am] 1970;52:1493–7.
24. Reynolds J. The "fallen fragment sign" in the diagnosis of unicameral bone cysts. Radiology 1969;92:949–53.
25. Ochsner SF. Eosinophilic granuloma of bone. Experience with 20 cases. Am J Roentgenol 1966;97:719–26.
26. Zinkham WH. Multifocal eosinophilitic granuloma. Natural history, etiology, and management. Am J Med 1976;60:457–63.
27. Lee ES. Osteosarcoma: a reconnaissance. Clin Radiol 1975;26:5–25.
28. Uribe-Botero G, Russell WO, Sutow WW, Martin RG. Primary osteosarcoma of bone. A clinicopathologic investigation of 243 cases, with necropsy studies in 54. Am J Clin Pathol 1977;67:427–35.
29. de Santos LA, Bernardino ME, Murray JA. Computed tomography in the evaluation of osteosarcoma: Experience with 25 cases. AJR 1979;132:535–42.
30. Fernandez CH, Lindberg RD, Sutow WW, Samuels ML. Localized Ewing's sarcoma—treatment and results. Cancer 1974;34:143–8.
31. Johnson RE, Pomeroy TC. Evaluation of therapeutic results in Ewing's sarcoma. Am J Roentgenol Radium Ther Nucl Med 1975;123:583–7.
32. Nance CL Jr, Roberts WM, Miller GR. Ewing's sarcoma mimicking osteomyelitis. South Med J 1967;60:1044–50.
33. Gootnick LT. Solitary myeloma: review of sixty-one cases. Radiology 1945;45:385–91.
34. Kyle RA, Elveback LR: Management and prognosis of multiple myeloma. Mayo Clin Proc 1976;51:751–60.
35. Cataldo E, Meyer L. Solitary and multiple plasma-cell tumors of the jaw and oral cavity. Oral Surg 1966;22:628–39.
36. Jacobson HG, Poppel MH, Shapiro JH, Grossberger S. The vertebral pedicle sign: a roentgen finding to differentiate metastatic carcinoma from multiple myeloma. Am J Roentgenol 1958;80:817–21.
37. Turner JW, Jaffe HL. Metastatic neoplasms; a clinical and roentgenological study of involvement of skeleton and lungs. Am J Roentgenol 1940;43:479–88.
38. Brady LW, Croll MN. The role of bone scanning in the cancer patient. Skeletal Radiol 1979;3:217–22.
39. Gerber FH, Goodreau JJ, Kirchner PT, Fouty WJ. The efficacy of preoperative and postoperative bone scanning in the management of breast cancer. N Engl J Med 1977;297:300–5.
40. Bloch C, Hermann G, Yu T-F. Radiologic re-evaluation of gout: study of 2,000 patients. AJR 1980;134:781–9.
41. Martel W, McCarter DK, Solsky MA, et al. Further observations on the arthropathy of calcium pyrophosphate crystal deposition disease. Radiology 1981;141:1–10.
42. Ling D, Murphy WA, Kyriakos M. Tophaceous pseudogout. AJR 1982;138:162–8.
43. Rohatgi PK. Radioisotope scanning in osseous sarcoidosis. AJR 1980;134:189–94.
44. Doppman JL, Marx SJ, Spiegel Am, et al. Differential diagnosis of known tumors vs. cystic osteitis by arteriography and computed tomography. Radiology 1979;131:339–46.
45. Resnick DL. Erosive arthritis of the hand and wrist in hyperparathyroidism. Radiology 1974;110:263–9.

NECK MASS

HOWARD LEVINE

☐ SYNONYM: Cervical mass

BACKGROUND

Neck masses in adults or children usually create worries in the patient or parent and physician. Any swelling noted by the patient or a family member nearly always raises anxiety about malignancy. Although while this particular diagnosis is often all the patient or parent thinks about, it is only one part of an extensive differential diagnosis that must be considered by the physician. To be sure that all possibilities are entertained, the diagnosis must be approached in an orderly and systematic fashion. Normal anatomic variants, infections, and congenital anomalies must be considered as well as benign and malignant neoplasms. Differential diagnosis of the neck mass is important, because it significantly affects the selection of the most effective mode of evaluation and therapy.[1]

The approach to the neck mass and to its evaluation depends upon patient's age and the location of and history related to the mass. Failure to approach the patient with a neck mass in an organized fashion may result in delay in diagnosis, inappropriate laboratory examinations, unnecessary surgery, untoward morbidity, and even mortality, depending upon the etiology.

Although there is no question that incisional or excisional biopsy is a relatively straightforward surgical procedure, biopsy is often not necessary and may even be contraindicated. Even when a biopsy is indicated, it is important to know exactly how to place the incisions so as not to compromise further treatment and even to know what tests to order on the tissue obtained at biopsy. This knowledge is available only through a complete understanding of the differential diagnosis of neck mass.

An injudicious, premature neck biopsy can result in surgical scarring, preventing performance of an adequate clean surgical dissection, if such a procedure is necessary at a later time. It also can delay proper treatment and, perhaps worst of all, give the patient a false sense of security, causing him or her to believe that the mass is gone and the disease is cured.[2] When one is dealing with metastatic squamous cell carcinoma in the adult, premature biopsy prior to definitive treatment significantly increases the chances of local recurrence, wound infection, and distant metastatic disease.[3]

Since the differential diagnoses of cervical masses in children and adults are considerably different, the approaches are not the same. In young children, congenital and inflammatory masses far outnumber neoplastic diseases, approximately 90 per cent of head and neck masses being congenital, infectious, or benign, and 10 per cent malignant. Twenty-seven per cent of malignant tumors in childhood occur in the region of the head and neck. Excluding the orbit and brain, cervical lymph nodes are the most common site of involvement.[4] Besides the hyperplastic cervical nodes that commonly result from upper respiratory infections, several other infectious processes need to be considered in children (Table 1).

The majority of the benign masses that appear in childhood are cervical lymphadenopathy, congenital cysts, lymphangiomas, or hemangiomas. About 80 per cent of the lymphangiomas and hemangiomas are present at birth or appear within the first few months of life.[4]

Although most neck masses in children are benign, the physician must consider malignancy when examining any child with such a mass. The differential diagnosis in an infant or child must include all of the seven neoplastic types that constitute 80 per cent of malignancies in children. The most common of these is lymphoid tumor, both Hodgkin's and non-Hodgkin's lymphomas, which account for 55 to 60 per cent of all childhood malignancies presenting in the head and neck.[4, 5] The chances are equal that neck mass in a child is either lymphosarcoma or Hodgkin's disease, even though in general lymphosarcoma is twice as common as Hodgkin's disease. Forty per cent of children with lymphosarcoma and 80 per cent of children with Hodgkin's disease have masses.[5] The next most common primary solid tumor of the head and neck in children is rhabdomyosarcoma. Although it often arises in the nasopharynx or auricular area, it can also present as a mass in the neck. Other tumor types appearing in children, in order of decreasing frequency, are fibrosarcoma, thyroid malignancies, neuroblastoma, and epidermoid carcinoma.[5] A solitary thyroid nodule in a child 10 years or younger has a greater than 70 per cent chance of being malignant.[6] Early recognition of these childhood neoplastic diseases is critical, because survival rates are markedly improved if appropriate therapy is initiated early.

Although only about a tenth of neck masses in children are malignant, approximately 80 per cent of cervical masses presenting in adults over the age of 40 are neoplasms, almost always cervical lymph node metastases. Approximately three-fourths of these are from a primary carcinoma above the clavicle. Asymptomatic enlargement of one or more cervical lymph nodes in the adult is

Table 1. DIFFERENTIAL DIAGNOSIS OF NECK MASSES IN CHILDREN

Inflammatory masses	Cervical adenitis (bacterial, viral) Atypical tuberculosis Sialadenitis (parotid, submandibular) Toxoplasmosis Infectious mononucleosis Cat-scratch disease Syphilis
Congenital cysts	Branchial cleft cyst Dermoid Thyroglossal duct cyst Cystic hygroma
Malignant masses	Lymphoma (Hodgkin's, non-Hodgkin's) Lymphosarcoma Rhabdomyosarcoma Fibrosarcoma Thyroid malignancies Neuroblastoma Epidermoid carcinoma

almost always cancerous and usually due to metastasis from a primary neoplasm in the mouth or pharynx. Benign inflammatory hyperplasia is one of the least likely causes. More than 90 per cent of cervical lymph node metastases are of ectodermal (squamous cell carcinoma) origin. In adults it is estimated that the primary site of metastatic carcinoma in the neck can be diagnosed in all but 10 to 15 per cent of cases if evaluation is properly performed. Enlargement of cervical lymph nodes in the adult demands a search for the primary growth of cancer.[2] Any nontender mass in the neck larger than 2 cm is significant enough to warrant further investigation and follow-up.[1]

It is interesting that the average duration of symptoms prior to the patient's consulting a physician is close to 3 months. Moreover, the average time from presentation to initiation of appropriate therapy is also 3 months, because of the delay between one physician's examination of the patient and subsequent referral to the appropriate treating physician. This diagnostic delay is common, but it is potentially avoidable.

The neck mass has life-threatening possibilities. As with many malignant neoplasms, early diagnosis often improves the cure rate and reduces the rates of morbidity and mortality associated with treatment. The diagnostic routine should be directed toward the diagnosis of the highest-priority, life-threatening disease (e.g., cancer), and it should be planned so as not to compromise the treatment of that disease. The diagnostic method should be broad enough to encompass other high-priority diseases simultaneously or subsequently without endangering the patient's life.

HISTORY

The history, although rarely diagnostic and occasionally confusing, may be revealing in many cases if the physician asks the appropriate questions. A lump in the neck may be the only complaint in many patients. When asking questions that might give clues to the cause of the neck mass, the physician should pay special attention to areas of specific head and neck malfunction, such as pain, deformity, bleeding, and changes in physiologic function. Physiologic changes might be difficulty in breathing or swallowing or change in voice quality. Family history, environmental history, and living habits are also important, and each is discussed separately.

Since the majority of patients present to the physician because of a lump in the neck, initial questioning usually involves the mass. Variation and fluctuation in size of the mass is often described by patients. Whereas in a child or young adult such fluctuation in size, especially a decrease, might suggest an inflammatory or congenital process, this assumption should not be made in an adult. Changes in size can be seen in malignant neoplasms, owing to the adjacent inflammatory response that can occur around tumors. Therefore, fluctuation in size should not engender a false sense of security. Perhaps the most important change in size is rapid enlargement over a short time, which suggests a growing neoplasm.

Pain and tenderness may also be confusing symptoms. They may indicate an inflammatory process or malignant invasion of adjacent bone or nervous structures. Such symptoms may also be seen in a neoplasm that has grown rapidly and whose center has become necrotic or hemorrhagic secondary to rapid growth with bleeding into the center.

The physician should inquire about drainage of mucus or pus from the neck mass, especially during an upper respiratory infection. This process can be seen with congenital branchial cleft cyst and cervical adenitis due to any infectious process. Although these are the most common causes of pus or mucus drainage from a neck mass, the physician must always be aware that malignant neoplasms can develop central necrosis, enlarge, and spontaneously drain pus. Therefore, when faced with a neck abscess, one cannot be satisfied merely with incision and drainage of the abscess; one must also consider culture and even biopsy of the mass.

A recent head or neck infection is important. A skin or scalp infection may be the cause of cervical adenopathy. Oral infections, such as tooth or gum infections, tonsillitis, and pharyngitis, and respiratory infections, such as adenitis, nasopharyngitis, rhinitis, and sinusitis, can also cause enlargement of cervical lymph nodes.

Because the majority of neck masses in adults are lymph node metastases, questions that may lead to the source of the primary tumor are important. Pain in another location might be extremely important, often giving a clue as to the the primary focus of disease. *Otalgia* (ear pain) is often a common symptom in head and neck problems. When the ear findings are normal, the otalgia is often referred pain. It is caused by stimulation of the vagus nerve felt through its branch in the ear, Arnold's nerve. Such referred pain can be caused by any problem anywhere in the course of the vagus nerve, but especially in the oropharynx, hypopharynx, or larynx. Otalgia is often associated with malignancy in the adult in whom the tumor has invaded a terminal branch of the vagus nerve. *Dysphagia* (difficulty in swallowing) can be due to any mass in the oropharynx, hypopharynx or esophagus. *Odynophagia* (pain on swallowing) can also be related to obstruction of the pharynx by a mass but is more often associated with a malignant neoplasm that has ulcerated, broken through the mucous membrane, and caused irritation of the vagus nerve or inflammatory masses. Therefore, otalgia, dysphagia, and odynophagia are extremely important to ask about. When accompanying a neck mass, such symptoms warrant further investigation of pharyngeal structures.

Another important area of inquiry concerning the pharyngolaryngeal complex is hoarseness, which usually indicates some type of disease at the level of the glottis, the true vocal cords. Hoarseness in an adult lasting longer than 2 weeks demands evaluation by a physician experienced in laryngeal disorders; when there is an accompanying neck mass, the cause of hoarseness will often be a squamous cell carcinoma of the pharyngolaryngeal area. Airway obstruction manifested by increasing dyspnea may also be a symptom of laryngeal carcinoma.

The physician should inquire about the presence or previous removal of skin or lip lesions. If such lesions have been removed within the last several years, their histologic features should be reviewed. One commonly thinks of squamous cell and basal cell carcinoma as metastasizing to cervical lymph nodes, but one should not neglect cutaneous basal cell carcinoma. In recent years, more and more lesions of cutaneous basal cell carcinoma have been found to have metastasized to cervical lymph nodes.[7]

When dealing with a cervical mass, one must know about the patient's general state of health. Questions must be asked about recent weight loss, fever, chills, night sweats, anorexia, and malaise. These symptoms may indicate a generalized infection, neoplastic processes, or systemic disease. Generalized neoplastic processes such as lymphoma and leukemia can manifest as cervical adenopathy. Previous lung, breast, gastrointestinal, renal, testicular, or pancreatic carcinoma can also cause cervical adenopathy. Systemic diseases such as sarcoid and systemic lupus erythematosus can also manifest within the head and neck.

Inquiry about travel, occupation, and habits is also important. With the ease of nationwide and worldwide travel, infectious processes like histoplasmosis, tuberculosis, coccidioidomycosis, toxoplasmosis, and plague are being seen. Many of these disorders may not have previously been considered to occur in this country or in certain regions of this country, but physicians are now reporting and seeing all of them in their practices. All of these infectious processes can cause neck masses.

Occupational exposure of individuals to carcinogenic chemicals or pollutants is now being recognized more frequently. Detailed questioning about the patient's past and present occupations has become extremely important in this highly industrialized age.

Tobacco and alcohol are known carcinogens and common causes of squamous cell carcinoma of the aerodigestive tract. The type and duration of exposure to both are extremely important to ask about.

Keeping and handling pets may also cause neck masses. Infections from rabbits, tularemia, cat-scratch disease, atypical tuberculosis, and spirotrichosis may manifest as enlargement of cervical lymph nodes.

It is also possible that additional questions should be asked concerning sexual habits and preferences. With a changing socioeconomic environment and an increase in homosexuality, patients now present new challenges in the form of infectious and neoplastic conditions. For this reason, the physician should be aware of the possibility of new and unusual diseases that may first appear in the head and neck area. It has long been known that both syphilis and gonorrhea can cause cervical adenopathy.

PHYSICAL EXAMINATION

The physical examination should focus on several areas. A thorough otolaryngologic–head and neck examination is mandatory prior to the initiation of invasive, expensive diagnostic studies or any surgical violation of a neck mass, because most of the time the cause of the mass will be found on such an examination. The head and neck examination is often neglected or inadequate because the examiner feels uncomfortable about performing it, but proficiency can be gained with practice and a minimum amount of equipment.

Using the head light or head mirror, one carefully examines the ears, nose, oral cavity, nasopharynx, larynx, and hypopharynx. In the external ear and the nose, crusting, ulceration, and unexplained inflammation should be noted and considered for biopsy in the office if it looks suspicious. The mucosal surfaces of the oral cavity and lips are carefully inspected. The examination must include palpation of oral surfaces and their recesses, with particular attention to the submucosal area of the base of the tongue. It is not at all unusual for lesions to occur beneath the mucosal surfaces and to be found only by careful palpation of those surfaces.

Inspection of the oropharynx should include palpation of the tonsils and lateral pharyngeal walls. It should be remembered that lymphomas may originate from lymphoid tissues of Waldeyer's ring, which is formed by the adenoids, tonsils, and base of the tongue. Parapharyngeal space tumor or deep lobe parotid neoplasm can extend into the lateral pharyngeal wall and present as a unilateral bulging mass in the pharynx. Indiscriminate biopsy of such lesions, whether incisional or by needle, is contraindicated and hazardous because of the possibility of injury to the carotid artery and jugular vein, which are adjacent to the parapharyngeal space.

Indirect visual examination and/or palpation of the nasopharynx is critical in evaluating all adults with cervical masses of unknown cause.

Indirect mirror examination of the laryngopharynx will reveal most lesions arising in this area, which are often the primary sources of midneck masses. Abnormalities that must be considered suspicious include not only fungating ulcerative lesions but also anatomic distortion and edema, which might suggest an occult tumor within an unseen recess such as the laryngeal ventricle, pyriform apex, or postcricoid region.

The neck should be examined last to avoid focusing on the mass and neglecting the other areas requiring attention. The size, consistency, degree of fixation, and, most important, location should be recorded accurately. Tenderness, necrosis, and suppuration of a metastatic lymph node may occur and must not be dismissed as evidence of a benign lesion. All seemingly uninvolved areas, such as the thyroid gland, salivary glands, posterior triangles of the neck, contralateral neck, and supraclavicular fossae, should be carefully palpated for further evidence of disease or its source.

The consistency of the neck mass often gives the examiner an idea of the etiology. The mass may feel cystic, as in congenital cysts (branchial cleft cyst, thyroglossal duct cyst, and cystic hygroma); firm and hard with occasional slight irregularity, as in metastatic lymph nodes; or firm but rubbery with smooth or matted surface, indicating multiple firm masses, as in lymphoma. The overlying skin may be erythematous, as in infectious processes, or invaded by neoplastic processes.

In children, the location of the mass usually indicates its cause. Most second and third branchial cleft cysts occur at the anterior border of the sternocleidomastoid muscle just inferior to the level of the hyoid bone (Fig. 1). They may enlarge slightly, just after or concomitant with an upper respiratory infection. Thyroglossal duct cysts are almost always in the midline, with two-thirds of them just beneath the hyoid bone (Fig. 2). Because of their embryologic association with the tongue base, thyroglossal duct cysts move upward in the neck when the tongue is protruded.

The precise location of the involved nodes may help determine the primary site, as seen in Figure 3. In adults, high digastric or posterior cervical nodes, particularly when bilateral, may be the result of occult nasopharyngeal carcinoma. Approximately one-fourth of all nasopharyngeal carcinomas manifest solely as a lump in the neck.[8] Lymph nodes in the supraclavicular fossae are

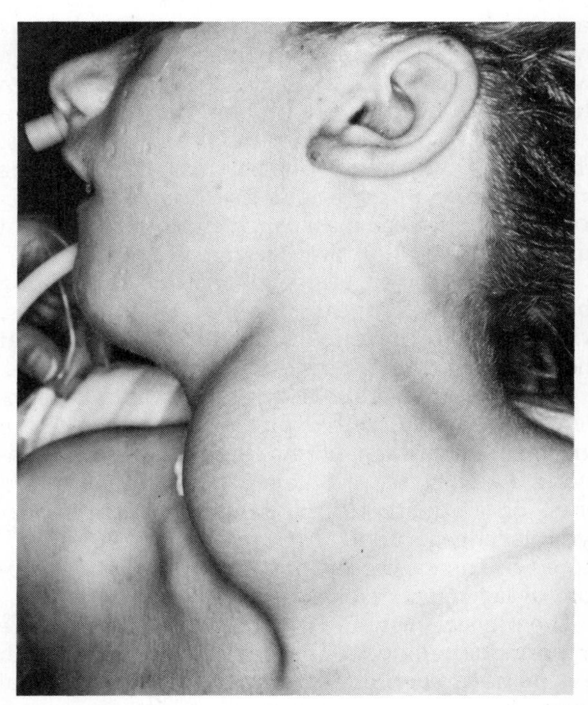

Figure 1. Second branchial cleft cyst anterior to border of sternocleidomastoid muscle.

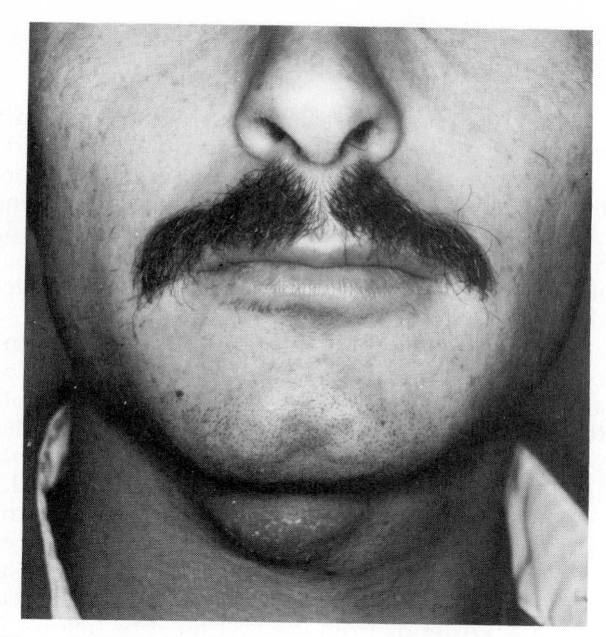

Figure 2. Thyroglossal duct cyst in midline of neck just beneath hyoid bone.

frequently metastatic from a primary tumor below the clavicles. Neck masses in the submental and submandibular triangles may arise from neoplasms in the lip, nose, anterior floor of the mouth, or anterior two-thirds of the tongue. Enlarged midjugular nodes may be due to neoplasms of the larynx, hypopharynx, or base of tongue, and enlarged low-jugular nodes may arise from thyroid or esophageal neoplasms.

It should always be remembered that normal anatomic structures can mimic neck masses. Common examples include the greater cornu of the hyoid bone, the carotid bulb, the transverse process of C1 cervical vertebra, normal lymph nodes in the neck, and normal submandibular salivary glands.

A complete physical examination of regions other than the head and neck should be done when there is the suggestion of symptoms referable to such regions.

DIAGNOSTIC STUDIES

Roentgenographic and laboratory studies should be used selectively. In most cases, a chest roentgenogram is all that is indicated in the adult with a painless lump in the midcervical region. Lateral soft-tissue roentgenograms or xeroradiograms of the nasopharynx are helpful in delineating nasopharyngeal space lesions. However, there is still no substitute for a good indirect mirror or direct visual examination of the nasopharynx. Roentgenographic studies of the paranasal sinuses may be fruitful in enlargement of superiorly or posteriorly located cervical lymph nodes, especially in cases with concomittant nasal obstruction, facial pain, or epistaxis. Thyroid scans may be useful but are no substitute for careful palpation of the thyroid gland; moreover, in the absence of palpable thyroid disease, the presence of a cold nodule on scan is not sufficient evidence of a thyroid disorder and is not necessarily related to the neck mass.

Laryngography, sialography, polytomography, and CT scanning are useful only as adjunctive tools, to determine the extent of already recognized disease but not to screen for occult disease. Selective angiography and digital subtraction angiography help to confirm the presence of a vascular tumor, such as a glomus jugulare or carotid body tumor, and to determine its extent.

The barium swallow is a useful roentgenographic study but should not be chosen over careful endoscopic examination. Although upper gastrointestinal series, barium enema, intravenous

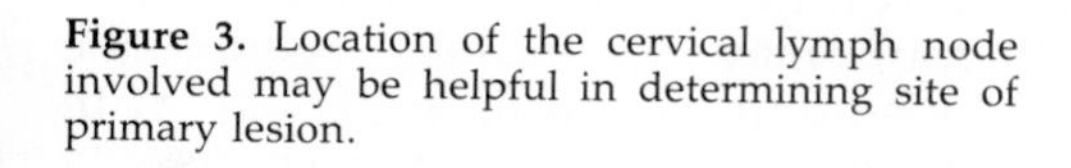

Figure 3. Location of the cervical lymph node involved may be helpful in determining site of primary lesion.

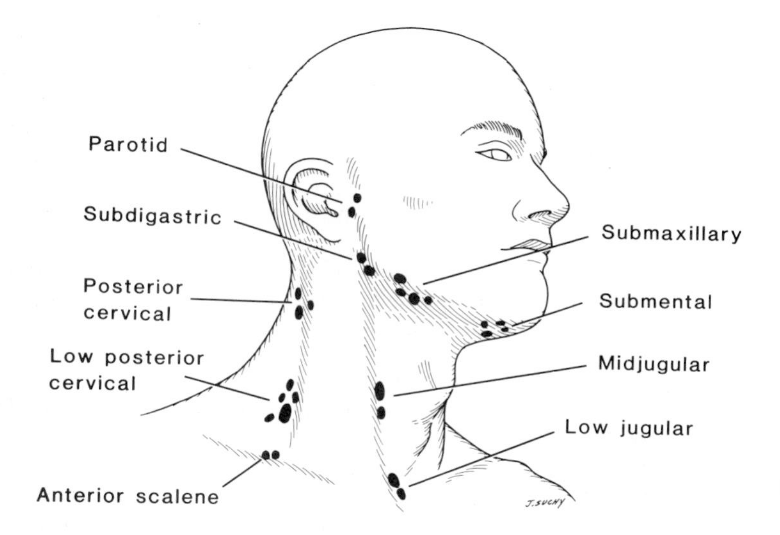

pyelography, abdominal CT scanning, and mammography may prove valuable, especially with supraclavicular masses, these particular roentgenographic studies are rarely indicated before a tissue diagnosis is made. Even if findings of one of these tests were positive, such a result would not completely rule out a second primary in the head and neck region.

In selected cases in which history and physical findings point toward a hematologic problem, complete blood count with differential counts, Monospot slide test, and heterophil antibody test are indicated. Epstein-Barr virus antibody titer determinations are useful in following patients with Burkitt's lymphoma, leukemia, and nasopharyngeal carcinoma but are rarely indicated prior to histologic examination. The antibody titer appears to increase with worsening of the disease.[8]

Following a carefully taken history, office physical examination, and selected roentgenographic studies, if the source of the neck mass has not been found, an endoscopic evaluation should be undertaken. Panendoscopy (laryngoscopy, bronchoscopy, nasopharyngoscopy, and esophagoscopy) *should* be performed in every patient with a lump in the neck that has a high probability of being a primary neoplasm in the upper aerodigestive tract. Although the use of random pharyngeal biopsy is controversial, biopsy of any suspicious area seen in the aerodigestive tract is certainly always indicated. Bronchoscopic washings for cytologic examination and, occasionally, culture should be obtained. Panendoscopy is almost always indicated prior to the performance of any open biopsy. Finding the primary tumor endoscopically enables one to perform endoscopic biopsy and avoid an open biopsy. As stated earlier, open neck biopsies have the potential for seeding adjacent tissue, destroying surgical neck planes, and increasing rates of morbidity and mortality.[2, 3] The patient with primary squamous cell carcinoma of the head and neck that is metastatic to cervical lymph nodes in whom a biopsy of the cervical lymph node is performed prior to definitive treatment has a much greater chance of local recurrence in the neck, distant metastatic disease, and wound infection.[2, 3] In addition to the primary source of the neck mass, one must seek other tumors in the aerodigestive tract, because the incidence of synchronous aerodigestive tract tumors is between 9 and 11 per cent.[9, 10]

If the neck mass is neither infectious nor congenital, but rather neoplastic, utilizing this comprehensive systematic approach enables the primary malignancy to be found in 85 per cent of the cases. In approximately 5 to 10 per cent of neck masses in adults ultimately found to be malignant, the primary is not found; roughly 90 per cent of the primaries are squamous cell carcinoma, one-third of which will subsequently be demonstrated either in the head and neck or the chest.[10]

MANAGEMENT OF THE NECK MASS: GENERAL CONCEPTS

When the clinician strongly suspects an inflammatory etiology, it is reasonable to try a short course of antibiotics under close observation prior to the definitive work-up. The antibiotic chosen should be effective against Staphylococcus and Streptococcus. No patient, however, with a mass that is not resolving should be given antibiotic therapy with follow-up at long intervals.

When the mass is suspected to be a neoplasm or has not resolved with antibiotics, the work-up already outlined should be undertaken. If none of the studies in the evaluation yield abnormal results or offer significant information as to the cause of the lump in the neck, excision may be considered. A good rule is that surgical excision is better than surgical incision. If a cyst is found, it should be excised completely. In excision of a congenital cyst of the branchial cleft or thyroglossal duct, the tract that often extends from the cyst must be followed surgically in accordance with the specific congenital abnormality.

If a lymph node containing pus is found, culture should be done for aerobic, anaerobic, fungal, and tuberculous organisms. The node should be removed totally, especially in the case of atypical tuberculosis, in which not only that node but all lymph nodes with atypical tuberculosis in the region should be removed. The treatment of choice for atypical tuberculosis in the lymph nodes is surgical excision.[11]

If the lymph node is so large that surgical excision would be difficult, a needle biopsy may be considered. Recently, at selected institutions, thin-needle aspiration biopsy with minimal risk of tumor seeding has been performed with excellent results. However, this technique necessitates an experienced pathologist capable of accurately interpreting the cytologic appearance of the aspirate.[12]

Most important, the physician performing the biopsy should be capable of performing a definitive surgical procedure at the same time. Because most neck masses in adults are metastatic malignancies from primary tumors within the head and neck, indiscriminate open biopsy that is not followed by some immediate therapy such as regional disease control with radical neck distention or radiotherapy may significantly reduce the chances of long-term survival, especially with lymph nodes larger than 4 cm (which usually means disease outside the capsule of the nodes).

ASSESSMENT

The physician must approach the cervical neck masses in a systematic fashion, with thorough knowledge of the possible causes and their consequences. He or she must also be aware of symptoms of neck masses that occur in other regions. There is a natural tendency to assume that a disease originates at the anatomic site where symptoms first appear. Although this is often true, in the case of the neck mass such a finding may only be a sign of distant or regional metastasis, or other disease elsewhere in the body. Therefore, a neck mass requires thorough history-taking, physical examination, and treatment.

Congenital neck masses are usually present from birth or arise and enlarge during upper respiratory infections. They grow slowly over 6 months or longer. Thyroglossal duct cyst usually manifests in the midline in association with the hyoid bone and rises in the neck when the tongue is protruded. The branchial cleft cyst tends to appear along the anterior border of the sternocleidomastoid muscle and may have an associated draining fistula site.

Metastatic carcinomas usually appear in adult smokers. Their location may give a clue to the site of origin, because the various common primary sites—nasopharynx, tonsil, oral cavity, base of tongue, larynx, and hypopharynx—drain to specific nodal locations.

Other symptoms apart from the lump in the neck often give clues to its etiology. Eustachian tube dysfunction may indicate nasopharyngeal disease. Otalgia may be associated with disease of the tonsils, base of the tongue, hypopharynx, or larynx. Hoarseness is associated with glottic disease. Dysphagia and odynophagia are associated with disease of the pyriform sinus and hypopharynx.

A mesenchymal malignancy in the neck is usually nontender, fixed, hard, matted, rubbery, rapidly enlarging, and larger than 4 cm. It often appears as a nondiscrete mass deep to the sternocleidomastoid muscle.

REFERENCES

1. Miller D, Ervin T, Weichselbaum R, Fabian RL. The differential diagnosis of mass in the neck. A fresh look. Laryngoscope 1981;91:140–5.
2. Martin H, Romieu C. Diagnostic significance of "lump in the neck." Postgrad Med 1952;11:491–500.
3. McGuirt W, McCabe BF. The significance of node biopsy before definitive treatment of cervical metastatic carcinoma. Laryngoscope 1978;88:594–7.
4. Conley J. Tumors of the head and neck in children. In: Conley J, ed. Concepts in head and neck surgery. New York: Grune & Stratton, 1970;181–92.
5. Jaffee BF. Pediatric head and neck tumors: a study of 178 cases. Laryngoscope 1973;83:1644–51.
6. Pigott JD. Management of thyroid nodule. Hosp Med 1:1, 1965;1:22–5.
7. Levine H. Cutaneous carcinoma of the head and neck: management of massive and previously uncontrolled lesions. Laryngoscope 1983;93:87–105.
8. Choa G. Cancer of the nasopharynx. In Suen JY, Myers EN, ed. Cancer of the head and neck. New York: Churchill Livingstone, 1981;372–414.
9. Vrabic D. Multiple primary malignancies of the upper aerodigestive tract. Ann Otol 1979;88:846–54.
10. Suen JY, Whitmore SJ. Cancer of the neck. In Suen JY, Myers EN, ed. Cancer of the head and neck. New York: Churchill Livingstone, 1981;185–211.
11. Olson N. Non-tuberculous mycobacterial infections of the face and neck; practical considerations. Laryngoscope 1981;91:1714–21.
12. Frable WJ, Frable MA. Thin-needle aspiration biopsy in the diagnosis of head and neck tumors. Laryngoscope 1974;84:1069–77.

OLIGURIA

MARC B. GOLDSTEIN

□ SYNONYMS: Low-output renal failure, antidiuresis

BACKGROUND

Definition

Oliguria is the state in which the urine output is less than 400 ml/day.

Rationale

There is an obligation to excrete at least 400 to 500 mOsm of solute in the urine daily. This obligate osmotic load represents the products of normal metabolism (urea, creatinine, uric acid, ammonium) and is increased by disease states resulting in higher catabolism, by glycosuria, and by increased intake of protein or salts. Because the maximum urine osmolality achievable by the normal human is approximately 1200 mOsm/kg, a urine volume of at least 400 ml is necessary to excrete the daily osmotic load. Hence, when the urine volume is less than 400 ml, normal needs are no longer being met, there is accumulation of nitrogenous wastes, and the patient is said to be oliguric.

CAUSES OF OLIGURIA

The problem of oliguria is best approached by the classification into prerenal, renal, and postrenal causes, with the fact that more than one cause may be present at any given time borne in mind (Table 1).

Prerenal Causes

Prerenal oliguria, the clinical situation in which low urine output results from underperfusion of the kidney, is the most common type of oliguria.[1] The most common cause of prerenal oliguria is extracellular fluid (ECF) volume contraction due to salt (sodium chloride) depletion. The sodium losses may occur via the gastrointestinal tract (vomiting, diarrhea, or nasogastric suction) or the urinary tract (diuretic use, sodium wasting secondary to osmotic diuresis as in glycosuria, or salt wasting due to intrinsic renal disease such as tubular necrosis or pyelonephritis or to mineralocorticoid deficiency). Skin losses of sodium may be substantial under hot environmental conditions (perspiration) or in extensive burns.

Circulating volume contraction due either to loss of circulating volume or to dilatation of the vascular tree leads to renal underperfusion. Loss of circulating volume occurs from either hemorrhage or hypoalbuminemia. In sepsis, there is also relative contraction of circulating volume owing to vasodilation, and in addition, loss of circulating volume may occur because of increased capillary permeability.

Cardiac failure is a common cause of prerenal oliguria, which is often also complicated by salt depletion secondary to aggressive diuretic therapy. Despite an expanded circulating volume in congestive heart failure, there is renal underperfusion owing to the reduction in cardiac output. In addition to myocardial disease (ischemic or inflammatory) and valvular disease, constrictive pericarditis and tamponade may result in prerenal oliguria.

Disease of either large or small vessels may cause prerenal oliguria. Renal artery stenosis (bilateral if the patient has both kidneys), a recognized cause of oliguria, is usually accompanied by hypertension; most other causes are accompanied by hypotension. Extensive nephrosclerosis for whatever reason—diabetes, hypertension, or atherosclerosis—may lead to prerenal oliguria. Similarly, inflammatory disease of the vessels leads to renal underperfusion.

Table 1. CAUSES OF OLIGURIA

Prerenal causes	*Extracellular fluid volume contraction due to sodium loss*
	Gastrointestinal tract
	Vomiting
	Nasogastric suction
	Diarrhea
	Urinary tract
	Diuretics
	Osmotic diuresis
	Salt-wasting renal disease
	Skin
	Perspiration
	Burns
	Circulating volume contraction
	Hemorrhage
	Hypoalbuminemia
	Sepsis
	Reduction in cardiac output
	Myocardial disease
	Valvular disease
	Constrictive pericarditis
	Tamponade
	Vascular disorders
	Renal artery disease
	Small-vessel disease
	Nephrosclerosis
	Vasculitis
Renal causes	*Glomerular disease*
	Glomerulonephritis (see Table 2)
	Tubulointerstitial diseases
	Acute tubular necrosis (see Table 3)
	Acute interstitial nephritis (see Table 4)
	Vascular diseases
	Embolism
	Atheromatous emboli
	Bacterial endocarditis
	Mural thrombi
	Systemic vasculitides
	Systemic vasculitis
	Scleroderma
	Malignant hypertension
	Hematologic disorders
	Thrombotic thrombocytopenic purpura
	Hemolytic uremic syndrome
Postrenal causes	*Ureteral obstruction*
	Calculi
	Blood clot
	Tumor
	Bladder
	Ureter
	Retroperitoneal compression
	Fibrosis
	Malignancy
	Urethral obstruction
	Prostatic disease
	Hyperplasia
	Carcinoma
	Cervical carcinoma
	Urethral stricture
	Meatal stenosis

Renal Causes

Renal oliguria is decreased urine output due to intrinsic renal disease. The renal causes of oliguria are best classified according to the various components of the kidney: the glomeruli, the tubulointerstitial area, and the blood vessels (see Table 1).

Glomerular Disease

A discussion of glomerulonephritis is beyond the scope of this section but a general classification is appropriate. Oliguria is most likely to be present in rapidly progressive glomerulonephritis, the causes of which are listed in Table 2. Primary glomerulonephritis may be caused by anti–glomerular basement membrane (anti-GBM) antibodies or circulating immune complexes, or it may be idiopathic (mechanism of injury unclear). Glomerulonephritis due to anti-GBM antibodies may occur solely as glomerulonephritis or in conjunction with intrapulmonary hemorrhage, in which case it is known as Goodpasture's syndrome. Except for the pulmonary hemorrhage, all three types may have identical clinical presentations.[2]

Rapidly progressive glomerulonephritis may follow infection with almost any bacteria or virus, and postinfectious glomerulonephritis has also been associated with intrapulmonary hemorrhage.[3] A large percentage of cases of polyarteritis nodosa are associated with hepatitis surface antigenemia and therefore the disorder may be classified as an "infectious" cause of rapidly progressive glomerulonephritis. Bacterial endocarditis can be associated with rapidly progressive glomerulonephritis on either an embolic or immunologic basis.

Several multisystem diseases are associated with rapidly progressive glomerulonephritis, systemic lupus erythematosus being the most common. Systemic vasculitides include Henoch-Schönlein purpura, Wegener's granulomatosis, polyarteritis nodosa, allergic angiitis, and systemic necrotizing vasculitis.

Table 2. CAUSES OF RAPIDLY PROGRESSIVE GLOMERULONEPHRITIS

Primary glomerular diseases	Due to anti–glomerular basement membrane antibodies Due to circulating immune complexes Idiopathic crescentic glomerulonephritis without immune deposits
Infections	Postinfectious rapidly progressive glomerulonephritis Vasculitis in association with hepatitis surface antigenemia Bacterial endocarditis
Multisystem diseases	Systemic lupus erythematosus Systemic vasculitides: Henoch-Schönlein purpura Polyarteritis Cryoglobulinemia Allergic angiitis Systemic necrotizing vasculitis

Table 3. CAUSES OF ACUTE TUBULAR NECROSIS

Type	Causes
Ischemic	Shock Trauma Sepsis Hypoxia
Toxic	*Antibiotics* Aminoglycosides Cephalosporins Amphotericin B Polymixin B *Heavy metals* Mercury Arsenic Platinum *Endogenous toxins* Endotoxin Myoglobin Hemoglobin Bence Jones protein Contrast media Fluorinated anesthetic agents Ethylene glycol Organic solvents Acetaminophen Mushrooms Paraquat

Tubulointerstitial Disease

Tubulointerstitial diseases are now being recognized more frequently as causes of oliguria, although it should be appreciated that the incidence of nonoliguric acute tubular necrosis is increasing. There are two common forms of tubulointerstitial disease—acute tubular necrosis (ATN) and acute interstitial nephritis (AIN). Often, ATN is used *incorrectly* as a synonym for acute renal failure.

Acute Tubular Necrosis. There are two major types of ATN, ischemic and toxic (Table 3).[4] The ischemic type occurs in states of hypovolemia due to either hemorrhage or large salt and water losses, in which prerenal failure due to renal underperfusion can progress to ischemic ATN. Ischemia may also result from trauma. *Ischemia* is reduced oxygen delivery. Therefore, sepsis, in which there is both relative hypovolemia and an inability to extract oxygen at the tissue level, is often associated with ischemia. Finally, severe hypoxia can result in ischemic acute tubular necrosis.

Antibiotics constitute the most common category of toxins causing ATN. Aminoglycosides are the major culprits, their toxicity being enhanced by advanced age, renal function impairment, and ECF volume contraction.[5] Although the early cephalosporins were severely nephrotoxic, the newer generations are much less so. Amphotericin B causes nephrotoxicity inevitably if a cumulative dose in excess of 5 gm is given.[6] The nephrotoxicity of the polymyxin group of antibiotics is so severe that it has markedly limited the use of these agents.

Heavy metal nephrotoxicity has also been recognized for many years, but it was encountered infrequently until the recent use of *cis*-platinum in the chemotherapy of solid tumors.

Endogenous toxins play a role in acute tubular necrosis, and some believe that endotoxin is the major basis for the ATN associated with sepsis. The toxic effect of myoglobin causes the ATN that occurs in rhabdomyolysis. Similarly, hemoglobin is a toxic pigment accounting for the ATN that may follow the transfusion of mismatched blood.

It is surprising that the nephrotoxicity of radiographic contrast agents has only recently become common knowledge, because these agents rank second only to antibiotics as causes of toxic ATN. The two groups of patients most susceptible to contrast media nephrotoxicity are diabetics, especially those with reduced renal function, and patients with chronic renal insufficiency.[7] Nephrotoxicity of contrast agents has been recognized for many years in patients with multiple myeloma, but it can probably be prevented by avoiding concomitant ECF volume contraction.

A number of other toxins also cause ATN (see Table 3). Repeated exposure to fluorinated anesthetics leads to more rapid metabolism as a result of the induction of enzymes, and the fluoride levels are consequently higher; the incidence of ATN correlates best with the free fluoride level. Ethylene glycol exerts its toxicity via metabolism to oxalate and subsequent crystalluria. The organic solvents that cause ATN as well as severe liver damage include carbon tetrachloride, tetrachloroethylene, and chloroform. Acetaminophen, which is associated generally with fulminant hepatic toxicity, also causes ATN, occasionally in the absence of severe liver injury. Certain mushrooms are extremely toxic, especially the members of the Amanita genus; resulting acute tubular necrosis is accompanied by profound hepatotoxicity. The toxicity of paraquat, a potent herbicide, is directed at the lung as well as the kidney.

Acute Interstitial Nephritis. Drug-induced acute interstitial nephritis (AIN) is becoming an increasingly common cause of acute renal failure and oliguria.[8] More than 40 drugs have now been incriminated (Table 4). The most common group are the β-lactam antibiotics,[9] which include penicillin G, methicillin, ampicillin, oxacillin, nafcillin, carbenicillin, amoxicillin, cephalothin, cephalexin, cephradine, and cefotaxime. A host of additional antibiotics that cause AIN are listed in Table 4. Chloramphenicol, gentamicin, and isoniazid have been suspected but not yet clearly proven to cause acute interstitial nephritis.

The nonsteroidal anti-inflammatory agents are another large family of drugs causing AIN.[10] They are somewhat unusual in that the patients in

Table 4. CAUSES OF ACUTE INTERSTITIAL NEPHRITIS

Drugs	
Antibiotics	Penicillins Cephalosporins Sulfonamides Trimethoprim-sulfamethoxazole Rifampin Polymixin Ethambutol Tetracyclines Vancomycin
Nonsteroidal anti-inflammatory agents	Indomethacin Phenylbutazone Fenoprofen Naproxen Ibuprofen Phenazone Mefenamic acid Tolmetin Diflunisal
Diuretics	Thiazides Furosemide Chlorthalidone Ticrynafen
Miscellaneous drugs	Phenindione Phenytoin Cimetidine Sulfinpyrazone Aspirin Allopurinol Carbamazepine Clofibrate Azathioprine Phenylpropanolamine Methyldopa Phenobarbital
Systemic infections	Streptococcal infections Leptospirosis Toxoplasmosis Infectious mononucleosis Measles Brucellosis Syphilis Mycoplasma infections Legionnaires' disease Rocky Mountain spotted fever
Idiopathic	

whom they cause the disorder tend to be older. Whether this tendency is due to a specific predisposition of the elderly to this disorder or merely to the fact that these drugs are primarily consumed by the elderly has not yet been established. The other distinctive feature of AIN due to nonsteroidal anti-inflammatory agents is that it may be associated with the nephrotic syndrome.

Diuretics have also been demonstrated to cause acute interstitial nephritis.[11] Despite the fact that these agents are so widely prescribed, diuretic-induced AIN is not a common phenomenon, suggesting that its incidence may be very low. The list of additional drugs capable of causing AIN continues to grow, and one should suspect any drug of having the capacity to cause AIN.

This disorder also occurs in two settings unrelated to drugs: systemic infection and circumstances in which no known etiologic factor is apparent (idiopathic).

Vascular Disease

The vascular factors of renal disease leading to oliguria are listed in Table 1. Embolisms have three major sources: atheromatous disease (often in association with an angiographic study), heart valves involved with subacute bacterial endocarditis, and thrombi within the atrial or ventricular cavities.

Several systemic diseases have an impact on the vessels of the kidney without involving the glomerulus. If the large vessels are involved, the effect resembles prerenal failure, because nephron underperfusion results. All the systemic vasculitides, scleroderma, and malignant hypertension are capable of such an effect. Also, both thrombotic thrombocytopenic purpura and the hemolytic uremic syndrome can cause oliguria if they involve the renal vessels.

Postrenal Causes

One should keep in mind that for obstruction to be the sole cause of oliguria, either the obstruction is bilateral, or the patient has only one kidney. Obstruction can occur at the level of the ureters or the urethra, as outlined in Table 1. Ureteral obstruction can be due to calculi, blood clots, or tumor of either the bladder or ureter. The ureter may be compressed in the retroperitoneal space by either retroperitoneal fibrosis or malignancy, which is usually lymphoma.

Obstruction at the level of the urethra causes bilateral obstruction with a single lesion. It usually results from either hyperplasia or carcinoma of the prostate or carcinoma of the cervix. Stricture of the urethra and meatal stenosis are the final considerations in postrenal oliguria.

Diagnosing the Basis of Oliguria

The major areas upon which to focus in pursuing the diagnosis of oliguria are: the history, a careful clinical assessment of ECF volume and circulating volume, and a good urinalysis. These areas are dealt with separately in the following pages.

HISTORY

If one suspects prerenal oliguria, one should look for a history of gastrointestinal fluid losses, diuretic exposure, or urine losses due to osmotic loads (mannitol, hyperglycemia, or catabolic state), all of which might cause ECF volume contraction. A history of overt bleeding should raise the question of circulating volume contraction. One should also inquire about symptoms of reduced cardiac output or intrinsic heart disease (angina, congestive heart failure, rheumatic fever).

The history often contains important clues to the presence of intrinsic renal disease. With glomerular disease, there may be a viral prodrome, a history of hematuria or hemoptysis (Goodpasture's syndrome), or symptoms of a systemic vasculitis or a collagen vascular disease (arthritis, rash, sun sensitivity, Raynaud's phenomenon, pleurisy, mouth ulcers, and alopecia). A history of purpura will raise the possibility of a systemic vasculitis, a collagen vascular disease, or thrombotic thrombocytopenic purpura. One should ask about upper respiratory problems (sinusitis or nosebleeds) to consider the possibility of Wegener's granulomatosis.

A drug history is critical, use of diuretics raising the possibilities of prerenal failure (ECF volume depletion) or AIN, and of antibiotics suggesting ATN or AIN. All drugs the patient is or has been taking should be regarded as having at least the potential to provoke AIN. One must also inquire about recent investigative or diagnostic procedures. Recent angiography, for example, raises the possibilities of atheromatous emboli and contrast-induced ATN. The presence of systemic infection points to ATN due to endotoxin, prerenal failure from vasodilatation, or AIN associated with infection.

Obstruction of the urinary tract is often asymptomatic, but the presence of gross hematuria should point to calculi, clots, or tumor, and the presence or absence of pain is a helpful distinguishing feature. Lower urinary tract symptoms in a male may signify urethral obstruction somewhere between the prostate and the meatus.

PHYSICAL EXAMINATION

The most important aspect of the physical examination in the oliguric patient is a careful assessment of the ECF, particularly the circulating volume status. This involves observing the blood pressure for a decrease in the erect position and the pulse rate for an increase in the erect position. The jugular venous pressure should be assessed by relating the height of the internal jugular venous pulsation to the sternal angle. Other, "softer" physical signs that can be used are tissue turgor and eyeball tension, but these are less reliable, particularly in the older patient. One should also keep in mind that the jugular venous pressure reflects the status on the *right* side of the heart and can be used to mirror the status in the left atrium. When right atrial pressure is elevated without relation to left atrial pressure (chronic lung disease, pulmonary hypertension, pulmonary or tricuspid valve disease) or when there is constrictive pericarditis or tamponade, the jugular venous pressure does *not* reflect the left atrial pressure. One should first ascertain that the cardiac status is normal, in order to rule out prerenal failure due to cardiac disorder as well as to exclude subacute bacterial endocarditis. The skin should be examined carefully for purpura (vasculitis, thrombotic thrombocytopenic purpura), rash (drug-induced AIN, collagen vascular disease), and livedo reticularis (atheromatous emboli). Pelvic and rectal examinations should always be done to rule out neoplasm and prostatic hyperplasia as possible sources of renal obstruction.

DIAGNOSTIC STUDIES

Laboratory Studies

Urinalysis. The most critical evaluation in oliguria is the urinalysis, which should be performed by a physician whenever possible. Relegating this important component of the evaluation to a technologist who may have a hundred other "routine" urinalyses to do is inappropriate. A urine specific gravity of greater than 1.020 suggests a prerenal cause of oliguria. On the other hand, in a patient with obvious physical signs of circulating volume contraction, a specific gravity less than 1.020 indicates tubular dysfunction. The presence of a large amount of protein (3+ or more) generally indicates a glomerular lesion, although occasionally a small amount of protein in very concentrated urine may give a 3+ reaction. Therefore, one should note the specific gravity as well and should be less inclined to assume 3+ proteinuria to be of glomerular origin if the specific gravity exceeds 1.020. It is more accurate to determine the 24-hour urine protein excretion rate; more than 3 gm/day is strongly suggestive of glomerular disease. The presence of red blood cells (RBC) in the sediment may indicate calculi, tumor, or glomerular disease. The presence of white blood cells (WBC) suggests inflammation and is consistent with AIN or infection. The presence of renal tubular cells, which are larger than white blood cells and have prominent eccentric nuclei, suggests ATN.

The most important finding is the presence of casts. RBC casts are strongly indicative of an active glomerulonephritis, whereas heme granular casts (mahogany-colored) are consistent with either glomerulonephritis or ATN. Granular casts indicate intrarenal disease and therefore make prerenal failure alone unlikely. The urine of patients with AIN may be shown to contain eosinophils when examined with Wright staining.

A number of additional tests can be performed on the urine to help differentiate between prerenal failure and ATN,[12] often a difficult distinction to establish. These tests, listed in Table 5, are based upon the following assumptions: (1) in prerenal failure, the tubules function well and are under a stimulus to remove as much sodium (Na) and water as possible; (2) because of this, any substance filtered but not reabsorbed (urea and cre-

Table 5. DIAGNOSTIC URINARY PARAMETERS IN OLIGURIA*

Parameter	Prerenal Cause	Renal Cause	Postrenal Cause
Urine osmolality (mOsm)	> 500	< 350 (ATN)	ND
Urine-plasma osmolality ratio	> 1.3	< 1.1	ND
Urine sodium concentration (mmol/L)	< 20	> 40	ND
Urine-plasma urea ratio	> 8	< 3 (ATN); > 8 (GN)	< 3
Urine-plasma creatinine ratio	> 40	< 20 (ATN); > 40 (GN)	< 20
FE_{Na} (%)	< 1	> 2 (ATN); < 1 (GN)	> 2
Renal failure index (%)†	< 1	> 2 (ATN); < 1 (GN)	> 2

*GN = glomerulonephritis; ATN = acute tabular necrosis; ND = nondiagnostic.
†See text for details.

atinine) will be concentrated in the urine in prerenal failure. The more the urine is concentrated, the higher is the ratio between the urine and the plasma concentrations of that substance.

Because the underperfused kidney is retaining sodium avidly, the fractional excretion of sodium (FE_{Na})—the fraction of the filtered sodium that is excreted—is low. Sodium filtration is defined by the product of the glomerular filtration rate (GFR)—or creatinine clearance rate—and the plasma sodium concentration: Filtered Na = GFR × P_{Na}. The fractional excretion of sodium (FE_{Na}) is calculated using the following equation:

$$FE_{Na} = \frac{U_{Na}\,V}{\frac{U_{cr}V}{P_{cr}} \cdot P_{Na}} \times 100$$

$$= \frac{U_{Na}/P_{Na}}{U_{cr}/P_{cr}} \times 100$$

where $U_{Na}V$ is excreted sodium, P_{Na} is plasma sodium, $U_{cr}V$ is excreted creatinine, and P_{cr} is plasma creatinine. FE_{Na} is expressed as a percentage. Note that a spot urine collection is sufficient for this calculation, because the urine volume "cancels out."[13]

The other derived parameter that may be useful is the Renal Failure Index (RFI), which expresses the urine sodium concentration (which is low in prerenal failure) as a function of the urine-plasma creatinine ratio (which is high in prerenal failure):

$$RFI\ (\%) = \frac{U_{Na}}{\frac{U_{cr}}{P_{cr}}} \times 100$$

The resultant ratio is very low in prerenal failure, further improving the predictive value of the individual parameters.[14] Several of these parameters will be the same in prerenal failure as in glomerulonephritis (GN), because in aggressive GN, the nephron is underperfused owing to the extensive inflammatory reaction in the glomerulus.

Other Studies. It is useful to evaluate the blood urea nitrogen–blood creatinine ratio in the oliguric patient. Although creatinine is not reabsorbed, in states of slow urine flow with good tubular function, urea is reabsorbable. Hence, the BUN–blood creatinine ratio, which is normally 10:1, is increased in prerenal failure and obstructive uropathy.[15] The eosinophil count may be increased in patients with AIN and polyarteritis nodosa.

The only other laboratory tests of value in assessing the oliguric patient are determinations of serologic abnormalities, which are helpful in separating the various forms of glomerulonephritis; they include measurements of ASO titer, serum complements, antinuclear factor, anti-GBM antibodies, anti-DNA antibodies, cryoglobulins, Bence Jones protein, and hepatitis-associated antigens, as well as urine protein electrophoresis and the VDRL test.

Imaging

Ultrasonography is a relatively simple, noninvasive way to rule out obstruction, which must be excluded if suspected. If ultrasonography is not available there are two options: intravenous pyelography (IVP) and retrograde pyelography, both of which carry risk. The chance that contrast-induced ATN may occur after IVP is significant if the serum creatinine level exceeds 4 mgm/100 ml, and one should first ensure that the patient does not have ECF volume contraction, which might enhance the dye's nephrotoxicity. Retrograde pyelography carries the risks associated with general anesthesia and is a very invasive procedure; it should not be done in the patient with urinary tract sepsis.

When calculi are suspected, a flat plate of the abdomen is useful, because 85 per cent of renal calculi are radiopaque.

When AIN is suspected, gallium scanning should be carried out. Results are positive in AIN owing to the active inflammatory process.[16] Of concern, however, is that gallium scan results are also positive in the nephrotic syndrome, making the procedure less helpful in cases of AIN due to nonsteroidal anti-inflammatory agents accompanied by nephrotic syndrome.

ASSESSMENT

When a patient presents with oliguria, there is an overwhelming urge to administer diuretics, as physicians seem to be mesmerized by the flow of urine. This compelling desire must be resisted, on two counts: (1) diuretic therapy is detrimental to the patient with prerenal failure, and (2) it eliminates several valuable clues to the differential diagnosis—urine sodium level, urinary-plasma creatinine and urea ratios, urine specific gravity and osmolality, fractional excretion of sodium, and RFI. Therefore, the physician should try to establish the basis of the oliguria prior to initiating therapeutic intervention.

One should begin by ruling out prerenal and postrenal causes, as these are easily reversible. As discussed previously, the history and physical findings should contain many clues if prerenal oliguria is present. If the physical findings are inconclusive and one suspects a prerenal problem, there are two options: a "fluid challenge" with

500 to 1000 ml of normal saline or its equivalent in tonicity (i.e., isotonic $NaHCO_3$ to the acidemic patient) or, if that procedure might be detrimental, more invasive techniques to establish the hemodynamic status of the patient (Swan-Ganz catheterization). Sometimes there is evidence of renal underperfusion (e.g., low urine sodium), but the circulating volume and cardiac output are normal. In that case, one should look for local causes of renal underperfusion (renal artery disease) or maldistribution of the cardiac output, which may occur in sepsis and the hepatorenal syndrome.[17]

A postrenal cause of oliguria may not be evident at the end of the history-taking, physical examination, and laboratory evaluation, because this type of diagnosis may be elusive. The physician is obliged at this point to rule out obstruction, which is easily reversed and may lead to permanent kidney damage if left untreated. Ultrasonography has totally eliminated morbid effects from the establishment of the presence or absence of urinary tract obstruction. If ultrasound evaluation is not available and the index of suspicion is high, either IVP or retrograde pyelography should be done.

Once prerenal and postrenal causes of oliguria have been ruled out, one is left with intrinsic renal disease as the possible diagnosis. The urinalysis is most helpful in separating the various causes of intrinsic renal disease. Heavy proteinuria and RBC casts implicate acute glomerulonephritis, whereas heme granular casts and renal tubular cells signify ATN. One may see white blood cells and WBC casts in AIN, but the urine sediment may be very "quiet" (i.e., absence of both cells and casts). Gallium scanning appears to be a useful and noninvasive means of establishing the diagnosis of AIN, providing the patient does not have the nephrotic syndrome. If ATN and AIN have been ruled out and the patient has undergone significant deterioration in renal function, a renal biopsy is indicated to establish the specific diagnosis. One must keep in mind that not infrequently, the basis of the oliguria is multifactorial (e.g., a patient with ATN may also have a prerenal component). Therefore, a complete clinical assessment must always be carried out, even after one has evidence for one cause of the oliguria.

REFERENCES

1. Anderson RJ, Schrier RW. Clinical spectrum of oliguric and non-oliguric acute renal failure. In: Brenner BM, Stein JH, ed. Acute renal failure. New York: Churchill Livingstone, 1980;1–16.
2. Glassock RL, Cohen AH, Bennett CM, Martinez-Maldonado M. Primary glomerular diseases—rapidly progressive glomerulonephritis. In: Brenner BM, Rector FC, ed. The kidney. 2nd ed. Philadelphia: WB Saunders, 1981;1385–98.
3. Aach R, Kissane J. Proliferative glomerulonephritis and pulmonary haemorrhage. Am J Med 1973;55:199–210.
4. Balslov JT, Jorgensen HE. A survey of 499 patients with acute anuric renal insufficiency. Am J Med 1963;34:753–64.
5. Bennett WM, Plamp CE, Porter GA. Drug-related syndromes in clinical nephrology. Ann Intern Med 1977;87:582–90.
6. Takacs FJ, Tomkiewicz ZM, Merrill JP. Amphotericin B nephrotoxicity with irreversible renal failure. Ann Intern Med 1963;59:716–24.
7. Van Zee BE, Hoy WE, Talley TE, Jaenike JR. Renal injury associated with intravenous pyelography in nondiabetic and diabetic patients. Ann Intern Med 1978;89:51–4.
8. Kleinknecht D, Vanhille PH, Morel-Maroger L, et al. Acute interstitial nephritis due to drug hypersensitivity. An up-to-date review with a report of 19 cases. Adv Nephrol 1982;12:277–308.
9. Appel GB, Neu HC. Nephrotoxicity of antimicrobial agents. N Engl J Med 1977;296:722–8.
10. Brezin JH, Katz SM, Schwartz AB, Chinitz JL. Reversible renal failure and nephrotic syndrome associated with nonsteroidal anti-inflammatory drugs. N Engl J Med 1979;301:1271–3.
11. Lyons H, Pinn VW, Cortell S, Cohen JJ, Harrington J. Allergic interstitial nephritis causing reversible renal failure in four patients with idiopathic nephrotic syndrome. N Engl J Med 1973;288:124–8.
12. Bastl CP, Rudnick MR, Narins RG. Diagnostic approaches to acute renal failure. In: Brenner BM, Stein JH, ed. Acute renal failure. New York: Churchill Livingstone, 1980;17–51.
13. Espinel CH. The FENa test. Use in the differential diagnosis of acute renal failure. JAMA 1976;236:579–81.
14. Miller TR, Henrich WL, Schrier RW. Urinary diagnostic indices in acute renal failure. A prospective study. Ann Intern Med 1978;89:47–50.
15. Perlmutter M, Grossman SL, Rothenberg S, Doblan G. Urine-serum urea nitrogen ratio. Simple test of renal function in acute azotemia and oliguria. JAMA 1959;170:1533–7.
16. Linton AL, Clark WF, Drieger AA, Turnbull DI, Lindsay RM. Acute interstitial nephritis due to drugs. Ann Intern Med 1980;93:735–41.
17. Levy M. The kidney in liver disease. In: Brenner BM, Stein JH, ed. Sodium and water homeostasis. New York: Churchill Livingstone, 1978;73–116.

PELVIC PAIN IN WOMEN

ROBERT McLELLAN □ MICHAEL R. SPENCE

BACKGROUND

Pelvic pain may be defined as discomfort that occurs in the lower abdomen, specifically in the area inferior to the umbilicus and medial and superior to the inguinal ligaments as they traverse toward the pubic symphysis. When pelvic pain occurs in the female, the differential diagnosis is complicated by the many pathologic alterations that may involve the female reproductive organs. This symptom accounts for approximately one-third of gynecologic consultations and is a prominent feature in many presentations to other physicians. The frequency of the complaint, however, does not detract from the necessity for proper evaluation and subsequent management. An accurate differential diagnosis is imperative, because pelvic pain frequently represents life-threatening catastrophes, including ectopic pregnancy, appendicitis, and even ovarian malignancy. The major responsibility for the initial evaluation and proper management lies with the primary care physician. Those clinicians "on the front line" must use readily available assessment tools in order to give appropriate treatment to the unhappy patient with pelvic pain. This chapter discusses the assessment of such a patient and, we hope, provides an efficient problem-oriented system of evaluation that enables the clinician to formulate an accurate differential diagnosis.

Anatomic Considerations

In order to treat pelvic pain, one must have a basic understanding of the anatomic and physiologic processes involved. The sensation of pain is carried to the cerebral cortex via both somatic and autonomic afferent fibers. These fibers enter the spinal cord through the posterior horn and ascend the lateral spinothalamic tract. Afferent fibers from the lower abdominal wall, perineum, and pelvic viscera enter the cord at the level of T10 and below. The abdominal wall below the umbilicus is supplied by segments T10 through L1, whereas the pelvic floor, outlet, and perineum are supplied by segments L4 through S4.[1] Hence, superficial and visceral pain sensations are established by a wide range of sensory fibers entering a comparatively small area of the cord.

We may divide the sensory innervation of the pelvis into two categories, the somatic system, which innervates all of the superficial and a few of the deep structures, and the autonomic system, which innervates all of the viscera and most of the deep structures.

The autonomic system is composed of sympathetic and parasympathetic plexuses. Pain stimuli from the deep pelvic viscera may pass along the following routes (Table 1). First, multiple afferent fibers passing into S2–S4 accumulate in the vicinity of the uterosacral ligaments, forming the pelvic plexus of the parasympathetic system. This plexus provides afferent fibers for the lower uterine segment, cervix, cervical ligaments, and upper one-third of the vagina, as well as sensory fibers for the lower portion of the ureters, their surrounding connective tissue, the trigone of the bladder, the posterior urethra, and the rectosigmoid colon. Second, the sympathetic system provides the majority of afferent fibers supplying the fundus of the uterus, the medial one-third of the fallopian tubes, the mesosalpinx, and the broad ligament. These fibers also serve the bladder, fundus, distal small bowel, cecum, appendix, and terminal end of the distal colon. These fibers pass to the hypogastric plexus, thence to the inferior mesenteric plexus, and subsequently to the posterior root of the spinal cord via the sympathetic chain. Third, the ovaries, lateral two-thirds of the fallopian tubes, a portion of the mesosalpinx, and the proximal pelvic ureter send sensory fibers to the superior mesenteric plexus and thence to the spinal cord segments T10–T12 via the sympathetic system.

This superficial review of pelvic innervation allows one to appreciate the wide range of afferent fibers entering any particular segment of the spinal cord. Pain from superficial structures is mediated via the somatic nervous system to well-developed foci in the cerebral cortex, but not visceral pain. In the human, cortical pain projections from deep pelvic structures are mediated through the autonomic system. The diffuse and nonspecific innervation, as just described, makes it difficult to locate the precise cause of pelvic pain. Certain generalizations, however, may be made regarding patterns of pain perception that, when present, offer a clue as to the location of pelvic disease. Pain from the cervix and lower uterine segment is frequently referred along the uterosacral ligaments to the lower back, buttocks, and posterior aspect of the lower extremities. Pain sensation from the medial fallopian tubes, uterine fundus, and fundus of the

Table 1. AUTONOMIC INNERVATION OF THE PELVIS AND VISCERA

Plexus	Spinal Cord Segment	Structures Innervated *Reproductive*	*Urinary*	*Gastrointestinal*
Pelvic	S2–S4	Vagina Upper one-third Cervix Cervical ligaments Cardinal ligaments Lower uterine segment	Trigone of bladder, pelvic ureter, and surrounding connective tissue Posterior urethra	Rectum and sigmoid
Hypogastric	(Posterior root)	Uterine fundus Fallopian tubes Medial one-third Mesosalpinx and broad ligament Connective tissue Vascular supply	Bladder fundus	Ileum Cecum and appendix Terminal end of distal colon
Aortic	T10–T12	Fallopian tubes Lateral two-thirds Ovaries Part of mesosalpinx	Proximal pelvic ureter and surrounding connective tissue	

bladder may be referred to the lower or middle abdominal wall, an area known as the "tubo-ovarian triangle." Pain from the ovaries, lateral fallopian tubes, and rectum is often referred to the anterior abdominal wall, lateral to and just below the umbilicus; this pain referral may become more localized and intensified with involvement of the parietal peritoneum. Unfortunately, pain referred to the periumbilical area may result from any process that irritates that position of parietal peritoneum, including acute appendicitis, diverticulitis, and mesenteric thrombosis. Pain from the ileum, cecum, appendix, and sigmoid colon may be referred to the substernal, epigastric, or lower abdominal areas. Pain sensation from the mesentery, pelvic connective tissue, and pelvic vessels tends to be deep-seated, dull, and poorly localized in the abdomen.

Causes of Pelvic Pain

The many causes of pelvic pain have been categorized in nearly as many ways. Pelvic pain may be of genital, nongenital, or psychogenic origin. One method of classification that may serve as a guide in the differential diagnosis is presented in Table 2. The various causes are dealt with in more detail under "Assessment."

HISTORY

The diagnostic armamentarium that may be employed in the evaluation of pelvic pain is described in Table 3. Although some of these tools may not be available to all practitioners (i.e., ultrasonography), the majority are readily at hand in most clinical settings. The value of the history and physical examination cannot be overemphasized. In well over 90 per cent of cases the correct diagnosis can be determined on the basis of a detailed history and a thorough physical examination.

To be adequate, the history must be complete and accurate. Good patient rapport is important to insure the quantity and quality of information. Patients must be reassured of the confidentiality of the conversation. Such reassurance is particularly important with the teen-age girl accompanied by one or both parents, whom it is mandatory to interview by herself.

Certain specific points should be included in the history. The pain should be characterized in terms of quality, location, duration, onset, and radiation. Is the pain steady or intermittent? Does it change with a change in position? A thorough menstrual history should be obtained, including the dates of the two most recent menstrual periods, their regularity, duration, and flow, and whether the patient believes the menses have been "normal" for her. Asking about the number of pads or tampons used per day is an informative method of quantitating the menstrual flow. Are the menses painful? The patient should be queried as to symptoms of pregnancy, such as breast tenderness, urinary frequency, nausea, vomiting, and a feeling of malaise. Does she "feel" pregnant? Usually, when a multiparous woman says that she "feels" pregnant, the urine pregnancy test will have a positive or false-negative result.

Information about sexual activity, parity, and use of contraception should be obtained. The number of different sexual partners or of symptomatic partners is of value when considering pelvic inflammatory disease (PID). The patient's reproduc-

Table 2. DIFFERENTIAL DIAGNOSIS OF PELVIC PAIN

Genital etiology	
Pathologic	Complications of pregnancy or abortion
	Ectopic pregnancy
	Endometritis
	Uterine rupture
	Abruptio placentae
	Septic abortion
	Spontaneous abortion
	Infection
	Pelvic inflammatory disease (PID)
	Pelvic abscess
	Neoplasia
	Benign
	Ovarian cyst (torsion, leakage, hemorrhage)
	Leiomyoma uteri (torsion, acute degeneration)
	Malignant
	Extension
	Peritoneal involvement
	Non-neoplastic disease
	Endometriosis
	Adenomyosis
	Pelvic congestion
	Torsion of normal adnexa
	Pelvic adhesions
	Other
	Malposition
	Dyspareunia
Physiologic	Mittelschmerz
	Dysmenorrhea
Nongenital etiology	
Urologic	Urinary tract infection
	Calculus
Enteric	Diverticular disease
	Appendicitis
	Mesenteric thrombosis
	Regional enteritis
	Volvulus
	Obstruction
	Enteric malignancies
Musculoskeletal	Hematoma of rectus muscle
Psychogenic etiology	

tive history is important, particularly if it includes ectopic pregnancy or tubal disease. Knowledge of the patient's contraceptive technique and the regularity of its use helps one decide whether to consider complications of pregnancy.

Are there associated symptoms, such as fever, chills, and rigors? Inquiries must be made regarding urologic symptoms such as dysuria, pyuria, and hematuria. A history of gastrointestinal symptoms, including melena, hematochesia, constipation, and diarrhea, is also important.

In addition to the history of present illness, a review of the previous medical history is essential. Obstetric and gynecologic information, including prior surgery, infections, and ovarian cysts, should be obtained as well as details of urologic or gastrointestinal diseases. Finally, after a review of systems is carried out, the entire history should be carefully reviewed with the patient. Frequently, inaccuracies may be corrected and additional information obtained during these last few, but essential, minutes of history-taking.

PHYSICAL EXAMINATION

Examination of the patient must always begin with inspection. Is she sitting comfortably, or does she have the pallor, sweating, and stupor of a patient with a ruptured ectopic pregnancy? The vital signs are a sensitive indicator of catastrophic events, but "normal" vital signs should not lull the examiner into a false sense of security. A patient with early appendicitis or a slowly leaking ectopic pregnancy may initially have unremarkable vital signs.

The acuteness of the patient's condition occasionally necessitates a more problem-oriented examination, but its thoroughness should never be compromised. Examination of conjunctiva and buccal mucosa can provide a reasonable assessment of the hematocrit level and state of hydra-

Table 3. COMPONENTS OF THE EVALUATION OF PELVIC PAIN

History	Last menstrual period (LMP)
	Parity
	Contraception
	Duration, location, and quality of pain
	Sexual activity
	Vaginal bleeding
	Associated urologic or gastrointestinal symptoms
	Symptoms of pregnancy
	Previous medical history
Physical examination	Inspection
	Vital signs
	Abdominal examination
	Pelvic examination
	Culdocentesis
Diagnostic studies	
Laboratory studies	Hematocrit
	White blood cell (WBC) count
	Differential leukocyte count
	Electrolyte measurements
	BUN level
	Creatinine level
	Sedimentation rate
	C-reactive protein test
	Urinalysis
	Urine culture
	Endocervical gram stain and culture
Imaging	Barium enema
	Pelvic ultrasonography
	Intravenous urography
	CT scanning

tion. Auscultation of the lungs may reveal a pleural effusion, as occurs in Meigs' syndrome.

Abdominal Examination. Abdominal examination should begin by having the patient point to where her pain is the most severe and then trace its radiation. This process is important, because gynecologic pain usually occurs significantly below the level of the umbilicus, and pain above the umbilicus is frequently from another cause. Radiation of pain to or from the costovertebral angle suggests urologic etiology. Pelvic pain is occasionally a prominent feature of upper urinary tract disease, but the correct diagnosis may be suspected when pain radiates in this manner. Radiation of pain to the costovertebral angle must not, however, be confused with radiation to the lower back or sacrum, to which gynecologic pain is frequently referred, particularly when it involves the cervix and lower uterine segment.

The abdomen should be auscultated prior to palpation. Bruits may occasionally be heard over the liver or abdominal aorta, suggesting hepatic adenoma or aneurysm. Characterizing the bowel sounds also contributes to the diagnosis. Are they high-pitched and occurring in loud rushes, as in an intestinal obstruction?

Percussion is the next step in the examination, to help determine the point of maximum tenderness. Percussion should be employed to compare localized tenderness in either lower quadrant, over the hypogastrium versus the adnexa, and over McBurney's point versus the adnexa. McBurney's point is several centimeters superior to the adnexa, so differentiating the two may be an important factor in making a diagnosis. Whether the pain is bilateral or unilateral is also important. Many patients present to the emergency room complaining of pain in both lower quadrants. However, on careful examination, the pain is found to be unilateral with radiation to the contralateral pelvis. Unilaterality is inconsistent with pelvic inflammatory disease and strongly suggests another diagnosis.

Palpation should start over an area away from the point of maximum tenderness. If a patient experiences significant discomfort early in the examination, the remainder of the examination will be more difficult.

Careful, gentle palpation from the upper abdomen toward the painful area may reveal a mass such as the firm irregular uterus of the acutely degenerated fibroid or the smooth round mass of a large ovarian cyst. However, in the exquisitely tender, acute abdomen, palpation of a mass may be impossible; in this instance, much more information may be gained by palpating for the degree of guarding and rebound tenderness.

Significant inflammation in the pelvis may irritate the psoas muscle, leading to elicitation of the psoas sign. Such patients often lie with the corresponding thigh flexed to ease the rigidity of the psoas muscle. Although this test is of value in acute inflammatory processes, it is less revealing when the symptoms are subacute.

Pelvic Examination. Pelvic examinations are dreaded by many patients because they are embarrassing and uncomfortable. This attitude is exacerbated if the patient has formerly experienced a prior painful examination, particularly when she presents with pelvic pain. Much more information may be gathered from a slow, gentle pelvic examination preceded by careful reassurance. During initial inspection of the perineum, the inguinal lymph nodes and Bartholin's glands may be palpated. Lymphadenopathy or cysts of Bartolin's gland ducts may be suggestive of prior infections related to the genital tract.

The speculum examination should follow. A Pedersen speculum, which has long narrow blades, is a good choice for young or nulliparous patients. When significant vaginal relaxation is present, however, the larger Graves speculum is more appropriate. The speculum should be warmed and moistened with water prior to insertion. Before touching the labia, the examiner should place the back of the hand against the inner aspect of the patient's thigh. This subtle maneuver helps prepare the patient for the next step, in which the fingers of the hand spread the labia minora. The speculum may then be rested on the forchet for a moment while the patient is instructed to breath deeply and slowly through her mouth. With minimal pressure toward the rectum, the speculum easily slides into the vagina. With the cervix in full view, one should look for (1) purulent endocervical discharge suggestive of a gonococcal or chlamydial infection, (2) bleeding from the cervical os, and (3) cyanosis suggestive of pregnancy (Chadwick's sign). An endocervical smear for Gram stain and gonococcal culture should be obtained at this time (see "Laboratory Studies").

The speculum is then removed and a manual examination is begun. Much can be learned by the gentle insertion of a *single*, well-lubricated finger into the vagina without exerting any pressure on the abdomen. The examiner may evaluate tenderness of the urethra, trigone, and bladder. Passing the finger upward, one reaches the cervix. The position and consistency of the cervix is noted. It is usually quite firm, but it becomes soft with pregnancy. The cervical os should be evaluated, to determine whether it will permit the passage of a finger; this evaluation is helpful in the patient who has had an incomplete abortion. Cervical motion tenderness is also a very important finding. Its presence suggests pelvic disease, but its absence does not necessarily rule out this cause of pelvic pain. When evaluating cervical motion tenderness, one should move the cervix gently from side to side with the single finger. If the patient complains of pain, she is asked to point to where on the abdomen she feels the pain. By gently performing this part of the examination, one can very accurately assess the presence and degree of genital disease.

Bimanual examination is then carried out by placing two fingers in the vagina and a hand on the patient's abdomen at the level of the umbilicus. The uterus and adnexa are evaluated with the fingers in the vagina, the hand on the abdomen being used to bring the pelvic structures within their reach. The hand exerts gentle pressure while it moves inferiorly toward the pubic symphysis. The uterus is evaluated for size, shape, consistency, and tenderness. The fingers in the vagina are then moved into the lateral fornices, and the adnexa is brought into reach by gentle abdominal pressure. Adnexal masses and tenderness are assessed in this manner, allowing one to determine whether the tenderness is coming from the adnexa itself or from a more superior area.

To complete the examination, one places the index finger in the vagina and a well-lubricated middle finger in the rectum. The cul-de-sac is evaluated for bulging, such as in hemoperitoneum .The uterosacral ligaments are also more easily palpated for implants due to endometriosis or cervical carcinoma. The uterus and adnexa are again palpated to confirm the findings of the vaginal examination. At the completion of the rectovaginal examination, any stool obtained should be tested for occult blood.

Culdocentesis. A valuable clinical study that may be performed in conjunction with the physical examination is the culdocentesis. This is a simple technique that permits evaluation of intraperitoneal fluid. It is most helpful in demonstrating hemoperitoneum in cases of possible ectopic pregnancy or ruptured corpus luteum cyst. As seen in Figure 1, the intraperitoneal cavity is separated from the posterior fornix of the vagina by the peritoneum, connective tissue, and vaginal mucosa. Culdocentesis should never be conducted until a bimanual examination has determined that there is not a cul-de-sac mass.

With the speculum in the vagina, the cervix is grasped with a tenaculum and lifted anteriorly. The posterior fornix can then be clearly visualized and cleaned with an antiseptic solution. The fornix is punctured in the midline with an 18-gauge spinal needle attached to a 20-cc syringe. Following injection of 5 ml of air to insure an intraperitoneal location, aspiration from the cul-de-sac (pouch of Douglas) is attempted. There are four possible results of this procedure; (1) a dry tap, in which no fluid is aspirated (approximately 30 per cent of cases); (2) straw-colored fluid; (3) frank pus; and (4) nonclotting blood. A few milliliters of clear, straw-colored fluid is considered normal. However, if nonclotting blood or pus is obtained, the nature of the patient's condition may be clari-

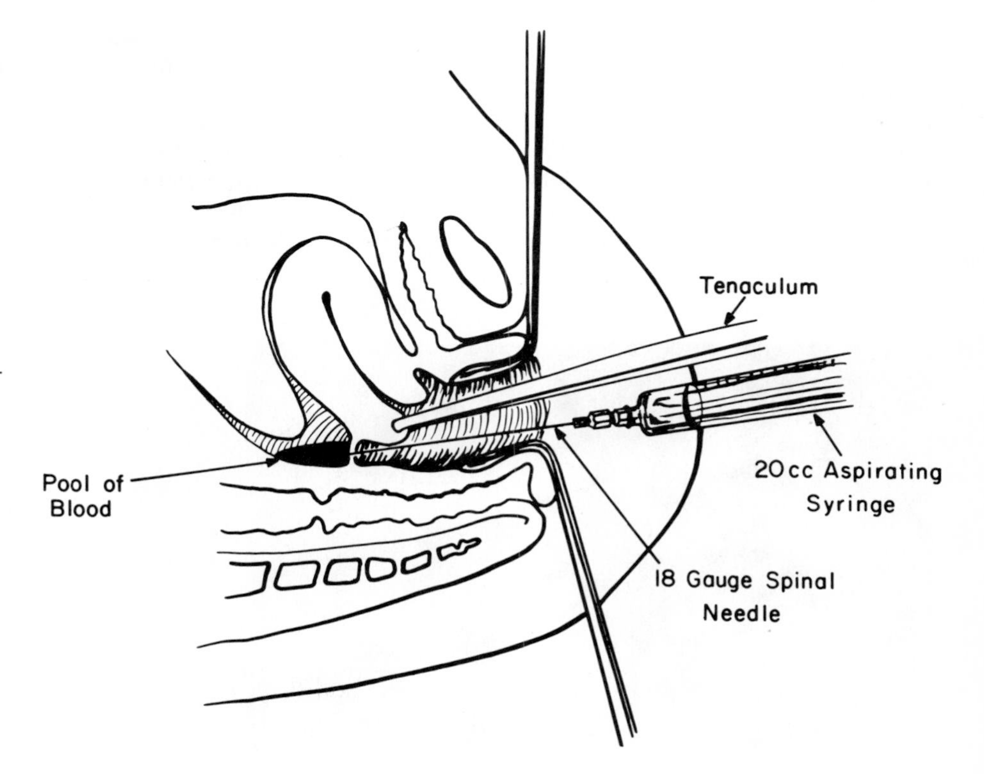

Figure 1. Culdocentesis technique.

fied. Culdocentesis is as safe as it is easy, if adequate care is taken in its performance.

DIAGNOSTIC STUDIES

Laboratory Studies

Table 3 indicates the many laboratory studies that may be obtained to evaluate pelvic pain. Hemoglobin and hematocrit values are always important regardless of the possible diagnosis. It is noteworthy, however, that "normal values" may exist prior to hemodilution in cases of intraperitoneal hemorrhage. Serial blood counts should be obtained whenever one is considering concealed hemorrhage.

An elevated white blood cell count may indicate an infectious cause, particularly when the differential leukocyte count demonstrates a shift. However, significant leukocytosis is common in many noninfectious conditions associated with acute stress, such as torsion of an ovarian cyst. The white blood cell count is therefore of value in substantiating the clinical impression of an acute process, but it is less helpful in differential diagnosis.

The endocervical Gram stain is a 3-minute procedure that demonstrates intracellular gram-negative diplococci from the endocervix in 60 per cent of cases of gonococcal PID.[2] When its result is positive, this simple procedure goes a long way toward differentiating PID from appendicitis and other causes of acute pelvic pain. The cervix is wiped with a clean gauze sponge. A cotton-tipped applicator is inserted into the endocervical canal and rotated 360 degrees. The applicator is rolled over a clean glass slide, which is dried and gram-stained in the usual manner. Observation on microscopic examination of sheets of white blood cells with gram-negative intracellular diplococci constitutes a positive result (Fig. 2).

A pregnancy test should be performed in all women with acute pelvic pain. Pregnancy tests as a whole are highly sensitive for intrauterine pregnancy but less so for ectopic pregnancy. Urine pregnancy tests can have a 50 per cent false-negative rate in ectopic pregnancy, and may have false-positive results in the presence of proteinuria.[3] Radioimmune assays for the beta-subunit of human chorionic gonadotropin (hCG) in serum are highly sensitive in ectopic pregnancy and may yield positive results before the first missed menstrual period.

Urinalysis should also be performed. The initial specimen may be mid-stream clean-catch urine. However, this type is easily contaminated with vaginal discharge or blood, so abnormal results of analysis of a clean-catch specimen should be confirmed by analysis of a catheter-obtained specimen. Pyuria mandates urine culture and sensitivity.

Gonorrhea culture of the endocervical smear is another study that should be obtained in all patients with pelvic pain. It has been demonstrated that under ideal circumstances endocervical culture for gonorrhea is only 80 per cent sensitive. Care must be taken to obtain the specimen with the proper technique. A cotton-tipped applicator should be inserted into the endocervical canal and rotated 360 degrees slowly for 30 seconds. The applicator should then be rolled onto a medium specifically designed for gonorrheal culture (Thayer-Martin or Martin-Lewis) that is at room temperature.

Nonspecific tests such as erythrocyte sedimentation rate and C-reactive protein have been of some value in following the progress of chronic pelvic infection, but they tend to be uniformly unhelpful in differential diagnosis. Other, more specific tests such as thick blood smears, sickle cell preparations, and tests for porphyria may be indicated if pain appears to be of a more obscure origin.

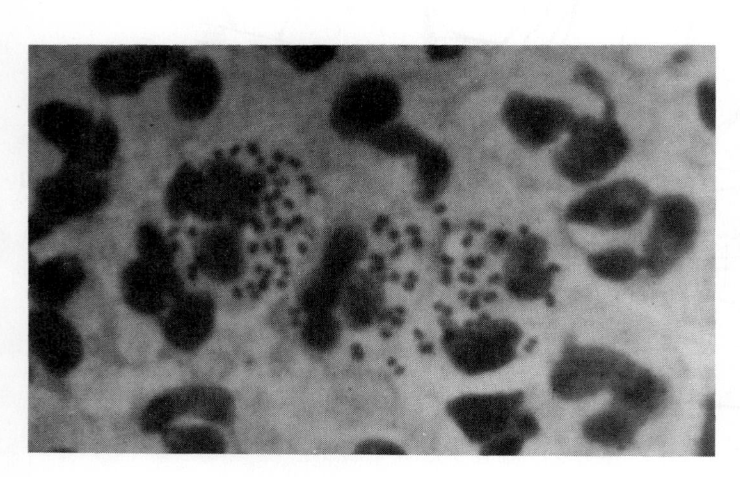

Figure 2. Intracellular *N. gonorrhoeae* from endocervical smear.

Imaging

One of the most significant advances in gynecology in recent times has been the development of ultrasonography. The technology of this procedure has improved to the point that it is the most popular radiologic procedure in the evaluation of pelvic pain. The sophistication of modern-day ultrasonography enables clinicians to non-invasively visualize ovarian follicles 1 to 2 cm in diameter. This procedure is of value in differentiating solid from cystic adnexal masses, ectopic from intrauterine pregnancies, and uterine fibroids from ovarian neoplasms. On our gynecologic services we have found that, aside from being less expensive and without radiation exposure, ultrasonography is superior to CT scanning in elucidating pelvic masses.

Other radiologic procedures, including abdominal radiography, intravenous pyelography, and barium enema, may be indicated when specific diagnoses are entertained, such as bowel obstruction, uterine perforation, ureteral calculus, and diverticulitis.

ASSESSMENT

To discuss every possible cause of pelvic pain is beyond the scope of this chapter, but a general review of the major causes is indicated.

Genital Etiology

Pathologic Causes

One should recall that, owing to the embryology and anatomy of the pelvis, many pathologic conditions may mimic one another. Eventual diagnosis is often made by exclusion, through employment of the wide range of diagnostic methods described. Pregnancy may be included or excluded on the basis of history, physical examination, and pregnancy testing; pelvic mass by physical examination and ultrasonography; hemoperitoneum by serial blood counts and culdocentesis. As the differential diagnosis becomes progressively more specific, the proper management may be instituted, whether it is immediate surgical intervention, close observation and antibiotic therapy, or outpatient treatment.

Complications of Pregnancy

As seen in Table 2, a myriad of complications of pregnancy may cause a patient to present with pelvic pain. Several of these can be life-threatening, and it is important to determine the pregnancy status of any woman complaining of pelvic pain. As noted previously, this determination may be made by noting any symptoms of pregnancy, eliciting Hegar's or Chadwick's sign or finding an enlarged uterus, and performing a pregnancy test. The slide or tube test for urine hCG is quick and inexpensive, but if this has a negative result, a serum test is indicated in patients with acute pain.

Ectopic Pregnancy. This disorder remains a major cause of maternal mortality.[4] Unfortunately, diagnosing an early or unrupted ectopic pregnancy is difficult, and most affected patients have been seen and examined several times before the correct diagnosis is made. A senior gynecologist in our department has a sticker on his locker in the operating suite that says, "ECTOPIC, STUPID!" One should always "think ectopic pregnancy" in evaluating women with acute pain. The classic presentation—missed menses, vaginal spotting, and acute abdominal pain referred to the shoulder followed by shock—is seldom seen. Patients more frequently complain of some menstrual irregularity followed by vaginal spotting, and they usually present 6 to 12 weeks after their last "normal" menstrual period. A history of PID or tubal ligation may be helpful; approximately 6 to 10 per cent of ectopic pregnancies occur following tubal ligation. The pain may vary from sharp to dull but is usually unilateral, unlike the cramping midline pain of spontaneous abortion. Hemoperitoneum can produce significant rigidity and rebound tenderness, but abdominal examination in the early stages of ectopic pregnancy may demonstrate only minimal localized tenderness. Cullen's sign, although described in some of the older texts as evidence of ectopic pregnancy, is usually a late finding. On pelvic examination the cervix may show the changes associated with pregnancy. Cervical motion tenderness is common. The uterus is usually only minimally enlarged if at all. Adnexal masses are palpable in approximately 40 per cent of cases. Serial blood counts may be helpful, but culdocentesis is particularly valuable and should be performed whenever this diagnosis is entertained. Ultrasound may also be of value, particularly in conjunction with quantitative serum hCG determinations. Pelvic ultrasonography is unreliable in detecting early extrauterine gestational sacs, but if the qualitative serum hCG level is 6000 units or more and an experienced examiner fails to detect an intrauterine gestational sac, ectopic pregnancy is highly likely. Serial quantitative hCG determinations may also provide evidence for ectopic pregnancy; the pregnancy in which the level does not double in 48 hours in the early stages is usually abnormal. Laparoscopy or laparotomy may eventually be required for a definitive diagnosis.

Abortion. Spontaneous abortion occurs in about 15 per cent of pregnancies.[3] Affected patients usually present between 6 and 12 weeks of gestation complaining of vaginal bleeding and cramping midline pelvic pain. It is important to differentiate this condition from ectopic pregnancy. The nature of the pain is a useful means of making the distinction. Bleeding is usually, but not always, much heavier than the spotting in ectopic pregnancy. Examination reveals a midline enlarged uterus and occasionally a dilated cervical os. Ultrasonography may demonstrate an intrauterine gestational sac, but histologic evidence of chorionic villi from passed tissue is diagnostic.

The incidence of septic abortion has decreased substantially since elective abortion was legalized in the United States. Although a history of attempted induction is certainly suggestive of the diagnosis, younger patients often refrain from volunteering, or even deny, this critical information. The diagnosis is further suggested by fever, an enlarged, boggy, exquisitely tender uterus, and occasionally a dilated cervical os with minor cervical lacerations suggestive of an attempt at induction. Leukocytosis with a shift to the left is common, and ultrasonography may demonstrate retained tissue in the uterine cavity. It is noteworthy that septic abortion must also be differentiated from ectopic pregnancy. Occasionally, the patient with the latter is given suction dilatation and curettage (D&C) in an attempt to terminate what is thought to be an early intrauterine pregnancy, only to become symptomatic later, when her ectopic pregnancy ruptures.

Other Complications. *Placental abruption* and uterine rupture generally occur late in pregnancy.[5] Abruption usually occurs in the third trimester and produces mild to severe uterine pain. Vaginal bleeding may or may not be present. Fetal and maternal tachycardia together with uterine irritability contribute to the diagnosis. Variable degrees of coagulopathy may be present in maternal blood, together with fetal cells demonstrated by an acid elution technique. The diagnosis is primarily clinical, because ultrasonography is unreliable in demonstrating a retroplacental hemorrhage.

Uterine rupture may occur at any time in pregnancy, most often in the third trimester, and is usually associated with a previous cesarean section or myomectomy. Approximately one-third of cases occur without labor and are associated with severe generalized abdominal pain; the fetus is usually in the upper abdomen in an unusual attitude, and dead. Rupture of a low transverse cesarean section scar is usually much less impressive. Separation may occur with only vague complaints of lower abdominal pain. Diagnosis in this situation is more difficult and is usually made at the time of second cesarean section.

Rupture of the unscarred uterus is rare in developed countries. It usually occurs following a prolonged, difficult, unattended labor or injudicious use of uterine stimulants such as pitocin.

Infections

Pelvic Inflammatory Disease. The incidence of pelvic inflammatory disease (PID), or acute salpingitis, has dramatically increased in recent years together with that of other sexually transmitted diseases. PID accounts for approxiamtely 250,000 hospital admissions annually, and three times that many affected patients are treated as outpatients. Young women are the most common victims, with a peak age range of 15 to 25 years.

PID is significant not only in terms of its incidence but also because of its many dire consequences. Infertility secondary to tubal occlusion is the most common complication. In a large study of patients with laparoscopically diagnosed PID, 13 per cent became involuntarily infertile following a single episode of PID, 35 per cent following two episodes, and 70 per cent following three or more.[7] Other complications are just as disastrous; the incidence of ectopic pregnancy is six-fold following PID, 17 per cent of patients subsequently develop chronic pelvic pain, and 5 to 10 per cent develop pelvic abscess.[6, 7]

The clinical diagnosis of PID is difficult to make, as Jacobsen and Westrom[8] documented in their classic study published in 1969. They performed laparoscopic examination of 814 consecutive patients with a clinical diagnosis of PID. Laparoscopy confirmed the diagnosis in only 65 per cent, 23 per cent had no discernible disease, and 12 per cent had other causes of pelvic pain—most often appendicitis, ectopic pregnancy, ovarian cyst, and endometriosis. It becomes clear not only that PID is disastrous in its effect but also that other life-threatening conditions are frequently missed when the diagnosis of PID is made.

A more accurate diagnosis of PID may be made by integrating the findings of a carefully taken history, physical examination, and several clinical and laboratory studies. A history of bilateral pelvic pain and vaginal discharge following the menses, together with multiple sexual partners and treatment for gonorrhea, should raise the index of suspicion. Furthermore, approximately 20 per cent of patients with PID complain of dysuria, a feature that helps differentiate this condition from appendicitis and ectopic pregnancy. Nausea and vomiting occur in about 40 per cent of patients with PID, and abnormal vaginal bleeding is seen in about one-third. Physical examination provides the most salient data for the diagnosis. Table 4 presents a set of clinical criteria required for the diagnosis of PID.[6] Three physical findings are required for the diagnosis: direct abdominal tenderness, cervical motion tenderness, and adnexal tenderness. Abdominal tenderness is generally bilateral, beginning over the adnexal areas. Adnexal tenderness elicited on bimanual palpation should also be bilateral. As shown in Table 4, at

Table 4. CLINICAL CRITERIA FOR THE DIAGNOSIS OF PID

Direct abdominal tenderness
Cervical motion tenderness
and
Adnexal tenderness
plus
At least one of the following features:
Fever (above 38°C [100.4°F])
Leukocytosis 10,000/mm^3
Pelvic abscess or inflammatory mass on pelvic examination or ultrasonography
Intracellular gram-negative diplococci on Gram stain of endocervical smear
Purulent material obtained on culdocentesis or laparoscopy

(Based on data from Spence MR. Pelvic inflammatory disease. Dermatol Clin 1983; 1:65–73.)

least one of five other factors must also be present. Gram stain of the endocervical smear demonstrates intracellular gram-negative diplococci in approximately 60 per cent of cases (see Fig. 2). Although the presence of fever may be helpful, it is found in only one-half of patients. Leukocytosis is also found in 50 per cent of patients with PID. Endocervical cultures for gonorrhea may be of value when their results are positive.

Employing these criteria may permit early and accurate diagnosis of PID. Considering the consequences of PID and the other conditions that may be overlooked, however, we believe that it is imperative to reevaluate every patient with a diagnosis of PID within 48 to 72 hours. In the last 3 years we have diagnosed over 50 cases of ectopic pregnancy at the Johns Hopkins Hospital Pelvic Infections Clinic on such a reevaluation.

Neoplasia

A variety of neoplastic processes involving the adnexa may lead to acute or subacute pelvic pain.

Ovarian Cyst. Ovarian cysts may be either benign or malignant and become acutely symptomatic by twisting on their pedicles or leaking their contents into the peritoneal cavity. They may be simple or functional cysts containing follicular fluid or blood, benign dermoid cysts or cystic adenomas, or malignant ovarian cysts. Obviously, the age of the patient is an important factor in the type of cyst, but regardless of its type the mechanism of pain appears to be the same. Distension of the cyst wall produces little or no pain unless it is sudden, as in a rapidly growing corpus luteum cyst. Occasionally, a basketball-sized cyst is discovered in a postmenopausal woman who had thought she was "just putting on some weight." This slow distension may, however, produce a gnawing, chronic pain, which if it occurs in such a patient must be promptly evaluated by physical examination and ultrasonography. Torsion and leakage of an ovarian cyst produce more acute symptoms. The symptoms of ovarian torsion are similar to those produced by the torsion of a testicle. The pain is usually abrupt in onset and severe in quality. It often becomes colicky and associated with vomiting. Examination reveals a tender cystic mass. This diagnosis may be confirmed by ultrasonography if necessary. It is not unusual for the patient to have a low-grade fever and severe leukocytosis secondary to the acuteness of ovarian torsion, which is a surgical emergency requiring prompt intervention.

Leakage of fluid from an ovarian cyst tends to be less dramatic but frequently is severe enough for the patient to seek medical attention. Even the physiologic event of a rupture of a follicular cyst at the time of ovulation may produce acute pain or "mittelschmerz." The rupture of other cysts, however, may require more aggressive management. A severe chemical peritonitis is produced by the rupture of a dermoid cyst, whereas rupture of a highly vascular corpus luteum cyst, particularly in pregnancy, may produce a significant hemoperitoneum. However, most cyst ruptures can be managed conservatively because symptoms usually defervesce within hours of onset. The diagnosis may be suggested by the sudden onset of sharp pain at midcycle, just before the menses, or during intercourse. The significant physical finding is localized tenderness in the lower abdomen. Pelvic examination may disclose a cystic, moderately tender adnexal mass and mild cervical motion tenderness. Ultrasonography may also contribute to the diagnosis by demonstrating an ovarian cyst or fluid in the cul-de-sac. Serum hCG determination is mandatory in premenopausal patients to rule out the possibility of an ectopic pregnancy, but laparoscopy may be required to differentiate between the hemoperitoneum produced by the rupture of a corpus luteum cyst in pregnancy from the rupture of an ectopic pregnancy.[9, 10]

Leiomyoma Uteri. Leiomyomas, or fibroids, are common neoplasias of the uterine myometrium.[11] They are usually asymptomatic and only rarely undergo malignant degeneration. A leiomyoma may produce acute pain, similar to that of a ruptured cyst, through acute central necrosis or torsion. Particularly in pregnancy, such tumors can grow so rapidly that they outgrow their blood supply. The subsequent "carneous degeneration" is acutely painful but requires only conservative management once the proper diagnosis is made. A leiomyoma may also be pedunculated and produce similar pain with torsion. The diagnosis may be suggested by a history of irregular, heavy vaginal bleeding. The condition is more common in blacks but can be found in all races. Abdominal and pelvic examinations may demonstrate a firm, irregular, large fibroid uterus. As with other pelvic masses, ultrasonography can be of value in demonstrating leiomyomas and may even suggest medial necrosis.

Malignancy. Gynecologic malignancies usually do not produce pain. An enlarging ovarian carcinoma may produce a gnawing discomfort, and malignant ascites may lead to vague abdominal discomfort and a feeling of fullness. Advanced carcinoma of the cervix may produce chronic low back pain through its involvement of the uterosacral ligaments. Unfortunately, however, most gynecologic malignancies remain relatively asymptomatic until they are quite advanced.

Non-Neoplastic Disorders

Endometriosis. Hormonally responsive endometrial tissue may occur anywhere in the abdominal cavity but is most common in the pelvis. Endometriosis is a common cause of dysmenorrhea and can be associated with dyspareunia, infertility, and pelvic adhesions.[12] With each menses, extrauterine endometrial implants bleed, producing peritoneal irritation and subsequent pain. An ovarian implant frequently becomes an "endometrioma" as blood collects within a cystic cavity. Endometriosis commonly causes chronic dysmenorrhea, but acute pain may occur with the rupture or torsion of an endometrioma. Typically, the pain begins a few days prior to menses and is worst on the first day of menstrual flow. Occasionally, premenstrual, brown vaginal spotting occurs. Physical examination may reveal nodular endometrial implants along the uterosacral ligaments or the tender cystic mass of an ovarian endometrioma, but frequently the findings are totally unremarkable. The pain of endometriosis is not proportional to the extent of the disease. A single implant may produce significant symptoms, whereas extensive disease may be asymptomatic. When endometriosis is suspected, a laparoscopy should be done in order to support the diagnosis prior to the institution of therapy.

Adenomyosis. The occurrence of endometrial tissue in the myometrium is known as adenomyosis.[13] This condition generally occurs after the age of 30 and is associated with prolonged menstrual periods and progressive dysmenorrhea. Pelvic examination often reveals an enlarged, somewhat tender, boggy uterus, particularly at the time of the menses. Definitive diagnosis, however, is made histologically following hysterectomy.

Physiologic Causes

Certain physiologic events may produce pelvic pain, particularly in young women.

Mittelschmerz. Ovulatory pain, or mittelschmerz, has already been described. Approximately one out of five women at some time experiences the pain of mittleschmerz, and in more than one woman a normal appendix has been removed following ovulation.[10]

Dysmenorrhea. Primary dysmenorrhea is common in adolescent women as their menstrual cycles become ovulatory. As with secondary dysmenorrhea, pain usually begins several days prior to the menses and is worst on the first 2 days of menstrual flow. It is not uncommon for teen-age girls to be bedridden because of the severity of pain. Endometriosis usually occurs after the age of 20, but it may be found in teenagers. Laparoscopy is frequently necessary to determine the etiology of dysmenorrhea.

Nongenital Causes

The vast array of nongenital causes of pelvic pain must be kept in mind whenever one is evaluating such a patient. Urologic, enteric, and musculoskeletal disorders all produce pelvic pain and must be ruled out by thorough evaluation.

Urologic Disorders

Urinary Tract Infection (UTI). Infections of the urinary tract, including cystitis and pyelonephritis, may produce pelvic pain that is frequently described as a midline pressure sensation or vague hypogastric discomfort. All women with pelvic pain should be questioned regarding dysuria, pyuria, urgency or frequency, hematuria, and prior history of UTI. Inspection may demonstrate an erythematous, inflamed urethra. Urethral and trigonal tenderness may be elicited by palpating these areas during vaginal examination. Definitive diagnosis is made by the presence of greater than 10^5 organisms/ml on urine culture, but UTI is strongly suggested by the presence of white blood cells in a catheter-obtained urine specimen.

Calculus. Ureteral calculi may also cause pelvic pain, in addition to its more common presentation as costovertebral angle (CVA) pain. Examination is remarkable for CVA tenderness. Hematuria is usually, but not always, found on urinalysis of a catheter-obtained specimen. Intravenous pyelogram usually provides the definitive diagnosis.

Enteric Diseases

Although many pathologic conditions of the bowel produce pelvic pain, the most common are appendicitis and diverticulitis.

Appendicitis. Appendicitis may mimic all other conditions heretofore discussed. A common dilemma is the differentiation between appendicitis and PID. When a pelvic appendix lies near the right adnexa, salpingitis may be produced secondary to appendiceal inflammation. In this instance, differentiation may be impossible without laparoscopy or laparotomy. In cases of suspected appendicitis, one must carefully consider the history prior to the onset of pain, symptoms of the attack, local signs, and the order of appearance of symptoms. Frequently, a history of "gastritis" precedes the actual onset of pain in an appendicitis. Some degree of unusual bowel irregularity, either constipation or diarrhea, is also common. The sequence of symptoms and signs is of the utmost importance in the diagnosis of appendicitis and frequently differentiates it from PID, ectopic pregnancy, ovarian cyst, and other pathologic processes. Cope[14] has stated that when the symptoms and signs do not occur in the proper sequence, the diagnosis of appendicitis must be questioned. The first to occur is periumbilical or epigastric pain. As the local parietal peritoneum becomes irritated by the inflammatory process, the pain gradually moves to the right lower quadrant, specifically McBurney's point. Subsequently, nausea with or without vomiting occurs. A loss of appetite or revulsion for food is common. Anyone previously in good health who develops abdominal pain followed by nausea or loss of appetite should be carefully observed for appendicitis. The next symptom is local iliac tenderness, which is frequently absent at the onset of other symptoms but gradually develops over the right lower quadrant. Abdominal examination reveals this tenderness, which may be further localized with gentle percussion over the affected area. Pelvic and rectal examinations will confirm iliac tenderness, which frequently appears to be localized above the right adnexa. Fever may develop but usually remains only 1 or 2°F above normal. Patients who present with abdominal pain and a fever of 103°F at the onset of symptoms rarely have acute appendicitis. Leukocytosis with a shift to the left is the last sign to occur. Generally it is mild, rarely above 20,000 cells/mm^3. In addition to the history and physical examination, a barium enema may be of value in ruling out appendicitis. If the appendix fills with contrast medium it is highly unlikely to be infected. In PID, the sequence of events is different. The pain is usually bilateral and slightly lower than McBurney's point, and it generally begins in the lower abdomen. Although evidence of nausea, tenderness, low-grade fever, and leukocytosis may variably exist, the sequence of events is usually altered. As previously noted, laparoscopy may be required to differentiate between the two conditions.

Diverticulitis. Another common condition that must be considered in patients with pelvic pain, diverticulitis generally occurs in middle-aged or older patients and most commonly involves the left lower quadrant. A history of bowel irregularity is not unusual. The pain, however, does not initiate in the epigastrium and frequently is unilateral. A history of prior episodes may be obtained. Nausea and vomiting may be present but are uncommon. Examination reveals localized tenderness in the left lower quadrant that is confirmed on pelvic examination. Occasionally, pelvic examination may reveal the exquisitely tender, left-sided mass of a diverticular abscess. The stool examination frequently demonstrates occult blood. Fever and leukocytosis are common. Ultrasonography may be helpful in diverticular abscess, but the most valuable radiologic procedure is the barium enema. False-negative barium enema results may occur infrequently. If diverticuli are not visualized radiographically, colonoscopy is indicated.

Other Disorders. Less common conditions that may produce pelvic pain include inflammatory bowel disease, colonic malignancies, bowel obstruction, and mesenteric thrombosis. Careful history-taking and physical examination together with the appropriate studies generally provide enough evidence to lead one to include these possibilities in the differential diagnosis.

Musculoskeletal Disorders

Rupture of a rectus muscle, although rare, may produce pelvic pain. A history of recent trauma together with superficial tenderness on examination will usually lead to the diagnosis.

Psychogenic Etiology

Finally, one must consider a psychosomatic cause of pelvic pain when an organic etiology cannot be demonstrated following a thorough evaluation. It must be pointed out, however, that a disastrous situation could result if organic disease were overlooked because a patient's symptoms were too enthusiastically ascribed to psychoneurosis. If no organic disease can be demonstrated, the patient should be interviewed regarding her lifestyle, behavior, attitudes, and interpersonal relationships. It has been demonstrated that patients without organic causes of pelvic pain tend to be more neurotic, have abnormal attitudes toward sexuality, and form less rewarding relationships.[15, 16, 17] These patients frequently benefit from psychotherapy and, once confronted with the lack of evidence for organic disease, may choose this alternative if it is offered in a reassuring manner.[17]

CONCLUSION

The anatomy and embryology of the female pelvic structures complicate the elucidation of specific reasons for pelvic pain. Similar signs and symptoms may be produced by the wide variety of possible causes, gynecologic, urologic, enteric, vascular, musculoskeletal, and psychogenic. A thorough evaluation requires the sequential performance of complete and accurate history-taking and physical examination. Specific clinical, laboratory, and radiologic studies are of value in narrowing the differential diagnosis. Although a specific diagnosis may not always be made, these tools permit the clinician to formulate an accurate differential diagnosis and institute the proper management.

REFERENCES

1. Guerriero WF, Guerriero CP, Edward RD, Stuart JA. Pelvic pain, gynecic and nongynecic: interpretation and management. South Med J 1971;64:1043–8.
2. Eschenbach DA, Holmes KK. Acute pelvic inflammatory disease: current concepts of pathogenesis, etiology and management. Clin Obstet Gynecol 1975;18:35–56.
3. Novak ER, Jones GS. Novak's Textbook of Gynecology. 6th ed. Baltimore: Williams & Wilkins, 1961;653–8.
4. DeCherney AH, Minkin MJ, Spangler S. Contemporary management of ectopic pregnancy. J Reprod Med 1981;26:519–3.
5. Cavanagh D, Woods RE, O'Connor TCF, et al. Obstetric Emergencies. 3rd ed. Philadelphia: JB Lippincott, 1982;177–216.
6. Spence MR. Pelvic inflammatory disease. Dermatol Clin 1983;1:65–73.
7. Westrom L. Incidence, prevalence and trends of acute pelvic inflammatory disease and its consequences in industrialized countries. Am J Obstet Gynecol 1980;138:880–92.
8. Jacobsen L, Westrom L. Objectionalized diagnosis of acute pelvic inflammatory disease. Am J Obstet Gynecol 1969;105:1088–98.
9. Liston WA, Bradford WP, Downie J. Laparoscopy in a general gynecologic unit. Am J Obstet Gynecol 1972;113:672–7.
10. Marsden DE, Cavanagh D. Differential diagnosis of pelvic pain. Contemp Obstet Gynecol 1983;21:69–87.
11. Mattingly RF. TeLinde's Operative Gynecology. 5th ed. Philadelphia: JB Lippincott, 1977;187–222.
12. Telinde RW. Endometriosis. Clin Obstet Gynecol 1961;4:738–806.
13. Israel SL, Woutersz TB. Adenomyosis: neglected diagnosis. Obstet Gynecol 1959;14:168–73.
14. Cope Z. The Early Diagnosis of the Acute Abdomen. 14th ed. London: Oxford University Press, 1972; 48–61.
15. Duncan GH, Taylor HC. A psychosomatic study of pelvic congestion. Am J Obstet Gynecol 1952;64:1–12.
16. Beard RW, Belsey EM, Liebertman BA, Wilkinson JCM. Pelvic pain in women. Am J Obstet Gynecol 1977;128:566–70.
17. Henker FO. Diagnosis and treatment of nonorganic pelvic pain. South Med J 1979;72:1132–4.

PLEURAL EFFUSION

SUSAN K. PINGLETON

□ SYNONYM: Pleural fluid

BACKGROUND

Pleural effusion is often a difficult diagnostic problem facing the clinician. A reasonable differential diagnosis can be constructed from clinical information and from pleural fluid examination findings. To maximize the information obtained from pleural fluid examination, the clinician should be aware of the physiology of pleural fluid formation. Additionally, the ability to analyze the cellular content and chemistry of the effusion, in conjunction with the history, physical findings, and ancillary laboratory data, should enable the clinician to reach a presumptive or definitive diagnosis in approximately 90 per cent of patients with pleural effusion. As with other laboratory tests, however, it should be noted that the pleural fluid examination most often supports a diagnostic impression rather than providing a specific diagnosis. Only when the pleural fluid contains malignant cells, organisms, or lupus erythematosus cells is a definitive diagnosis made on that basis alone.

Anatomy of the Pleural Space

The pleural membrane covers the lungs and lines the inner aspect of the chest wall. Composed of loose connective tissue and covered by a single layer of mesothelial cells, it is divided into visceral pleura and parietal pleura. Visceral pleura covers the surface of both lungs, and parietal pleura lines the internal surface of the chest wall, the superior surface of the diaphragm, and the mediastinum.

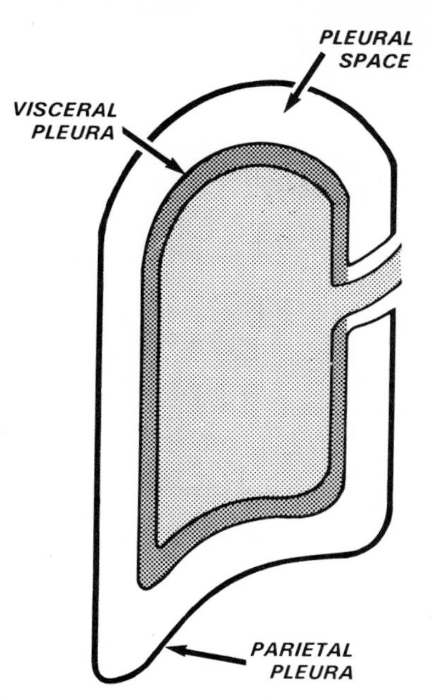

Figure 1. Anatomy of the lung and pleural space. Visceral pleura covers the lung; parietal pleura lines the chest wall, diaphragm, and mediastinum. They join at the hilum of the lung.

Visceral pleura and parietal pleura join at the hilum of the lung (Fig. 1). Although the two types are similar histologically, they differ in two important features. First, the parietal pleura has sensory nerve receptors and the visceral pleura has none. Second, the parietal pleura can be stripped easily from the chest wall, and the visceral pleura is strongly adherent to the lung.

Between the visceral pleura and parietal pleura is an enclosed, potential space—the pleural space. Pressure in the pleural space is normally subatmospheric during inspiration because of the balance between the inward elastic recoil of the lung and the outward elastic recoil of the chest wall. The pleural space normally contains 3 to 5 ml of pleural fluid, which serves as a lubricant during inspiration and expiration. In disease states, the pleural space can accommodate several liters of fluid or air.

Physiology of Pleural Fluid Formation

Pathologic accumulation of pleural fluid, or pleural effusion, results from an alteration of normal pleural fluid dynamics.[1] The movement of pleural fluid in and out of the pleural space is governed by principles of Starling's equation. That equation is as follows:

$$F = K\,[(HP_{cap}\ HP_{pl}) - (COP_{cap} - COP_{pl})]$$

where F is fluid movement, K is pleural fluid filtration coefficient, HP_{cap} is capillary hydrostatic pressure, COP_{cap} is capillary oncotic pressure, and COP_{pl} is pleural oncotic pressure.

Hydrostatic pressures in the parietal pleura are systemic, because branches of the intercostal arteries supply the parietal pleura and venous drainage is to the right atrium via the azygos system. Hydrostatic pressures in the visceral pleura are pressures of the pulmonary circulation, because branches of the pulmonary artery supply visceral pleura and venous drainage is to the left atrium via the pulmonary veins. Colloid osmotic pressure in both beds is related to the protein concentration. In addition, lymphatics located in the pleura normally absorb the small amount of protein that leaks from the pleural capillaries. Permeability of the pleural capillaries is governed by the filtration coefficient (K). Increases in permeability increase the pleural fluid protein content.

From Starling's equation, we can see that hydrostatic and oncotic pressures primarily govern fluid movement in and out of the pleural space. Pleural fluid moves along a pressure gradient from systemic parietal pleural vessels into the pleural space and is then reabsorbed into the pulmonary visceral pleural vessels (Fig. 2). It is estimated that 5 to 10 liters of pleural fluid pass through the pleural space in 24 hours.

As normal pleural fluid dynamics are understood, several points become clear. With the normally large amounts of fluid formed and reabsorbed each day, potential for abnormal fluid accumulation arises with any imbalance in the system. Also, the mechanisms for abnormal pleural fluid accumulation are, in essence, only two: (1) abnormalities of pressure, that is, changes in hydrostatic and/or oncotic pressure (congestive heart failure, severe hypoproteinemia), and (2) diseases of the pleural surface altering capillary permeability (pneumonia, tumor) or affecting lymphatic reabsorption of protein (mediastinal carcinomatosis). On the basis of these pathophysiologic mechanisms, we can classify pleural effusions as either transudates (abnormalities of pressure) or exudates (conditions of altered permeability).

HISTORY

Although symptoms of pleural effusion are varied and most often relate to the primary disease process, most patients complain of dyspnea to some degree.[2] Patients with severe underlying heart and lung disease will become more symptomatic with smaller amounts of fluid than patients with otherwise normal lungs. A patient with pleural effusion may be aware of a heavy or tight feeling in the chest. Pain is more likely to precede pleural effusion than to accompany it. With pleural effusion resulting from pleural inflammation, the rubbing of the visceral pleura and parietal pleura

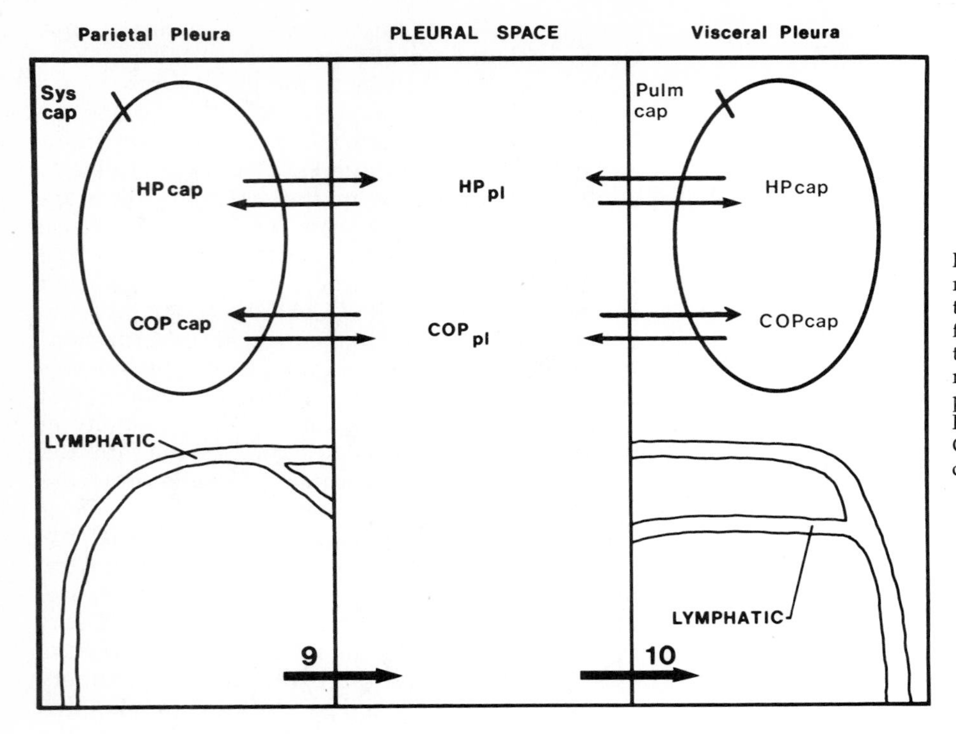

Figure 2. Normal pleural fluid movement from parietal capillaries to visceral capillaries. The net forces of 9 and 10 cm H_2O across the parietal and visceral pleura, respectively, favor absorption of pleural fluid. Driving pressure = $K \cdot (HP_{cap} - HP_{pl}) - (COP_{cap} - COP_{pl})$, where K is the filtration coefficient.

against each other may cause sharp pleuritic pain. Cough may occur with pleural effusion but is more likely to result from underlying lung involvement.

PHYSICAL EXAMINATION

Characteristic physical findings are associated with pleural effusion. When pleural effusion develops, the lung is separated from the chest wall by a layer of fluid that interferes with sound transmission. Except in very small pleural effusions (less than 300 ml), decreased fremitus and breath sounds are noted as well as dullness to percussion on the affected side. With massive pleural effusion (more than 2,000 ml), a contralateral mediastinal shift can occur. Several important points should be remembered about the physical findings in pleural fluid.

1. Decreased fremitus may result with an extensive postobstructive pneumonia when the obstruction is due to endobronchial tumor. The anticipated increased fremitus usually found with pneumonia is less in this case, because the transmitted sound waves are blocked by the obstructed bronchus.
2. Physical findings may be normal with a pleural effusion of less than 300 ml.
3. More than 2,000 ml of fluid is required to produce a contralateral mediastinal shift.
4. When a contralateral mediastinal shift does not occur with an apparent massive pleural effusion, several diagnoses should be considered: carcinoma of the mainstem bronchus with atelectasis of the ipsilateral lung, a fixed mediastinum due to neoplastic lymph nodes, malignant mesothelioma, and pronounced infiltration of the ipsilateral lung, usually by tumor.

DIAGNOSTIC STUDIES

Roentgenographic Appearance of Pleural Fluid

Roentgenographic examination of the chest is essential to confirm the presence of pleural effusion.[3] The first abnormality seen on a routine PA chest roentgenogram will be a blunting of the costophrenic angle in a typical meniscus configuration (Fig. 3). About 250 ml of fluid must be present, however, before this occurs. Free pleural fluid in a lesser quantity may accumulate between the lung and the diaphragm. Infrapulmonic or subpulmonic effusion is suggested by an apparent elevation of one hemidiaphragm, a shallow costophrenic sinus, or a great distance between the stomach air bubble and the top of the diaphragm (Fig. 4). A lateral decubitus view is used to confirm the diagnosis of infrapulmonic effusion (Fig. 5). This view may demonstrate as little as 10 to 15 ml of fluid with special maneuvers. A lateral decubitus view is also essential to establish that a larger pleural effusion is free-running and not loculated. Pleural fluid may also loculate in the intralobar fissure, producing a pseudotumor. Newer radio-

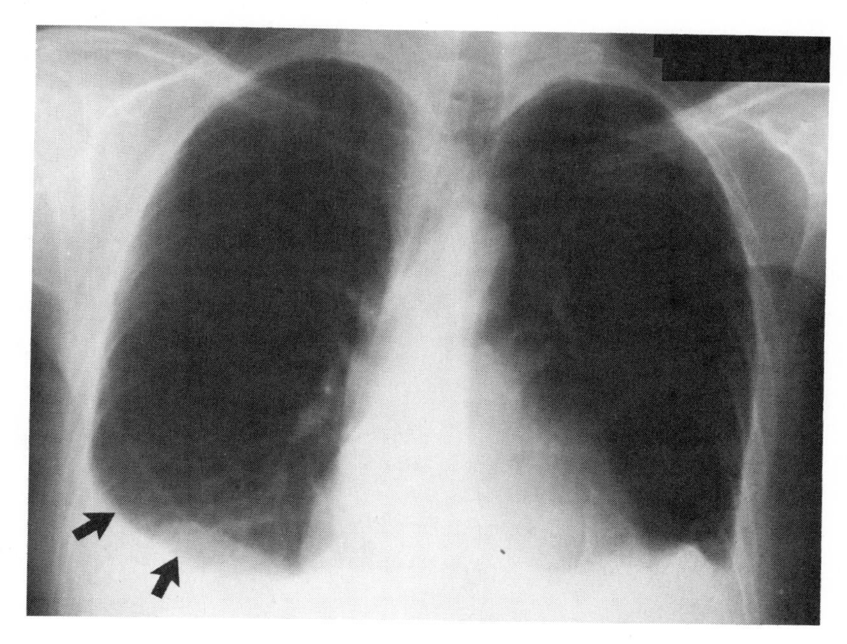

Figure 3. Blunting of costophrenic angle on the right *(arrows)* with a typical meniscus sign from a pleural effusion.

logic approaches to the diagnosis of pleural disease include ultrasonography and computerized tomography (CT scanning). The CT scan has proved extremely helpful in differentiating pleural from parenchymal disease.

Thoracentesis

Detection of pleural effusion most often requires a thoracentesis for diagnosis. Only when the diagnosis is definite, when a small amount of fluid is present, or when pleural fluid is found in a patient with uncomplicated congestive heart failure is observation without thoracentesis warranted. As thoracentesis is a relatively simple technique, however, the clinician should not hesitate to perform it if the clinical circumstances change.

Thoracentesis may also be performed in a therapeutic manner in a patient with a large pleural effusion who is dyspneic because of the effusion.

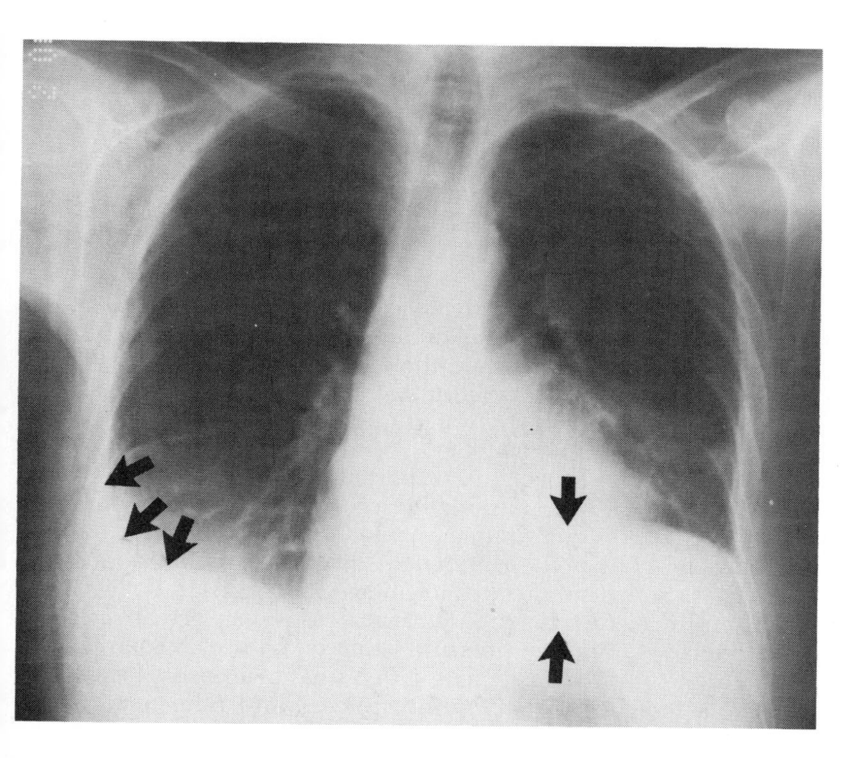

Figure 4. Infrapulmonic effusion on left (*arrows*). Note the great distance between the diaphragm and stomach air bubble. There is also a small pleural effusion on the right (*arrows*).

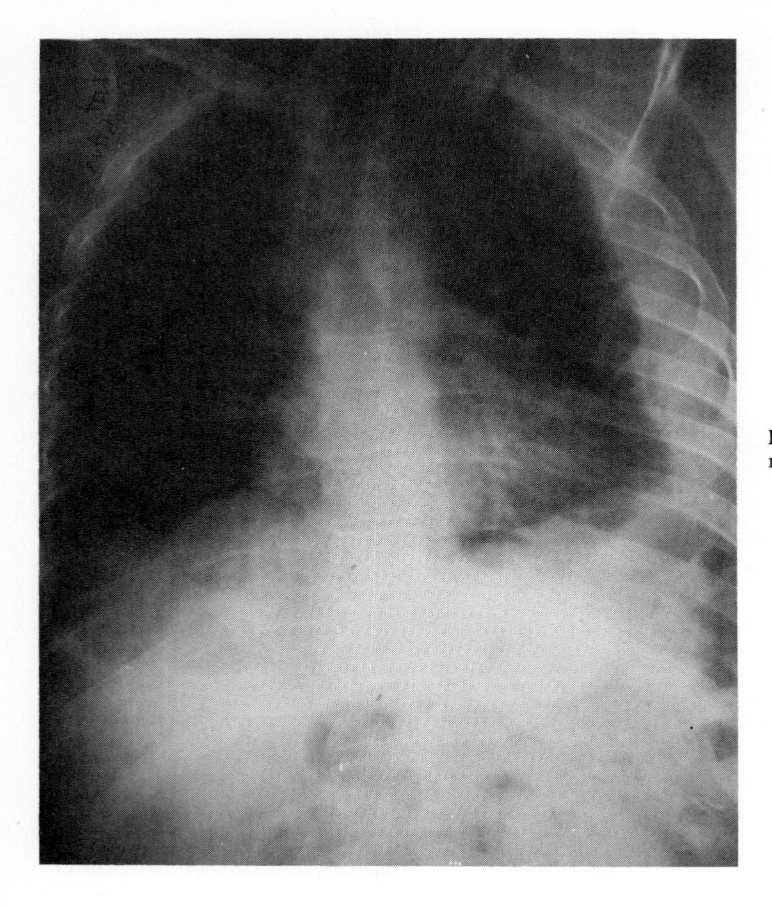

Figure 5. Lateral decubitus view demonstrating freely moving pleural fluid.

The dyspnea probably relates more to the neurogenic factors in compressed lung tissue than to oxygen receptors, because most patients have relief of dyspnea even if the Po_2 falls.[4] The clinician should not remove more than 1,000 ml of pleural fluid at any one time.[5]

Pleural Fluid Analysis

Pleural fluid should be analyzed in several different ways: appearance, cell count, chemistry, and culture. However, the first and most important step in the diagnosis of pleural effusion is determining whether the fluid is a transudate or an exudate.[6]

Transudative effusion occurs when systemic factors alter capillary hydrostatic pressure or colloid osmotic pressure. Increased capillary hydrostatic pressure is seen in congestive heart failure. Decreased plasma oncotic pressure is exemplified by hypoproteinemic states such as cirrhosis. Both processes favor the accumulation of a low-protein pleural fluid.

In contrast, an exudative effusion results from any disease of the pleural surface that produces increased capillary permeability or lymphatic obstruction. Pleural infection or tumor can damage the pleural surfaces, thus allowing for the formation of a protein-rich pleural fluid.

Traditionally, an effusion has been classified as an exudate if the *protein concentration* exceeds 3.0 gm. Recent studies note that using the 3.0-gm protein limit to define an exudative effusion results in inaccurate classification of over 10 per cent of effusions.[6] Evidence has accumulated suggesting that the most accurate classification of exudative effusion results when three criteria are met: (1) the pleural fluid protein–serum protein ratio is greater than 0.5; (2) the pleural fluid LDH–serum LDH ratio exceeds 0.6; and (3) the pleural fluid LDH ($>$ 200 IU) is more than two-thirds of the upper normal limit of serum LDH. If none of these criteria is met, the effusion is transudative. Therefore, the criteria are believed to be most accurate in correctly classifying exudative and transudative effusions.

Table 1 is a partial list of causes of pleural effusions divided according to whether the effusion is transudative or exudative. It can be seen that the differential diagnosis of transudative effusion relates to clinical states caused by increased capillary hydrostatic pressure or decreased colloid osmotic pressure—that is, hypoproteinemia from any cause. The differential diagnosis of exudative effusion is more protean, and other analyses of

Table 1. DIFFERENTIAL DIAGNOSIS OF PLEURAL EFFUSION

Transudative pleural effusion	Congestive heart failure Cirrhosis with ascites Nephrotic syndrome Hypoalbuminemia Peritoneal dialysis Atelectasis, acute
Exudative pleural effusion	Malignancy Pulmonary infarction Parapneumonic effusion Tuberculosis Collagen vascular disease (SLE, rheumatoid pleuritis) Pancreatitis Esophageal rupture Trauma (hemothorax) Drug sensitivity (nitrofurantoin) Asbestosis Chylothorax Uremic pleurisy

pleural fluid will help narrow the list of possible causes.

The *gross appearance* of the fluid at times yields useful information. The color, turbidity, odor, and presence or absence of blood should be noted. A majority of exudative effusions and all transudative effusions are clear and straw-colored. A white milky fluid indicates chylothorax or chyloform pleural effusion. Frank pus indicates empyema. A foul-smelling effusion is highly suggestive of anaerobic empyema. A very viscous fluid that is hemorrhagic suggests malignant mesothelioma.

The *white and red blood cell counts* of pleural fluid may at times be helpful in narrowing the differential diagnosis of an exudate.[7] Grossly bloody effusions often have red blood cell counts greater than 100,000 cells/mm^3. Essentially only three disease processes cause this finding: trauma (hemothorax), malignancy, and pulmonary embolization. The presence of only 5,000 to 10,000 erythrocytes/mm^3 causes fluid to appear hemorrhagic. Only 1 ml of blood is required to impart the bloody tinge to pleural fluid. Therefore, a blood-tinged effusion with a red blood cell count of less than 100,000 cells/mm^3 offers essentially no specific diagnostic help. Transudative effusions are rarely sanguineous, and the finding of a bloody effusion in the setting of congestive heart failure should prompt a search for another diagnosis, especially pulmonary emboli with infarction. A traumatic tap also causes bloody fluid. There are two bedside tests that can be used to determine whether the thoracentesis is traumatic or the pleural fluid is actually bloody: One can measure the hematocrit of the fluid and compare it with the blood hematocrit. Identical hematocrit ranges usually indicate traumatic thoracentesis, but this finding can also be seen with chest trauma and, rarely, with malignancy. Alternatively, one can note whether the pleural fluid clots. Fluid from a traumatic thoracentesis should clot within several minutes, whereas blood that has been present in pleural fluid for several hours to days will become defibrinated and will not form a good clot.

The absolute *white blood cell count* is less helpful, although a leukocyte count of less than 1,000 cells/mm^3 suggests a transudate, and higher than 1,000 cells/mm^3 suggests an exudate. The differential white cell count, however, is helpful in two instances: a neutrophilic predominance (> 75 per cent) suggests a primary inflammatory process; a lymphocytic predominance (> 50 per cent) is a strong indication of chronic exudative effusion (caused, for example, by tuberculosis, uremic pleurisy, or rheumatoid pleurisy) or malignancy, especially lymphoma.[8] The reason these effusions are mononuclear-predominant is that patients with these diseases are not usually seen early in the acute infectious process. At the time of thoracentesis, the acute neutrophilic predominance has changed to a mononuclear predominance.

Pleural fluid *eosinophilia* (> 10 eosinophils/mm^3) is not helpful in a specific diagnosis but does appear to indicate that the effusion is probably self-limited and will have a favorable outcome. Also, the presence of eosinophils makes the diagnosis of tuberculosis unlikely. Eosinophils may be found when blood or air has entered the thorax. Eosinophilic pleural fluid may be seen in pulmonary infarction, polyarteritis nodosa, and parasitic and fungal diseases.[9]

The *glucose level* of pleural fluid most often parallels that of serum. A low pleural fluid glucose level (< 60 mg/100 ml) narrows the differential diagnosis of an exudative effusion.[10] Six disease processes are reported to cause a low pleural fluid glucose: (1) parapneumonic effusion, especially empyema, in which the glucose level is almost always low; (2) rheumatoid pleural effusion (< 30 mg/100 ml); (3) tuberculous pleural effusion; a minority (< 20 per cent) of cases have a low glucose level; (4) malignant effusion; approximately one-third of patients have glucose levels between 20 and 60 mg/100 ml; (5) lupus pleuritis, in which decreased glucose is usually transient; (6) and esophageal rupture, in which low glucose level is usually related to empyema.

The mechanism responsible for a low pleural fluid glucose level appears to be a combination of increased glycolysis by pleural fluid cells, bacteria, or pleural tissue impairment and by glucose transport from blood to pleural fluid.[11, 12] For the most accurate glucose determinations, the patient should be fasting and the serum glucose level should be measured at the same time.

Pleural fluid *amylase* is elevated (> 160 Somogyi units/100 ml) in cases of pleural effusion associated with pancreatitis.[10] It can also be high in esophageal rupture and, rarely, in malignancies in which the primary tumor is often not in the pancreas.[13]

Measurement of pleural fluid *pH* has generated much interest in the past few years. A reading of less than 7.30 limits the differential diagnosis to empyema, malignancy, collagen vascular disease, tuberculosis, esophageal rupture, and hemothorax.[14] A pH of less than 7.0 has been found only in empyema, collagen vascular disease, and esophageal rupture. Thus low pleural fluid pH ($<$ 7.30) in a patient with pneumonia and an associated effusion suggests that the fluid either is an empyema or will behave clinically like an empyema and therefore will probably require chest tube drainage.[15] Fluid for pH determination must be collected anaerobically in a heparin-rinsed syringe and iced for accurate determination.

Other more specific tests of pleural fluid include the *lupus erythematosus preparation* to look for LE cells in patients with lupus pleuritis. *Rheumatoid factor* level, although increased in rheumatoid effusion, may also be increased in a variety of other nonrheumatoid effusions; therefore the test is not specific for the diagnosis of rheumatoid effusion. *Lipid analysis* should be performed on milky fluid. A chylous effusion reveals high levels of triglycerides and low cholesterol, whereas a chyloform effusion demonstrates an elevated cholesterol level and normal triglyceride levels.[16]

Cytologic Examination

Pleural fluid should be sent for cytologic examination when the clinical suspicion of malignancy is high. A small amount of heparin should be added to the specimen to inhibit clotting. Results are positive in 50 to 75 per cent of patients with malignancy.[17] False-negative results may be due to chronic effusion with resultant degenerative cells, lack of adequate pathologic expertise, or improper handling. Additionally, not all metastatic pleural effusions result directly from a carcinomatous involvement of pleura; some may be due to lymphatic obstruction, especially at the mediastinal level, or endobronchial obstruction with pneumonia or atelectasis. If the initial cytologic results are negative, data suggests that a repeat cytologic examination will increase the diagnostic yield.

Bacteriologic examination of the pleural fluid is essential. Fluid should undergo Gram staining, smear to look for acid-fast bacilli, and culture for aerobic and anaerobic organisms. Fungal culture is also indicated.

Pleural biopsy with either the Cope or Abrams pleural biopsy needle is helpful in the differential diagnosis of exudative effusion, but not in transudative effusions. The pathophysiologic mechanism in transudative effusion is pressure change, and therefore no abnormalities would be expected to be found in the pleura. Pleural biopsy should be performed in exudative effusions only when there is a strong suspicion of either granulomatous or malignant disease. The probability of positive diagnosis from pleural biopsy depends on the suspected disease process, the number of biopsies performed (yield increases with each of up to three separate biopsies), and ancillary procedures performed in conjunction with biopsy. When tuberculous effusion is suspected, culture of the pleural biopsy specimen as well as histologic examination for acid-fast microorganisms will increase the chance of a diagnosis to more than 95 per cent.[18] The yield in malignant effusion increases to 90 per cent if cytologic examination is combined with biopsy.[17] Contraindications to pleural biopsy include a bleeding diathesis with a prothrombin consumption of less than 50 per cent, a platelet count of less than 100,000 cells/mm^3, and abnormal bleeding or clotting time.

ASSESSMENT: CLINICAL CAUSES OF PLEURAL EFFUSION

Empyema. Empyema is simply defined as pus in the pleural cavity. Occasionally, fluid that is not grossly purulent may still be an empyema. In this instance, a positive pleural fluid culture result suggests empyema even though the fluid is serous. This finding probably represents early empyema. Causes of empyema are multiple. Frequently, it occurs as a complication of pneumonia in which the infectious process extends from the parenchyma to the pleura.[19] Common pathogens include *Staphylococcus aureus, Streptococcus pneumoniae*, gram-negative bacilli, and anaerobic organisms.[20] Empyema may also be a sequela of surgery, especially a thoracic procedure, trauma, and pneumothorax.

Symptoms at presentation are consistent with the primary disease. Patients with pneumonia and empyema are often febrile, tachycardic, and tachypneic. Many appear toxic. Physical findings are those of pleural effusion.

Empyema is suggested by the history and physical examination, but the diagnosis is confirmed by findings on thoracentesis and roentgenography. Thoracentesis usually reveals an exudative effusion that has a high leukocyte count ($>$ 10,000 cells/mm^3 with neutrophilic predominance ($>$ 80 per cent). The pleural fluid glucose level is usually low. Organisms may be seen on Gram staining and are usually cultured from the pleural fluid.

The effusion may appear free-running but also may be loculated at presentation or may become loculated. (*Loculation* refers to fluid encapsulated by adhesions between the parietal and visceral pleura.) Loculated fluid by definition is not free-

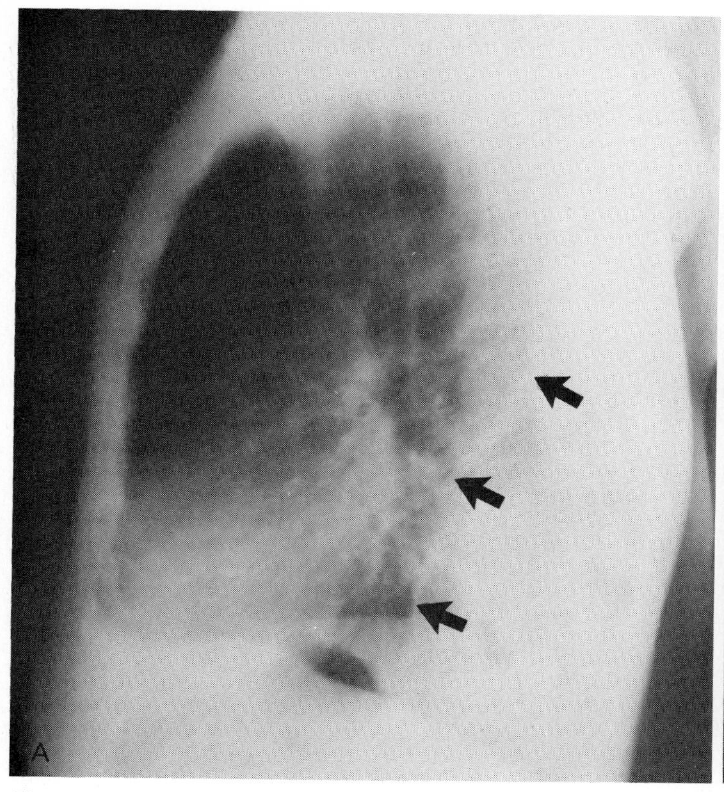

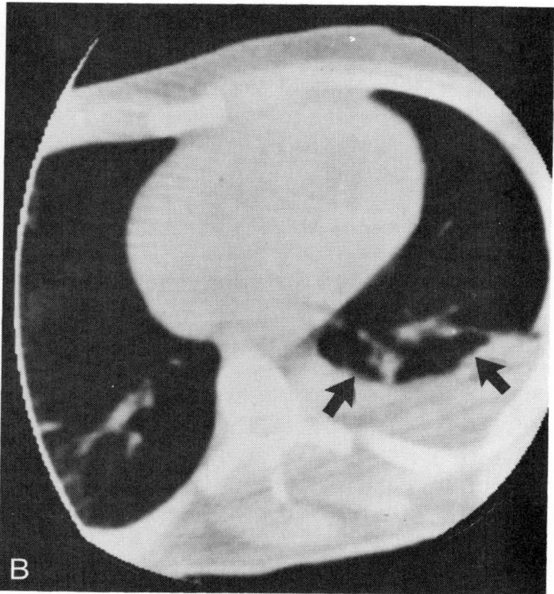

Figure 6. Lateral chest roentgenogram showing posterior loculated density (*arrows*). *B*, CAT scan revealed density to be a loculated pleural effusion *(arrows)*.

running and therefore does not change position on the lateral decubitus film. Fluid commonly loculates posteriorly, where it may appear as a smooth, sharply demarcated, homogeneous density protruding into the hemithorax (Fig. 6*A*). A CT scan is extremely helpful in differentiating loculated pleural effusion from lower lobe parenchymal disease (Fig. 6*B*).

Treatment of empyema includes treatment of the inciting disease process, usually pneumonia. If thoracentesis reveals grossly purulent fluid, immediate chest tube drainage is required. If nonpurulent fluid is obtained that meets the criteria for empyema, laboratory analysis may be helpful for selection of therapy. A pleural fluid pH greater than 7.30 suggests that no further specific therapy is needed and that the empyema will resolve spontaneously with systemic antibiotic therapy. If the pleural fluid pH is less than 7.20, closed chest tube drainage should be performed to evacuate the pleural space. Without drainage, complications such as loculations may occur. When loculated effusion or signs of infection such as fever or chills persist, closed chest tube drainage should be converted to open drainage with rib resection thoracotomy. Occasionally, the empyema persists in a chronic manner, until ultimately the pleural space is replaced by fibrous tissue and the lung is encased or trapped by a fibrin peel. More aggressive surgical procedures are indicated; that is, decortication of the lung and parietal pleura.

The goal of empyema therapy is early adequate evacuation of the pleural space to hasten the resolution of infection and to prevent chronic problems of loculation, fibrothorax, and trapped lung.

Congestive Heart Failure. Pleural effusion secondary to congestive heart failure is usually a transudative effusion in a patient with clinical evidence of right and left heart failure.[21] Therefore, the patient most often will have obvious physical signs of edema, hepatojugular reflux, crackles, and a left ventricular gallup. The effusion is not usually massive, although it can be a source of significant symptoms in a patient with underlying lung disease. Most often such effusions are bilateral, although when unilateral, they are found more commonly on the right side.

Malignant Pleural Effusion. The most common sites of tumors metastasizing to the pleura are lung, breast, stomach, and ovary.[22] A documented metastatic effusion represents an incurable lesion. Malignant pleural effusion is usually large and is the most common type of massive pleural effusion. A bloody massive effusion in the absence of trauma strongly suggests a malignant effusion.

When both cytologic examination and pleural biopsy are performed, the diagnostic yield is approximately 90 per cent.

Pulmonary Infarction. Pleural effusion after thromboembolic disease that results in a pulmonary infarction is usually small, bilateral, and exudative.[23] For the patient in the appropriate clinical setting (bed rest, oral contraceptive use, etc.) in whom the radiograph demonstrates a basal pulmonary infiltrate, elevation of the hemidiaphragm, and small pleural effusion, pulmonary infarction should be very strongly considered, even if the ventilation/perfusion lung scan indicates a low probability of such a diagnosis. Patients with pulmonary emboli without infarction rarely develop effusion.

Tuberculous Effusion. Tuberculous effusion occurs most often without other radiographic evidence of tuberculosis. Effusion secondary to tuberculosis is most commonly an early manifestation of the disease (primary) and may be the result of hypersensitivity to the tuberculous protein.[24] The tuberculous effusion is usually exudative with a mononuclear predominance. The diagnosis depends on the findings of: (1) a positive result of acid-fast bacilli (AFB) smear of the fluid (< 20 per cent of cases), (2) a positive AFB pleural fluid culture result (20–70 per cent), (3) the finding of caseating granuloma (25–40 per cent), and (4) culture of *Mycobacterium tuberculosis* from pleural tissue (55–80 per cent). Therefore when tuberculous effusion is considered, pleural biopsy must include *culture* of the biopsy specimen.

REFERENCES

1. Black LR. The pleural space and pleural fluid. Mayo Clin Proc 1972; 47:493–503.
2. Sahebjami H, Louden RG. Pleural effusion: pathophysiology and clinical features. Semin Roentgenol 1977;12:269–75.
3. Felson B. Roentgenographic recognition of pleural effusion. JAMA 1974;229:695–98.
4. Brandstetter RD, Cohen RP. Hypoxemia after thoracentesis. A predictable and treatable condition. JAMA 1959;242:1060–1.
5. Light RW, Jenkinson SG, Minh VD, George RB. Observations on pleural fluid pressures as fluid is withdrawn during thoracentesis. Am Rev Resp Dis 1980;121:799–804.
6. Light RW, MacGregor I, Luchsinger PC, Ball WC Jr. Pleural effusions: the diagnostic separation of transudates and exudates. Arch Intern Med 1972;77:507–13.
7. Light RW, Erozan YC, Ball WC Jr. Cells in the pleural fluid: their value in differential diagnosis. Arch Intern Med 1973;132:854–60.
8. Yam L. Diagnostic significance of lymphocytes in pleural effusions. Arch Intern Med 1967;66:972–82.
9. Campbell GD, Webb UR. Eosinophilic pleural effusion. Am Rev Resp Dis 1964;90:194–201.
10. Light RW, Ball WC Jr. Glucose and amylase in pleural effusions. JAMA 1973;225:257–9.
11. Potts DE, Willcox M, Good JT Jr, Taryle DA, Sahn SA. The acidosis of low glucose pleural effusions. Am Rev Resp Dis 1978;117:665–71.
12. Good JT Jr, Taryle DA, Kaplan RL, Maulitz RM, Saha SA. Pathogenesis of low glucose—low pH malignant effusion. Am Rev Resp Dis 1979;119:119.
13. Sherr HP, Light RW, Merson MH, Wolf RO, Taylor LL, Hendrix TR. Origin of pleural fluid amylase in esophageal rupture. Ann Intern Med 1972;76:985–6.
14. Good JT Jr, Taryle DA, Maulitz RM, Kaplan RL, Sahn SA. The diagnostic value of pleural fluid pH. Chest 1980;78:55–9.
15. Potts DE, Levin DC, Sahn SA: Pleural fluid pH in parapneumonic effusions. Chest 1976;70:328–31.
16. Seriff NS, Cohen ML, Samuel P, et al. Chylothorax: Diagnosis by lipoprotein electrophoresis of serum and pleural fluid. Thorax 1977;32:98–100.
17. Salyer WA, Eggleston JC, Erozan YS. Efficacy of pleural needle biopsy and pleural fluid cytopathology in the diagnosis of malignant neoplasm involving the pleura. Chest 1975;67:536–9.
18. Levine H, Metzger W, Lacera D, Kay L. Diagnosis of tuberculous pleurisy by culture of pleural biopsy specimen. Arch Intern Med 1970;126:269–71.
19. Light RW, Girard WM, Jenkinson SG, George RB. Parapneumonic effusions. Am J Med 1980;69:507–12.
20. Bartlett JG, Gorbach SL, Thadepalli H, Finegold SF. Bacteriology of empyema. Lancet 1974;1:338–40.
21. Race G, Scherfey C, Edward J. Hydrothorax in congestive heart failure. Am J Med 1957;22:83–90.
22. Leff A, Hopewell PC, Costello J. Pleural effusion from malignancy. Arch Intern Med 1978;88:532–7.
23. Bynum LJ, Wilson JE III. Radiographic features of pleural effusions in pulmonary embolism. Am Rev Resp Dis 1978;117:829–34.
24. Berger HW, Mejia E. Tuberculous pleurisy. Chest 1973;63:88–92.

PNEUMONIA, POORLY RESOLVED

EDWARD TSOU

☐ SYNONYMS: Pneumonitis, lung infection

BACKGROUND

Definitions and Origins

Pneumonia is an inflammation of the lungs most commonly caused by microbial agents. Although the term is also used to describe lung injury of other etiologies (hypersensitivity, eosinophilic, lipoid, radiation), this chapter concentrates on infectious pneumonia.

Pneumonia was the most common cause of death in the pre-antibiotic era. Recognized etiologies were tuberculosis, some aerobic and anaerobic bacteria, and influenza virus. Atypical pneumonia was described in 1942, and the infectious agent, *Mycoplasma pneumoniae,* was isolated in 1944. Gram-negative pneumonias, especially nosocomial, emerged in the early 1960s and continue to proliferate in the setting of extensive use of antimicrobial agents, corticosteroids, mechanical ventilation, inhalation therapy, and intensive care units. Beginning in the late 1960s, the introduction of antineoplastic chemotherapy and organ transplantation resulted in pneumonia caused by a variety of previously harmless viruses, fungi, and parasites, which usually required lung biopsy for diagnosis. In 1976, *Legionella pneumophila* was recognized as a cause of epidemic pneumonia and subsequently as an opportunistic, nosocomial, and increasingly common pathogen in sporadic pneumonia.[1] In 1981, a brand new form of opportunistic infection caused by *Pneumocystis carinii,* atypical mycobacteria, viruses (cytomegalovirus, herpes simplex virus), fungi *(Cryptococcus, Aspergillus, Candida)* and *Toxoplasma gondii* was found to occur in male homosexuals, drug addicts, and Haitians, possibly owing to lymphopenia and a change in the helper-suppressor T lymphocyte ratio.[2] These infections together with Kaposi's sarcoma, benign lymphadenopathy, lymphoma, and autoimmune thrombocytopenic purpura in this population have been termed the acquired immune deficiency syndrome (AIDS). The spectrum, and therefore the differential diagnosis, of pneumonia has widened tremendously in the past 20 years and promises to continue to do so.

Following the diagnosis and initiation of antimicrobial therapy for pneumonia, generally one of four clinical patterns emerges: (1) a convincing etiology is determined by culture, biopsy, or serologic analysis, and improvement occurs with specific therapy; (2) no etiology is discovered, but the patient improves when given antibiotics; (3) an alternative cause such as pulmonary infarction, lupus erythematosus, or drug-induced lung disease is diagnosed; or (4) the pneumonia persists, increases, or recurs in spite of treatment and no diagnosis is made. Because the focus of this chapter is on the last category, both common and uncommon lung infections and some features of nonmicrobial lung disease are presented to aid the clinician in solving the problem of poorly responsive pneumonia.

Incidence and Causes

Pneumonia, the fifth leading cause of death, is seen in about 10 per cent of hospitalized patients in the United States. It is estimated that 15 per cent of all deaths in hospital are due to nosocomial infection of the lower respiratory tract, and that two-thirds of these victims have a disease that probably would have been fatal within 6 months.[3] Up to 51 per cent of adult Asian refugees tested have been found to have intermediate-strength PPD skin reactions greater than 10 mm, 5 per cent have chest x-ray abnormalities consistent with active or inactive tuberculosis, and 1 per cent have active tuberculosis (rate 100 times higher than in American population) despite screening efforts. This increase in cases of tuberculosis (often drug-resistant) and parasitic infections of the lung have also been detected in refugees from the Caribbean. A substantial increase in opportunistic infections has occurred in patients with neoplasms, organ transplants, and AIDS, but the incidence of other pneumonias has otherwise remained relatively stable over the past 10 to 15 years.

The clinical features of pneumonia are variable but, in general, not difficult to recognize. What is difficult is to determine the exact microbial or nonmicrobial etiology of the lung inflammation at the time of presentation or when it is apparent that the pneumonia is responding poorly to initial therapy. The reasons for the difficulty are that findings of the history, physical examination, initial laboratory studies, sputum Gram stain, and chest roentgenogram are commonly not specific or sensitive enough for the physician to be confident of the cause. Perhaps the majority of known human-pathogenic microbes can involve the lung. Therefore, in order to substantially narrow the diagnostic possibilities from the myriad of causes

Table 1. CAUSES OF PNEUMONIA IN IMMUNOCOMPETENT PATIENTS*

Type of Pneumonia	Patients Without Underlying Disease	Patients With Underlying Disease
Bacterial		
Common	*Streptococcus pneumoniae*	*Streptococcus pneumoniae* *Hemophilus influenzae* *Staphylococcus aureus* *Klebsiella pneumoniae*
Less common	*Hemophilus influenzae* *Staphylococcus aureus* *Streptococcus pyogenes*	Aerobic gram-negatives Bacillus, especially in drug users *B. cereus* *B. sphaericus* *B. subtilis*
Unusual	*Klebsiella pneumoniae* *Neisseria meningitidis* *Francisella tularensis* Yersinia *Y. pestis* *Y. enterocolitica* Salmonella *S. typhosa* *S. choleraesuis* *S. typhimurium* and others *Bacillus anthracis*	Same as in those without underlying disease, except *Klebsiella pneumoniae*
Nonbacterial pneumonia simulating bacterial pneumonia	*Entamoeba histolytica*[5] *Blastomyces dermatitidis*	None
Atypical		
Common	*Mycoplasma pneumoniae*	Same as in those without underlying disease
Less common	*Legionella pneumophila* and other Legionella species[1, 20] Viruses Influenza Adenovirus Varicella Rubeola	
Unusual	Rickettsiae *R. rickettsii*[9] *R. prowazekii* *R. tsutsugamushi* *Coxiella burnetii* Viruses Coxsackie A and B ECHO Epstein-Barr Fungi *Histoplasma* (acute) *Coccidioides* (primary pulmonary) *Blastomyces* (acute)	
Aspiration[24]	Anaerobic bacteria, most commonly: *Bacteroides melaninogenicus* *Fusobacterium nucleatum* Anaerobic streptococci	Aerobic gram-negatives Anaerobes *Staphylococcus aureus*
Chronic	*Mycobacterium tuberculosis* Fungi *Coccidioides* *Blastomyces* *Cryptococcus* *Sporothrix schenckii* Bacteria *Actinomyces* *Nocardia* *Brucella* *Pseudomonas pseudomallei* Parasites *Paragonimus westermani*	Chronic obstructive lung disease due to: Mycobacterium *M. kansasii* *M. intracellulare*, and others *Histoplasma capsulatum*, chronic cavitary form
Nosocomial[3]	None	Aerobic gram-negatives *Staphylococcus aureus* *Streptococcus pneumoniae* *Staphylococcus epidermidis* (especially with IV lines)[16] *Legionella pneumophila* and other Legionella species[1, 20] *Listeria monocytogenes*

*Superscript numbers indicate chapter references.

of infectious pneumonia, separation based on epidemiologic and clinical patterns of disease is helpful. Initially, patients can be classified as immunocompetent (Table 1) or immunocompromised (Table 2). Immunocompromised persons in this discussion constitute patients with defects in cell-mediated immunity such as those with lymphoreticular malignancy, those receiving corticosteroid or cytotoxic drugs, and male homosexuals. Some drug addicts, hemophiliacs, and Haitians may also be in this category. Immunocompetent patients are separable into those who are healthy at the onset of pneumonia and those with underlying disease. All causes of lung infection may be found in those with underlying disease. However, pharyngeal colonization patterns make gram-negative bacteria much more likely in debilitated, diabetic, alcoholic, and hospitalized patients than in healthy ones. Further categorizing of patients into those with bacterial, atypical, aspiration, nosocomial, chronic, and recurrent pneumonias is helpful because these groups are commonly clinically separable, the responsible pathogens distinct, and the choices of antimicrobials for each group relatively limited.

HISTORY

Subjective Data

History of the Present Illness. The severity of symptoms in pneumonia ranges from asymptomatic to fulminant and life-threatening. True rigors are fairly specific for bacterial pneumonia, but fever, chilliness, sweats, night sweats, chest pain, cough, sputum production, and hemoptysis as well as constitutional symptoms such as malaise, anorexia, and myalgias, may be present in most, if not all, types of pneumonia. Assignment of cases of pneumonia to specific categories or etiologies is usually related to four broad historical features, as follows:

1. *Relative severity of symptoms.* In classic bacterial pneumonia, cough and purulent sputum production commonly predominate, whereas in atypical pneumonia, the cough is usually dry, minimally productive, and hacking and constitutional symptoms are relatively severe. In fact, in a patient with minimal or no cough, the diagnosis of mycoplasmal pneumonia should be questioned. Chest discomfort is not uncommon in viral, mycoplasmal, or chlamydial pneumonias, but true pleuritic chest pain is more often a feature of bacterial pneumonia.

2. *Time factors.* The abrupt onset of viral pneumonias can distinguish an influenza or adenovirus pneumonia from mycoplasmal pneumonia, which commonly has an insidious progression of symptoms. The definition of *chronic* is arbitrary. However, the presence of slowly increasing symptoms over a period of 3 weeks or longer would reasonably suggest a chronic pneumonia. For example, patients with chronic granulomatous infections of the lung such as tuberculosis, chronic histoplasmosis, and melioidosis may be initially asymptomatic, but with progression of infiltrates, nonspecific constitutional symptoms such as fever, anorexia, fatigue, and night sweats may be present. It is not uncommon for these symptoms to be poorly recognized by the patient, who may appear nontoxic in spite of documented fever. As the disease continues, cough—which may be mild or severe, productive or nonproductive, and with or without blood—may appear and may progress with extension of lung infiltrates. A *recurrent* pneumonia is one that has definitely improved or resolved, with or without treatment, only to reappear or worsen. The known seasonal occurrence of some pneumonias is occasionally helpful. Viral pneumonias predominate in the winter, legionnaires' disease occurs mainly in summer and fall, but mycoplasmal infections occur all year round.

3. *Underlying health status.* In the patient with a history of depressed central nervous system (e.g., anesthesia, cardiopulmonary arrest, drug overdose, seizure disorder), disturbance of swallowing (e.g., achalasia, Zenker's diverticulum, esophageal scleroderma or carcinoma), or severe neuromuscular weakness or paralysis (e.g., amyotrophic lateral sclerosis, quadriplegia), aspiration is a leading cause of pneumonia. Influenza pneumonia is ordinarily restricted to gravidas and to patients with pulmonary or cardiac disease, especially rheumatic heart disease with mitral stenosis.

Table 2. CAUSES OF PNEUMONIA IN IMMUNOCOMPROMISED PATIENTS

Bacterial pneumonia	Aerobic gram-negatives[22] *Streptococcus pneumoniae* *Nocardia asteroides* *Listeria monocytogenes*
Atypical pneumonia	*Pneumocystis carinii* *Legionella* species Cytomegalovirus Varicella Herpes simplex[15] *Toxoplasma gondii* *Cryptococcus neoformans* *Strongyloides stercoralis*
Fungal pneumonia (with clinical features of pulmonary infarction)	*Aspergillus* *Mucor*
Chronic pneumonia	*Mycobacterium tuberculosis* Atypical mycobacteria (many species) Fungi *Cryptococcus* *Coccidioides* *Histoplasma*

Table 3. SOME NONINFECTIOUS DISEASES THAT SIMULATE PNEUMONIA DUE TO MICROBIAL AGENTS

Diseases simulating bacterial, atypical, or recurrent pneumonia	Pulmonary infarction[4] Fat embolism Congestive heart failure Hypersensitivity pneumonia (e.g., farmer's lung, pigeon-breeder's lung) Bronchopulmonary aspergillosis Loeffler's syndrome Eosinophilic pneumonia Sickle cell lung disease[6] Systemic lupus erythematosus Drug-induced lung disease (e.g., nitrofurantoin lung) Pulmonary hemorrhage (e.g., Goodpasture's syndrome, idiopathic hemosiderosis, systemic lupus erythematosus) Pulmonary vasculitis (e.g., Wegener's granulomatosis)[7] Pulmonary contusion or hemorrhage
Diseases simulating chronic pneumonia	Alveolar cell carcinoma Pulmonary alveolar proteinosis Aspiration lipoid pneumonia

4. *Place of origin of pneumonia.* Acquisition of pneumonia by a patient in the hospital defines the pneumonia as nosocomial. It is usually gram-negative or staphylococcal.[3]

Symptoms unrelated to infectious disease may be crucial, because nonmicrobial disease may closely mimic pneumonia and does not respond to antibiotics (Table 3). In a recent study, autopsy examination showed 31 per cent of patients with pulmonary embolism to have pulmonary infarction.[4] Clinical features of pulmonary infarction commonly resemble those of acute pneumonia. Abrupt onset, recurrent chest pain and dyspnea, underlying cardiovascular disease or malignancy, bedridden or postoperative status, and symptoms of lower extremity phlebitis suggest this diagnosis. In patients with coexisting pneumonia and elderly patients, however, pulmonary embolism is rarely diagnosed. The presence of wheezing and eosinophilia suggests that symptoms of pneumonia are being caused by bronchopulmonary aspergillosis, allergic parasitic lung disease due to nematodes, microfilariae, and schistosomes,[5] or eosinophilic pneumonia. Sickle cell lung disease due to in situ thrombosis may mimic classic or atypical pneumonia in every way.[6] On the other hand, the incidence of pneumococcal pneumonia and the severity of mycoplasmal pneumonia are increased in sickle cell disease. Overt renal disease is seen in Goodpasture's syndrome, systemic lupus erythematosus, and Wegener's granulomatosis, all of which may have the clinical features of infectious pneumonia. Other multisystem symptoms may indicate that a patient with fever and chest infiltrates has pulmonary vasculitis.[7] Congestive heart failure can produce local infiltrates suggesting pneumonia, especially in patients with underlying lung disease.

Family History. About half of patients with common bacterial pneumonia and most patients with mycoplasmal or viral pneumonia have symptoms related to upper respiratory tract infection. Under conditions of household association, approximately 10 per cent of adults acquire viral respiratory tract infections from index cases. Therefore, concurrent respiratory tract infection in the household increases suspicion that pneumonia is pneumococcal, mycoplasmal, or viral. Present or remote tuberculosis in family members should be ascertained. The United States Public Health Service estimated that about 28 per cent of household contacts of tuberculous patients acquire infection, 5 to 15 per cent of whom develop clinically active tuberculosis within 5 years, and 3 to 5 per cent more after 5 years.[8]

Personal History. The incidences of bacterial pneumonia, legionnaires' disease, and postoperative pneumonia are higher in smokers, especially those with chronic airways obstruction. The likelihood that a locally recurrent pneumonia is due to an obstructing bronchogenic carcinoma increases with age and amount and duration of tobacco use. Heavy alcohol ingestion correlates with pneumonias due to *Streptococcus pneumoniae, Hemophilus influenzae*, anaerobes, and *Mycobacterium tuberculosis*.

Drug History. A variety of medications may produce pulmonary edema, pulmonary infiltrates with eosinophilia, drug-induced lupus, vasculitis, embolic phenomena, and interstitial pneumonitis, all of which may mimic infectious lung disease. Aspiration of mineral oil, lip balm, and petroleum jelly may cause lipoid infiltrates that resemble chronic infectious pneumonia. Fever and lung infiltrates indistinguishable from *Pneumocystis carinii* or viral pneumonia can result from use of antineoplastic drugs and other medications of many types (e.g., nitrofurantoin, phenytoin).

Social and Occupational History. A number of outdoor recreational activities and occupations are associated with uncommon pneumonias, including hunting (tularemia, plague), poultry farming (histoplasmosis, ornithosis), ranching (Q fever, brucellosis), spelunking (histoplasmosis), and wood-chopping (blastomycosis). Tick bites have resulted in pneumonia due to Rocky Mountain spotted fever,[9] Q fever, and tularemia. Occupational exposure to animal hides is a key historical point in the rare case of anthrax pneumonia. Even brief inhalation of dried psittacine bird excreta or handling of feathers or tissues of infected birds (which may appear healthy or minimally ill) can result in psittacosis pneumonia. Pulmonary cryptococcosis has been traced to pigeons, and pet dogs and cats have been the source of pneumonia due to *Pasteurella multocida, Blastomyces, Toxoplasma,* and *Toxocara*.

History of Overseas Travel or Residence. Tuberculosis is extremely prevalent in most areas of the world outside North America, Europe, and Australia. Parasitic pulmonary disease, including falciparum malaria pneumonia, roundworm allergic reactions of the lung (*Ascaris*, hookworm, *Strongyloides, Toxocara*), pulmonary amebiasis, and paragonimiasis are commonly acquired outside the United States.[5] Besides tuberculosis and paragonimiasis, the possibility of melioidosis (caused by *Pseudomonas pseudomallei*) should be considered in anyone with chronic infection of the lung resembling tuberculosis who has recently or in the remote past resided in Southeast Asia. Travel through the Southwest United States always suggests that a pneumonia is due to *Coccidioides immitis*.

High-Payoff Queries

1. *Did you have a chronic cough prior to the onset of pneumonia?* Patients with pneumonia due to obstruction, bronchiectasis, cystic fibrosis,[10] and alveolar proteinosis commonly have a chronic cough. Increased cough or wheeze with change in body position suggests a pneumonia due to obstruction, esophagobronchial fistula, or aspiration.

2. *What does your sputum look like? Does it have odor or taste? Is it bloody?* Although rarely diagnostic in themselves, classic sputum characteristics are related to specific etiologies. Hence, sputum has been described variously as "rusty" in pneumococcal pneumonia and paragonimiasis, "currant jelly" in Klebsiella pneumonia, creamy yellow or salmon-colored in staphylococcus pneumonia, "raspberry syrup" in plague, "anchovy paste" or "chocolate sauce" in amebiasis, three-layered in bronchiectasis, foul-smelling and foul-tasting in anaerobic infections, and pink and frothy in pulmonary edema. Sputum streaked or mixed with blood suggests microbial infections, whereas pure blood may be due to pulmonary infarction, lung hemorrhage (Goodpasture's syndrome, lung contusion) or infection (tuberculous Rasmussen's aneurysm.)

3. *Have you noted a skin rash, nodule, ulcer, abscess, or cold sore?* Although infrequent in most pneumonias, abnormalities of the skin and mucous membranes can suggest specific diagnoses (to be discussed under "Physical Examination").

4. *Do you have diarrhea?* Diarrhea may be a prominent early manifestation of legionnaires' disease and is seen in pneumonia due to *Salmonella*, amebiasis, and roundworm infections. Diarrhea and steatorrhea are clues to the diagnosis of cystic fibrosis in any young patient with recurrent pulmonary infections.[10]

5. *Have you had a headache, drowsiness, confusion, stiff neck, visual disturbance, weakness or numbness of an extremity, or a seizure?* Although meningitis can be seen uncommonly in many pneumonias, focal symptoms of brain abscess should always suggest *Nocardia, Staphylococcus,* or anaerobic infection. Coexistent central nervous system symptoms in an immunocompromised patient with pneumonia raise the possibilities of toxoplasmosis, cryptococcosis, nocardiosis, and legionnaires' disease.

6. *Have you received any antibiotics? What type and dosage, and for how long?* Antibiotic usage is extremely common in poorly resolved pneumonia, and knowledge of the pharmacology, spectrum, and resistance patterns of antimicrobials is helpful in eliminating or incriminating specific causes of pneumonia, suggesting the possibility of superinfection, or raising the question of recurrent pneumonia due to inadequate therapy.

PHYSICAL EXAMINATION

The presence or absence of physical signs is contributory to the evaluation of pneumonia but in most cases does not define the etiology. For example, in one series of 200 consecutive roentgenographically demonstrated pneumonias, 26 per cent of patients had rales in the area of abnormality and only 41 per cent had any significant physical findings.[11] Some physical findings that may be specifically helpful in diagnosis are listed in Table 4.

DIAGNOSTIC STUDIES

Usually, the diagnostic studies whose results are available to the physician at the time of presentation or when it is recognized that a case of pneumonia is poorly resolved include respiratory secretion staining by the Gram, acid-fast, and potassium hydroxide methods, chest reontgenogram, blood cell counts, urinalysis, routine blood chemistries, and, occasionally, pleural fluid analysis. Only after days or weeks do results of cultures, skin tests, serologic tests, and biopsy examination become available.

Laboratory Studies

Examination of Respiratory Secretions. Examination of deep respiratory secretions, if obtainable, should be performed in all poorly resolved pneumonias. The specificity and sensitivity of *sputum* Gram *staining*, however, remains controversial. A

Table 4. PHYSICAL FINDINGS AND THEIR SIGNIFICANCE IN POORLY RESOLVED PNEUMONIA*

Physical Finding	Significance and Possible Etiology
Vital Signs	
Relative bradycardia	Legionnaires' disease, psittacosis, typhoid
Skin	
Pruritic vesicles in crops	*Varicella*
Reddish-brown macules beginning on the face and spreading to trunk and extremities	Measles
Erythematous or maculopapular rash progressing to petechial, vesicular, or purpuric rash	Atypical measles (patients given inactivated measles vaccine who subsequently become infected with live measles vaccine or wild virus)[12]
Pink macules beginning on the wrists and ankles and spreading to the body	Rocky Mountain spotted fever[9]
Mottled pink to red-blue erythema	Meningococcus
Deep red 2- to 4-mm macules on the anterior abdominal wall and thorax	Psittacosis (Horder's spots), typhoid (Rose spots)
Erythema nodosum	Mycoplasma,[13] tuberculosis, coccidioidomycosis, histoplasmosis, blastomycosis
Erythema multiforme, including Stevens-Johnson syndrome	Mycoplasma,[13] coccidioidomycosis
Ecthyma gangrenosum	*Pseudomonas*
Papule, ulcer, warty lesion, subcutaneous abscess	Blastomycosis, cryptococcosis, nocardiosis, sporotrichosis
Eschar at site of tick bite	Tularemia, plague
Head and neck	
Bullous myringitis	Mycoplasma (uncommon in viral or bacterial infection)[13]
Choroidal tubercles	Tuberculosis
Fluffy white retinal exudates	*Candida* (disseminated)
Nasal ulceration, pansinusitis, periorbital cellulitis (in immunocompromised patient)	Aspergillosis (invasive), mucormycosis
Herpes labiales, or other mucocutaneous herpes	Pneumococcal pneumonia (seen in 10 per cent), herpes simplex pneumonia in immunocompromised individuals[15]
Oropharyngeal ulcers	Histoplasmosis (disseminated)
Koplik spots	Measles
Periodontitis, gingivitis	Anaerobes, actinomycosis
Exudative pharyngitis	beta-Hemolytic streptococcus (50 per cent of pneumonias), adenovirus, Epstein-Barr virus
Chest	
Intercostal muscle swelling and tenderness	Pleurodynia (coxsackie B virus inflammation of chest wall muscles, which may mimic pneumonia)
Chest wall sinus tracts	Actinomycosis, uncommon in nocardiosis, blastomycosis, and tuberculosis
Consolidation	Favors bacteria over uncomplicated virus, mycoplasma, and chlamydia
Abdomen	
Hepatomegaly and/or splenomegaly (uncommon in most pneumonias)	Amebiasis, psittacosis, brucellosis, disseminated histoplasmosis, miliary tuberculosis, cytomegalovirus, Epstein-Barr virus
Extremities	
Thrombophlebitis	Psittacosis, brucellosis
Infected intravenous line, catheter site, shunt, or fistula	*Staphylococcus aureus* or *S. epidermidis*[16]
Genitals	
Swelling of prostate, epididymis, or seminal vesicles	Blastomycosis (15 per cent of cases), tuberculosis
Neurologic	
Focal neurologic signs	*Nocardia*, anaerobes, *Staphylococcus*

*Superscript numbers indicate chapter references.

recent study found that the presence of more than 10 gram-positive, lancet-shaped diplococci per oil immersion field yielded a 90 per cent specificity for *Streptococcus pneumoniae* as detected by culture, Quellung reaction, or mouse inoculation, but failed to identify 38 per cent of the total cases of pneumococcal pneumonia.[17] Similar studies in gram-negative pneumonia showed specificity and sensitivity of about 75 per cent for Gram stains, which increased to 80 to 90 per cent when large numbers of organisms were cultured.[18] Currently, observations of numerous typical, lancet-shaped, gram-positive encapsulated diplococci, gram-positive cocci in clusters, gram-negative coccobacilli, and gram-negative rods are presumptive, but not definitive, evidence of pneumonia due to *Streptococcus pneumoniae, Staphylococcus aureus* or *S. epidermidis, Hemophilus influenzae,* and gram-negative pathogens of many species, respectively. Commonly, gram-stained sputum preparations in nonbacterial pneumonias show mononuclear and some segmented cells with no organisms or mixed gram-positive and gram-negative bacteria. Rarely the presence of *Nocardia, Actinomyces,* and *Aspergillus* can be detected by Gram staining. Acid-fast staining may detect *Mycobacterium, Nocardia,* and *Legionella micdadei. Nocardia* will not fluoresce with auramine O–rhodamine B staining. Direct immunofluorescent staining can detect *Legionella.*

Results of *bacterial culture* of expectorated sputum should similarly be considered presumptive evidence of infection, but the results should be dismissed when response to therapy is poor because of contamination by organisms colonizing the pharynx. One-half of some healthy populations may be colonized by *Streptococcus pneumoniae* or *Hemophilus influenzae* during winter months, and the incidence of gram-negative colonization increases with the degree of underlying illness owing to adherence of gram-negative bacteria to the pharyngeal mucosa, such that the rate of gram-negative colonization approaches 75 per cent in some intensive care units. The report of heavy growth or pure culture of organisms is suggestive of specific etiologies, but the true value of such reports is not known. It must be remembered that in only 50 per cent of patients whose blood cultures are positive for pneumococcus or *Hemophilus influenzae* do these organisms grow in sputum cultures. Once such an organism is suspected, the laboratory must be instructed accordingly, i.e., to culture anaerobically for *Actinomyces,* to look specifically for *Nocardia* (owing to its resemblance to *Mycobacterium*), to culture for *Legionella* (charcoal yeast extract agar, Mueller-Hinton agar), to hold cultures for fungi, especially *Histoplasma* (growth 8 to 14 days), and to take precautions for organisms such as *Coccidioides, Brucella, Francisella tularensis* and *Yersinia pestis* (danger to laboratory personnel).

When expectorated sputum cannot be obtained or interpreted because of colonization, consideration should be given to *translaryngeal aspiration* (TLA), *fiberoptic bronchoscopy* (FOB) using a shielded brush, or direct percutaneous *needle aspiration* to evalute respiratory secretions for microbes. Despite its proven value, translaryngeal aspiration is frightening to most alert patients, may be hazardous, and can produce false-positive results in 20 per cent of patients, especially bronchitics. Although not a routine procedure, it is useful in selected patients, especially those who are mentally unresponsive. The value of fiberoptic bronchoscopy in diagnosing tuberculosis when expectorated sputum examination has been unrevealing is established.[19] However, routine bacterial cultures of specimens obtained through the bronchoscope do not escape oropharyngeal contamination, and the value of using the shielded brush is controversial. If the shielded brush method has proved reliable at the physician's institution, it may be performed in poorly resolved pneumonia in which sputum examination appears essential. Transthoracic needle aspiration has not yet been systematically evaluated in the diagnosis of acute or chronic pneumonias, but when the hazards of pneumothorax and bleeding are minimal and the expertise exists, evaluation of material from direct needle puncture into the site of lung infiltration may enable one to avoid open lung biopsy.

Other Studies. Unfortunately, blood cell counts, urinalysis, and liver and renal function tests rarely provide specific diagnostic information. In general, a white blood cell count greater than 15,000 cells/mm^3 favors bacterial over viral or mycoplasmal infection. Abnormal results of urinalysis and liver function tests and the finding of hypophosphatemia and especially hyponatremia should make legionnaires' disease a prime consideration.[20] Cold agglutinins, which are present in one-half to two-thirds of patients with mycoplasmal pneumonia,[13] can be evaluated at the bedside by observing agglutination of red blood cells on the glass of a tube after it has been placed in ice and noticing the disappearance of agglutination with hand-warming of the tube. Titers must be in excess of 1:64 for the result of bedside evaluation to be positive.[21] Counterimmunoelectrophoresis rapidly detects pneumococcal antigen in the serum or urine in about 50 per cent and in the sputum in 90 per cent of patients with lobar pneumonia due to *Streptococcus pneumoniae. Hemophilus influenzae* and *Staphylococcus* have also been evaluated by this technique. Where available and reliable, counterimmunoelectrophoresis for bacterial antigens may be useful in typical bacterial pneumonias, especially in patients treated with antibiotics. Other serologic tests that may ultimately be diagnostically helpful include those for *Legionella, Mycoplasma,* influenza, cytomegalovirus, Epstein-Barr virus, psittacosis, Q fever, *Cryptococcus, Coccidioides, Histoplasma,* tularemia, and *Brucella.*

Imaging

Patterns on Chest Roentgenogram. Although in rare exceptions pneumonia may be diagnosed in the absence of radiographically demonstrated chest infiltrates (notably in leukopenic patients),[22] the presence of infiltrates on chest roentgenogram is generally considered the *sine qua non* of pneumonia. Radiographic features of bacterial pneumonia include lobar or segmental distribution, cavitation, microabscesses, bulging fissures, and large, rapidly loculating or later-appearing pleural effusion. Although some features are considered characteristic, such as pneumatocele formation in staphylococcal pneumonia, bulging fissures in *Klebsiella* pneumonia, small irregular oval opacities with hilar adenopathy in tularemia, and mediastinal widening (hemorrhagic mediastinitis) in anthrax, most specific causes of pneumonia cannot be discerned by roentgenographic patterns. Radiographic findings in viral pneumonia include nodular, reticular, diffuse, and perihilar infiltrates. Small pleural effusions are present in some patients. Radiographic findings in mycoplasmal pneumonia are protean, but segmental or patchy consolidation and centrally dense infiltrates are said to be helpful features.[13] Regrettably, the diagnosis of bacterial versus nonbacterial causes by means of roentgenographic criteria is only about 66 per cent accurate and is especially poor in mycoplasmal infections, which are mostly mistaken for bacterial pneumonia.[23] In immunocompromised patients, although segmental infiltrates are common in bacterial and fungal infections and findings indicative of pulmonary infarction should suggest the diagnosis of *Aspergillus* or *Mucor* infections, roentgenographic patterns are nonspecific. Alveolar cell carcinoma, alveolar proteinosis, and lipoid aspiration pneumonia are prime considerations in patients with chronic alveolar infiltrates but without clinical manifestations of pneumonia.

Anatomic Distribution of Pulmonary Infiltrates. Specific locations of infiltrates are typical in some pneumonias. For example, an infiltrate in the upper lobe (Fig. 1) may be seen in *Mycobacteria* pneumonia, chronic pulmonary histoplasmosis, infections by other fungi, melioidosis and the pneumonia of cystic fibrosis (right upper lobe). An infiltrate in the posterior segments of the upper lobes and superior segments of the lower lobes (Fig. 2) suggests aspiration lung abscess or necrotizing pneumonia. Recurrent infection in bronchopulmonary sequestration causes an infiltrate in the posterior basal segments of the lower lobes. In amebiasis, especially with liver enlargement, an infiltrate may be seen in the right lower lobe.

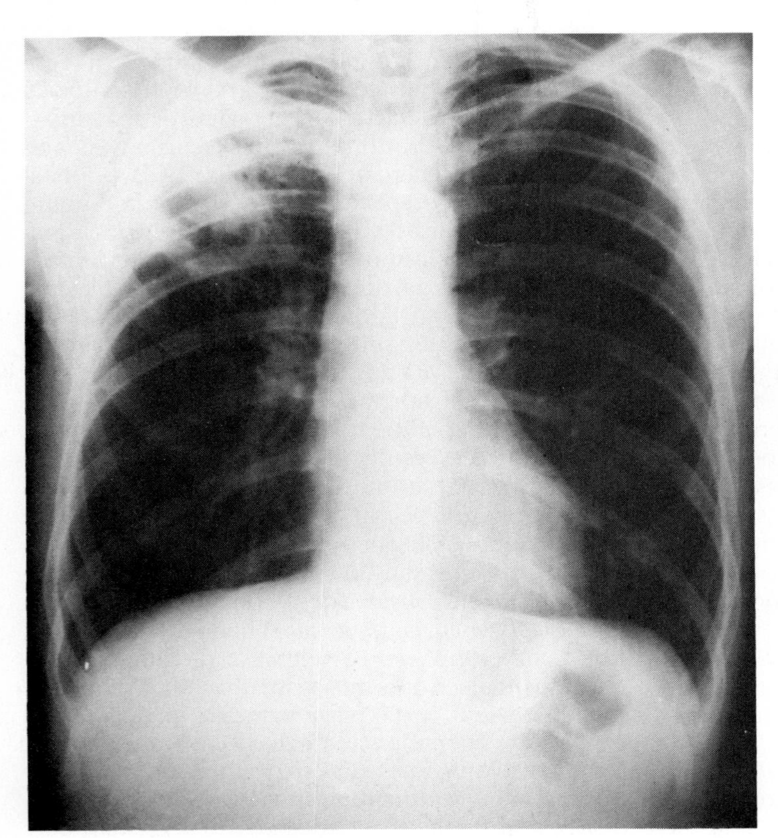

Figure 1. Chest roentgenogram demonstrating the typical location of a chronic granulomatous cavitary infiltrate in the right upper lobe in a 62-year-old male with severe chronic emphysema. Multiple cultures of sputum and the right upper lobe following lobectomy grew *Mycobacterium intracellulare.*

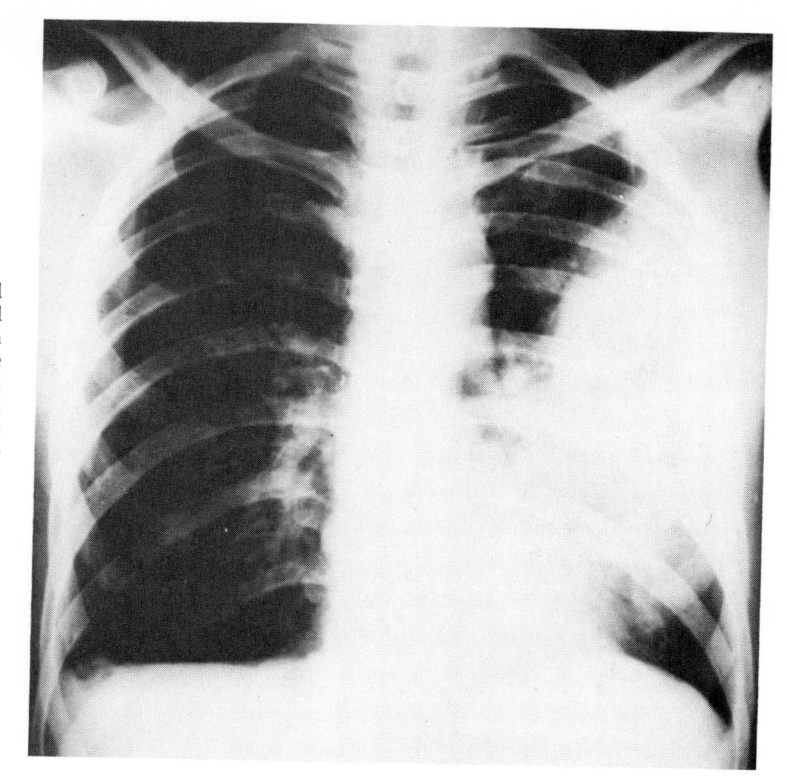

Figure 2. Chest roentgenogram of a 45-year-old alcoholic with a seizure disorder and poor oral hygiene, showing a characteristic location of an anaerobic necrotizing aspiration pneumonia in the posterior segment of the upper lobe, lingula, and superior segment of the left lower lobe. The small infiltrate in the right lower lobe and blunting of the right costophrenic angle are residua of a prior aspiration pneumonia.

Hilar Adenopathy. The presence of hilar node enlargement is distinctly uncommon in most adult pneumonias. This finding should prompt one to suspect tuberculosis, fungal infections (histoplasmosis, coccidiomycosis, blastomycosis), tularemia, anthrax, mononucleosis, or coexisting neoplasm (Fig. 3).

Patterns of Progression and Resolution. Extremely rapid progression of infiltrates may occur in many pneumonias, sometimes owing to accompanying adult respiratory distress syndrome. Influenza and plague pneumonia are notorious for rapid progression. An infiltrate beginning in one lobe and moving rapidly to multilobar, bilateral involvement is characteristic of legionnaires' disease,[20] but staphylococcal, gram-negative, and even pneumococcal pneumonia may have such a pattern. Delayed resolution of infiltrates is seen most often in patients with underlying anatomic abnormalities or metabolic diseases such as emphysema, obstruction, bronchiectasis, heart failure, and diabetes. The resolution of localized chest infiltrates by contraction and increased density suggests pulmonary infarction, though some pneumonias result in fibrosis and produce this roentgenographic finding.

Other Findings. The chest roentgenogram should be searched carefully for rib abnormalities (actinomycosis, nocardiosis, blastomycosis), endobronchial masses (bronchial adenoma, foreign body) (Fig. 4), lobar volume loss (obstruction), and coexisting mass lesions (tumor, esophageal diverticulum). Specialized examinations such as bronchography, tomography, esophagography, and CT scanning may be necessary to confirm abnormalities suspected on plain film.

Biopsy Examination of Lung Tissue

If the patient is deteriorating on empiric antimicrobial therapy and the diagnosis of pneumonia eludes the preceding diagnostic techniques, transbronchial or open lung biopsy should be performed. Because of the smallness of biopsy specimens and sampling errors, nondiagnostic transbronchial biopsy results should not be accepted, and open lung biopsy should be planned subsequent to receiving complete information on stains and sections of the transbronchial specimen. The decision to perform transbronchial or open biopsy is made earlier in immunocompromised patients owing to the potential for rapid progression. If the patient is stable, progression of pneumonia is slow, and facilities for rapid processing of specimens are available, transbronchial biopsy may obviate thoracotomy. However, if progression is rapid and the bleeding potential is high, immediate open lung biopsy is indicated.

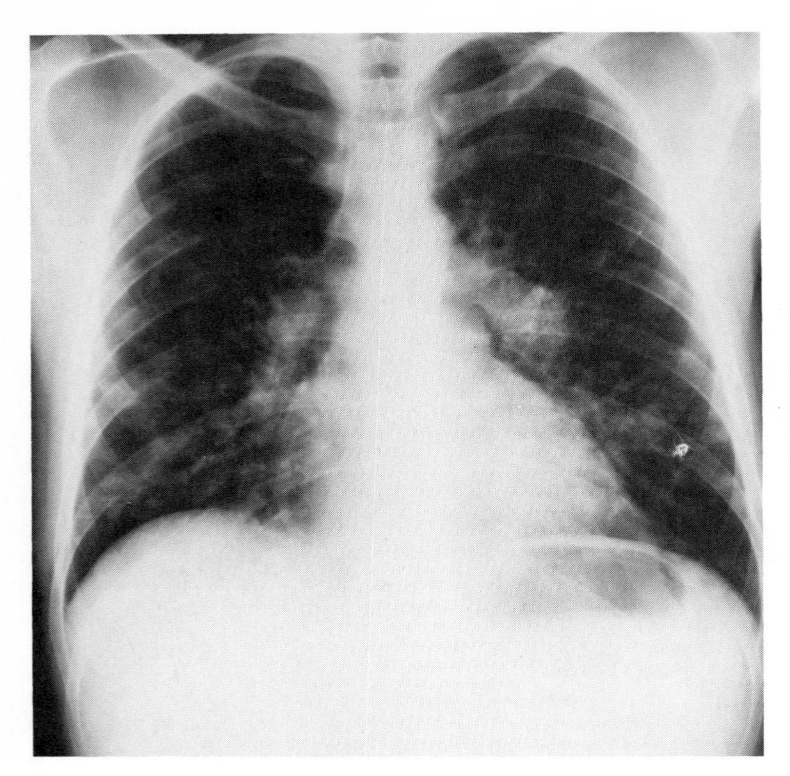

Figure 3. Chest roentgenogram of a 32-year-old male who had symptoms of an atypical pneumonia for 12 days. Note the large hilar lymph nodes and soft nodular parenchymal infiltrates. Five weeks previously he had cleaned out a chimney filled with birds' nests. Sputum cultures yielded *Histoplasma capsulatum*.

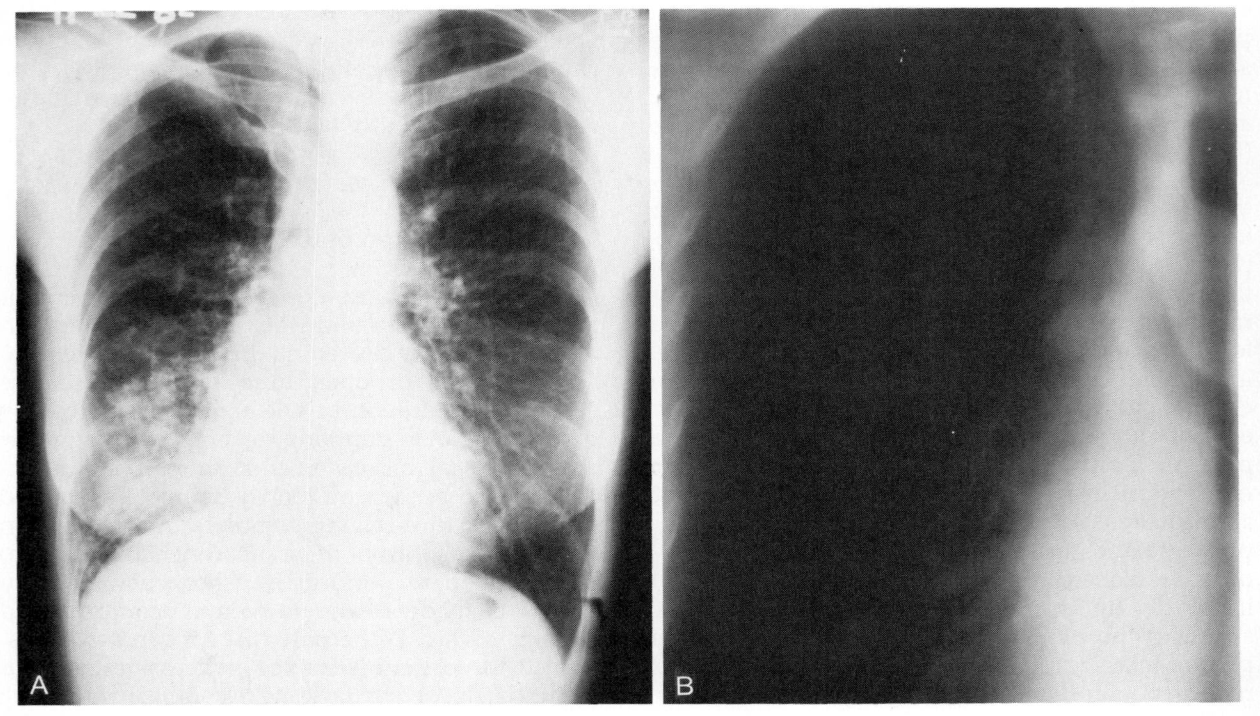

Figure 4. *A,* Chest roentgenogram demonstrating the third episode of acute right middle and lower lobe pneumonia within a 5-month period in a 56-year-old woman. A density is visible in the right main bronchus. The left heart border is indistinct. *B,* Tomogram demonstrating a mass lesion in the right main bronchus. A carcinoid tumor was found at bronchoscopy and thoracotomy.

ASSESSMENT

Constellations of Findings

Most cases can be classified as to main type of pneumonia through assessment of the constellation of findings. Some patients, however, have indistinct, changing, overlapping, and coexisting clinical features that require constant reevaluation. Key findings in specific types of pneumonia are printed in italics.

Bacterial Pneumonia. The most common cause of pneumonia, bacterial infections are characterized by abrupt onset, *shaking chills,* and *purulent sputum production.*

Atypical Pneumonia. Within this group are pneumonias due to mycoplasmas, viruses, rickettsiae, *Chlamydia psittaci,* and the *Legionella* bacillus. Patients typically have a *nonproductive cough* and relatively severe constitutional symptoms.

Aspiration Pneumonia. Anaerobic bacteria usually predominate in community-acquired aspiration pneumonia, whereas gram-negative pathogens are found in about three-quarters of hospital-acquired cases.[24] The presence of *disturbed swallowing, depressed consciousness,* and severe neuromuscular weakness is usually observed in this group.

Nosocomial Pneumonia. Any pneumonia *acquired in hospital* has a high probability of being gram-negative (60 per cent), but may be due to staphylococcus (11 per cent) or pneumococcus (5 per cent).[3]

Chronic Pneumonia. Pathogens such as *Mycobacterium* (typical and atypical), fungi, some bacteria *(Pseudomonas pseudomallei, Brucella)* and rarely parasites *(Paragonimus)* are found in this group. *Slowly progressive* symptoms, physical signs, and roentgenographic findings are common.

Recurrent Pneumonia. Interference with mechanical clearance (obstruction, bronchiectasis, bronchopulmonary sequestration), immune or phagocytic defects (hypogammaglobulinemia, Job's syndrome), superinfection, reactivation of latent tuberculosis by a pneumonic infiltrate, continued aspiration, and inadequate antimicrobial therapy are some causes of pneumonia that *improves* only to *reappear* (Table 5).[25]

Table 5. CAUSES OF RECURRENT PNEUMONIA

Airways obstruction (e.g., carcinoma, bronchial adenoma, foreign body)
Bronchiectasis
Cystic fibrosis*
Immune deficiency (e.g., AIDS, hypogammaglobulinemia)
Phagocytic defect (e.g., Job's syndrome)
Bronchopulmonary sequestration
Recurrent aspiration (e.g., achalasia, carcinoma of the esophagus, tracheoesophageal fistula)
Superinfection by resistant organism
Reactivation of latent tuberculosis by pneumonia
Inadequate antimicrobial therapy

*Chapter reference 10.

Pneumonia in the Immunocompromised Patient. Lymphoreticular *malignancy,* use of *corticosteroid* or *antineoplastic drugs, male homosexuality,* and *drug addiction* are some historic features in this category. A wide variety of pathogenic and nonpathogenic organisms cause life-threatening lung infections in immunocompromised patients (see Table 2).

Diagnostic Approach

Pathogens and causes of lung infection in the previously listed categories are reasonably specific. After initial classification, diagnostic evaluation should concentrate on isolation or identification of a specific organism or disease process within the category by means of respiratory secretion analysis, determinations of specific serologic features, globulins, and white blood cells, biopsy examination, and skin tests. Assessment of underlying diseases and of types, doses, and responses in antimicrobial therapy also aids in this assessment (see algorithm).

The clinician should constantly ask himself or herself the following ten questions when assessing a patient with poorly responsive pneumonia:

1. Is there an anatomic cause (e.g., carcinoma obstructing a bronchus, bronchiectasis, sequestration)?
2. Is there an immunologic or phagocytic defect (e.g., AIDS, common variable hypogammaglobulinemia, Job's syndrome)?
3. Is the pneumonia due to organisms not responsive to the antibiotics administered? Viruses, rickettsia, mycoplasma, tuberculosis, fungi and parasites may not respond to many commonly administered antibiotics.
4. Is the selection, dosage, or administration of antibiotic adequate? Noncompliance, inadequate dosage, or selection of a third-line drug may lead to poor resolution of a common pneumonia.
5. Is there resistance to the antibiotic administered? Methicillin-resistant staphylococcus, aminoglycoside-resistant gram-negative organisms in some institutions, and drug-resistant tuberculosis in Southeast Asian refugees are a few examples.
6. Is the disease merely responding slowly to antimicrobials? Necrotizing pneumonia, mycoplasmal pneumonia, and actinomycosis are notoriously slow responders to antibiotics.
7. Is superinfection present? Bacterial pneumonia commonly complicates viral illness but is seen infrequently following mycoplasmal, chlamydial, and rickettsial infections. Gram-negative infection may follow high-dosage penicillin therapy for pneumococcal pneumonia.

DIAGNOSTIC ASSESSMENT OF POORLY RESOLVED CLINICAL PNEUMONIA

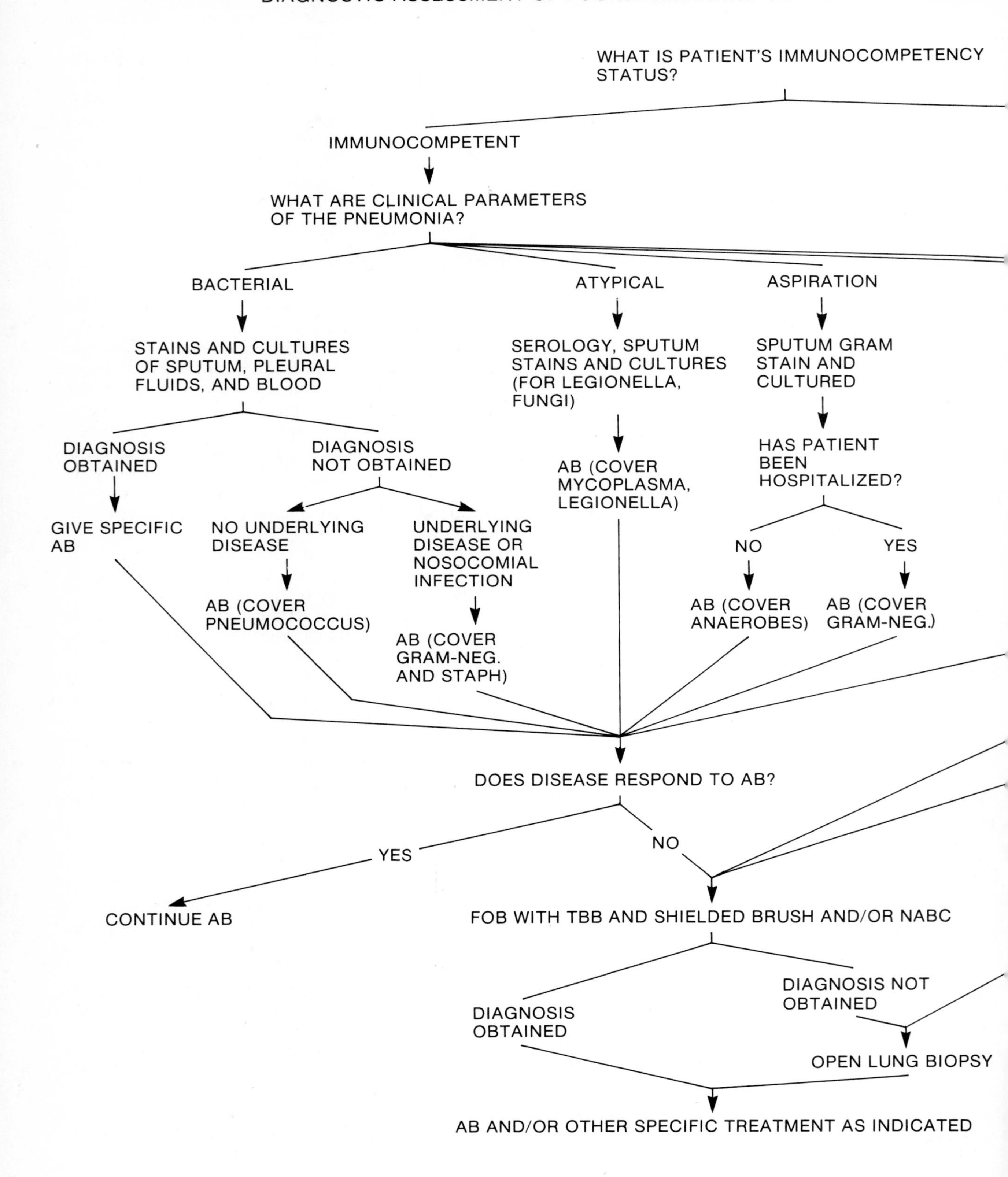

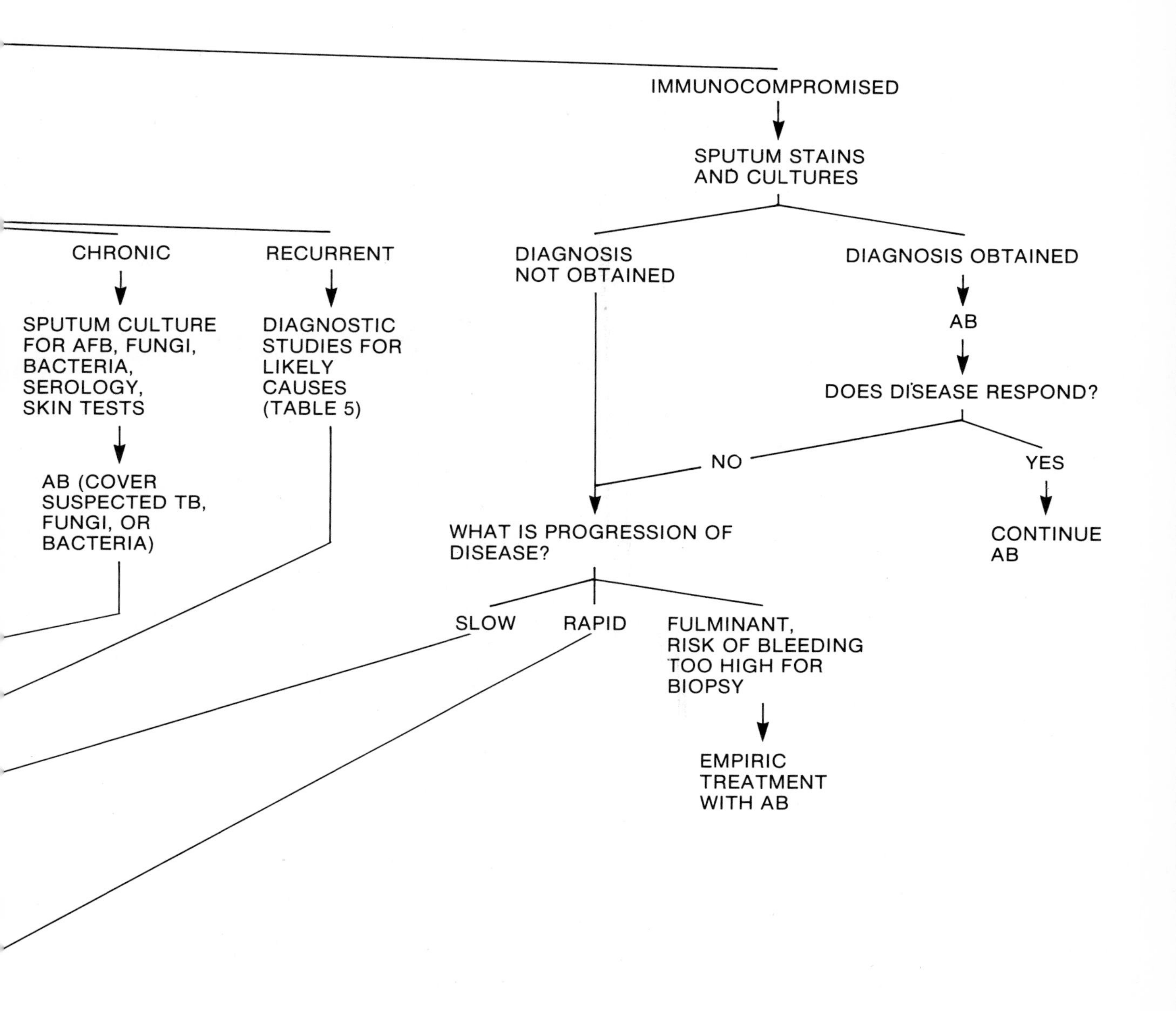

FOB: fiberoptic bronchoscopy
TBB: transbronchial biopsy
NABC: needle aspiration biopsy and culture
TB: tuberculosis
AB antibiotics

8. Is there a feeding focus? Does the patient have an infected intravenous line, abdominal abscess, pelvic infection, esophagobronchial fistula, or disturbance in swallowing?

9. Is the infection due to an unusual organism? Many rare causes are related to occupation (Q fever, anthrax, psittacosis), outdoor recreation (tularemia, sporotrichosis), or foreign travel or immigrant status (melioidosis, paragonimiasis).

10. Could the disease be due to noninfectious causes (see Table 3)? Answering these ten questions and using the diagnostic approach described in this chapter should allow the physician to identify the cause of most poorly resolved pneumonias.

REFERENCES

1. Yu VL, Kroboth FJ, Shonnard J, Brown A, McDearman S, Magnussen M. Legionnaires' disease: new clinical perspective from a prospective pneumonia study. Am J Med 1982;73:357–61.
2. Mildvan D, Mathur U, Enlow RW, et al. Opportunistic infections and immune deficiency in homosexual men. Ann Intern Med 1982;96:700–4.
3. LaForce FM. Hospital-acquired gram-negative rod pneumonias: an overview. Am J Med 1981;70:664–9.
4. Tsao M, Schraufnagel D, Wang N. Pathogenesis of pulmonary infarction. Am J Med 1982;72:599–606.
5. Barrett-Connor E. Parasitic pulmonary disease. Am Rev Resp Dis 1982;126:558–63.
6. Haupt HM, Moore GW, Bauer TW, Hutchins GM. The lung in sickle cell disease. Chest 1982;81:332–7.
7. Fulmer JD, Kaltreider HB. The pulmonary vasculitides. Chest 1982;82:615–24.
8. Johnston RF, Wildrick KH. The impact of chemotherapy on the care of patients with tuberculosis. Am Rev Resp Dis 1974;109:636–64.
9. Donohue JF. Lower respiratory tract involvement in Rocky Mountain spotted fever. Arch Intern Med 1980;140:223–7.
10. Wood RE, Boat RF, Doershuk CF. Cystic fibrosis. Am Rev Resp Dis 1976;113:833–78.
11. Osmer JC, Cole BK. The stethoscope and roentgenogram in acute pneumonia. South Med J 1966;59:75–7.
12. Martin DB, Weiner LB, Nieburg PI, Blair DC. Atypical measles in adolescents and young adults. Ann Intern Med 1979;90:877–81.
13. Murray HW, Masur H, Senterfit LB, Roberts RB. The protean manifestations of *Mycoplasma pneumoniae* infection in adults. Am J Med 1975;58:229–42.
14. Herbert PA, Bayer AS. Invasive pulmonary aspergillosis. Chest 1981;80:220–5.
15. Ramsey PG, Fife KH, Hackman RC, Meyers JD, Corey L. Herpes simplex virus pneumonia. Ann Intern Med 1982;97:813–20.
16. Christensen GD, Bisno Al, Parisi JT, McLaughlin B, Hester MG, Luther RW. Nosocomial septicemia due to multiply antibiotic resistant *Staphylococcus epidermidis*. Ann Intern Med 1982;96:1–10.
17. Rein MF, Gwaltney JM, O'Brien WM, Jennings Rh, Mandell Gl. Accuracy of Gram's stain in identifying pneumococci in sputum. JAMA 1978;239:2671–3.
18. Guckian JC, Christensen WD. Quantitative culture and Gram stain of sputum in pneumonia. Am Rev Dis 1978;118:997–1006.
19. Wallace JM, Deutsch AL, Harrell JH, Moser KM. Bronchoscopy and transbronchial biopsy in evaluation of patients with suspected active tuberculosis. Am J Med 1981;70:1189–94.
20. Cordes LG, Fraser DW. Legionellosis. Med Clin North Am 1980;64:395–416.
21. Griffin JP. Rapid screening for cold agglutinins in pneumonia. Ann Intern Med 1969;70:701–5.
22. Valdivieso M, Gil-Extremera B, Zornoza J, Rodriguez V, Bodey GP. Gram-negative bacillary pneumonia in the compromised host. Medicine 1977;56:241–54.
23. Tew J, Calenoff L, Berlin BS. Bacterial or nonbacterial pneumonia; accuracy of radiographic diagnosis. Radiology 1977;124:607–12.
24. Wynne JW, Modell JH. Respiratory aspiration of stomach contents. Ann Intern Med 1977;87:466–74.
25. Winterbauer RH, Bedon GA, Ball WC. Recurrent pneumonia. Ann Intern Med 1969;70:689–700.

POLYURIA

ANDREW S. LEVEY □ JOHN T. HARRINGTON

□ SYNONYM: Excessive urination

BACKGROUND

Polyuria is a dramatic and often puzzling problem occurring in a wide variety of clinical settings. It may be simply a normal homeostatic response, or it may reflect a profound metabolic disturbance. The polyuria that results from oral ingestion or intravenous infusion of large amounts of water and solute is benign and transient, and should pose no difficulty in diagnosis. On the other hand, persistent polyuria due to primary polydipsia, diabetes insipidus (DI), acquired renal diseases, or osmotic diuresis can be diagnostically challenging and life-threatening. Accurate differential diagnosis of polyuria requires detailed understanding of the physiologic mechanisms of water excretion.

The importance of this background information, which is essential to the recognition and management of the many disturbances that may result in polyuria, accounts for our emphasizing the basic physiology of water excretion.

Definition

Polyuria, the excretion of an excessive amount of urine, is usually evident to both patient and practitioner. Because there is no generally accepted definition of polyuria, we have arbitrarily selected a urine volume greater than 3.5 liters/day, or greater than 150 ml/hour, as excessive. Usual urine volume in normal adults is from 1 to 2 liters/day and obviously depends on oral fluid intake. Given that the urge to void is sensed after urinary bladder volume is 100 to 200 ml and that bladder capacity is 300 to 450 ml, urination typically occurs four to seven times daily in adults. If urine volume rises to 3.5 liters/day or greater, voiding increases in frequency to ten or more times daily. Increased frequency of urination and nocturia without an increase in urine volume do not constitute polyuria and are not discussed in this chapter.

Determinants of Urine Flow Rate

Urine formation begins with the elaboration of 150 liters/day of glomerular filtrate in a normal 70-kg adult. Some 80 per cent of this filtered salt and water is reabsorbed by proximal portions of the nephron. The major determinant of final urine volume is the fraction of water reabsorbed from the remaining 20 per cent of the filtrate, as it passes through the distal portions of the nephron, by processes regulated by the renal concentration mechanism and pituitary secretion of antidiuretic hormone (ADH). If ADH is present, more water is reabsorbed from the distal nephron, resulting in a smaller volume of concentrated urine. Conversely, if ADH is absent, less water is reabsorbed, leading to a larger volume of dilute urine.

The physiologic range of urine concentration is from 50 to 1400 mOsm/kg (specific gravity ≅ 1.000–1.040). This range allows for more than a 25-fold change in urine volume, if urinary solute excretion is constant (Fig. 1). The rate of urinary solute and water excretion by the kidneys is regulated to maintain the overall constancy of body fluid solute composition and volume.[1] In health, the composition and volume of the urine reflect the dietary intake and extrarenal losses of solute and water.

Solute balance

The solutes requiring renal excretion are sodium, potassium, chloride, and the end-products of protein catabolism (nitrogenous wastes such as urea, creatinine, uric acid, and ammonia, and inorganic acids such as phosphoric and sulfuric acids). For example, a diet containing 6 gm sodium chloride and 60 gm protein results in the generation of approximately 600 mOsm/day of solute requiring renal excretion. Given the physiologic range of urine concentration, this solute load can be excreted in a urine volume ranging between 12 liters/day and 400 ml/day (see Fig. 1). Despite wide variation in food intake, the solute load requiring renal excretion is usually within the range of 400 to 1200 mOsm/day. It is apparent therefore that distal nephron water reabsorption, as determined by the rate of ADH secretion and the renal concentration mechanism, is a clinically more important determinant of urine volume than is the amount of solute requiring renal excretion.

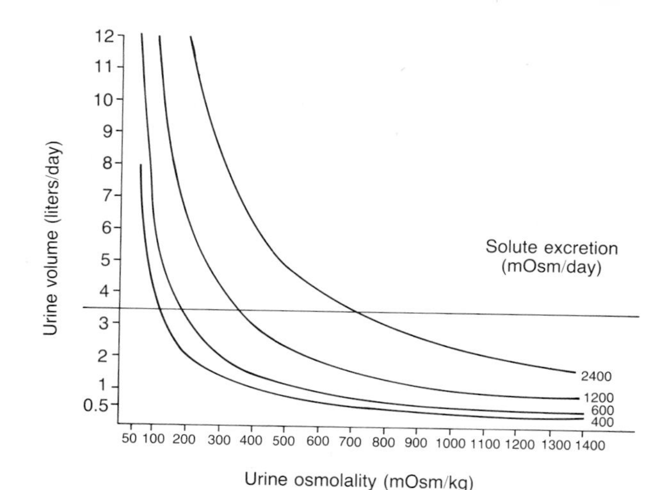

Figure 1. Urine flow rate at different solute concentrations for a variety of solute excretion rates. An osmole (Osm) is defined as a mole of solute divided by the number of ions or particles formed upon its dissociation in solution. For example a 1-millimolal solution of sodium chloride (NaCl) has an osmolality of 3 mOsm/kg. Urine volume greater than 3.5 liter/day (as indicated by the *horizontal line*) is defined arbitrarily as polyuria.

Water Balance

Overall water balance is regulated to maintain a normal plasma osmolality of 280 to 295 mOsm/kg. Within this range, water balance is adjusted principally by alterations in the rate of renal water excretion under the influence of ADH and the renal concentration mechanism.[2] The relationships among plasma osmolality, ADH concentration, and urinary osmolality are depicted in Figure 2. The major stimulus to alterations in the rate of pituitary ADH secretion is a change in body fluid osmolality. Given an initial plasma osmolality of 287 mOsm/kg (*solid arrow* in Fig. 2*A*), ingestion of 0.5 liters water, an amount sufficient to lower plasma osmolality by only 1 per cent (3 mOsm/

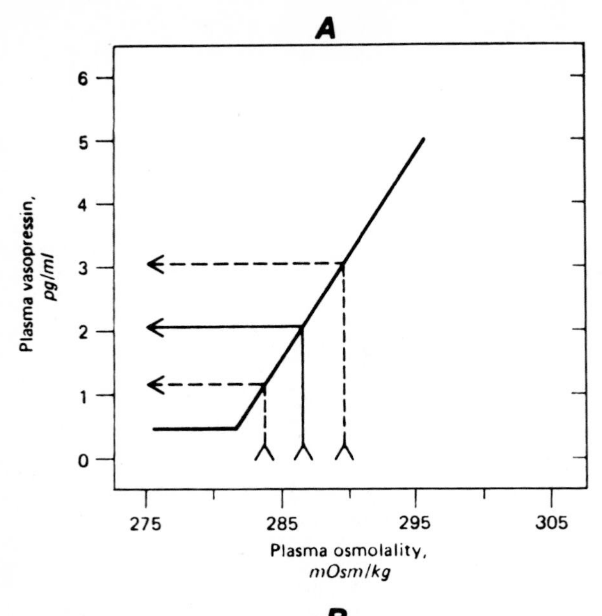

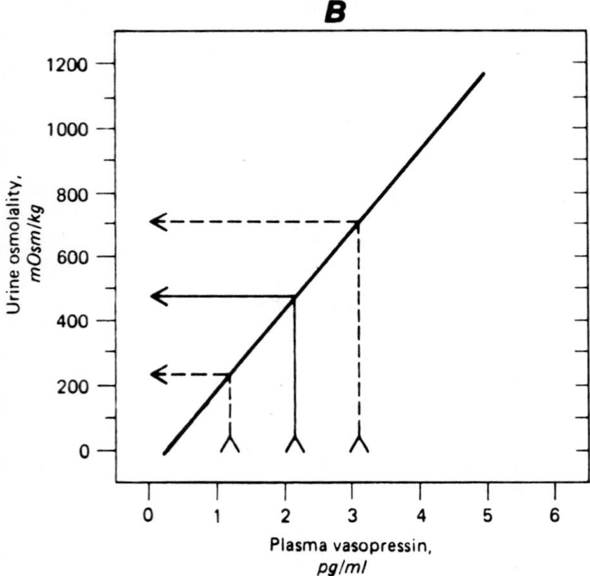

Figure 2. Schematic representation of the effect of small alterations in basal plasma osmolality on plasma vasopressin (ADH) and urine osmolality in healthy adults. For explanation, see text. (From Robertson GL, Shelton RL, Athar SH: The osmoregulation of vasopressin. Kidney International 10:25–37, 1976. Reprinted with permission.)

kg), is recognized by osmoreceptors in the anterior hypothalamus and results in decreased posterior pituitary ADH secretion and a fall in plasma ADH concentration from 2 to 1 pg/ml. Urinary concentration declines from approximately 500 to 250 mOsm/kg (Fig. 2*B*). If we assume a constant solute load of 600 mOsm/day, urine volume doubles from 1.2 to 2.4 liters/day (see Fig. 1).

Conversely, if sufficient water is lost to raise plasma osmolality by 1 per cent, plasma ADH rises by 1 pg/ml, urine concentration increases from 500 to approximately 700 mOsm/kg, and urine volume falls from 1.2 liters/day to 850 ml/day. If plasma osmolality rises above the normal range, thirst is stimulated, leading to increased water drinking. The ingested water, retained because of the increase in ADH levels, dilutes body fluids and ultimately restores plasma osmolality to normal.

Within the normal range of plasma osmolality, water ingestion is determined by social and cultural custom rather than by thirst.[3] The alterations in plasma osmolality resulting from ingestion of water in turn lead to alterations in ADH secretion, urinary concentration, and urine volume. Therefore, under normal circumstances, it is apparent that water intake is the principal determinant of urine volume.

Renal Concentration Mechanism

The wide physiologic range of water excretion is attributable to the wide range of urine concentration, from 50 to 1400 mOsm/kg. In order for one to appreciate fully the clinical problem of polyuria, a clear understanding of this mechanism is mandatory. Urine formation begins with the elaboration of an isotonic ultrafiltrate of plasma at the glomerulus. Selective reabsorption of solute and water modifies the composition and osmolality of tubular fluid as it passes through subsequent segments of the nephron. Within the medullary thick ascending limb of the loop of Henle, sodium and chloride are reabsorbed without accompanying water reabsorption, resulting both in hypotonicity of the tubular fluid entering the cortical distal convoluted tubule and in hypertonicity of the interstitium of the renal medulla. This critical selective reabsorption of solute without water is known as the "single effect" leading to generation of medullary hypertonicity. This effect is magnified by the parallel and countercurrent arrangement of ascending and descending limbs of Henle known as the "countercurrent multiplier."

A highly schematic representation of the operation of the countercurrent mechanism is shown in Figure 3. The loop in Figure 3*A*, an example of a countercurrent multiplier, illustrates the mechanism whereby increasing medullary concentration is achieved by the loop of Henle. In this model, solute is transported out of the ascending limb unaccompanied by water. Because the descending limb is permeable to both solute and water, the solute concentration in this limb progressively increases as tubular fluid approaches the hairpin turn. In actuality, solute transport from the ascending limb is not directly into the descending limb but rather into the medullary interstitium surrounding the loop. Furthermore, tubular fluid tonicity rises in the descending limb, probably as a result of water reabsorption from that segment

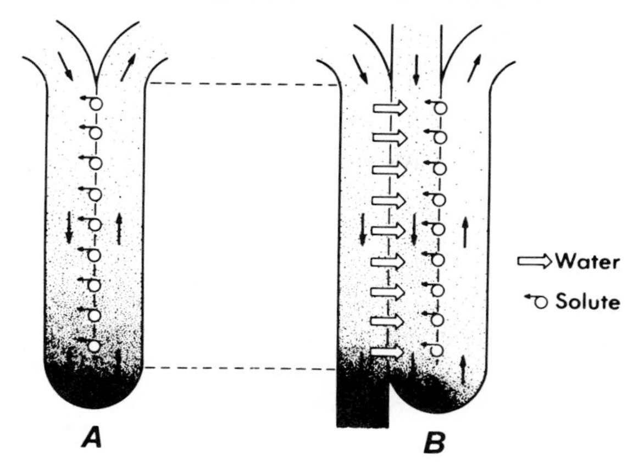

Figure 3. Renal concentration mechanism. *A*, Pump mechanism within water-impermeable membrane transports solute from ascending limb of the loop to the descending limb (the single effect). *B*, A "flow-through element," representing the medullary collecting tubule, is juxtaposed to the countercurrent system shown in *A*. Fluid flowing down the collecting tubule is progressively concentrated as water is drawn by osmosis into the countercurrent loop. (From Marsh D: Osmotic concentration and dilution of the urine. *In* Rouiller C, Muller AF (ed): The Kidney: Morphology, Biochemistry and Physiology. New York, Academic Press, 1971. Reprinted with permission.)

into the hypertonic medulla.[1] The overall effect of this arrangement is to establish a concentration gradient along the renal medullary interstitium from isotonicity at the corticomedullary junction to maximal concentration at the papilla. The osmolality at the tip of the papilla is 1,200 to 1,400 mOsm/kg. In Figure 3*B*, the collecting tubule (the "flow-through element") containing hypotonic fluid is depicted as lying immediately next to the loop. Permeability of the collecting tubule to water is enhanced by ADH. In the presence of ADH, water is reabsorbed from tubular fluid by osmosis as it passes through the hypertonic medulla. If ADH is absent the collecting duct is relatively impermeable to water, which remains within the tubule and is excreted in the urine.

A simplified illustration of the operation of nephron solute and water transport is shown in Figure 4; filtrate formed at the glomerulus is isotonic with plasma (≈ 300 mOsm/kg). Of the approximately 150 liters formed each day, some 120 liters are absorbed isotonically by the proximal tubule. Hence, 30 liters of isotonic fluid enter the descending limb of Henle. Water is absorbed as it descends within the hypertonic medulla; tubular fluid osmolality is maximal at the hairpin turn. Thereafter, solute is absorbed by primary active chloride transport and passive sodium reabsorption. As a result of solute reabsorption, the tubular fluid reentering the cortical nephron is hypotonic. As shown in Figure 4*A*, if ADH is present, tubular fluid equilibrates with renal interstitium, resulting in maximal urine concentration. If ADH is not present (Fig. 4*B*), the distal nephron is relatively impermeable to water. Urine osmolality declines progressively owing to further reabsorption of sodium, reaching a minimal value of 50 to 60 mOsm/kg in the collecting tubule.

In summary, urine concentration requires the establishment and maintenance of medullary hypertonicity and the presence of ADH. Polyuria arises in circumstances in which secretion of ADH or tubular sensitivity to ADH is reduced, or nephron solute transport is impaired, leading to diminished medullary hypertonicity.[4]

Relationship Among Urine Concentration, Solute Load, and Urine Volume

Figure 1 depicts urine volume for various values of urine osmolality and solute load. If solute load

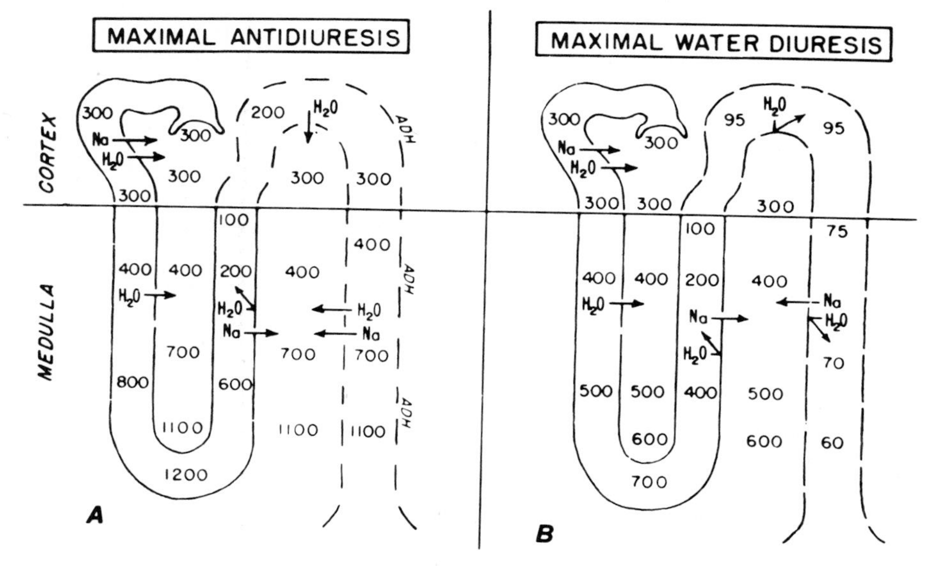

Figure 4. Simplified version of the renal concentration mechanism. *A*, Maximal antidiuresis; alterations in tubular fluid and interstitial osmolality when ADH is present. *B*, Maximal water diuresis; same system when ADH is absent. For explanation, see text. (From Harrington JT, Cohen JJ: Clinical disorders of urine concentration and dilution. Arch Intern Med 131:810–825. Copyright 1973, American Medical Association. Reprinted with permission.)

is normal (≈ 600 mOsm/day), urine volume does not exceed 3.5 liters unless urinary osmolality is less than 200 mOsm/kg. In such cases urinary losses are predominantly water with no excess solute, i.e., a "water diuresis." If urinary concentration is partially impaired so that maximal urinary osmolality is 300 mOsm/kg, polyuria results only if the daily solute load is well above the usual 600 mOsm. In this setting, urinary losses are solute and water together, i.e., a "solute diuresis." Urine volumes greater than 5 liters/day are seen only if urine concentration is very low (50 to 100 mOsm/kg) or if the solute load is extremely high (> 1500 mOsm/day).

Causes of Polyuria

Water Diuresis

Polyuria due to water diuresis is usually characterized by a urinary osmolality of 200 mOsm/kg or less without excess solute loss. Large volumes of urine may result, and in some cases, the high rate of urine flow may lead to hydronephrosis and bladder enlargement.

Water Administration or Compulsive Water Drinking (Primary Polydipsia). Expansion of total body water during water administration dilutes solute concentration, thereby lowering plasma osmolality transiently. Suppression of ADH secretion lowers plasma ADH concentration and reduces water reabsorption by the distal nephron. The result is the excretion of a large volume of dilute urine until plasma osmolality rises to normal. Given that insensible water loss in adults is approximately 500 ml daily, water ingestion must be greater than 4 liters/day for polyuria (as defined here) to result. Plasma hypo-osmolality does not occur unless the intake of water exceeds the normal capacity to excrete it, approximately 12 liters daily. Patients with psychiatric disorders, however, may drink enormous amounts of water within a short time and thus overwhelm even normal renal water excretory capacity. In these patients, plasma osmolality ranges from approximately 240 to 290 mOsm/kg.[5] Severe hypo-osmolality may result in abdominal cramps, nausea, vomiting, diarrhea, and metabolic encephalopathy characterized by headache, depression of consciousness, irritability, and seizures.[5,6] The syndrome may be difficult to recognize because these seriously ill patients may deny having ingested water. Furthermore, if the patient becomes comatose (and water intake thus ceases), normal renal water excretion may restore plasma osmolality to normal by the time the patient is seen by the clinician.

Neurogenic Diabetes Insipidus (DI); Complete and Partial Defects. Polyuria can result from absolute or relative lack of ADH due to central nervous system disorders.[7] As discussed earlier, given a normal solute load, urine volume exceeds 3.5 liters/day only if urinary osmolality is less than 200 mOsm/kg, indicating a plasma ADH concentration of less than 1 pg/ml (see Figs. 1 and 2). Such severe reduction in ADH levels appears to require a loss of more than 90 per cent of ADH-producing cells in the hypothalamus.[8] Lesser degrees of damage result in partial defects in urinary concentrating ability and smaller increases in urine volume.

Water diuresis in excess of intake leads to concentration of body fluids. The resulting hypertonicity stimulates thirst, however, and the increased water ingestion replaces losses. The patient with neurogenic DI with an adequate thirst mechanism and access to water thus has polyuria, polydipsia, and a plasma osmolality within the normal range. If water is not available, however, progressive water depletion results in severe hypertonicity and metabolic encephalopathy.[6,9] Intravascular volume depletion is mild because less than 10 per cent of the water lost is from this compartment.

The major disorders causing neurogenic DI are listed in Table 1. Most can be recognized by their associated neurologic or endocrinologic abnormalities, such as headaches and visual field defects or hypopituitarism. Probably the most common cause of DI is head trauma or a neurosurgical procedure near the pituitary or hypothalamus.[10] DI occurs in from 28 to 84 per cent of patients following hypophysectomy. Impairment of ADH secretion is due to retrograde degeneration of neurons of the supraoptic and paraventricular nuclei in the hypothalamus after transection of the pituitary stalk.[11] Defects appear to be less common and are more likely to be transient after transection low in the pituitary stalk, whereas permanent damage is more likely to result after high stalk section.[11] Idiopathic DI, still one of the most common diagnostic entities, is most often found in young adults, although it may occur at any age. Pathologic examination of the brain in a few cases

Table 1. CAUSES OF NEUROGENIC DIABETES INSIPIDUS

Cause
Head trauma, including neurosurgery
Idiopathic
Brain tumor
Pituitary adenoma
Craniopharyngioma
Metastases
Infiltrative disorders
Sarcoidosis
Hand-Schüller-Christian disease
Drugs (ethanol)
Postpartum pituitary necrosis
Encephalitis
Familial

of idiopathic DI has disclosed selective and virtually complete destruction of ADH-producing neurons in the hypothalamus.[12] Familial neurogenic DI accounts for only 2 per cent of cases.

Ethanol ingestion results in reversible suppression of ADH secretion and transient polyuria.[13] Water diuresis occurs within 30 to 60 minutes after ingestion of 25 gm alcohol (equivalent to 2 ounces of 100-proof whiskey), which results in blood alcohol levels ranging from 50 to 80 mg/100 ml. The urine volume is dependent upon the amount of alcohol ingested in a single dose. Continued ingestion does not result in a persistent diuresis even though the blood alcohol concentration may be sustained.[14]

Nephrogenic Diabetes Insipidus. In contrast to neurogenic DI, plasma ADH concentration is appropriate for the plasma osmolality in patients with nephrogenic DI. The cause of polyuria in these disorders is either impermeability of the renal collecting tubule to water despite the presence of ADH or failure of the renal concentration mechanism to sustain adequate medullary hypertonicity. The renal functional defects in these disorders range from a selective impairment in ADH response to a global disruption of nephron function. Except for congenital nephrogenic DI, the urinary concentration defect is incomplete, enabling patients to raise urine osmolality above plasma osmolality. Therefore, at normal solute loads, these patients usually do *not* have a urine volume in excess of 3.5 liters/day, nor the marked polydipsia characteristic of patients with complete neurogenic DI.

Congenital Nephrogenic DI. In this rare inherited disease, males are affected predominantly. Striking polyuria and polydipsia are apparent shortly after birth ("water babies") and episodes of hypertonic dehydration are frequent in infancy. Mental and physical retardation commonly occur in association with this disease.[15]

Metabolic Disturbances. Hypokalemia or hypercalcemia from any cause is associated with a mild concentrating defect[4, 16] that is reversible after the underlying electrolyte disorder has been corrected. In either instance, mild tubulointerstitial alterations are present that may be important in the pathogenesis of the concentrating disorder.

Parenchymal Renal Diseases. A number of renal diseases result in prominent damage to tubules and interstitium before severe reductions in glomerular filtration rate (GFR) occur (Table 2). Urine volume is usually less than 3.5 liters/day, and polyuria is seen only when there is increased water intake. The causes of the urinary concentration mechanism impairment are multifactorial, including reduced solute transport in the loop of Henle, structural alterations in the countercurrent arrangement of medullary tubules and vessels, impaired permeability of the collecting duct to water,

Table 2. PARENCHYMAL RENAL DISEASES CAUSING NEPHROGENIC DIABETES INSIPIDUS

Diseases causing prominent tubulointerstitial damage	Acute pyelonephritis Obstructive nephropathy Sickle-cell nephropathy Sjögren's syndrome Myeloma kidney and light-chain nephropathy Amyloidosis Lead nephropathy
Diseases causing progressive renal failure	Chronic glomerulonephritis Chronic interstitial nephritis Nephrosclerosis Diabetic glomerulosclerosis

and diminished responsiveness to ADH.[4] In the glomerular and tubulointerstitial diseases causing progressive renal failure, urinary concentrating ability is diminished, in addition, by the reduced delivery of solute to the loop of Henle as a result of a lower GFR. Although it is unusual for parenchymal renal diseases to lead to a urine volume greater than 3.5 liters/day, they do represent the most common cause of nephrogenic DI.

Drugs. Lithium and demeclocycline impair the responsiveness of collecting tubules to ADH.[4, 17] Marked reduction in urinary concentrating ability has been noted in 10 per cent of patients treated with lithium. After prolonged administration, irreversible interstitial fibrosis and renal insufficiency have been found in some patients.[18] Diminished urinary concentration due to the tetracycline derivative demeclocycline is dose-related and reversible; in fact, this drug's side effect has been successfully exploited in the long-term management of the syndrome of inappropriate ADH secretion.[4, 17]

Amphotericin B and the anesthetic agent methoxyflurane cause diminished urinary concentrating ability in most patients. Use of these agents in higher doses can lead to disturbances in multiple tubular functions and acute renal failure.[4, 17]

Solute Diuresis

Polyuria due to solute diuresis is characterized by urinary osmolality that approximates 300 mOsm/kg and marked solute and water losses.

Solute Administration. In contrast to polyuria due to a water load, plasma osmolality in patients undergoing a solute diuresis is typically high-normal or frankly elevated.[19] Addition of solute increases plasma osmolality, thereby stimulating thirst and causing water ingestion. The resulting expansion of extracellular fluid volume increases renal blood flow and glomerular filtration rate and decreases proximal tubular reabsorption. The result is a higher solute delivery to the distal nephron. As demonstrated in Figure 1, if urinary osmolality is 300 mOsm/kg, urine volume exceeds 3.5 liters/day only if solute load exceeds 1,200 mOsm/day.

Administration of large volumes of saline or protein-containing solutions (e.g., in total parenteral nutrition) is a common cause of polyuria in hospitalized patients. The increased load of sodium chloride, sodium bicarbonate, or nitrogenous compounds is excreted in the final urine. Careful examination of affected patients and their laboratory data will reveal extracellular fluid (ECF) volume excess, metabolic alkalosis (or alkaline urine), or azotemia, respectively. Usually the urine is not more concentrated than plasma because there is no stimulus to conserve either water or solute. It is apparent that polyuria in these settings is simply a normal homeostatic response designed to preserve overall solute balance, and that increased urine volume will continue only as long as solute administration continues. Difficulty in diagnosis occurs if polyuria is thought to reflect a primary renal defect in conservation of sodium, and if intravenous infusions are continued in an effort to avoid ECF volume depletion. As discussed later, renal sodium wasting sufficient to lead to polyuria (as defined here) is rare.

Osmotic Diuresis. Diabetic hyperglycemia (either ketoacidosis or nonketotic hyperosmolar coma) and continuous mannitol infusion are the two clinically important causes of prolonged osmotic diuresis. The properties of the osmotic agents are central to the pathophysiology. Mannitol is an inert sugar that cannot cross cell membranes. Similarly, the transport and metabolism of glucose occur only slowly in the absence of insulin. These low-molecular-weight compounds are freely filtered by the glomerulus and delivered directly from plasma into tubular fluid. Mannitol is not reabsorbed at all by the renal tubule, and tubular glucose reabsorption is easily overwhelmed by the high filtered load when blood glucose is elevated. The poorly permeant solute (either glucose or mannitol) increases tubular fluid osmolality and reduces both water and solute reabsorption from the proximal tubule, thereby increasing solute and water delivery to the distal nephron and final urine. Furthermore, the impermeant solute and the high tubular fluid flow rate limit solute and water reabsorption in the distal nephron, thereby dissipating medullary hypertonicity and preventing both concentration and dilution of the urine.[19] As a result, urine osmolality approaches plasma osmolality—typically 310 to 340 mOsm/kg—and large quantities of water and sodium chloride (as well as the glucose or mannitol) are lost in the urine. Extreme ECF volume depletion and hypertonicity can result. ECF hypertonicity is the result of two factors: (1) the presence of the glucose or mannitol in high concentration, and (2) the impairment of urinary concentrating ability, leading to increased renal water losses. Although hypertonicity may be blunted by the rise in water ingestion stimulated by increased thirst, progressive loss of solute from the ECF usually leads to severe volume depletion. Clinical expressions of this situation include metabolic encephalopathy, hypotension, tachycardia, poor skin turgor, and prerenal azotemia.

Renal Disease. Inability to conserve sodium (salt-wasting) is a feature of some renal diseases with prominent tubulointerstitial damage and of all diseases causing progressive renal failure. However, sodium losses are rarely sufficient to result in urinary volumes greater than 3.5 liters/day (see Fig. 1). A solute diuresis of this magnitude may be observed, however, in medullary cystic renal disease, during recovery from acute tubular necrosis (ATN), and after relief of bilateral renal obstruction. In these circumstances, solute diuresis may result in rapid depletion of ECF volume. It is also important to note that the tubular response to ADH is impaired in these disorders. Thus, excessive water losses may accompany the solute diuresis and result in plasma hypertonicity.

Medullary Cystic Disease (Hereditary Nephronophthisis). This rare genetic disease affects young adults and leads to progressive renal failure. The kidney contains numerous small cysts at the corticomedullary junction, and renal biopsy reveals interstitial fibrosis. Typically, salt-wasting is an early and prominent feature of the disorder and often provides a clue to the diagnosis.[20]

Recovery from ATN. As the GFR improves, a marked solute diuresis may occur, with urine volumes as high as 6 to 8 liters/day ("diuretic phase" of ATN). The polyuria probably is due to excretion of solutes retained during the oliguric phase and usually subsides within a week or so. A mild concentrating defect can, however, be demonstrated for many months after ATN; it generally resolves within a year.[21]

Postobstructive Diuresis. The pathogenesis of the marked solute diuresis that may occur following relief of bilateral obstruction remains uncertain. At least three factors are involved: (1) ECF volume expansion due to salt retention during the period of urinary obstruction; (2) osmotic diuresis due to excretion of retained urea and other nitrogenous wastes; and (3) persistent tubular dysfunction. Marked salt wasting does not occur following relief of experimental unilateral ureteral obstruction, suggesting that retention of solutes is the primary factor in clinical postobstructive diuresis.[22]

Diuretics. Sodium and water losses are the desired and predictable effects of diuretic administration. Severe volume depletion usually does not occur, because reduction in ECF volume reduces renal blood flow and glomerular filtration rate, increases renal tubular reabsorption, and limits the delivery of sodium and chloride to the final urine. Sodium and chloride losses may continue, however, if osmotic diuretics (such as mannitol, as described) or the potent loop diuretics (furosemide and ethracrynic acid) are used. Although use of osmotic diuretics results in plasma hyperosmolality, administration of loop diuretics can result in increased urinary concentration (via volume depletion), water retention, and plasma hypo-osmolality.

HISTORY

By identifying the clinical setting in which polyuria appears, one can narrow the range of diagnostic possibilities rapidly. Important facts to determine are whether polyuria is the sole problem or only one of many clinical problems present, whether it exceeds 5 or 6 liters/day, and whether it is transient or persistent.

The most important historical factor in patients with polyuria is detailed knowledge of the specific clinical setting. Polyuria following head trauma or neurosurgery is likely to be due to neurogenic DI, as is polyuria in a patient with focal neurologic symptoms or findings indicative of pituitary disease. Polyuria in patients receiving large volumes of intravenous infusions, such as parenteral nutrition or saline, is probably caused by the solute and/or water loads. In patients with known renal disease, polyuria usually represents nephrogenic DI, and in patients recovering from ATN or bilateral renal obstruction, it is probably due to excretion of previously retained solutes. In the diabetic patient, polyuria usually is caused by hyperglycemia and glycosuria. Polyuria in patients being treated for manic-depressive illness is usually the result of lithium administration. Polyuria in newborn infants is likely to be caused by familial neurogenic or nephrogenic DI.

Urine volume in excess of 5 to 6 liters/day is uncommon even in conditions with significant impairment of urinary concentration. Polyuria of this magnitude is most often due to primary polydipsia, saline infusions, complete neurogenic DI, or osmotic diuresis. Of course, these disorders may be responsible for polyuria with urine volumes between 3.5 and 5 liters/day.

Transient polyuria, which occurs after ingestion of any large water and solute load, is most familiar as the diuresis following a large, salty, high-protein meal with many alcoholic drinks. Administration of diuretics or radiographic contrast medium usually leads to a brief period of polyuria. Diabetes insipidus following head trauma or neurosurgery also may be transient.

Persistent moderate polyuria (urine volume between 3.5 and 5 liters/day) in the absence of obvious manifestations of associated disease is the most difficult to diagnose. The differential diagnosis includes recent onset of diabetes, pituitary or renal disease, hypokalemia, hypercalcemia, and primary polydipsia.

PHYSICAL EXAMINATION

Abnormal physical findings in patients with polyuria may be either primary, due to the disorder causing the polyuria, or secondary, due to the fluid and electrolyte disturbances caused by the water and solute losses.

Acute weight loss, hypotension, tachycardia, decreased skin turgor, and postural changes in pulse and blood pressure indicate depletion of intravascular fluid volume. Under these circumstances, the appropriate renal response is to conserve salt and water. Thus, the hypotensive patient with polyuria has seriously impaired urinary concentrating ability. Volume depletion is most marked in the patient who has osmotic diuresis, is recovering from ATN or bilateral obstruction, or has medullary cystic disease. Weight loss without alterations in blood pressure or pulse often indicates water loss without solute, as occurs in diabetes insipidus, hypercalcemia, hypokalemia, and most parenchymal renal diseases. Extreme water depletion does not occur in these patients unless the thirst mechanism is disordered or the patient does not have access to water.

Acute weight gain, hypertension, and edema indicate extracellular fluid excess, suggesting solute administration. Weight gain without hypertension or edema may be due to either solute or water administration.

Focal neurologic symptoms suggest that the polyuria is due to neurogenic DI secondary to a mass lesion such as a pituitary tumor or an infiltrative disease. Generalized symptoms such as lethargy, confusion, and agitation are not diagnostically helpful.

DIAGNOSTIC STUDIES AND ASSESSMENT

Laboratory evaluation of the patient with polyuria requires only a small number of routinely available blood and urine measurements. Careful consideration of the clinical facts coupled with an appropriate interpretation of the laboratory data provides the final diagnosis in patients with polyuria, with few exceptions. Occasionally, performance of an overnight water deprivation test and measurement of plasma ADH levels are required.

Urinalysis

Glycosuria in a patient with polyuria (with or without ketonuria) suggests hyperglycemia and an osmotic diuresis. Proteinuria and the presence of renal tubular cells and cellular or coarse granular casts indicate parenchymal renal disease. The principal value of the urinalysis in the polyuric patient, however, is the measurement of specific gravity, an index of urine osmolality. The relationship between urine osmolality and specific gravity is shown in Figure 5. Urinary osmolality of 300 mOsm/kg (corresponding approximately to 0.3 osm/liter), a value virtually isotonic to normal plasma, indicates no concentration of glomerular filtrate and corresponds to a specific gravity of approximately 1.010. The molecular weight of glucose (180 daltons) is higher than osmotically active substances normally present in urine (urea 60 daltons, NaCl 58 daltons); thus, in patients with glycosuria, urinary specific gravity (by hygrometer) overestimates osmolality throughout the entire range of values. In practice it is not always necessary to measure urine osmolality. In most cases of polyuria, the diagnosis can be established by proper interpretation of the specific gravity value, especially if determined by refractometer.

A specific gravity greater than 1.012 (urine osmolality > 300 mOsm/kg) in a patient with polyuria indicates excretion of a large solute load, as in polyuria due to solute administration (saline or TPN), osmotic diuresis, use of diuretics, medullary cystic disease, or recovery from ATN or bilateral obstruction. A specific gravity less than 1.005 (urine osmolality < 150 mOsm/kg) in a patient with polyuria indicates virtual absence of ADH secretion, as seen in patients with complete neurogenic DI or primary polydipsia and in babies with congenital nephrogenic DI. Specific gravity values between 1.005 and 1.012 (urine osmolality 200–300 mOsm/kg) may be due to any of the causes of polyuria.

Blood Tests

The necessary determinations are of Na^+, K^+, Cl^-, total CO_2, blood urea nitrogen (BUN), creatinine, glucose, and calcium, and plasma osmolality. If solutes such as radiographic contrast medium, mannitol, ethanol, methanol, and ethylene glycol are not present in the patient's blood, plasma osmolality may be estimated using the following calculation:

$$\text{Plasma osmolality} = 2\,(\text{Na}^+) + \frac{\text{BUN}}{2.8} + \frac{\text{glucose}}{18}$$

Osmolality is measured in mOsm/kg, Na^+ in mEq/liter, and BUN and glucose in mg/100 ml. Osmolality calculated in this manner is usually within 10 to 15 mOsm/kg of measured osmolality.

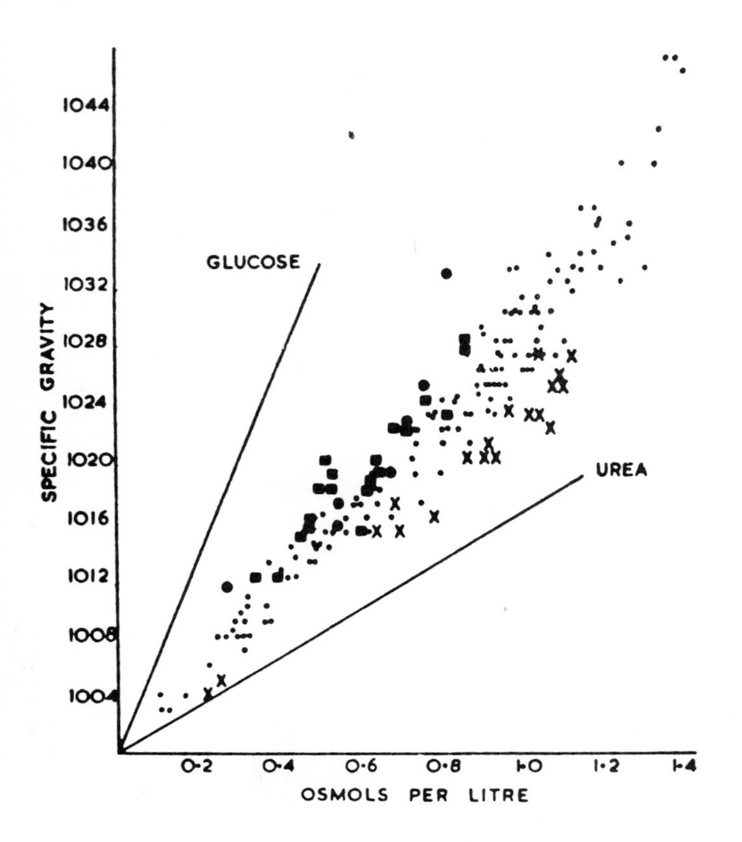

Figure 5. Relationship between specific gravity and osmolality of urine. Different urine samples are shown as follows: *small dots*, with no sugar or protein; *large dots*, 3+ sugar; *squares*, 3+ protein; *X*, after 25 g urea by mouth. The lines show the relation between specific gravity and osmolality for glucose and urea solutions. (From Miles BE, Paton A, de Wardener HE: Maximal urine concentration. Br Med J 2:901–905, 1954. Reprinted with permission.)

Plasma hyperosmolality in the polyuric patient signifies loss of water and impairment of the thirst mechanism or lack of access to water, indicating that primary polydipsia cannot be the cause of the polyuria. If plasma hyperosmolality is present, identifying the solute present in excess provides important diagnostic information. Hyperosmolality due to hyperglycemia indicates uncontrolled diabetes and osmotic diuresis, whereas hyperosmolality due to hypernatremia indicates water loss or addition of hypertonic saline. Azotemia (elevated BUN) suggests that hyperosmolality is due to administration of high-protein nutrients (e.g., enteral tube feedings or TPN) and also that renal insufficiency is present. If the measured plasma osmolality exceeds calculated osmolality by more than 15 mOsm/kg, an unidentified solute, such as mannitol or alcohol, must be present in plasma and may be responsible for the polyuria.

If plasma osmoality is normal in the polyuric patient, the patient has adequate thirst sensation and access to water. The finding of normal plasma osmolality is of little diagnostic value, however, unless the measured osmolality exceeds the calculated value, in which case an unidentified solute in plasma may be responsible for the polyuria.

Plasma hypo-osmolality in the polyuric patient indicates dilution of body fluids due to administration and retention of water. The finding of plasma hypo-osmolality is diagnostically very helpful because it narrows the possibilities to either primary polydipsia or iatrogenic water administration.

In addition to calculation of plasma osmolality, measurement of electrolytes permits the identification of hypokalemia and hypercalcemia as possible causes of polyuria. Serum creatinine should be measured in all patients with polyuria in order to assess renal function.

Overnight Water Deprivation Test

The primary utility of this test is to determine the integrated response of both pituitary ADH secretion and the renal concentrating mechanism to water deprivation. Insensible water losses during water deprivation raise plasma osmolality slightly, leading to increases in ADH secretion and urine concentration in normal individuals. During 12 to 16 hours of water deprivation, insensible losses of 300 to 400 ml normally result in a 1 per cent rise in plasma osmolality, a stimulus sufficient to increase ADH secretion markedly.[2] Of course, any urinary water loss during this time would lead to an even greater increase in plasma osmolality and ADH secretion. In normal subjects, urine volume declines and urine osmolality rises steadily throughout the period of water deprivation, reaching a plateau of 900 to 1400 mOsm/kg, representing maximal urinary concentrating ability.[23] Weight loss is usually less than 1 kg, and plasma osmolality at this time remains within the normal range. On the basis of the relationship shown in Figure 2, one would predict plasma ADH to be in the range of 3 to 5 pg/ml. Indeed, administration of exogenous ADH—5 units of aqueous vasopressin (Pitressin)—at this juncture results in no further rise in urine concentration in normal persons. In hospitalized patients, maximal urinary osmolality is less, rising to only 400 to 1,200 mOsm/kg, as in normal subjects, however, maximal urine concentration is not increased further by the injection of 5 units of aqueous vasopressin.

In practice, a water deprivation test may be conducted in the outpatient clinic or office if a patient's urine volume is 4 to 5 liters/day or less. Water deprivation begins at 8 P.M. on the first day; starting 12 hours later (8 A.M. the next day), urine specimens are collected hourly for measurement of specific gravity. In patients with severe polyuria (urine volume more than 5 liters/day), the water deprivation test should be undertaken in the hospital and should begin in the morning rather than at night. Blood pressure, pulse, and weight are measured frequently. Weight loss (an estimate of fluid loss) should not be permitted to exceed 3 per cent of body weight. After the urinary specific gravity reaches a maximal value, plasma and urine are collected for measurement of osmolality, and 5 units of aqueous vasopressin are injected subcutaneously. One hour later, urine is again collected for measurement of osmolality. Failure of urinary osmolality or specific gravity to rise despite a weight loss of 3 per cent or a rise in plasma osmolality of similar magnitude is abnormal and indicates a defect in the hypothalamic-pituitary-renal system.

In the following section, we describe the response to water deprivation in patients with polyuria of various causes.

Solute or Water Administration. Polyuria due to solute administration is usually easily recognized by the clinical circumstances and a urine specific gravity of approximately 1.010; it is usually not necessary to perform a water deprivation test in affected patients. Polyuria due to water ingestion is often difficult to recognize, however, because patients frequently deny excessive water ingestion or complain of increased thirst. The response of patients with primary polydipsia to water deprivation is qualitatively similar to that of normal individuals, with the following exceptions. First, a longer period may be required for urinary osmolality to reach maximal values (usually 16 hours), and weight loss during the test may be greater (approximately 2 kg), as a result of prior overhydration. Second, maximal urinary concentration is less than normal (500–900 mOsm/kg). As in normal subjects, plasma osmolality remains

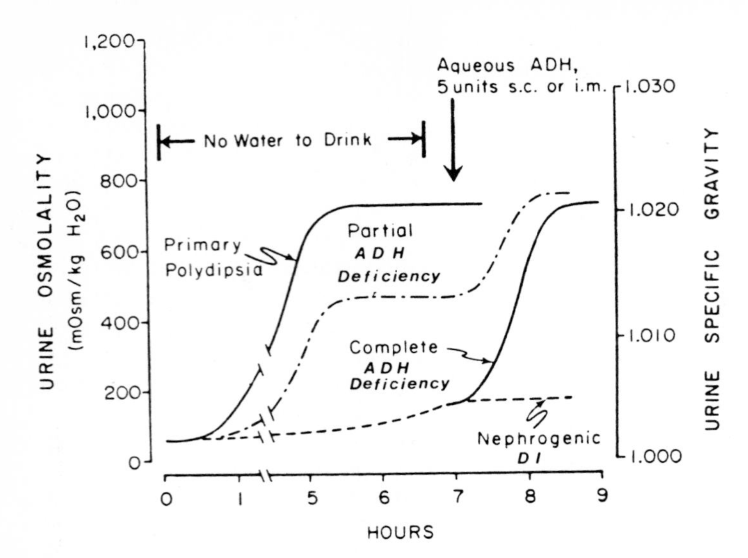

Figure 6. Urinary osmolality and specific gravity during water deprivation in patients with polyuria due to various disorders. For explanation, see text. (From Valtin H: Renal Dysfunction. Mechanisms Involved in Fluid and Solute Imbalance. Boston, Little, Brown, 1979. Reprinted with permission.)

within the normal range, and addition of exogenous ADH does not increase urine osmolality further (Fig. 6).

Neurogenic DI. Patients with severe neurogenic DI experience rapid dehydration, with urinary osmolality reaching maximal values of only 100 to 250 mOsm/kg within 4 to 12 hours (see Fig. 6). Weight loss during this time is 2 to 3 kg, and plasma osmolality rises to approximately 300 mOsm/kg. Despite these changes, plasma ADH levels remain low. The response to the administration of exogenous ADH is diagnostic. Urine osmolality increases, on average, to twice its pre-ADH value, indicating that the cause of the polyuria is ADH deficiency, not renal tubular dysfunction. The rapid dehydration possible in these patients underscores the need for close medical supervision during the water deprivation test.

In patients with partial ADH deficiency, maximal urinary osmolality is higher (300–600 mOsm/kg) than in patients with complete ADH deficiency and is reached after a longer period of water

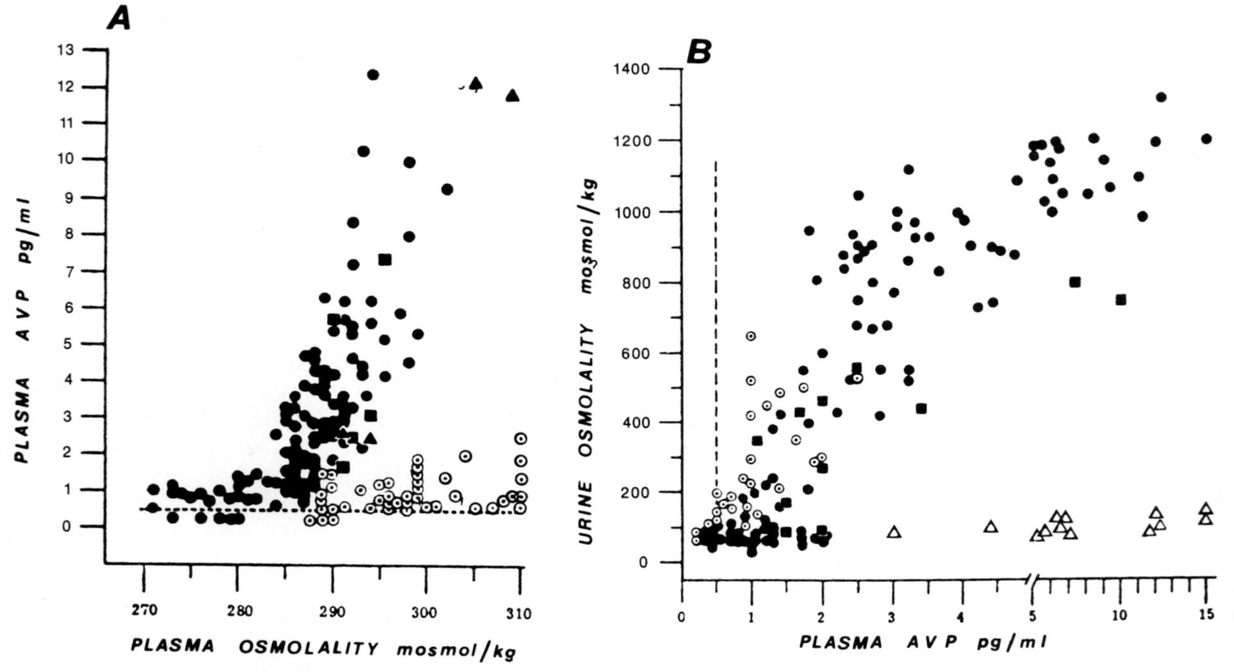

Figure 7. Relationship among plasma AVP, plasma osmolality, and urinary osmolality in normal adults in various states of hydration and in patients with polyuria due to various disorders (see text). *Solid circles,* normal (n = 25); *squares,* primary polydipsia (n = 2); *triangles,* nephrogenic diabetes insipidus; *dotted circles,* neurogenic diabetes insipidus (n = 8). (From Robertson GL, et al: Development and clinical application of a new method for the radioimmunoassay of arginine vasopressin in human plasma. J Clin Invest 52:2340–2352, 1973. Used by copyright permission of the American Society for Clinical Investigation.)

deprivation, normally 8 to 16 hours (see Fig. 6). Weight loss is usually less than 2 kg, and plasma osmolality is only slightly elevated, to approximately 295 mOsm/kg.[23]

Nephrogenic DI. As discussed before, except for those with the congenital form, most patients with nephrogenic DI have mild urinary concentration defects and are able to raise urinary osmolality above plasma osmolality. Administration of ADH does not lead to a further increase in urine concentration, thus differentiating this group from patients with partial neurogenic DI. The largest subgroup of patients with nephrogenic DI are those with tubulointerstitial renal disease, a diagnosis that is usually apparent after examination of urine sediment and measurement of serum creatinine and electrolytes. In these patients, a water deprivation test is usually not necessary to establish the diagnosis of nephrogenic DI.

Osmotic Diuresis. Because disorders causing osmotic diuresis are usually easily recognized (diabetic hyperglycemia and prolonged mannitol administration), the water deprivation test is rarely performed in such patients. Characteristically, urine osmolality is similar to plasma osmolality (usually 310–340 mOsm/kg), rises little or not at all as water deprivation continues, and fails to rise further after exogenous ADH is given.

Solute Diuresis Due to Renal Disease or Diuretics. A water deprivation test is usually not necessary in patients with solute diuresis because they are usually easily recognized on the basis of the clinical setting, examination of urine sediment, and measurement of serum creatinine. Urine osmolality would be expected to increase minimally if at all following water deprivation and ADH administration in such patients.

Plasma ADH (AVP) Measurement

Plasma ADH can be directly measured by radioimmunoassay utilizing antibodies to the active antidiuretic hormone in humans. Although not routinely performed by most clinical chemistry laboratories at this time, this procedure is likely to be widely available in the near future. Furthermore, preliminary use suggests that patients with polyuria can be classified more accurately if this measurement is combined with results of the overnight water deprivation test.[24]

Plasma AVP is assayed in patients with polyuria after urinary specific gravity or osmolality reaches a plateau during water deprivation (Fig. 7). If plasma AVP does not rise appropriately for the plasma osmolality, the patient likely has neurogenic DI. If plasma AVP rises but urinary osmolality does not, nephrogenic DI is present. Appropriate rises in both plasma AVP and urinary osmolality during water deprivation are taken to indicate primary polydipsia. Classification of polyuria due to water diuresis by measurement of plasma AVP concurs with results of standard water deprivation tests in patients with complete neurogenic DI. However, differences in classification may arise in one-third to one-half of patients with partial neurogenic DI, nephrogenic DI, and primary polydipsia.[24] When plasma AVP measurement becomes routinely available, its use in combination with the standard water deprivation test will lead to more accurate diagnosis of polyuria.

REFERENCES

1. Berliner RW. Mechanisms of urine concentration. Kidney Int 1982;22:202–11.
2. Robertson GL, Shelton RL, Athar SH. The osmoregulation of vasopressin. Kidney Int 1976;10:25–37.
3. Fitzsimons JC. Thirst. Physiology Rev 1972;52:468–561.
4. Jamison RL, Oliver RE. Disorders of urinary concentration and dilution. Am J Med 1982;72:308–22.
5. Barlow ED, de Wardener HE. Compulsive water drinking. Q J Med 1959;28:235–58.
6. Arieff AI, Guisado R. Effects on the central nervous system of hypernatremic and hyponatremic states. Kidney Int 1976;10:104–16.
7. Leaf A. Neurogenic diabetes insipidus. Kidney Int 1979;15:572–80.
8. Heinbecker P, White HL. Hypothalamicohypophysial system and its relationship to water balance in the dog. Am J Physiol 1941;133:582–93.
9. Feig PU, McCurdy DK. The hypertonic state. N Engl J Med 1977;297:1444–54.
10. Tan MH. Changing factors in the etiology of diabetes insipidus. Nova Scotia Med Bull 1971;50:153–60.
11. Sharkey PC, Perry JH, Ehni G. Diabetes insipidus following section of the hypothalamic stalk. J Neurosurg 1961;18:445–60.
12. Blotner H. Primary or idiopathic diabetes insipidus: a system disease. Metabolism 1958;7:191–200.
13. Strauss MB, Rosenbaum JD, Nelson WP. Effect of alcohol on the renal excretion of water and electrolyte. J Clin Invest 1950;29:1053–58.
14. Eggleton MD. The diuretic action of alcohol in man. J Physiol 1942;101:172–91.
15. Bode HH, Crawford JD. Nephrogenic diabetes insipidus in North America: the Hopewell hypothesis. N Engl J Med 1969;280:750–4.
16. Bennett CM. Urine concentration and dilution in hypokalemic and hypercalcemic dogs. J Clin Invest 1970;49:1447–57.
17. Singer I, Forrest JN. Drug-induced states of nephrogenic diabetes insipidus. Kidney Int 1976;10:82–95.
18. Singer I. Lithium and the kidney. Kidney Int 1981;19:374–87.
19. Gennari FJ, Kassirer JP. Osmotic diuresis. N Engl J Med 1974; 291:714–20.
20. Steele BT, Lirenman DS, Beattie CW. Nephronophthisis. Am J Med 1980;68:531–38.
21. Levers DT, Matthew TH, Haher JF, Schreiner GE. Long-term follow-up of renal function and histology after acute tubular necrosis. Ann Intern Med 1970;73:523–9.
22. Wilson DR. Pathophysiology of obstructive nephropathy. Kidney Int 1980;18:281–92.
23. Miller M, Dalakos T, Moses AM, Fellerman H, Streeten DHP. Recognition of partial defects in antidiuretic hormone secretion. Ann Intern Med 1970;73:721–9.
24. Zerbe RL, Robertson GL. A comparison of plasma vasopressin measurements with a standard indirect test in the differential diagnosis of polyuria. N Engl J Med 1981;305:1539–46.

PRENATAL DETECTION OF GENETIC DISORDERS

ALBERT B. GERBIE □ SHERMAN ELIAS

□ SYNONYMS: Antenatal diagnosis of genetic disease, human genetic diagnosis

BACKGROUND

The prenatal diagnosis of genetic diseases is of concern not only to obstetrician-gynecologists and pediatricians, but to all physicians who take care of couples in their reproductive years. Because of their knowledge of a family's medical history and because they are aware of the first occurrence of an abnormality in the family, physicians can and must assume the responsibility for genetic counseling. Some aspects of genetic counseling are sufficiently complex to necessitate consultation with a medical geneticist; however, a number of routine problems can be managed by the well-informed physician. Currently available diagnostic modalities permit the prenatal diagnosis of essentially all chromosomal disorders, many mendelian disorders, and some polygenic/multifactorial disorders.

In order to counsel properly, the physician should: (1) obtain an accurate family history, (2) have an understanding of the genetic principles involved, (3) have an accurate diagnosis of the abnormality in question, (4) understand the potential effect of environmental factors on the developing fetus, and (5) be aware of current diagnostic capabilities.[1, 2]

GENETIC AMNIOCENTESIS

Counseling

The couple should be carefully counseled regarding the genetic risks of their fetus and the prognosis for a child affected with the disorder in question. Ideally, a couple should have the opportunity to discuss their risks for having a child with a congenital anomaly either prior to pregnancy or before the end of the first trimester. They should be made aware of the diagnostic capabilities as well as the risks of the amniocentesis procedure. Risks to the mother include bleeding, infection, and blood group sensitization. Fetal risks include abortion and injury. (These risks are discussed in detail later.) It is important to emphasize that the time needed to perform the analysis is usually between 3 and 5 weeks, so that unnecessary emotional tension will not be created by expectation of earlier results.

Technique of Amniocentesis

Genetic amniocentesis should be performed by an obstetrician who is experienced in the procedure and is in a position to act on the results.[2] The laboratory processing the samples should be experienced in culturing amniotic fluid cells and performing the necessary analyses. The procedure is usually performed in an outpatient facility. It is best done at about the 15th to the 16th week of gestation, which is sufficiently early that pregnancy termination remains an option. At this time the uterus is easily accessible and there is a sufficient volume of amniotic fluid to permit the procedure to be performed safely. It is important to conduct an ultrasonographic examination preceding amniocentesis to: (1) verify fetal viability, (2) confirm gestation age, (3) diagnose multiple gestation, (4) localize the placenta, (5) detect gross fetal malformations or hydatid mole, (6) detect uterine or adnexal abnormalities, and (7) potentially reduce the risk of blood group sensitization.[3]

In preparation for amniocentesis the patient voids. The actual procedure is performed under strict aseptic conditions. A local anesthetic, 1 per cent lidocaine solution, is injected at the proposed puncture site. A 22- or 20-gauge, 3½-inch, disposable spinal needle with stylet is inserted percutaneously into the amniotic cavity. The stylet is then removed and the needle is cleared into a syringe to minimize the possibility of maternal cell contamination. If a bloody sample is obtained in the initial several milliliters of fluid, the needle is cleared by aspiration into additional syringes. Between 20 and 30 ml of amniotic fluid are aspirated into a second or third syringe, after which the needle is withdrawn. The sample is then transferred to the laboratory either in the syringes or in sterile siliconized glass or plastic tubes. It is crucial that all specimens be properly labeled and transported at room temperature. Immediate preparation of the amniotic fluid in the laboratory is preferred, because samples transported over large distances have yielded less optimal results. Following amniocentesis, the patient is observed and given postprocedure instructions. She may continue her normal activities; however, strenuous exercise (e.g., running) is to be avoided for at least several days. She must report any fluid loss, bleeding, uterine cramps, or fever immediately. Finally, all aborted fetuses and all newborn infants should be evaluated by the physician for disorders.

Urine and amniotic fluid are often indistinguishable in appearance, and analysis of cells derived from maternal tissues could obviously lead to erroneous diagnoses. Inadvertent aspiration of maternal urine is of particular concern because amniocentesis is usually performed at a suprapubic site. We have found that the crystalline arborization pattern characteristic of amniotic fluid is observed if the fluid is allowed to dry on an acid-cleaned slide and examined under low (× 100) magnification. With this method one can quickly differentiate amniotic fluid from urine with a high degree of accuracy.[4]

Multiple gestation may be clinically suspected when the uterine size is larger than expected according to the women's last menstrual period; however, the diagnosis may be missed, especially in an obese woman. Ultrasonography will exclude multiple gestation before amniocentesis. Separate amniocentesis of each amniotic sac is necessary in order to determine the status of each fetus. If twins are detected, separate sacs may be distinguished by injecting a dye, e.g., indigocarmine, after aspiration of the first fluid sample. A second amniocentesis is then performed in the ultrasonographically determined location of the second fetus. Withdrawal of clear amniotic fluid indicates a successful entry into the second amniotic sac, whereas aspiration of blue-tinged amniotic fluid indicates that the first sac was reentered. Using such techniques, we have been successful in obtaining information regarding both fetuses in approximately 90 per cent of twin gestations.[5] This technique of multiple amniocentesis does not appear to pose a significant risk for the patient or her fetuses beyond that seen with amniocentesis in the singleton pregnancy. Finally, the parents and physician must be prepared to face the possible dilemma of having one normal fetus and one abnormal fetus.

Because of the theoretical risks of Rh sensitization, it is our policy to administer anti-D immune globulin following second-trimester amniocentesis to Rh-negative women.

Risks of Amniocentesis

Amniocentesis with culture of amniotic fluid cells is relatively safe and highly accurate (> 99 per cent). Nonetheless, no surgical procedure is without risk. Indeed, the rationale underlying antenatal diagnosis limits application of the procedure to cases in which potential diagnostic benefits outweigh known risks (i.e., favorable benefits-risks ratio).

The various risks of amniocentesis may be divided into those affecting the fetus and those affecting the mother. Fetal risks include abortion, needle injury, infection, and possible injury due to withdrawal of amniotic fluid or to defects in the amniotic membranes (e.g., fetal joint contractures or amniotic bands). Karp and Hayden[6] have estimated that minor skin injuries (dimpling and linear scars) occur in about 3 per cent of infants whose mothers have had midtrimester amniocentesis. However, the risk of serious fetal injury appears to be remote, probably less than one per 1,000 procedures.[7]

Several collaborative studies have attempted to assess the risks of amniocentesis. The first major prospective study, coordinated by the National Institutes of Child Health and Human Development, comprised 1,040 subjects and 992 controls.[8] The incidence of immediate complications (e.g., bleeding, leakage of amniotic fluid, and abortion) was about 2 per cent, a figure only slightly higher than in the control group. Moreover, only a few of the immediate complications were serious. Overall, 3.5 per cent of pregnant women who underwent amniocentesis experienced fetal loss subsequent to the procedure, compared with 3.2 per cent of controls. There was some suggestion of higher incidence of fetal loss with a larger number of attempts at amniocentesis. Only one case of fetal puncture was recognized. Amnionitis was not reported in relation to the amniocentesis in this study. A Canadian study reached a similar conclusion.[9] However, a British collaborative study showed a significantly higher fetal loss rate in the study group (2.6 per cent) than in the controls (1.1 per cent) and an unexplained increase in rate of neonatal respiratory distress syndrome.[10] Some biases may have affected this study, inasmuch as the controls were significantly older and of greater parity than the study subjects.

When differences in study designs are taken into account, however, differences among these three studies are minimized. Accordingly, we can make the following conclusions:

1. The increased risk of fetal loss following amniocentesis is in the range of 0.5 per cent.
2. The risk of serious fetal injury is remote.
3. The risk of small needle marks is low.
4. The risk of maternal injuries is minimal, with amnionitis being the only real consideration.

Indications for Prenatal Diagnosis by Genetic Amniocentesis

Amniocentesis with appropriate genetic studies of amniotic fluid cells makes possible the antenatal diagnosis of all known chromosomal disorders, many mendelian disorders, and open neural tube defects. In addition, other diagnostic modalities such as fetoscopy and ultrasonography have expanded diagnostic capabilities. For example, ultrasonography has been successfully utilized for the prenatal detection of certain gross congenital anomalies (e.g., advanced hydrocephalus, skeletal dysplasias). A detailed discussion of the many disorders currently diagnosable before birth is beyond the scope of this chapter; however, we shall highlight those conditions with which the practicing physician should be familiar.

Chromosomal Abnormalities

Chromosomal abnormalities represent a major cause of aberrant human development. Although technically feasible, it is not appropriate to determine the chromosome complement of every fetus, because for many couples the risk of amniocentesis may outweigh the potential diagnostic benefits. The following conditions are the currently acceptable indications for prenatal diagnosis of chromosome disorders: advanced parental age; a parent with balanced translocation, inversion, or other chromosomal abnormality; and a previous child with a chromosome abnormality, particularly an autosomal trisomy. Other possible cytogenetic indications are also discussed briefly.

Advanced Parental Age. The most common indication for genetic amniocentesis is *advanced maternal age.* In our unit, about 85 per cent of all such procedures are performed solely for this reason. The incidence of trisomy 21 is about one per 800 live births. By contrast, a woman 35 years old at the birth of her child has a one in 385 likelihood of having a child with Down's syndrome. At age 39, the risk is one in 137, and at age 45 one in 30 (Table 1).[11] However, trisomy 21 is not the only chromosomal abnormality whose incidence increases with maternal age. Trisomy 13, trisomy 18, 47,XXX, and 47,XXY also demonstrate an increased mean maternal age.[12, 13] Thus, the likelihood of delivering a child with any chromosomal abnormality at age 35 is one in 204, at age 39 one in 82, and at age 45 one in 20. From these data, it is clear that no absolute definition of advanced maternal age can be given. It is now standard medical practice in this country, however, that all women aged 35 and older (i.e., at the time of delivery) be counseled concerning the risk of having a child with a chromosomal abnormality and the availability of genetic amniocentesis. Moreover, we suggest physician flexibility when younger women inquire about prenatal diagnosis.

Advanced paternal age is also worth mentioning, although its relationship with chromosomal abnormalities is not as well established as that of advanced maternal age. Studies have shown that the likelihood of a man's fathering a child with trisomy 21 doubles after about the age of 55.[14, 15] On the basis of antenatal diagnosis data from Europe, Stene[16] has recently also demonstrated a paternal age effect above age 40. In our unit, it is therefore the practice to double the maternal age risks when the father is older. For example, if the mother is 35 years old and the father 55, we would quote the risk for Down's syndrome as about one in 190 and the risk for any type of chromosome abnormality as about one in 100.

Table 1. RISK OF HAVING A LIVE-BORN CHILD WITH DOWN'S SYNDROME OR OTHER CHROMOSOME ABNORMALITY ACCORDING TO MATERNAL AGE*

Maternal Age	Risk of Down's Syndrome	Total Risk for All Chromosome Abnormalities†
20	1 in 1,667	1 in 526
21	1,667	526
22	1,429	500
23	1,429	500
24	1,250	476
25	1,250	476
26	1,176	476
27	1,111	455
28	1,053	435
29	1,000	417
30	952	384
31	909	384
32	769	322
33	625	317
34	500	260
35	385	204
36	294	164
37	227	130
38	175	103
39	137	82
40	106	65
41	82	51
42	64	40
43	50	32
44	38	25
45	30	20
46	23	15
47	18	12
48	14	10
49	11	7

*Because sample size for some ages is relatively small, 95 per cent confidence limits are sometimes relatively large.

†Risk of 47,XXX excluded for ages 20 through 32 (data not reported).

(Data from Hook and Chambers,[11] Hook and Linsjo,[12] and Hook et al.[13])

Previous Child with a Chromosome Abnormality. Genetic amniocentesis is frequently recommended to couples who have already had a child with a chromosome abnormality. However, the risk for having a second child with Down's syndrome is probably not as great as usually stated. Specifically, only mothers who give birth to a Down's syndrome infant while under age 25 appear to be at a higher risk than that expected on the basis of maternal age alone.[17] Information regarding the chance of recurrence following births of live-borns with chromosome abnormalities other than trisomy 21 is very limited; however, it appears that the risk is approximately 1 to 2 per cent for either the same or for a different chromosome abnormality.[17] Nonetheless, although the data may not suggest a particularly increased risk, such couples frequently request genetic amniocentesis to relieve their anxiety.

Structural Chromosome Rearrangement in a Parent. An important indication for prenatal diagnosis is the presence of either a balanced translocation or an inversion in a parent. (*Translocation* is the transfer of a segment of one chromosome to a nonhomologous chromosome; *inversion* is a chromosomal aberration in which a segment of a chromosome is reversed end-to-end.) For example, 2 to 3 per cent of individuals with Down's syndrome have a translocation, usually between chromosomes 14 and 21. About 25 per cent of these translocations are inherited, the remaining occurring de novo (i.e., not detected in either parent). Such situations are usually ascertained after the birth of an abnormal child. After the birth of a child with Down's syndrome due to a de novo translocation, the recurrence risk is probably no greater than the risk of Down's syndrome in the general population. By contrast, if one parent carries the translocation, the empiric risk depends upon the type of translocation and which parent carries it. Specifically, if the mother carries a 14/21 translocation (the most common form) the risk is about 10 per cent, whereas if the father carries it, the risk is only about 2 per cent.[18, 19] These empiric figures are less than the theoretical risks (33 per cent), probably because of selection against abnormal gametes or conceptuses. Other translocations do not necessarily carry similar risks for recurrence. For example, in the rare situation in which one parent carries a 21/21 translocation, pregnancies lead to either nonviable monosomic zygotes or zygotes with Down's syndrome. Thus, all offspring of a parent with a 21/21 translocation will have Down's syndrome. Finally, individuals with a chromosomal inversion may also produce chromosomally unbalanced gametes. Empiric data are not available for specific inversion, but pooled data for all inversions indicate about a 5 per cent risk for abnormal progeny, with maternal carriers at a greater risk than paternal carriers. Counseling in such situations is usually complex and is best offered by an experienced geneticist. A noteworthy exception involves an inversion in chromosome 9, a common variant that is thought to be without clinical significance.

Other Indications. Couples experiencing repetitive spontaneous abortion should be evaluated cytogenetically to exclude a translocation or inversion, either of which would justify prenatal cytogenetic studies in subsequent pregnancies. Finally, prenatal diagnosis might be extended to couples who have had a chromosomally abnormal spontaneous abortus or stillborn infant, depending upon the specific chromosome abnormality detected.

Mendelian Disorders

Diseases produced by a single mutant gene, whether transmitted as dominant, recessive, autosomal, or X-linked, are generally uncommon, with an upper limit of frequency of about 1 in 2,000. Depending upon the specific disorder and its mode of inheritance, the risk of having an affected offspring ranges from 25 to 50 per cent. Unfortunately, methods are available for prenatal diagnosis in only a relative few of the more than 1,200 mendelian disorders.[20]

The specific enzymatic defects have been identified in over 150 of the more than 400 catalogued inborn errors of metabolism. For the majority of disorders, the underlying defect is deficiency of an enzymatic activity that normally mediates a metabolic process. Affected infants usually show vomiting, failure to thrive, protein intolerance, hypotonia and/or hypertonia, lethargy or coma, and unusual odor. Such disorders usually result in severe disability and death in early childhood. Prenatal detection of a metabolic disorder usually requires that the enzymatic or metabolic reaction be expressed in amniotic fluid fiberblasts in the midtrimester. The inborn errors of metabolism may generally be subdivided into several categories: (1) mucopolysaccharidoses, (2) mucolipidoses and other disorders of carbohydrate metabolism, (3) lipidoses, (4) amino acid disorders, and (5) miscellaneous biochemical disorders. Table 2 lists those inborn errors of metabolism that are prenatally detectable. Because this list is under continuous revision, absence of a particular disorder from the table does not necessarily mean that its detection is not possible.

At present, most couples are identified as being at increased risk for having a child with a mendelian disorder only after having an affected child. One important exception is Tay-Sachs disease, which results from a deficiency of the enzyme hexosaminidase A. Affected children show psychomotor deterioration beginning at 1 year of age with progressive deterioration resulting in deafness, blindness, seizures, and a decerebrate state. The frequency of Tay-Sachs disease is one per 3,600 Ashkenazi Jews; one of every 30 Ashkenazi Jews is a carrier. Because of this high frequency, all Jewish couples should be screened by an assay of serum hexosaminidase A activity. Antenatal diagnosis of Tay-Sachs disease by measurement of hexosaminidase A activity in cultured amniotic fluid cells is an option available to the identified carrier couple, for whom the risk of having an affected child is 25 per cent. Because it is technically difficult to determine the carrier state in a pregnant woman, such screening should be performed prior to conception. However, screening can be performed during pregnancy using a leukocyte assay. Successful screening programs for

Table 2. INHERITED METABOLIC DISORDERS DETECTABLE IN THE SECOND TRIMESTER OF PREGNANCY

Disorders of lipid metabolism	Cholesterol ester storage disease Fabry's disease Familial hypercholesterolemia Farber's disease Gaucher's disease (infantile and adult types) GM_1 gangliosidosis, types I and II GM_2 gangliosidosis type I (Tay-Sachs disease) type II (Sandhoff's disease) type III GM_3 gangliosidosis Krabbe's disease (globoid cell leukodystrophy) Metachromatic leukodystrophy (infantile, juvenile, and adult types) Multiple sulfatase deficiency Neuraminidase deficiency Niemann-Pick disease, types A, B, and C Refsum's disease Wolman's disease
Disorders of carbohydrate or glycoprotein metabolism	Aspartylglucosaminuria Fucosidosis Galactokinase deficiency Galactosemia Glucose-6-phosphate dehydrogenase (G-6-PD) deficiency Glycogen storage disease, types II, III, IV, VI, and VIII Mannosidosis Pyruvate carboxylase deficiency Pyruvate decarboxylase deficiency Pyruvate dehydrogenase deficiency
Disorders of mucopolysaccharide (MPS) metabolism	Hurler's syndrome (MPS IH) Scheie's syndrome (MPS IS) Hunter's syndrome (MPS IIA and IIB) Sanfilippo's syndrome (MPS IIIA and IIIB) Morquio's syndrome (MPS IV) Maroteaux-Lamy syndrome (MPS VI A and VI B) beta-Glucuronidase deficiency (MPS VII)
Mucolipidoses	Mucolipidosis type I type II (I-cell disease) type III type IV
Disorders of amino acid and organic acid metabolism	Arginase deficiency Argininosuccinicaciduria Citrullinemia Cystathioninuria Cystinosis Dihydropteridine reductase deficiency (phenylketonuria variant) Glutaric acidemia Histidinemia Homocystinuria (both vitamin B_{12}–responsive and vitamin B_{12}–nonresponsive types) 3-Hydroxy-3-methylglutaryl-coenzyme lyase deficiency Hyperornithinemia (gyrate atrophy of the choroid and retina) Hypervalinemia Isovalericacidemia Maple syrup urine disease (severe and intermittent types) Methylenetetrahydrofolate reductase deficiency Methylmalonic acidemia (vitamin B_{12}–responsive and vitamin B_{12}–nonresponsive types) Prolidase deficiency Propionic acidemia (ketotic hyperglycinemia) Saccharopinuria Sulfite oxidase deficiency
Miscellaneous	Acute intermittent porphyria Adenosine deaminase deficiency $Alpha_1$-antitrypsin deficiency Chronic granulomatous disease Congenital adrenal hyperplasia Contenital erythropoietic porphyria Congenital nephrotic syndrome Cystic fibrosis Hypophosphatasia Ichthyosis (X-linked type) (steroid sulfatase deficiency) Lesch-Nyhan syndrome Lysosomal acid phosphatase deficiency Menke's syndrome (kinky-hair syndrome) Orotic aciduria Xeroderma pigmentosum

(Adapted from Burton BK, Nadler HL. Antenatal diagnosis of metabolic disorders. Clin Obstet Gynaecol 1981;24:1041–54.)

this disorder have been developed in a number of communities in the United States and have led to the identification of couples at risk prior to the tragedy of having an affected child. The experience with Tay-Sachs disease may serve as a model for the implementation of carrier detection programs for other inborn errors of metabolism in selected high-risk populations.[21]

With relatively few exceptions (see Table 2), prenatal diagnosis is not possible in most X-linked recessive disorders. For those disorders not amenable to specific diagnosis, couples can elect prenatal sex determination with termination of all male fetuses, who would have a 50 per cent chance of being affected. Fetal sex should be determined on the basis of a karyotype from cultured amniotic fluid cells, not by the presence or absence of X chromatin or Y chromatin in fetal interphase cells.

Until recently, human genetic diagnosis has been necessarily indirect. Genetic alterations have been analyzable only through ascertaining secondary changes (e.g., abnormal gene products or phenotypes) resulting from the primary mutation. Newer methods applicable in certain mendelian disorders employ restriction endonucleases, enzymes that recognize and incise DNA strands at precisely defined short nucleotide sequences. DNA fragments from fetal cells may be examined for detection of a primary lesion or some associated disease marker (e.g., sickle cell disease, beta^0-thalassemia, hereditary persistence of fetal hemoglobin). Hopefully, with the discovery of more polymorphisms that can serve as markers for deleterious genes, the number of genetic diseases that are prenatally diagnosable will increase. The reader is referred to the recent review by Kurnit and associates[22] for additional details.

Polygenic/Multifactorial Disorders

Thus far, the disorders discussed in this chapter are the results of either chromosomal errors or single-gene mutations. However, these factors cannot explain every congenital abnormality, nor can they explain the heritability of normal anatomic and physiologic variations such as height. The recurrence risk of many anatomic anomalies indicates a heritable tendency. One explanation for a trait whose recurrence risk is 2 to 5 per cent is that the trait is influenced by the cumulative effects of several genes (polygenic) or possibly by their interaction with environmental factors (multifactorial). Because their recurrence risk is relatively low, most individuals with these disorders have no affected relatives. Examples of disorders inherited in polygenic/multifactorial fashion include cleft palate, certain cardiac defects, pyloric stenosis, talipes equinovarus, and neural tube defects.

Neural Tube Defects. Approximately 6,000 infants with neural tube defects (anencephaly and spina bifida) are born each year in the United States. The estimated incidence varies, from six to eight per 1,000 births in Northern Ireland to one to two per 1,000 births in the United States. Embryologically and genetically, spina bifida and anencephaly appear to be related, the etiology in both cases being failure of neural tube closure. Other neural tube anomalies include exencephaly and encephalocele. Hydrocephalus in the presence of spina bifida should be considered a secondary manifestation of the spinal defect; hydrocephalus without spina bifida is etiologically distinct. Anencephaly is incompatible with life; however, spina bifida is not and frequently results in hemiparesis, urinary incontinence, and sometimes hydrocephalus. It is important to establish a definitive diagnosis before offering recurrence risks. Although most neural tube defects are a consequence of polygenic/multifactorial inheritance, a few may be caused by single mutant genes (e.g., Meckel's syndrome, median cleft face syndrome), chromosomal abnormalities (e.g., trisomy 13, trisomy 18, triploidy), or teratogens (e.g., aminopterin, thalidomide).

The primary diagnostic test in pregnancies at risk for neural tube defects is analysis of amniotic fluid alpha-fetoprotein (AFP) concentration. AFP is the major serum protein during fetal life and is similar to albumin in size and amino acid composition. The concentration gradient between fetal serum and amniotic fluid AFP is about 100:1. If the fetal circulation communicates with the amniotic fluid, as in a neural tube defect, amniotic fluid levels of AFP are elevated. Abnormalities other than neural tube defects have been associated with elevated amniotic fluid AFP, including congenital nephrosis, duodenal atresia, fetal death, gastroschisis, omphalocele, nuchal cysts, severe Rh disease, and teratomas.

In reviewing publications reporting major experiences with the amniotic fluid AFP assay, Milunsky[23] calculated that the detection rates were approximately 98 per cent for anencephaly and 85 per cent for spina bifida. In about 10 per cent of cases of spina bifida the defect is closed (i.e., skin covers it), resulting in normal AFP values (false-negative results). False-positive results (AFP elevations) occur, although the most experienced laboratories report the phenomenon rarely (0.1 per cent). Many false-positive results can be explained by admixture of fetal blood and amniotic fluid. Because fetal blood levels of AFP are at least 100 times amniotic fluid AFP levels, even small amounts of contamination may raise amniotic fluid AFP values into the abnormal range. Accordingly, in cases in which the fluid is contaminated with fetal blood, measurement of amniotic fluid acetylcholinesterase is particularly useful.[24] Finally, another approach for the prenatal diagnosis of neural tube defects is ultrasonography. This technique can definitely exclude anencephaly before 20 weeks gestation, and a few investigators are capable of detecting spina bifida by ultrasound scanning of the vertebral column.[25]

Only about 10 per cent of neural tube defects occur in families with previously affected offspring. Therefore, a method to screen pregnant women to identify the other 90 per cent would be desirable, particularly in high-risk population areas such as Britain. After it was demonstrated that neural tube defects could be identified by maternal serum screening, a collaborative study was initiated in the United Kingdom.[26] This study demonstrated that between 16 and 18 weeks gestation, 88 per cent of fetuses with anencephaly and 79 per cent of fetuses with spina bifida can be identified by elevated maternal serum AFP level. However, a major problem with serum AFP level as a screening test for neural tube defects is the high rate of false-positive results, which occur in 1.7 to 7.8 per cent of all pregnant women. In addition to neural tube defects, maternal serum AFP values can be elevated in the following situations: underestimation of gestational age, multiple gestation, threatened abortion, fetal distress, Rh disease, ectopic pregnancy, preeclampsia, and fetal growth retardation. The number of amniocenteses required to detect a single neural tube defect will depend on the upper limits of normal selected by the laboratory, the detection efficiency of the assay, and the incidence of neural tube defects in the screened population. In the United States, 5 to 10 per cent of amniocenteses performed because of an unexplained maternal serum AFP elevation identify fetuses affected with neural tube defects. In the United States, mass screening of maternal serum AFP must await appropriate public and professional education regarding the goals and problems of such screening, and the availability of facilities for follow-up prenatal diagnosis and potential termination of affected pregnancies. Whether or not the diagnostic benefits justify the cost of serum AFP screening in this country is still controversial.

OTHER TECHNIQUES FOR PRENATAL DIAGNOSIS

Ultrasonography

Many mendelian disorders and most multifactorially inherited congenital abnormalities are not associated with biochemical or chromosomal abnormalities. In certain disorders, ultrasonography may be a useful means of prenatal diagnosis.

In addition to neural tube defects, hydrocephalus and certain renal anomalies can be diagnosed with ultrasound. Hydrocephalus is usually inherited in polygenic/multifactorial fashion, but X-linked recessive (aqueductal stenosis) and autosomal recessive (Dandy-Walker syndrome) forms exist. Prognosis based solely on head size, i.e., biparietal diameter, is not sufficiently sensitive, because an increase in biparietal diameter may not become evident until the late second or the third trimester; however, measurements of the lateral ventricles can identify some affected fetuses by 20 to 24 weeks gestation. Bilateral renal agenesis also usually has polygenic/multifactorial inheritance. The presence of fetal urine excludes bilateral, but not unilateral, renal agenesis; however, absence of urine does not necessarily identify an affected fetus, for the fetus may have recently voided.

Reports of other congenital abnormalities diagnosable via ultrasonography include skeletal dysplasias, certain cardiac anomalies, polycystic kidneys, omphalocele, urethral obstruction, and microcephaly.[25, 27] However, additional data are required to establish the sensitivity and specificity of ultrasonography in the prenatal diagnosis of various fetal malformations. Caution is particularly necessary before committing oneself to the clinical diagnosis of disorders that as yet are only theoretically detectable.

Radiography

Certain fetal abnormalities may be amenable to diagnosis by x-ray studies. Examples include the thrombocytopenia–absent radius (TAR) syndrome, the Ellis–van Creveld syndrome (on the basis of polydactyly), and certain short limb dysplasias such as achondroplasia. In the future, it is expected that most of these disorders may be consistently detectable by ultrasonography.

Fetoscopy

Fetoscopy may be defined as the transabdominal introduction of an instrument into the amniotic cavity to allow direct visualization of the fetus and sampling of fetal tissues, including blood and skin, for the prenatal diagnosis of certain genetic disorders. The overall rate of spontaneous abortion following fetoscopy is about 6 per cent, of perinatal loss about 1.5 per cent, and of prematurity about 8 per cent. Prenatal diagnosis of certain hemoglobinopathies (e.g., sickle cell disease, and beta-thalassemia) can be accomplished by analysis of fetal blood samples. Such diagnosis is feasible because reticulocytes of affected fetuses manifest effects of the mutant genes early in gestation, and heterozygotes can be accurately distinguished from homozygotes. Recent developments in molecular genetics now permit the diagnosis of some hemoglobinopathies using amniotic fluid fibroblasts rather than fetal blood (see earlier discussion). Other disorders that can be detected prenatally using fetal blood samples include hemophilia A (classic hemophilia), hemophilia B (Christmas disease), von Willebrand's disease, and chronic granulomatous disease. Initial reports suggested that fetal blood creatinine phosphokinase levels could be used for antenatal diagnosis of Duchenne muscular dystrophy; however, the reliability of this assay in distinguishing an affected from an unaffected fetus has subsequently proved to be unreliable. Fetoscopically directed fetal skin sampling has been utilized for the prenatal detection of hereditary skin diseases (genodermatoses) such as harlequin ichthyosis, epidermolytic hyperkeratosis, epidermolysis bullosa letalis, epidermolysis bullosa dystrophica, and albinism. Interested readers are referred to a recent review.[28]

REFERENCES

1. Nadler HL, Gerbie AB. Role of amniocentesis in the intrauterine detection of genetic disorders. N Engl J Med 1970;283:596–9.
2. Gerbie AB, Elias S. Amniocentesis for antenatal diagnosis of genetic defects. Clin Obstet Gynaecol 1980;7:5–12.
3. Elias S, Simpson JL. The role of ultrasonography in amniocentesis. In: Sabbagha RE, (ed.) Diagnostic ultrasound applied to obstetrics and gynecology. Hagerstown, Harper & Row, 1980; 165–77.
4. Elias S, Martin AO, Patel VA, Gerbie AB, Simpson JL. Analysis for amniotic fluid crystallization in second trimester amniocentesis. Am J Obstet Gynecol 1978;133:401–4.
5. Elias S, Gerbie AB, Simpson JL, Nadler HL, Sabbagha RE, Shkolnik A. Genetic amniocentesis in twin gestations. Am J Obstet Gynecol 1980;138:169–73.
6. Karp LE, Hayden PW. Fetal puncture during midtrimester amniocentesis. Obstet Gynecol 1977;49:115–7.
7. Gerbie AB, Nadler HL, Gerbie MV. Amniocentesis in genetic counseling. Safety and reliability in early pregnancy. Am J Obstet Gynecol 1971;109:765–8.
8. NICHD National Registry for Amniocentesis Study Group. Midtrimester amniocentesis for prenatal diagnosis. JAMA 1976;236:1471–6.
9. Simpson NE, Dallaire L, Miller J, et al. Prenatal diagnosis of genetic disease in Canada: report of a collaborative study. Can Med Assoc J 1976;115:739–48.
10. Report to the Medical Research Council by their Working Party on Amniocentesis. Br J Obstet and Gynaecol 1978;85 Suppl 2:1–41.
11. Hook EB, Chambers GC. Estimated rates of Down syndrome in live births by one year maternal age intervals for mothers aged 20–49 in a New York State study—implications of the risk figures for genetic counseling and cost-benefit analysis of prenatal diagnosis programs. Birth Defects 1977;13:123–41.
12. Hook EB, Linsjo A. Down syndrome in live births by single year maternal age interval in a Swedish study: comparison with results from a New York State study. Am J Hum Genet 1978;30:17–27.
13. Hook EB, Cross PK, Schreinemachers DM. Contemporary estimates of maternal age specific rates of Down's syndrome and trisomies in live births (in absence of selective abortions) using regression-smoothed rates from prenatal diagnosis studies adjusted for spontaneous fetal death after amniocentesis. Presented at the 1982 Annual Meeting, American Society of Human Genetics, Detroit, Sept 28–Oct 2, 1982.
14. Stene J, Fisher B, Stene E, Mikkelsen M, Petersen E. Paternal age in Down's syndrome. Ann Hum Genet 1977;40:299–306.
15. Matsunga E, Tonomura A, Oishi H, Kikuch Y. Reexamination of paternal age effect in Down's syndrome. Hum Genet 1978;40:259–68.
16. Stene J. Presentation at the Sixth International Congress of Human Genetics, Jerusalem, 1981.
17. Mikkelsen M, Stene J. Previous child with Down's syndrome and other chromosome aberrations. In: Prenatal diagnosis: proceedings 3rd European conference on prenatal diagnosis of genetic disorders. Stuttgart, Ferdinand Enke, 1979; 22–9.
18. Mikkelsen M. Down's syndrome: current state of cytogenetic research. Humangenetik 1971;12:1–28.
19. Simpson JL. Antenatal diagnosis of chromosomal disorders. Clin Obstet Gynaecol 1980;7:13–26.
20. Burton BK, Nadler HL. Antenatal diagnosis of metabolic disorders. Clin Obstet Gynaecol 1981;24:1041–54.
21. Kaback MM. Tay-Sachs disease: prenatal diagnosis and heterozygote screening, 1969–1976. Pediatr Res 1977;11:458.
22. Kurnit D, Orkin S, White R. Prenatal analysis of human DNA-sequence variation. In: Latt S, Darlington GJ, eds. Methods in cell biology. New York: Academic Press, 1982;311–30.
23. Milunksy A. Prenatal diagnosis of neural tube defects. In: Genetic disorders and the fetus. New York: Plenum Press, 1979;379–430.
24. Milunksy A, Blusztajn JK, Zeisel SH. Amniotic-fluid cholinesterase and neural-tube defects. Lancet 1979;2:36.
25. Sabbagha RE, Tamura RK, Dal Compo S. Antenatal ultrasonic diagnosis of genetic defects. Present status. Clin Obstet Gynaecol 1981;24:1103–20.
26. U.K. Collaborative Study of alpha-fetoprotein in relation to neural tube defects. Maternal serum alpha-fetoprotein measurement in antenatal screening for anencephaly and spina bifida in early pregnancy. Lancet 1977;1:1324.
27. Hobbins JC, Venus I, Mahoney MJ. Ultrasonography and fetoscopy in the prenatal detection of hereditary diseases. In: Kaback MM, ed. Genetic issues in pediatric and obstetric practice. Chicago: Year Book Medical Publishers, 1981; 517–24.
28. Elias S. Fetoscopy: Use in prenatal diagnosis. Clin Perinatol 1983;10:357–67.

PRIAPISM

JOHN A. BELIS

☐ SYNONYM: Persistent erection of the penis

BACKGROUND

Definition and Origin

Priapism is a persistent erection of the penis that may occur with or without prior sexual stimulation (Fig. 1). It is a complex disease with many causes, and determining the cause in individual cases is necessary for appropriate therapy.[1, 2] Because priapism is painful and often results in impotence, immediate therapy is necessary. Urination may be difficult, and urethral catheterization may be required.

The term priapism is derived from the name for the ancient Greco-Roman god of fertility and harvest, Priapus. Images of the god were made in the form of a crude pillar with a club, sickle, and an exaggerated phallic symbol. These images were placed in the gardens and fields to insure fertility and growth of the crops, flocks, and family.[3]

The first medical description of priapism was made by Tripe in 1845.[4] In a 1914 review of the condition, Hinman[5] discussed the fundamental observations of deGraff, who had demonstrated in 1668 that erection could be obtained in the cadaver by injecting water into the dorsal artery of the penis.

Physiology of Erection

Erection occurs by a complex neurovascular mechanism that may be initiated by local penile stimulation or by erotic stimulation through the central nervous system. Sensory fibers of the pudendal nerve transmit impulses to the sacral spinal cord after local stimulation of the penis. Subsequently, erection is produced by a reflex mechanism with impulses transmitted through the parasympathetic nerves originating from S2 through S4 (nervi erigentes). Erotic stimulation of the central nervous system produces erection through impulses traveling through the thoracolumbar sympathetic pathways and sacral parasympathetic fibers.

During erection the corpora cavernosa and the corpus spongiosum fill with blood from the branches of the internal pudendal artery (Figs. 2 and 3). The mechanism by which arterial inflow is maintained at a level exceeding venous outflow during erection and the mechanism of subsequent penile detumescence are incompletely understood.[6]

Pathophysiology of Priapism

A patient with priapism has complete erection in both corpora cavernosa, but the corpus spongiosum is not turgid as in a normal erection.[1] It has been postulated that when an erection is abnormally prolonged, the blood in the corpora cavernosa loses oxygen, accumulates carbon dioxide, and increases in viscosity. Venous outflow may be obstructed by cellular aggregation, edema, or inflammation, any of which may contribute to a prolonged erection.[1] A drug-induced or toxic influence on the neurovascular system may also produce erection by increasing arterial blood flow to the corpora cavernosa. If priapism lasts for more than a few days, fibrosis of the corpora cavernosa occurs, leading to impotence.

Incidence and Causes

Although priapism can usually be readily diagnosed, determination of its underlying cause can be difficult. Emergency management is needed to prevent the major sequela, impotence secondary to fibrosis. Priapism can occur in patients at any age, including newborns, but the highest incidence is in patients between 16 and 50 years old.[1]

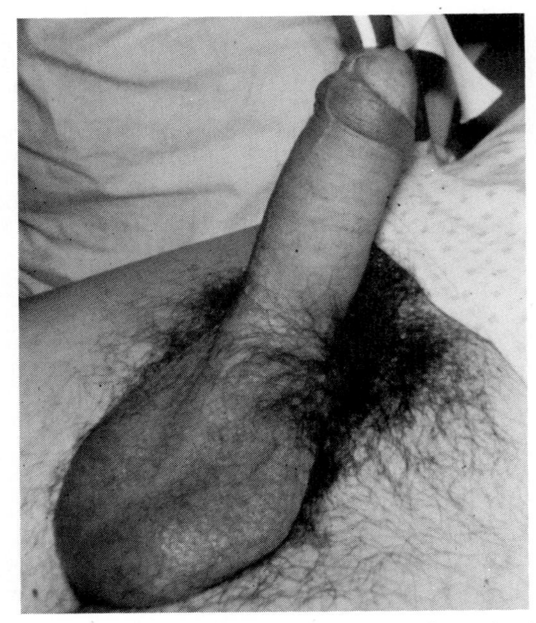

Figure 1. Appearance of priapism on physical examination.

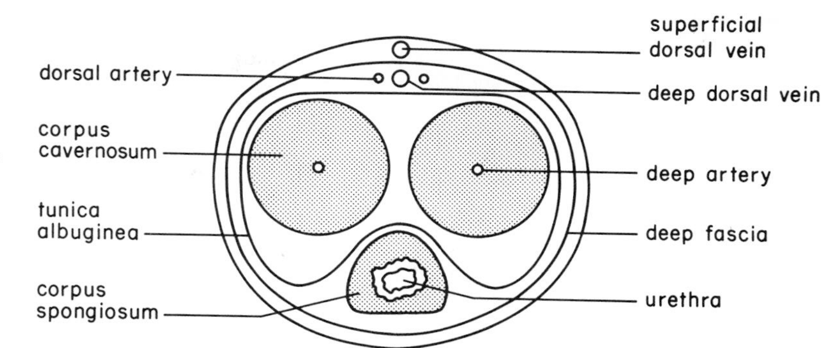

Figure 2. Transverse section of the penis showing arteries and veins.

The etiology varies in different age groups. Priapism is rare in children, in whom most cases are caused by sickle cell disease or leukemia.[1,2] The pathogenesis of priapism in sickle cell disease probably involves stagnation of blood during normal erection, which causes decreased oxygen tension with increased blood viscosity, leading to sickling of red blood cells with further stagnation. Children with sickle cell disease often have multiple episodes of priapism. Prolonged erection in leukemia can be caused by sludging of leukocytes, local infiltration, or impairment of venous flow by leukemic thrombosis.[1,2,7]

The cause of priapism in an adult may not be apparent, in which case it is classified as primary or idiopathic.[1,2] Priapism is secondary when an underlying condition can be shown to be directly or indirectly responsible for the prolonged erection.

The initial episode of priapism brings most patients to a physician, but in sickle cell disease, there may be a history of previous attacks of short duration.[8]

Conditions that have been associated with priapism are listed in Table 1. The majority of cases of secondary priapism can be classified into six major categories: neurogenic, toxic (including drug-induced), traumatic, hematologic, inflammatory, and neoplastic.

Neurogenic Causes

Lesions that effect neural pathways involved in the psychogenic and reflexogenic mechanisms of erection may be involved pathophysiologically in the development of priapism.

Direct central nervous system stimulation may also cause priapism. The disorder has been reported to occur in spinal cord tumors, injuries, and compression, vertebral tuberculosis, cauda equina compression,[9] multiple sclerosis, tabes dorsalis, damage to the cerebral hemispheres, encephalitis, and meningitis.[2]

Toxic or Chemical Exposure

An increasing number of drugs have been reported to induce priapism. Any drug that effects the central nervous system or neurovascular system may induce priapism. Drugs may account for as many as 25 per cent of new cases.[1] Most prominent are phenothiazines, antihypertensive agents, anticoagulants, marijuana, and alcohol.[1,2] Priapism has also been reported in association with ingestion of androgens, tetanus antitoxin,[3] adrenal steroids, methaqualone, and tolbutamide.[10]

Specific toxic agents that have been reported to be associated with priapism include cantharides,

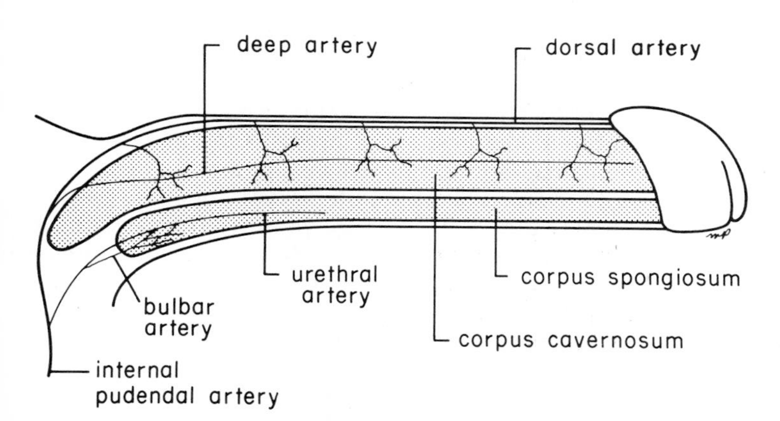

Figure 3. Longitudinal section of the penis showing arterial blood supply.

Table 1. CONDITIONS ASSOCIATED WITH PRIAPISM

Neurogenic disorders	Trauma to the brain or spinal cord Tumor of the brain or spinal cord Multiple sclerosis Tabes dorsalis Encephalitis Meningitis Compression of the spinal cord or cauda equina Vertebral tuberculosis
Toxic or chemical exposure	Drugs Antihypertensives Anticoagulants Phenothiazines Hormones Adrenal steroids Tolbutamide Tetanus antitoxin Methaqualone Alcohol Marijuana Poisons Aphrodisiac mixtures, including cantharides, yohimbine, and turpentine Carbon monoxide Carbon dioxide Lead Strychnine Red scorpion sting Black widow spider bite
Trauma	Excessive sexual activity External trauma to the penis, perineum, or scrotum Pelvic and retroperitoneal hemorrhage, including aneurysm Genital thrombophlebitis from local trauma
Hematologic conditions	Sickle cell disease or trait Leukemia Coagulopathy Multiple myeloma Anticoagulation during hemodialysis or filtration leukapheresis Primary thrombocythemia Hyperfibrinogenemia
Inflammatory disorders	Periurethral abscess Appendicitis Prostatitis Pelvic thrombophlebitis Syphilis Mumps Typhoid fever Rabies Rocky Mountain spotted fever Tularemia
Neoplasms	Primary carcinoma of the penis or urethra Obstruction of venous drainage or corpora cavernosa by tumor Metastatic tumor Extension of prostatic, bladder, or rectal neoplasm
Idiopathic priapism	

yohimbine, turpentine, lead, carbon monoxide, carbon dioxide, strychnine, and muscarine.[2] Priapism had also occurred during the reactions to toxins from red scorpion stings[11] and black widow spider bites.[12]

Trauma

Trauma to the penis in patients of all ages accounts for 5 per cent of the cases of priapism.[10] Hemorrhage or hematoma after trauma to the perineum or urethra or direct injury to the penis or scrotum may produce thrombosis of veins, leading to priapism. Pelvic and retroperitoneal hemorrhages with venous obstruction have also been known to cause persistent erections.[3] The percentage of cases caused by trauma would be larger if excessive sexual activity were included.[1]

Hematologic Conditions

Approximately 30 per cent of all cases of priapism are due to various hematologic conditions.[10] Several pathologic processes that may affect blood viscosity apparently are responsible, such as sickle cell disease, primary thrombocythemia, anticoagulant therapy, coagulopathy, hyperfibrinogenemia, leukemia, and multiple myeloma.[1, 2, 10, 13–15] Priapism has also been reported during hemodialysis and filtration leukapheresis.[15, 16] Heparin is administered during both procedures, which have also been associated with enhanced granulocyte adhesion and aggregation.

Most hematologic causes of priapism are due to sickle cell disease or sickle cell trait in black patients. Physiologic erections apparently result in increased consumption of oxygen and increased carbon dioxide content of blood in the cavernous sinuses accompanied by increased blood viscosity. These events cause sickling of red blood cells, which is believed to lead to obstruction of the venous outflow from the corpora cavernosa and development of priapism.

Sickle cell disease has been reported to account for 50 per cent of priapism cases in blacks. More than 60 per cent of affected patients are children.[10] A report of Jamaican patients with homozygous sickle cell disease demonstrated a 42 per cent incidence rate, with a median age at onset of 21 years.[13] This study isolated two predominantly different patterns of priapism. One group of patients had short episodes lasting less than 3 hours, with normal subsequent sexual function, and a second group had severe prolonged attacks usually lasting more than 24 hours and commonly followed by impotence. Most patients who had a major attack had previous episodes of short attacks. Seventy-five percent of attacks occurred between midnight and 6:00 a.m. The relative dehydration and metabolic acidosis existing during sleep may contribute to sickling of erythrocytes in the corpora cavernosa, which impairs venous drainage and may cause a physiologic spontaneous nocturnal erection to develop into an attack of priapism.

Priapism occurring in patients with primary thrombocythemia is possibly caused by platelet sludging in the corpora cavernosa, analogous to erythrocyte sludging in sickle cell disease and white blood cell sludging in leukemia. Ongoing thrombogenesis has been demonstrated in the corpora cavernosa in this condition.[14]

Whereas priapism has been described in association with anticoagulant therapy, a direct cause-and-effect relationship has not been established. The mechanism by which anticoagulants may contribute to priapism is incompletely understood but has been attributed to possible intermittent hypercoagulability or to heparin-dependent antiplatelet antibodies with immunologically induced platelet aggregation.[16] The development of priapism during hemodialysis or filtration leukapheresis suggests that anticoagulation may indeed rarely play a role.[3, 16] It has been postulated that inadequate heparinization with a subsequent rebound hypercoagulability may be the predisposing factor in these patients.[16, 17]

In patients with leukemia, priapism most likely occurs as a result of leukostasis, although leukemic infiltration of the corpora cavernosa and dorsal veins of the penis has also been reported. In 5 per cent of adults and 18 per cent of children with priapism, leukemia has been found to be the cause.[10]

Inflammatory Disorders

Priapism has been associated with several inflammatory conditions, including prostatitis, appendicitis, and periurethral abscess, causing local suppuration leading to genital thrombophlebitis. Systemic inflammatory disease such as tularemia, typhoid fever, rabies, and Rocky Mountain spotted fever have been associated with priapism, possibly on the basis of pelvic thrombophlebitis.[1, 2, 15] Other infectious diseases causing priapism include syphilis and mumps.[2]

Neoplasms

Primary carcinoma of the penis and urethra and metastatic tumors to the pelvis, perineum, or external genitalia may be responsible for priapism through infiltration and subsequent obstruction of venous drainage of the corpora cavernosa. Infiltration of the penis by other materials may produce obstruction in a similar fashion. These include amyloid[15, 18] and glycosphingolipids, which may be deposited in tissues in Fabry's disease.[3]

Idiopathic Priapism

In approximately 50 per cent of all patients, a cause of priapism cannot be determined. Most of these patients give a history of sexual activity, in many instances excessive, prior to the onset of priapism. Trauma may be important in this group. Many patients do not reveal all contributing factors, particularly use of drugs, and therefore the idiopathic category tends to be large.[1]

HISTORY

Although the diagnosis of priapism is not difficult, a careful history is important to determine the probable cause.

Subjective Data

History of the Present Illness. The time of onset of the attack of priapism should be recorded, along with descriptions of previous (prodromal) episodes of priapism that were short in duration.[13, 14] The patient with a prodromal history should be questioned about having some degree of impotence, which occurs in more than 25 per cent of patients who have had short episodes.[13] If a patient has had short episodes, how long were they, and how often did they occur? For how long have the prodromal episodes been happening? What activities precipitated or relieved them? What precipitated the present episode? It should be determined whether the patient has had prolonged sexual activity or trauma to the penis prior to the onset of the current attack of priapism.

Information should be obtained regarding the patient's mental and psychiatric status. The patient should be questioned regarding pain on intercourse or difficulty with urination since the onset of priapism.

The evaluation should include a medication history and a search for specific diseases or possible etiologic factors. The questions would cover use of any drugs or medications, including alcohol. Have there been recent infections in the abdomen, pelvis, or genital area? Has the patient had unexplained sweats, chills, or fever? Has there been exposure to toxins such as carbon monoxide or insect venom at work or at home?

Family History. The family history may be important in blacks, in whom there is a higher incidence of sickle cell disease or trait. Other questions should focus upon recent febrile illnesses in the family, neurologic diseases, drug abuse, and Fabry's disease.

Social and Occupational History. What is the patient's job and what exposures to chemical toxins does the patient encounter? What are the patient's habits regarding sexual activity?

Drug History. The history of drug use may be valuable in determining a possible cause for priapism. Questions should be asked about antihypertensives, phenothiazines, antidepressants, anticoagulants, adrenal steroids, and hormones. The drug history should also include the patient's use of alcohol and marijuana.

Previous Medical History. Have there been previous episodes of priapism that were of short duration? Has the patient ever suffered any injury in the area of the external genitalia and perineum? Has he had tuberculosis, syphilis, hematologic disorders, or cancer?

General History. Other questions that may help to determine the etiology of priapism should focus on complaints of neurologic deficits, including numbness, weakness, or pain in the legs and difficulty with bowel or bladder control.

High-Payoff Queries

1. *Do you have numbness, weakness or pain in your legs?* Neurologic deficits may reflect disease processes in the brain and spinal cord that may effect the neurogenic mechanism of erection, resulting in priapism.

2. *Have you had any sweats, chills, or fever?* A careful history may reveal exposure to tularemia, tuberculosis, or Rocky Mountain spotted fever. These symptoms may also reflect inflammatory conditions in the abdomen, pelvis, perineum, or external genitalia that may be associated with priapism.

3. *Have you had pain or burning on urination?* The patient may have bladder calculi, prostatitis, or periurethral abscess. In addition to inflammatory changes that may be associated with these conditions, there may be an irritative effect on the neurovascular mechanism of penile erection.

4. *Have you been exposed to toxic chemicals at home or work?* One should not overlook use of insecticides or herbicides around the home.

5. *Have you injured your genitals, hips, or rectal area?* This consideration should also include episodes of trauma that occurred long before the present episode of priapism and may have led to fibrosis in the corpora cavernosa or thrombosis of pelvic veins. A history of prolonged or vigorous intercourse may also be a traumatic etiology for priapism.

6. *Do you or does anyone in your family have sickle cell disease or other blood disease?* In as many as 40 per cent of black male patients, sickle cell disease is the cause of priapism.[1]

7. *Have you ever had cancer?* Metastatic deposits in the pelvis, perineum, or penis may cause obstruction of venous drainage.

8. *What prescribed or over-the-counter drugs have you taken?* An association between drugs and priapism is being elicited with increasing frequency and may be responsible for the large number of patients whose disease was previously categorized as idiopathic.

9. *Have you recently drunk alcohol or used marijuana?* There is increasing evidence for use of social drugs in the etiology of priapism.[1]

10. *Have you had sexual fantasies or a lot of erotic stimulation lately?* Aberrant mental states may result in autoeroticism and priapism.[2]

PHYSICAL EXAMINATION

Physical examination should include examination of the penis and general examination for specific physical findings that may be related to the diagnosis of priapism.

Temperature. Unexplained fever has been noted in 60 per cent of patients with priapism.[10]

Penis. In most cases of priapism turgor is noted only in the corpora cavernosa and not in the corpus spongiosum and glans penis.[1] The examination may also reveal the occasional rare case of partial priapism.[19, 20] There may be evidence of primary or secondary neoplasms in the area of the penis and perineum.

Abdomen. Evaluation for abdominal or pelvic masses, including aortic and iliac aneurysms, should be performed. One should carefully note signs of venous obstruction with collateral venous drainage on the abdominal wall.

Rectum and Prostate. The consistency, size, and tenderness of the prostate should be noted. The quality of the rectal sphincter tone and the presence or absence of a bulbocavernosus reflex should be determined.

Neurologic Status. The extent of this examination will depend on the neurologic history, but examination of the lower extremities, perineum, and external genitalia should be complete. Important factors include sensory examination, determination of motor strength, and reflex changes. Vibratory sensation, proprioception, and temperature perception should be checked. A straight leg raising test should be performed. Abnormal findings should also be sought in the perineal and perianal areas.

Lower Extremities. An evaluation should include peripheral vascular pulses in the lower extremities and signs of thrombophlebitis or leg edema, which may reflect venous occlusion.

DIAGNOSTIC STUDIES

Laboratory Studies

The laboratory evaluation can be used to determine causes of secondary priapism. The white blood count and platelet count may reveal leukemia or primary thrombocythemia. The erythrocyte sedimentation rate may reflect underlying inflammatory, toxic, or neoplastic conditions.

Blood chemistry studies and a serologic test for syphilis should be performed. If the patient has received anticoagulants or is suspected of having a bleeding disorder, specific coagulation studies should be performed.

Special assays for drugs may be ordered if there is suspicion of drug use or abuse contributing to the development of priapism.

A urinalysis should be done to check for possible urinary tract infection, including prostatitis.

A sickle cell smear and hemoglobin electrophoresis should be performed in blacks with priapism because of the high incidence of sickle cell disease in such patients. Comparison of hematologic indices in patients with sickle cell disease with or without history of priapism indicates a lower average hemoglobin F level in the priapism group.[13]

Imaging

A chest x-ray should be obtained to look for primary or metastatic tumors, inflammatory diseases including tuberculosis, and changes caused by toxic chemicals that may affect the lungs.

Lumbar spine x-rays and myelography may be indicated if the patient's history and physical findings suggest a neurogenic cause.

Additional x-rays, radionuclide scans, CT-scans, and ultrasound studies may be obtained as indicated by results of the history and physical examination and the preliminary laboratory tests. These studies should focus upon specific neurologic, neoplastic, or inflammatory diseases.

^{125}I-fibrinogen scanning has been used to detect ongoing thrombogenesis in the corpora cavernosa in patients with primary thrombocythemia. This technique can differentiate between blood clot and fibrosis in the corpora cavernosa.[14] Although acute priapism requires emergency treatment that should not be delayed for ^{125}I-fibrinogen scanning, cases of priapism of several days' duration may benefit from this information in the selection of therapy.[14]

ASSESSMENT

Constellations of Findings

The following findings characterize the most common causes for priapism. Significant findings are printed in italics.

Neurogenic Conditions. Central nervous system or peripheral nervous system diseases may contribute to the development of priapism. They may produce abnormal neurologic findings by affecting neural pathways involved in the psychogenic or reflexogenic mechanisms of erection. The patient may have *back pain, leg pain, numbness or weakness* of the legs, or *changes in voiding* or *bowel habits.* Symptoms referable to the central nervous system may be present if the cause of priapism is a neurologic intracranial process.

Toxic or Chemical Exposure. If priapism has been caused by a poison, the patient may have other associated symptoms, such as *headache, malaise, dizziness, syncope, nausea, vomiting, abdominal pain, cough,* or *hemoptysis.* There may be no significant side effects other than priapism if the patient is taking phenothiazines or antihypertensive agents in recommended doses. History and physical examination may yield evidence of *illicit drug use* or *excessive alcohol ingestion.*

Trauma. There is often a history of vigorous, *prolonged sexual activity.* The patient may have an *aberrant mental state* with fantasy syndromes and unusual sexual behavior. There may be physical findings of *trauma to the genitalia* or perineum with hemorrhage or hematoma formation.

Hematologic Conditions. A patient in this category may have a *history of intermittent episodes of priapism* of short duration often occurring at night or of *sickle cell crises. Fever* or *sore throat* may be associated with *leukemia.* Specific laboratory evaluation for sickle cell disease or leukemia will lead to diagnosis in the majority of patients with a hematologic cause for priapism.

Inflammatory Disorders. This group of patients may have *fever, sweats,* or *chills.* There may be signs and symptoms of *abdominal, pelvic,* or *external genital infection.* There may be symptoms of *urinary tract infection* or *prostatitis,* including *urinary frequency, dysuria, perineal pain,* and *pain on intercourse.* Urinary infection may be confirmed by urinalysis and urine culture.

The chest x-ray may reveal inflammatory diseases such as tuberculosis. The patient may have been hunting or traveling in areas of endemic infectious diseases. Syphilis may be suggested by history and physical findings and confirmed by serologic tests. The white blood cell and differential blood cell counts and the erythrocyte sedimentation rate may reflect the presence of an inflammatory process of either bacterial or viral etiology.

Neoplasms. The patient may have had a malignancy and may now have metastases. Examination of the perineum and external genitalia may demonstrate *primary* or *metastatic neoplasms* obstructing the venous drainage from the corpora cavernosa. Examination of lymph node–bearing areas and the abdomen may suggest neoplastic disease.

Primary or metastatic tumor may appear on chest x-ray. Blood chemistry evaluations may show hepatic or renal involvement by neoplasm. A genitourinary tumor may cause *microhematuria* to appear on urinalysis. A tumor of the central or peripheral nervous system may be found by CT scan.

Idiopathic Priapism. Although this category accounts for about one-half of all cases of priapism, a diligent history, physical examination, and laboratory evaluation should focus upon *excessive sexual activity, unrevealed trauma,* or *unrevealed drug usage.*

Implications of Priapism

Identifying the underlying cause of priapism can pose considerable diagnostic difficulty for the physician. The disorder itself should be managed as an emergency because of the subsequent development of impotence in patients who are untreated or whose priapism is unresponsive to treatment.

Determination of the etiology of priapism may contribute to the selection of therapy. A diagnosis of leukemia or primary solid neoplasm will require evaluation and therapy. Inflammatory causes may evolve into further serious complications, including sepsis and shock, if not properly diagnosed and treated.

Therefore, priapism itself needs to be treated, but it may also be a symptom of an underlying disease process of significant magnitude. Using the evaluation outlined in this discussion, the physician should be able to differentiate among the conditions that may be associated with priapism.

REFERENCES

1. Winter CC. Priapism. Urol Survey 1978;28:163–6.
2. Becker LE, Mitchell AD. Priapism. Surg Clin North Am 1965;45:1523–34.
3. Stein JJ, Martin DC. Priapism. Urology 1974;3:8–14.
4. Tripe JW. Priapism. Lancet 1845;1:8–13.
5. Himan F. Priapism. Report of cases and a clinical study of the literature with reference to pathogenesis and surgical treatment. Ann Surg 1914;60:689–716.
6. Krane RJ, Siroky MB. Neurophysiology of erection. Urol Clin North Am 1981;8:91–102.
7. Amlie RN, Bourgeois B, Huxtable RF. Priapism in preterm infant. Urology 1977;9:558–9.
8. Ihekwaba FN, Lawani J. Caverno-saphenous shunt in the treatment of priapism. Postgrad Med J 1981;57:132–5.
9. Ravindran M. Cauda-equina compression presenting as spontaneous priapism. J Neurol Neurosurg Pysch 1979;42:280–2.
10. Nelson JH, Winter CC. Priapism: evolution of management in 48 patients in a 22-year series. J Urol 1977;117:455–8.
11. Bawasker HS. Diagnostic cardiac premonitory signs and symptoms of red scorpion sting. Lancet 1982;1:552–4.
12. Stiles AD. Priapism following a black widow spider bite. Clin Pediatr 1982;21:174–5.
13. Emond AM, Hulman R, Serjant GR. Priapism and impotence in homozygous sickle cell disease. Arch Intern Med 1980;140:1434–7.
14. Welford C, Spies SM, Green D. Priapism in primary thrombocythemia. Arch Intern Med 1981;141:807–8.
15. Wasmer JM, Carrion HM, Mekras G, Politano VA. Evaluation and treatment of priapism. J Urol 1981;125:204–7.
16. Dahlke MB, Shah SL, Sherwood WC, Shafer AW, Brownstein PK. Priapism during filtration leukapheresis. Transfusion 1979;19:482–6.
17. Port FK, Hecking E, Fiegel P, Kohler H, Distler A. Priapism during regular haemodialysis. Lancet 1974;2:1287–8.
18. Lapan DI, Graham AR, Bangert JL, Boyer JT, Conner WT. Amyloidosis presenting as priapism. Urology 1980;15:167–70.
19. Llado J, Peterson LJ, Fair WR. Priapism of the proximal penis. J Urol 1980;123:779–80.
20. Johnson GR, Corriere JN Jr. Partial priapism. J Urol 1980;124:147–8.

PRURITUS, GENERALIZED

BARBARA A. GILCHREST

☐ SYNONYM: Itching

BACKGROUND

Definition

Itching is a sensation perceived only in the skin that by definition is unpleasant and provokes an urge to scratch. It may be "sharp" and well-localized (epicritic) or "burning" and poorly localized (protopathic). Many different stimuli and almost certainly different mechanisms are responsible.

Pathophysiology

Cutaneous nerves form a finely arborizing network just immediately below the epidermis. Nerves may terminate in tapered or slighly bulbous unmyelinated fibers or in very intricate encapsuled sensory receptors. It is currently believed that none of the endings is uniquely adapted to itch perception, but rather that the spatial and temporal pattern of neural excitation determines whether itch, pain, touch, or pressure is registered centrally. From the skin, itch impulses are conducted primarily by myelinated fibers 5 to 10 μ in diameter to the ipsilatreal dorsal root ganglia, immediately cross over to the opposite anterolateral spinothalmic tract, continue to the thalamus, and then travel via the internal capsule to the sensory cortex. There, factors such as anxiety or boredom, mental distraction, and competing cutaneous sensations may magnify or reduce the perceived pruritus.

Pruritus shares many features and pathways with pain but is unequivocably a separate sensation with its own precipitants, blockers, and potentiators and a full range of severity.

The cutaneous mediators of pruritus are unknown in all but a few experimental systems. "Itch powder," or cowhage, which is made from spicules of the plant *Mucuna pruriens*, contains an endopeptidase, mucunain, that is extremely pruritogenic for human skin. Trypsin, papain, epidermal protease, and a number of other endopeptidases as well as kallikrein have also been reported to induce itching, leading many investigators to conclude that proteases released from keratinocytes or leukocytes during inflammation may be directly responsible for the pruritus so frequently seen in various dermatoses. In this regard, it is interesting that many systemic disorders associated with generalized pruritus, such as chronic renal failure, biliary cirrhosis, and hyperthyroidism, are also charactreized by hyperpigmentation, and that proteases themselves can induce melanin production. Intradermal injection of histamine, normally present in mast cells throughout the dermis, consistently produces itching, and antihistamines successfully block this form of experimental pruritus. The mechanism appears to be a direct effect of histamine on cutaneous nerves. Despite direct and indirect evidence implicating histamine in the pathogenesis of pruritus, however, antihistamines are minimally effective in most pruritic diseases, suggesting that histamine is not the only clinically relevant mediator of pruritus.

Substance P is a peptide previously implicated in pain sensation and detectable both in the central nervous system and in peripheral nerves, including those in the skin. Intracutaneous injection of substance P in concentrations as low as 10^{-6} molar has been found to evoke itching in human subjects. The reaction appears to be mediated through histamine, because it is inhibited by prior administration of an antihistamine and by local histamine depletion with compound 48/80, a mast cell degranulator. Whether substance P is responsible for the pruritus associated with any clinical disease state remains to be determined.

Intravenous administration of the opiate antagonist naloxone has been found to block pruritus induced by either intrathecal injection of opiates[2] or intradermal injection of histamine[3] and to temporarily abolish otherwise intractable pruritus in a patient with primary biliary cirrhosis.[4] These observations suggest that opiate receptors in the central nervous system and possibly the naturally occurring endorphins or enkephalins mediate at least some forms of pruritus.

Prostaglandins of the E series, believed to be generated in the course of many inflammatory dermatoses, are not themselves pruritogenic but can potentiate itch due to other factors. Less well-defined factors—such as heating or vasodilation, "dehydration," proximity to another itchy focus, and previous inflammation of the target area—may also increase the pruritus perceived after a standardized stimulus.

Incidence and Causes

Pruritus is the most common symptom of dermatologic disease and is second only to disfigurement as a source of distress to patients. Moreover, many patients presenting solely because of pruri-

Table 1. SYSTEMIC DISORDERS ASSOCIATED WITH PRURITUS

Renal	Chronic renal failure
Hepatic	Primary biliary cirrhosis Cholestasis of pregnancy Extrahepatic biliary obstruction Hepatitis Drug ingestion
Hematopoietic	Polycythemia vera Hodgkin's disease Other lymphomas and leukemias Multiple myeloma Mastocytosis Iron deficiency anemia
Endocrine	Hyperthyroidism Carcinoid syndrome Diabetes mellitus
Miscellaneous	Visceral malignancies Neurologic syndromes Opiate ingestion Drug allergy or toxicity Psychosis Parasitic infestations Advanced age

(Reproduced with permission from Gilchrest BA. Pruritus: pathogenesis, therapy and significance in systemic disease states. Arch Intern Med 1982;142:101–5. Copyright 1982, American Medical Association.)

tus in fact have an eruption that is responsible for the symptom, although its other manifestations may be so subtle that the patient and even the physician do not notice the rash.[5, 6] Because they are readily treatable or preventable, rashes should be carefully sought before undertaking the evaluation and therapy of generalized pruritus.

Table 1 lists the systemic disorders associated with generalized pruritus. Among all patients seeking medical attention for pruritus, the prevalence of underlying systemic disease has been reported as 10 to 50 per cent, the percentage depending on patient selection, diagnostic evaluation, and period of follow-up.[5–8]

Chronic Renal Failure

Numerically, perhaps the most important known cause of persistent generalized pruritus is chronic renal failure. Since the inception of maintenance hemodialysis in the 1960s, survival of uremic patients has greatly increased, and currently more than 60,000 Americans undergo maintenance hemodialysis.[9] Fifty years ago, pruritus was estimated to affect 10 to 30 per cent of uremics.[1] Two small surveys in the early 1970s suggested a prevalence of 80 to 90 per cent, but a more recent analysis based on the responses of patients at four dialysis centers yielded a point prevalence of 37 per cent and a cumulative prevalence of 77 per cent for "prolonged bothersome itchiness" in this population.[10] Patient age, sex, and duration of participation in the dialysis program had no influence on these figures.

Hyperparathyroidism has been suggested as the abnormality in uremia responsible for pruritus, because hyperparathyroidism may result in elevated serum histamine levels[11] and because subtotal parathyroidectomy often produces dramatic, if temporary relief from itching.[1] In addition, mast cell hyperplasia, another possible source of histamine, has been reported in the skin and other organs of uremic patients. However, the ineffectiveness of antihistamines, both H_1 and H_2 blockers, in the treatment of uremic pruritus has led other investigators to implicate endopeptidases or kinins, pruritogenic substances that may accumulate in uremia. A circulating mediator is suggested by the finding that phototherapy restricted to half the body decreases pruritus evenly over the entire surface and by the apparent effectiveness of both oral cholestyramine[1] and oral charcoal[12] in some patients. Peripheral neuropathy has also been proposed as the mechanism for uremic pruritus.

Hepatic Cholestasis

Pruritus is probably the most distressing and consistent symptom of chronic cholestasis, which underlies all the hepatic disorders listed in Table 1. Overall, pruritus occurs in approximately 20 to 25 per cent of jaundiced patients[11] but is rare in those who do not have cholestasis.

Pruritus affects virtually 100 per cent of patients with primary biliary cirrhosis and is the presenting symptom in nearly 50 per cent.[11, 13] Generalized pruritus occurs in one per 500 to one per 300,000 pregnancies in some studies, but in as many as 1.5 to 3 per cent in others, apparently varying with different seleciton criteria.[1] It is most common in the third trimester and does not necessarily affect all pregnancies of predisposed women. In one report of 42 cases of obstetric cholestasis, 15 patients had pruritus only; the remainder were also juandiced, although pruritus preceded the jaundice in most of these cases.[14] Pruritus secondary to cholestasis may also occur in users of oral contraceptives, with symptoms appearing during the first menstrual cycle for 50 per cent of affected women and within six cycles for 90 per cent.[15] There is a single case report of a woman who repeatedly experienced pruritus premenstrually as well as during two pregnancies.[1]

Extrahepatic biliary obstruction of any etiology is often associated with pruritus. For example, in one series of 38 patients with carcinoma of the ampulla of Vater, 19 presented with pruritus.[16] Generalized pruritus has also been reported in patients with cholestasis due to viral or syphilitic hepatitis and ulcerative colitis.[1] Drugs that can cause pruritus by inducing cholestasis include phenothiazines, tolbutamide, erythromycin, and anabolic hormones as well as estrogens and progestins, as mentioned.

The pruritus associated with cholestasis almost certainly is related to the accumulation of bile salts. Evidence in favor of this hypothesis includes the unquestioned efficacy of treatments directed toward removal of bile acids from the body. The best documentation derives from the oral administration of the anion exchange resin cholestyramine, but plasma perfusion with charcoal-coated glass beads has also been reported to relieve pruritus due to cholestasis.[1] Early studies suggested a close correlation of severity of pruritus with total bile salt content of the skin and a lesser correlation with serum concentration. More recently, however, two well-controlled investigations of patients with partial biliary obstruction, some with and some without pruritus, revealed no correlation between severity of pruritus and concentration of bile salts in the serum, skin, or stratum corneum.[17, 18] Both total and individual bile salt concentrations were measured. In support of their findings, both groups of authors noted that pruritus is common in extrahepatic biliary obstruction, which causes relatively little elevation of bile salts, and rare in the blind loop syndrome, which often causes far greater elevations. Furthermore, cholestyramine has also been reported to relieve the pruritus associated with polycythemia vera and uremia, conditions without marked elevations of bile salts, whereas androgens, which are often useful in the treatment of pruritus due to biliary obstruction, actually increase serum levels of bile salts. The authors of these studies conclude that pruritus cannot be due directly to bile salts in any body compartment but may be mediated through proteases, which are known to be liberated in the skin by bile salts.

Hematopoietic Disorders

A number of apparently unrelated hematopoietic malignancies are associated with generalized pruritus. Approximately 50 per cent of patients with polycythemia vera experience pruritus that is classically exacerbated by hot baths,[19] and up to 30 per cent of patients with Hodgkin's disease are also affected.[20] The incidence of pruritus in other lymphomas and leukemia is unknown,[17] but the occasional association cannot be disputed.[1] Generalized pruritus has been reported as a presenting symptom in two patients with multiple myeloma and in one with Waldenström's macroglobulinemia as well as in several with benign gammopathies.[1] Systemic mastocytosis may also be associated with generalized pruritus in the absence of clinical skin lesions; the pruritus in this instance is presumably due to histamine release from dermal mast cells. Finally, iron deficiency anemia has been reported to cause generalized pruritus in more than 90 patients[1] and was strongly implicated as the proximate cause in all of six symptomatic patients with polycythemia vera.[21]

Histamine has been suggested as the mediator for pruritus associated with lymphoproliferative diseases. The compound is normally released from circulating basophils, which are often numerous in these disorders, and the activity of histidine decarboxylase, the enzyme responsible for production of histamine, is commonly elevated in the abnormal cells. Circulating histamine levels in polycythemia vera, for example, may reach five times the normal value, although not all patients with elevated histamine levels experience pruritus. Leukopeptidases, also released from abnormal lymphocytes and granulocytes, are a second candidate.

Endocrine Disorders

Generalized pruritus is said to occur in 4 to 11 per cent of patients with thyrotoxicosis, especially Graves' disease, and is probably more common in patients with long-standing untreated disease.[22] Increased kinin activity in the presence of a slightly elevated skin temperature (itself known to reduce the itch threshold) has been postulated to induce pruritus in these patients. The pruritus occasionally associated with hypothyroidism appears to be due to accompanying xerosis rather than the endocrine disorder itself.[1]

Diabetes mellitus is a frequently quoted but poorly documented cause of generalized pruritus; the least anecdotal data derive from a survey of 500 patients in 1927, approximately 3 per cent of whom reported generalized pruritus at some time after diagnosis of their diabetes.[23] There are no recent publications on the subject. In contrast, pruritus vulvae and pruritus ani secondary to *Candida albicans* infections are indisputably common among diabetics.

Generalized pruritus has been reported rarely as a manifestation of carcinoid syndrome. Tumor cell release of histamine or kallikrein, which later releases bradykinin, may be responsible for the discomfort in these patients.[1] As in thyrotoxicosis, peripheral vasodilation may decrease the threshold for perception of pruritus.

Miscellaneous Disorders

Generalized pruritus may occur in association with adenocarcinoma and squamous cell carcinomas of many viscera.[5] Advanced brain tumors are characteristically responsible for pruritus restricted to the nostrils.[1] There is a single case report of severe paroxysmal itching in a patient with multiple sclerosis, and pruritus in a dermatomal distribution may rarely result from herpes zoster in a manner analogous to postherpetic neuralgia.[1]

Opiate ingestion can provoke generalized pruritus via a central mechanism or peripherally by degranulation of mast cells, and pruritus is a presenting complaint of many heroin addicts.[24] Other drugs may rarely cause pruritus without a rash as a manifestation of allergic sensitization.[1, 5] Methoxsalen photochemotherapy (PUVA) produces intense localized or generalized pruritus in nearly 15 per cent of regularly treated patients,[1] probably by a toxic rather than immunologic mechanism.

Psychotic individuals occasionally suffer from severe generalized pruritus for which no etiology is apparent. Many of these patients have delusions of parasitosis.

Intestinal, pulmonary, and systemic parasitosis may produce generalized pruritus, presumably as a manifestation of allergic sensitization of the host to the organism.

Finally, many elderly individuals experience generalized pruritus. For some, xerosis or one of the previously described disorders can account for the symptom.[5] For others, however, there is no apparent explanation, and one must either accept a higher incidence of idiopathic pruritus with advancing age or infer the existence of an entity, "senile pruritus," which may be the result of age-associated degenerative changes in peripheral nerve endings.

Medical Significance of Pruritus

The medical significance of generalized pruritus is two-fold. First, like its analog, pain, pruritus can destroy the quality of life for affected individuals. It can prevent sleep, interfere with concentration, and become a constant preoccupation. It has literally driven patients to suicide. Second, pruritus may be a symptom of occult disease. In some disorders, such as obstetric jaundice[14] and lymphoma,[25, 26] it appears to be of prognostic as well as diagnostic value. For all these reasons, a specific etiology for generalized pruritus should be vigorously sought in each patient at the time of initial presentation.

HISTORY

Statements in the literature that suggest that the character of pruritus depends to some degree on its precipitants are poorly substantiated. Duration of pruritus did not distinguish those with idiopathic symptoms from those with an identifiable etiology in one recent series,[8] and there is no evidence that severity of pruritus, which is always subjective, differentiates between these groups.

The following questions are often helpful in determining the cause of generalized pruritus, however.

1. *Do you have any known medical illness?* The most commonly identified causes of generalized pruritus are chronic renal failure, chronic cholestatic liver disease, and myeloproliferative disorders. Visceral malignancies may also be responsible.

2. *Do you use any medications or recreational drugs?* Medication requirements may indicate an underlying disease, and drug allergies may rarely manifest as pruritus in the absence of a rash. Aspirin, morphine-like drugs, and certain antibiotics may exacerbate pruritus by facilitating histamine release from mast cells. Opiates may also act directly on the central nervous system. Other drugs cause pruritus by inducing cholestasis.

3. *Have you traveled recently?* Parasitic infestations may manifest as pruritus.

4. *What do you think causes the itching?* Psychotic patients with delusions of parasitosis will usually describe their imagined tormentors in lurid detail.

5. *Is the itching related to your menstrual cycle, use of oral contraceptatives, or pregnancies?* The mild hepatic cholestasis induced by elevated estrogen and progestin levels may cause pruritus.

6. *Do you have heat intolerance, increased nervousness, palpitations, recent weight loss [or other symptoms of hyperthyroidism]?* Hyperthyroidism is occasionally associated with generalized pruritus.

7. *Is your skin very dry?* Xerosis itself may cause or exacerbate pruritus. "Dry skin" may also indicate a subtle irritant reaction or other dermatosis.

8. *Have you recently been exposed to fiber glass?* Fiber glass particles imbedded in the skin may be intensely pruritic, but produce little or no "rash."

9. *Is the itching precipitated by hot baths or showers?* This feature is said to be classic for pruritus due to polycythemia vera but may in fact occur in patients with pruritus of any etiology.

PHYSICAL EXAMINATION

The physical examination should be directed toward (1) excluding a "rash" as the cause of pruritus and (2) detecting an underlying systemic disease that may explain the pruritus.

The patient must disrobe to permit thorough examination of the skin. "Peeking" down the back of the shirt, at the beltline, or around the ankles of a fully or partially clothed patient is an unwise economy of time and poor medical practice. The color, texture, and temperature of the skin may provide clues regarding systemic disease (Table 2).

An attempt should be made to elicit dermatographism, indicative of exaggerated histamine release. To obtain a positive response, the skin must

Table 2. EXAMINATION OF THE SKIN

Attribute	Abnormality	Possible Etiology	Associated Disease(s)
Color	Yellow (jaundice)	Bilirubin retention	Primary biliary cirrhosis Extrahepatic biliary obstruction Hepatitis
	Red (plethora)	Increased hemoglobin	Polycythemia vera Carcinoid syndrome (facial flush)
	White (anemia)	Decreased hemoglobin	Iron deficiency anemia Lymphoma or leukemia
	Yellow-brown	Decreased hemoglobin, increased melanization	Chronic renal failure
	Brown	Increased melanization	Hyperthyroidism
Texture	Very smooth	Increased epidermal turnover (postulated)	Hyperthyroidism
	Rough	Increased, irregular stratum corneum	Xerosis (dry skin) Hypothyroidism Certain malignancies (associated with acquired ichthyosis)
Temperature	Warm	Increased basal metabolism	Hyperthyroidism Pregnancy
Response to trauma	Dermatographism	Excessive histamine release	Mastocytosis Urticaria (drug-induced or idiopathic)

be firmly stroked with a nearly sharp object such as the closed tip of a ballpoint pen. The stroke should be sufficiently hard to cause some redness in the skin and slight discomfort to the patient. The immediate response in both normal and involved skin is macular erythema along the stroke line. After several minutes, patients with dermatographism develop a pale wheal in the area that persists for several minutes more. It is wise to reexamine an apparently negative test response site at the very end of the physical examination so as to avoid false-negative results due to slow evolution of the response.

Primary skin lesions responsible for pruritus may be sufficiently subtle to escape the patient's notice. Table 3 lists possible findings and their significance. Excoriations are common and when present usually indicate the most symptomatic areas. It should be noted, however, that the correlation between the patient's subjective evaluation of the severity of pruritus and the number or character of excoriations is poor. Absence of excoriations does not imply absence of itching, only absence of forceful scratching.

Atopic dermatitis is associated with a reduced threshold for perception of pruritus from several stimuli even in noninvolved skin. Physical findings suggestive of atopy include Dennie-Morgan lines (prominent infraorbital folds), hyperlinear palms (increased number of palmar creases), and

Table 3. SUBTLE PRIMARY SKIN LESIONS THAT SUGGEST A CAUSE FOR PRURITUS

Lesion	Possible Significance
Pinpoint scars, crusts, or ecchymoses over veins ("tracks")	Opiate abuse
Minute insects ("crabs") in pubic or other body hair	Pediculosis pubis
Small excoriations and excoriated papules in body creases, digital webspaces, glans penis	Scabies
Small grouped vesicles or crusted erosions, especially over elbows and sacral area	Dermatitis herpetiformis

Table 4. LABORATORY EVALUATION FOR GENERALIZED PRURITUS

Procedure	Disorders Detected
Blood Studies	
Complete blood count	Anemia (due to iron deficiency or chronic disease) Polycythemia Leukemia Certain allergies (eosinophilia)
BUN* and creatinine levels	Chronic renal failure
SGOT,† bilirubin, and alkaline phosphatase levels	Primary biliary cirrhosis Cholestasis Hepatitis
Fasting blood glucose level	Diabetes mellitus
Thyroxine level	Hyperthyroidism
Urine Studies	
5-hydroxyindolacetic acid	Carcinoid syndrome
Drug profile (serum or urine)	Opiate ingestion Drug allergy
Histamine metabolites	Mastocytosis
Fecal examination for ova and parasites	Parasitic infestation
Chest x-ray	Lymphoma Metastatic malignancies

*Blood urea nitrogen.
†Serum glutamine oxalotransferase.

keratosis pilaris (a "sandpaper" texture of skin usually in the deltoid areas and/or lateral thighs, due to perifollicular retention of scale). Fair complexion, "rosy cheeks," and cool hands and feet are much less specific but frequent findings in young atopic individuals.

DIAGNOSTIC STUDIES

Generalized pruritus has been attributed to an underlying systemic disease in 10 to 30 per cent of patients in four published series.[5-8] Laboratory tests directed at detecting these disorders are listed in Table 4. Components of the initial laboratory evaluation should obviously be determined by the patient population under consideration as well as any leads obtained from the history and physical examination. In most settings, a complete blood count, measurements of creatinine, blood urea nitrogen, hepatic enzyme and thyroxine levels, and routine chest x-ray are probably sufficient.[8] Any positive results in this screening battery should be pursued until a definitive diagnosis is achieved.

REFERENCES

1. Gilchrest BA. Pruritus: pathogenesis, therapy, and significance in systemic disease states. Arch Intern Med 1982;142:101–5.
2. Scott PV, Fischer HBJ. Intraspinal opiates and itching: a new reflex? Br Med J 1982;284:1015–6.
3. Berstein JE, Swift RM, Solteni K, Lorincz AL. Antipruritic effect of an opiate antagonist, naloxone hydrochloride. J Invest Dermatol 1982;78:82–3.
4. Berstein JE, Swift RM. Relief of intractable pruritus with naloxone. Arch Dermatol 1979;115:1366–7.
5. Lyell A. The itching patient: a review of the causes of pruritus. Scot Med J 1972;17:334–47.
6. Beare JM. Generalized pruritus: a study of 43 cases. Clin Exp Dermatol 1976;1:343–52.
7. Rajka G. Investigation of patients suffering from generalized pruritus, with special reference to systemic disease. Acta Dermatol Venerol (Stockh) 1966;49:190–4.
8. Kantor GR, Lookingbill DP. Generalized pruritus and systemic disease. J Am Acad Dermatol, 1984.
9. Muse DN, Sawyer D. Medicare and Medicaid data book, 1981. Washington, DC: U.S. Dept. Health, and Human Services, 1982; USDHHS publication no. (HCFA) 82–03128.
10. Gilchrest BA, Stern RS, Steinman TI, Brown RS, Arndt KA, Anderson WW. Clinical features of pruritus among patients undergoing maintenance hemodialysis. Arch Dermatol 1982;118:154–6.
11. Botero F. Pruritus as a manifestation of systemic disorders. Cutis 1978;21:873–80.
12. Pederson JA, Matter BJ, Czerwinski AW, et al. Relief of idiopathic generalized pruritus in dialysis patients treated with activated oral charcoal. Ann Intern Med 1980;32:446–8.
13. Ahrens EH, Payne MA, Kunkel HG et al. Primary biliary cirrhosis. Medicine 1950;29:299–364.
14. Johnston WG, Baskett TK. Obstetric cholestasis. A 14-year review. Am J Obstet Gynecol 1979;133:299–301.
15. Drill VA. Benign cholestatic jaundice of pregnancy and benign cholestatic jaundice from oral contraceptives. Am J Obstet Gynecol 1974;119:165–74.
16. Makipour H, Cooperman A, Danzi JT, Farmer RG. Carcinoma of the ampulla of Vater. Review of 38 cases with emphasis on treatment and prognostic factors. Ann Surg 1976;183:341–4.
17. Ghent CN, Bloomer JR, Klatskin G. Elevations in skin tissue levels of bile acids in human cholestasis. Relation to serum levels and to pruritus. Gastroenterology 1977;73:1125–30.
18. Freedman MR, Holzbach RT, Ferguson DR. Pruritus in cholestasis: no direct causative role for bile acid retention. Am J Med 1981;70:1011–6.
19. Klein H. Polycythemia: theory and management. Springfield: Charles C Thomas, 1973:96.
20. Bluefarb SM: Cutaneous manifestations of malignant lymphomas. Springfield. Charles C Thomas, 1959:534.
21. Salem HH, van der Weyden MB, Young IF, Wiley JS. Pruritus and severe iron deficiency in polycythaemia vera. Br Med J 1982;285:91–2.
22. Barnes HM, Sarkany I, Calnan CD. Pruritus and thyrotoxicosis. Trans St Johns Hosp Derm Soc 1974;60:59–62.
23. Greenwood AM. A study of the skin in 500 cases of diabetes. JAMA 1927;89:774–6.
24. Young AW Jr, Sweeney EW. Cutaneous clues to heroin addiction. Am Fam Physician 1973;7:79–87.
25. Feiner AS, Mahmood T, Willner SF. Prognostic importance of pruritus in Hodgkin's disease. JAMA 1978;240:2738–40.
26. Lamberg ST, Green SB, Byar DP et al. Status report of 376 mycosis fungoides patients at 4 years: Mycosis Fungoides Cooperative Group. Cancer Treat Rep 1979;63:701–7.

PUBERTY, DELAYED

HERBERT S. KUPPERMAN

☐ SYNONYMS: Delayed sexual maturation, hypogonadism

BACKGROUND

In any treatment of delayed puberty, it is essential to discuss those factors that are responsible for initiation of the process of sexual maturation, which is also dependent upon the increase in secretion of hypothalamic gonadotropic releasing hormones. There appears to be a critical level of central nervous system maturity necessary for the hypothalamic-pituitary-gonadal axis to become activated.[1] Part of this maturity is associated with an increased sensitivity of the luteinizing hormone to gonadotropic releasing substances.[2] It has been suggested that there are several periods of activity of hypothalamic-pituitary-gonadal activity in the human. The first one occurs during pregnancy, with respect to sexual differentiation, the second in early infancy, and the third in adolescence. Apparently, there is an increased sensitivity of these centers to the inhibiting effects of circulating sex steroids.[1] The sensitivity decreases as one approaches puberty, so that finally, release of the secretion of hypothalamic regulating hormones occurs.[2–4] It now appears that there is an increase in importance of the biogenic amines of the central nervous system, including noradrenaline and dopamine, which act as neurotransmitters for the hypothalamic-pituitary-gonadotropic regulation and secretion.[5] These amines seem to be necessary for the control and elaboration of pituitary FSH and LH secretion. The role of serotonin in antagonizing these agents is unclear.

Silman and associates[6] have reported that there may be a drop in plasma melatonin in connection with the onset of puberty in boys. Melatonin may act as an inhibitor, thus suppressing prepubertal initiation of sexual maturation.

My colleagues and I have described some experimental evidence in rodents and fetal mammals that still leaves much to be explained.[7–11] We administered to immature 1-day-old rats sheep antigonadotropic hormone in rabbit serum obtained from rabbits chronically treated with crude sheep gonadotropic hormone. When injected subcutaneously this substance produced a decrease in size of both the ovaries and uterus during the 10 days of administration. When the antihormone was discontinued, a marked increase in endogenous gonadotropic hormone secretion occurred so that sexual precocity actually took place in these animals. They began to show vaginal openings and cyclic estrous changes at the age of 22 to 25 days, compared with the normal age of 45 to 50 days in untreated litter mate controls.

The gonadotropic content of the pituitary glands of the animals treated for 10 days with antihormone was markedly increased and was comparable to that seen in the litter mate controls that had been castrated for the same 10-day period.[8, 11] We also demonstrated that the pituitary gland of the fetal calf is relatively potent as far as gonadotropic content is concerned when compared with that of the young bull or mature cow. It would appear then that the pituitary gland of the immature animal or fetus contains a high level of gonadotropins and is capable of secreting gonadotropic hormones under appropriate stimulation. However, the gonadotropin secretion from these hypophyses is held in abeyance primarily by inhibitory substances of gonadal origin. These substances appear to be estrogen-like and may well be secreted directly by the immature ovary.

The hormonal secretory potential of the ovary was demonstrated experimentally when we gave sheep antigonadotropic hormone to 1-day-old rats for 10 days and castration was performed in 1-day-old litter mates.[8] At autopsy on the morning of the 11th day after castration and/or initiation of antihormone treatment, the uteri of both groups of animals as well as the ovaries of the antihormone-treated animals were significantly smaller than those of the untreated, noncastrated litter mate controls. This finding establishes that there are ovarian substances with a uterotrophic effect. The ovarian effect enhancing uterine growth is apparently maintained by the pituitary itself, because the ovaries of the antihormone- treated animals were considerably smaller than those of the untreated controls. With the increasing age of the hypothalamus, synthesis and elaboration of the hypothalamic gonadotropic releasing hormones occur, and sexual maturation can take place. In other words, the hypothalamus loses its ability to be inhibited by the gonadal hormone as it matures with the passage of time alone.[2–4]

Causes of Delayed Puberty

In our discussion of the problem of delayed puberty, the following etiologic classification is offered as a relatively simple guide. Causes of delayed puberty may be divided into constitutional causes, nonendocrine systemic diseases, and endocrine dysfunction.

Constitutional Causes

This classification comprises patients who usually show delayed growth and retardation of bone age and genital development. There may well be a familial tendency, in that several siblings may show a similar pattern at the same age. One can theorize that the delay is due in part to a failure of appropriate maturation of the central nervous system, so that the hypothalamic-pituitary-gonadal axis has not reached its full state of maturation or development. Delayed growth is usually accompanied by a lack of responsiveness of the hypothalamic gonadotropic releasing factor to those stimuli that are normally responsible for the release or secretion of the hypothalamic hormone. It may also be due to an aging factor whereby the central nervous system, with its ultimate secretion of neurohormones, has not sufficiently developed to respond adequately.

The patient with constitutional delay in puberty should not be summarily dismissed without due consideration of the effect that the disorder may have upon his or her psychological development. This concern is particularly appropriate in boys. The external position of their genitalia may make them objects of ridicule by their peers because of their hypoplastic genitalia.

Nonendocrine Systemic

Malnutrition. Puberty is markedly retarded in patients who are poorly nourished because of malabsorption syndrome, starvation, or anorexia nervosa. In contrast, puberty in the female may take place early in an obese child, owing in part to increased storage of estrogen in the fat depots of the body as well as to increased production of estrogen from androstenedione in adipose tissue.

Renal Disease. Mucopolysaccharidosis and galactosemia have been associated with ovarian follicular destruction due to accumulation of toxic substances within the ovary, which is not uncommon in women. In the male, however, galactosemia does not result in infertility.

Other Disorders. Other systemic causes of delayed puberty include: severe cardiac distress and impairment including congenital defects, gastrointestinal disease, cystic fibrosis, ileitis and/or severe parasitic infestation, chronic pulmonary disease, and liver disease.

In any illness of a chronic nature onset of puberty may be delayed because of the debilitating effect of the illness per se, which results indirectly in inappropriate hormonal transport and possible reduction of essential hormone receptor sites.

Endocrine Causes

Endogenous Causes. This classification includes most patients with marked hypothyroidism or hyperthyroidism, panhypopituitarianism usually associated with a craniopharyngioma, hyperprolactinemia (as a result of microadenoma or macroadenoma), and adrenocortical hyperplasia of the Cushing type.

Exogenous Causes. High doses of corticoids, which have been used for the treatment of asthma and other serious allergic manifestations as well as for certain dermatologic conditions, can inhibit the gonadotropic hormones and, thus, delay maturation or prevent normal gonadal development.

Gonadal Abnormalities

Hypogonadotropic Syndromes. Hypogonadotropism in the male or female with delayed sexual maturation may be due to selective gonadotropic deficiency or failure of response by the pituitary gland to hypothalamic gonadotropic releasing hormones. Central nervous system disease, such as sarcoidosis, may interfere with the transmission of the stimuli of the hypothalamic releasing factor to the pituitary gland itself if the involved area can interfere with the normal hypothalamic-hypophyseal relationship. Included in this classification would also be gonadotropic releasing deficiency per se, as seen in Kallmann's syndrome, in which there is a dysplasia of the olfactogenital system resulting in a failure of transmission of gonadotropic releasing factor. Hyposomia or anosmia secondary to relative agenesis of the olfactory lobe of the brain is characteristic of the syndrome. In affected males, gynecomastia may or may not be present with or without cryptorchidism. It is interesting to note that Kallmann's syndrome is one of the few hypogonadotropic hypogonadisms that may be associated with gynecomastia in the adult male. Normally, gynecomastia is seen in patients with hypergonadotropism. In the female, Kallmann's syndrome may result in failure of labial fusion. There may also be an accompanying failure of fusion of the palate and associated deafness. The use of gonadotropic releasing hormones in both males and females with Kallmann's syndrome frequently results in marked increase in FSH and LH levels, indicating that there is no loss of responsiveness of the hypophyseal gonadotropic system.[12]

The Laurence-Moon-Biedl syndrome may have an associated hypothalamic dysfunction. However, the most devastating characteristic is retinitis pigmentosa, usually accompanied by polydactylism, marked obesity, mental retardation, and, of course, hypogonadotropic hypogonadism. This is an autosomal recessive disease. Occasionally, affected patients may have diabetes mellitus.

Another syndrome in this classification is holoprosencephaly, also known as Prader-Willi syndrome. It is due to a hypothalamic defect that is associated with excessive ingestion of food (bulimia) resulting in severe obesity and hypogonadism. The affected patient has a characteristically round face, small but broad hands and feet, infantile hypotonia, and mental retardation. Usually, an isolated FSH and LH insufficiency exists, which may result in delayed sexual maturation and gonadal infantilism.

Anorexia nervosa and severe stress, as seen in competitive sports and various types of severe chronic disease, may also result in delayed puberty owing to the adverse effects of such conditions upon the hypothalamic-hypophyseal-thyroid relationship.

Hypergonadotropic Syndromes. The hypergonadotropic syndromes associated with delay or absence of puberty in the female include Turner's syndrome or gonadal dysgenesis, pure gonadal dysgenesis, ovarian resistance syndrome (Savage syndrome), and the insensitivity reaction to androgens. The androgen insensitivity syndrome is normally seen in individuals with well-developed breasts but no uterus. These individuals have a normal male karyotype and usually lack pubic and axillary hair. There may be a short rudimentary vagina. There is a variant of this syndrome in which there is no breast development but the same male karyotype, with normal testosterone levels for the female, in contrast to the insensitivity syndrome, in which the testosterone levels may be normal for the male but high for the female. Also in the variant, the gonadotropic levels are high, whereas in the pure insensitivity syndrome, they are low or normal. This syndrome differs from gonadal dysgenesis in that patients with androgen insensitivity have no uterus, in contrast to Turner's syndrome, in which the uterus is present. The etiology of the insensitivity syndrome probably relates to 17,20-desmolase deficiency associated with testicular regression. Other examples of hypergonadotropisms include premature ovarian failure due primarily to genetic factors causing ovarian immune disease. In affected patients, there may be multiple endocrine dysfunctions such as adrenal and parathyroid insufficiency as well as Hashimoto's thyroiditis. In addition, there may be myasthenia gravis, lupus erythematosus, and systemic candidasis. Also, 172α-hydroxylase deficiency, 5α-reductase deficiency, and 17-keto-reductase deficiency all result in gross abnormalities of the external genitalia of the female. Affected patients usually present with indeterminant external genitalia but have a normal internal female reproductive tract.

In the male, there are several types of hypergonadotropic syndromes. One requires immediate, prompt medical investigation: bilateral undescended testicles in an infant. If cryptorchism is the cause, there will be no increase in gonadotropic secretion. If instead anorchism is the prime factor, the gonadotropic secretion level may be high. Hence, it is essential not to wait until puberty to establish a more precise differential diagnosis but rather to ascertain as soon as possible whether or not the testes are present, capable of function, or absent. In affected children, human chorionic gonadotropin should be administered as early as possible in doses of 500 to 2000 IU (depending upon the age and size of the patient) three times per week for 4 to 5 weeks. If penile rubor and turgidity occur during the course of therapy, testes are no doubt present and functioning, and therapy may be discontinued. During therapy, one should measure blood testosterone and estradiol levels. Increases in these substances obviously substantiate the presence of testes capable of responding to the chorionic gonadotropin to induce the rubor and turgidity. If no penile response is noted, one should continue therapy for the full 5 weeks and then measure blood hormone levels. A failure of response would be associated with no change in blood testosterone and estrogen levels, indicating an anorchid state (Fig. 1). One would then expect to treat the patient with androgens at the time puberty normally takes place. These androgens should be administered in gradually increasing doses in an attempt to ape the endogenous secretion of testicular hormone during normal puberty. Because there is always a possibility of gonadal dysgenesis in such a patient, surgical exploration would be indicated to be certain that no abnormalities with anaplastic poten-

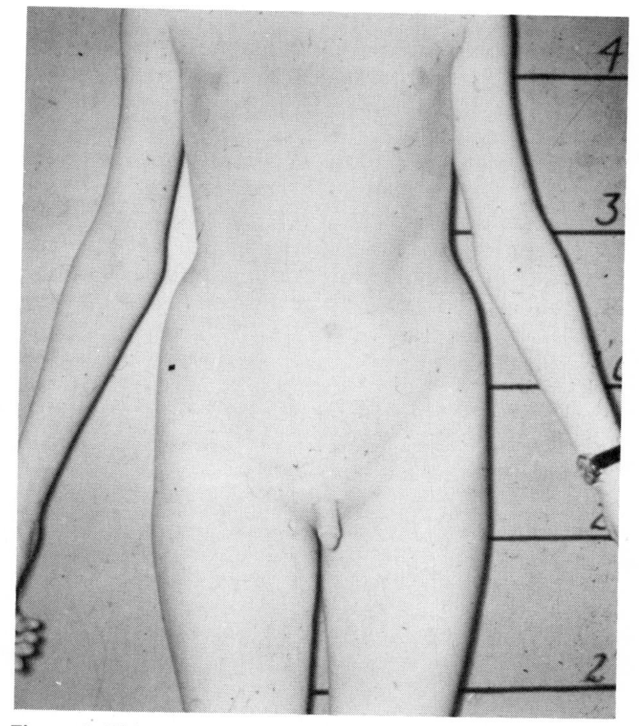

Figure 1. This 14-year-old chromatin-negative male presented with bilateral cryptorchism. He showed no response to human chorionic gonadotropin. Surgical exploration confirmed the diagnosis of anorchism. Androgen therapy was initiated at the time when puberty would normally occur. Puberty took place without any adverse effects. Without therapy, this patient would not have shown spontaneous sexual development.

tials are present. Obtaining a karyotype would be well worthwhile in all such patients.

In those patients in whom there is a penile response and an increase in sex hormone levels is noted, one can assume that undescended testes are present. Orchiopexy should be done as soon as possible, before the age of 3 or 4 years, or sooner if it can be achieved. The treatment with human chorionic gonadotropin should make the surgical procedure somewhat easier to accomplish. Orchiopexy is necessary for two major reasons. First, it is well known and accepted that the testes in cryptorchism have a propensity to become malignant. One must recognize the fact that bringing the testes down into the scrotum does not minimize their malignant potential; nevertheless, it does make them readily available for palpation and examination and early recognition of malignancy or abnormal growth. Second, irreparable damage to the seminiferous tubules can occur as long as the testes are intra-abdominal. Such damage may be minimized with early orchiopexy, and infertility later in life due to faulty spermatogenesis may thereby be prevented.

Turner's syndrome, associated with an abnormal karyotype, and Noonan's syndrome, in which there is a normal karyotype but an increase of gonadotropic hormones, are examples of hypergonadotropic delay in puberty. Boys with the typical findings of Turner's syndrome but without the accompanying chromosomal abnormalities occasionally have characteristic right-sided cardiac anomalies. Invariably, the testes are hypoplastic or cryptorchism may be present. There is a characteristic defect in germ cell and androgen production. Occasionally, these patients with the characteristic physical features of Turner's syndrome may show no evidence of delayed puberty.

Klinefelter's syndrome, or seminiferous tubular dysgenesis, is signified by the presence of unusually small testes in a patient with a relatively normal or slightly hypoplastic penis. The dichotomy between the micro-testes and the lack of comparable decrease in penile size is characteristic of seminiferous tubular dysgenesis. Affected patients may present with gynecomastia and eunuchoid characteristics; most are azospermic. Some may have sperm, either seen in the ejaculate or confirmed by testicular biopsy, but fertility has not been reported. As the patient ages, a greater destruction of the cytoarchitecture of the testes takes place, so that eventually all the tubules are hyalinized and azospermia is absolute (Figs. 2 and 3). The Leydig cells appear to be histologically normal, but there is actually a decrease in their numbers. At puberty, there is relatively poor secondary sexual development and inadequate testicular growth. A karyotype will usually show XXY chromosomes, although there may be variations in which three or more X chromosomes are associated with a single Y chromosome.

Stages of Genital Development

The therapeutic approach to patients with delayed puberty requires knowledge of what to expect in the normal development of the male and female. Genital development may be divided into five major levels based on the various stages of total body development in both males and females:

Stage I, prepubertal; Stage II, peripubertal; Stage III, neopubertal; Stage IV, Puberty; Stage V, postpubertal. They are discussed separately according to sex.

Genital Development in the Male

Stage I: Less Than 7 Years. In the prepubertal male, who is usually below the age of 7 years,

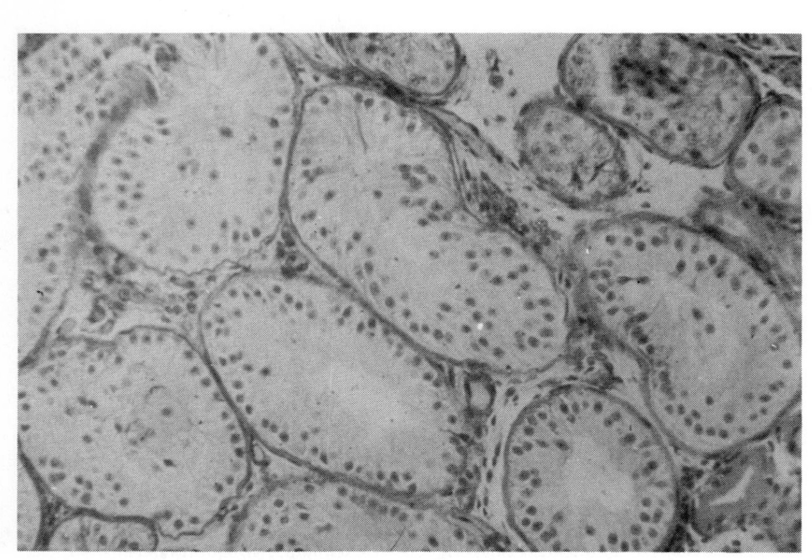

Figure 2. Histologic section of testis from a 12-year-old XXY male with Klinefelter's syndrome, showing no disturbance of the cytoarchitecture of the testes. However, there is almost complete absence of primary spermatocytes. Leydig cells are normal for the patient's age.

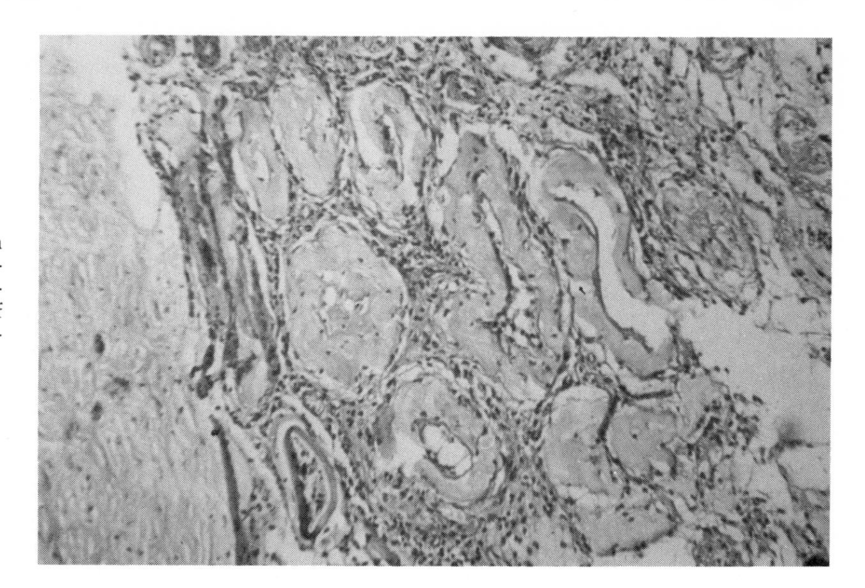

Figure 3. Histologic section of testis from a 32-year-old XXY male with Klinefelter's syndrome, showing complete destruction of cytoarchitecture and complete hyalinization of the tubules. Obviously, there is no spermatogenic function in such testes.

there is no secondary sex hair development. The testes are spherical rather than elongated and measure approximately 1 to 1.5 cm in diameter. The scrotum has no pigmentation or rugae. The penis, which lacks rubor, may measure 2 to 3 cm in length and 1 to 2 cm or less in diameter.

Stage II: 7 to 9 Years. The *peripubertal* stage, which usually occurs between 7 and 9 years, is characterized by elongation of the testicles. They become cylindrical and may reach a length of approximately 2 to 4 cm with an increase in diameter. The penis only slightly increases in size, measuring more than 3 to 5 cm in length with a diameter greater than 2 cm. Pubic and axillary hair are still absent, as is body hair growth. There is no increase in body odor. The scrotum is smooth, having no rugae.

Stage III: 9 to 11 Years. In the *neopubertal* stage, further elongation of the testes occurs, so they measure approximately 3.5 to 5 cm in length and are cylindrical. The penis has also increased to approximately 5 to 8 cm in length. There is no evidence of significant prostatic development (which was also absent in the prepubertal and peripubertal phases). Body odor is now noted, as well as some cracking of the voice. Formation of rugae begins in the scrotum, as does pigmentation of the scrotal area. Redundancy of the scrotum would depend primarily upon the temperature of the external environment. Axillary hair is absent, but pubic hair has begun to develop in the form of a very fine fuzz. At this time, as well as in Stage IV, gynecomastia can develop, usually occurring in 90 to 95 per cent of all males going through puberty. In Stage III, it is represented by a small amount of tissue approximately 1 cm thick over the chest wall and 1 to 2 cm in diameter, directly below the areolae. The firmness may be a cause of some concern to the parents as well as the patient, if tenderness is readily elicited. The patient and parent should be reassured as to the innocuousness of the situation, but injury to the tissue should be avoided.

Stage IV: 10 to 14 Years. At *puberty,* there is further elongation of the penis and testes; the testes now measure approximately 4 to 6 cm in length and 2 to 3 cm in diameter. The penis measures 6 to 9 cm in length with a diameter of about 3 to 4 cm. Pubic hair is present, as is axillary hair. There is practically no beard except for a fine fuzz, and body hair growth is now seen but is minimal. Ejaculation and erection may now take place either spontaneously or when induced. Gynecomastia may progress or subside; it can progress to the size of the Stage III female breast.

Stage V: 15 Years or Older. In the *postpubertal* stage, a boy is approaching adult size and the rest of his body develops as well as the size of his penis. Rugae and increased pigmentation of the scrotum are seen, pubic hair is present, axillary hair is formed, and facial hair has begun to show more significantly. Body odor is present to a notable degree. The testes usually are more than 5 to 7 cm in their largest diameter, and the penis is more than 8 to 12 cm in length and 4 cm in diameter. The voice has deepened and is adult-like in tone.

Genital Development in the Female

Stage I: Less Than 7 or 8 Years. In the *prepubertal* female, there is no breast development, nor is there axillary or pubic hair growth. The vulvae are still immature. The distinction between the labia majora and labia minora is not readily noticeable.

Stage II: 8 to 11 Years. In the *peripubertal* stage, breast development is beginning. There are small, nodular knobs of tissue beneath the areolae, which have pigmentation and measure approximately 2 cm in diameter. There is a greater differentiation between the labia majora and labia minora, and fine labial hair may be seen, but pubic hair is still absent. Significant body odor is absent.

Stage III: 10 to 12 Years. In the *neopubertal* stage, breast development has increased, so that glandular development extends beyond the border of the areolae, which still show no significant increase in pigmentation. The breast tissue increases to about 2 to 4 cm above the level of the chest wall and 3 to 8 cm in diameter. Axillary and pubic hair are now present, although only minimal. Vulvar hair is more extensive, and body odor is apparent.

Stage IV: 11 to 13 Years. *Puberty* is associated with the onset of menses, which may be somewhat irregular and can be ovulatory or anovulatory. Breasts now measure some 3 to 6 cm or more above the chest wall and 8 to 12 cm in diameter. The areolae are slightly pigmented. Axillary hair is now present, as is pubic hair in the form of a female escutcheon.

Stage V: 14 to 16 Years or Older. There is now adult breast formation, a female escutcheon consisting of an adequate amount of pubic hair growth, and some increase of hair in the perineal area with mucus-like vaginal secretion, and definite body odor. Menses are occurring at regular or irregular intervals with or without dysmenorrhea and premenstrual molimina.

MANAGEMENT

The therapeutic approach to the management of the patient with delayed puberty depends upon several major factors. One, of course, is the psychological overtones that may prevail in these individuals because of their lack of sexual development. They may be exposed to ridicule, particularly boys who, as a result of the external location of their genitalia, may be the objects of coarse gibes and criticism from their better-developed peers.

It is also important to note, however, that premature therapy may have adverse effects and that lack of therapy may also cause a detrimental reaction that may lead to psychological and physical aberrations in the adult patient. Because delayed puberty has different causes, obviously there are those for whom no type of therapy would be effective in creating spontaneous development and maturation. In these individuals, complete replacement therapy will be necessary at a stage of life when development of secondary sexual characteristics is essential. In these individuals, too, however, the use of gonadotropins or sex steroids must be tempered by the degree of growth and development, inasmuch as sex steroids, particularly estrogens, may have an adverse effect upon epiphyseal closure.

In female patients in whom there is no possibility of spontaneous ovarian function, the use of sex steroid replacement therapy should not be initiated until full growth has been achieved. On the other hand, if the patient becomes desperate about her lack of sexual development and is not concerned about eventual height, replacement therapy with estrogen and progesterone may be initiated. At no time should an estrogen be given without cyclic progestins. The progestins prevent nuclear atypia from occurring on organs that respond to estrogens. The major problem as far as therapy for delayed puberty would be in those patients with a constitutional cause in whom the delay in puberty may be due to factors other than absolute absence of ovarian function or gonadal activity. In these patients, the initation of gonadal function may take place in the late teens. However, the psychic trauma caused by such delay in maturation may necessitate early initiation of replacement therapy or at least an investigation of the possible causes for the delay.[13, 14]

The underdeveloped male with delayed puberty usually withdraws from normal physical activity and may fail to appear in physical education classes, where he would have to expose his body to his peers when dressing or showering. As a result of the fear of ridicule, many a young patient has refused to continue gymnastic activities and, when told that attendance is compulsory, may even drop out of school. School work suffers and the young man may become a social rebel, exhibiting unusual behavior which may be generated primarily to obtain attention. These males usually have low gonadotropic levels and low gonadal function. The testes may not elongate at the anticipated time, remaining spherical and hypoplastic. I see no contraindication in these individuals to the use of human chorionic gonadotropin in an attempt to produce maturation of the testes and improve sexual development (Fig. 4). My colleagues and I have never found such therapy to have an adverse effect upon epiphyseal closure. I know much has been said in the literature about such an effect, but in our review of hundreds of boys so treated, there has been no evidence of accelerated epiphyseal closure or maturation. When the developmental progress has improved following the use of human chorionic gonadotropin, the aberrant behavior rapidly subsides (Figs. 5 and 6).

CONCLUSION

The management of a patient with delayed puberty requires appropriate diagnosis and the phy-

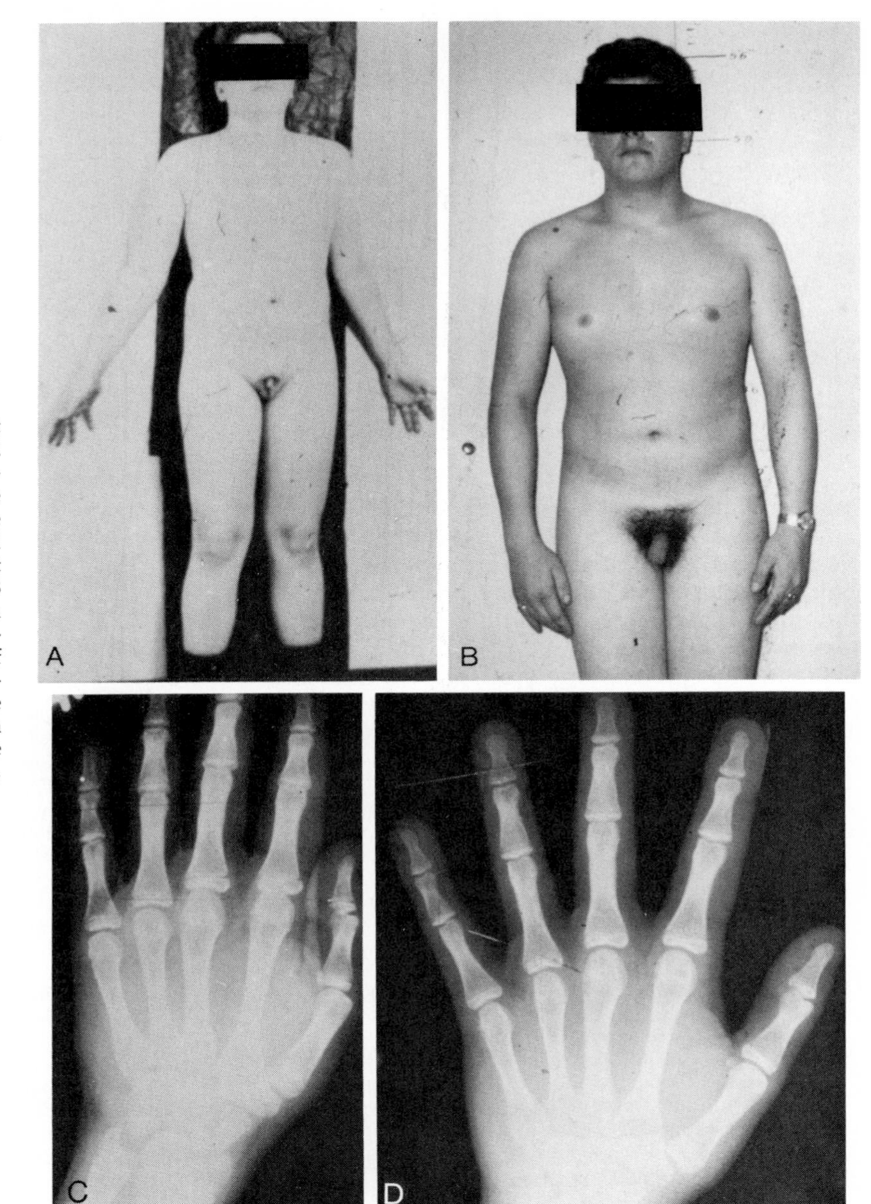

Figure 4. Patient with delayed puberty at 21 years *(A)*, before treatment, and at 22 years *(B)*, after treatment with gonadotropin. Maturation was satisfactory, but he was still somewhat abashed by the size of his genitalia, even though they had increased enormously over pretreatment size. X-rays taken at 21 years *(C)* and 23 years *(D)* show the epiphyses to be open before therapy and after sexual maturation had occurred; there is a difference of approximately 1.5 years between these x-rays. As long as the epiphyses of the patient aged 20 or more are open when treatment is begun, penile growth can be anticipated. If the epiphyses are closed, little or no penile growth will occur.

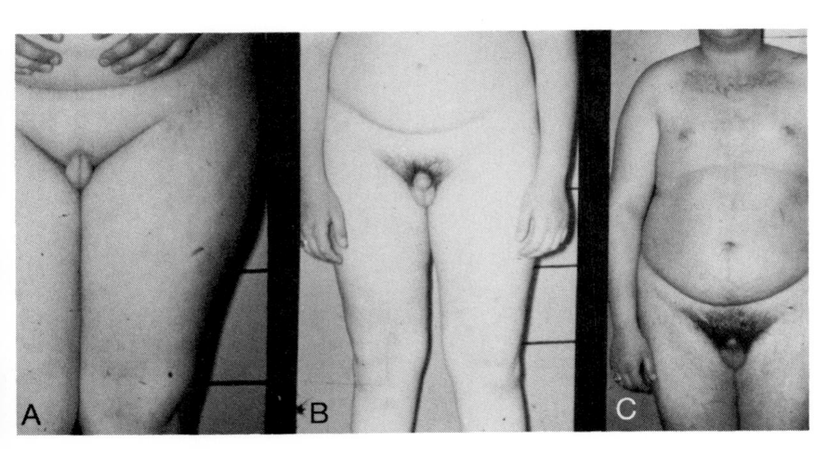

Figure 5. Patient shown at 15 years *(A)*, 16 years *(B)*, and 20 years *(C)*. He received a course of gonadotropic therapy between the ages of 15 and 16 years, with excellent results. No further therapy was given and there was no further maturation. By the age of 20, epiphyseal closure had taken place and little further penile growth could be accomplished. Without the initial therapy he would have had markedly hypoplastic genitalia as an adult.

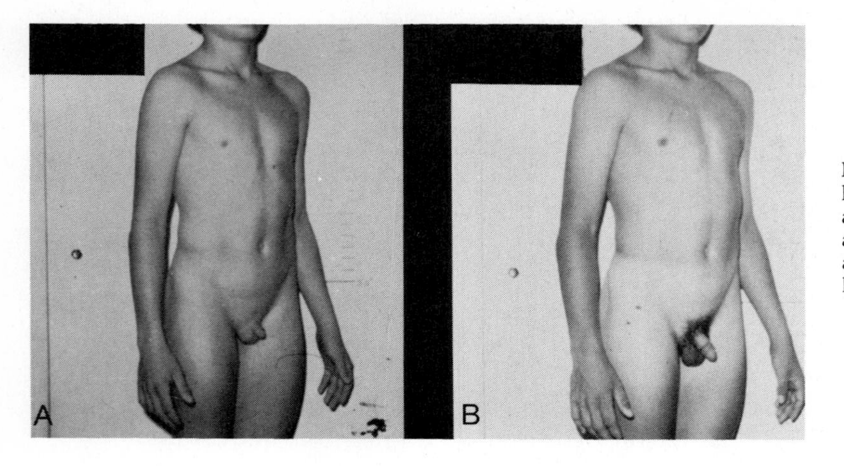

Figure 6. Patient at 17 years 11 months, before hCG therapy *(A)*, and at 18 years 6 months, after therapy *(B)*. Note the excellent response and improved sexual maturation. There was also enormous improvement with respect to his association with peers.

sician's willingness to understand that such a patient is in a sensitive stage of physical and psychological development. The adverse psychological effects of delayed puberty are enormous and may lead to social aberrations that can be stemmed by appropriate use of gonadotropic therapy with no adverse effect on growth and later reproductive potential. Therefore, it is imperative that an appropriate diagnosis be made and proper therapeutic measures be taken.

REFERENCES

1. Beck W, Wuttke W. Diurnal variation of plasma luteinizing hormone, follicule stimulating hormone and prolactin in boys and girls from birth to puberty. J Clin Endocrinol Metab 1980;50:635–9.
2. Kulin HE, Grumbach MM, Kaplan SI. Changing sensitivity of the pubertal gonadal hypothalamic feedback mechanism in man. Science 1969;166:1012–3.
3. Forst MG, Saez JM, Bertrand J. Present concept in the initiation of puberty and prepubertal hormonal influences. In: Some aspects of hypothalamic regulation of endocrine functions. Stuttgart: FK Schattawer, 1973;339–67.
4. Winter SSD, Hughes IA, Reyes FI, Faiman C. Pituitary-gonadal relations in infancy; patterns of serum gonadal steroid concentration in man from birth to two years of age. J Clin Endocrinol Metab 1976;42:679–86.
5. Collu R. Neuroendocrine control of pituitary hormone secretion. In: Collu R, Ducharme JR, Guyda H, eds. Pediatric endocrinology. New York: Raven Press, 1981; 1–28.
6. Silman RE, Leone RM, Hooper RJL, Preece MD. Melatonin, the pineal gland and puberty. Nature 1977;282:301–3.
7. Kupperman HS, Meyer RK, Hertz R. The effect of antigonadotropic sera upon gonadotropic secretion in parabiotic rats. Endocrinology 1939;24:115–8.
8. Meyer RK, Kupperman HS. Hypersecretion of gonadotropic hormone of pituitary gland of rats resulting from treatment with antigonadotropic serum. Proc Soc Exper Biol Med 1939;42:285–8.
9. Finerty JC, Kupperman HS, Meyer RK. Quantitative studies of cell types in rat hypophysis following administration of antigonadotropic serum. Proc Soc Exper Biol Med 1940;44:551–3.
10. Kupperman HS, Meyer RK, Finerty JC. Precocious gonadal development occurring in immature rats following a short-time treatment with antigonadotropic serum. Am J Physiol 1942;135:293–8.
11. Meyer RK, Kupperman HS, Finerty JC. Increase in gonadotropic content of pituitary glands of female rats treated with antigonadotropic serum. Endocrinology 1942;30:662–6.
12. Jacobson RI, Seyler LF, Tamborlane WV, Gertner JM, Genel M. Pulsatile subcutaneous nocturnal administration of GnRH by portable infusion pump in hypogonadotrophic hypogonadism: initiation of gonadotropin responsiveness. J Clin Endocrinol Metab 1979;49:652–54.
13. Kupperman HS, Epstein JA. Hormonal therapy versus watchful waiting in hypogonadism: the male. J Geriatr Soc 1958;6:87–98.
14. Spitz IM, Hirsch HJ, Trestian S. The prolactin response to thyrotropin-releasing hormone differentiates isolated gonadotropin deficiency from delayed puberty. N Engl J Med 1983;308:575–9.

PUBERTY, PRECOCIOUS

RICHARD E. BLACKWELL □ J. BENJAMIN YOUNGER

□ SYNONYMS: Isosexual precocity, heterosexual precocity, true precocious puberty

BACKGROUND

The acquisition of reproductive potential and adult stature is an expression of the interaction of many endogenous and exogenous factors. The age of onset of normal puberty is subject to such processes as stress, nutritional status, and environmental factors.

The onset of puberty is usually heralded by the beginning of the growth spurt. One may expect to see this spurt as well as adrenarche (the development of sexual hair) or thelarche (breast development) between 8 and 13 years of age, with a mean of 11 years. Most young women reach menarche (the onset of cyclic menstrual bleeding) by age 12 or 13. Young men achieve puberty by age 14. The acquisition of secondary sexual characteristics is usually completed in approximately 4.2 years (mean range 1.5 to 6 years) (Table 1).[1, 2]

Definitions

The accepted definition for *precocious puberty* is the appearance of signs of secondary sexual maturation at an age that is two standard deviations below the mean (8 years for girls, 9 years for boys). It is essential to establish an accurate diagnosis for the patient who presents with physical findings of premature development. One must attempt to differentiate between the various forms of complete and incomplete precocity and processes that are self-limited, such as premature adrenarche or premature thelarche.

Precocious puberty is usually classified as *complete isosexual precocity* (true precocious puberty) if there is premature maturation of the hypothalamic pituitary gonadal axis, and as *incomplete isosexual precocity* if there is a nonpituitary source of gonadotropins or sex steroids. The term heterosexual precocity is reserved for premature puberty associated with masculinization of the female.

Table 1. DEVELOPMENTAL CHANGES IN NORMAL PUBERTY

Change	Age (years)
Axillary hair	9–16
Breast development (thelarche)	8–13
Menses (menarche)	9–16
Pubic hair development (pubarche)	8–14
Peak and growth spurt	9½–14

Causes of Precocious Puberty

Table 2 summarizes the causes of precocious puberty.

Complete Isosexual Precocity

Idiopathic (Constitutional) Precocious Puberty. Complete isosexual precocity is generally idiopathic or may result from a central nervous system disorder. The patient with idiopathic precocity, who is usually female, may begin pubescence extremely early. This type of precocity is associated with certain electroencephalographic abnormalities. Such patients usually present with the appearance of pubic hair, breast development, or perhaps enlargement of the labia minora. It should be noted that the addition of secondary sexual characteristics will progress in a normal pattern of pubertal maturation. There is some suggestion that various types of constitutional

Table 2. CAUSES OF PRECOCIOUS PUBERTY

Complete isosexual precocity (true precocious puberty)	Constitutional (idiopathic)
	Central nervous system tumor or trauma
	Epilepsy
	Prenatal or perinatal infection
	Encephalopathy or meningitis
	Neurofibromatosis
	McCune-Albright syndrome
	Granulomatous disease (sarcoid, syphilis, tuberculosis)
Incomplete isosexual precocity	Increased estrogen levels
	Ovarian cyst
	Ovarian tumor
	Tumors producing hCG
	Increased androgen levels
	Congenital adrenal hyperplasia
	Ovarian neoplasm
	Adrenal neoplasm
Exogenous steroids	
Pseudo–precocious puberty	

precocious puberty may be transmitted as either autosomal recessive or x-linked dominant traits. However, the majority of patients with constitutional precocious puberty have no familial tendency for early development.[3, 4]

Central Nervous System Disorders. A number of central nervous system disorders can lead to complete isosexual precocity, including tumor, sarcoidosis, head trauma, brain abscess, encephalitis, tuberculosis, the McCune-Albright syndrome, neurofibromatosis, severe hypothyroidism, and various forms of epilepsy.

Various tumors of the central nervous system are associated with the development of complete isosexual precocity, such as ependymoma, astrocytoma, optic glioma, germinoma, hypothalamic teratoma, and hemartoma. Such tumors generally impinge on the hypothalamic region, disrupting neurochemical outflow to the pituitary gland. In general, they occur more commonly in males than females and may or may not be endocrine-active.[5]

Although not generally thought of as true tumors, various granulomas, such as those associated with sarcoidosis and tuberculosis, can cause hypothalamic compression that results in precocious puberty.

Likewise, in neurofibromatosis (von Recklinghausen's disease), gliomas or neurofibromas can develop in the central nervous system and affect hypothalamic function. Neurofibromatosis is an autosomal dominant disorder with a variable degree of penetrance. Findings in affected patients include mental retardation, seizure disorders, visual defects, and café au lait spots. It should be remembered that neurofibromatosis may manifest as either precocious or delayed puberty.[6]

The McCune-Albright syndrome (polyostotic fibrous dysplasia) has been associated with precocious puberty more frequently in boys than in girls. Presenting features are café au lait spots, cyst formation in the long bones and skull, and fibrous dysplasia. The mechanism by which this disorder causes precocious puberty is unknown.[7]

Primary Hypothyroidism. Finally, hypothyroidism in its primary form has been rarely mentioned as a cause of precocious puberty. The mechanism by which the precocity is brought about is unclear. It has been speculated that thyrotropin-releasing factor (TRF) has the capacity to release follicle-stimulating hormone (FSH) in primary hypothyroidism. This concept is somewhat of a paradox, because TRF is known to release thyroid-stimulating hormone (TSH) and prolactin in vivo and in vitro in all animal species, and does not release gonadotropins in the euthyroid state. In fact, hyperprolactinemia in vivo is thought to increase the turnover of hypothalamic dopamine, therefore inhibiting LRF production and subsequently LH and FSH secretion and resulting in the state of hypogonadotropic hypogonadism. It should also be remembered that hypothroidism may manifest as delay in the onset of puberty or menarche.[8]

Incomplete Isosexual Precocity

Incomplete isosexual precocity is caused by an increase in secretion of estrogen in the female or testosterone in the male. The increase may be secondary to direct production of human chorionic gonadotropin (hCG) by various tumors, such as teratoma and teratocarcinoma. Therefore, males present with precocious puberty and females may present with precocious puberty and/or masculinization.

Inappropriate hCG Secretion. The glycoproteins FSH, LH, TSH, and hCG are composed of alpha and beta chains. The alpha chains are the same in all of these proteins, whereas the beta chains are different and confer specificity. LH and hCG, however, have very similar alpha and beta chains; therefore, each of these compounds can stimulate Leydig cells in the male to produce testosterone and the granulosa and theca cells in the female to produce androstenedione, testosterone, and estradiol. Secretion of hCG is detected in the presence of a teratoma. Teratomas and chorioepitheliomas have been found in the mediastinum, gonad, retroperitoneum, pineal gland, and hypothalamus. Likewise, hCG can be produced from hepatomas or hepatoblastomas. Production of hCG in males is sometimes extremely difficult to differentiate from constitutional precocious puberty. In the female, however, gonads are usually stimulated to produce estrogen and subsequent breast development, and bleeding will occur.[9]

Adrenal Enzymatic Defects. Various partial deficiencies of adrenal enzyme metabolism may result in precocious puberty. The most notable is 21-hydroxylase deficiency, which metabolizes the conversion of progesterone to 11-deoxycorticosterone and 17α-hydroxyprogesterone to 11-deoxycortisol. The latter blockage decreases the production of cortisol, thereby breaking the negative feedback to the pituitary hypothalamic axis. Subsequently, there are increases in production of dihydroepiandrosterone (DHEAS) and androstenedione with resulting virilism. Although less common than the 21-hydroxylase defect, partial deficiency of 11β-hydroxylase blocks the conversion of 11-deoxycortisol to cortisol. Therefore, production of the precursor androgens, dihydroepiandrosterone and androstenedione, is increased. Both of these forms of congenital adrenal hyperplasia are inherited as autosomal recessive traits, although there is extreme variability of penetrance. The various adrenal tumors that can secrete androgens, primarily DHEAS, are generally classified as adrenal carcinomas.[10, 11]

Ovarian Tumors. A wide variety of ovarian tumors, ranging from simple follicle cyst to malignant germ cell tumor, have been associated with isosexual precocity in the female. The common follicle cyst is frequently seen as a cause of precocious puberty and secretes enough steroid to cause periodic bleeding and incomplete isosexual precocity.[12] Follicle cysts must be differentiated from the germ cell tumors, a group of ovarian neoplasms composed of different histologic tumor types and derived from primitive germ cells of the embryonic gonad. These tumors make up 59 per cent of the ovarian cancers found in patients less than 20 years old. Pain is the most frequently reported symptom, and a palpable abdominal mass is found in half the patients with a neoplasm. Approximately 10 per cent of patients present with incomplete isosexual precocity, the symptoms of which include vaginal bleeding, breast development, and areolar pigmentation. These changes completely regress with surgical extirpation of the tumor.[13] Although the granulosa-theca cell tumor is by far the most common ovarian tumor found in the child with isosexual precocity, other endocrine tumors in pure and mixed forms may cause this problem. The benign cystic teratoma is the most common germ cell tumor found in the pediatric age group, followed by the malignant teratoma, mixed germinal tumor, intradermal sinus tumor, and Sertoli-Leydig cell tumor.[14] Only 5 per cent of the granulosa cell tumors and theca cell tumors are found before puberty. Although the majority of these tumors produce estrogen, a few are androgenic. Fortunately, 80 to 85 per cent of such tumors are palpable on either abdominal or pelvic examination. The granulosa cell tumor is found bilaterally in 2 to 5 per cent of patients, whereas the theca cell tumor is almost always confined to a single ovary. It should be noted that 15 per cent of patients with granulosa cell tumors present with an acute abdomen secondary to hematoperitoneum.[15, 16, 17]

Sertoli-Leydig cell tumor is synonymous with androblastoma and arrhenoblastoma. Many of these tumors are associated with androgen production, but some of them have no endocrine function and others secrete estrogen.[18] These are extremely rare lesions, accounting for 0.5 per cent of all ovarian tumors. Although in the older female these tumors are thought to be associated with progressive masculinization (hirsutism, temporal balding, voice change, and clitoromegaly), it should be remembered that they are occasionally found in pediatric patients.[19, 20]

Choriocarcinoma is a very rare and highly malignant tumor. It can be associated with sexual precocity and the production of hCG. The tumor is found in children and young adults, and 50 per cent of the cases have been reported in children who have not reached puberty. Because of the malignant nature of this tumor, precocious puberty in the female should be aggressively evaluated.[21, 22, 23]

An equally malignant ovarian tumor is the embryonal cell carcinoma. Fortunately, it represents only 4 per cent of malignant ovarian germ cell tumors. The mean age of occurrence is 15 years, and half the affected patients have hormonal abnormalities, including precocious puberty, irregular uterine bleeding, amenorrhea, and hirsutism. Embryonal cell carcinoma secretes both human chorionic gonadotropin and alpha-fetoprotein, both of which may be used as markers in tumor treatment. In two studies of patients with such tumors, the most common finding was vaginal bleeding (33 per cent) and survival for patients with stage I tumors was 50 per cent.[24, 25]

Exogenous Steroids

An often overlooked cause of precocious puberty is ingestion of exogenous sex steroids. Creams, lotions, and tonics contain estrogens, and consumption of these agents by a child may lead to any of the manifestations of precocity.

Pseudo–Precocious Puberty

There are other variations of pubertal development that are neither complete nor incomplete forms of isosexual precocity. In chronic perineal irritation by either a yeast infection or diarrhea, for example, one may see the development of hair along the inner aspect of the labia minora. The bone age of a child with this finding is not advanced, and it does not represent a form of true precocious puberty. Similarly, one may encounter premature thelarche with either unilateral or bilateral breast development without other signs of estrogen stimulation. Although breast enlargement may regress, it can persist for years. This usually benign and self-limited disorder is not associated with a significant elevation in estrogen. Premature adrenarche may also occur without other signs of virilization. The appearance of axillary or pubic hair is very common in girls less than 6 years of age and, like premature thelarche, is a nonprogressive disorder. Likewide, one may encounter gynecomastia in prepubertal boys with an inappropriate estradiol-testosterone ratio; the condition is benign and usually resolves within 2 years. However, one must remember that gynecomastia is a component of some of the syndromes of the intersex state, most notably Reifenstein's syndrome and other forms of incomplete testicular feminization. Also, a rare estrogen-secreting adrenal adenoma or chorioepithelioma may cause gynecomastia, and disorders of extraglandular aromatization have been reported.[26, 27]

HISTORY

Information should be obtained about the mother's *obstetric history,* with emphasis placed on the possibility of *traumatic delivery.* One should inquire whether the mother was septic at the time of delivery, or whether the child had a subsequent *perinatal or neonatal infection.* A history of *childhood illnesses* should be obtained with emphasis on various viremias that may have resulted in *encephalopathy* or aseptic *meningitis.* Childhood head or *central nervous system trauma* should be excluded, as well as a history of epilepsy. The parent and child should be questioned with regard to various childhood habits, such as the oral *ingestion of cosmetics* or medications that might contain steroids. A history of *chronic diarrhea, incontinence,* or perineal pruritus should be sought to rule out chronic peritoneal irritation and stimulation of hair cells. One should also ask about *abdominal pain* or *swelling.* Inquiry should be made as to the age of *onset of puberty in* other *family members* in order to rule out a hereditary basis for precocity.

PHYSICAL EXAMINATION

Initially, *height* and *weight* should be plotted on a sex-corrected *growth curve,* and *head circumference* should be measured. The *skin* should be examined for the presence of café au lait spots and neurofibromas. *Development* of breasts and pubic hair, as well as external genitalia, should be *staged* according to the method of Marshall and Tanner (Table 3).[2] A complete *neurologic examination,* including funduscopy and visual field evaluation, should be performed. Finally, *vaginal inspection* and *transrectal palpation* should be performed to rule out the presence of pelvic mass.

DIAGNOSTIC STUDIES

Initially, serum LH and FSH determinations should be carried out to ascertain whether the patient has complete or incomplete isosexual precocity. In the normal prepubertal individual, gonadotropin levels are decreased, and the FSH level is generally slightly higher than the LH level. The child with complete isosexual precocity will have adult gonadotropin levels, with the LH level greater than the FSH level. Both levels are decreased in the presence of a tumor secreting either hCG or estrogen. Therefore, it is often convenient to obtain *LH, FSH, hCG, and estradiol* (E_2) measurements as an initial endocrine screen. If one suspects hypothyroidism, *T_4 and TSH* measurements should be obtained; markedly depressed T_4 level and increased TSH secretion confirm the presence of hypothyroidism. If adrenal disease is suspected, *DHEAS* or *17-ketosteroids* can be determined. It should be noted that DHEAS, like cortisol, shows a diurnal variation, with blood levels being highest in the morning and lowest in the late evening. When 24-hour urinary 17-ketosteroid levels are measured, a 24-hour *creatinine* determination should also be carried out to indicate the adequacy of collection. A *17-hydroxyprogesterone* blood determination can be made to rule out the presence of the 21-hydroxylase deficiency; 24-hour urinary pregnanetriol measurement will give similar information.

If a central nervous system disorder is suspected, an *electroencephalogram* should be obtained, as should radiologic evaluation of the skull. PA and lateral *skull films* have traditionally been used, as well as linear and hypocycloidal *tomograms,* both methods being effective in detecting bone-eroding central nervous system tumors, such as craniopharyngioma. On the other hand, *CT scanning* is thought to be superior for evaluation of soft tissue masses. Bone age should be determined on *x-rays of* the *hands* and *wrists.* Development of these bones is usually be found to be advanced compared with chronologic age. Finally, a *vaginal smear* can be used as an index of maturation and measurement of estrogen secretion, if serum estradiol assays are not available. *Abdominal ultrasonography* (gray-scale, reactive, or sector) is also useful in

Table 3. DEVELOPMENT OF BREASTS, GENITALIA, AND PUBIC HAIR AS DESCRIBED BY MARSHALL-TANNER STAGING

Stage	Female Breast	Female Pubic Hair	Male Genitalia
I	Preadolescent; elevation of papilla	Preadolescent; no pubic hair	Preadolescent; child-like testes, scrotum, and penis
II	Breast bud, elevation of breast and papilla, enlargement of areolar diameter	Slight growth along labia, some increased pigmentation	Spreading of scrotal skin, enlargement of genitalia
III	Continued enlargement of breast and areola, but no separation of contour	Sparsely spread, dark, coarse, curly hair at junction of pubis	Increased breadth and length of penis, further rugation of scrotum
IV	Projection of areola, secondary mound formation	Adult type with no spread onto the medial aspects of the thighs	Penile enlargement with glans development, testes enlarged, scrotal skin darkened
V	Mature stage	Adult type, spread onto thigh with inverse triangle formation	Adult genitalia with hair growth onto the abdominal wall

screening for the presence of a pelvic mass and may be as effective as transrectal palpation.

ASSESSMENT AND DIAGNOSTIC APPROACH

The algorithm summarizes the diagnostic approach to precocious puberty.

The vast majority of patients with signs of pubertal precocity have a self-limited process, such as premature adrenarche or thelarche, or constitutional precocity. Premature adrenarche or thelarche can be easily ruled out by the finding of only one sign of precocious puberty. The constitutional form can be diagnosed by the finding of a slightly advanced bone age associated with adult LH and FSH levels (LH greater than FSH) and adult estrogen level. The patient with either premature menarche or thelarche or constitutional precocity requires no treatment other than adequate psychological support for herself and her family.

Potentially life-threatening conditions are usually associated with a decreased gonadotropin level and an increase in either hCG or estrogen level. This finding should prompt the physician to look for various forms of tumor, primarily with radiologic techniques. If premature adrenarche is associated with an advanced bone age, the physician should look for adrenal hyperplasia or tumor, or ovarian disease. An elevated 17-ketosteroid level points to adrenal disease, whereas an elevated free testosterone level might suggest ovarian disease. If adrenal disease is suspected, the dexamethasone suppression test can be used to differentiate adrenal hyperplasia from adenoma or carcinoma. Suppression testing in conjunction with adrenal CT scanning will usually isolate the tumor.

Although the diagnosis and medical treatment of precocious puberty is not complex, psychological support for affected children is essential. Because of their advanced physical appearance, unrealistic expectations and demands are frequently made of them. They are subject to immense peer pressure and stress, and every effort should be made to help them through a difficult life transition.

DIAGNOSTIC ASSESSMENT OF PRECOCIOUS PUBERTY

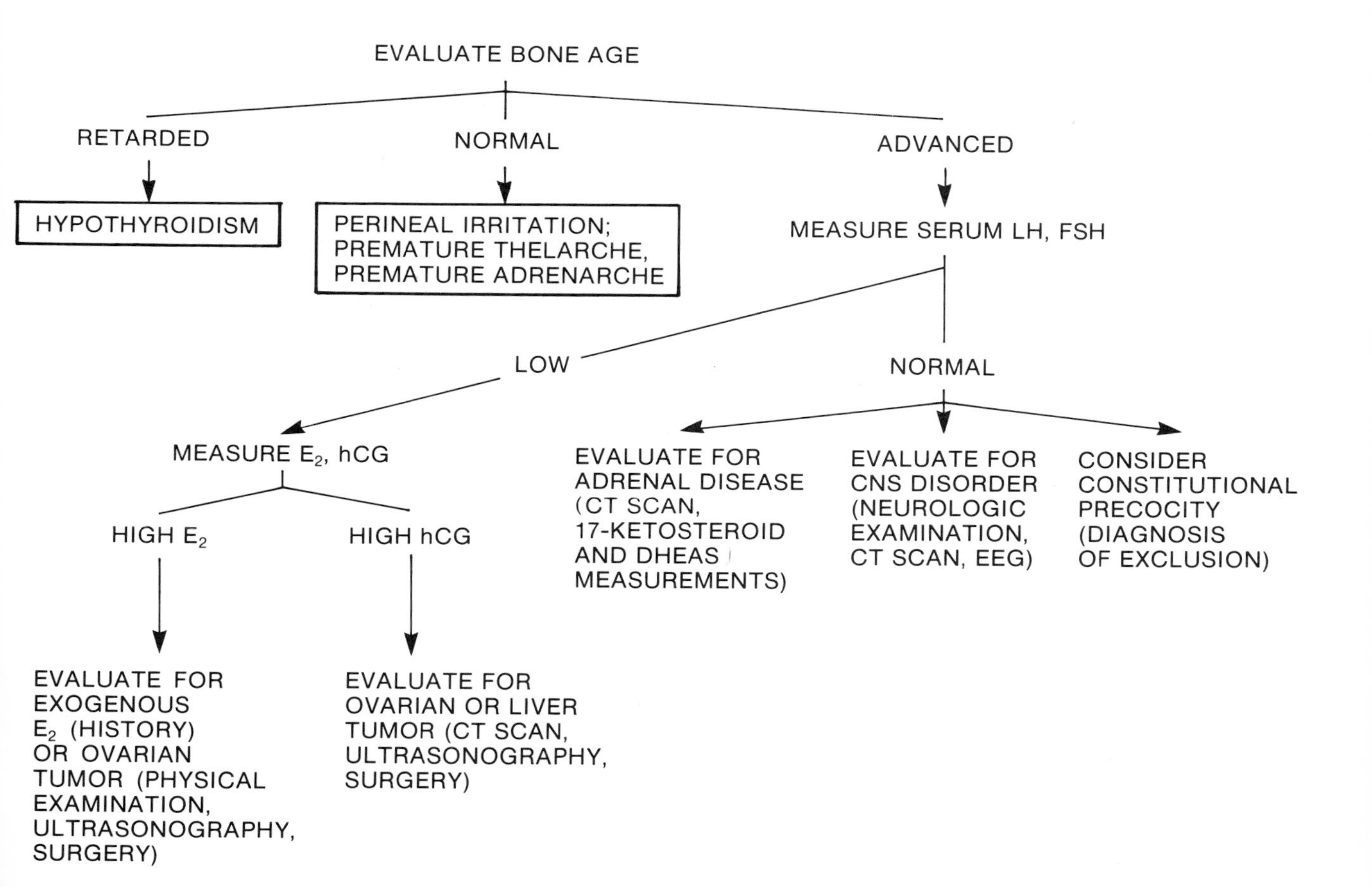

REFERENCES

1. Zacharias L, Wurtman RJ. Age at menarche. N Engl J Med 1969;280:868–75.
2. Marshall WA, Tanner JM. Variations in pattern of pubertal changes in girls. Arch Dis Child 1969;44:291–303.
3. Liu N, Grumbach MM, de Napoli RA, Morishima A. Prevalence of electroencephalographic abnormalities in idiopathic precocious puberty and premature pubarche: bearing on pathogenesis and neuroendocrine regulation of puberty. J Clin Endocrinol Metab 1965;25:1296–1308.
4. Bierich JR. Sexual precocity; disorders of puberty. J Clin Endocrinol Metab 1975;4:107–42.
5. Sigurjonsdottir TJ, Hayles AB. Precocious puberty: a report of 96 cases. Am J Dis Child 1968;115:309–21.
6. Saxena KM. Endocrine manifestations of neurofibromatosis in children. Am J Dis Child 1970;120:265–71.
7. Benedict PH. Sex precocity and polyostotic fibrous dysplasia. Am J Dis Child 1966;111:426–9.
8. Van Wyk JJ, Grumbach MM. Syndrome of precocious menstruation and galactorrhea in juvenile hypothyroidism: an example of hormonal overlap in pituitary feedback. J Pediatr 1960;57:416–35.
9. Styne DM, Grumbach MM. Puberty in the male and female: its physiology and disorders. In: Yen SSC, Jaffe RB, eds., Reproductive endocrinology. Philadelphia: WB Saunders, 1978;189–240.
10. Wilkins L. The diagnosis and treatment of endocrine disorders in childhood and adolescence. 3rd ed. Springfield, Ill: Charles C Thomas, 1965;619.
11. Conte FA, Grumbach MM. Pathogenesis, classification, diagnosis, and treatment of anomalies of sex. In: DeGroot L, Martini L, Potts J, et al., eds. Metabolic basis of endocrinology. New York: Grune & Stratton, 1977.
12. Towne BH, Mahour GH, Woolley MM, Isaacs H Jr. Ovarian cysts and tumors in infancy and childhood. J Pediatr Surg 1975;10:311–20.
13. DiSaia PJ, Creasman WT. Germ cell, stromal, and other ovarian tumors. In: Clinical gynecologic oncology. St Louis: CV Mosby, 1981;321–50.
14. Cangir A, Smith J, van Eys J. Improved prognosis in children with ovarian cancers following modified VAC (vincristine sulfate, dactinomycin, and cyclophosphamide) chemotherapy. Cancer 1978;42:1234–8.
15. Thompson JP, Dockerty MB, Symmonds RE, Hayles AB. Ovarian and parovarian tumors in infants and children. Am J Obstet Gynecol 1967;97:1059–65.
16. Eberlein WR, Bongiovanni AM, Jones IT, Yakovac WC. Ovarian tumors and cysts associated with sexual precocity. J Pediatr 1960;57:484–97.
17. Abell MR, Johnson VJ, Holtz F. Ovarian neoplasms in childhood and adolescence. I. Tumors of germ cell origin. Am J Obstet Gynecol 1965;92:1059–81.
18. Anderson WR, Levine AJ, MacMillan D. Granulosa-thecal cell tumors; clinical and pathologic study. Am J Obstet Gynecol 1971;110:32–5.
19. Novak ER, Long JH. Arrhenoblastoma of the ovary: a review of the Ovarian Tumor Registry. Am J Obstet Gynecol 1965;92:1082–93.
20. O'Hern TM, Neubecker RD. Arrhenoblastoma. Obstet Gynecol 1962;19:758–70.
21. Acosta A, Kaplan AL, Kaufman RH. Gynecologic cancer in children. Am J Obstet Gynecol 1972;112:944–52.
22. Barber HRK, Graber EA. Gynecological tumors in childhood and adolescence. Obstet Gynecol Surv 1973;28:357–81.
23. Groeber WR. Ovarian tumors during infancy and childhood. Am J Obstet Gynecol 1963;86:1021–35.
24. Neubecker RD, Breen JL. Embryonal carcinoma of the ovary. Cancer 1962;15:546–56.
25. Santesson L, Marrubini G. Clinical and pathological survey of ovarian embryonal carcinomas, including so-called "mesonephromas" (Schiller) or "mesoblastomas" (Teilum), treated at the Radiumhemmet. Acta Obstet Gynecol Scand 1957;36:399–419.
26. LaFranchi SH, Parlow AF, Lippe BM, Coyotupa J, Kaplan SA. Pubertal gynecomastia and transient elevation of serum estradiol level. Am J Dis Child 1975;129:927–31.
27. Hemsell DL, Edman CD, Marks JF, Siiteri PK, MacDonald PC. Massive extraglandular aromatization of plasma androstenedione resulting in feminization of a prepubertal boy. J Clin Invest 1977;60:455–64.

PULMONARY NODULE, SOLITARY

MICHAEL G. CORBETT □ GLEN A. LILLINGTON

□ SYNONYM: Coin lesion

BACKGROUND

Definition

The solitary pulmonary nodule is radiologically defined as a single circumscribed spherical intrapulmonary lesion (Fig. 1). Its margins may be smooth or irregular but should be distinct enough to define the contour of the lesion and allow measurement of its diameter in two or more dimensions. The surrounding lung parenchyma should also be relatively normal. Calcification may be seen within the lesion. The nodule may cavitate but usually does so only to a minor degree. If the majority of the lesional volume is involved in the cavitary process, reclassification as a cyst or thin-walled cavity is advisable for purposes of differential diagnosis.

Size is also an integral part of the definition of a pulmonary nodule. We believe that the term solitary nodule should be restricted to lesions less than 4 cm in diameter. Lesions with diameters greater than 4 cm have a much greater likelihood of malignancy. The differential diagnosis and decision process in these large mass lesions are sufficiently different to warrant separate consideration. The choice of 4 cm as the dividing point is clearly somewhat arbitrary.

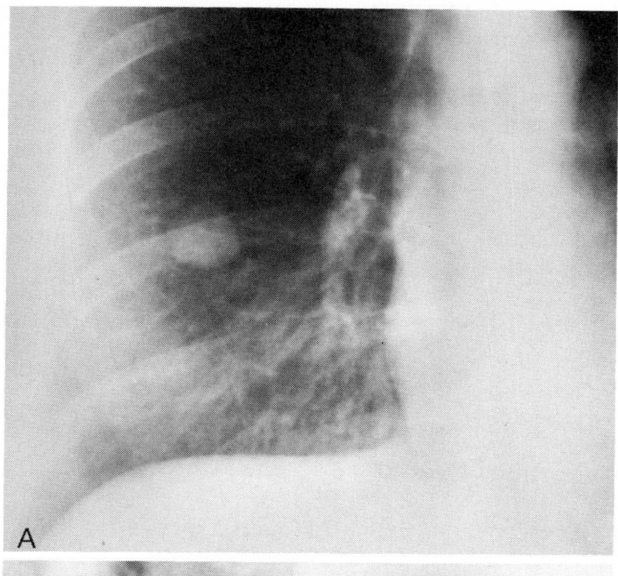

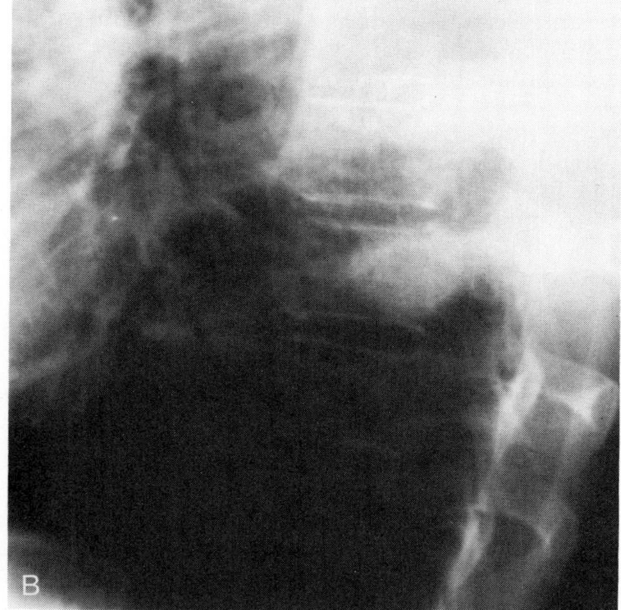

Figure 1. PA *(A)* and lateral *(B)* views of a well-circumscribed solitary nodule in a 40-year-old woman. Previous roentgenograms showed no change in size over a 10-year period. The nodule was considered benign and was not resected.

Etiology and Incidence

The causes of solitary pulmonary nodules are varied but generally can be divided into two basic groups, benign and malignant (Table 1). The most commonly occurring benign lesions are granulomas caused by tuberculosis, coccidioidomycosis, and histoplasmosis.[1] The malignant lesions of major concern are primary bronchogenic carcinomas and metastatic tumors from the kidney, colon, and breast. The percentage of nodules proven to be malignant in various series ranges between 20 and 40 per cent.[2–5] The reasons for this observed variability are multiple. Surgical series, which usually exclude calcified lesions, have a higher percentage of malignancies than those studies in which such lesions were not excluded.[3, 5] Studies originating in geographical areas endemic for coccidioidomycosis or histoplasmosis will, understandably, have a higher percentage of benign lesions. Age is also an important factor, in that malignancy is rare (1 per cent or less) in a person 35 years of age or younger but is quite common in older patients.[2, 4, 5] Larger pulmonary nodules are more likely to be malignant than smaller nodules.

Table 1. CAUSES OF THE SOLITARY PULMONARY NODULE

Malignant (20–40%)	Bronchogenic carcinoma (majority)
	Alveolar cell carcinoma
	Metastatic carcinoma
	Bronchial adenoma
Benign (60–80%)	Infectious granuloma (majority)
	Noninfectious granuloma
	Benign tumors
	Miscellaneous (healed infarct, arteriovenous aneurysm, pulmonary hematoma, echinococcal cyst, etc.)

HISTORY

Most patients with pulmonary nodules are asymptomatic. However, certain clues may be obtained in a thorough patient interview that may help in the management process. Pulmonary symptoms occur more commonly in patients with malignant nodules than in those with benign nodules.

History of Present Illness. A history of a recent upper respiratory tract infection, flu-like illness, or pneumonia is important, because pneumonic infiltrations occasionally are spherical. The presence of chronic cough, sputum production, weight loss, or hemoptysis increases the likelihood that the nodule is malignant.

Review of Systems. Evidence of the presence of nonmetastatic paraneoplastic syndromes may become apparent with appropriate questioning. Such syndromes may include clubbing with hypertrophic pulmonary osteoarthropathy, ectopic hormone production, migratory thrombophlebitis, and a variety of neurologic abnormalities.[6] All of these, however, are rare in association with pulmonary malignancy presenting as a solitary nodule. The main importance of the review of systems relates to the possibility that extrapulmonary symptoms may provide clues to the presence of a primary extrathoracic malignancy or of metastases from a primary pulmonary neoplasm. Symptoms such as a change in bowel habits, blood in the stool or urine, the finding of a breast lump, and discharge from the nipples are particularly suggestive of an extrapulmonary neoplasm.

Previous Medical History. Strong clues to the possible etiology of a solitary pulmonary nodule are provided by a previous extrapulmonary malignancy or proven granulomatous infection (tuberculous or fungal). Other systemic diseases that may be associated with the appearance of a solitary nodule include rheumatoid arthritis and opportunistic infections due to compromised immunity.

Social, Travel, and Work History. A significant smoking history markedly increases the chance that a pulmonary malignancy is present. Alcoholism is associated with an increased incidence of tuberculosis. Residence or travel in certain geographic areas (fungal endemic areas) may provide clues to the possible presence of some of the more common (coccidioidomycosis, histoplasmosis) and uncommon (echinococcosis, dirofilariasis) causes of lung nodules.[1] A thorough work history should be obtained, because certain industrial employees, such as asbestos workers and uranium and nickel miners, have an increased incidence of pulmonary malignancy.

PHYSICAL EXAMINATION

In the evaluation of the patient with a solitary pulmonary nodule, a complete and comprehensive physical examination is mandatory. On occasion, it may even obviate invasive diagnostic procedures and their associated morbidity and mortality. As with the history, the physical examination will usually be unrevealing, but specific features of diagnostic value are sometimes found. Lymphadenopathy should be carefully sought, as it may represent metastatic disease. Telangiectases of the skin and mucous membranes suggest that the pulmonary lesion is an arteriovenous malformation. The extremities should be checked for the presence of clubbing or osteoarthropathy and also for joint manifestations of rheumatoid arthritis. Any breast lumps or nipple discharge should be noted. Physical signs referable to the lungs are not commonly detected and, when present, are usually a reflection of an unrelated disease process such as asthma or emphysema. Hepatosplenomegaly, rectal masses, testicular irregularities, and guaiac-positive stools suggest that the lung nodule may be a metastasis from an extrapulmonary malignancy. In rare instances, the head and neck examination in the patient with an apical lung nodule may reveal evidence of Horner's syndrome owing to tumor involvement of the cervical sympathetic plexus. A careful neurologic examination should also be done to look for the paraneoplastic and metastatic neuromuscular abnormalities associated with bronchogenic carcinoma.

DIAGNOSTIC STUDIES

Certain basic laboratory studies are advisable in most patients in whom a solitary pulmonary nodule has been detected on chest roentgenogram. An exception can be made if the clinical and radiographic evidence indicates that the lesion is benign. (The criteria that must be satisfied to make such a judgment are outlined later.) Certain individuals require more specialized laboratory tests or procedures as indicated by the information obtained from the history and physical examination.

Laboratory Tests

Every patient in whom malignancy is a consideration should have a complete blood count, serum electrolyte measurements (including calcium), liver function studies, a urinalysis, and a coagulation profile. These basic studies help to detect some of the paraneoplastic syndromes associated with bronchogenic cardinoma and may provide evidence of possible metastatic spread to the liver or bones. They are also needed as a preliminary screening before invasive diagnostic procedures are undertaken.

Other studies of limited value include cytologic examination of the sputum and skin tests for tuberculosis, coccidioidomycosis and histoplasmosis. Results of the cytologic sputum study for cancer will be positive in less than 20 per cent of primary malignant nodules,[7] but this test has the advantages of high specificity and ease of performance. Positive skin test results provide clues as to possible etiologies but do not rule out malignancy. Sputum cultures and serologic studies for fungal antibodies are indicated only if opportunistic infection is suspected.

Pulmonary Function Tests

Comprehensive pulmonary function testing, including spirometry and measurements of lung volumes, diffusing capacity, and arterial blood gases, is indicated in many cases, particularly if invasive diagnostic procedures or surgical resection is contemplated. Information of this type helps in assessment of the risk of diagnostic procedures (bronchoscopy, needle biopsy, exploratory thoracotomy) and is critical to preoperative determination of the feasibility of pulmonary resection.[8]

Imaging

The standard PA and lateral chest roentgenograms establish the presence of the solitary nodule and provide information on the size, shape, position, and degree of calcification of the lesion. Serial roentgenograms indicate changes in size and permit calculation of growth rate, expressed as the "doubling time," which is the number of days required for the nodule to double its volume.

Chest tomography is indicated in many cases. Tomograms define the position of the nodule in instances in which the lesion is seen in only one of the two standard projections and sometimes demonstrate the presence of intranodular calcification that was not clearly detectable on the standard films.

Fluoroscopy is useful only as a guide for the passage of bronchoscopic biopsy forceps toward the lesion and for the placement of the needle tip within the lesion during percutaneous needle aspiration biopsy (Fig. 2).

The computed tomographic (CT) scan has limited usefulness in the patient with a solitary nodule. It may demonstrate the presence of multiple pulmonary nodules in the patient considered to have a solitary intrapulmonary metastatic deposit. Although CT measurements of the density of apparently uncalcified nodules have been reported to provide proof of benignity in some cases, such results have been difficult to confirm in most centers.[7]

The gallium-67 scan has some utility in the detection of occult mediastinal metastases, but it does not differentiate benign from malignant lesions.

Because radiographic and radioisotopic studies of other structures (brain, liver, bone) for metastatic lesions are usually normal in the absence of signs or symptoms referable to these structures, such studies are not indicated unless there is clinical or laboratory evidence of abnormality or dysfunction. Similarly, performance of such studies in a search for an occult extrathoracic primary is not indicated in the absence of localizing clinical abnormalities.

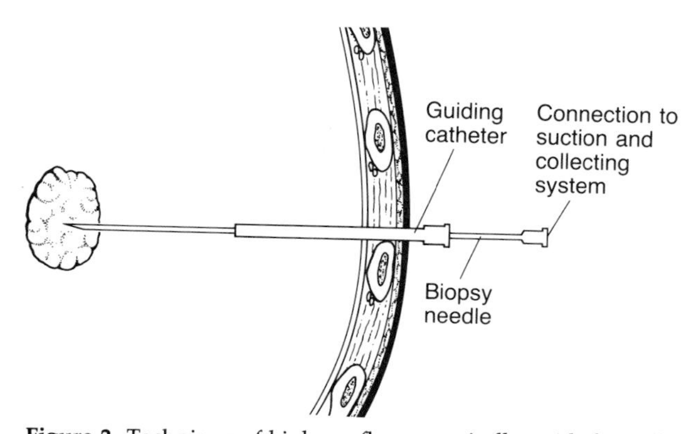

Figure 2. Technique of biplane, fluoroscopically guided needle aspiration biopsy using a small (18-gauge or less), long, beveled biopsy needle and negative pressure for specimen withdrawal. Various types of needles can be employed. In the technique shown here, a plastic catheter (Jelco needle) was passed initially to act as a transpleural conduit for the biopsy needle.

ASSESSMENT

The justification for a prompt and vigorous diagnostic assessment of the patient with a solitary pulmonary nodule is based upon the following premises:

1. A significant percentage of solitary pulmonary nodules are malignant neoplasms.
2. Prompt resection of solitary nodular bronchogenic carcinomas results in a 5-year survival rate of 50 per cent,[9] with rates as high as 80 per cent if the nodules are slow-growing[10] or small.[4, 11] It is presumed that the 5-year survival rate would be significantly reduced if there are prolonged delays between discovery of the nodule and surgical resection.[7]
3. All nodules should be regarded as potentially malignant unless strict criteria for benignity are satisfied. If they do not meet such criteria, all nodules should be subjected to resection unless other contraindications to surgery are present.

Resective lung surgery is accompanied by appreciable morbidity and a mortality rate varying from 0.5 to 10 per cent, so the chief goal of the clinical assessment and decision process is to reduce the number of resections for lesions that prove to be benign while avoiding inordinate delays in the resection of nodules that prove to be malignant. The development in the past two decades of more sensitive methods for the presurgical identification of benign lesions represents a major advance in the rational management of pulmonary nodules.

Determination of Benignity

The presence of *calcification* within the nodules is a highly reliable indication of benignity,[12, 13] particularly if its pattern is diffuse, lamellar, speckled, or central. In rare instances, eccentric flecks of calcium have been noted in malignant nodules, presumably because the cancer is arising from or adjacent to a previously calcified scar. Lung tomography is quite sensitive in detecting calcification and should be performed when standard chest roentgenograms fail to show any lesional

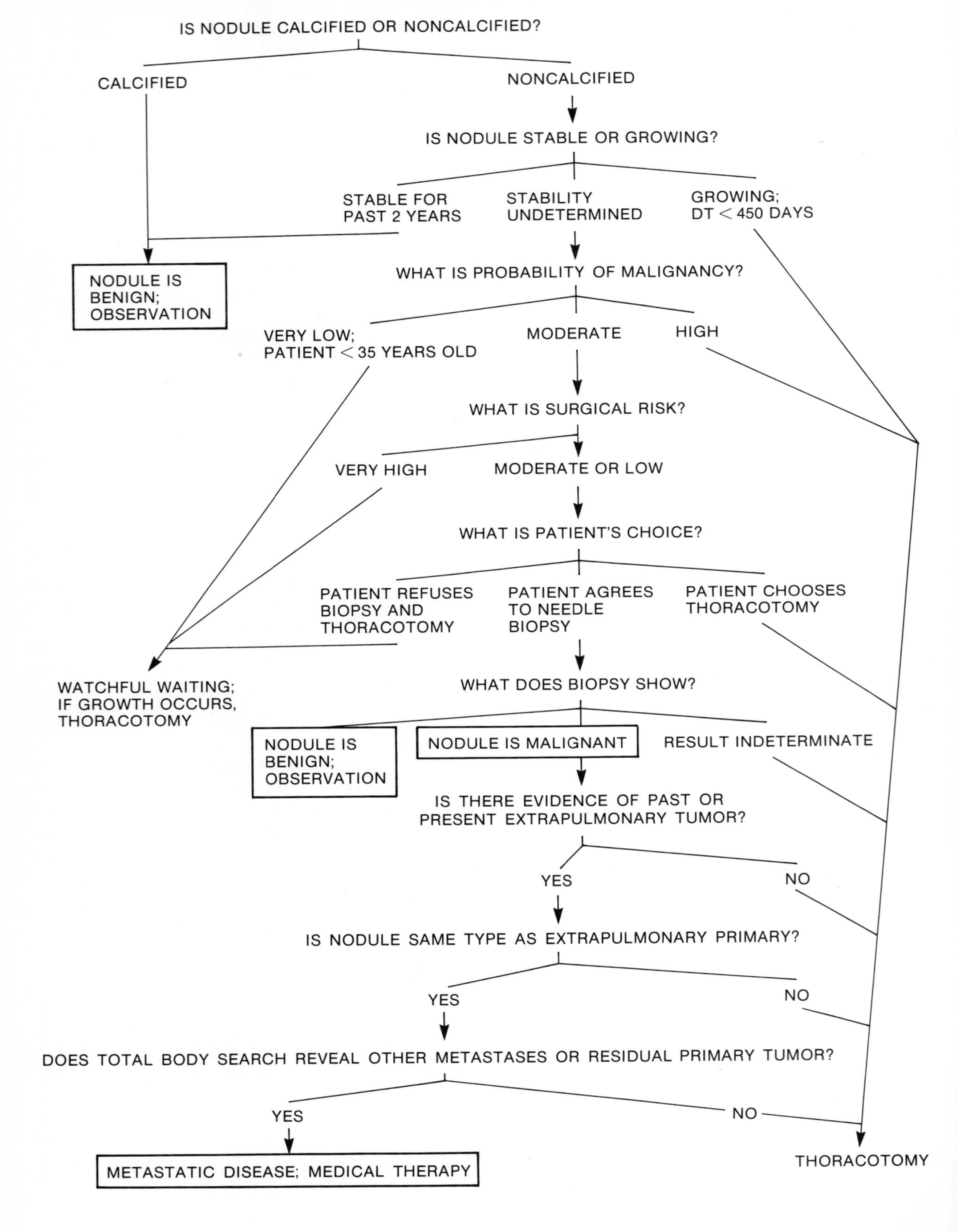
DIAGNOSTIC ASSESSMENT OF SOLITARY PULMONARY NODULE
IS NODULE CALCIFIED OR NONCALCIFIED?
CALCIFIED
NONCALCIFIED
IS NODULE STABLE OR GROWING?
STABLE FOR PAST 2 YEARS
STABILITY UNDETERMINED
GROWING; DT < 450 DAYS
NODULE IS BENIGN; OBSERVATION
WHAT IS PROBABILITY OF MALIGNANCY?
VERY LOW; PATIENT < 35 YEARS OLD
MODERATE
HIGH
WHAT IS SURGICAL RISK?
VERY HIGH
MODERATE OR LOW
WHAT IS PATIENT'S CHOICE?
PATIENT REFUSES BIOPSY AND THORACOTOMY
PATIENT AGREES TO NEEDLE BIOPSY
PATIENT CHOOSES THORACOTOMY
WATCHFUL WAITING; IF GROWTH OCCURS, THORACOTOMY
WHAT DOES BIOPSY SHOW?
NODULE IS BENIGN; OBSERVATION
NODULE IS MALIGNANT
RESULT INDETERMINATE
IS THERE EVIDENCE OF PAST OR PRESENT EXTRAPULMONARY TUMOR?
YES
NO
IS NODULE SAME TYPE AS EXTRAPULMONARY PRIMARY?
YES
NO
DOES TOTAL BODY SEARCH REVEAL OTHER METASTASES OR RESIDUAL PRIMARY TUMOR?
YES
NO
METASTATIC DISEASE; MEDICAL THERAPY
THORACOTOMY

calcium deposition. Recently, CT scanning has been used in assessing the density of pulmonary nodules shown to be uncalcified by routine radiologic means.[14] It was found that the density numbers generated by the computer correlated well with the pathologic nature of the lesion, with malignant lesions being less dense than benign ones. Although intriguing, this method remains unproven and should not be included in the standard diagnostic evaluation of pulmonary nodules.

Stability of the lesion, defined as an absence of growth over a period of 2 or more years, is a highly reliable indicator of benignity.[1, 15] This assessment is retrospective and depends upon the availability of prior chest roentgenograms. Every effort should be made to obtain old chest roentgenograms for direct comparison with the current films; reliance should never be placed on "negative" reports, no matter how distinguished the radiologist or prestigious the institution.

The prospective determination of stability, by means of obtaining serial chest roentgenograms at intervals of 6 to 12 weeks after the discovery of the solitary nodule, is called *watchful waiting*.[7, 10, 16] This policy has been condemned in the past, on the reasonable presumption that the delay in resection of nodules that are eventually proven to be growing, and therefore malignant, would reduce the surgical cure rate.

In our opinion, watchful waiting is a reasonable management alternative in three situations: (1) the patient with a very high surgical risk due to coronary disease or COPD, (2) the patient who refuses exploratory thoracotomy or other biopsy procedures, and (3) the patient who is less than 35 years of age and has no history or current evidence of an extrapulmonary primary malignancy. In such cases, the likelihood that the nodule is a primary lung tumor or a solitary metastasis is less than 1.0 per cent. The choice of watchful waiting in situations other than these three is highly controversial and requires further study.

Watchful waiting permits the calculation of the "doubling time," which is the interval in which the nodule doubles its volume. Malignant tumors usually have doubling times between 20 and 450 days, and if the calculated doubling time (prospective or retrospective) falls in this range, early thoracotomy is advisable.

Invasive Diagnostic Procedures

The criteria of calcification and stability, although important, are useful in establishing benignity in only a minority of cases. A tissue diagnosis is required for the ultimate proof. Recent years have seen the development of biopsy procedures that are less invasive than exploratory thoracotomy. Because many noncalcified nodules are benign,[2, 4, 5] such procedures will reduce the number of unnecessary thoracotomies.

Flexible Fiberoptic Bronchoscopy. Flexible fiberoptic bronchoscopy with fluoroscopically guided biopsy and brushing of the lesion has been carried out with some success.[17, 18] Diagnostic accuracy for nodular bronchogenic tumors approaches 60 per cent for lesions that are larger than 2 cm and centrally located. The yield is markedly lower, however, for benign processes and for metastatic nodules, as these conditions usually do not arise from bronchial mucosa. This procedure is least helpful in the situation in which we most need help, i.e., the histologic identification of benign nodules.

Needle Aspiration Biopsy. Short of thoracotomy, needle aspiration biopsy is the most accurate diagnostic method available for evaluating the solitary pulmonary nodule (see Fig. 2). Numerous studies report a diagnostic accuracy for malignant nodules, either primary or metastatic, of approximately 80 to 85 per cent.[19, 20] Although aspiration biopsy is less accurate for benign lesions, 40 to 60 per cent of these were correctly diagnosed with this procedure.[7, 19, 20] The advantages become evident. Not all benign lesions are correctly diagnosed, but those patients in whom benign lesions are diagnosed will be saved the morbidity and expense of unnecessary thoracotomy. If the needle biopsy shows the presence of carcinoma and the cell type, the physician is better able to assess the advisability of curative resection in high-risk individuals.[21] The patients themselves may also feel more comfortable about accepting surgery when the diagnosis of cancer is definitely proven.

Complications occur in approximately one-third of patients undergoing needle aspiration biopsy,[20, 22] including pneumothorax (30 per cent), local bleeding (11 per cent), and limited hemoptysis (2 to 4 per cent). Although their incidences are relatively high, the seriousness of the complications is slight and most require no specific therapy. Approximately 4 to 8 per cent of the pneumothoraces require exsufflation.[20, 22] The incidence of adverse side effects does appear to correlate with increasing age and the presence of abnormal lung compliance.[23]

The main contraindication to needle biopsy is advanced emphysema.

Thoracotomy. The purpose of thoracotomy is three-fold: (1) to rule out malignancy in those patients previously undiagnosed by prior methods, (2) for curative resection of primary lung tumors that show no evidence of mediastinal, pleural, or systemic metastases at the time of exploration, and (3) for occasional removal of solitary metastatic lung lesions secondary to extrapulmonary primary malignant tumors.

Metastatic disease from a primary lung lesion contraindicates operative therapy. Pleural and systemic involvement is unusual in nodular bronchogenic carcinoma, except in the relatively rare instances in which a small-cell carcinoma presents as a solitary nodule. Mediastinal involvement, however, is more common and may occur in as many as 50 to 60 per cent of cases, depending on tumor size, location, and cell type.[21] For this reason, mediastinoscopy, gallium-67 scanning, and computerized tomography have been used to assess tumor extension into the mediastinum.[24, 25, 26] Except in specific instances, these studies add little to the management of the peripheral nodules. The majority of the tumors (70 to 85 per cent) are adenocarcinoma or squamous cell carcinoma, which in the presence of a normal hilum or mediastinum on chest x-ray have a low incidence (3 to 16 per cent) of occult mediastinal involvement.[21, 24] Mediastinoscopy or gallium-67 scanning may be useful in determining operability in established cases of undifferentiated carcinoma, in which a high incidence (> 50 per cent) of mediastinal metastases is expected.[25] CT scanning is most useful in finding metastatic nodules to the lung that are not visible with standard roentgenographic techniques.[26]

Diagnostic Approach

Given the potential for cure, a significant number of patients with solitary pulmonary nodules come to surgical resection. The decision to proceed not only incorporates the previously discussed data but must also include a consideration of the wide range of risks involved (Table 2) and the mental preparedness of the patient. The algorithm attempts to offer guidelines for the work-up of these difficult cases.

Calcified nodules require little if any follow-up, but if the calcification is scanty, we suggest one or two repeat films at 3-month intervals for extra reassurance. Similarly, the stable nodule deserves at least one additional film in 6 months as a matter of prudence.

Watchful waiting requires follow-up films at intervals of 1½ to 3 months for a year, then every 6 months for another year. If growth occurs, with a doubling time of less than 450 days, needle biopsy or prompt resection is required.

Table 2. RISK FACTORS FOR INVASIVE DIAGNOSTIC PROCEDURES AND THORACOTOMY

Increasing age
Presence of impaired pulmonary function
Other unstable systemic illnesses
Bleeding diatheses
Altered mental status
Negative patient attitude
Significant coronary artery disease

Table 3. FACTORS INDICATING HIGH PROBABILITY OF BRONCHOGENIC CARCINOMA

Age > 45 years
Presence of pulmonary symptoms
Uncalcified nodule with blurred or fuzzy margins
Significant smoking history
Nodule diameter > 2 cm
Growth of nodule (doubling time < 450 days)

If there is a history (or current evidence) of an extrapulmonary primary malignancy, needle biopsy is advisable. It the tissue obtained is the same type as that of the primary tumor, resection of the nodule may still be considered but should be preceded by a "total body search" for other metastases.

If the needle biopsy reveals a benign disease, follow-up should comprise one or two additional films at 6-month intervals.

In the patient with an uncalcified nodule, the presence of one or more factors suggesting a high probability of primary lung cancer is an indication for exploratory thoracotomy (Table 3). Conversely, if the factors suggest a low probability of malignancy, needle aspiration biopsy would be the preferable action. In such situations, the wishes of the patient play an important and legitimate role in the decision process.

REFERENCES

1. Lillington GA, Jamplis RW. A diagnostic approach to chest diseases: differential diagnoses based on roentgenographic patterns. 2nd ed. Baltimore: Williams & Wilkins, 1977:131–44.
2. Trunk G, Gracey, DR, Byrd RB. The management and evaluation of the solitary pulmonary nodule. Chest 1974:66:236–9.
3. Nolim SM, Dwork RE, Glaser S, Rikli AE, Stocklen JD. Solitary pulmonary nodules found in a community wide chest roentgenographic survey. Am Rev Tuberc 1959:427–39.
4. Jefferson FR, Lawton BR, Magnin GE, et al. The coin lesion story: update 1976. Twenty years experience with early thoracotomy for 179 suspected malignant coin lesions. Chest 1976;70:332–6.
5. Higgins GA, Shields TW, Keehn RJ. The solitary pulmonary nodule: ten year follow-up of Veterans Administration–Armed Forces cooperative study. Arch Surg 1975;110:570–5.
6. Stolinsky DC. Paraneoplastic syndromes (medical progress). West J Med 1980;132:189–208.
7. Lillington GA. Pulmonary nodules: solitary and multiple. Clin Chest Med 1982;3:361–7.
8. Tisi GM. Preoperative evaluation of pulmonary function: validity, indication, and benefits. Am Rev Resp Dis 1979;119:293–309.
9. Jackman RJ, Good CA, Clagett OT, Woolmer LB. Survival rates in peripheral bronchogenic carcinomas up to four centimeters in diameter presenting as solitary pulmonary nodules. J Thorac Cardiovasc Surg 1969;57:1–8.
10. Meyer JA. Growth rate versus prognosis in resected primary bronchogenic carcinomas. Cancer 1973;31:1468–72.
11. Buell PE. The importance of tumor size in prognosis for

resected bronchogenic carcinoma. J Surg Oncol 1971;3:539–51.
12. Bateson EM. An analyses of 155 solitary lung lesions illustrating the differential diagnosis of mixed tumors of the lung. Clin Radiol 1965;16:51.
13. O'Keefe ME, Good CA, McDonald JR. Calcification in solitary pulmonary nodules of the lung. Am J Roentgenol 1957;77:1023.
14. Siegelman SS, Zerhouni EA, Leo FP, Khouri NF, Stitik FP. CT of the solitary pulmonary nodule. AJR 1980;135:1–13.
15. Nathan MD, Collins VP, Adams RA. Differentiation of benign and malignant nodules by growth rate. Radiology 1962;79:221–32.
16. Nathan MH. Management of solitary pulmonary nodules: an organized approach based on growth rate and statistics. JAMA 1974;227:1141–4.
17. Cortese DA, McDougall JC. Biopsy and brushing of peripheral lung cancer with fluoroscopic guidance. Chest 1979;75:141–5.
18. Radke JR, Conway WA, Eyler WK, Kvale PA. Diagnostic accuracy in peripheral lung lesions: factors predicting success with flexible fiberoptic bronchoscopy. Chest 1979;76:176–9.
19. Sinner WN. Transthoracic needle biopsy of small peripheral malignant lung lesions. Invest Radiol 1973:8:305–14.
20. Lalli AF, McCormack LJ, Zelch M, Reich NE, Belovich D. Aspiration biopsies of chest lesions. Radiology 1978;127:35–40.
21. Whitcomb ME, Barham E, Goldman AL, Greene DC. Indications for mediastinoscopy in bronchogenic carcinoma. Am Rev Resp Dis 1976;113:189–95.
22. Sinner WN. Complications of percutaneous transthoracic needle aspiration biopsy. Acta Radiol [Diagn] (Stockh) 1976;17:813–28.
23. Berquist TH, Bailey PB, Cortese OA, Miller WE. Transthoracic needle biopsy: accuracy and complications in relation to location and type of lesion. Mayo Clin Proc 1980;55:475–81.
24. Hirleman MT, Yiu-Chiu VS, Chiu LC, Schapiro RL. The resectability of primary lung carcinoma: a diagnostic staging review. CT 1980;4:146–63.
25. Shanti LL, Ruckdeschel JC, McKneally MF, et al. Noninvasive evaluation of mediastinal metastases in bronchogenic carcinoma: a prospective comparison of chest radiography and gallium-67 scanning. Cancer 1981;47:672–9.
26. Muhm JR, Brown LR, Crowe JK. Use of computed tomography in the detection of pulmonary nodules. Mayo Clin Proc 1977;52:345–8.

PURPURA

ROBERT R. CARROLL □ CRAIG S. KITCHENS

□ SYNONYMS: Petechiae, ecchymoses

BACKGROUND

Purpura is discoloration of skin or mucous membrane caused by the extravasation of red blood cells from intravascular, usually capillary, spaces. When these extravasations are minute—resembling paprika sprinkled on skin—they are referred to as *petechiae;* when larger than 3 mm, they are considered *ecchymoses*. When a large amount of blood extravasates into subcutaneous tissue or a fascial plane, the palpable extravascular mass is considered a *hematoma*. Petechiae are originally bright red and fade to brown within several days. Ecchymoses in healthy skin may originally be purple or blue-black, but as the blood is phagocytized and catabolized by tissue macrophages, the color changes to brown, then yellow-brown. Purpuric lesions in sun-damaged or very old, tissue-paper–thin skin initially appear red-purple and may seem very superficial; they may persist for a prolonged time.

When purpura is caused by extravasation of red cells through uninflamed vessels, as is the case when purpura is caused by deficiencies in platelet number or function or by weakness of vessel walls (as in scurvy or amyloidosis), the lesions are not palpable; the examiner cannot discern normal from purpuric skin by touch alone. An exception to this rule occurs if enough red cells extravasate to produce blood-filled blebs. These blebs have a soft, fluctuant consistency, and are usually seen only in severe thrombocytopenia. When purpura is caused by inflammatory destruction of vessel walls, the perivascular infiltrate of leukocytes causes the tissue to feel firm or nodular; such palpable purpura is usually caused by vasculitis. The inflammation may cause these lesions to be urticarial and erythematous as well as purpuric.

Purpura should be distinguished from vascular anomalies in the skin. Small cherry angiomas, the telangiectases of Osler-Weber-Rendu disease, and, at times, the malignant lesions of Kaposi's sarcoma may mimic purpura. Since the blood in these lesions is intravascular, pressure applied over them with a microscope slide allows the observer to see them blanch, whereas petechiae and ecchymoses remain unchanged; this maneuver is helpful but not infallible, because it is difficult to express blood from some vascular anomalies. Also, Kaposi's sarcoma may leak erythrocytes into surrounding tissue, causing true purpura. Observations over time may help; vascular abnormalities remain unchanged, the lesions of Kaposi's sarcoma may enlarge and become nodular, but petechiae and ecchymoses gradually resolve.

Causes

Possible causes of purpura are legion, but they can be arranged into groups according to pathophysiologic mechanism (Table 1).[1] This classification facilitates the physician's approach to the diagnosis and permits rational ordering of laboratory tests.

Purpura Not Associated with Any Known Disease

Mechanical Purpura. Purpura can result from direct trauma to skin capillaries. Familiar examples include the precordial lesions produced by the suction cups of electrocardiograph electrodes and those caused by an unduly sharp needle used to evaluate a patient's sensory perception. Increases in intravascular pressure can overwhelm normal capillary wall intergrity, producing petechiae over the face and neck of postictal patients, children who have been vomiting, and persons who practice hanging upside-down as therapy for back pain.[2] Purpura may be caused surreptitiously using a number of means, usually in an effort to gain attention; self-inflicted lesions are most often found on easily accessible areas of skin.

Progressive Pigmented Purpura. On occasion, an otherwise healthy patient may develop purpuric skin lesions that may continue to occur for years. They may be pruritic and are often described in the dermatologic literature as having a characteristic "cayenne pepper" color; they occur most often in men, usually on the legs. Biopsy of these lesions shows only a perivascular lymphocytic infiltrate (not the granulocytic infiltrate of leukocytoclastic vasculitis).[3] Depending on minor clinical criteria, a variety of names have been attached to variations of this condition, including Schamberg's disease, pigmented purpuric lichenoid dermatosis of Gougerot and Blum, lichen purpuricas, purpura annularis telangiectodes or Majocchi's disease, and purpura telangiectatica arciformis.

No underlying disease is present, and, by definition, none develops. Results of laboratory tests such as the erythrocyte sedimentation rate, platelet count, bleeding time, serum protein electrophoresis, and rheumatoid factor are normal. The diagnosis is made on clinical appearance, accompanied by a compatible skin biopsy specimen and the chronic, benign course.

Table 1. CLASSIFICATION OF PURPURA LISTED ACCORDING TO PATHOPHYSIOLOGIC MECHANISM

Not associated with any known disease	Mechanical purpura Progressive pigmented purpura
Abnormalities of platelet number or function	Thrombocytopenic purpura Thrombocytopathic purpura
Leukocytoclastic vasculitis	Underlying disease (see text) Specific agents
Direct endothelial cell damage	Chemical injury Injury by microorganisms
Decreased mechanical strength of the microcirculation	Scurvy Hypercortisolism Hereditable diseases of connective tissue Amyloidosis Senile or atrophic purpura
Microthrombi	Fat embolism Disseminated intravascular coagulation (DIC) Thrombotic thrombocytopenic purpura (TTP) Myloblastemia Cholesterol embolization
Psychogenic causes	Psychogenic purpura

(Adapted from Kitchens CS. The anatomic basis of purpura. Prog Hemost Thromb 1980; 5:211–44.)

Purpura Due to Abnormalities of Platelet Number or Function

Thrombocytopenic Purpura. Severe thrombocytopenia causes capillary fragility, which is easily demonstrated by the Rumpel-Leede or Hess capillary test and is evidenced by the petechiae seen on the legs in patients with a low platelet count. The mechanism by which platelets maintain normal capillary integrity is not known. Either decreased platelet production or unduly rapid removal of platelets from the circulation may account for thrombocytopenia; an estimate of the megakaryocyte numbers seen in a bone marrow aspirate is most helpful in differentiating between these two mechanisms. A normal or increased number of megakaryocytes in a bone marrow aspirate from a patient with thrombocytopenia would suggest a condition such as hypersplenism, immunologic destruction of platelets (which can be idiopathic or drug-induced), or thrombotic thrombocytopenic purpura. Diminished numbers of megakaryocytes imply difficulties with platelet production, as seen in amegakaryocytic thrombocytopenia, metastatic carcinoma, aplastic anemia, leukemia, drug-induced marrow damage, thrombocytopenia with absent radius syndrome, and other primary disorders of bone marrow.

Thrombocytopathic Purpura. Dysfunctional

platelet syndromes are common. Patients with platelet dysfunction rarely notice petechiae; their most common complaint is "easy bruising." Minimal, often unnoticed trauma may cause ecchymotic lesions, and bleeding from minor skin or mucous membrane wounds may be excessive. Characteristically, the bleeding time is prolonged in the presence of adequate numbers of platelets. Dysfunctional platelets are found in both hereditary syndromes and acquired diseases. Congenital causes of platelet dysfunction include Bernard-Soulier syndrome, May-Hegglin anomaly, and Glanzmann's disease, as well as the very common "intermediate platelet dysfunction" syndromes, in which platelets behave as though they had been exposed to aspirin and are unable to properly release intraplatelet contents owing to defects in arachidonic acid metabolism.[4] Also, although platelets themselves are normal in von Willebrand's disease, deficiency of the plasma von Willebrand factor prevents platelets from functioning normally. Actual exposure to aspirin may worsen the platelet dysfunction in any of the preceding disorders. The myeloproliferative diseases may cause very high platelet counts, but the platelets are often dysfunctional and the patient may develop purpura even when the platelet count is elevated.[5]

Purpura Associated with Leukocytoclastic Vasculitis. Leukocytoclastic vasculitis is defined as collections of granulocytes surrounding the microvasculature. The granulocytes may be normal-appearing or in varying stages of disintegration. This condition may be initiated by leakage of immune complexes through capillary walls. The extravascular immune complexes then activate complement, producing chemotactic factors and causing the neutrophilic infiltration. Vessel wall destruction results from release of neutrophilic enzymes. Leukocytoclastic vasculitis is associated with an extensive list of diseases, including Waldenström's macroglobulinemia, systemic lupus erythematosus, lymphomas, cryoglobulinemia, Wegener's granulomatosis, subacute bacterial endocarditis, rheumatoid arthritis, polyarteritis nodosa, and Henoch-Schönlein purpura. Also, leukocytoclastic vasculitis is seen in some drug reactions, including reactions to penicillin, iodides, isoniazid, aspirin, azo dyes, benzoic acid, thiazides, oxytetracycline, colchicine, carbromal, and phenothiazines. Immune complexes due to infection with hepatitis B virus may cause a leukocytoclastic vasculitis, sometimes occurring as a prodrome to overt hepatitis.[6]

Purpura Due to Direct Endothelial Cell Damage

Chemical Injury. Acute hemorrhagic fat necrosis may be caused by coumarin derivatives. This reaction occurs idiosyncratically, most often in women, and usually over the breast or buttocks. It is thought to be due to a direct toxic effect on endothelium. The lesions are initially purpuric and may progress to skin necrosis.[7]

Microbial Injury. Rickettsiae invade endothelial cells. Presumably, the purpura of Rocky Mountain spotted fever and other rickettsioses are due to direct endothelial cell invasion and disruption. Meningococci can also be found in endothelium and are directly toxic to these cells. The coagulation abnormalities caused by meningococcal endotoxin may account for the extensive purpura seen in some cases of meningococcemia.[8]

Purpura Associated with Decreased Mechanical Strength of the Microcirculation

Scurvy. Ascorbic acid is necessary for the production of both hydroxyproline, an amino acid peculiar to collagen, and chondroitin sulfate, the ground substance of collagen. The pathologic changes in scurvy are thought to be due to defective collagen production. As collagen affords the capillaries tensile strength, the scorbutic capillaries become fragile, resulting in petechiae, ecchymoses, and hematomas. Perifollicular petechiae are distinctive and are most commonly seen on the abdomen, extensor surface of the forearms, and posterior thighs. Ecchymoses may appear in areas of pressure or irritation. Results of platelet function tests, including platelet aggregation and bleeding time, are normal.

Hypercortisolism. Long-term exposure to excessive levels of glucocorticosteroids, from either Cushing's disease or exogenous administration, results in thinning of skin and the propensity to develop purpura, particularly over the extensor surfaces of the extremities. Corticosteroids diminish collagen production, and the cause of the purpura is similar to that in scurvy.[9]

Heritable Diseases of Connective Tissue. The various forms of Ehlers-Danlos syndrome are manifested by hyperextensible joints, hyperelastic, often thin and friable skin, and a propensity to form purpura and ecchymoses. The defect is due to abnormal synthesis of collagen with a resulting decrease in vessel wall strength.[10]

Amyloidosis. Amyloid involvement in skin is found frequently in so-called primary amyloidosis and in multiple myeloma. The amyloid deposits appear to replace the vessel walls in capillaries and small arterioles, and purpura results when these weakened vessels are subjected to even minimal trauma. For unknown reasons, eyelid and periorbital purpura are common in amyloidosis.[11]

Senile or Atrophic Purpura. Aging and chronic sunlight exposure result in thin skin due to destruction of collagen. This skin is friable and quickly develops superficial-appearing ecchymoses with minimal trauma. Purpura are most common over extensor surfaces of forearms and lower legs. Platelet function is normal. This common form of purpura is also seen in debilitated patients regardless of age.[12]

Purpura Associated with Microthrombi

Fat Embolism. Severe trauma, with fractures of the pelvis or long bones, may release marrow fat into the circulation. Petechiae may be caused either by the fat droplets themselves or by toxic effects on endothelium produced as the neutral fat is metabolized to free fatty acids. This syndrome is accompanied by respiratory distress, diffuse pulmonary infiltrates, and fever, in addition to petechiae, and usually occurs within 48 hours of the injury. The petechiae are commonly seen over the face, neck, chest, and axillary folds and in the conjunctivae. Results of clotting studies and platelet counts are usually normal or nearly so; fat embolization itself does not usually cause disseminated intravascular coagulation.[13]

Disseminated Intravascular Coagulation (DIC). DIC from any cause (endotoxins, retained dead fetus, presence of necrotic tissue, tumor, etc.) results in the production of thrombin, activation of plasminogen and fibrinogen, consumption of other coagulation proteins, and aggregation of platelets in the circulation, as platelet and fibrin microthrombi are formed in small vessels. Microvascular occlusion may cause necrosis of vessel walls and surrounding tissue with the production of petechiae and purpura. The thrombocytopenia produced by platelet destruction adds to the production of petechiae.

Thrombotic Thrombocytopenic Purpura (TTP). The pathologic hallmark of TTP is occlusion of the microcirculation by platelet plugs. Early in the course of the disease the patient may notice "easy bruising" even though the platelet count may be only minimally diminished; the concept of "platelet exhaustion" is thought to account for this platelet dysfunction. Later, petechiae and purpura may be produced by the dual mechanisms of severe thrombocytopenia and microinfarction due to platelet thrombi.[14]

Myeloblastemia. Leukemic blast cell counts of greater than 100,000/mm^3 may be associated with leukostasis syndromes, producing central nervous system dysfunction, hypoxia with pulmonary infiltrates, and purura. The cause is mechanical obstruction of capillaries by the "sticky" myeloblasts, with resulting necrosis of the walls of the vessels.[15]

Cholesterol Embolization. Cholesterol crystals may embolize from ulcerated atherosclerotic plaques to the microvascular circulation. Usually the legs and kidneys are involved. Purpuric lesions may be produced in the skin of the lower legs; livedo reticularis is commonly seen. Pulses in the large arteries are not directly compromised. Cholesterol crystals can be seen in skin biopsy specimens.[16]

Psychogenic Purpura

This bizarre and uncommon type of purpura deserves mention, as it can cause great diagnostic confusion. It seems to originate as a form of factitious purpura, but later, autoantibodies to erythrocyte stroma apparently develop. At this point, the patient often tells of tingling or burning at the site of the skin lesions. Indeed, an inflammatory component, including a wheal-and-flare reaction, may be witnessed. This disorder is seen nearly exclusively in women who have psychiatric difficulties.[17]

HISTORY

The following questions regarding the history of the patient's purpura are helpful in arriving at a diagnosis of the underlying cause.

How Old Is the Patient? Some causes of purpura are more likely to affect a certain age group than others. Neonates are susceptible to gram-negative sepsis with its attendant DIC; they may also develop purpura from thrombocytopenia caused by the Wiskott-Aldrich syndrome, by thrombocytopenia with absent radius syndrome, or by placental crossing of maternal antibodies to fetal platelets, which may occur when the mother has immune thrombocytopenic purpura (ITP) or when she becomes sensitized to fetal platelets that possess an antigen not present on her own platelets.[18] Scurvy, though rare, might also be considered as a possible cause of purpura in a malnourished infant. Scurvy is now a disease of the extremes of age. Other diseases occurring in childhood that may manifest as purpura include acute ITP, acute lymphoblastic leukemia (the peak age incidence of childhood leukemia is 3 years), and Henoch-Schönlein purpura. The rheumatic diseases are most common in the middle years, whereas myeloma, amyloidosis, the myeloproliferative diseases, and other primary disorders of bone marrow tend to occur most frequently in late adulthood. Senile purpura is exceedingly common in older adults.

How Long Has Purpura Been Present? Depending on the underlying causes, purpura may be chronic, subacute, acute, or, rarely, fulminant. The patient may have first noted purpura months or even years before seeking medical advice, a delay that suggests a relatively benign cause of the problem. Purpuras due to chronic dermatologic conditions—senile purpura, Schamberg's disease and its congeners—fall into this category. Many of the diseases underlying a leukocytoclastic vasculitis tend to be chronic. The patient with chronic ITP, whose platelet count may typically be 15,000 to 20,000/mm³, being otherwise healthy, may not seek medical attention until months after petechiae and ecchymoses have been first noted. Certainly, if the patient has had lifelong purpura, congenital causes of thrombocytopenia or platelet dysfunction should be considered.

Illnesses that cause a more abrupt onset of purpura, often with other associated symptoms, include acute ITP, TTP, drug reactions, acute derangements of bone marrow function, rickettsial and meningococcal infections, and Henoch-Schönlein purpura. Patients with acute ITP typically have platelet counts below 10,000/mm³, and may be bothered by overt hemorrhage. Fever may be a prominent symptom of TTP or septicemia. The patient may report that the lesions of Henoch-Schönlein purpura were erythematous and pruritic before becoming purpuric, and that they occurred in crops appearing over several weeks.

Rarely, purpura may appear with dramatic suddenness, within a few hours of the patient's becoming ill. This occurrence is most often due to fulminant meningococcal sepsis, though it may happen in drug-induced thrombocytopenia, such as is sometimes seen following quinine or quinidine ingestion.

Has the Patient Had Abnormal Bleeding? As a rule, menorrhagia and mucosal surface bleeding implicate thrombocytopenia or, less often, platelet dysfunction. On occasion, the leukocytoclastic vasculitis of Henoch-Schönlein purupura may cause gastrointestinal bleeding due to infarctions of gut mucosa.[19] Interestingly, although classic hemophilia may cause severe bleeding, it usually causes fascial plane hematomas and hemarthroses rather than purpuric lesions.

Does the Patient Have Symptoms Other Than Purpura? Patients with dermatologic conditions causing purpura are generally healthy. Likewise, patients with ITP, unless thay have symptoms specifically caused by bleeding, are well and do not otherwise have complaints referable to the hematologic disorder. Malaise and fever should suggest an infectious disorder or TTP. Clues to the presence of a rheumatic illness (history of joint or abdominal pain, pleurisy, pericarditis) should be noted. Back pain (or other bone pain) can be seen with myeloma or related diseases, with or without amyloidosis. Some of the diseases causing a leukocytoclastic vasculitis (e.g., lupus) are equally capable of causing vasculitis in any organ.

Has the Patient Recently Been Severely Ill, Been Injured, or Undergone Surgery? Such a patient may be at risk of developing gram-negative sepsis, with its attendant DIC and purpura. Many of the technological devices of medicine, including indwelling catheters in bladder or vessels and endotracheal tubes, predispose to sepsis. Severe injuries, such as pelvic or long bone fractures, may cause fat embolization. Recent blood transfusions may cause post-transfusion purpura due to thrombocytopenia.[20]

Is the Patient Pregnant? Both ITP and TTP occur with higher frequency in pregnancy. Complications of pregnancy such as retained placental fragments, a retained dead fetus, abruptio placentae, toxemia, septic abortion, and postpartum sepsis may cause DIC.

Is the Patient Taking Drugs That Might Cause Purpura? Corticosteroids taken over long periods may cause skin damage that predisposes to purpura. Numerous drugs are capable of causing thrombocytopenia by decreasing production of platelets by the marrow, increasing platelet destruction by immunologic means, or inciting a vasculitis. Many drugs are capable of interfering with platelet function; this effect rarely causes purpura by itself, although it may contribute to other inadequacies of platelet number or function. Aspirin is certainly the most common offender in this regard.[21]

Is There a Family History of Purpura or Easy Bruising? Whereas some dysfunctional platelet syndromes (Bernard-Soulier syndrome, Glanzmann's disease) are transmitted in autosomal recessive fashion, von Willebrand's disease and the "intermediate platelet dysfunction" syndromes are commonly inherited as autosomal dominant traits.

Are There Influencing Psychiatric or Social Circumstances? Factitious illnesses, including purpura, are difficult to diagnose unless the possibility enters the physician's mind. ITP has been described as a component of the acquired immunodeficiency syndrome (AIDS) that has now been found in homosexual males, Haitians, hemophiliacs, and drug addicts.[22] Another component of this syndrome, Kaposi's sarcoma, may mimic purpura or may actually be purpuric before becoming nodular.

PHYSICAL EXAMINATION

The general appearance of the patient may provide the first clue to the etiology of purpura. The patient with purpura as a manifestation of a dermatologic phenomenon will appear well, as will a patient with uncomplicated ITP. Should the patient be tachypneic, tachycardic, febrile, prostrate, or otherwise acutely ill, TTP or sepsis (Neisseria, Rickettsia, or other organism) with DIC should be considered. Wasting, inanition, or pallor may be a clue to an underlying process such as myeloma, Waldenström's disease, or a related illness.

The location and characteristics of the purpura may give some insight into the cause. "Wet" purpura on skin or mucous membranes is almost always caused by severe thrombocytopenia and is accompained by epistaxis and gum bleeding. Lesser degrees of thrombocytopenia will cause fine petechiae, usually first seen over the legs. Firm, nodular purpura, sometimes pruritic or with surrounding erythema, denotes a vasculitis. Vasculitic purpura may cause areas of skin necrosis. Henoch-Schönlein purpura usually occurs symmetrically on the legs and buttocks. The purpura of hemorrhagic fat necrosis from anticoagulants occurs most often over the breasts and buttocks in women. Purpura in Schamberg's disease may be accompanied by hyperpigmentation of the skin in the involved areas. Amyloid purpura commonly occurs over the face and neck.

The physical examination may disclose other features of particular diseases associated with purpura, such as the macroglossia, hepatosplenomegaly, and Tinel's sign of amyloidosis; the splenomegaly of Waldenström's disease, other lymphoproliferative and myeloproliferative diseases, and hypersplenism; the joint changes of rheumatoid arthritis; and the butterfly rash of systemic lupus erythematosus.

DIAGNOSTIC STUDIES

The first task of the laboratory evaluation is to separate thrombocytopenic from nonthrombocytopenic purpura. Other information provided by complete blood counts and examination of a peripheral blood smear might include: abnormal numbers or varieties of leukocytes (myeloproliferative diseases, leukemia), fragmented red cells (DIC, TTP), unusually large platelets (some dysfunctional platelet syndromes), and evidence of rouleaux formation (myeloma, rheumatic diseases). Low platelet counts are the result of rapid peripheral destruction (DIC, idiopathic or drug-induced ITP, TTP, hypersplenism) or decreased production (primary marrow disorders) of platelets; examination of a bone marrow aspirate for the presence of adequate numbers of megakaryocytes may help distinguish between these two processes.

If the platelet count is greater than 100,000/mm^3, the bleeding time should be normal; a normal bleeding time, which is the best clinical test of platelet function, eliminates consideration of dysfunctional platelets as a cause of purpura in most cases, though occasionally a "post-aspirin bleeding time" may be required to reveal mild degrees of platelet dysfunction.[23]

Further tests useful in defining the cause of nonthrombocytopenic purpura include erythrocyte sedimentation rate, serum protein electrophoresis, and tests for rheumatoid factor and antinuclear antibodies. Kidneys as well as skin may be involved by vasculitis; proteinuria and diminished creatinine clearance may be present. Biopsy of involved skin may be necessary to prove the existence of a vasculitis.

ASSESSMENT

History, physical examination, and a few laboratory tests quickly provide a proximate cause, or at least narrow the field of possibilities, in most cases of purpura. Although in some cases the examiner may feel relatively confident of the presence of a particular cause after history and physical examination, it is often the platelet count that points most clearly to the direction the further evaluation should take. A reasonable approach to the diagnosis of purpura, incorporating points gleaned from the patient's history, findings of the physical examination, and laboratory data, would proceed as follows:

If the patient is thrombocytopenic, a bone marrow aspirate should be examined to separate those diseases associated with increased platelet destruction from those associated with decreased platelet production. If megakaryocytes are present in normal to increased numbers in the marrow aspirate, increased platelet destruction may be assumed, and the following possibilities should be considered:

Is the patient febrile or acutely ill? Is there an actual or potential source of infection or other known cause of DIC present? Do clotting studies confirm the presence of intravascular coagulation? Are schistocytes present in peripheral blood? Could the patient have TTP? Are other parts of the classic pentad—fever, microangiopathic hemolytic anemia, neurologic signs, renal disease—present?

If the patient appears well, and thrombocytopenia is the only abnormal laboratory result, could the underlying disease be ITP? Is there a history of abnormal bleeding (menorrhagia, bleeding from gums, etc)? Are other autoimmune phenomena present in the patient (or patient's family)? The spleen should not be palpable in ITP. What drugs has the patient taken?

If the spleen is palpable, is hypersplenism present? Does the patient have an underlying disease known to be associated with splenomegaly?

If the megakaryocyte count is decreased, other possibilities come to mind:

Is drug-induced megakaryocyte damage present? A careful history of drug ingestion is essential. One should inquire about over-the-counter medications. Is some type of primary bone marrow disorder evident? Is other evidence of marrow disease present (megaloblastic changes, aplasia, fibrosis, abnormal maturation of other cell lines)? Were malformations found on physical examination that indicate a congenital cause of thrombocytopenia (radial anomalies)?

If the platelet count is normal, the examiner should proceed along the following lines:

If the purpura are not palpable, is there any evidence of underlying disease, or is the patient well? Could the purpura have been produced by physical means or caused by a dermatologic condition? Is the bleeding time normal, eliminating platelet dysfunction as a cause? Is the patient elderly or suffering from the effects of chronic exposure to glucocorticosteroids? Is the patient malnourished enough to be a candidate for vitamin C deficiency? Does the patient have abnormal skin, consistent with the Ehlers-Danlos syndrome? Are features such as macroglossia, hepatosplenomegaly, and neuropathy present, which might be due to amyloidosis? Has the patient just suffered severe injury including fractures of bone? Does he or she appear ill or "toxic" and have fever, as might be found with meningococcemia (direct endothelial injury, not necessarily accompanied by thrombocytopenia) or rickettsial disease? Finally, does the patient have a history of psychiatric disease?

Palpable purpura, on the other hand, should invite the investigator to pursue the possibility of the various vasculitic diseases. Are the lesions on the legs and buttocks, as typically seen in Henoch-Schönlein purpura? Have they been erythematous or pruritic? Is there evidence of renal disease—proteinuria, an abnormal urinary sediment, or elevated serum creatinine level? Is the erythrocyte sedimentation rate elevated? Is a skin biopsy needed to confirm the suspicion of a leukocytoclastic vasculitis? Does the patient have a known immunologic or malignant disease? Has he or she been given drugs known to cause a hypersensitivity vasculitis? Is there overt evidence of hepatitis, liver enzyme abnormalities, or serologic proof of hepatitis B virus infection? Are cryoglobulins present in the serum? Are serum complement levels low, as seen with hypocomplementemic vasculitis? Does the patient have pulmonary infiltrates or evidence of sinusitis, as in Wegener's granulomatosis? The examiner should remember that some causes of vasculitis in skin may be equally adept at producing vasculitis in other organs. For example, Henoch-Schönlein vasculitis has been shown to cause testicular and myocardial infarctions, as well as eye and neurologic disease.

The preceding suggestions for assessing the patient with purpura should provide a diagnosis in most cases.

REFERENCES

1. Kitchens CS. The anatomic basis of purpura. Prog Hemo Thromb 1980;5:211–44.
2. Pitt PW. Purpura associated with vomiting. Br Med J 1973;2:667.
3. Carpentieri U, Gustavson LP, Crim CB, Haggard ME. Purpura and Schamberg's disease. South Med J 1978;71:1168–70.
4. Weiss HJ. Congenital disorders of platelet dysfunction. Semin Hematol 1980;17:228–41.
5. Malpass TW, Harker LA. Acquired disorders of platelet dysfunction. Semin Hematol 1980;17:242–58.
6. Fauci AS, Haynes BF, Katz P. The spectrum of vasculitis. Ann Intern Med 1978;89:660–76.
7. Koch-Weser J. Coumarin necrosis. Ann Intern Med 1968;68:1365–7.
8. Chu DZ, Blaisdell FW. Purpura fulminans. Am J Surg 1982;143:356–62.
9. Scarborough H, Shuster A. Corticosteroid purpura. Lancet 1960;1:93–4.
10. McKusick VA. Heritable disorders of connective tissue. 4th ed. St. Louis: C V Mosby, 1972; 292–371.
11. Kyle RA, Bayrd ED. Amyloidosis: review of 236 cases. Medicine 1975;54:271–99.
12. Tattersall RN, Seville R. Senile purpura. Q J Med 1961;19:151–9.
13. Moreau JP. Fat embolism: a review and report of 100 cases. Can J Surg 1974;17:196–9.
14. Kitchens CS. Studies of a patient with recurring thrombotic thrombocytopenic purpura. Am J Hematol 1982;13:259–67.
15. McKee LC, Collins RD. Intravascular leukocyte thrombi and aggregates as a cause of morbidity and mortality in leukemia. Medicine 1974;53:463–78.
16. Pierce JR, Wren MV, Cousar JB. Cholesterol embolism: diagnosis antemortem by bone marrow biopsy. Ann Intern Med 1978;89:937–8.
17. Ratnoff OD. The psychogenic purpuras: a review of autoerythrocyte sensitization, autosensitization to DNA, "hysterical" and factitial bleeding, and religious stigmata. Semin Hematol 1980;17:192–213.
18. Cines DB, Dusak B, Tomaski A, Mennuti M, Schreiber AD. Immune thrombocytopenic purpura and pregnancy. N Engl J Med 1982;306:826–31.
19. Morichau-Beauchant M, Touchard G, Maire P, et al. Jejunal IgA and C_3 deposition in adult Henoch-Schönlein purpura with severe intestinal manifestations. Gastroenterology 1982;82:1438–42.
20. Slichter SJ. Post transfusion purpura: response to steroids and association with red blood cell and lymphocytotoxic antibodies. Br J Hematol 1982;50:599–605.
21. Carroll RR, Kitchens CS. Drugs and drug-drug interactions affecting platelets. In: Petrie J, Cluff LE, eds. Clinically important adverse drug reactions. Gastroenterology, Hematology and Infectious Disease Therapy, Vol. 3. New York: Elsevier, 1984.
22. Ratnoff OD, Menitove JE, Aster RH, Lederman MM. Coincident classic hemophilia and "idiopathic" thrombocytopenic purpura in patients under treatment with concentrates of antihemophilic factor (factor VIII). N Engl J Med 1983;308:439–42.
23. Bachmann F. Diagnostic approach to mild bleeding disorders. Semin Hematol 1980;17:292–305.

RESPIRATORY FAILURE, ACUTE

WARREN C. MILLER

☐ SYNONYMS: Hypoxia, hypercapnia, carbon dioxide retention, cyanosis, respiratory acidosis, asphyxiation, suffocation

BACKGROUND

Definition and Origins

Strictly speaking, respiratory failure is concerned with malfunction of the entire process of *respiration,* including entry of oxygen into the body, its distribution to body tissues, and its utilization with food substrate at the cellular level, and the production and excretion of carbon dioxide. Although this chapter's emphasis is on the pulmonary aspects of this process, several clinical disorders that involve the nonpulmonary areas—e.g., cyanide poisoning respiration at the mitochondrial level ("gray cyanosis"), carbon monoxide poisoning of the oxygen-carrying capacity of blood ("cherry red cyanosis"), and circulatory shock ("peripheral cyanosis")—are, in fact, respiratory failures. Also, as is shown subsequently, metabolism and circulation play a vital role in the physiologic consequences of gas exchange in the lungs.

In the clinical sphere, *acute respiratory failure* means the relatively sudden derangement of one or both of the primary lung functions, oxygenation of systemic arterial blood and elimination of carbon dioxide, creating *hypoxia* and *hypercapnia,* respectively. In the absence of breathing supplemental oxygen, the presence of significant carbon dioxide retention in the alveoli reduces the alveolar oxygen and begets simultaneous hypoxia.

Conventionally, medical students have been taught that the physiologic causes of hypoxia are:

1. Global *hypoventilation,* in which the elevated partial pressure of CO_2 in the alveoli displaces oxygen. With less alveolar oxygen, there is necessarily less blood oxygen, even if complete equilibrium between blood gases and alveolae occurs.

2. *Shunting,* in which oxygen-poor systemic venous blood either bypasses the pulmonary circulation entirely (e.g., in intracardiac defects) or passes through vascular channels in the lung that are not adjacent to gas-exchanging spaces (e.g., in arteriovenous malformations or vessels within areas of complete atelectasis).

3. *Ventilation-perfusion imbalance,* in which there is regional mismatching of varying amounts of ventilation and perfusion; for example, a large amount of blood flow to a small area of lung that is poorly ventilated and hence relatively deficient in oxygen. One extreme of ventilation-perfusion imbalance is the shunting previously mentioned (full perfusion, no ventilation). Another is dead space ventilaiton (no perfusion, full ventilation), which, because blood is not directly affected, does not contribute to hypoxia but may add to the patient's work of breathing. Ventilation-perfusion imbalance is proably the major mechanism of hypoxemia in most disease states.

4. *Diffusion defects,* in which, conceptually, the barrier to diffusion between blood and alveolar gases is widened so that full equilibrium does not occur during the transit time of blood through the pulmonary capillary. The histopathologic correlate would therefore be the thickened, fibrotic alveolar walls seen in pulmonary fibrosis. Since the transit time of blood in the lung would be critical, with exercise the decrease in transit time due to the increase in cardiac output would aggravate hypoxia. These phenomena were once referred to as the "alveolar-capillary block syndrome." More recent knowledge, based on morphometric measurements of postmorten lung specimens and mathematical models of blood flow and gas diffusion, have suggested that diffusion defects are not a significant factor in clinical disease states. Nevertheless, it remains difficult to explain the exercise-induced hypoxia seen in many chronic lung diseases.

Although these classic pathophysiologic mechanisms are the building blocks of our understanding of hypoxia, clinical circumstances and new observations may modify our concepts. To give a clinical example: In the presence of shunt, the degree of hypoxia produced is, obviously, related to the amount of blood shunted from the right side of the circulation to the left, but it is not so apparent that the degree of hypoxia is also related to the degree of oxygen desaturation of the venous blood. The patient in shock with a sluggish peripheral circualtion will extract a great deal of oxygen from the blood that is to become venous blood and subsequently shunted, and such a patient will have proportionally worse hypoxemia.[1] A similar case might be made for hypermetabolic states requiring increased oxygen consumption with a relative circulatory impairment such that blood flow is inadequate to provide oxygen without excessive extraction by the peripheral tissues. As an example of new concepts, consider that if the thickened-membrane concept of diffusion defects is not tenable, there is new evidence that certain diseases may have a defect of radial diffusion, i.e., the movement of gases from the wall of the capillary to its center. Patients so affected appear to have enlarged pulmonary capillaries. Considerable time is required for oxygen to diffuse from the endothelial inner surface to the hemoglobin in the center of such a capillary.[2] If the transit time of the red blood cell in the center of an enlarged pulmonary capillary is rapid, it may exit the capillary deficient in oxygen. Such a mechanism would easily explain exercise-induced hypoxia, but further study is required before its role in clinical disease is established.

Ventilatory failure with rising carbon dioxide (CO_2) tension results when the effective alveolar ventilation is insufficient to excrete the carbon dioxide load presented to the lungs. The effectiveness of the alveolar ventilation is in turn dependent upon the bellows or pump function of the chest and the matching of ventilation and perfusion, as already described. In most clinical circumstances, ventilation-perfusion mismatching is not a significant contribution to carbon dioxide retention because (1) carbon dioxide is considerably more diffusible than oxygen, and the problems of hypoxia are often manifest at a lesser degree of pulmonary impairment, (2) CO_2 retention is to some extent self-limiting, in that in the face of CO_2 retention each exhaled breath has a relatively higher concentration of CO_2 and hence excretion of CO_2 is augmented, and (3) even in very damaged lungs in which dead space or wasted ventilation is 70 to 80 per cent of total ventilation, if the pump function of the chest is preserved intact, total ventilation can be increased sufficient to maintain CO_2 homeostasis. Rather, the pathophysiology of ventilatory failure with carbon dioxide retention may be thought of as either an overwhelming work of breathing that the patient's efforts cannot sustain ("can't breathe") or failure of the respiratory center in the brain to properly direct the bellows ("won't breathe").

The carbon dioxide load presented to the lungs is higher with increased metabolism (e.g., exercise, fever, stress, other hypermetabolic states), metabolic acidosis (with bicarbonate buffering), and food substrate high in carbohydrate,[3] (e.g., in intravenous hyperalimentation)—all recognizable clinical aberrations.

The work of breathing is a mechanical phenomenon including *resistive* work, which increases in airway obstructive diseases, and *elastic* work, which increases in restrictive lung diseases. Restrictive disease may be intrinsic to the lung (e.g., the stiff lungs of pulmonary fibrosis and other parenchymal lung diseases) or extrinsic to the lung (e.g., the heavy chest wall of the morbidly obese and pleural diseases such as mesothelioma and pleural effusion).

The patient's ability to cope with stress to the ventilatory apparatus is a function of the integrity and coordination of the chain of nerves, neuromuscular junctions, respiratory muscles, and chest cage that provide ventilation. Clinical disorders such as degenerative neurologic diseases, myasthenia gravis, muscular dystrophies, and flail chest, respectively, can impair the integrity of the links of the chain. Recent evidence suggests that exhaustion and discoordination of respiratory muscles may play a major role in acute respiratory failure superimposed on severe chronic lung disease.[4]

As the central controller, the respiratory center is pivotal in balancing ventilatory needs with ventilatory efforts. The respiratory center itself may malfunction because of a direct influence such as trauma or sedation, because of congenital weakness (perhaps the etiology of sudden infant death syndrome), or because of hyperadaptiveness permitting ever-rising CO_2 tension without stimulating augumented ventilatory efforts.[5] Hyperadaptiveness may determine whether a given patient with an increased work of breathing has hypercapnic ventilatory failure or not. For example, among equally morbidly obese patients, some maintain near normal blood gas levels and others develop pickwickian syndrome, and among patients with chronic obstructive pulmonary disease and seemingly equal degrees of increased airway resistance, some present as normocapnic "pink puffers" and others as hypercapnic "blue bloaters."

Historical Perspective

Modern medicine's experience with large numbers of patients with acute respiratory failure began with the polio epidemics of about five decades ago. This was, of course, failure of the neuromuscular bellows apparatus and was pure hypercapnic ventilatory failure, with hypoxia occurring only secondarily or with complications such as atelectasis or pneumonia. This type of respiratory failure occurs today in the form of acute neurologic paralysis such as in Guillain-Barré syndrome and myasthenia gravis. As immunization conquered polio in civilized countries, a new form of epidemic respiratory failure took its place because of the smoking habits in those countries. During the 1950s and 1960s acute respiratory failure due to chronic obstructive pulmonary disease became commonplace.[6] This was respiratory failure due to airways disease, in which the bellows apparatus and the lung per se were relatively intact. In the early stages hypoxic failure was preeminent, but as the disease progressed hypercapnic failure frequently supervened. Chronic obstructive pulmonary disease remains a major cause of acute respiratory failure today. During the last 15 to 20 years another form of respiratory failure has occupied considerable clinical interest. Generally it has come to be called "adult respiratory distress syndrome."[7] Although evolving as a consequence of modern resuscitation and life support systems, the term may be applied to any acute diffuse lung injury characterized by diffuse damage to pulmonary parenchyma such that the lungs are edematous (not due to back-pressure from left heart failure but rather to vascular damage), and microatelectasis and disordered ventilation-perfusion relationships predominate.[8] Such a disorder spares the bellows and the airway and directly affects lung parenchyma. In the early stages, hypoxic failure predominates, and only terminally—if mechanical ventilation has not been instituted—does hypercapnia occur.

Although respiratory failure is conventionally viewed in terms of pulmonary gas exchange, it is not necessarily synonymous with lung failure in the definitive sense. The lung has important nonrespiratory functions, most notably biochemical functions such as inactivation of certain vasoactive amines and other substances and activation of certain circulating enzymes, which may in the future be found to play a major role in disease processes.

HISTORY

The nervous system response to hypoxia and hypercapnia produces the most common symptoms of acute respiratory failure (Table 1). Although the clinical diagnosis may be evident in such extreme circumstance as apnea and gross cyanosis, in most cases the signs and symptoms are subtle and the diagnosis is made only by means of arterial blood gas analysis (see "Laboratory Tests"). Perhaps the symptom of dyspnea is the most common chief complaint and may be reliable in the presence of intact respiratory drive. Although dyspnea may be psychogenic in origin, blood gas measurements should be performed if there is the slightest clinical suspicion of acute respiratory failure or if the patient has a known predisposing condition, such as: impaired mental function, drug or alcohol abuse, head or chest trauma, neuromuscular disease, obstructive airway disease, chest pain, lower respiratory tract infection, circulatory collapse, or congestive heart failure.

Table 1. SIGNS AND SYMPTOMS OF ACUTE RESPIRATORY FAILURE

Hypoxia	Altered mental function
	Hypotension and tachycardia (rarely) *or* Hypertension and tachycardia (commonly)
	No sensation of distress
	Tachypnea and hyperpnea
Hypercapnia	Decreased level of consciousness
	Headache and flushing
	Hypertension and tachycardia
	Dyspnea (sometimes)
	Tachypnea and hyperpnea

PHYSICAL EXAMINATION

The physical examination may by necessity be undertaken after interventional respiratory support has been instituted or may be more leisurely, depending on the situation. In either case its value is not diminished. Bilateral rales are the hallmark of the adult respiratory distress syndrome (noncardiogenic pulmonary edema). Cyanosis is one of the most unreliable signs. Because it usually requires 5 grams/100 ml of deoxygenated hemoglobin for cyanosis to be detectable, patients with normal hemoglobin concentrations must have very severe desaturation before cyanosis is observed, whereas patients with anemia may never develop cyanosis.

The physical examination in cases of obstructive airway disease may be almost as accurate as arterial blood gas analysis, because the degree of airway obstruction may be determined therewith.[9] The adage, "Beware the quiet chest," applies. A wheeze is produced by air flow through an obstructed orifice. It increases proportionately to obstruction until it becomes so severe that air flow is reduced, after which wheezing may not be heard. Retractions may be a better index of airway obstruction in this context.

DIAGNOSTIC STUDIES

Laboratory Tests

The single mandatory and diagnostic laboratory test for acute respiratory failure is determination of arterial blood gases. Blood for gas analysis is obtained by direct arterial puncture utilizing a small-gauge needle and heparinized syringe. Technical personnel may safely perform this procedure with proper training and due caution to apply direct pressure to the puncture site, especially in patients receiving anticoagulants. The blood gas levels should be measured immediately; otherwise, the specimen should be iced for a short delay. If the patient is receiving supplemental oxygen, it is helpful to record the inspired oxygen concentration (F_IO_2).

Arbitrarily, *hypercapnic respiratory failure* is said to be present if the partial pressure of carbon dioxide (P_aCO_2) is greater than 50 mm Hg.[10] Almost invariably this will be accompanied by a decrease in pH owing to respiratory acidosis. One rare exception is seen in the occasional patient who hypoventilates dramatically in a compensatory response to metabolic alkalosis. As a rough approximation, in acute hypoventilation pH will decrease from a normal 7.40 by .0075 pH unit for each 1 mm Hg of CO_2 retention above a normal of 40 mm Hg; e.g., acute CO_2 retention with P_aCO_2 rising from 40 to 60 mm Hg may be expected to produce a pH of about 7.25. Substantial deviations from this expected value suggest additional superimposed acid-base aberrations.

Hypoxic respiratory failure is present when the arterial partial pressure of oxygen (P_aCO_2) is less than 60 mm Hg. This level of hypoxemia is somewhat arbitrary but is based on the rationale that because of the nature of the oxyhemoglobin dissociation curve, in lesser degrees of hypoxia hemoglobin is still 85 to 90 per cent saturated with oxygen and therefore a reasonably good content of oxygen is in the blood available to tissues. Conversely, more severe hypoxia leads to a progressive oxyhemoglobin desaturation and a marked decrease in arterial oxygen content.

In addition to permitting the instant diagnosis of acute respiratory failure, arterial blood gases can be further interpreted to aid in differential diagnosis.[11] This interpretation requires the computation of the *alveolar partial pressure* (P_AO_2) of oxygen, the short computation for which is:

$$P_AO_2 = P_IO_2 - \frac{P_aO_2}{.8}$$

where P_IO_2 is the *inspired partial pressure of oxygen.* This parameter is derived in turn from the oxygen concentration in inspired air and the barometric pressure (P_B) using the equation:

$$P_IO_2 = F_IO_2 \times P_B$$

For example, in a person breathing room air at sea level, the P_IO_2 would be 0.21 × 713, or 150 torr; in a person breathing 35 per cent oxygen 5,000 feet above sea level, it would be 0.21 × 518, or 170 torr.

With knowledge of the P_AO_2, one can determine the *alveolar-arterial oxygen difference,* $(A\text{–}a)P_{O2}$, using the following equation:

$$(A\text{–}a)P_{O2} = P_AO_2 - P_aO_2$$

and the *arterial-alveolar oxygen ratio* (a-AO_2) with this equation:

$$a/AO_2 = \frac{P_aO_2}{P_AO_2}$$

The $(A\text{–}a)P_{O2}$ is especially useful in a patient breathing room air. It reflects the degree of severity of all of the classic mechanisms of hypoxia except hypoventilation, including shunts, diffusion defects, and ventilation-perfusion imbalance. The larger the discrepancy between alveolar and arterial oxygen pressures, the larger the shunt, the greater the diffusion defect, or the more disordered the ventilation-perfusion relationships. As a rough rule, in room air, any $(A\text{–}a)P_{O2}$ value greater than half the patient's age in years is abnormal. The immediate clinical applicability of this ruleis to discriminate, in the presence of hypoventilation, hypoxia due solely to the hypoventilation from hypoxia due to both hypoventilation and additional gas exchange problems. The a/AO_2 is used largely when the patient is breathing supplemental oxygen (because normal values of $(A\text{–}a)P_{O2}$ are difficult to define when the subject is breathing supplemental oxygen).[12] Usually, an a/AO_2 value less than 0.74 is considered abnormal.

In the future, arterial blood gas analysis may be replaced or supplemented by noninvasive tests of the same or related parameters, such as transcutaneous measurement of carbon dioxide or oximetry of oxygen saturation.

Diagnostic Imaging

The other most useful and immediately available tool in the differential diagnosis of acute respiratory failure is the chest x-ray. Sophisticated radiologic interpretation is often not required in the emergency setting, in which the fundamental role of the chest x-ray is to determine the presence or absence of many of the restrictive disorders. The presence of restrictive parenchymal lung disease or obvious chest wall disease may be seen as gray-white infiltrates or pleural haziness; an exception to this generality is pneumothorax. In the absence of pneumothorax, chest wall haziness, and parenchymal infiltrates, one can by exclusion infer that the problems lie in the areas not seen on the conventional x-ray i.e., the airways (as in asthma), the neuromuscular system, or the cardiovascular system.

Pulmonary Function Testing

If the patient is alert and cooperative, screening tests of pulmonary function may provide diagnostic information and baseline data for following the response to therapy. Simple spirometry or measurement of peak expiratory flow with a peak flow meter is useful for demonstrating the presence of airway obstructive disease. The measurement of maximum negative inspiratory pressure gives information regarding neuromuscular weakness.

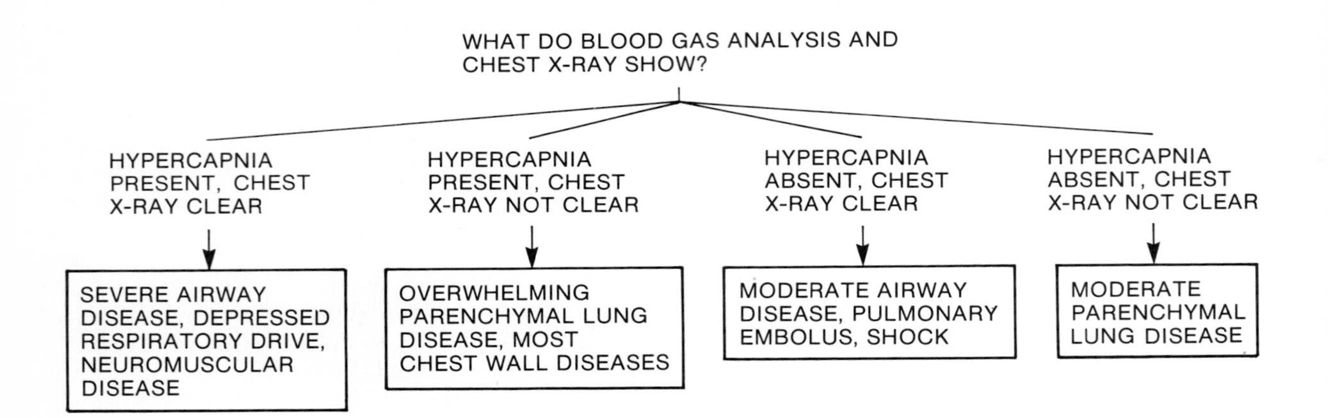

Table 2. CAUSES OF ACUTE RESPIRATORY FAILURE*

Causes	Depressed Respiratory Drive	Neuromuscular Disease	Chest Wall Disease[27]	Airway Disease	Lung Disease
Traumatic	Head trauma[13] Sedative overdose[14]	Spinal cord trauma[18] Drugs/poisons[19]	Thoracoplasty Flail chest Burn eschar	Foreign body aspiration Hanging[28]	Contusion Inhalation injury Fat embolism syndrome[30] Cytotoxic drugs[31]
Vascular	Cerebrovascular accidents	Transverse myelitis	Pleural effusion	Aortic aneurysm[29]	Congestive heart failure Pulmonary embolus Shock
Neoplastic	Primary or metastatic carcinoma	Paraneoplastic syndromes	Mesothelioma	Laryngeal carcinoma Bronchial adenoma	Lymphangitic spread of carcinoma Diffuse lymphoma[32]
Infectious	Meningitis Brain abscess Encephalitis	Poliomyelitis Guillain-Barré syndrome Tetanus[21] Botulism[22]	Empyema	Bronchitis	Pneumonias†
Congenital	Primary alveolar hypoventilation	Muscular dystrophies Acid-maltase deficiency[23]	Scoliosis	Cystic fibrosis	Alpha$_1$-antitrypsin deficiency
Idiopathic	CNS degenerative diseases	Diaphragmatic paralysis[24] Amyotrophic lateral sclerosis[25] Multiple sclerosis	Spontaneous pneumothorax	Chronic obstructive lung disease	Adult respiratory distress syndrome Pulmonary fibrosis
Metabolic	Coma Myxedema[15] Alkalosis[16]	Hypophosphatemia[26]	Obesity	Laryngospasm	Carbonic anhydrous inhibition[33] Hypoxemia of cirrhosis[2]
Immunologic	Sleep apnea with allergic rhinitis[17]	Myasthenia gravis	Scleroderma Ankylosing spondylitis	Allergic asthma Crycoarytenoiditis in rheumatoid arthritis	Hypersensitivity pneumonitis Transfusion reaction[34]

*Superscript numbers refer to chapter references.
†Including viral and mycoplasmal pneumonias, legionnaires' disease, bacterial pneumonia (esp. streptococcus and gram-negatives), miliary tuberculosis, overwhelming fungal disease (histoplasmosis, blastomycosis), and parasites (in immunologically impaired patients).

Other Tests

Additional initial laboratory tests that may be helpful in the differential diagnosis of acute respiratory failure include liver function tests and determination of serum calcium, phosphorus, and hemoglobin concentrations. Liver function tests are helpful because liver disease may alter pulmonary gas exchange (although usually not to the point of respiratory failure). Calcium and phosphorus are vital to muscular function and hemoglobin is fundamental to oxygen delivery to tissues. Once a specific cause of respiratory failure is suspected, specialized testing may be required to confirm the diagnosis.

ASSESSMENT

Because acute respiratory failure is a life-threatening emergency, the initial approach to diagnosis is initially simplified and limited to broad areas. The algorithm illustrates an emergency approach to the problem utilizing the most simple tools—the chest x-ray and blood gas analysis. The premises of this approach are: (1) that hypercapnia does not occur unless the chain of respiratory drive–neuromuscular bellows function is disrupted or the work of breathing is overwhelming and (2) that the chest x-ray will demonstrate most significant chest wall diseases and infiltration of pulmonary parenchyma, and if it is largely clear, the nonvisualized areas (airways, vasculature, bellows) are implicated by exclusion. Once the overall nature of the disorder is defined, features of the entire clinical setting and ancillary testing can be brought to bear for an exact etiologic diagnosis. Table 2 presents an approach based on the aforementioned algorithm and classic pathologic mechanisms—trauma, vascular disorders, neoplasia, infection, congenital disorders, idiopathic causes, metabolic derangements, and immunologic abnormalities. Although any individual case may fall into one or several of these catagories, the majority of cases will be due to common disorders such as postoperative respiratory failure, chronic obstructive pulmonary disease, drug overdoses, the adult respiratory distress syndrome, and neuromuscular diseases. Often, interventional respiratory support is undertaken with supplemental oxygen or mechanical ventilation while precise diagnostic evaluation is in progress.

REFERENCES

1. Pontoppidan H, Geffin G, Lowenstein E. Acute respiratory failure in the adult. 1 and 2. N Engl J Med 1972;287:690–5 and 743–52.
2. Wolfe JD, Tashkin DP, Holly FE, Brachman MB, Genovesi M. Hypoxemia of cirrhosis. Detection of abnormal small pulmonary vascular channels by a quantitative radionuclide method. Am J Med 1977;63:746–53.
3. Covelli HD, Black JW, Olsen MS, Beekman JF. Respiratory failure precipitated by high carbohydrate loads. Ann Intern Med 1981;95:579–81.
4. Macklem PT. Respiratory muscles: the vital pump. Chest 1980;78:753–8.
5. Ahmad M, Cressman M, Tomashefski JF. Central alveolar hypoventilation syndromes. Arch Intern Med 1980;140:29–30.
6. Moser KM, Shibel EM, Beamon AJ. Acute respiratory failure in obstructive lung disease. JAMA 1973;225:705–7.
7. Wilson RF, Sibbold WJ. Acute respiratory failure. Crit Care Med 1976;4:79–89.
8. Staub NC. "State of the art" review. Pathogenesis of pulmonary edema. Am Rev Respir Dis 1974;109:358–72.
9. McFadden ER, Kiser R, DeGroot WJ. Acute bronchial asthma. Relations between clinical and physiologic manifestations. N Engl J Med 1973;288:221–5.
10. Murry JF. Mechanism of acute respiratory failure. Am Rev Respir Dis 1977;115:1071–8.
11. Snider GL. Interpretation of the arterial oxygen and carbon dioxide partial pressures. A simplified approach for bedside use. Chest 1973;63:801–6.
12. Gilbert R, Keighley JF. The arterial/alveolar oxygen tension ratio. An index of gas exchange applicable to varying inspired oxygen concentrations. Am Rev Respir Dis 1974;109:142–5.
13. Schumacher PT, Rhodes GR, Nervell JC, et al. Ventilation-perfusion imbalance after head trauma. Am Rev Respir Dis 1979;119:33–43.
14. Jay SJ, Johanson WG, Pierce AK. Respiratory complications of overdose with sedative drugs. Am Rev Respir Dis 1975;112:591–8.
15. Domm BM, Vassollo CL. Myxedema coma with respiratory failure. Am Rev Respir Dis 1973;107:842–5.
16. Janaheri S, Shore NS, Rose B, Kayemi H. Compensatory hypoventilation in metabolic alkalosis. Chest 1982;81:296–301.
17. McNicholas WT, Tarlo S, Cole P, et al. Obstructive apneas during sleep in patients with seasonal allergic rhinitis. Am Rev Respir Dis 1982;126:625–8.
18. McMicham JC, Michel L, Westbrook PP. Pulmonary dysfunction following traumatic quadriplegia. JAMA 1980;243:528–31.
19. Greenberg C, Davies S, McGowan T, Schorer A, Drage C. Acute respiratory failure following severe arsenic poisoning. Chest 1979;76:596–8.
20. Massam M, Jones RS. Ventilatory failure in the Guillain-Barré syndrome. Thorax 1980;35:557–8.
21. Trujillo MJ, Castillo A, Espana JV, Guerara P, Eganey H. Tetanus in the adult. Crit Care Med 1980;8:419–23.
22. Lernos SW, Pierson DJ, Cary JM, Hudson LD. Prolonged respiratory paralysis in wound botulism. Chest 1979;75:59–61.
23. Rosenow EC, Engel AG. Acid maltase deficiency in adults presenting as respiratory failure. Am J Med 1978;64:485–91.
24. Sandham JD, Shaw DT, Guenter CA. Acute supine respiratory failure due to bilateral diaphragmatic paralysis. Chest 1977;72:96–8.
25. Fromm GB, Wisdom PJ, Black AJ. Amyotrophic lateral sclerosis presenting with respiratory failure. Chest 1977;71:612–4.
26. Newman JH, Neff TA, Ziporin P. Acute respiratory failure associated with hypophosphatemia. N Engl J Med 1977;296:1101–3.
27. Bergofsky EH, Respiratory failure in disorders of the thoracic cage. Am Rev Respir Dis 1979;119:643–69.

28. Fischman CM, Goldstein MS, Gardner LB. Suicidal hanging. Chest 1977;71:225–7.
29. Gothe B, Harris L. Thoracic aortic aneurysm causing acute bronchospasm. Crit Care Med 1981;9:496–7.
30. Gossling HR, Donohue TA. The fat embolism syndrome. JAMA 1979;241:2740–2.
31. Weiss RB, Muggia FM. Cytotoxic drug-induced pulmonary disease. Am J Med 1980;68:259–66.
32. Sahebjami H, Vassallo CL. Rapidly progressive lymphoma of the lung appearing as the adult respiratory distress syndrome. Chest 1975;68:741–2.
33. Condon WL, Black AJ. Acute respiratory failure precipitated by a carbonic anhyrdase inhibitor. Chest 1976;69: 112–3.
34. Dubois M, Lotze MT, Diamond WJ, Kim YD, Flye MW, Macnamara TE. Pulmonary shunting during leukoagglutinin-induced noncardiac pulmonary edema. JAMA 1980;244:2186–9.

SALIVARY GLAND ENLARGEMENT

JONAS T. JOHNSON

□ SYNONYMS: Parotitis, sialoadenitis, ranula

BACKGROUND

The upper aerodigestive tract is plentifully supplied with salivary gland tissue. The major salivary glands are the parotid, submandibular, and sublingual glands. Of equal importance, however, are the minor salivary glands, microscopic foci of glandular tissue that lie submucosally throughout the upper aerodigestive tract.

Enlargement of any single salivary gland may be caused by inflammation, neoplasm, or obstruction of the duct. Careful development of the history, physical examination, and associated laboratory tests can usually lead the practitioner to the proper diagnosis. Diffuse enlargement of multiple salivary glands is most commonly a sign of systemic disease.

Parotitis may be viral or bacterial. The most common viral pathogen is the mumps virus. Mumps is highly contagious, but at least 25 per cent of infected persons may not have clinically apparent disease. Eighty to 90 per cent of the adult population has serologic evidence of previous infection. The peak age incidence of mumps is 6 to 10 years, although adult cases do occur. The peak of infectivity is just after the onset of the parotitis; however, saliva may be infectious several days before then and for as long as 2 weeks afterward.

Typically, parotitis begins suddenly, although it may be preceded by malaise, anorexia, sore throat, and fever. In some cases parotid swelling may be the first indication of illness. The swelling generally resolves within a week following the maximal enlargement. In mumps, the parotid gland is diffusely swollen and the gland is not usually warm or erythematous. On occasion, submandibular gland involvement may exist without parotid involvement, causing difficulty in diagnosis. It is of interest that parotitis may be unilateral in approximately one-third of individuals with mumps, which may also involve the testes, pancreas, and central nervous system in unusual cases.

The clinical diagnosis can generally be made on clinical grounds alone although a definite diagnosis of mumps depends upon isolation of the virus. Immunofluorescent methods can detect positive cell cultures. Complement-fixing (CF) antibodies reach a peak titer within 2 to 3 weeks after onset and may remain elevated for 6 weeks and then persist at lower levels for many years to come. Paired serum samples taken 2 to 3 weeks apart are tested for CF antibodies. The skin test for mumps is useless in the diagnosis of acute mumps.

Bacterial parotitis may be seen in all age groups. Recurrent infection in infancy commonly indicates an abnormality of the collecting ducts with resultant stasis that leads to recurring infection. Conversely, parotitis may also be seen in the elderly and in debilitated patients as a complication of dehydration. Involvement of the glands by autoimmune disease may result in glandular destruction and saccular dilatation of the ducts (sialectasia). The resultant stasis and pooling of saliva lead to recurrent parotitis. Similarly, occlusion of the duct by stones (sialolithiasis) may cause acute enlargement and pain, especially when accompanied by infection. In all cases, the most commonly isolated organism in acute bacterial parotitis is *Staphylococcus aureus.*[1]

Most cases of acute infection may be readily diagnosed (Fig. 1). Chronic inflammatory disease with glandular enlargement may commonly cause problems of differential diagnosis. Confusion exists regarding chronic non-neoplastic enlargement of the salivary glands. Although various terms are employed (e.g., Mikulicz's disease), it is probably best to use *benign lymphoepithelial disease.*[1, 2] This disease is most common in middle-aged females. Diffuse swelling of the salivary glands is associated with mild pain and tenderness. There may be intermittent attacks of more acute pain with glandular enlargement. With progression of the disease, atrophy of the acini and periductal infiltration of lymphocytes develop. Wide dilatation of the ducts then results in poor emptying and retained secretions, which may be demonstrated on sialography as punctate sialectasis (Fig. 2). With progression of the disease, actual cavities may develop.

Sjögren emphasized the frequent association of salivary and lacrimal gland enlargement with keratoconjunctivitis sicca and xerostomia. It is now apparent that many other collagen disorders may be associated with benign lymphoepithelial disease.[3, 4] These include systemic lupus erythematosus, scleroderma, polyarteritis nodosa, and polymyositis. Affected patients may have a variety of other manifestations, such as leukopenia, hemolytic anemia, and splenomegaly. The chronicity of such a process in an adult makes confusion with mumps unlikely.

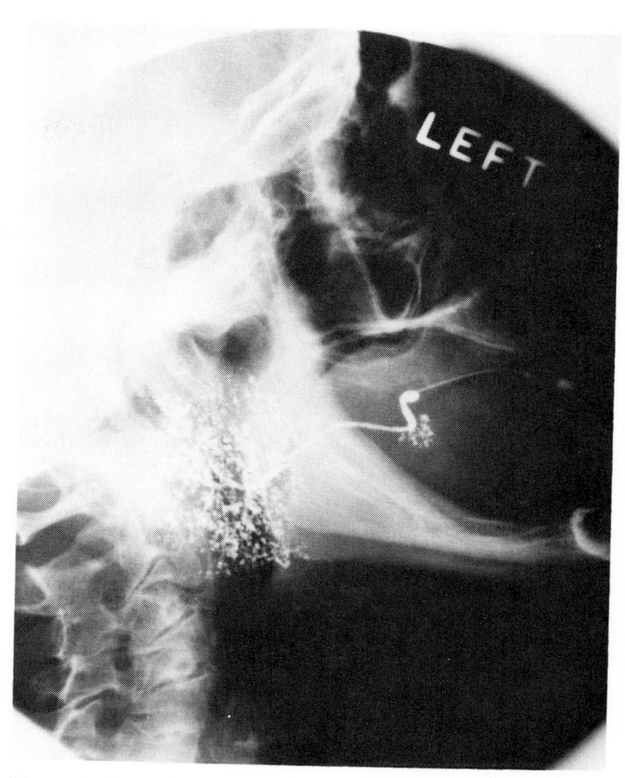

Figure 2. Parotid sialogram demonstrates punctate sialectasis, an early manifestation of benign lymphoepithelial disease. As the disease progresses there may be further destruction of the ductal structures with resultant retention of saliva.

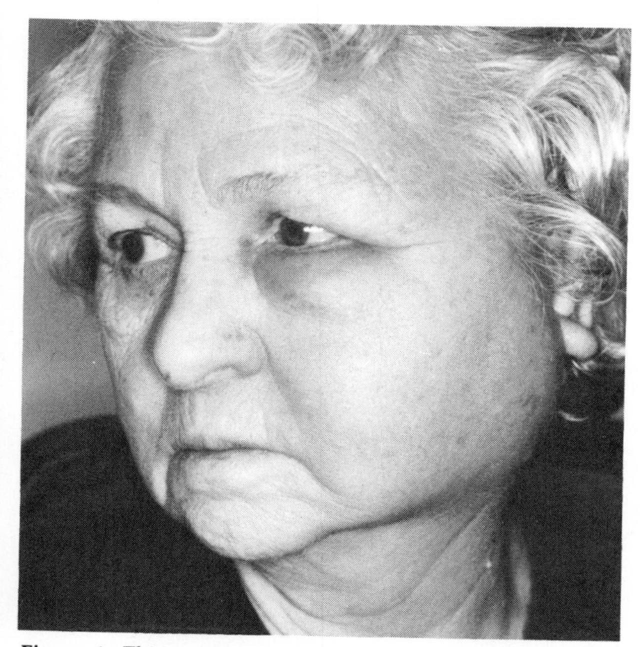

Figure 1. This woman presented with the sudden onset of painful swelling, diffuse erythema, and induration in the left parotid area. She had an accompanying fever and leukocytosis. Purulent debris was expressed from Stensen's duct on palpation. The parotitis subsequently required intravenous antibiotics and surgical drainage.

Histologically, the salivary gland lesions associated with the autoimmune diseases are identical. In most circumstances all of the salivary glands are equally affected, including the minor glands; however, the parotid glands, being the largest and most prominent, are most easily noticed.

In many cases of salivary gland enlargement, a diagnosis cannot be made without obtaining a specimen for histologic evaluation. The parotid is the salivary gland most commonly involved by neoplasms, but fortunately, approximately three-fourths of the tumors are benign.[5] Recently, the histologic features in 140 patients undergoing parotidectomy at the Eye and Ear Hospital of Pittsburgh were reviewed retrospectively.[6] Seventy-three per cent of the parotid masses were found to be neoplastic. The remaining 27 per cent were inflammatory or cystic. Approximately 80 per cent of parotid neoplasms were benign, and the remaining 15 to 20 per cent were malignant.

Submandibular gland enlargement is usually caused by ductal obstruction by stones, concretions, or chronic inflammation (Fig. 3). This tendency may be due in part to the antigravitational flow of saliva through the ducts. Neoplasm is much less common in the submandibular gland than in the parotid.

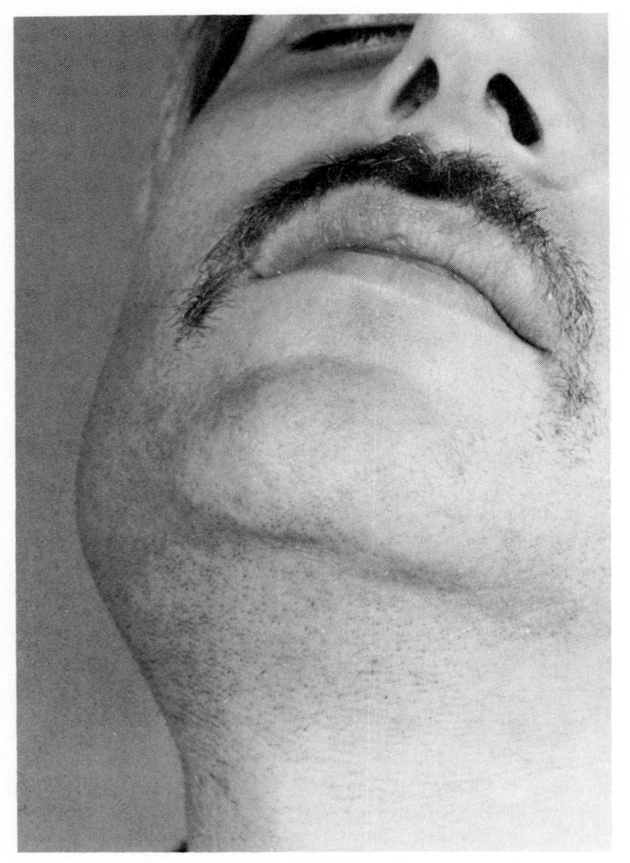

Figure 3. This patient complained of painful swelling under the jaw on eating. Subsequent evaluation revealed a stone in the submandibular duct.

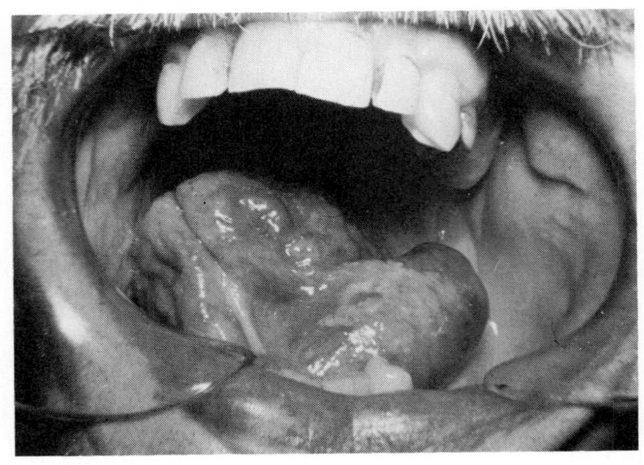

Figure 4. A ranula may develop when there is obstruction of the duct of the submandibular gland. The diagnosis is apparent when the thin-walled cystic cavity is palpated and inspected.

In a review of the pathologic features of 110 patients who underwent submandibular gland excision because of a persistent mass, 85 per cent of the lesions were non-neoplastic.[6] The overwhelming majority of these were inflammatory. The submandibular gland is rarely affected by neoplasm, although approximately 50 per cent of the neoplasms involving the submandibular glands are malignant.

The sublingual glands are rarely involved by tumor or inflammation. Interestingly, however, approximately 80 per cent of neoplasms in sublingual glands are malignant.[7] Needless to say, the finding of a mass in the floor of the mouth requires early and aggressive investigation, which generally involves surgical exploration and removal. Sublingual glands are rarely affected by inflammation, probably owing to their very short ductal system. Obstruction does occasionally occur, manifesting as a fluid-filled cyst with a thin, translucent membrane. These lesions are found in the floor of the mouth and are called ranula (Fig. 4).

The mucosa of the entire upper aerodigestive tract contains tiny foci of glandular tissue called minor salivary glands. It is estimated that most people have between 500 and 1,000 such glands. The palate and tongue have the highest density, and these glands also occur in the nose, paranasal sinuses, pharynx, larynx, lips, and buccal mucosa. Obstruction of a minor gland results in a "cyst," which may be observed in many asymptomatic individuals.

Neoplasms occur infrequently in the minor salivary glands. Most authors agree, however, that approximately 50 per cent of such neoplasms are malignant.[8, 9] The other 50 per cent tend to be benign pleomorphic adenomas (Fig. 5).

HISTORY

The history may aid in the development of a differential diagnosis of salivary gland enlarge-

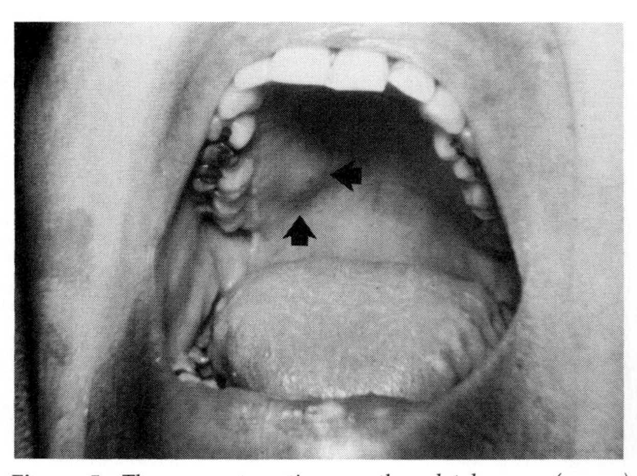

Figure 5. The asymptomatic smooth palatal mass *(arrows)* should be carefully inspected and palpated. This firm soft tissue mass was a benign pleomorphic adenoma, which must be differentiated from the midline, bony-hard torsus palatinus.

ment. Several aspects are important: Are the symptoms acute or chronic? Has the process been progressive or intermittent? Is there swelling and pain with eating? Is a single gland involved or are multiple glands involved? Are there associated systemic symptoms?

The hallmark of salivary gland obstruction due to stone formation is intermittent swelling with eating. From a pathophysiologic standpoint this is easy to understand. The salivary glands are stimulated by eating, and when the duct is obstructed, stimulation of the gland causes swelling and resultant pain.

Infected salivary glands generally hurt continuously. Neoplasms of the salivary gland tend to be relatively asymptomatic. The exception to this is the aggressive neoplasm that produces pain by invasion of adjacent structures.

Patients with bilateral parotid hypertrophy should be questioned about having had mumps, the most common cause of bilateral parotid enlargement. Recent exposure to a person with mumps and a negative history of the disease would be highly suspicious. When multiple salivary glands are enlarged, the patient should be queried about other systemic complaints. Has the patient noticed dry, itching eyes or a dry mouth? Is there a history of arthritis or recent arthralgias? A positive answer to these questions may lead the physician to suspect a collagen vascular disease (Fig. 6). Glandular enlargement may also be seen with infiltration by sarcoid. Similarly, an occasional patient is encountered with parotid hypertrophy secondary to chronic disease, such as cirrhosis, bronchiectasis, diabetes mellitus, hypertriglyceridemia, or severe malnutrition (Fig. 7).[1, 10, 11]

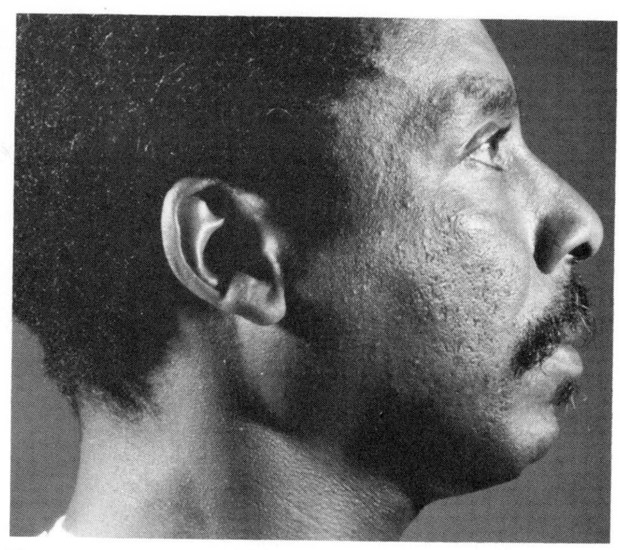

Figure 7. Bilateral parotid hypertrophy is evident in this 38-year-old man with cirrhosis of the liver.

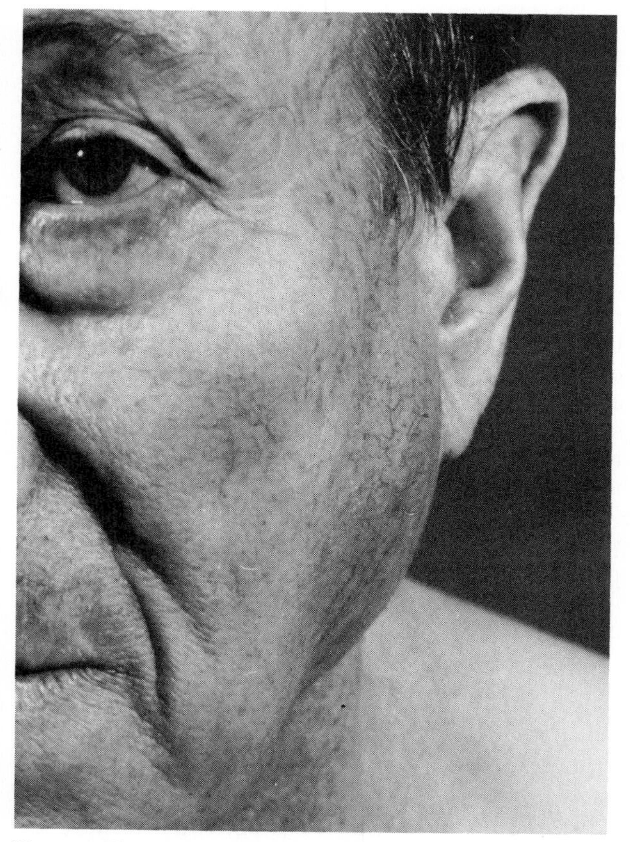

Figure 6. This 68-year-old man presented with bilateral parotid hypertrophy, dry eyes, and arthralgia. Serologic testing and subsequent lip biopsy confirmed the diagnosis of Sjögren's syndrome.

PHYSICAL EXAMINATION

A detailed anatomic description is not the primary focus of this discussion; however, it is important to stress that an understanding of the normal location and variation of the salivary glands is important to facilitate interpretation of physical findings. The first undertaking in evaluating patients with salivary gland enlargement is to distinguish whether, in fact, the patient has enlargement of a salivary gland or of an adjacent structure. This distinction may, at times, be difficult even in the most experienced hands. A small lymph node or cyst may lie adjacent to the parotid parenchyma or actually lie within it.

Parotid Gland. It is important to know that the parotid gland is frequently thought of as existing in three segments that are anatomically connected without real boundaries. However, the location of each segment in relation to adjoining structures often dictates how a mass will manifest. The "superficial lobe" of the parotid gland is that tissue lateral to the facial nerve. A mass in this tissue

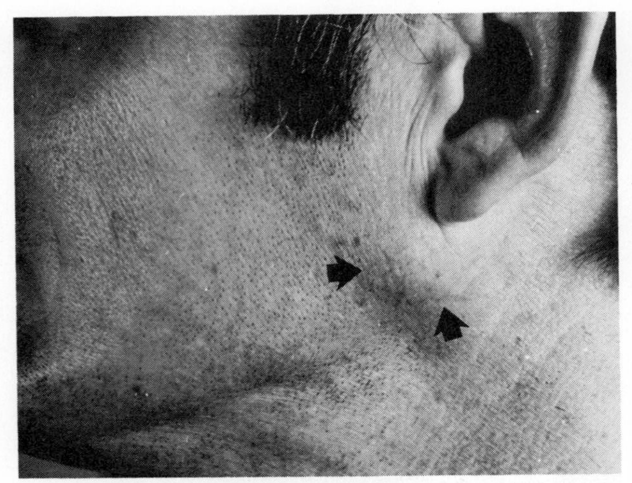

Figure 8. This asymptomatic mass in the superficial lobe of the parotid had been present for many months. It was subsequently found to be a benign pleomorphic adenoma.

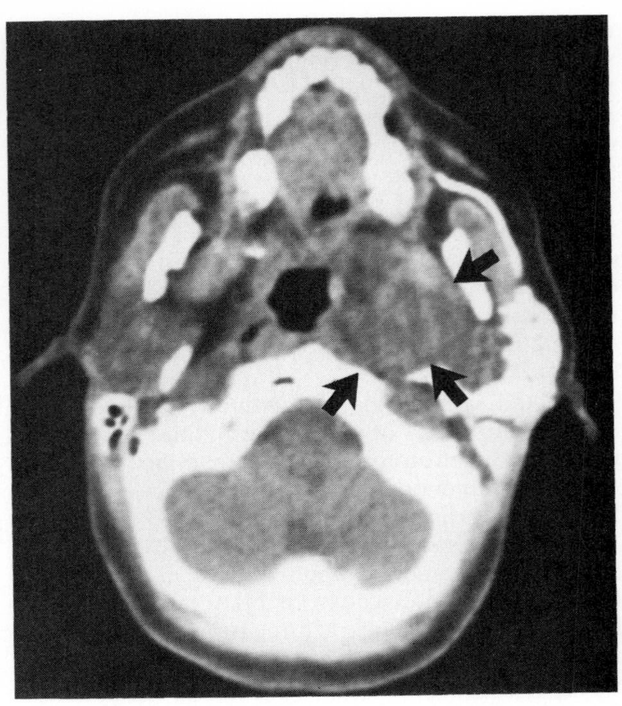

Figure 10. An enhanced computed tomogram demonstrates the anatomic limits of a lesion of the deep lobe of the parotid *(arrows)*. Note that a sialogram has been performed simultaneously, demonstrating a rim of normal parotid tissue lateral to the neoplasm. The medial aspect of the lesion compromises the pharyngeal airway.

always occurs as a lump overlying the angle and ascending ramus of the mandible (Fig. 8). The "tail" of the parotid is a small segment of glandular tissue lying posterior to the angle of the mandible. This tissue may most frequently be confused with a lymph node in the neck. The "deep lobe" of the parotid gland is that tissue medial to the facial nerve. Under normal circumstances this lobe lies just posterior to the ascending ramus of the mandible. Neoplastic formation in the deep lobe may cause expansion into the parapharyngeal space and many manifest as an intraoral mass (Fig. 9). Bimanual palpation of such a mass will lead the astute observer to realize that, in fact, an intraoral mass may be externally connected to the gland (Fig. 10).

It is important for the examiner to distinguish between diffuse enlargement of the parotid gland and a discrete mass or lump. Diffuse enlargement is non-noeplastic under most circumstances, and a discrete mass is frequently neoplastic. The most common neoplasm is the pleomorphic adenoma.

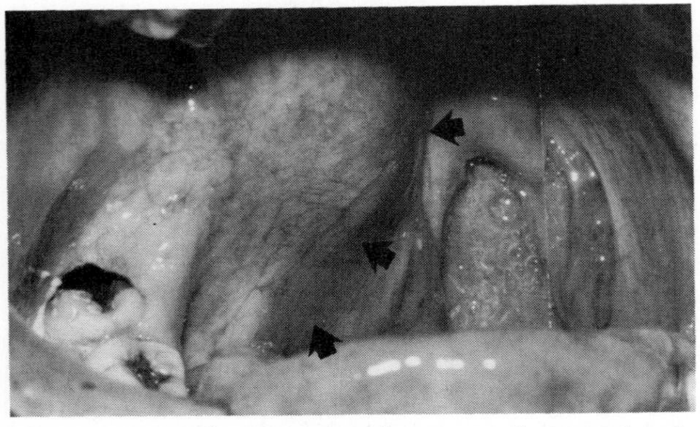

Figure 9. Intraoral examination demonstrated a smooth submucosal mass in the left soft palate *(arrows)*. Bimanual palpation led the clinician to suspect that the mass was, in fact, attached to the parotid gland.

One cannot always make a precise histologic diagnosis at the bedside, although a few clues can lead one in the proper direction. As noted, the most common parotid tumor is benign. Malignant tumors may mimic a benign growth, but subtle differences may be detected. Rapid growth, pain, and fixation to skin or deep structures are danger signs. The most consistent hallmark of malignancy is facial nerve paresis or paralysis. Facial nerve involvement with a parotid mass is "almost always" a sign of malignancy. Conversely, however, most malignant tumors do not manifest as facial paralysis.

Physical examination of the parotid gland is not complete without examination of its secretions. Stensen's duct, located adjacent to the second maxillary molar, should be observed as the gland is milked from posterior to anterior (Fig. 11). Purulent secretions are an indication of infection. The absence of secretions is an important observation and may indicate duct obstruction.

Submandibular Gland. Frequently it may be difficult to distinguish enlargement of the submandibular gland from an adjacent mass such as a lymph node. This determination is facilitated if

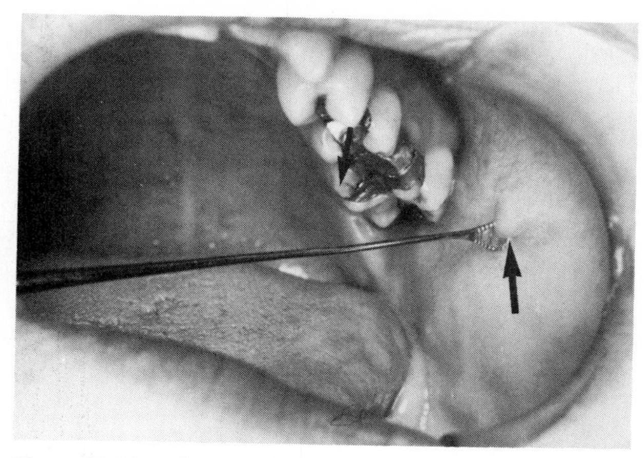

Figure 11. Note the normal location of Stensen's duct, adjacent to the second maxillary molar.

the patient is examined bimanually. One gloved finger can palpate the gland intraorally while the second hand palpates it externally (Fig. 12). With experience, the ductal structures can be clearly identified and the gland isolated. In this way the observer can decide whether, in fact, the mass is glandular or nodal (Fig. 13).

The nature of the submandibular secretions should be observed. Stones in the collecting system can frequently be palpated.

Infection in the submandibular or parotid gland characteristically causes pain, fever, tenderness, and induration and erythema of the overlying skin.

Sublingual and Minor Glands. Proper physical evaluation of the sublingual and minor salivary glands requires some facility in examination of the upper aerodigestive tract. Palpation is frequently possible and should be employed. Minor salivary gland cysts can be identified when encountered.

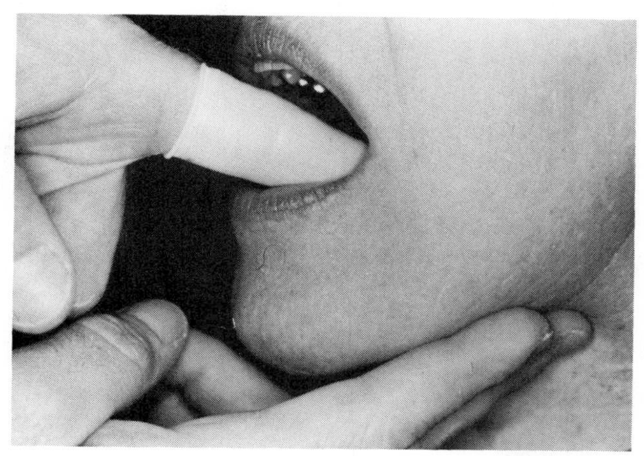

Figure 12. Bimanual palpation of the submandibular gland is an important part of the physical examination. In this way the clinician can distinguish whether a mass is arising in or adjacent to the gland. Similarly, stones in the duct may be evaluated.

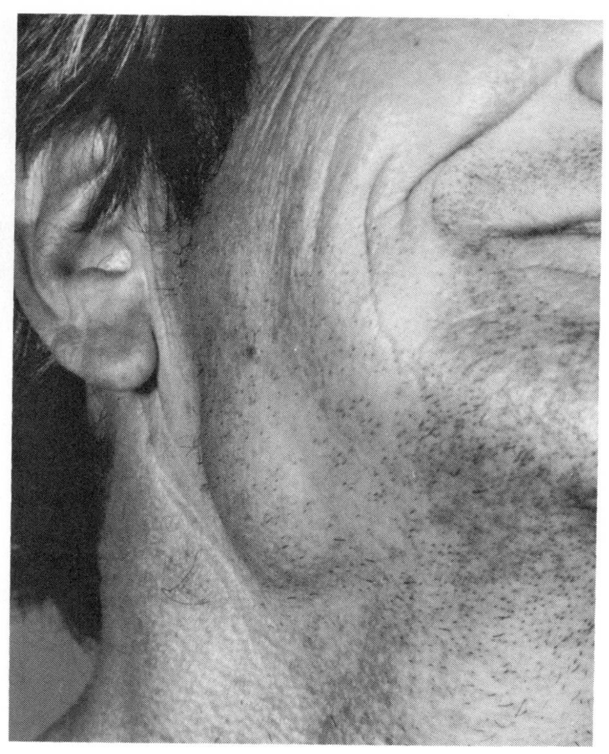

Figure 13. This 46-year-old man presented with an asymptomatic right submandibular mass. Bimanual palpation indicated that the mass was, in fact, adjacent to the submandibular gland, which seemed normal on palpation. Excision subsequently demonstrated the mass to be a lipoma.

Neoplasms may be suspected when a firm submucosal nodule is found.

DIAGNOSTIC STUDIES

Culture

Whenever purulent infection of the salivary gland is encountered a culture should be made of material expressed from the ducts. The most common organism encountered is *Staphylococcus aureus*. When circumstances dictate, empiric therapy should be started with antistaphylococcal drugs.

Imaging

Plain Radiography. Suspicion of stone formation in the salivary gland ducts may sometimes be confirmed using plain radiographic evaluation. It is important to note, however, that only 80 per cent of submandibular stones are calcific (Fig. 14).[1] The remaining 20 per cent are noncalcific and radiolucent. Parotid stones are much less commonly radiopaque; approximately 80 per cent are not demonstrated on x-ray. Under most circum-

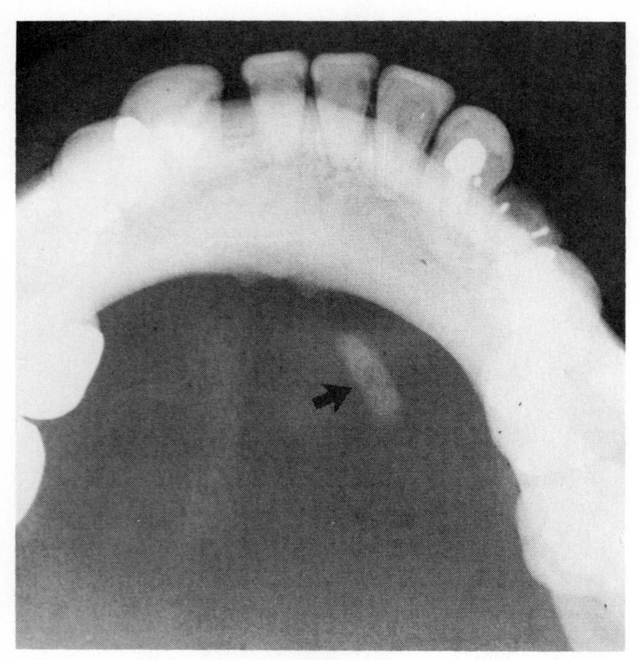

Figure 14. This submental radiograph demonstrates a calcific submandibular stone in Wharton's duct.

stances, if the stone can be palpated, radiographic confirmation is unnecessary.

Sialography. Sialography may be helpful in evaluating salivary gland enlargement.[12] The ducts of the parotid and submandibular glands are cannulated with a small catheter and dye is instilled under low pressure. Plain radiographs are then made (Fig. 15). Sialography is rarely helpful in distinguishing neoplastic from inflammatory disease but may be useful in differentiating a glandular from a nonglandular mass. Patients with suspected autoimmune salivary gland disease may demonstrate the classic findings of saccular dilatation of the ductal system, called sialectasia (see Fig. 2). Sialography of an acutely infected gland should not be undertaken.

Computed Tomography. CT scanning may be an invaluable aid in ascertaining the extent of parotid neoplasms, particularly when they involve the deep lobe. Some have advocated that CT scanning may be accompanied by sialography to maximize the information obtained (see Fig. 10). The addition of contrast material to routine CT scanning has, in fact, made the routine use of sialography rarely necessary.

Biopsy

Biopsy of salivary lesions may be necessary for accurate diagnosis.

Fine-Needle Aspiration. Now under investigation in many sections of the country, fine-needle aspiration is appealing because of its low morbidity; however, the practitioner must recognize the limitations of this diagnostic procedure. First, fine-needle aspiration produces a small cytologic specimen, and microscopic evaluation of the cellular morphology may not be diagnostic. The pleomorphic nature of many salivary gland tumors may make interpretation of fine-needle aspirates exceedingly difficult. Second, the proper area must be sampled with the needle. Negative results must be very closely correlated with clinical findings before they are accepted.

Surgical Biopsy. Open biopsy of small salivary gland lesions usually means complete removal. In this way, the surgeon achieves histologic diagnosis and treatment simultaneously. Incisional or wedge biopsy is discouraged, because it has been associated with frequent seeding of the surrounding

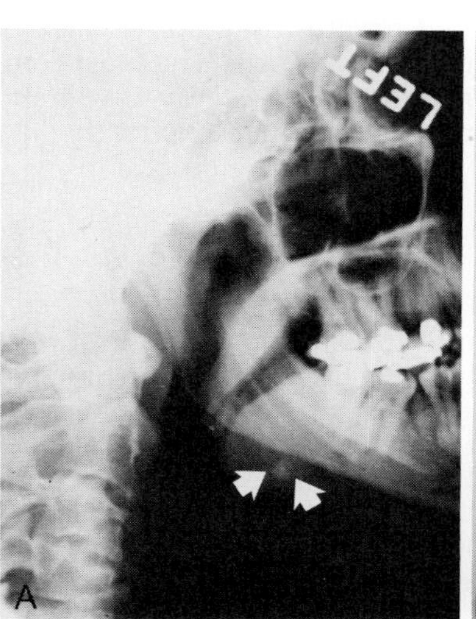

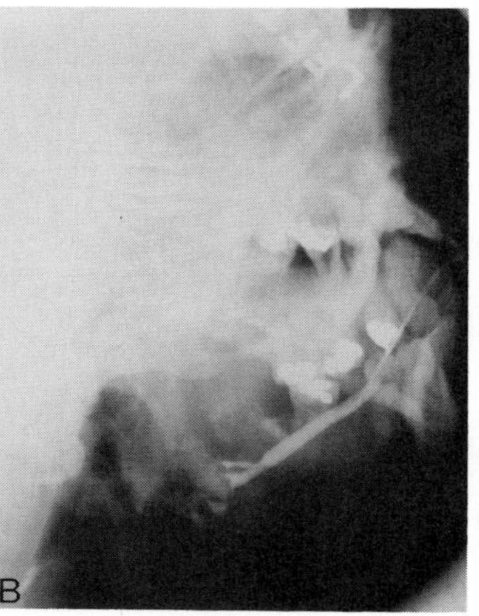

Figure 15. *A,* A plain radiograph demonstrates a small calcific density in the area of the enlarged submandibular gland. *B,* Subsequent sialogram more clearly demonstrates a stone in the hilum of the submandibular gland.

mucosa and subsequent recurrence if tumor is encountered. In this regard, biopsy of neoplasms involving the superficial lobe of the parotid gland should be accomplished by removal of all glandular tissue lateral to the facial nerve. A superficial lobe parotidectomy affords the surgeon an opportunity to identify and preserve the facial nerve while removing the lesion. A diagnosis can be made, and under most circumstances treatment has been completed.

Incisional biopsy of the submandibular gland is rarely, if ever, indicated. Total gland excision is the method of choice when a histologic diagnosis is deemed appropriate. The abundance of salivary gland material of the head and neck precludes the development of symptomatic dryness following glandular removal.

The diagnosis of autoimmune disease may require a sampling of glandular tissue. The structures that are easiest to sample with the lowest morbidity are the minor salivary glands of the lip.[13] These glands may be identified by making a superficial incision through the mucosa of the inner aspect of the lip. The glands will then pout through and may be easily excised for histologic evaluation.

ASSESSMENT

The differential diagnosis of salivary gland enlargement may be long and complex. Careful integration of the history, physical findings, and demographic data allows the physician to greatly narrow the differential diagnosis and guides the decision-making relative to necessary laboratory tests.

Under most circumstances, the diagnosis of viral or bacterial parotitis can be made in a straightforward way. Appropriate treatment can then be embarked upon.

Similarly, the finding of a discrete mass in one of the salivary glands frequently is an indication of a neoplasm, and in most instances tissue must be obtained for pathologic evaluation.

Obstructive diseases of the salivary glands in most cases have a characteristic history. Physical examination may frequently reveal the source of the obstruction. Plain radiography and, occasionally, sialography can be used to confirm the diagnosis. Conversely, chronic asymptomatic swelling of the salivary glands should make the practitioner suspicious of systemic disease. Careful inquiry into other complaints as well as a complete physical examination is mandatory.

REFERENCES

1. Batsakis JG. Non-neoplastic disease of the salivary glands. In: Batsakis JG, ed: Tumors of the head and neck. 2nd ed. Baltimore: Williams & Wilkins, 1979;100–20.
2. Bark CJ, Perzik SL. Mikulicz's disease, sialoangiectasis, and autoimmunity based upon a study of parotid lesions. Am J Clin Pathol 1968;49:683–9.
3. Cipoletti JF, Buckingham RB, Barnes EL, et al. Sjögren's syndrome in progressive systemic sclerosis. Ann Intern Med 1977;87:535–41.
4. Deegan MJ. Immunologic disease of the salivary glands. Otolaryngol Clin North Am 1977;10:351–61.
5. Conley J, Baker DC. Cancer of the salivary glands. In: Suen JY, Myers EN eds. Cancer of the head and neck. New York: Churchill Livingstone, 1981;524–56.
6. Gallia LJ, Johnson JT. The incidence of neoplastic versus inflammatory disease in major salivary gland masses diagnosed by surgery. Laryngoscope 1981;91:512–6.
7. Rankow RM, Mignogna F. Cancer of the sublingual salivary gland. Am J Surg 1969;118:790–5.
8. Chaudhry AP, Vickers RA, Gorlin RJ. Intraoral minor salivary gland tumors. An analysis of 1,414 cases. Oral Surg, Oral Med, Oral Pathol 1961;14:1194–226.
9. Johnson JT, Edwards PR. The asymptomatic smooth palate mass: a dangerously deceptive growth. Postgrad Med 1980;68:96–104.
10. Ray GC, Petersdorf RG. Mumps. In: Isselbacher KJ, Adams RD, Braunwald E, Petersdoref RG, Wilson JD eds. Harrison's principles of internal medicine. 9th ed. New York: McGraw-Hill, 1980;815–8.
11. DuPlessis DJ. Parotid enlargement in malnutrition. S Afr Med J 1956;30:700–3.
12. Gates GF. Sialography and scanning of salivary glands. Otolaryngol Clin North Am 1977;10:379–90.
13. Chisholm DM, Mason D. Labial salivary gland biopsy in Sjögren's disease. J Clin Pathol 1968;21:656–60.

SCROTAL MASS

MARK T. TSUANG

☐ SYNONYMS: Swelling seed, swollen testicle

BACKGROUND

Definition

Scrotal mass is defined as any abnormally enlarged swelling or mass that is related to the structures of the scrotum itself or its contents. It can be a presenting symptom or a physical finding. Scrotal masses have a variety of possible causes. Accurate diagnosis is necessary to prevent the loss of the testicle and to initiate proper treatment for a possible neoplasm. This chapter discusses the diagnostic approach to scrotal masses.

Anatomic Consideration of Scrotal Contents

Scrotal masses can arise in any structure in the scrotum. Understanding the anatomic relationship of the structures is important to the differential diagnosis of the origin of such masses. The scrotum is a cutaneous pouch containing the testes, epididymides, and parts of the spermatic cords (Fig. 1). It develops from the skin of the abdominal wall in the region of the genital swellings. The scrotal layers are identical to the abdominal wall layers but they are identified by different names (Table 1). The scrotum has the vital role of protected site for the testes outside the abdominal cavity with proper temperature regulation for spermatogenesis.

The testes are paired, ovoid bodies. Each testis is about 4 to 5 cm in length and 2 to 3 cm in width. The lateral and medial surfaces of the testis are flattened, the anterior border is free, and on the posterior border lies the epididymis.

The epididymis is a comma-shaped structure. The head of the comma is represented by the head of the epididymis. It gradually becomes smaller toward the back of the testis; this portion is called the body of the epididymis. The tail of the epididymis is the inferior end. The sharp upward turn of the tail is the vas deferens.

On the upper pole of the testis is a minute oval remnant of the paramesonephric duct (müllerian duct) called the appendix testis. On the head of the epididymis is a second small appendage, a remnant of the mesonephric duct (wolffian duct), which is usually regarded as the appendix epididymis.

The testicular artery, which supplies blood to the testis, arises from the aorta below the renal artery. The epididymis is supplied by the defer-

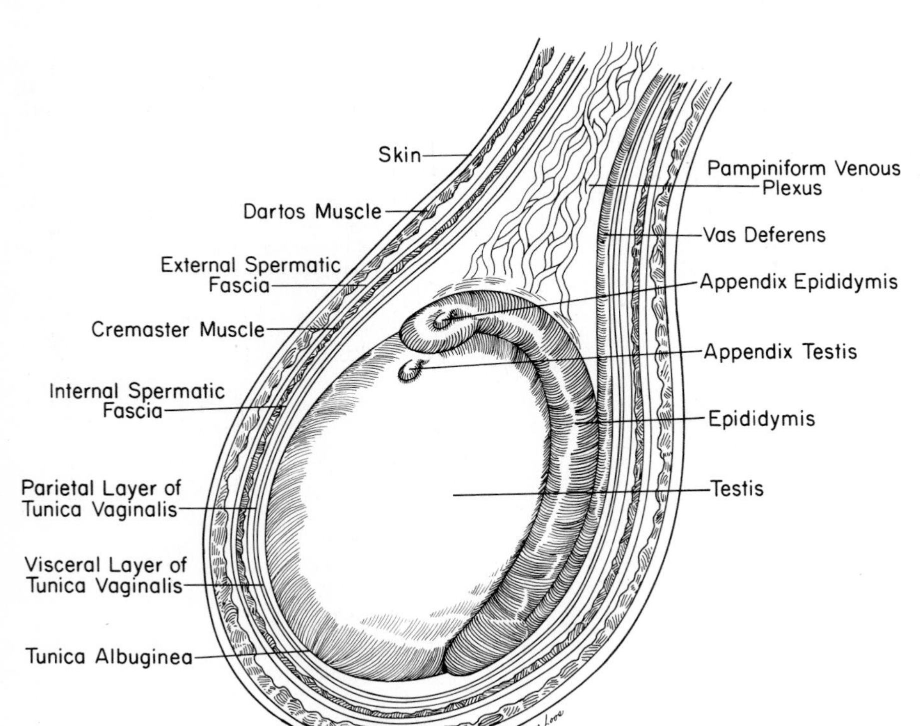

Figure 1. Anatomy of the scrotum and its contents.

Table 1. THE RELATIONSHIP OF ABDOMINAL LAYERS AND SCROTAL LAYERS

Scrotum	Abdomen
Skin	Skin
Dartos	Scarpa's fascia
External spermatic fascia	External oblique muscle
Cremasteric muscle	Internal oblique muscle
Internal spermatic fascia	Transversalis
Tunica vaginalis	Peritoneum

ential artery, which arises from the inferior vesical artery. The venous drainage forms the convoluted venous pampiniform plexus above the upper pole of the testis. This plexus proceeds up the cord to the internal inguinal ring, where it becomes a single vein, the internal spermatic vein. On the right side, this vein joins the vena cava, and on the left side it joins the left renal vein.

The primary lymphatic drainage of the testis and epididymis is to their area of origin, the preaortic lymph nodes.

The spermatic cord is a fascia-covered structure containing blood vessel, lymph, nerves, and vas deferens. It suspends the testicle in the scrotum and provides involuntary testicular contraction via the cremasteric muscle for protection against testicular trauma.

Incidence and Causes

The relative incidence of scrotal diseases requiring hospital admission is about 63 patients per 1,000 urologic hospital admissions.[1] The principal causes of scrotal masses according to anatomic structure are listed in Table 2. Many of the causes discussed here are encountered infrequently, but if one understands the anatomic structures, the differential diagnosis is not difficult to make. In my daily practice the most common entities are: torsion of the spermatic cord, epididymo-orchitis, hydrocele, testicular neoplasm, inguinal hernia, spermatocele, varicocele, and torsion of the appendix testis or epididymis. Torsion of the spermatic cord, testicular neoplasms, and strangulated hernias are associated with significant morbidity and mortality. Careful evaluation of these conditions is necessary.

Age Incidence

Some intrascrotal and extrascrotal masses may occur more frequently in certain age groups. Differential diagnosis should consider the age of the patient. Table 3 classifies scrotal masses according to age groups; the peak age incidences of the principal entities are shown in Table 4.

Table 2. CAUSES OF SCROTAL MASSES ACCORDING TO ANATOMIC STRUCTURE

Structures	Causes
Testis	Orchitis Contusion Tumor, primary or secondary
Tunica albuginea	Cyst Tumor
Tunica vaginalis	Hydrocele
Epididymis	Epididymitis Spermatocele Tumor
Appendix epididymis or testis	Torsion
Spermatic cord	Torsion Varicocele Hernia
Vas deferens	Spermatocele Sperm granuloma
Scrotum	Edema

In newborn infants, hydrocele is frequently encountered, but it resolves spontaneously after closure of the processus vaginalis. Healed meconium peritonitis can present as a mass in the scrotum. After 1 month of age, abdominal examination will reveal calcification in the mass as well as in the scrotum.[2] The incidence of hydrocele is also high in older patients, perhaps owing to a chronic inflammatory process that causes accumulation of fluid in the layers of the tunica vaginalis.

The peak age range for torsion of the cord is lower than that for testicular neoplasms, but the

Table 3. OCCURRENCE OF SCROTAL MASSES ACCORDING TO AGE GROUP

Neonatal period	Torsion of spermatic cord Incarcerated inguinal hernia Hydrocele Healed meconium peritonitis
Childhood and adolescence	Torsion of spermatic cord Torsion of appendix testis or epididymis Contusion Mumps orchitis Epididymitis Hydrocele Spermatocele Tumor Varicocele Edema
Adulthood	Epididymitis Hydrocele Inguinal hernia Tumor Varicocele

Table 4. PEAK AGE INCIDENCES OF SCROTAL MASSES

Mass	Peak Age Incidence (years)
Hydrocele	1–9 and 50–69
Epididymo-orchitis	30–59
Spermatocele	40–59
Testicular neoplasm	20–49
Torsion of spermatic cord	10–19
Varicocele	10–19
Malignant neoplasm	30–59

Table 5. PAINFUL VERSUS NONPAINFUL SCROTAL MASSES

Painful scrotal masses	Torsion of spermatic cord Torsion of appendix testis or epididymis Contusion Epididymitis Strangulated hernia Orchitis Tumor
Nonpainful scrotal masses	Edema Tumor Cyst Hydrocele Spermatocele Hernia Varicocele Sperm granuloma

range may overlap. Careful evaluation for both possible causes is necessary in some patients. Neonatal torsion of the spermatic cord is in an extravaginal fashion, i.e., the testis, epididymis, and tunica vaginalis, which are all enveloped in the spermatic fascia, twist together in a vertical axis on the cord. This is different from childhood torsion, which occurs in an intravaginal manner, whereby the twisting involves only the testicle and epididymis without the tunica vaginalis. Extravaginal torsion rarely occurs also on the contralateral side, whereas with intravaginal torsion, the contralateral side may undergo torsion later.

HISTORY

History of the Present Illness

Types of Onset. The acute onset of swelling of the scrotum needs immediate attention because of the risk of testicular torsion. The patient with torsion can pinpoint the exact time of onset of pain. A gradual onset of swelling may be due to an inflammatory process or neoplasm. Most commonly, masses in the scrotum that occur during straining are varicoceles or sliding inguinal hernias to the scrotum.

Duration. Long duration (3 to 4 days) without any change in clinical signs can help us rule out the possibility of torsion. Long-standing masses should be considered neoplasms until proven otherwise.

Pain. Scrotal masses should be classified into two groups by their presentation—painful or nonpainful (Table 5). Of the painful masses, torsion and strangulated hernia need immediate attention; however, it is important to make a prompt diagnosis of testicular tumor in a nonpainful presentation. The term acute scrotum is used for sudden, severe, painful swelling of the scrotum without definitive diagnosis.

Voiding Symptoms. Voiding symptoms in the presence of scrotal masses imply associated urinary tract infection. This is a helpful means of differentiating torsion from acute epididymitis.

Previous Medical History

Trauma. A history of trauma to the scrotum may confuse the differential diagnosis. A recent injury may lead to an impression of testicular contusion. However, prolonged swelling after a specific injury should prompt the physician to consider the possibility of testicular neoplasm. Thompson and colleagues[3] reported that 21 per cent of their patients with testicular tumors had a definite history of trauma. The enlarged testis is more vulnerable to injury. Patients with acute torsion may have a previous history of attacks of testicular pain owing to intermittent torsion. Incarcerated hernia may develop from a previously known hernia.

Surgery. A history of vasectomy may suggest sperm granuloma at the surgical site.

Infection. Onset of orchitis is usually seen 5 to 6 days after parotitis, but mumps orchitis rarely occurs prior to puberty. The swelling of the testicle will subside in 7 to 10 days.

High-Payoff Queries

The following questions are helpful in evaluating scrotal masses:

1. *Did the swelling in your scrotum happen suddenly or gradually?*
2. *How long has your scrotal mass been present?*
3. *Is it painful?*
4. *Do you have any trouble urinating?*
5. *Have you had an operation or an injury in the area of your scrotum?*

PHYSICAL EXAMINATION

The examination of scrotal masses consists of inspection, palpation, transillumination, and, if indicated, Doppler blood flow studies.

Inspection of Scrotum. The size and shape of the mass should be noted. Scrotal edema will cause the disappearance of the characteristic wrinkles of scrotal skin. Edema may occur in congestive heart failure, nephrotic syndrome, or ascites. With idiopathic edema, Henoch-Schönlein purpura should be included in the differential diagnosis.[4] The color of the scrotal skin and masses should be observed. The "blue dot" sign is representative of torsion of the testicle or epididymal appendage when visible through the skin.[5]

Palpation of Scrotum. The best approach to differential diagnosis of scrotal masses is to palpate the anatomic structure and its relationship to the scrotal contents (Fig. 1). The testes, epididymides, and spermatic cords are palpated separately. The testes are ovoid bodies. Their size should be measured. Each testis is about 4 to 5 cm in length and 2 to 3 cm in width. The examiner should note the consistency and the surface. Masses that arise from the testis or tunica albuginea can be easily detected by palpation. Tenderness of the testis itself is an indication of orchitis. One should remember that the epididymis lies on the posterior border of the testis, an important indicator of the axis of the testis. In patients with torsion of the spermatic cord, the postion of the epididymis will be changed owing to the twisting. Tenderness of the epididymis on palpation is indicative of epididymitis. Masses that arise from the testis and epididymis should not be confused. Palpation alone can distinguish intratesticular from extratesticular masses.

Intratesticular masses should be surgically explored through the inguinal approach. Tumors of the testis account for 1 per cent of all malignant neoplasms in males.[6] The incidence is 2.1 to 2.2 per 100,000 males per year in the United States.[7] No biopsy of the testis can be performed through a scrotal incision if the mass is intratesticular. The differential diagnosis in extratesticular masses includes epididymitis, spermatocele, and solid tumor of the epididymis (see Table 2). The most common solid tumors of the epididymis are adenomatoid tumors, followed by leiomyomas.

Cystic dilatation in the scrotum is the characteristic sign of hydrocele. Light transillumination in the dark examining room is helpful in differentiating cystic from solid masses. Eleven per cent of patients with testicular tumor present with the symptoms of hydrocele.[3]

A palpable, irregular, worm-like mass overlying the spermatic cord and above the upper pole of the testis is the physical finding in varicocele, which occurs more commonly on the left side because of the right angle of the venous return of the spermatic vein to the left renal vein. The varicocele becomes larger during Valsalva maneuver in the standing position and decreases in the supine position.

Sperm granulomas occasionally occur at the vasectomy site. They are firm, indurated nodules that may be tender on palpation.

Beading of the vas deferens is a classic sign of tuberculosis of the vas deferens. This condition is very rare in recent clinical practice.

Doppler Ultrasound Stethoscope Examination. The ultrasound Doppler stethoscope has been used to assess the blood flow in the acute scrotum.[8] The distinguishing feature of torsion of the testis is the loss of testicular blood flow, which the Doppler stethoscope can demonstrate. It is helpful, but at present the results of ultrasound Doppler examination of blood flow are unreliable in the diagnosis of acute scrotal disease.[9]

DIAGNOSTIC STUDIES

Laboratory Tests

Routine laboratory investigation includes a complete blood count and urinalysis. If a testicular tumor is suspected, tumor markers can be sought.

Complete Blood Count. In the patient with a painful scrotal mass, such as torsion, epididymo-orchitis, or strangulated hernia, there may be some evidence of leukocytosis, but this finding is not reliable. In early stages of acute scrotum, the white blood cell count may be normal.

Urinalysis. In order to differentiate torsion of the spermatic cord from epididymitis, one should look for signs of infection in the urine, which may indicate epididymitis. Sequential collection of voided urine can help localize lower urinary tract infections.[10] The first-voided 5 to 10 ml of a urine specimen represents washings from the urethra. The second-voided specimen, the midstream catch, represents the urine from the bladder or upper tract. Prostatic massage is then performed to collect the prostatic fluid. The third-voided urine, collected after prostatic massage is performed, represents the prostatic elements. The sequentially collected urine specimens are examined under the microscope; the diagnostic significance of the results are listed in Table 6. This procedure, which takes only a few more minutes of the physician's time and can be done in the office or during an emergency room visit, yields very valuable information.

Tumor Marker Evaluations. Neoplasms of the testis can be detected by tests for tumor markers, substances generally found only in the presence of tumors. Alpha-fetoprotein is produced by the yolk sac.[11] It does not occur in adults except in pathologic states. This marker has been found commonly in patients with hepatocellular carcinoma as well as in those with testicular tumor. The beta subunit of human chorionic gonadotropin (HCG-β) appears to be manufactured in the

Table 6. SEQUENTIAL COLLECTION OF URINE FOR LOCALIZING LOWER URINARY TRACT INFECTION

First-Voided Specimen	Second-Voided Specimen	Prostatic Fluid	Third-Voided Specimen	Diagnosis
++	–	–	–	Urethritis
+	++	–	++	Cystitis, upper tract infections
–	–	++	++	Prostatitis

+Evidence of infection.
++Strong evidence of infection.

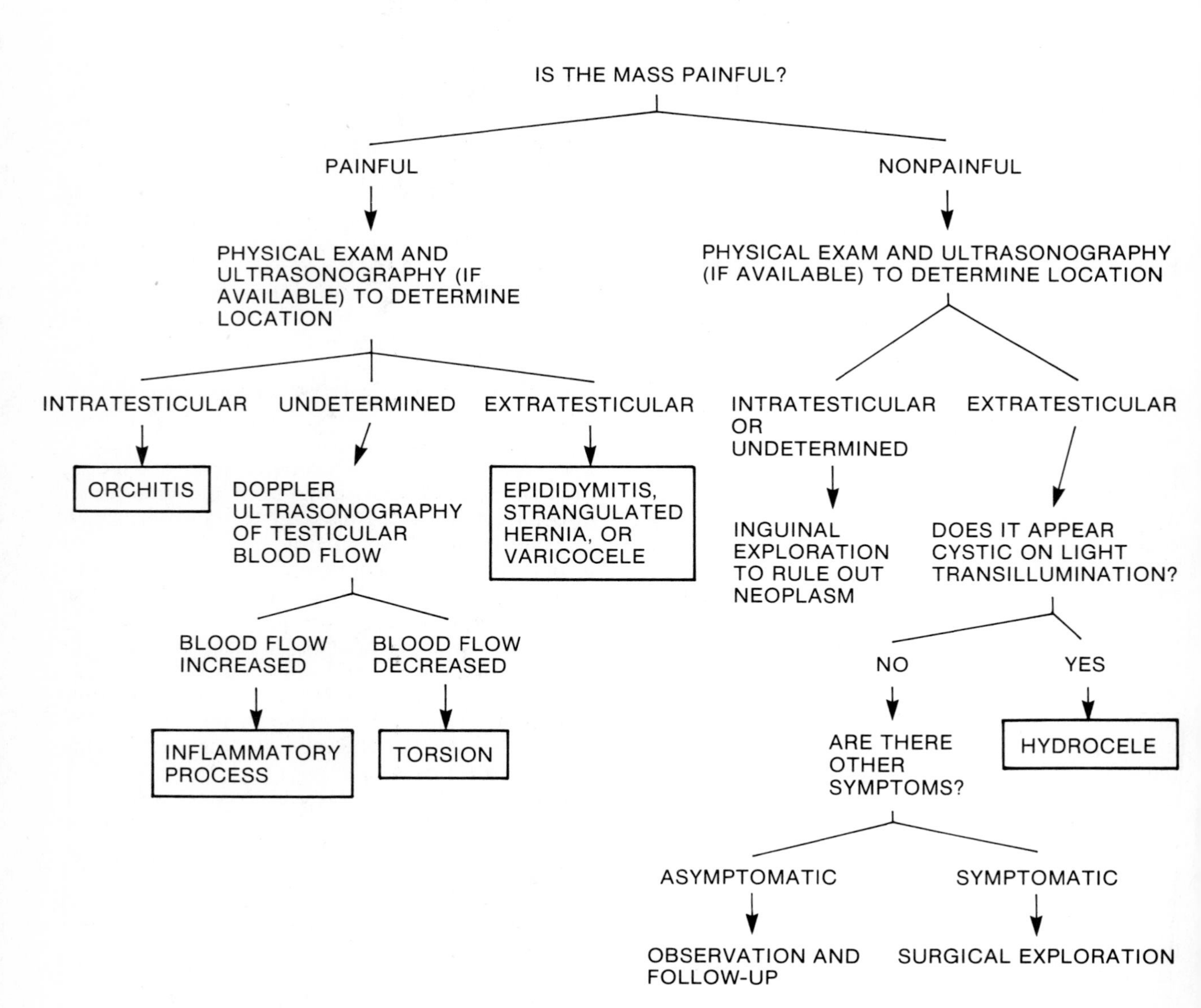

syncytiotrophoblastic element of testicular tumors.[12] The value of tumor marker evaluation in regard to prognosis and response to therapy of testicular tumors is significant.

Imaging

Nuclear Imaging. Nuclear imaging techniques were introduced in 1973 as an additional method to evaluate the blood perfusion of the testes.[13] Decreased testicular perfusion (cold scan) is seen in torsion of the spermatic cord. Increased perfusion (hot scan) is seen in inflammation and torsion of the appendages. Hydrocele sometimes can produce a diagnostic challenge by scan. The overall accuracy for diagnosis is 86 per cent.[14] Of course, the timing of scanning is important only when the procedure is immediately available. A delay to perform scanning only increases the ischemic period in torsion of the spermatic cord, in which testicular function is preserved for only 6 to 10 hours after the onset of vascular compromise.[15]

Varicocele can be easily diagnosed by radionuclide scanning, a new technique using red cell labeling and blood pool imaging of the scrotum that has a sensitivity rate of 90 per cent.[16]

Ultrasonography of the Scrotum. Ultrasonography is a helpful adjunct for determining whether a palpable mass is intratesticular or extratesticular, a benefit in nonpainful scrotal masses in which normal anatomic structures are not clearly distinguishable. Ultrasonography can be used to differentiate cystic from solid masses, and to enhance the impression obtained on physical examination, thereby prompting either medical or surgical treatment.[17]

ASSESSMENT

Scrotal mass is a presenting symptom or sign with various causes, as already described. The physician should carefully analyze the aggregate history, physical findings, and laboratory data to make a correct diagnosis or to choose further diagnostic procedures.

Diagnostic Approach

The algorithm illustrates the diagnostic approach to the scrotal mass, according to whether it is painful or nonpainful. Physical examination, especially scrotal palpation, is very important to define the anatomic location of the scrotal mass (see Fig. 1), particularly as to whether it is intratesticular or extratesticular. The purpose of the approach shown in the algorithm is to differentiate the mass with significant morbidity from the mass with a benign prognosis. Some benign scrotal masses can be followed without surgical exploration as long as they are asymptomatic.

Implications of Scrotal Mass

Any mass lesion arising in the scrotum needs careful evaluation. Accurate diagnosis is important for the initiation of proper management. Scrotal masses that have significant morbidity should be recognized and treated immediately, and those with a benign prognosis can be followed carefully. Laboratory tests, scrotal scans, ultrasonography, and Doppler blood flow studies may assist in the differential diagnosis, but if diagnosis is uncertain after such tools have been used, surgical exploration is necessary.

REFERENCES

1. Clark BG. Relative frequency and age incidence of principal urologic diagnosis. J Urol 1967;87:701–5.
2. Thompson RB, Rosen DI, Gross DM. Healed meconium peritonitis presenting as an inguinal mass. J Urol 1973;110:364–5.
3. Thompson IM, Wear J, Almond C, Schewe EJ, Sala J. An analytical survey of one hundred and seventy-eight testicular tumors. J Urol 1961;85:173–9.
4. Meredith GE, Long W, Karzon DT. Scrotal swelling. South Med J 1979;72:56.
5. Hemalatha V, Rickwood AMK. The diagnosis and management of acute scrotal conditions in boys. Br J Urol 1981;53:455–9.
6. Rubin P. Cancer of urogenital tract: testicular tumors. JAMA 1970;213:89–90.
7. Mostofi FK. Testicular tumors: epidemiology, etiology and pathologic features. Cancer 1973;32:1186–1201.
8. Milleret R, Liaras H. Ultrasonic diagnosis and therapy of torsion of the testis. J Chir (Paris) 1974;107:35–8.
9. Brereton RJ. Limitations of the Doppler flow meter in the diagnosis of the "acute scrotum" in boys. Br J Urol 1981;53:380–3.
10. Meares EM Jr, Stamey TA. Bacteriologic localization patterns in bacterial prostatitis and urethritis. Invest Urol 1968;5:492–518.
11. Bergstrand CG, Czar B. Determination of new protein fraction in serum from human fetus. Scand J Clin Lab Invest 1956;8:174–7.
12. Vaitukaitis JL, Ross GT. Recent advances in the elevation of gonadotropic hormone. Annu Rev Med 1973;24:295–302.
13. Nadel NS, Gitter MH, Hahn LC, Vernon AR. Preoperative diagnosis of testicular torsion. Urol 1973;1:478–9.
14. Abu-Sleiman R, Ho JE, Gregory JG. Scrotal scanning—present value and limits of interpretation. Urology 1979;13:326–30.
15. Smith GI. Cellular changes from graded testicular ischemia. J Urol 1955;73:355–62.
16. Freund J, Handelsman DJ, Bautovich GJ, Conway AJ, Morris JG. Detection of varicocele by radionuclide blood-pool scanning. Radiology 1980;137:227–30.
17. DiGiacinto TM, Patten D, Willscher M, Daly K. Sonography of the scrotum. Med Ultrasound 1982;6:95–101.

SEIZURES OF RECENT ONSET

BERNARD J. D'SOUZA □ JEROME V. MURPHY

□ SYNONYMS: Fits, convulsions, spells, falling spells, epilepsy

BACKGROUND

Terminology

Owing to the variable clinical manifestations of *seizures*,[1, 2] a good definition is lacking. The physiologic basis of all seizures is a spontaneous discharge of cerebral neurons that produces an uncontrolled change in the affected individual. As the neuronal discharge is spontaneous, the individual has no control over the seizure itself. The clinical manifestation depends on the location of the originally discharging neurons, the number of neurons involved, and the electrical spread of this activity. The result is an alteration in motor activity, sensation, behavior, or level of consciousness. Although the expression of seizures varies from one person to another, seizures are clinically similar in the same person when they recur.

The word epilepsy is derived from the Greek word *epilambanein*, meaning "to seize," suggesting that a spirit seized a person and caused a convulsion. *Epilepsy* is used today to refer to recurrent seizures, generally in the absence of any known underlying anatomic or metabolic abnormality; the term would therefore not be used to describe recurrent seizures in a patient with bacterial meningitis or a brain tumor.

Status epilepticus indicates a single prolonged (> 20 minutes) seizure, or seizures occurring so frequently that the patient does not regain alertness between them. As the mortality rate of status epilepticus is 10 to 20 per cent, affected patients require emergency medical attention for immediate control of their seizures.

Classically a seizure has three phases: the aura, the ictus, and postictus. The *aura*, or warning, is probably the most important part. It may indicate the anatomic origin of the neuronal discharge producing the seizure and may give the patient time to prepare for it. Bizarre odors or tastes suggest a temporal lobe focus and herald the onset of a partial complex seizure. In *The Idiot*, Dostoyevsky described the aura of his own seizures, which was characterized by a satisfying sense of well-being and intelligence, suggesting a temporal lobe origin. An aura consisting of weakness in one leg would indicate a frontal lesion in the contralateral motor strip, near the midline. *Ictus* refers to the seizure itself. A patient is generally not aware of events occurring during the ictus unless it is focal. When the seizure is focal, e.g., clonus of the right arm, only a restricted neuronal pool is actively discharging. In such a situation the uninvolved areas of brain might be functioning normally, and the patient may retain awareness and may be responsive. During the ictus, tonic activity (extensor rigidity) and clonic activity (recurrent and rhythmic flexor movement) may occur.

The *postictus* commonly consists of resolving lethargy or confusion after the seizure. During this time the patient may have Todd's paralysis—a hemiparesis or weakness of one limb. Postictal states can last several hours or as long as a day. In a prolonged postictal paralysis, it may be difficult to determine whether the weakness is due to the seizure or damage to the brain has produced both the seizure and the weakness. Certain seizures are not accompanied by postictal states, and the patient is immediately alert after the seizure, e.g., an absence (petit mal) seizure.

Classification

Like most disorders, a complete classification of seizures that is satisfactory to everyone is not available. The classification of the International League Against Epilepsy, presented in the following outline, is the most popular. The basic division is seizures of focal onset (i.e., partial seizures), which therefore are likely to be associated with a correspondingly focal area of abnormal brain, and seizures that appear to be generalized at their onset.

I. Partial epilepsy
  A. Partial seizures with elementary symptomatology and retention of consciousness
    1. With motor symptoms such as clonic activity in one arm, or spreading up one arm (a Jacksonian seizure)
    2. With sensory or somatosensory symptoms
    3. With autonomic symptoms (e.g., pallor, diaphoresis)
    4. Compound forms
  B. Partial seizures with complex symptomatology (formerly called temporal lobe or psychomotor seizures)
    1. With impairment of consciousness only
    2. With cognitive symptomatology

3. With affective symptomatology
4. With "psychosensory" symptomatology
5. With psychomotor symptomatology (automatisms)
6. Compound forms

C. Secondarily generalized seizures

II. Generalized seizures (bilateral and symmetric at onset)

A. Absence (formerly petit mal)
B. Bilateral massive epileptic myoclonus
C. Infantile spasms (salaam seizures)
D. Clonic seizures
E. Tonic seizures
F. Tonic-clonic seizures (grand mal)
G. Atonic seizures

III. Unilateral seizures

IV. Unclassified epileptic seizures

Epidemiology of Seizures

According to the Epilepsy Foundation of America[3] the prevalence rate (number of patients in a specific population at a specific time) of epilepsy is 2 per cent, making it the most common neurologic disease in the general population. Thirty per cent of affected patients are less than 5 years old. In 1972 it was estimated that 4.37 billion dollars were spent in the United States annually on epilepsy by both federal and private organization as well as private individuals.[3]

The intelligence quotients of noninstitutionalized epileptics is comparable to those of the normal population. In patients with both mental impairment and epilepsy, either an associated brain abnormality is causing the seizures and the impairment, or the mental impairment is a drug-related effect that is therefore avoidable. Epilepsy itself generally does not cause brain dysfunction between seizures. Incessantly recurrent seizures or prolonged status epilepticus may cause primary brain damage resulting in mental impairment.

Despite the findings of normal intellect in patients with epilepsy, this diagnosis has been a major barrier to employment. Forty to 50 per cent of adults with epilepsy have difficulties getting jobs, difficulties that are attributed to the epilepsy itself. This situation has led to the withholding of information about the disease by the individual when seeking employment. Similarly, epilepsy is a disqualification for enlistment in the military; the basis for this policy is that recruits must be physically fit to serve anywhere, even in remote outposts without access to medical support. These consequences should lead the physician to restrict the diagnosis of epilepsy to patients in whom it is certain.

All states have regulations governing the issuance of driver's licenses to people with seizures. Most require a variable period of seizure control, as well as an assurance of fitness to drive from a physician, before a license can be issued. Considering the stigma of being known to have these kinds of spells, as well as the frequent necessity to hold a driver's license, it is not surprising that patients with epilepsy do not always disclose their disorder. If failure to make such a disclosure is discovered, the patient's automobile insurance may not be valid.

Although the prevalence rate of epilepsy in the American population is 2 per cent the risk of a seizure disorder in first-degree relatives (siblings, parents, and offspring) of patients with epilepsy is about 12 per cent. In more distant relatives the risk is no more than that in the general population.

If a person has a single seizure and no prior neurologic deficit, the likelihood of recurrence is about 25 per cent in the 36 months after the seizure. Seizures will not recur after this period. Recurrences are seen in about one-third of children following a single seizure. If a spike and slow wave pattern is observed on the initial EEG, the risk of recurrence after a single seizure increases to 50 per cent.[4]

Seizures Peculiar to Specific Situations

Although the majority of seizures are idiopathic, a seizure can be a symptom of central nervous system disease. By eliciting the pertinent information indicated under "History" and "Physical Examination," the examiner should be able to determine whether the seizure is a symptom of underlying disease or represents an idiopathic event. Table 1 lists the causes of seizures according to age at onset, in approximate order of frequency.

These factors do not, however, apply to all seizure types. In well over 50 per cent of cases in both children and adults, no cause can be established (idiopathic seizures).[1, 2, 5]

Neonatal Seizures. Seizures occurring in the newborn may require the attention of specialists experienced in such disorders. At this age seizures can be extremely subtle, e.g., bicycling movements, tonic eye deviation, repetitive blinking, and they can reflect catastrophic illness. Table 2 lists the causes of neonatal seizures.

Infection. In children a seizure can be a very early sign of meningitis. Therefore it is imperative for the physician to determine rapidly whether a febrile child who has had a seizure has meningitis. This determination may require only a clinical assessment of the patient or may necessitate a lumbar puncture and an analysis of cerebrospinal fluid. In children less than 24 months of age, a lumbar puncture is a routine procedure after the first febrile convulsion, because meningismus may not be present in meningitis at this age.

If a child between the ages of 3 months and 5

Table 1. CAUSES OF SEIZURES ACCORDING TO AGE GROUP

Children	Idiopathic
	Infections
	  Meningitis
	  Viral encephalitis
	Genetic disorders
	Metabolic disorders
	  Hypoglycemia
	  Hyponatremia
	  Hypocalcemia
	  Aminoacidopathies
	Trauma
	Toxins
	Neurodegenerative disorders
	Arteriovenous malformation
	Tumor

Adults	Idiopathic
	Infections
	  Meningitis
	  Viral encephalitis
	  Abscess
	  Syphilis
	  Parasites
	Trauma
	Metabolic disorders
	Alcohol withdrawal
	Toxins or drug withdrawal
	Cerebrovascular lesion
	Tumor

Elderly	Cerebrovascular lesion
	Infections
	  Meningitis
	  Viral encephalitis
	  Abscess
	  Syphilis
	Metabolic disorders
	Tumor
	Trauma
	Toxins of drugs
	Neurodegenerative diseases

Table 2. CAUSES OF NEONATAL SEIZURES

Anoxia

Metabolic disorders
  Hypoglycemia
  Hyponatremia
  Hypernatremia
  Hypocalcemia
  Hyperbilirubinemia
  Pyridoxine dependency or deficiency
  Aminoacidurias
  Maternal drug withdrawal

Infections
  Bacterial
  Viral encephalitis
  TORCHS (toxoplasmosis, rubella, cytomegalovirus, herpes, syphilis)

Trauma
Developmental anomalies

years has a generalized convulsion with a fever and no infection of the central nervous system, the physician assumes that the seizure was a febrile convulsion.[6] In an otherwise well child, this is a benign event and is the most common cause of seizures in children. Febrile seizures do recur in the same individual and tend to occur in first-degree relatives. The child with febrile convulsions has no greater risk for spontaneous (afebrile) seizures or neurologic handicap than other children. However, the physician *must* differentiate between a febrile convulsion and a convulsion due to bacterial meningitis.

Infantile Myoclonic Spasms. Very brief, generalized, myoclonic jerks occurring in the first year of life carry an ominous prognosis for intellectual development. In such an attack, the infant typically extends and adducts the arms and legs and flexes at the hip. The descriptive name for this seizure is "salaam seizure." The mother may see them as spontaneous startles, and the physician, witnessing no untoward event, may dismiss her description of them as a sign of excessive maternal concern or may attribute them to infant colic. The EEG pattern in this type of seizure is unique, demonstrating disorganized high-voltage slow waves and spikes and periodic electrical suppression, called hypsarrhythmia (Fig. 1).

One reason for recognizing these events as seizures is that more than one-half of infants with infantile myoclonic spasms are mentally retarded, but prompt and specific treatment may reduce this number. Causes of infantile spasms are numerous and include central nervous system infections, asphyxia, tuberous sclerosis, phenylketonuria and other aminoacidurias, and hypoglycemia.

Post–Pertussis Vaccine Seizures. Another cause of seizures during the first year of life is immunization with pertussis vaccine (the P of DPT).[7] Most such seizures occur within 24 hours of immunization, although there is some increased risk for several days thereafter. The risk of a seizure in the 24 hours following a DPT vaccine is one per 1,750 immunizations. Most such seizures are benign and may be febrile seizures. In about one in 310,000 immunizations, permanent cerebral damage occurs, for unknown reasons. Because permanent damage may occur, albeit rarely, any patient experiencing a seizure within 24 hours of a DPT immunization should avoid subsequent exposure to the pertussis antigen; i.e., subsequent immunizations should be with DT rather than DPT.

Head Trauma. Patients experiencing severe head trauma are at increased risk for seizures.[8] Mild head trauma—such as injury that produces unconsciousness or amnesia of less than 30 minutes' duration—carries no increased risk of epilepsy.

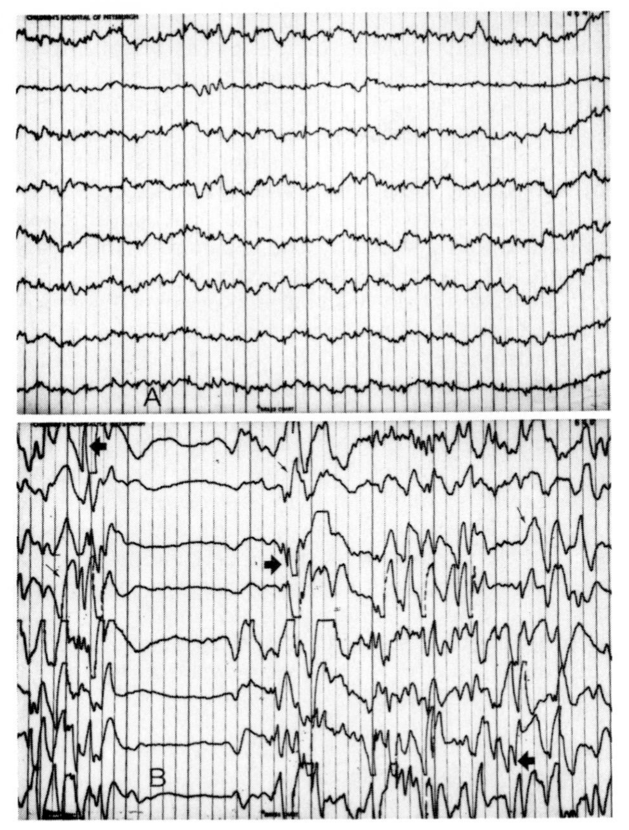

Figure 1. EEGs from a normal 8-month-old infant *(A)* and from a similarly aged patient with hypsarrhythmia *(B)*. Time (one second between dark lines) is measured on the horizontal axis and voltage on the vertical axis. Key features of hypsarrhythmia are the high voltage slow waves *(small arrows)* and spikes *(large arrows)*.

Absence Seizures. Such seizures typically start in childhood and consist of a brief and sudden staring, without preceding aura or subsequent depression. Eye-blinking and/or lip-smacking may accompany the seizure. The patient is aware only of having missed something that occurred during the absence. A classic clinical presentation is deteriorating scholastic performance with frequent daydreaming in a first-grade child.

Such a spell can often be precipitated during the clinical evaluation by having the patient hyperventilate for several minutes. In this type of seizure, the EEG is diagnostic, showing generalized 3 to 4 per second spike and slow wave pattern during a seizure (Fig. 2). Almost one-half of patients with absence seizures subsequently have generalized tonic and/or clonic seizures.

Partial Complex Seizures with Psychomotor Symptomatology. These seizures can be the most difficult to diagnose and, once diagnosed, the hardest to treat satisfactorily. Lee Harvey Oswald, President Kennedy's assassin, was in turn killed by Jack Ruby in what Mr. Ruby's attorneys tried and failed to prove was a partial complex seizure. Although criminal behavior probably never occurs as part of a specific partial complex seizure, the bizarre behaviors that are seen frequently suggest psychiatric illness. Examples of these unusual psychomotor seizures include: sudden and unprovoked rage; peculiar, sustained, inappropriate, and unusual laughter; and the sudden onset of sexually specific language and behavior at a sedate gathering. One might suspect this kind of seizure on the basis of its sudden and unprovoked onset and the patient's postictal depression. Because these seizures have an underlying anatomic temporal lobe abnormality, they may be amenable to neurosurgical intervention, if medical control is unsatisfactory.

Abdominal Epilepsy. Abdominal epilepsy is a common term but, in fact, a rare event. A person with recurrent abdominal pain who has an abnormal electroencephalogram does not have abdomi-

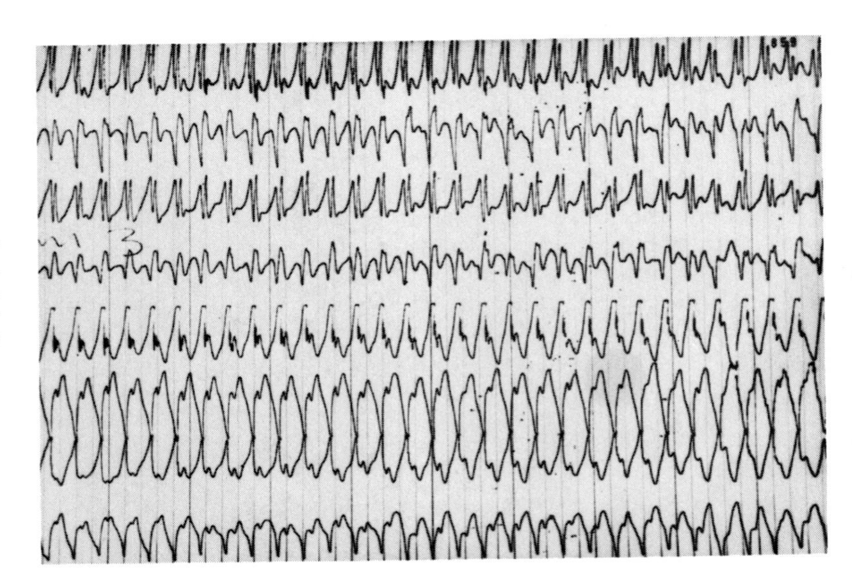

Figure 2. Spike and slow wave with frequency of 3 to 4 per second. The pattern occurred during prolonged hyperventilation and was accompanied by unresponsive staring. This pattern is diagnostic of absence seizures.

nal epilepsy per se. Occasionally, periods of episodic abdominal pain with autonomic accompaniments may reflect an epileptic phenomenon. The discharges arise from the limbic areas and temporal lobe. One should differentiate these episodes from functional disorders.

HISTORY

The most important aspect of the diagnosis is the history. It will indicate whether or not the event for which the patient seeks medical attention is a seizure. The observations of a witness to the event are crucial to this determination. The patient may understand only that he or she is suddenly and inexplicably lethargic and lying on the floor in a pool of urine. The patient's teacher, parent, fellow worker, or spouse may have to be interviewed to obtain an accurate description of the event.

The differential diagnosis of recurring spells includes syncope, cerebrovascular accidents, narcolepsy, breath-holding attacks in children, paroxysmal vertigo, tics, myoclonus, organic mental syndromes, and hysteria. Episodes that can masquerade as seizures vary with the age of the patient and include breath-holding spells in an infant and transient ischemic attacks in an adult. Breath-holding spells are not uncommon in children between 6 months and 3 years of age. Generally the episode is triggered by a child's being frustrated, followed by incessant crying and holding of the breath. The period of apnea is usually brief. The child turns blue and is unconscious and usually limp, and a short, clonic convulsion may be noted. These episodes are usually self-limited and the child outgrows them. Anticonvulsants are not effective in their control.

Hysterical seizures are usually not seen until later in childhood or adolescence and may be difficult to differentiate from epilepsy. Generally, there is some secondary gain to be derived by the patient. The episodes are often not physiologic. The patient usually is not injured or postictal. The EEG is usually normal, especially during such a spell.

Syncopal attacks are seen in young people and may be caused by abnormal vascular reflexes leading to hypotension and cardiac arrhythmias[9] or asystole associated with heart disease (e.g., Stokes-Adams disease). Syncope can also be seen in vertebrobasilar artery insufficiency. In one series of patients referred to a neurologic department with possible idiopathic epilepsy, cardiac arrhythmias were eventually believed to be the cause of symptoms in 20 per cent.[9]

Next, one must identify the type of seizure, which may vary with the age of patient (see Table 1). The type of seizure may help in determining the cause, extent of investigations, prognosis, and choice of drugs. Other factors of historical importance include frequency and time of day of seizures, duration, and presence or absence of a postictal state. Seizures can be precipitated by certain factors, such as flashing lights, reading, music, touch, loud sounds, menstruation, stress, and lack of sleep. If the specific provocations can be determined, avoiding them can contribute significantly to seizure management.

If the description of the spell suggests a seizure, events in the patient's previous history that might be contributory should be sought. Key events would include unusual head trauma, early morning headaches (a sign of increased intracranial pressure), recent intellectual decline (suggesting a degenerative process), recurring fevers, and occurrence of similar events in first-degree relatives. A family history of seizures is important because there is an increased risk, particularly with absence (petit mal) seizures, febrile seizures, and focal (rolandic spike) epilepsy. Additionally, certain metabolic and degenerative diseases have a familial pattern in which seizures may be a part of the neurologic manifestation.

PHYSICAL EXAMINATION

A complete general physical examination may offer evidence as to the underlying cause. Table 3 offers a few clues.

Vital Signs. The presence of *fever* suggests an infectious process involving the brain, a febrile seizure if the patient is a child, or a predisposition to seizure aggravated by the fever. The finding of *elevated blood pressure* raises the possibility of hypertensive encephalopathy or an intracerebral hemorrhage. If the pulse is low, the blood pressure is high, and the patient is poorly responsive, herniation of the brain is suspected and death may be imminent.

Skin. As in many disorders, examination of the skin will yield clues to the primary disease process. *Petechiae* might be a sign of a defect in coagulation or subacute bacterial endocarditis. *Adenoma sebaceum,* firm oily nodules on the malar eminences of the face, are diagnostic of tuberous sclerosis. The young child with this disease will not have the adenoma, but a careful examination of the skin may disclose discrete hypopigmented lesions, or ash leaf spots. In a fair-skinned individual these may be seen only on ultraviolet illumination. Computed tomography (CT scanning) of the head should show periventricular calcification. A *port wine stain* over the forehead suggests Sturge-Weber-Dimitri disease, the impression of which can be confirmed by finding appropriate cortical calcifications on a CT scan of the head.

Head and Neck. In any child with a neurologic

Table 3. PHYSICAL SIGNS SUGGESTING CAUSES OF SEIZURES

Aspect of Examination	Sign	Possible Disease(s)
Temperature	Fever	Meningitis, encephalitis, brain abscess
Hair	Friable or white hair (patchy)	Menkes' syndrome, argininosuccinicaciduria, tuberous sclerosis
Skin	Petechiae	Subacute bacterial endocarditis, blood dyscrasia, leukemia, thrombocytopenic purpura, fat emboli
	Cyanosis	Cyanotic congenital heart disease, pulmonary disease
	Adenoma sebaceum	Tuberous sclerosis
	Malar skin rash	Systemic lupus erythematosus, homocystinuria
	Facial port wine stain	Sturge-Weber-Dimitri disease
Head	Large head circumference	Hydrocephalus, microcephaly
	Bruit	Arteriovenous malformation
Eye	Cataracts	Lowe's syndrome (oculocerebral syndrome), prenatal rubella, pseudohypoparathyroidism
	Cherry-red spot in macular area	Ganglioside storage disease
	Chorioretinitis	Congenital infection
	Retinitis pigmentosa	Chronic neuronal ceroid lipofuscinosis
	Papilledema	Brain tumor, subdural hematoma, brain abscess
	Nystagmus	Drug toxicity
Neck	Stiff neck	Meningitis, subarachnoid hemorrhage, fractured odontoid, herniated cerebellar tonsils
Circulation	Carotid pulses or bruit	Cerebrovascular disease
	Hypertension	Hypertensive encephalopathy
	Arrhythmia	Congenital or arteriosclerotic heart disease
Abdomen	Hepatosplenomegaly	Ganglioside storage disease, mucopolysaccharidoses
Bones and joints	Clubbing	Lung carcinoma, cyanotic congenital heart disease
Neurologic	Ataxia	Argininosuccinicaciduria, urea cycle defects, mass lesion, drug toxicity
	Hemiparesis	Stroke, tumor, trauma

disorder the *head circumference* should be measured and compared with easily available normal values. Auscultation of the head in a focal seizure may yield the *bruit* of an arteriovenous malformation.

Nuchal rigidity carries the differential diagnosis of inflammatory disease of the central nervous system, blood in the subarachnoid space, and neck trauma.

Circulation. A carotid bruit suggests turbulent flow, which could be due to an (embolizing) arteriosclerotic plaque. A *heart murmur* raises the possibility of embolization to brain of fibrin or bacteria.

Abdomen. *Enlargement of the abdominal viscera* suggests abnormal storage. Ganglioside storage diseases may first manifest as seizures.

Neurologic. A complete neurologic examination is essential in the evaluation of a patient with suspected seizures, from two standpoints. Deficits demonstrated on testing indicate an underlying cerebral abnormality and the need for further laboratory studies. Additionally, the initial examination will serve as a basis for future comparison, i.e., the development of nystagmus would suggest a drug effect, but a new, later-discovered Babinski sign might be the first indicator of a slowly growing brain tumor. As part of the assessment, the patient should be asked to hyperventilate for 2 minutes; if the patient has a seizure, the physician will have the opportunity to witness the event firsthand.

DIAGNOSTIC STUDIES

No single laboratory test is helpful in establishing a diagnosis of a seizure disorder. The history almost always provides the diagnosis. However, further investigations may indicate the cause of the disorder.

Basic Laboratory Studies

The usefulness of routine complete blood counts, blood urea nitrogen, glucose, electrolytes, and calcium measurements, and liver function studies is limited. Appropriate tests should be done if clinically indicated. An ECG may be helpful in ruling out an arrhythmia leading to syncope. However, transient ST-T wave changes can occur in the immediate postictal state. A toxicologic screen may be helpful in certain circumstances.

Electroencephalogram (EEG)

The EEG is useful but has been abused in the management of patients with seizures.[10] A normal EEG does not rule out the diagnosis of epilepsy, and conversely, an abnormal EEG does not establish the diagnosis. When there is a conflict between the history and the EEG, the clinician should rely on the history.

In the event of equivocal information, a repeat EEG, a 24-hour recording with accompanying video monitoring, the use of special recordings, such as sleep deprivation, hyperventilation, and photic stimulation, and the use of nasopharyngeal leads, may be necessary. The EEG may show focal or generalized abnormalities. It is often helpful in confirming the diagnosis, for example, of hypsarrhythmia in infantile spasms (see Fig. 1), or 3 to 4 per second spike and wave discharges in absence (petit mal) seizures (see Fig. 2).

The presence of focal slowing should raise strong suspicion of a structural abnormality or space-occupying lesion and may necessitate further radiologic studies.

Follow-up electroencephalograms in a patient with an established seizure disorder are indicated only in the following circumstances: (1) poor control despite good anticonvulsant compliance, (2) change in behavior or intellect unrelated to anticonvulsants, (3) neurologic deficits in a previously normal patient, and (4) consideration of discontinuation of anticonvulsants in a patient with well-controlled seizures.

Imaging

Computed Tomography. With the advent of this relatively new diagnostic tool there has been a tendency for excessive utilization. In one study, routine CT scanning was normal in 94 per cent of all patients with seizures. However, 50 per cent of patients with focal neurologic findings or a slow wave focus on EEG had CT abnormalities. Of the focal abnormalities on CT scans, 25 per cent were potentially treatable by surgery. In children with seizure disorders routine CT scanning revealed a 30 per cent incidence of nonspecific abnormalities such as atrophy. In less than 2 per cent of patients did these findings affect management.

A detailed history and careful clinical examination supported by an EEG constitute the essentials in managing patients with seizures. CT scanning should be done only for patients with: (1) focal neurologic deficits, (2) evidence of increased intracranial pressure, (3) focal slowing on EEG, (4) presence of a neurocutaneous lesion as in tuberous sclerosis or Sturge-Weber disease, (5) suspicion of brain abscess, and (6) severe head trauma.

Other Studies

Skull x-rays, radionuclide brain scanning, pneumoencephalography, and arteriography are rarely indicated but may be necessary in individual situations. Lumbar puncture for examination of the cerebrospinal fluid is necessary if meningitis is a possibility; otherwise it is rarely helpful.

ASSESSMENT

The final assessment of a patient with spells is rational and easy, if all the pertinent information

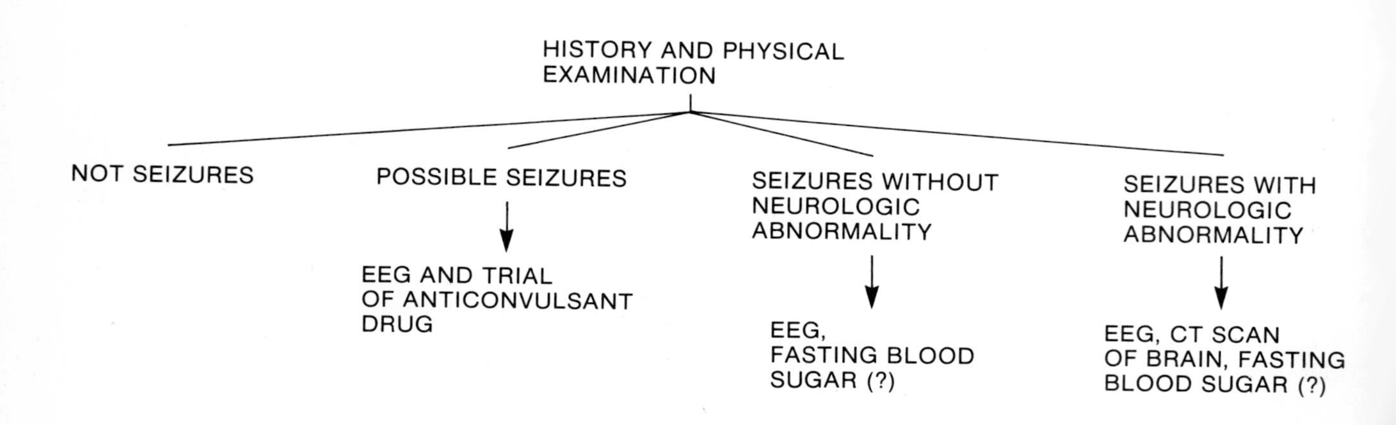

has been collected. The algorithm illustrates a diagnostic approach to the patient who may have seizures. If despite a complete evaluation, the presence of seizures is still uncertain, a trial of anticonvulsant therapy may be indicated. If the spells are controlled by an anticonvulsant and recur when placebo is given, the patient has seizures. Obviously, witnessing the event is the most helpful observation for the physician.

If seizures are diagnosed, the next major question is, Does the patient have an idiopathic seizure disorder (epilepsy) or are the seizures a manifestation of an anatomic abnormality of the brain? Most seizures are idiopathic, but one must never become too comfortable with this diagnosis. Physicians experienced in epilepsy have been humbled by encounters with a few patients whose underlying brain tumors were not evident, even on CT scanning, for several years after the onset of seizures. Fortunately such situations are rare.

Once the physician is convinced that the patient has seizures, appropriate therapy should be started. It is not necessary to withhold therapy pending the EEG or other laboratory studies if the diagnosis is certain.

REFERENCES

1. So EL, Penry JK. Epilepsy in adults. Ann Neurol 1981;9:3–16.
2. Gomez MR, Klass DW. Epilepsies of infancy and childhood. Ann Neurol 1983;13:113–25.
3. Epilepsy Foundation of America. Basic statistics on the epilepsies. Philadelphia: FA Davis, 1975.
4. Hauser WA, Anderson VE, Lowenson RB, McRoberts SM. Seizure recurrence after a first unprovoked seizure, 1982. N Engl J Med 1982;307:522–8.
5. Kolden KR, Mellits ED, Freeman JM. Neonatal seizures. Correlation of prenatal and perinatal events with outcome. Pediatrics 1982;70:165.
6. Nelson KB, Ellenberg JH, eds. Febrile seizures, New York: Raven, 1981.
7. Cody CL, Baraff LJ, Cherry JD, et al. Nature and rates of adverse reactions associated with DPT and DT immunizations in infants and children. Pediatrics 1981;68:650.
8. Young B, Rapp RP, Norton JA, Haack D, Tibbs PA, Bean JR. Failure of prophylactically administered phenytoin to prevent early post traumatic seizures. J Neurosurg 1983;58:231–41.
9. Schott GD, McLeod AA, Jewitt DE. Cardiac arrhythmias that masquerade as epilepsy. Br Med J 1977;1:1454–7.
10. Lewis DV, Freeman JM. The use and abuse of the electroencephalogram in pediatrics. Pediatrics 1977;60:324–30.
11. Young AC, Constanz JB, Mohr PD, Forbes W, St Clairr. Is routine computerized axial tomography in epilepsy worthwhile? Lancet 1982;2:1446–7.

SHORT STATURE

WILLIAM L. JAFFEE

□ SYNONYMS: Growth retardation, growth delay, growth failure, pituitary dwarfism

BACKGROUND

Linear growth occurs at a predictable rate in any given population. The National Center for Health Statistics[1] has collected growth data from a large population of children in this country, some of which is presented graphically in Figures 1 and 2. One could arbitrarily state that all children with heights below the fifth percentile have short stature. However, most of these children are growing at rates determined by familial factors and should not be considered abnormal. In this chapter, *short stature* is considered to be the consequence of a pathologic process that slows or stops normal linear growth.

Just as short stature cannot be diagnosed on the basis of arbitrary measurements, height above the fifth percentile does not exclude disease in a child genetically predetermined to be tall. The heterogeneity of our population means that growth abnormalities cannot be identified by simple measurements alone. Instead, the examiner must have some knowledge of the mechanisms that control linear development as well as the disorders that can modify normal patterns.

Although pituitary hormones mediate growth, genetic factors control the ultimate capacity for height. This capacity can be roughly estimated for an individual on the basis of parental stature. By taking an average of the parents' height, one can arrive at an estimation of the child's expected growth percentile. For instance, if the father is 181 cm tall (75th percentile) and the mother is 160 cm tall (25th percentile), the child might be expected to grow with the cohort of children in the 50th percentile. Because this crude estimate ignores the effect of nongenetic factors that may have affected parental stature during their formative years, it may underestimate growth potential. Furthermore, stature is polygenic with variable expres-

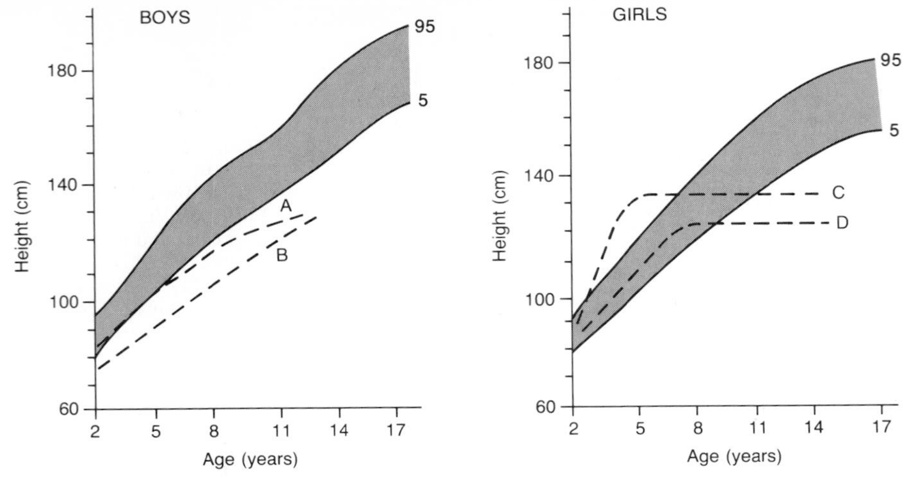

Figure 1. The range of normal for juvenile height correlated with age is graphically presented. In pattern A, the child starts out at the lower end of the normal range and later falls below the range of normal; this pattern is consistent with several genetic disorders as well as with constitutional growth delay. In pattern B, the child is below the range of normal, but the rate of growth is relatively constant; this pattern would be seen in familial short stature. In pattern C, accelerated growth raises the child transiently above normal, followed by no further growth; this pattern is typical of precocious puberty. In pattern D, normal growth rate is suddenly arrested, suggesting an acquired insult such as a pituitary tumor. (Normal range data adapted from Hamill PVV, Drizd TA, Johnson CL, et al: Physical growth: National Center for Health Statistics Percentiles. Am J Clin Nutr 1979; 32:607–629.)

sion, so that growth potential for any individual is not completely predictable.

Intrauterine growth seems relatively less dependent on pituitary function than on maternal and uteroplacental health. Thus, a small-for-dates neonate should not be thought to have pituitary insufficiency, but rather maternal or neonatal illness or placental insufficiency should be suspected.

The average birth length is approximately 50 cm, and most children grow 25 cm in the first year. Linear growth slows to an average of 12.5 cm during the second year and to 6 cm per year subsequently. Height velocity charts, as suggested by Tanner and Whitehouse,[2] accentuate acquired growth abnormalities and are useful for monitoring development (Fig. 3). Linear growth tends to be episodic and seasonal, so that average growth

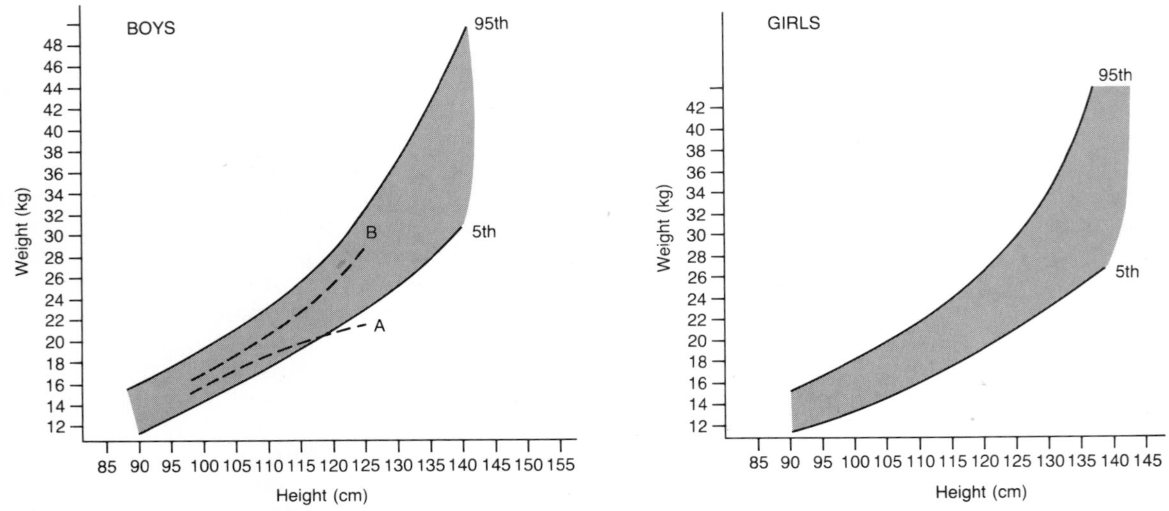

Figure 2. Weight versus height (stature) in a juvenile population. In pattern A, the child's growth pattern falls into a lower percentile, as is seen in malnutrition and many systemic illnesses. In pattern B, the body weight is normal or increased for height; such a pattern would be seen in idiopathic growth hormone deficiency. (Normal range data adapted from Hamill PVV, Drizd TA, Johnson CL, et al: Physical growth: National Center for Health Statistics Percentiles. Am J Clin Nutr 1979; 32:607–629.)

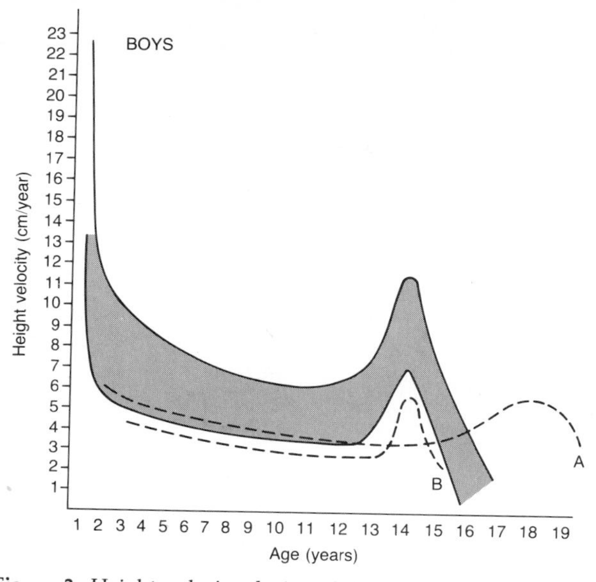

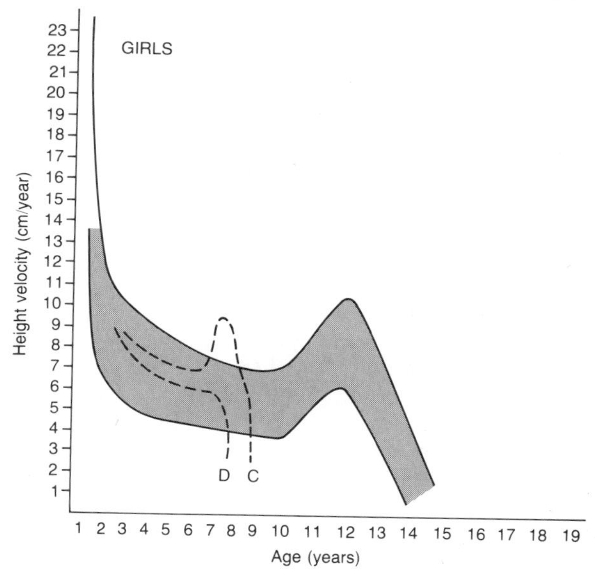

Figure 3. Height velocity during childhood and adolescence in boys and girls (3rd to 93rd percentiles represented). Pattern A represents constitutional growth delay, with borderline low height velocity and a delayed pubertal growth spurt. Pattern B would be characteristic of familial short stature, with puberty occurring at the normal time. Pattern C shows an early growth spurt followed by arrested further growth, characteristic of precocious puberty. Pattern D shows sudden arrest of normal growth, consistent with an acquired disease or pituitary insufficiency. (Normal range data adapted from Tanner JM, Whitehouse RH: Clinical longitudinal standards for height, weight, height velocity, weight velocity, and the stages of puberty. Arch Dis Child 1976;51:170–179.)

over 1-year periods should be considered rather than shorter intervals. From age 3 years until puberty, growth rate is relatively constant. At puberty, rising levels of gonadal sex steroids cause epiphyseal closure and accelerated growth. The growth spurt seems to occur earlier in females, at Tanner stage II or III (12–13 years), versus Tanner stage IV or V (14–15 years) in males. During the pubertal growth spurt, the rate of growth may exceed 10 cm per year.

Normal growth depends upon normal endocrine function and especially upon the presence of growth hormone (GH) and the somatomedins. Central nervous system control of GH release from the pituitary is mediated through hypothalamic neurons. Alpha-adrenergic and serotonergic stimulation within the hypothalamus is known to cause GH secretion, whereas beta-adrenergic stimulation is inhibitory. In addition to the aforementioned factors modifying GH release at the hypothalamic level, a variety of peptides, amino acids (including arginine), and dopamine act directly on the pituitary to cause GH secretion.[3]

Because ablative central nervous system lesions result in GH deficiency, it was thought that there must be a hypothalamic growth hormone–releasing factor (GHRF). Ironically, the first somatotroph-active peptide isolated was somatostatin, or GH release–inhibiting hormone. This 14–amino acid peptide, described by Guillemin's group during the early 1970s, blocks the release of GH. The same group of investigators has recently tentatively identified GHRF.[4]

GH is known to have anabolic effects on bone and muscle, as well as modifying glucose and intermediary metabolism by its anti-insulin effects. Although GH could act on tissue directly, the majority of its effects are mediated by the somatomedins.[5] Somatomedins are large (molecular weight 5,000–10,000 daltons) polypeptides produced in response to GH. A variety of somatomedins have been identified, and several commercial laboratories offer an assay for somatomedin-C determinations. Unlike GH, somatomedins are protein-bound in the circulation, so that their levels do not fluctuate during the day. Likewise, somatomedin levels do not respond immediately to growth hormone stimulation tests. Therefore, a single random somatomedin-C level may be more useful than several random GH determinations.

In addition to the growth hormone-somatomedin axis, other hormones are important in modifying growth. As described earlier, the pubertal increase in secretion of testosterone or estradiol by the gonads is responsible for epiphyseal closure and the normal adolescent growth spurt. Sex steroids also accelerate bone age as measured radiographically. In children with precocious puberty, early epiphyseal closure ultimately results in short stature with mature bone appearance on x-ray.

Thyroid hormone is known to be necessary for normal development of many organs. Prenatal deficiency of thyroid hormone results in the pathologic state known as cretinism. Postnatal onset of hypothyroidism is noted for causing short stature and delayed intellectual development. Thyroid hormone deficiency results in delayed bone maturation in relation to bone length.

Causes

The causes of short stature are myriad. A classification scheme for major categories is shown in Table 1. Although it would be difficult for any one practitioner to be familiar with all of the hundreds of obscure syndromes that can manifest principally as short stature, it should be possible to identify phenotypic characteristics that suggest a *genetic illness*. Identification of such a disorder is important, not in the least because it usually renders further evaluation for alternative causes of short stature unnecessary.

The presence of a *systemic illness* causing short stature is usually obvious. On occasion, short stature may be a presenting complaint for previously undiagnosed renal or inflammatory bowel disease. Likewise, alteration of normal growth may be the initial manifestation of juvenile-onset hypothyroidism or Cushing's disease. GH and somatomedin levels are low in most of these disorders, although in chronic renal failure GH levels may be elevated and wide variations are reported for somatomedin-C levels.[5]

Familial or hereditary short stature is characterized by a family history of short stature. Growth velocity tends to be within the normal range, and comparison with growth charts adjusted for parental height shows the growth rate to be normal for this population.[6] Children with familial short stature have normal bone age on x-ray and go through puberty at the expected age. The concept of familial short stature must take into account environmental influences on parental height. For example, orientals were previously thought to be genetically shorter than caucasians, but improved nutrition in Japan has resulted in the present generation's being significantly taller than their parents, correcting this "genetic" defect.

GH deficiency is an important cause of short stature, especially because it is now treatable. It may be part of the spectrum of pituitary insufficiency or an isolated hormone deficiency; may be caused by a destructive central nervous system lesion or occur in the absence of a detectable cause; may be absolute or partial; and may cause either severe or mild growth retardation. Somatomedin-C levels are low in GH deficiency.[5]

Constitutional delay of growth is a diagnosis made in children (usually males) with linear growth at the bottom of the normal range. Onset of adolescence is delayed, so that subjects frequently come to medical attention when the pubertal growth spurt of their peers emphasizes the abnormality. Affected children eventually undergo normal pubertal development and growth several years later and reach an adult height somewhat below the normal range. Bone age is usually retarded although appropriate for height. Frequently there is a family history of similar problems. Although constitutional delay of growth is commonly re-

Table 1. CAUSES OF SHORT STATURE

Prenatal and neonatal causes	Fetal growth delay
	  Maternal systemic illness
	  Placental insufficiency
	Neonatal infection
	  Cytomegalovirus
	  Toxoplasmosis
	Prenatal illness/birth defect/trauma

Genetic causes	Familial or hereditary short stature
	Identifiable chromosome disorders
	  Down's syndrome
	  Turner's syndrome
	Genetic skeletal disorders (over 50 described; achondroplasia probably best-known)
	Dwarfism of unknown cause
	  Progeria
	  Noonan's syndrome
	  Leprechaunism
	Inborn errors of metabolism
	  Glycogen storage disease
	  Cystinosis

Systemic causes	Organ failure
	  Renal
	  Pulmonary
	  Hepatic
	  Cardiac
	Systemic illness
	  Inflammatory bowel disease
	  Tuberculosis
	Therapy for systemic illness
	  Glucocorticoids for malignancy or asthma
	Endocrine insufficiency or excess
	  Hypothyroidism
	  Cushing's disease
	  Diabetes mellitus

Hypothalamic-pituitary causes	Destructive lesions
	  Pituitary tumors
	  Craniopharyngiomas
	  Other CNS tumors
	  Infiltrative disorders (e.g., sarcoidosis)
	Trauma

Resistance to growth hormone	Laron type dwarfism Protein-calorie malnutrition Anorexia nervosa Abnormal forms of growth hormone

garded as a normal, non–endocrine-related variant, some investigators believe that affected children can benefit from GH treatment.

The complexities of neuroendocrine growth control are emphasized in children with *psychosocial deprivation*. These children from disturbed homes are physically and intellectually immature. Early evaluation demonstrates GH deficiency. After placement in a healthy environment with normal social input, the endocrine abnormalities resolve, and accelerated ("catch-up") growth occurs. Chronic malnutrition or starvation also impairs growth. GH levels may be normal or elevated, but somatomedin levels are low. Normal or accelerated growth and normal somatomedin levels are restored by feeding.

Abnormal forms of GH have occasionally been reported. Affected children would be expected to have short stature and normal or elevated GH levels on immunoassay but diminished GH activity in a bioassay.[7] Somatomedin-C levels are low and increase in response to exogenous GH. In Laron type dwarfism, the GH level is increased but a receptor or postreceptor defect is present. Affected children have short stature and low somatomedin-C levels unresponsive to exogenous GH.[8] Other variants of GH or GH receptor dysfunction probably exist.

Incidence

The incidence of short stature is impossible to estimate, even with arbitrary definitions. Although some authorities like to classify all children whose height is more than two standard deviations below normal as having short stature, many of these subjects come from short families and do not have an otherwise identifiable disorder. Other children whose height falls in the range of normal may have an easily identifiable illness and subsequent accelerated growth after therapy.

As one of the major treatable causes of short stature, GH deficiency is diagnosed much more frequently now than in times past. One group of investigators examined all children more than 2.5 standard deviations below the mean height for age and identified 5 per cent to be GH-deficient. Even if the possibility of GH deficiency in the taller children not tested is ignored, the prevalence in this population was at least one in 4,000.[9]

Other investigators have suggested that subtle forms of GH deficiency may be much more common. A recent study of GH treatment in children thought to have normal variant or familial short stature has shown that a significant percentage respond to GH treatment with increases in both plasma somatomedin-C levels and growth velocity.[7] This controversial study emphasizes the difficulty in diagnosing GH deficiency as well as a possible role for GH therapy even in children without obvious hormonal abnormalities.

HISTORY

Given the large number of disorders that can result in short stature, the history and physical examination are both extremely important in narrowing the diagnostic possibilities. Were there problems during gestation or the perinatal period? Maternal illness or neonatal infections can retard growth. Difficult labor and delivery can be associated with subtle pituitary damage and short stature.[10]

The ages of achieving standard milestones of infancy and childhood should be recorded. Did the child begin to crawl, walk, and talk at the expected ages? The most important historical information is a record of heights and weights for given ages. It is mandatory that a graph for each subject be made and compared with that for a normal peer group. As illustrated in Figures 1, 2, and 3, growth patterns may give a clue as to the etiology of short stature.

The history should also concentrate on recording symptoms of major organ system disease and systemic illness. Although the presence of cardiac or pulmonary disease can usually be documented by obvious historical and physical findings, in renal diseases such as renal tubular acidosis and occult nontropical sprue (celiac disease), short stature may be the only obvious finding.

In a similar manner, diseases of the central nervous system that persist for a sufficient time to result in short stature may manifest few localizing symptoms. Features of the history such as headaches, seizures, and visual disturbances should be elicited. Diabetes insipidus may signify either histiocytosis X or other infiltrative diseases of the central nervous system.

Obesity and hypertension in a child with impaired growth suggest Cushing's disease; frequently, however, these findings are not present.[11] Juvenile-onset hypothyroidism, although often accompanied by modest intellectual deficit, may give none of the typical clues—constipation, cold intolerance, obesity, and change in voice.

As the child grows to adolescence, pubertal milestones become important. Children with pituitary insufficiency may have loss of gonadotropins and subsequent failure to go through puberty. Constitutional delay of growth and many systemic illnesses are accompanied by delayed onset of puberty. Children with isolated growth hormone deficiency and those with familial short stature usually go through puberty at the normal age. Precocious puberty of any etiology will result in the premature onset of pubertal progression and accelerated growth, followed in subsequent years by arrested growth and ultimate short stature.

Family history is extremely important. Growth patterns, including age of puberty in parents and siblings, help to establish familial norms. A family history of hereditary inborn errors of metabolism or genetic disorders is useful. Social history is important, because psychological and social deprivation can cause severe disturbance in growth. Nutritional information is also important in children from both indigent and affluent environments. Juvenile or adolescent onset of anorexia nervosa may be accompanied by growth delay.

The previous medical history should include information about all medications. Adrenal steroid (glucocorticoid) therapy is a classic cause of growth retardation. Such therapy, used for asthma or inflammatory bowel disease, may turn out to be a more significant factor in short stature than the original illness.

PHYSICAL EXAMINATION

Physical examination concentrates on eliciting signs of major organ system illnesses, systemic illnesses, and genetic disorders. Identification of abnormal facies or skeletal abnormalities suggesting a congenital or genetic disorder should prompt the examiner to consult a reference atlas to aid definitive diagnosis; either the more succinct text by Smith[12] or Warkany's larger work[13] is recommended.

Arm span and crown–pubic symphysis–foot distances (upper to lower body segment dimensions) should be recorded. Disorders characterized by defective long bone growth result in arm span significantly less than expected for height, as well as an increased upper-lower body segment ratio. Normally, this ratio is 1.5 at 18 months, 1.33 at 3 years, and 1.0 or less at 10 years. Premature puberty, early-onset hypothyroidism (cretinism), and many genetic disorders are associated with short extremities and an increased upper-lower body segment ratio as well as decreased relative arm span. Disorders characterized by late epiphyseal closure may have greater long bone growth and a low upper-lower ratio.

Special emphasis should be given to recording secondary sexual characteristics. The level of pubertal progression should be compared with that of the normal peer group (Table 2).[14] A careful neurologic examination should be performed on all affected children.

Table 2. AGE RANGES FOR ONSET AND COMPLETION OF PUBERTAL DEVELOPMENT

	Males		Females	
	Year of Onset	*Year of Completion*	*Year of Onset*	*Year of Completion*
Gonadal enlargement	10–14	14–18	—	—
Penile development	11–14	13–17	—	—
Pubic hair	10–15	14–18	8–14	11–16
Growth spurt	10–16	13–19	9–14	12–17
Breasts	—	—	8–13	11–16
Menarche	—	—	10–16	—

(Modified from Tanner JM. Growth at adolescence. 2nd ed. Oxford:Blackwell Scientific, 1962.)

DIAGNOSTIC STUDIES

Laboratory Studies

The diagnostic evaluation of patients with short stature must be considered in two sections. First, laboratory tests should be directed toward excluding systemic illness and endocrine disorders that can cause aberrations in growth. Only after such disorders are excluded can testing for GH deficiency be carried out. This timing is critical, because most systemic illnesses secondarily cause abnormalities in GH and somatomedin metabolism, and evaluation of the GH axis in this situation provides misleading information.

Testing should include a blood count, urinalysis, liver enzyme tests, renal function tests, and glucose, calcium, phosphate, and sedimentation rate determinations. Evaluation for nutritional status and malabsorption is appropriate in children who appear thin. Thyroid function values must be obtained in every patient with short stature. Although rare, Cushing's disease should be excluded by an overnight dexamethasone suppression test in all children with unexplained growth delay. In this test, 1 mg of dexamethasone is given by mouth at bedtime and the cortisol level is measured in the morning; failure of cortisol suppression to less than 5 mcg/100 ml is abnormal and mandates further evaluation for Cushing's disease.

Chromosomal evaluation should be performed in patients with phenotypic abnormalities suggestive of genetic disorders. Although a buccal smear examination for Barr bodies is adequate to detect Turner's syndrome, cytogenetic banding studies are required for diagnosis of many other problems. A variety of special tests are available for the multiple inborn errors of metabolism.[15]

Imaging

Radiologic evaluations are of use in many subjects with short stature. X-ray of the wrists and hands for measurement of bone age are important in making a differential diagnosis. Familial short stature is characterized by similarity between bone age and chronologic age. Constitutional growth delay results in bone age that is proportional to height age but retarded in comparison with chronologic age. Hypothyroidism is unique in that it often causes bone age to be delayed compared with height. Skeletal x-rays are of obvious importance in diagnosing the numerous skeletal dysplasias. X-rays are also useful for evaluation of the gastrointestinal tract for inflammatory bowel disease and malabsorption. Central nervous system lesions including pituitary tumors are relatively easy to detect on skull x-rays and CT scans of the head.

Testing for Disorders of Growth Hormone Release and Metabolism

At this point in the work-up, major organ system illnesses and genetic and metabolic disorders should be excluded. The differential diagnosis should consist of familial short stature, constitutional growth delay, and GH deficiency. Diagnosis at the earliest age possible is of major importance, because GH deficiency can now be treated.

A screening test commonly employed is GH stimulation through physical exercise. Normally, 20 minutes of brisk exertion, such as running up and down stairs, is accompanied by an elevation in GH level to more than 7 ng/ml. Children who are unable to mount such a response should be subjected to provocative testing for GH reserve.

In addition to GH levels, a resting somatomedin-C level should be obtained. Somatomedin-C levels increase with age, so the results must be interpreted by comparison with those of the patient's peer group. Unfortunately, a normal somatomedin-C level does not exclude growth hormone deficiency completely.[16] Most serious illnesses and malnutrition cause somatomedin-C levels to be low, falsely suggesting growth hormone deficiency.

Provocative testing for growth hormone reserve has been carried out with many agents, including oral levodopa and clonidine as well as combinations of glucagon and propranolol.[17] The most widely used and best-standardized tests are insulin hypoglycemia stimulation and arginine infusion. Insulin hypoglycemia stimulation, usually regarded as the most reliable, is also potentially the most dangerous test. An intravenous line is started, and a resting GH level is obtained. Then, 0.1 U/kg of insulin is given by intravenous injection, and serial blood sugar and GH levels are obtained over the next hour. For the result to be significant, the blood sugar level must fall by more than 50 per cent, preferably reaching a level of 30 mg/100 ml or less, and GH levels should be stimulated to more than 10 ng/ml.

In arginine infusion, 0.5 gm/kg of L-arginine monohydrochloride is infused over 30 minutes. GH levels are recorded over a 2-hour period. Many investigators require both the arginine infusion and insulin hypoglycemia tests to demonstrate absence of GH response before they will diagnose deficiency.

In the evaluation for this disorder, associated deficiency of other pituitary hormones is considered strongly supportive evidence. Absence of thyroid-stimulating hormone (TSH) and ACTH responses to stimulation tests[17] in conjunction with GH deficiency makes the diagnosis of hypopituitary dwarfism certain. In addition, treatment of all pituitary hormone deficiencies—for example, thyroxine replacement for TSH deficiency and cortisol replacement for ACTH deficiency—may be necessary to restore normal growth.

ASSESSMENT

The history and physical findings in most patients will strongly suggest the cause of short stature. Laboratory assessment should be used to document illnesses that cause short stature or to demonstrate GH deficiency. If the latter is proven, additional tests of pituitary function are needed to exclude pituitary insufficiency. Radiologic studies to detect a CNS or pituitary lesion should also be performed.

In some children, a certain diagnosis of growth retardation cannot be arrived at during the initial evaluation. These children should be followed for determination of growth patterns and should be evaluated prospectively for disorders that can result in short stature.

REFERENCES

1. Hamill PVV, Drizd TA, Johnson CL, Reed RB, Roche AF, Moore WM. Physical growth: National Center for Health Statistics Percentiles. Am J Clin Nutr 1979;32:607–29.
2. Tanner JM, Whitehouse RH. Clinical longitudinal standards for height, weight, height velocity, weight velocity and the stages of puberty. Arch Dis Child 1976;51:170–9.
3. Martin JB. Neuronal regulation of GH secretion. Med Clin North Am 1978;62:327.
4. Guillemin R, Brazeau P, Bohlen P, Esch F, Ling N, Wehrenberg WB. Growth hormone-releasing factor from a human pancreatic tumor that caused acromegaly. Science 1982;218:585–7.
5. Underwood LE, D'Ercole AJ, Van Wyk JJ. Somatomedin-C and the assessment of growth. Pediatr Clin North Am 1980;27:771–82.
6. Tanner JM, Whitehouse RH, Marshall WA, Carter BS. Prediction of adult height from height, bone age and occurrence of menarche at ages 4–16 with allowance for midparent height. Arch Dis Child 1975;50:14–26.
7. Rudman D, Kutner MH, Blackston RD, Cushman RA, Bain RP, Patterson JH. Children with normal-variant short stature: treatment with human growth hormone for six months. New Engl J Med 1981;305:123–31.
8. Golde DW, Bersch N, Kaplan SA, Rimoin DL, Li CH. Peripheral unresponsiveness to human growth hormone in Laron dwarfism. New Engl J Med 1980;303:1156–8.

9. Vimpani GV, Vimpani AF, Lidgard GP, Cameron EHD, Farquhar JW. Prevalence of severe growth hormone deficiency. Br Med J 1977;2:427–30.
10. Craft WH, Underwood LE, Van Wyk JJ. High incidence of perinatal insult in children with idiopathic hypopituitarism. J Pediatr 1980;96:397–402.
11. Lee PA, Weldon VV, Migeon CJ. Short stature as the only clinical sign of Cushing's syndrome. J Pediatr 1975;86:89–91.
12. Smith DW. Recognizable patterns of human malformation. 2nd ed. Philadelphia: WB Saunders, 1976.
13. Warkany J. Congenital malformations: notes and comments. Chicago: Year Book, 1971.
14. Tanner JM. Growth at adolescence. 2nd ed. Oxford: Blackwell Scientific, 1962.
15. Stanbury JB, Wyngaarden JB, Fredrickson DS, Goldstein JL, Brown MS, eds. The metabolic basis of inherited disease. 5th ed. New York: McGraw-Hill, 1983.
16. Dean HJ, Kellett JG, Bala RM, Guyda HJ, Bhaumick B, Posner BI, Friesen HG. The effect of growth hormone treatment on somatomedin levels in growth hormone-deficient children. J Clin Endocrinol Metab 1982;55:1167–73.
17. Abboud CF, Laws ER. Clinical endocrinologic approach to hypothalamic-pituitary disease. J Neurosurg 1979;51:271–90.

SMELL AND TASTE DISTURBANCES

PEAK WOO □ COLLIN S. KARMODY

□ SYNONYMS: Dysosmia and dysgeusia

BACKGROUND

Separation of the senses of smell and taste is often impossible, and for this reason, they are usually considered together. They are, however, anatomically separate entities that respond to completely different stimuli; fusion of sensation occurs centrally. Clinically, separation is sometimes extremely difficult. In a general medical practice, evaluation of disorders of sense of smell might be technically problematic because of the inaccessibility of the olfactory sensory end organ. The delicate qualitative nature of the senses involved and the difficulty with quantifying test stimuli have resulted in a comparative paucity of relevant medical literature. Smell and taste have, therefore, become somewhat "neglected senses."[1] Our ability to smell and taste, however, contributes greatly to our daily perceptions of the environment and is mandatory for appreciation of food and drink. These senses also help us to avoid unacceptable and dangerous stimuli. Disorders of smell and taste are mainly annoying but they can represent the first symptoms of more serious problems.

Taste is generally considered to be a combination of several sensory perceptions, primarily the chemical senses of taste and olfaction with some input from vision. There are no reliable objective tests for taste and smell. Evaluation of disorders of these senses is therefore based on clinical factors and requires a careful history, thorough physical examination with emphasis on the upper aerodigestive tract, and a few clinical tests.

An estimated 2 million American adults suffer from loss or impairment of olfactory or gustatory senses.[1] Complaints about smell and taste should not be regarded as "trivial" or "neurotic," but should be approached positively and systematically.

Definitions and Origins

Smell

It is important for the clinician to differentiate among the afferent pathways of the nasal cavity. The somatic sensory afferent fibers of the trigeminal nerve innervate the mucosa of the nasal cavity and respond to tactile stimuli and to irritating volatile gases such as ammonia and acids. Odors, however, are perceived through the finely specialized olfactory epithelium and the olfactory nerve, which are situated in the roof of the nasal cavity and together form the organ of olfaction. Smell is the interpretation of stimulation of the olfactory organ by some of the gaseous molecules that enter the nasal passages.

In humans, the olfactory neuroepithelium covers an area about the size of an adult's thumbnail. The afferent nerve fibers that constitute the first cranial nerve perforate the cribriform plate of the ethmoid bone and ultimately connect centrally with the cerebral cortex. Because humans can differentiate thousands of subtle odors, there is no general consensus on the concept of basic odors. Amoore[2] has listed primary and complex odors. The primary odors such as camphor and almond extracts are used to test for the presence or absence of the sense of smell. Adaptation, however, is an important characteristic of olfaction, and the more one is exposed to an odor, the less one notes its presence.

Taste

The peripheral organs of taste are the taste buds, specialized sensory cells that respond to chemical substances dissolved in a water base such as saliva. The receptors to taste are predominantly on the dorsal and lateral surfaces of the anterior two-thirds of the tongue and are concentrated on the fungiform and circumvallate papillae. Other taste buds are scattered over the hard and soft palates, posterior third of the tongue, and tip of the epiglottis. A taste stimulus is relayed to the central nervous system by different peripheral nerves. The chorda tympani, a branch of the facial nerve (seventh cranial nerve), carries taste sensation from the anterior two-thirds of the tongue. The glossopharyngeal nerve (ninth cranial nerve) supplies much of the remaining taste fibers on the posterior tongue and pharynx.

Taste occurs in the moist, finely balanced environment of the oral cavity, which is well-lubricated by secretions of the parotid, submandibular, sublingual, and innumerable minor salivary glands. The acuity and full range of sensation depends upon the preservation of the oral milieu. In the young, taste buds are numerous and evenly distributed, but with increasing age there is atrophy and reduction in the number of sensory units. Acuity decreases with age.[3]

Four primary sensations of taste are recognized—sweet, sour, bitter, and salt—but infinite combinations of these sensations are possible.

Causes

Disorders of Smell

There is considerable variation of olfactory acuity in otherwise normal individuals that may be attributed to local and hormonal factors and to age.

Olfactory disorders are usually described as being qualitative or quantitative. The quantitative disorders are hyperosmia, hyposmia, and anosmia. *Hyperosmia* is an increased sensitivity to odors. *Hyposmia* is a decreased ability to detect the presence of odors. *Anosmia* is complete loss of the sense of smell. The qualitative disorders of smell are cacosmia, dysosmia, and parosmia. *Cacosmia* is the presence of a subjective and usually objective foul smell that is caused by an organic problem. *Dysosmia* refers to a distorted sense of smell. *Parosmia* is the sensation of smell in the absence of a stimulus.[4] The sense of smell is generally more sensitive in women than in men and is heightened during pregnancy and ovulation. Gradually progressive hyposmia is usual in aging, whereas hyperosmia is experienced in hunger, nausea, and obesity. Certain professions, such as perfumer and chef, require a finely developed sense of smell, which is usually inherent and cannot be acquired.

Quantitative Disorders of Smell

Congenital Causes. Kallmann's syndrome is a combination of hypogonadism and anosmia caused by agenesis of the olfactory organ. It is a hereditary recessive disorder.[5]

Inflammatory Causes. By far, the most common causes of loss of smell are local conditions in the nose, the most frequent being the common cold, in which nasal obstruction causes transient hyposmia or anosmia. Other types of rhinitis often result in transient nasal obstruction with hyposmia. In allergic rhinitis, seasonal exacerbations occur with temporary loss of smell. If there are associated allergic polyps, which are usually bilateral, loss of smell might be constant and long-term, as also occurs in vasomotor rhinitis from prolonged use of topical vasoconstrictors. In atrophic rhinitis and Sjögren's syndrome the nasal mucosa and olfactory epithelium are virtually nonfunctional, and affected patients are therefore unaware of the presence of malodorous crusts that form in the nose. Influenza causes areas of damage and repair of the olfactory epithelium, accounting for the frequent complaints of hyposmia in this disease. Henkin and associates[6] have described irreversible hyposmia after influenza.

Traumatic Causes. The neuroepithelium of the olfactory organ is damaged by a variety of chemicals, and hyposmia is common in cocaine users and workers exposed to petroleum products, heavy metals, and formaldehydes.

Mechanical damage to the olfactory nerve is common after head trauma. About 40 per cent of patients with frontal and occipital injuries and 4 per cent with facial fractures have post-traumatic anosmia. The delicate olfactory fibers are torn by fractures through the cribriform plate or by sudden violent motion of the brain as occurs in occipital injuries (contrecoup).

Localized nasal trauma is frequently associated with transient anosmia, and smell returns after resolution of local edema. Anosmia and hyposmia are rare after elective nasal surgery.

Neoplastic Causes. Tumors of the nasal cavity and paranasal sinuses produce gradual nasal obstruction and loss of smell, but certain rare intranasal tumors that originate in the olfactory cleft, e.g., esthesioneuroblastoma, might cause olfactory dysfunction without complete nasal obstruction.

Intracranial neoplasms may press on or invade the olfactory tract. Midline osteomas, meningiomas of the olfactory groove and sphenoid ridges, neoplasms of the optic chiasm, and tumors of the frontal lobe may cause decreased sense of smell through pressure on the olfactory bulb.

Miscellaneous Causes. *Pollutants* in the working environment, such as sulfurous vapors and tobacco smoke, can cause edema of the nasal mucosa and secondary hyposmia. Some *medicants* used for non-nasal diseases, specifically the antihypertensives, might cause vasomotor-like reactions in the nose. These reactions are reversible, and discontinuing the drug usually confirms the diagnosis. Many *systemic diseases* are associated with abnormalities of smell. Hyperosmia is comparatively infrequent and is encountered in untreated Addison's disease and in mucoviscidosis. Hyposmia is more frequent and often occurs in hormonal imbalances such as hypogonadism, hypothyroidism, and diabetes mellitus, after hypophysectomy, and in renal failure and avitaminosis.

Table 1. CAUSES OF DISORDERS OF SMELL OTHER THAN LOCAL NASAL AND CRANIAL LESIONS

Psychogenic	Depressive illness Schizophrenia Malingering
Drugs	Amphetamines Levodopa Thiazides
Iatrogenic	Post-laryngectomy
Diseases	Hepatitis Vitamin A deficiency Hypogonadism in a female Kallmann's syndrome (congenital hypogonadotrophic eunuchoidism) Turner's syndrome Familial dysautonomia Diabetes mellitus Hypothyroidism Pseudohyperparathyroidism

Qualitative Disorders of Smell

Cacosmia is a common symptom of sinusitis, nasal vestibulitis, carcinoma of the sinuses, midline granuloma, and infective rhinitis. Drugs such as tetracycline, penicillamine, and chloramphenicol may cause parosmia; therefore, all medications in use must be noted when evaluating disorders of olfaction.

More deeply sited cerebral disorders might cause olfactory symptoms. Temporal lobe seizures may have an olfactory aura such as pleasant or unpleasant parosmia or hyposmia. Contusion and concussion of the brain may also distort the sense of smell by a process that is still unclear. A number of disorders that are outside the nasal intracranial axis may also cause disturbances of smell; these are listed in Table 1. Unfortunately, even after the most thorough investigation, some problems remain unexplained.

Disorders of Taste

Abnormalities of taste, collectively known as *dysgeusia,* are subdivided into ageusia, hypogeusia, dissociated hypogeusia, parageusia, and phantageusia. *Ageusia* is the absence of one or all of the primary sensations of taste., *Hypogeusia* is a quantitative reduction in the sensitivity of taste. A decrease in only a single modality is called *dissociated hypogeusia. Parageusia* refers to the confusion of one taste for another. *Phantageusia* is the presence of an abnormal, usually metallic taste, which is frequently a side effect of medication.[7]

Abnormalities of taste in humans are modified by many local factors in the oral cavity. Diminished acuity of taste due to loss of taste buds is caused by aging and is accelerated by excessive smoking or irritants and trauma. Any disease process that alters the local structure, changes the salivary flow, or affects the taste receptors produces a disturbance of taste. Genetic, hormonal, and metabolic disorders frequently affect taste. Nutritional deficiencies and the abuse of drugs are also common contributory factors.

A thick, furred tongue often causes hypogeusia. The surface coating of the tongue might be thickened by mouth breathing, mild gastritis, or dehydration. In the elderly, the surface of the tongue is thickened owing to diminished production of saliva. The taste receptor areas may be blocked by black hairy tongue or by new maxillary dentures. Transient disorders of taste occur in lichen planus, thrush, and infections of the tonsils and pharynx.

Glossitis is often accompanied by alterations of taste. For instance, a smooth red tongue devoid of taste buds is seen in iron deficiency anemia and Plummer-Vinson syndrome. Pellagrous glossitis and the red beefy tongue of vitamin A deficiency cause disturbances of taste. Prolonged treatment with antibiotics resulting in fungal superinfection and burns from hot fluids may damage the papillae and cause concomitant loss of taste. Irradiation of the oral cavity with ionizing rays dries the mouth by damaging the salivary glands and taste receptors; recovery of salivation and taste after such therapy is slow and often incomplete.[8]

Surgical procedures or intrinsic lesions of the seventh and ninth cranial nerves may compromise the afferent pathways of taste. For instance, trauma to the chorda tympani during surgery causes a metallic taste that subsides gradually.

Patients with Ramsay Hunt syndrome (herpes oticus) or Bell's palsy may complain of diminished taste. An acoustic neuroma can cause ipsilateral loss of taste before the development of facial paralysis or impairment of hearing. In the evaluation of facial paralysis, the testing of taste sensation provides information in three dimensions: (1) topographic—taste is lost in lesions proximal to the chorda tympani nerve; (2) etiologic—a metallic taste occurring 48 hours prior to the onset of facial paralysis is symptomatic of a viral infection of the nerve; and (3) prognostic—return of taste thresholds indicates impending return of motor function.

In familial dysautonomia (Riley-Day syndrome) ageusia is due to absence of the fungiform and circumvallate papillae. Aberrations of metabolism and endocrinopathies frequently cause disturbances of taste.Hypothyroid patients show diminished sensitivity of taste, whereas hyperthyroid patients show slight hypersensitivity; these symptoms resolve with appropriate treatment. Diabetics may have hypogeusia of all four basic tastes, which is supposedly caused by peripheral neuropathy and is more marked when diabetes is unstable and accompanied by other degenerative complications.[9] In adrenal-cortical insufficiency (Addison's disease) there is considerable increase in the acuity of taste that resolves with replacement therapy. Generally, the sensitivity of taste is directly proportional to the level of female hormones; however, testosterone-producing, virilizing adrenal tumors cause hypertrophy of the taste buds and an increase in taste sensitivity.

Many medications cause abnormalities of taste by mechanisms that are poorly understood. Possibly there is a direct effect on the taste buds or an indirect effect on the cortical taste centers. Metallic phantageusia and reduced perception of sweetness are common side effects of drug therapy.[10] Prolonged administration of medication may cause progression of dissociated hypogeusia to ageusia. Drugs known to produce alteration in taste include antibiotics (cefamandole, tetracycline, ethambutol), antifungal agents, gold, chelating agents (penicillamine), levodopa, lithium carbonate, and cytotoxic agents.[11]

HISTORY

Definitive diagnosis of smell and taste disturbances requires obtaining a careful history that includes details of recent medical problems and medications with specific discussion of otolaryngologic and neurological disorders. The examiner should note the time of onset of the disorder and determine whether one or both senses are affected. Is the abnormality quantitative; for example, are taste and smell the same but diminished? Alternatively, is there a qualitative difference? Is there a subjective odor when none is present (parosmia)? Is the disturbance constant or does it vary? Are certain tastes more difficult than others (dissociated hypogeusia)? Are the symptoms changing? Is there a history of sinusitis, nasal obstruction, rhinorrhea, allergy, trauma, or self-medication? Is the patient using topical nasal medications? The details of oral and dental hygiene are relevant. Prior surgery on the tonsils, sinuses, and ear must be documented. Has the appearance of the tongue changed? Pain on eating or complaints of a hot, burning tongue are symptoms of glossitis or mucosal ulceration.

Is there epistaxis, which occurs with tumors of the nasal cavity and sinusitis? Has the patient experienced cranial or facial injury? Does the patient have headaches or changes in personality and/or vision, as occur in tumors of the frontal lobe and optic chiasma? Has there been recent loss or gain of weight or intolerance to heat and cold, which might suggest thyroid disease?

In patients with disorders of taste, one should enquire about flu-like syndromes (post-influenza hypogeusia). Is there dysphagia, as occurs in Plummer-Vinson syndrome? Does the patient have new dentures? Is there associated facial pain or facial asymmetry, which suggests lesions of the fifth or seventh cranial nerve, respectively?

A family history of endocrine disorders must be explored. Note must also be taken of the patient's occupation, specifically for the presence and duration of exposure to noxious or toxic gases or volatile liquids. The examiner should inquire about the use of tobacco, alcohol, cocaine, and snuff. All medications in use should be noted, including prescription, nonprescription, local, and systemic drugs. The patient should be asked specifically whether there is a noticeable change in taste or smell with the beginning or stopping of medications.

Is there cause for anxiety or depression? Recent pregnancy or symptoms of menopause are relevant. Has the patient been generally unwell or lethargic? Finally, the initial assessment of the pattern of symptoms should provide a clue as to diagnosis. Are the complaints specific or detailed? Are details reproducible or do the accounts vary considerably? Is the history vague and coupled with a myriad of other nonspecific complaints? In general, the more specific the history, the more likely there is an organic problem.

High-Payoff Queries

The following questions will elicit pertinent information in a smell or taste disturbance:

1. *What medications are you taking?*
2. *What medical conditions are you being treated for? Do you have any chronic ailments?*

3. *Are you able to smell perfume? Ammonia? Coffee?*
4. *Have you noticed any change in the appearance of your tongue?*
5. *Have you had any pain in your throat or tongue?*
6. *Have you lost weight? Have your preferences for food changed recently?*
7. *Can you breathe through your nose?*
8. *Have you recently had flu-like symptoms or a cold?*
9. *Have you ever been in an automobile accident or fractured your skull, nose, or facial bones?*
10. *Have you had any surgery on your ears, nose, or throat? Have you had sinus infections that would not clear up?*
11. *Do you have a headache or facial pain that is new?*

PHYSICAL EXAMINATION

The level of physical examination is determined by the tools and skills of the examiner, but the basic examination should include a thorough inspection of the upper aerodigestive and respiratory tracts, a neurologic examination, and a general physical examination. The ears should be checked for evidence of surgery and infectious processes. The external nose should be assessed for widening, as might be seen with long-standing polyps. Deviation of the nasal septum may manifest as displacement of the nasal tip, whereas a recent fracture of the nasal bones is evidenced by swelling, tenderness, and a palpable irregularity. Having the patient inhale and exhale through each nostril separately demonstrates the characteristic turbulent noises heard in narrowing and obstruction.

One should inspect the nasal cavity carefully, noting the condition of the mucosa. In allergic rhinitis, the nasal mucosa is pale, violaceous, and edematous with clear watery secretions. In suppurative rhinitis it is erythematous and boggy and there is purulent discharge that might be crusted. Pus emanating from a specific part of the nose indicates suppurative sinusitis, and percussion of the forehead and cheek will elicit tenderness over an inflamed sinus. Deviation and perforations of the septum are noted. Polypoid masses that occlude the airway are usually seen low in the nasal cavity and have the appearance and consistency of grapes. Smaller polyps high in the nasal cavity are less visible but can cause anosmia.

The oral cavity should be examined with a bright, focused light and a tongue blade and should be palpated with a finger. The oral mucosa is checked for moistness. The tongue is examined for the presence and distribution of papillae, excessive coating, leukoplakia, fissures, ulcerations, and swellings. Suspected neoplasms and infiltrates must be palpated. Is the palate normal, highly arched, or cleft? One should examine the faucial tonsils for deep crypts and evidence of inflammation. The posterior wall of the pharynx should be inspected for purulent exudate that usually comes from the nasal cavity. The submaxillary and parotid glands should be assessed for inflammation or infection; these glands might be swollen or tender from infection, Sjögren's syndrome, or neoplasia.

The ability to smell is tested with three discrete stimuli. Oil of cloves, spirit of peppermint, and ammonia in separate vials are presented one at a time. A true anosmic identifies the ammonia, which stimulates the tactile sensory endings, whereas a malingerer denies recognition of all three. The Elsberg test is a simple quantitative test of smell in which phenol-ethyl alcohol is placed in an Erlenmeyer flask and thresholds of smell are tested incrementally.[12]

Taste is tested by placing, one at a time, solutions of salt, vinegar, sugar, and bitter quinine on the dorsum of the tongue. The patient identifies the primary taste. The mouth is rinsed thoroughly with water between tests. For unilateral problems the test is performed on the protruded tongue and drops are carefully placed on the afflicted side. In clinical practice, electrogustometry has been cumbersome and is not in common use.

A general physical examination may provide evidence of systemic disease. Sjögren's syndrome, avitaminosis, diabetes mellitus, and Addison's disease all have physical features that are not restricted to the head and neck. A general neurologic examination, particularly for peripheral neuropathy and function of cranial nerves I, V, VII, IX, and X, is indicated. The distribution of body hair and virilizing features suggests the association of a disorder of smell and taste with a hormonal imbalance.

Some common physical findings in patients with smell and taste disorders and their diagnostic significance are shown in Table 2.

DIAGNOSTIC STUDIES

Laboratory Studies

Laboratory tests may provide supportive evidence of clinical diagnoses or, alternatively might indicate the direction of further investigation.

A hematologic profile and a differential count of the leukocytes help distinguish viral, bacterial, and allergic diseases. Iron deficiency or sideropenia is determined by the indices of the hematologic profile. The levels of serum electrolytes and glucose after fasting may indicate mineralocorticosteroid deficiency or diabetes mellitus. Thyroid function tests and other specialized proce-

Table 2. COMMON PHYSICAL FINDINGS IN SMELL AND TASTE DISORDERS

Finding	Likely Diagnosis
Moist, boggy nasal mucosa with obstruction	Viral rhinitis, cold
Crusted, purulent discharge in the anterior nares	Vestibulitis
Moist, grape-like mass in the nasal cavity	Nasal polyp
Pus in the middle or superior turbinates	Sinusitis
Obstructed air flow through one side of the nose from deformed septal cartilage	Nasal septal deviation
Red velvety nasal mucosa	Rhinitis medicamentosa
Excessive black tongue cover	Black hairy tongue
Patches of white on the tongue and buccal mucosa	Thrush (*c. albicans* infection)
Foul, cheesy material from tonsil crypts	Large tonsillar crypts
Red, painful tongue with smooth surface	Glossitis with atrophy of papillae
Firmly adherent white plaques	Leukoplakia of the tongue

dures are performed when there is clinical suspicion of specific disorders. Serum levels of zinc and copper should be assayed in patients on renal dialysis, alcoholics with nutritional deficiencies, and patients receiving penicillamine.

Imaging

Roentgenograms will confirm the diagnosis of sinusitis, and films of the skull may show a fracture involving the cribriform plate, identifying the cause of post-traumatic anosmia. An expanded sella turcica, eroded clinoid processes, or localized calcifications may be evidence of an intracranial neoplasm. A specialized procedure such as angiography, tomography, or CT scanning should be used only when there is strong clinical suspicion of a condition that such a technique would demonstrate.

Other Studies

If a patient presents with symptoms involving the seventh and eighth cranial nerves, electronystagmography and detailed hearing tests and roentgenograms are indicated. These procedures are best directed by an otolaryngologist.

A simple, efficient, and possibly diagnostic test is to change the patient's medications whenever possible. In general, 2 or 3 weeks after withdrawal of medication are needed for a subjective change to be noted.

DIAGNOSTIC APPROACH

Not unusually no obvious cause for a disorder of smell or taste is found at the patient's first visit.

Table 3. DIAGNOSTIC APPROACH TO A DISORDER OF SMELL

I. Local Causes.
  A. Nasal cavity:
    1. Is it adequately visualized?
    2. Is there an anatomic abnormality, edema or obstruction?
    3. Evaluate for polyps, septal deviation, tumor, allergic rhinitis.
    4. Is there a mucosal abnormality?
    5. Evaluate for: toxin, pollutants.
      a. Damage by toxins or pollutants.
      b. Atrophic rhinitis.
      c. Infection (sinusitis).
      d. Rhinitis medicamentosa.
  B. Neural ending:
    1. Is there evidence of a recent viral or systemic illness?
  C. Intracranial:
    1. Is there intracranial disease?
    2. Evaluate cranial nerves and optic discs.
    3. Evaluate for head trauma and fractures of the skull.
    4. Neurologic examination
II. General causes.
  A. Could the problem be endocrine?
  B. Could the problem be metabolic?
  C. Could it be caused by medication?
  D. Could it be psychogenic?

An honest and sympathetic approach to the patient's problem is warranted, and re-examination in 2 to 4 weeks is often helpful. Transient and self-limiting processes can then be differentiated from those that are progressive and unremitting and require further, aggressive investigation.

Table 4. DIAGNOSTIC APPROACH TO A DISORDER OF TASTE

I. Local Causes.
  A. Is the tongue coated?
  B. Evaluate for:
    1. Recent illness.
    2. Antibiotic use and thrush.
    3. Mouth breathing.
    4. Dental abnormalities
    5. Tonsil enlargement and infection.
    6. Hypertrophic, deep tonsillar crypts.
    7. Is there a tongue abnormality?
    8. Examine the tongue for leukoplakia, glossitis, and signs of nutritional changes.
    9. Evaluate for xerostomia, radiation, medication, and Sjögren's syndrome.
  C. Peripheral nerve(s):
    1. Has there been surgery of the ear, nose, or throat?
    2. Evaluate for disorders of hearing and balance via specialized tests and consultation with an otolaryngologist.
II. General Causes.
  A. Could the problem be nasal? If so, evaluate smell (see Table 3).
  B. Could the problem be iatrogenic?
  C. Is there evidence of diabetes, thyroid, endocrine, or metabolic disorder, renal failure, carcinomatosis, or multiple sclerosis?

The difficulties encountered in dealing with abnormalities of taste and smell cause many patients to seek second and third opinions and eventually to be considered neurotics. A planned scheme for diagnosis should be to evaluate local factors and then to investigate systemic conditions (Tables 3 and 4).

Fortunately, disorders of smell and taste are seldom caused by life-threatening problems. The etiology might be obvious after one has taken careful history and performed a physical examination. The more difficult cases require repeated evaluations. There is tremendous satisfaction in making a correct diagnosis, which is worth the effort to both patient and physician.

REFERENCES

1. Zioryn T. Taste and smell. The neglected senses. JAMA 1982;237:277–85.
2. Amoore JE. Toilet Goods Association: Special Supplement. Proc Sci Sec 1962;37:1.
3. Variation of taste thresholds with human aging. JAMA 1982:247:775.
4. Zilstorff K, Herbild O. Parosmia. Acta Otolaryngol 1979;360:40–1.
5. Gregson RAM, Smith DAR. The clinical assessment of olfaction: differential diagnoses including Kallmann's syndrome. J Psychosomat Res 1981;25:165–74.
6. Henkin RI, Larson AL, Powell RD. Hypogeusia, dysgeusia, hyposmia, and dysosmia following influenza-like infection. Ann Otol Rhinol Laryngol 1975;84:672–82.
7. Rollin H. Drug related gustatory disorders. Ann Otol 1978;87:37–42.
8. Zusho H. Post-traumatic anosmia. Arch Otolaryngol 1982;103:90–2.
9. Griffith IP. Abnormalities of smell and taste. Practitioner 1976;217:907–14.
10. Geurrier Y, Uziel A. Clinical aspects of taste disorders. Acta Otolaryngol 1979;87:232–5.
11. Thawley S. Disorders of taste and smell. South Med J 1978;71:267–70.
12. Strauss EL. A study on olfactory acuity. Ann Otol Rhinol Laryngol 1970;79:95–104.

SPLENOMEGALY

EDWARD R. EICHNER

□ SYNONYMS: Hypersplenism, Banti's syndrome (congestive splenomegaly)

BACKGROUND

Definitions and Origins

The variation in weight of the normal spleen, a two-fold range, is greater than that of any other major organ of the body, making the threshold for *splenomegaly* somewhat arbitrary. Normal spleens in adults usually weigh 100 to 150 gm, however, and most physicians would agree that splenomegaly begins at 200 gm. The point at which splenomegaly results in hypersplenism is also imprecise. Classically, *hypersplenism* is defined as: (1) splenomegaly, (2) any combination of anemia, leukopenia, and/or thrombocytopenia, (3) compensatory bone marrow hyperplasia, and (4) "cure" by splenectomy. Different diseases cause different forms of hypersplenism, however, and perhaps hypersplenism should be redefined to mean that the spleen in question is doing more harm than good.[1] *Banti's syndrome* is an old term that should be discarded, except for historical interest. It is still occasionally applied to the congestive splenomegaly that occurs with cirrhosis of the liver or with occlusion of the portal or splenic vein.

Splenomegaly has many diverse origins; indeed, perusal of a textbook table of the causes of splenomegaly could give the impression that the challenge of correct diagnosis is formidable. Frequently, however, the spleen becomes palpable as a consequence of performing its normal functions, a form of "work hypertrophy." In general terms, the spleen performs a three-fold function: it is the most elegant blood filter in the body, it is the largest single compact mass of reticuloendothelial tissue in the body, and it is the largest lymph node in the body. As an elegant filter (described in more detail elsewhere),[1] with its nearby reticuloendothelial cells and lymphocytes, the spleen is a primary site for the clearance from the blood of microorganisms, particulate antigens, effete or abnormal red blood cells, and immune complexes, as well as for an early immune response, such as the production of immunoglobulin and properdin factors. The most common causes of splenomegaly in clinical practice are, first, types of "work hypertrophy" as the spleen performs its normal filtering, phagocytic, and immune-response functions in acute infections, hemolytic anemias, and immune complex diseases, and, second, "congestive" splenomegaly, because the unique microcirculation that makes it an elegant filter also causes it to expand in response to portal hypertension. A fourth function of the spleen is embryonic hematopoiesis, which can reactivate as extramedullary hematopoiesis in certain myeloproliferative diseases. Other general mechanisms of splenomegaly include neoplasia, infiltration, trauma, and developmental defects.

A comprehensive, but not exhaustive, list of causes of splenomegaly in adolescents and adults in the United States is offered in Table 1, grouped according to the functions and mechanisms just described. As can be surmised from the list, splenomegaly usually reflects a reaction to systemic disease and only occasionally results from a primary disease of the spleen. The entity of primary hypersplenism, or nontropical, idiopathic splenomegaly, is real but rare. So far, only 46 cases have been reported, and at least 20 per cent of the affected patients have developed lymphoma on follow-up.[2] Another general rule of thumb is: the larger the spleen, the smaller the list of possible causes. In fact, in the United States, giant splenomegaly (defined as ten times or more the usual upper limit of normal weight, which is 200 gm) as a presenting or early feature is limited mainly to: agnogenic myeloid metaplasia, chronic myelocytic leukemia, hairy cell leukemia, isolated splenic lymphoma, Gaucher's disease, non-tropical, idiopathic splenomegaly, splenic cyst (usually epidermoid), and sarcoidosis.[3]

The incidence of splenomegaly can be estimated from a composite analysis of the studies on the incidence of palpable spleens, even though not all palpable spleens are enlarged. In one study, almost 3 per cent of 2,200 healthy college freshmen had palpable spleens that could not easily be accounted for by infectious mononucleosis or body habitus; they remained healthy 10 years later.[4] In another study, 2 per cent of almost 6,000 unselected adult outpatients seen in 1 year had palpable spleens.[5] In neither study, however, was splenomegaly verified by spleen scan. In the first study, there was a sharp, significant fall in the incidence of "palpable" spleens (3.7 to 1.4 per cent) in the third year, when different physicians were the examiners, and the authors said that rates of "palpability" might vary with the examiner and with the ability of some subjects to relax and breathe deeply, making a normal-sized spleen palpable. Conversely, clinical techniques for detecting minimal splenomegaly are not especially reliable. In one study in a teaching hospital, splenomegaly measured by radioisotopic scan was detected by examining physicians only 28 per cent of the time, but when the examining physicians were certain splenomegaly was present, they were wrong only 1.4 per cent of the time.[6] In another study of spleen size detection by scan versus physical examination, one examiner correctly identified splenomegaly 88 per cent of the time using both palpation and percussion, but also "called"

Table 1. CLASSIFICATION OF SPLENOMEGALY

"Work hypertrophy" splenomegaly	
As an immune response	Acute or subacute causes
	Infectious mononucleosis
	Infectious hepatitis
	Toxoplasmosis
	Cytomegalovirus
	Septicemia
	Bacterial endocarditis
	Typhoid fever
	Tularemia
	Pyogenic abscess
	Serum sickness
	Chronic causes
	Tuberculosis
	Sarcoidosis
	Brucellosis
	Malaria
	Histoplasmosis
	Felty's syndrome
	Systemic lupus erythematosus
In response to blood cell destruction	Hereditary spherocytosis
	Autoimmune hemolytic anemia
	Sickle cell disorders
	Thalassemias and other hemoglobinopathies
	Pernicious anemia (occasionally)
	Autoimmune neutropenia
	Autoimmune thrombocytopenia (rarely)
	Chronic hemodialysis
Congestive splenomegaly	Cirrhosis of liver
	Splenic vein thrombosis
	Obstruction of portal vein
	Chronic heart failure (rarer now)
Myeloproliferative splenomegaly	Agnogenic myeloid metaplasia
	Chronic myelocytic leukemia
	Polycythemia vera
Neoplastic splenomegaly	Lymphomas; hairy cell leukemia
	Acute lymphocytic or monocytic leukemia
	Chronic lymphocytic leukemia
	Metastatic carcinoma (rare)
	Angiosarcoma (rare)
	Macroglobulinemia
Infiltrative splenomegaly	Gaucher's disease
	Amyloidosis
	Hystiocytosis X
Miscellaneous	Cysts (true, false, parasitic)
	Occult splenic rupture
	Thyrotoxicosis
	Nontropical, idiopathic splenomegaly

it when it was not present 10 per cent of the time using palpation alone and slightly more frequently using percussion alone.[7] All things considered, it seems reasonable to estimate that "true" splenomegaly is present in 1 to 2 per cent of unselected medical outpatients.

HISTORY

Although sometimes splenomegaly is asymptomatic,[8] a careful history will often suggest the correct diagnosis of the cause of splenomegaly.

General Queries

Splenomegaly usually reflects systemic illness. One should inquire about the patient's general sense of well-being, strength, endurance, energy, and appetite. One should ask about general symptoms of illness: fever, night sweats, weight loss, weakness, and malaise. A history of long-standing heart failure may suggest congestive cirrhosis and splenomegaly. This disorder used to be a major cause of splenomegaly,[5] but it is seen less often these days. One should ask about a history of cancer, especially blood disease and lymphoma. Family and occupational history is less important, but one should ask about medications the patient is taking, because hypersensitivity reactions to drugs such as phenytoin, sulindac, and many others can cause splenomegaly. If the patient is aware of the splenomegaly, one should ask about its rate of growth. Especially rapid growth occurs after traumatic hematoma and with large-cell lymphomas, whereas epidermoid cysts enlarge slowly over many years and, in fact, are usually asymptomatic. In one report, other common causes of asymptomatic splenomegaly at the Mayo Clinic were cryptic cirrhosis, agnogenic myeloid metaplasia, and Gaucher's disease.[8]

High-Payoff Queries

The following ten questions are especially likely to elicit helpful data:

1. *Have you had a recent blow or other injury to your abdomen?* Blunt abdominal trauma raises the possibility of subcapsular hematoma, traumatic cyst, or occult rupture of the spleen. Rarely (1 per cent of the time), traumatic rupture of the spleen may occur without acute symptoms and may manifest months or even years later as splenomegaly and a confusing variety of symptoms.[9]

2. *Have you recently had pain in your left upper abdomen, left side, or left shoulder?* Acute pain suggests spontaneous or traumatic subcapsular hematoma, splenic rupture, infarct, or abscess. Splenic abscesses are usually seen after peritonitis or abdominal surgery, with bacterial endocarditis, or with disease in a contiguous organ.[10]

3. *Have you recently had an illness with a fever?* Probably the most common cause of minimal splenomegaly is a "work hypertrophy" response to infectious diseases due to viral, bacterial, or other agents. The most common single example, at least in adolescents, is infectious mononucleosis.

4. *Do you have anemia or a blood disease such as sickle cell disease?* A positive reply raises the possibility of "work hypertrophy" from red blood cell destruction in hemolytic anemias or of splenic infarct or sequestration syndrome in certain hemoglobinopathies. Some patients undergoing long-term hemodialysis for renal failure get a "work hypertrophy" splenomegaly that seems to combine immune response to infections such as hepatitis with accelerated red blood cell destruction and with a splenic foreign-body reaction to fragments of silicone from the dialysis tubing. Transient, painful splenomegaly from splenic infarct can occur rarely in white persons with sickle cell trait who have been exercising at altitude.

5. *Have you had liver disease, hepatitis, or jaundice?* Cirrhosis, sometimes rather covert, is a common cause of splenomegaly.

6. *Have you noticed swollen lymph glands?* Lymphadenopathy in the neck suggests infectious mononucleosis; generalized lymphadenopathy suggests chronic lymphocytic leukemia or certain lymphomas.

7. *Have you had arthritis or hip or leg pain?* Active rheumatoid arthritis alone or with Felty's syndrome causes splenomegaly. Gaucher's disease, although often relatively asymptomatic, can manifest as hip or leg pain if the bone marrow is packed with Gaucher's cells.

8. *Have you recently found that you tire easily or have trouble breathing on exertion, or have your friends said you looked pale?* Such symptoms may reflect the anemia of autoimmune hemolysis or leukemia.

9. *Have you or your friends noticed your complexion getting redder or ruddier? Have you ever been told your blood was "too thick?" Have you recently had itching after a warm bath?* These features suggest polycythemia vera.

10. *Have you ever had pancreatitis?* Pancreatitis is probably the most common cause of splenic vein thrombosis; carcinoma of the pancreas is probably the next most common.[11]

PHYSICAL EXAMINATION

Inasmuch as splenomegaly has many diverse causes, a comprehensive physical examination is usually necessary. Sometimes, of course, the history and readily apparent physical features allow an early, tentative diagnosis, in which case an exhaustive physical examination is not essential. Examples of this situation include infectious mononucleosis, cirrhosis, Felty's syndrome, chronic lymphocytic leukemia, and polycythemia vera.

First of all, one should make sure that the left upper quadrant mass is really an enlarged spleen. Almost every clinician with extensive experience can recall patients in whom a large kidney, the left lobe of the liver, a pancreatic pseudocyst, or a retroperitoneal tumor was mistaken for splenomegaly. The patient should lie supine on a firm surface. The examiner's right hand is placed in the left upper quadrant, gently but firmly, and the patient slowly takes a deep breath. The examiner's hand is not moved; if the spleen is enlarged, it will descend to meet the hand. In doubtful splenomegaly, the patient should lie in the right lateral decubitus position with the knees up. The position of the spleen varies considerably; it may be superficial and thus may be missed by deep palpation. It may enlarge toward the umbilicus or the epigastrium or down the left flank; it may be so large that it extends into the pelvis and can thus be missed if the examiner's hand is placed too high. An exquisitely tender spleen with a friction rub suggests an infarct or hematoma. Sometimes, even careful palpation fails to identify the organ as the spleen with certainty. Even the splenic "notch" can be mimicked by lobulated pancreatic cysts or renal tumors. In these cases, one must proceed to splenic scanning, ultrasonography, or CT scanning (see "Diagnostic Studies").

High-Payoff Physical Findings

The following physical features are especially helpful to specific diagnosis of the cause of splenomegaly.

1. *A ruddy complexion,* perhaps with acrocyanosis, suggests polycythemia vera.
2. *Generalized lymphadenopathy* suggests an infectious disease, chronic lymphocytic leukemia, or a collagen vascular disorder such as systemic lupus erythematosus. Localized lymphadenopathy can suggest infectious mononucleosis or lymphoma.
3. *Signs of current or recent infection or inflammation* (fever, pharyngitis) suggest the splenomegaly is from "work hypertrophy."
4. *Cardiac enlargement, murmur, or gallop* may suggest congestive cirrhosis with splenomegaly, or splenomegaly as part of the "work hypertrophy" or complications of subacute bacterial endocarditis.
5. *Signs of cirrhosis or portal hypertension*—large or small firm liver, varices, ascites, spider angiomas, red palms, testicular atrophy—suggest congestive splenomegaly from cirrhosis, formerly called Banti's syndrome.
6. *Pallor, tachycardia, and tachypnea, especially with exertion,* suggest anemia of autoimmune hemolysis or other origin, such as leukemia.
7. *Arthritis of rheumatoid pattern* suggests the associated splenomegaly and should evoke consideration of Felty's syndrome.
8. *Petechiae and purpura* suggest thrombocytopenia, which can occur from hypersplenism, per se, but is more severe with the coagulation abnormalities of, for example, cirrhosis or leukemia.

DIAGNOSTIC STUDIES

The proper use of selected laboratory tests is critical to the diagnosis of the cause of splenomegaly. No sequence of testing is right for all instances of splenomegaly. If there is doubt that the mass is the spleen, useful imaging studies include barium gastrointestinal examination, radioisotope liver-spleen scanning, ultrasonography, excretory urography with nephrotomography, CT scanning, and angiography. In general, the gastrointestinal and urographic examinations are too nonspecific and angiography is too invasive for initial use; the test of first choice is liver-spleen scanning in most cases. Ultrasonography can help identify the organ and is especially useful for demonstrating splenic cysts. In the United States, parasitic cysts are rare, so most splenic cysts are either post-traumatic pseudocysts (75 per cent) or, especially in asymptomatic young women, epidermoid cysts.[12, 13] Angiography, besides its invasive risks, has limits in defining relatively avascular masses. All things considered, I agree with the view recently expressed by Amis and colleagues[14] that CT scanning is the best test to identify unusual left upper quadrant masses; their report describes cases in which only CT scanning, of all the tests listed here, correctly identified the mass.[14] In more routine cases, however, one may merely want to visualize the spleen to see if it is indeed enlarged; the radioisotopic spleen scan, using ^{99m}technetium sulfur colloid and gamma scintillation camera, gives an excellent index of spleen size, providing that careful measurements are made in both the lateral and posterior projections.[15] Further use of the laboratory for the etiologic diagnosis of splenomegaly is discussed in the next section.

ASSESSMENT

An algorithmic approach has recently been described for the use of the laboratory in the approach to splenomegaly.[16]

In the face of *acute left upper quadrant pain with tender splenomegaly* and a history of trauma, heart disease, or sickling hemoglobinopathy, one should obtain a spleen scan or a CT scan to look for splenic rupture, subcapsular hematoma,[17] embolic infarct or abscess from the heart, infarct from in situ sickling, or an unusual disorder such as hemorrhage into a splenic cyst or, very rarely, carcinoma metastatic to the spleen. Apparently, CT scanning is fast becoming the procedure of choice to evaluate splenic trauma; it is more sensitive than radioisotopic scanning and is less invasive and perhaps more sensitive than angiography.[18]

In the face of *acute or subacute febrile illness,* the first tests should be complete blood count, differential cell counts, and inspection of a peripheral blood smear for atypical lymphocytes. Infectious mononucleosis can be confirmed with a Monospot test. The chest roentgenogram and skin testing can help exclude tuberculosis and sarcoidosis, whereas blood cultures can exclude subacute bacterial endocarditis. Biopsy of enlarged peripheral lymph nodes might be considered for suspicion of sarcoidosis or Hodgkin's disease. Especially with rash and arthralgias, one should look for antinuclear antibody titers and other serologic evidence of systemic lupus erythematosus. With recent medication use, one should consider a drug hypersensitivity like serum sickness.

With *acute pallor, easy tiring, and dyspnea on exertion,* the complete blood count, reticulocyte count, and inspection of the peripheral blood smear should be ordered first. Anemia, reticulocytosis, spherocytes, and polychromasia call for a Coombs' test to confirm autoimmune hemolytic anemia; however, anemia, leukocytosis or leukopenia, and thrombocytopenia with or without blasts in the peripheral smear call for a bone marrow aspiration to confirm acute lymphocytic or monocytic leukemia.

Splenomegaly with chronic illness or asymptomatic splenomegaly requires a different approach. If the history or physical findings suggest *chronic liver disease,* the first evaluation should be of serum chemistry, followed by nuclear liver-spleen scanning, which together should confirm congestive splenomegaly from cirrhosis; in rare cases, liver biopsy is necessary for confirmation of cirrhosis. *Features of rheumatoid arthritis or Felty's syndrome* should prompt confirmatory serologic tests such as the rheumatoid factor titer. For *lymphadenopathy,* a complete blood count, differential cell count, and inspection of the peripheral smear for the mature lymphocytosis of chronic lymphocytic leukemia should be performed. Biopsy of a node may be necessary to diagnose lymphoma or a granulomatous disease. A *ruddy complexion* calls for a complete blood count to detect the increased hemoglobin concentration and variably increased white blood cell and platelet counts of polycythemia vera, which can then be confirmed by ^{51}chromium-labeled red cell mass determination and a bone marrow biopsy.

With *weight loss and other signs of chronic illness,* the first tests are a complete blood count, differential cell count, and inspection of the peripheral blood smear. Leukocytosis, a full spectrum of myeloid cells in the smear, and variable thrombocytosis would suggest chronic myelocytic leukemia, which could be confirmed by a low leukocyte alkaline phosphatase score and a bone marrow biopsy with karyotyping. Anemia, leukopenia, and thrombocytopenia (pancytopenia) with a few "hairy" lymphocytes on smear would suggest hairy cell leukemia, which could be confirmed by demonstration that the hairy lymphocytes contain a tartrate-resistant acid phosphatase and by bone marrow aspiration (usually "dry") and biopsy showing heavy infiltration by characteristic hairy cells. Anemia, poikilocytosis, nucleated red blood cells, and some young myeloid cells would suggest agnogenic myeloid metaplasia, which could be confirmed by finding myelofibrosis on marrow biopsy.

If the patient has *only mild to moderate fatigue,* the complete blood count and peripheral smear may show the mild hemolytic anemia and spherocytes of hereditary spherocytosis, or the characteristic red blood cell abnormalities of one of the sickling disorders, another hemoglobinopathy, or thalassemia, all of which can be confirmed by hemoglobin electrophoresis and other special tests.

If all the previously described tests fail to reveal the cause of splenomegaly, bone marrow aspiration and biopsy, with cultures and special stains, should be done. This may reveal Gaucher's disease, tuberculosis, histoplasmosis or other fungal disease, or amyloidosis. CT scanning or angiography may reveal a primary disease of the spleen, such as a cyst or angiosarcoma, or may show that the splenomegaly is due to splenic vein thrombosis. Finally, after careful investigation and thought and allowing time to observe the course and to await resolution of splenomegaly, if the patient is obviously ill, with such symptoms as fever, sweats, and major weight loss, and the spleen remains large, one might consider laparotomy and diagnostic splenectomy for identification of possible isolated splenic lymphoma, abdominal Hodgkin's disease, or other diseases.[19, 20]

Splenic Rupture. The enlarged spleen may rupture while the patient is under observation. Rupture has been reported most often in infectious mononucleosis, but considering the frequency of infectious mononucleosis, it must be an extremely rare complication. When it occurs in infectious mononucleosis, it does so usually after the second week of illness, usually is "spontaneous," occurring during normal activity, and seems more common in men. Unduly vigorous or repeated palpation of the enlarged spleen in infectious mononucleosis should, of course, be avoided, but rupture of such a spleen by palpation has been recorded only twice.[21] The range of disorders in which a pathologic spleen has ruptured is almost as wide as the range of causes of splenomegaly.[22] Pathologic splenic rupture has been reported in virtually all the infections, hematologic disorders, infiltrative diseases, and malignancies covered in this chapter, sometimes as the presenting feature of illness.[22, 23] In the hematologic malignancies, rupture is a rare event that usually occurs spontaneously; it is generally accompanied by abdominal pain, a left upper quadrant mass, hypotension, and fever, and the correct preoperative diagnosis is made in only a minority of cases.[23] In an occasional report, the sequence of events suggests that palpation of the enlarged spleen by the physician may have played a role in the rupture.[24] A final "iatrogenic" cause of splenic rupture is left-sided thoracentesis or pleural biopsy. In this case, rupture can manifest within hours as shock or weeks later as fatigue, anemia, pain in the abdomen, chest, or shoulder, and a left upper quadrant mass—the syndrome of "occult" rupture of the spleen, which can mimic many other disorders.[25]

REFERENCES

1. Eichner ER. Splenic function: normal, too much and too little. Am J Med 1979;66:311–20.
2. Manoharan A, Bader LV, Pitney WR. Non-tropical idiopathic splenomegaly (Dacie's syndrome). Scand J Haematol 1982;28:175–9.
3. Dill JE, Pilot R. Sarcoidosis presenting as giant splenomegaly. South Med J 1982;75:1430–1.
4. Ebaugh FG Jr, McIntyre OR. Palpable spleens: ten-year follow-up. Ann Intern Med 1979;90:130–1.
5. Schloesser LL. The diagnostic significance of splenomegaly. Am J Med Sci 1963;245:84–90.
6. Halpern S, Coel M, Ashburn W, et al. Correlation of liver and spleen size. Arch Intern Med 1974;134:123–4.
7. Sullivan S, Williams R. Reliability of clinical techniques for detecting splenic enlargement. Br Med J 1976;4:1043–4.
8. Silverstein MN, Maldonado JE. Asymptomatic splenomegaly. Postgrad Med 1970;60:80–5.
9. Budd DC, Fouty WJ, Johnson RB, Lukash WM. Occult rupture of the spleen. JAMA 1976;236:2884–6.
10. Chun CH, Raff MJ, Contreras L, et al. Splenic Abscess. Medicine 1980;59:50–65.
11. Salam AA, Warren WD, Tyras DH. Splenic vein thrombosis: a diagnosable and curable form of portal hypertension. Surgery 1973;74:961–72.
12. Faer MJ, Lynch RD, Lichtenstein JE, Madewell JE, Feigin DS. Traumatic splenic cyst. Radiology 1980;134:371–6.
13. Robbins FG, Yellin AE, Lingua RW, et al. Splenic epidermoid cysts. Ann Surg 1978;187:231–5.
14. Amis ES, Cronan JJ, Pfister RC, Althausen AF, Dretler SP. Role of abdominal computed tomography in evaluating left upper quadrant masses. Postgrad Med 1982;72:131–6.
15. Westin J, Lanner LO, Weinfeld A. Spleen size in polycythemia. Acta Med Scand 1972;191:263–71.
16. Eichner ER, Whitfield CL. Splenomegaly. An algorithmic approach to diagnosis. JAMA 1981;246:2858–61.
17. Patel JM, Rizzolo E, Hinshaw JR. Spontaneous subcapsular splenic hematoma as the only clinical manifestation of infectious mononucleosis. JAMA 1982;247:3243–4.
18. Mall JC, Kaiser JA. CT diagnosis of splenic laceration. AJR 1980;134:265–9.
19. Long JC, Aisenberg AC. Malignant lymphoma diagnosed at splenectomy and idiopathic splenomegaly. Cancer 1974;33:1054–61.
20. Hermann RE, DeHaven KE, Hawk WA. Splenectomy for the diagnosis of splenomegaly. Ann Surg 1968;168:896–900.
21. Rutkow IM. Rupture of the spleen in infectious mononucleosis. Arch Surg 1978;113:718–20.
22. Keaton BF. Pathologic splenic rupture in a child. Ann Emerg Med 1982;11:429–32.
23. Bauer TW, Haskins GE, Armitage JO. Splenic rupture in patients with hematologic malignancies. Cancer 1981;48:2729–33.
24. Andrews DF, Hernandez R, Grafton W, Williams DM. Pathologic rupture of the spleen in non-Hodgkin's lymphoma. Arch Intern Med 1980;140:119–20.
25. Mearns AJ. Iatrogenic rupture of the spleen. Br Med J 1973;1:395–6.

SYNCOPE

WISHWA N. KAPOOR □ MICHAEL KARPF □ GERALD S. LEVEY

□ SYNONYMS: Fainting, blackout

BACKGROUND

Definition and Incidence

Syncope is defined as a transient loss of consciousness associated with loss of postural tone.[1] Syncope must be distinguished from other states of altered consciousness such as seizure, coma, vertigo, narcolepsy, drop attack, and dizziness. Presyncope, dizziness, and near-syncope are less well-defined entities that at times may represent lesser degrees of the same disorder.

Syncope is a common symptom; up to 30 percent of normal adults report at least one episode of loss of consciousness.[2] The spectrum of diseases causing syncope is broad, ranging from common, benign problems to severe, life-threatening disorders.[3, 4, 5] Syncope in certain groups of patients, especially those with cardiovascular disease, may be a premonitory symptom of sudden death; therefore, patients with this symptom require a thorough diagnostic work-up.

Causes

Syncope can be classified according to the three general categories of causes: noncardiovascular, cardiovascular, and unknown causes (Table 1).

Noncardiovascular Causes

Vasodepressor Syncope. The most common noncardiovascular syncope, vasodepressor or vasovagal syncope (the common faint), occurs in all ages, although it is more common early in life and rare in the elderly. Vasodepressor syncope occurs in response to sudden emotional stress or in a setting of real, threatened, or fancied injury. Some of the situations commonly leading to vasodepressor syncope include pain, sight of blood, instrumentation, and venipuncture. This event occurs primarily in the standing position and less frequently in the sitting position. It is usually characterized by several minutes of prodromal symptoms, including weakness, pallor, sweating, nausea, increased peristalsis, yawning, belching, and dimming of vision followed by a loss of consciousness associated with hypotension and bradycardia. The patient generally appears pale and diaphoretic; if he or she is kept recumbent, blood pressure, pulse, and mental status return to normal within minutes. Syncope may recur upon regaining of an upright position.

A hemodynamic mechanism may be responsible for vasodepressor syncope, because the vascular resistance in the skeletal muscle bed and other major vascular areas such as the mesentery, renal, and cerebral vessels is markedly reduced. The fall in total peripheral resistance is not compensated by the rise in cardiac output found in normal individuals in the presence of widespread vascular dilatation. Why the cardiac output fails to respond to this stimulus is unknown. Vagal inhibition is probably not a contributory factor, since blockade by atropine does not prevent vasodepressor syncope.

Table 1. CAUSES AND TYPES OF SYNCOPE

Noncardiovascular causes	Vasodepressor (vasovagal) syncope
	Situational syncope
	Micturition syncope
	Defecation syncope
	Cough syncope
	Swallow syncope
	Orthostatic hypotension
	Drug-induced syncope
	Cerebrovascular disease
	Carotid sinus syncope
Cardiovascular causes	Reduced cardiac output
	Arrhythmia
Unknown cause	Syncope of unknown origin

Situational Syncope. Syncope may occur in response to usually normal body functions.

Micturition Syncope. Micturition syncope is reported in healthy young to middle-aged men. Syncope usually occurs in the middle of the night during or immediately following voiding, often without premonitory symptoms.[6] Episodes are usually not repeated, and many persons report having drunk large quantities of alcoholic beverages before retiring or having had a viral infection, fatigue, or reduced food intake shortly before the episode. Recurrent micturition syncope has been reported with bladder neck obstruction, pheochromocytoma of the bladder wall, and severe chronic orthostatic hypotension and as a manifestation of psychomotor epilepsy occurring during micturition. The mechanism of micturition syncope is not well-known, and in the majority of patients the underlying cause is not determined.

Defecation Syncope. The occurrence of syncope during defecation has been reported in elderly patients and usually does not recur.[7] The mechanism of defecation syncope is unknown.

Cough Syncope. Syncope that occurs following a paroxysm of severe coughing is termed cough syncope.[8] Affected patients are usually middle-aged men who are mildly obese and heavy alcohol users. Cough syncope can occur with acute processes leading to severe cough but more commonly is associated with chronic lung diseases such as chronic obstructive pulmonary disease, asthma, bronchiectasis, pneumoconiosis, sarcoidosis, and tuberculosis. It has also been associated with hypertrophic cardiomyopathy and herniation of cerebellar tonsils. The mechanism of cough syncope is poorly understood. It may be due to a prolonged Valsalva maneuver or to a rapid rise in CSF pressure with a resulting internal concussion–like effect.

Swallow Syncope. Syncope has been rarely reported during initiation of swallowing. Usually, an esophageal lesion or rapid gastric distension is responsible.[9]

Orthostatic Hypotension. Marked orthostatic hypotension can lead to syncope. Orthostatic hypotension is seen in a variety of clinical situations associated with volume depletion or decreased venous return. Various pharmacologic agents and diseases of central and peripheral nervous systems may also induce orthostatic hypotension (Table 2).

Drug-Induced Syncope. Drugs are a common

Table 2. CAUSES OF ORTHOSTATIC HYPOTENSION

Volume depletion or venous pooling	Prolonged bed rest
	Prolonged standing
	Dehydration
	Bleeding
	Severe varicose veins
	Adrenal insufficiency
Pharmacologic agents	Antihypertensives
	Diuretics
	Nitrates
	Arterial vasodilators
	Calcium channel–blocking agents
	Levodopa
	Phenothiazines and other tranquilizers
Neurogenic hypotension	Peripheral neuropathy
	Spinal cord disease
	Surgical sympathectomy
	Idiopathic postural hypotension
	Shy-Drager syndrome

cause of syncope, and a history of drug ingestion is important in determining the etiology of a syncopal episode. Drugs can lead to syncope by at least four different mechanisms:

1. Postural hypotension. Drugs such as antihypertensives, diuretics, nitrates, other arterial vasodilators, levodopa, phenothiazines, and other tranquilizers may induce postural hypotension and syncope.
2. Anaphylactic reaction. Any type of drug can lead to an anaphylactic reaction, and associated symptoms of anaphylaxis should be sought.
3. Drug overdose.
4. Drug-induced ventricular tachycardia. Agents in this group include drugs that lead to Q-T interval prolongation and torsade de pointes.[10] Those most commonly implicated are quinidine, disopyramide, procainamide, psychotropic drugs, phenothiazines, and tricyclic antidepressants. In addition, drug-induced hypokalemia and hypomagnesemia may lead to prolonged Q-T interval and development of torsade de pointes.

Cerebrovascular Disease. Cerebrovascular disease is an uncommon cause of syncope. Disorders that potentially lead to syncope include subclavian steal syndrome, vertebrobasilar transient ischemic attacks, cerebral vasculitis, and Takayasu's disease. Syncope in patients with subclavian steal syndrome occurs in association with other symptoms of vertebrobasilar artery ischemia. The important finding in this disease is the differences in blood pressures and pulses in the patient's arms, which should lead to further evaluation for the presence of subclavian steal syndrome. The diagnosis of transient ischemic attacks should be made when neurologic symptoms of vertebrobasilar ischemia accompany a syncopal episode and when no other cause for syncope is evident.

Carotid Sinus Syncope. Carotid sinus hypersensitivity may produce bradycardia and/or hypotension leading to syncope.[11] The bradycardia can be blocked by atropine, but hypotension without bradycardia has been reported to be unresponsive to atropine.

Although elderly patients frequently have hyperactive carotid sinus reflexes, actual carotid sinus syncope is rare, occurring in only 5 to 20 per cent of persons with a hyperactive reflex. Carotid sinus syncope occurs more often in men in the seventh and eighth decades of life. In most patients, a trigger mechanism cannot be demonstrated, but in some patients hyperextension of the neck, head turning, wearing tight collars, carrying shoulder loads, and other postural changes may lead to syncope. Occasionally, thyroid tumors, carotid body tumors, and inflammatory and malignant lymph nodes may precipitate carotid sinus syncope, as may drugs such as digoxin, propranolol, and methyldopa. The unequivocal diagnosis of carotid sinus syncope is difficult to establish but is probably justified in an individual with a hyperactive carotid sinus reflex in whom syncope is clearly related to activities that press on or stretch the sinus or in whom recurrent syncope has no other cause.

Cardiovascular Causes

Cardiovascular causes of syncope may be related to reduced cardiac output or to disturbances of cardiac rhythm (Table 3). The diseases producing decreased cardiac output can generally be diagnosed on the basis of history and physical exami-

Table 3. CARDIOVASCULAR CAUSES OF SYNCOPE

Reduced cardiac output	Obstruction to left ventricular outflow
	Aortic stenosis and hypertrophic cardiomyopathy
	Prosthetic valve malfunction
	Obstruction to pulmonary flow
	Pulmonary stenosis
	Pulmonary hypertension
	Pulmonary embolism
	Tetralogy of Fallot
	Pump failure
	Massive myocardial infarct
	Cardiac tamponade
	Atrial myxoma
	Ball valve thrombus
	Aortic dissection
Arrhythmia	Bradyarrhythmia
	Second- and third-degree atrioventricular block
	Ventricular asystole
	Sick sinus syndrome
	Tachyarrhythmia
	Ventricular tachycardia
	Supraventricular tachycardia

nation with appropriate noninvasive and invasive testing, but the diagnosis of arrhythmia may be more difficult.

Syncope Due to Reduced Cardiac Output. Structural abnormalities leading to decreased cardiac output include aortic stenosis, hypertrophic cardiomyopathy, prosthetic valve malfunction, and left atrial myxoma. Pulmonic stenosis, pulmonary hypertension, pulmonary embolism, and tetralogy of Fallot, which produce obstruction to the pulmonary flow, also cause syncope. Patients with aortic stenosis may present with exertional syncope owing to a reflex fall in peripheral vascular resistance with exercise in combination with a failure of the cardiac output to increase adequately. Transient arrhythmias have been reported to cause syncope in patients with aortic stenosis and hypertrophic cardiomyopathy. Pulmonary hypertension may cause syncope related to effort; in this circumstance the limitation to right ventricular outflow markedly inhibits the cardiac output response during increased peripheral demand. A similar mechanism is probably responsible for syncope in patients with pulmonary valvular stenosis. Syncope due to aortic dissection may on occasion be caused by an obstruction of cerebral circulation by aortic dissection.

Arrhythmias. Severe bradycardia as well as tachycardia can depress cardiac output to the point of hypotension and syncope. Arrhythmia as a cause of syncope frequently poses a difficult diagnostic problem, which is discussed further under "Assessment."

HISTORY

Meticulous history and physical examination are invaluable in investigating the cause of syncope. Vasodepressor syncope can be diagnosed if there is a history of a precipitating factor and the presence of characteristic premonitory symptoms. The sole presence of premonitory symptoms without a precipitating factor is not sufficient for diagnosis of vasodepressor syncope. Various types of situational syncope (micturition, cough, defecation, swallow) can be recognized only with a careful history. The underlying mechanism and the disease responsible for these syncopal events frequently will need to be determined, but an appropriate history may eliminate the need for extensive diagnostic evaluation.

Historical information may also be useful in limiting the differential diagnosis (Table 4). Syncope with exertion is classically described in severe aortic stenosis but may also occur with hypertrophic cardiomyopathy, pulmonary hypertension, and cyanotic congenital heart disease. Syncope associated with lateral movement of the head may indicate carotid sinus hypersensitivity or a mechanical obstruction such as a cervical rib. Syncope with arm exercise may indicate the presence of a subclavian steal syndrome.

Table 4. CLINICAL CLUES TO A POSSIBLE CAUSE OF SYNCOPE

Clinical Presentation	Possible Cause
Historical feature associated with syncope:	
Fearful or emotional situations	Vasodepressor syncope
Exertional	Aortic stenosis Pulmonary hypertension Pulmonic stenosis Congenital heart disease
Lateral movements of neck	Carotid sinus syncope
Arm exercise	Subclavian steal syndrome
Neurologic symptoms	TIAs Subclavian steal syndrome
Physical finding:	
Orthostatic hypotension	Orthostatic hypotension
Differences in blood pressures or pulse in two arms	Subclavian steal syndrome Aortic dissection
Abnormal carotid pulse and cardiac murmur	Left ventricular outflow obstruction
Carotid sinus hypersensitivity	Carotid sinus syncope

A complete medication history is essential, because diuretics and antihypertensive drugs are well-recognized causes of syncope secondary to the development of orthostatic hypotension. In addition, anaphylactic reactions may manifest as hypotension and syncope. Antiarrhythmic drugs such as quinidine, procainamide, and disopyramide are known to produce Q-T interval prolongation, predisposing to torsade de pointes and resulting in recurrent syncope.

PHYSICAL EXAMINATION

The physical examination may be helpful in defining the cause of syncope in a variety of situations (see Table 4). Postural hypotension with concurrent symptoms suggests a differential diagnosis including drugs, volume depletion, and neuropathy. Significant differences in pulses and blood pressures (greater than 20 mm Hg systolic) of the patient's arms may signify subclavian steal syndrome. Auscultatory cardiovascular findings may indicate aortic stenosis, hypertrophic cardiomyopathy, pulmonary hypertension, or congenital heart disease. Objective neurologic findings help focus the evaluation on the central nervous system.

DIAGNOSTIC STUDIES

Commonly employed diagnostic studies are as follows.

Carotid Sinus Massage. Carotid sinus massage should be performed in elderly patients only if other diagnostic studies have not been helpful, because in rare cases, transient and permanent neurologic deficits have been precipitated by this maneuver. The test should be done with electrocardiographic monitoring, and blood pressure should be determined frequently during the procedure. The massage is performed with the patient in the supine position and is repeated with the patient sitting and standing. An asystolic pause of 3 seconds or more or a decrease in systolic pressure of more than 50 mm Hg with no significant decrease in pulse represents a positive result diagnostic of hypersensitive carotid sinus.[11] Cardiac asystole lasting 2 seconds or a decrease of 30 mm Hg in systolic pressure is a borderline response. The diagnosis of carotid sinus syncope is justified in (1) the patient with a hyperactive carotid sinus reflex whose syncope is clearly related to activities that press on or stretch the sinus and (2) the patient with recurrent syncope and without another defined etiology who has demonstrated carotid sinus hypersensitivity.

Electrocardiogram. The electrocardiogram (ECG) is essential in the diagnostic evaluation of syncope, especially if the initial history and physical examination do not disclose a definite cause. The incidence of diagnostic abnormalities on an initial ECG is low, but when found such abnormalities may eliminate the need for extensive evaluation. Significant findings derived from both the initial ECG and prolonged electrocardiographic monitoring are similar and are discussed in the next paragraph.

Prolonged Electrocardiographic Monitoring. Prolonged electrocardiographic (Holter) monitoring is indicated when the initial evaluation, including an ECG, is suggestive but not diagnostic of an arrhythmia or a conduction disturbance, or when no cause can be determined from the initial evaluation. However, the following limitations should be recognized: First, cardiac electrical abnormalities may be episodic, and thus, may not be detected on a single 24-hour monitor recording. Second, brief episodes of bradyarrhythmias and tachyarrhythmias may remain unnoticed by patients. Thus, there is a poor correlation between symptoms (dizziness, syncope, palpitations, chest pain) during monitoring and the presence of dysrhythmias. Despite these shortcomings, prolonged electrocardiographic monitoring is the single most useful diagnostic test in the evaluation of patients with syncope of unknown origin.[12] The information derived from monitoring can be classified in the following manner:

Syncope with Transient Asymptomatic Serious Dysrhythmias. The majority of patients with syncope have no complaints during the monitoring period; therefore, presumptions regarding the etiology of syncope often need to be made from monitor results obtained during asymptomatic periods.[13] Transient sinus arrests longer than 2 seconds are rarely seen in normal asymptomatic individuals.[14] Consequently, pauses of more than 2 seconds in a patient with recurrent syncope should be considered indicative of sinus node dysfunction. A single episode of syncope and pauses of less than 3 seconds may require repeated monitoring or, possibly, electrophysiologic studies to ascertain the presence of sick sinus syndrome. Brief runs of supraventricular tachycardia have been reported in up to 50 per cent of the normal population and thus cannot be considered diagnostic of the cause of syncope unless they are sustained or are accompanied by alterations of consciousness.[14, 15] Similarly, severe sinus bradycardia (< 40 beats/min) has been noted in approximately 25 per cent of normal adults undergoing 24-hour Holter monitoring; therefore, if asymptomatic, such a finding may be physiologic and may not reflect the cause of syncope. Supraventricular extrasystoles and premature ventricular extrasystoles (reported in 50 to 75 per cent of males) do not aid in the diagnosis of the cause of syncope. Although frequent (> 30/hour) bigeminal, trigeminal, or multiform ventricular extrasystoles have a low incidence in the normal population, they should not be considered the cause of syncope unless they are associated with symptoms.

First-degree atrioventricular (AV) block and Mobitz I AV block are not considered to be causes of syncope. When present, Mobitz II AV block should be considered diagnostic of the cause of syncope because it occurs so rarely in normal individuals. Similarly, findings of third-degree AV block in a patient presenting with syncope should be considered diagnostic.

The finding of a fascicular block on Holter monitoring is generally not helpful in defining the cause of syncope. Patients with chronic or intermittent bifascicular block may require further evaluation, including electrophysiologic studies.

An episode of sustained ventricular tachycardia should be considered diagnostic of the cause of syncope. When ventricular tachycardia is isolated and comprises 3 to 5 beats, further monitoring may be needed to determine whether more prolonged episodes occur.

Exclusion of Cardiac Dysrhythmias as a Cause of Syncope. Rarely, electrocardiographic monitoring may provide objective evidence to exclude dysrhythmias, e.g., when the patient has a syncopal episode during an unrevealing period of monitoring.

Electrophysiologic Studies. Electrophysiologic studies are commonly performed in patients with recurrent syncope who have ECG or Holter findings suggestive of a conduction disturbance or arrhythmia. In some centers, patients with syncope of unknown origin without definitive findings on prolonged monitoring undergo electrophysiologic studies,[16] which include His bundle recordings, measurement of the sinus node recovery time, and attempts at induction of supraventricular or ventricular tachycardia.[17, 18] These procedures require a specialized facility as well as an experienced cardiologist. The indications for, and the utility of, results obtained from this study are controversial and are not completely established. These studies may be useful in patients with the following features:

1. Recurrent syncope with severe sinus bradycardia (rate < 40 beats/min) in order to document prolonged sinus node recovery time as evidence for sick sinus syndrome. For this purpose, the test seems to be very specific (90 per cent) but not very sensitive (40 to 60 per cent).[19]
2. Syncope of unknown origin (after thorough evaluation) when bifascicular block is documented on an electrocardiogram.
3. Recurrent syncope of unknown origin.

Echocardiography and Cardiac Catheterization. These studies do not in themselves establish the cause of syncope. They are helpful in defining the significance of abnormalities detected on initial clinical evaluation, are *not* a routine part of the evaluation of patients with syncope, and should be reserved for patients with appropriate physical features. For example, in a patient with syncope and the murmur of aortic stenosis an echocardiogram may be required to better define the evidence for aortic stenosis, and cardiac catheterization to assess the hemodynamic significance of the aortic stenosis.

Electroencephalography (EEG). Differentiating between syncope and a seizure disorder can occasionally be very difficult, especially if the episode has not been witnessed. An EEG is indicated when a seizure disorder is suspected clinically, when there is a neurologic deficit on physical examination, or when the patient has recurrent syncope of unknown origin. The EEG can provide information regarding only a convulsive tendency or the possibility of a focal abnormality. If such features are detected, further testing with head CT scanning and angiography may be needed.

Brain Scans, Head CT Scans, and Cerebral Angiography. If a seizure disorder or other neurologic disorder is suspected on the basis of clinical findings and EEG features, further evaluation with these tests is warranted. The finding of cerebrovascular atherosclerotic disease on cerebral angiography does not help to establish the cause of syncope, because such disease may be common in elderly asymptomatic patients. The diagnosis of subclavian steal syndrome requires cerebral angiography.

Glucose Tolerance Test. Hypoglycemia can lead to gradual changes in sensorium but does not generally lead to syncope as defined by usual criteria. There are no data demonstrating that a 5-hour glucose tolerance test is useful in the evaluation of the etiology of syncope.

ASSESSMENT

A pragmatic approach to the evaluation of patients with syncope is shown in the algorithm. The majority of the causes of syncope are established on the basis of initial history and physical examination.[20] Results of these procedures may also suggest potential causes that need further evaluation. For example, the diagnosis of vasodepressor syncope or situational syncope is made through the initial history and physical examination, and extensive evaluation is generally not necessary. In patients with exertional syncope, the initial evaluation should center on resolving the differential diagnosis of that symptom. A history suggestive of a seizure disorder may require neurologic evaluation with EEG and head CT scanning in order to clarify and determine the cause of the episodes. The evaluation of symptomatic orthostatic hypotension should be directed at defining the cause and improving orthostasis, in hopes of alleviating the symptoms and explaining the syncopal episode. Patients with auscultatory findings of cardiovascular disease should undergo further evaluation via appropriate studies such as echocardiography, stress testing, and cardiac catheterization. Patients with objective acute neurologic findings require investigation directed toward the central nervous system by means of such procedures as CT scanning and electroencephalography.

A 12-lead electrocardiogram obtained on admission is only rarely helpful in defining the cause of syncope.[20] An electrocardiogram, however, is needed to evaluate most patients with syncope, because a detected abnormality may obviate further extensive diagnostic testing. For example, if Mobitz II AV block, complete heart block, or a symptomatic episode of either supraventricular or ventricular tachycardia is present, an appropriate diagnostic and therapeutic plan can be established. In approximately 30 per cent of patients who present with syncope, a well-documented cause can be defined on the basis of history, physical examination, or initial electrocardiogram. Carotid sinus massage is useful when symptoms of carotid sinus syncope are obtained and may also be useful in patients with recurrent syncope of unknown origin.

The remainder of patients should initially undergo prolonged electrocardiographic monitoring either by telemetry or ambulatory monitoring

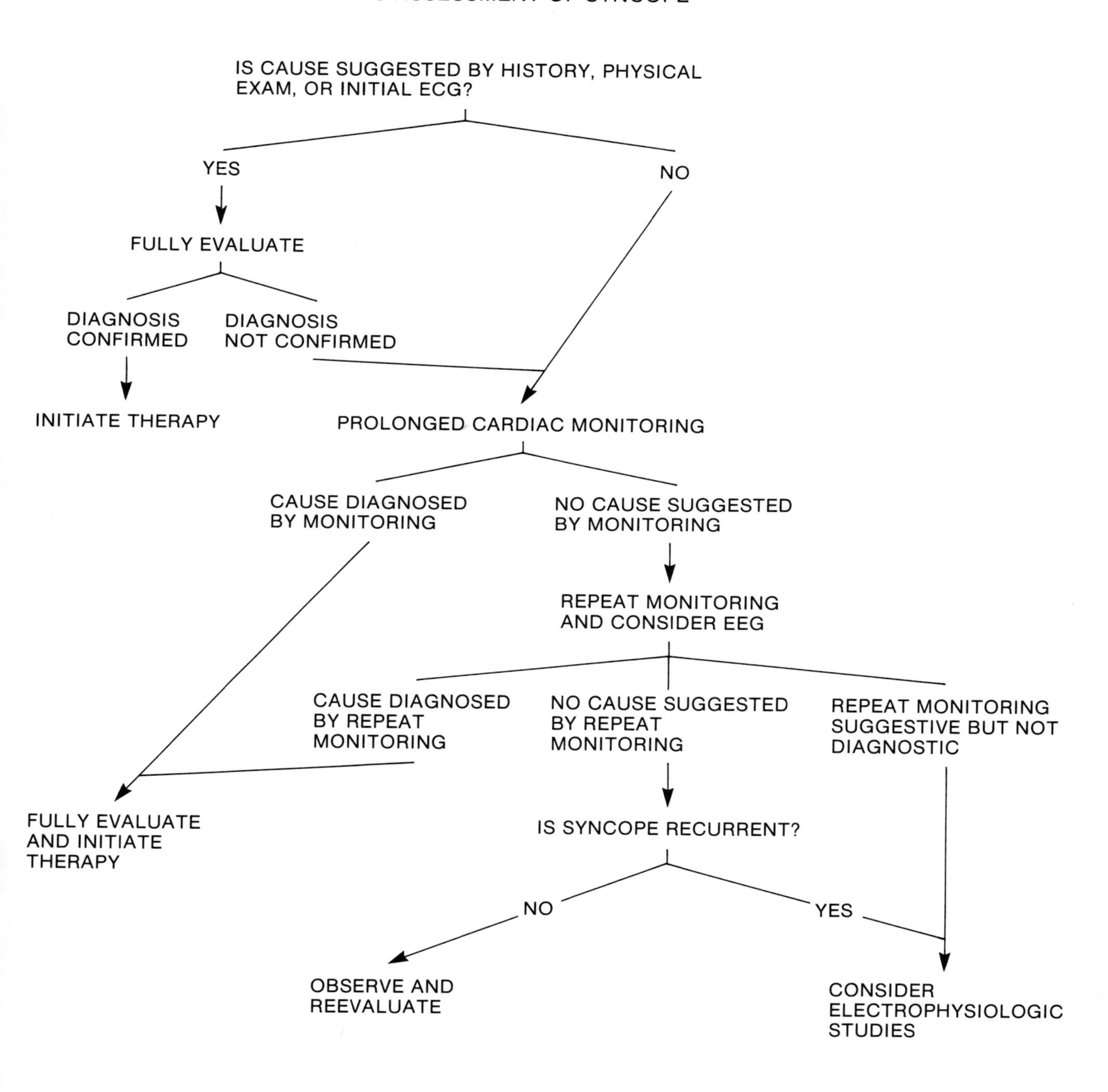
DIAGNOSTIC ASSESSMENT OF SYNCOPE
IS CAUSE SUGGESTED BY HISTORY, PHYSICAL EXAM, OR INITIAL ECG?
YES
NO
FULLY EVALUATE
DIAGNOSIS CONFIRMED
DIAGNOSIS NOT CONFIRMED
INITIATE THERAPY
PROLONGED CARDIAC MONITORING
CAUSE DIAGNOSED BY MONITORING
NO CAUSE SUGGESTED BY MONITORING
REPEAT MONITORING AND CONSIDER EEG
CAUSE DIAGNOSED BY REPEAT MONITORING
NO CAUSE SUGGESTED BY REPEAT MONITORING
REPEAT MONITORING SUGGESTIVE BUT NOT DIAGNOSTIC
FULLY EVALUATE AND INITIATE THERAPY
IS SYNCOPE RECURRENT?
NO
YES
OBSERVE AND REEVALUATE
CONSIDER ELECTROPHYSIOLOGIC STUDIES

(Holter). In approximately 15 per cent of patients, the results are either diagnostic or very suggestive of a cause of syncope.[20] If the findings are suggestive but not diagnostic, repeat electrocardiographic monitoring may be of value. If the patient has recurrent syncope and repeated Holter monitoring results are suggestive but not diagnostic of sick sinus syndrome, conduction system disease, or arrhythmias, then electrophysiologic studies may have value in management.

Those patients in whom a diagnosis cannot be established should be periodically re-evaluated for new clues as to the etiology of syncope. Patients having recurrent episodes of syncope of unknown cause may require an EEG and repetitive ambulatory monitoring. Patients who have recurrent syncope with nondiagnostic prolonged electrocardiographic monitoring results and no evidence of a seizure disorder should undergo electrophysiologic studies, which may also be useful in subgroups of patients with organic heart disease and recurrent syncope of unknown origin.

Utilizing this approach, a cause can be established in approximately 50 to 60 per cent of patients who present with syncope. The experience at our medical center indicates that using these various diagnostic modalities in a less goal-directed fashion does not increase the diagnostic yield, but only increases potential cost and duration of hospitalization.[21]

REFERENCES

1. Weissler AM, Warren JV. Syncope. In: Hurst JW, ed. The heart. 4th ed. New York: McGraw-Hill, 1978;705.
2. Dermksian G, Lamb LE. Syncope in a population of healthy young adults: incidence, mechanisms, and significance. JAMA 1958;168:1200–7.
3. Friedberg DK. Syncope: pathologic physiology, differential diagnosis and treatment. Mod Concepts Cardiovasc Dis 1971;40:55–63.
4. Wright KE Jr, McIntosh HD. Syncope: a review of pathophysiological mechanisms. Prog Cardiovasc Dis 1971;13:580–94.
5. Shillingford JP. Syncope. Am J Cardiol 1970;26:609–12.
6. Proudfit WL, Forteza ME. Micturition syncope. N Engl J Med 1959;260:328–31.
7. Patby, MS. Defecation syncope. Age Ageing 1972;7:233–6.
8. Aaronson DW, Rovner RN, Patterson R. Cough syncope: case presentation and review. J Allergy 1970;46:359–63.
9. Levin B, Posner JB. Swallow syncope: report of a case and review of literature. Neurology 1972;22:1086–93.
10. Reynolds EW, Vander Ark CR. Quinidine syncope and the delayed repolarization syndromes. Mod Concepts Cardiovasc Dis 1976;45:117–21.
11. Thomas JE. Hyperactive carotid sinus reflex and carotid sinus syncope. Mayo Clin Proc 1969;44:127–39.
12. Kennedy HL, Caralis DG. Ambulatory electrocardiography: a clinical perspective. Ann Intern Med 1977;87:729–39.
13. Kapoor W, Peterson J, Karpf M. Ambulatory monitoring in patients with syncope: lack of correlation between symptoms and simultaneous cardiographic findings. Clin Res 1982;30:196A.
14. Brodsky M, Wu D, Denes P, et al. Arrhythmias documented by 24-hour continuous electrocardiographic monitoring in 50 male medical students without apparent heart disease. Am J Cardiol 1977;39:390–5.
15. Barrett PA, Petter CT, Swan HJC, et al. The frequency and prognostic significance of electrocardiographic abnormalities in clinically normal individuals. Prog Cardiovasc Dis 1981;23:299–319.
16. DiMarco JP, Garen H, Harthorne JW, et al. Intracardiac electrophysiologic techniques in recurrent syncope of unknown cause. Ann Intern Med 1981;95:542–8.
17. Narula OS, Shantha N, Narula LK, Alboni P. Clinical and electrophysiological evaluation of sinus node function. In: Narula OS, ed. Cardiac arrhythmias: electrophysiology, diagnosis and management. Baltimore: Williams & Wilkins, 1979:176–206.
18. Josephson ME, Seides SF. Clinical cardiac electrophysiology: techniques and interpretations. Philadelphia: Lea & Febiger, 1979.
19. Vera Z, Mason DT. Detection of sinus node dysfunction: consideration of clinical application of testing methods. Am Heart J 1981;102:308–12.
20. Kapoor W, Peterson J, Levey G, Karpf M. A Prospective evaluation and followup of patients with syncope. N. Engl J Med 1983; 309:197–204.
21. Kapoor W, Karpf M, Maher Y, Miller R, Levey G. Syncope of unknown origin. The need for a more cost-effective approach. JAMA 1982:247:2687–91.

TINNITUS

JOHN A. McCURDY, JR.

☐ SYNONYMS: Tinnitus aurium, head noise, ringing in the ear

BACKGROUND

Definitions and General Considerations

Tinnitus—a sensation of sound in the ears or head in the absence of external acoustic stimulation—is one of the most challenging complaints in otology. Because tinnitus is a symptom, not a disease or definitive diagnosis, a comprehensive effort should be directed toward determination of the underlying pathophysiologic process. A myriad of conditions may result in tinnitus, and although most are benign, the physician must be alert to certain cardinal findings that warrant extensive evaluation in an effort to detect a serious underlying abnormality. The extent of diagnostic evaluation, especially with regard to the multitude of ancillary clinical studies currently available, is a function of the severity of each patient's tinnitus as well as the findings of the initial history, physical examination, and basic screening studies.

Tinnitus is generally described as a single noise, e.g., ringing, hissing, whistling, roaring, or buzzing, and should be distinguished from complex sounds such as bells, chimes, music, or voices, which fall into the classification of auditory hallucinations rather than tinnitus and suggest a psychiatric disturbance or drug intoxication.

Most patients are able to adjust to their tinnitus, but many associate the symptom with insomnia, inability to concentrate, and interference with the performance of daily routines. Although some patients state that the sound is so loud that it interferes with hearing, in most such cases tinnitus is of relatively low intensity, and the complaint is usually found to be a consequence of associated hearing loss rather than tinnitus per se.

Tinnitus is often classified as objective or subjective. *Objective tinnitus* consists of noises that are heard by both patient and examiner; this type is relatively uncommon. *Subjective tinnitus* encompasses those sounds that are perceived only by the patient; the vast majority of tinnitus cases fall into this category.

Tinnitus may also be classified as vibratory or nonvibratory. *Vibratory tinnitus* consists of sounds of mechanical origin that arise within or adjacent to the ear. Such sounds usually originate from vascular or neuromuscular structures and on occasion are of sufficient intensity to be appreciated by the examiner as well as the patient (i.e., objective tinnitus). *Nonvibratory tinnitus* consists of perceptions of sound resulting from neural excitation within the inner ear, auditory nerve, or central auditory pathways. Such tinnitus is always subjective. Nonvibratory tinnitus can be further classified into peripheral and central varieties. In general, *peripheral tinnitus* is perceived as originating in one or both ears, whereas *central tinnitus* is localized in the center of the head. In many cases, nonvibratory tinnitus has both peripheral and central components. The observation that many patients who undergo cochlear nerve section note persistent tinnitus following this procedure suggests that tinnitus originating in the auditory periphery often becomes imprinted in the central auditory pathways.

Most cases of tinnitus encountered in clinical practice are nonvibratory, i.e., subjective and the result of abnormal excitation in the peripheral or central auditory pathways. The diagnostic challenge, then, is to rule out the possibility that a serious disorder is affecting these pathways.

Incidence

Virtually all adults have experienced tinnitus at some time during their lives. Ninety five per cent of adults placed in anechoic environments experience tinnitus of some type, probably secondary to perception of neural activity in the auditory periphery that is masked by ambient noise in the normal environment.[1] Given the universality of this condition, the exact incidence of symptomatic tinnitus is difficult to ascertain. Investigations suggest that between 15 and 30 per cent of the population experiences intermittent tinnitus, and that approximately 20 per cent of these patients consider the symptom to be severe.[2]

Other studies have shown that approximately 85 per cent of patients with otologic disorders manifest tinnitus as an associated symptom and that severe tinnitus is almost always (92.5 per cent) associated with hearing loss.[3] Tinnitus is most common in patients aged 40 through 80, and the incidences are approximately equal in women and men. Severe tinnitus, however, is more common in men; this fact is consistent with the observation that hearing loss is more common in males because of more frequent exposure to industrial and recreational noise. Approximately 50 per cent of patients state that their tinnitus is bilateral.[6]

In spite of the fact that approximately 20 per cent of patients with tinnitus consider their symptoms to be severe, there is little difference in the intensity of tinnitus, as measured with audiometric matching techniques, in patients with severe and mild tinnitus. In both groups, the average intensity of tinnitus approximates 15 decibels above the hearing threshold level (i.e., 15 db SL) observed at the maximum tinnitus frequency.[4]

Tinnitus frequently becomes more troublesome when associated with anxiety, stress, and fatigue, and many patients with severe tinnitus demonstrate evidence of chronic anxiety and/or depression.[5] The great variability in individual response to tinnitus is often a manifestation of such psychiatric conditions rather than an indication that tinnitus is of abnormal intensity.

Factors that often precipitate or exacerbate tinnitus are: noise, head injury, age, stress, fatigue, anxiety, tobacco use, caffeine use, and use of some medications (see Table 3).

Etiology

A multitude of disorders is associated with the symptom of tinnitus, an etiologic classification of which is presented in Tables 1 and 2. Again it is stressed that in evaluating tinnitus, the physician should attempt to rule out serious underlying disease by maintaining a high index of suspicion about cardinal symptoms and findings that suggest such disease and that therefore warrant more extensive evaluation.

Table 1. AN ETIOLOGIC CLASSIFICATION OF VIBRATORY TINNITUS

Neuromuscular	Myoclonus
	Palatal myoclonus
	Tensor tympani myoclonus
	Stapedius myoclonus
	Temporomandibular joint crepitus
Vascular	Neoplasms
	Glomus tympanicum
	Glomus jugulare
	Arteriovenous malformations
	Aneurysms of internal carotid artery
	Arterial stenosis (atherosclerosis)
	Common carotid artery
	Internal carotid
	Dehiscence of jugular bulb
	Venous hum
	High cardiac output
	Fever
	Hyperthyroidism
	Anemia
	Aortic insufficiency
	Aberrant vessels
	Internal carotid artery
	Persistent stapedial artery
Inflammatory	Otitis media
	Acute suppurative
	Chronic suppurative
	With effusion
Miscellaneous	Patulous eustachian tube
	Otosclerosis (early stages with increased vascularity)

Table 2. AN ETIOLOGIC CLASSIFICATION OF NONVIBRATORY TINNITUS

Degenerative	Presbycusis
	Noise-induced hearing loss
	Endolymphatic hydrops (Meniere's syndrome)
	Hypertension
	Atherosclerotic vascular disease
Metabolic	Hypothyroidism
	Diabetes or hypoglycemia
Toxic	Ototoxic drugs
Inflammatory	Otitis externa
	Otitis media
	Labyrinthitis
	Cochlear "neuritis"
	Influenza
	Hepatitis
Traumatic	Acoustic trauma
	Head injury
	Whiplash
	Perilymphatic fistula
Neoplastic	Acoustic neuroma
	Tumor of the cerebellopontine angle
	Meningioma
	Epidermoid tumor
	Neoplasm of temporal lobe or brain stem
Mechanical	External canal stenosis
	Cerumen
	Foreign body
	Exostosis/osteomas

HISTORY

Evaluation of the patient with tinnitus begins with a thorough history.

Subjective Data

History of the Present Illness. Each patient should be encouraged to describe the type of sound he or she hears. Is it similar to ringing, whistling, pulsating, buzzing, clicking, roaring, etc.? Where is the tinnitus located? Is it constant or intermittent? If intermittent, are there any precipitating factors, such as noise exposure, stress, anxiety, use of certain medications, and various body positions? Does tinnitus vary with respiration? The severity of tinnitus should also be determined by inquiring as to the degree with which this symptom interferes with daily activities.

After obtaining a description of the characteristics of tinnitus, the patient should be questioned regarding the other *six cardinal symptoms* of otologic disease:

1. *Hearing loss.* If present, is it unilateral or bilateral, fluctuating or constant, high-pitched or low-pitched? What is the relationship of the hearing loss to tinnitus, i.e., has the tinnitus become more noticeable as hearing loss increases, or is

there no definite relationship between hearing loss and tinnitus?

2. *Vertigo.* If vertigo is present, its relationship to tinnitus should be ascertained.

3. *Aural fullness.* Does the patient complain of pressure or fullness in the ears? If so, is this sensation constant or intermittent? What is the relationship of this pressure or fullness to the onset and persistence of tinnitus? Is the aural fullness associated with decreased hearing or vertigo? When the fullness or pressure is present, does the patient note a change in the sound of his or her own voice (autophony)?

4. *Otalgia.* If ear pain is present, what is its precise location? Is the pain constant or intermittent? Are there any precipitating or exacerbating factors? Does it occur at any particular time of the day? What is the relationship of the pain to the tinnitus?

5. *Otorrhea.* What is the character of the aural discharge? How long has it been present? Is it constant or intermittent? Are there precipitating or exacerbating factors? What is the relationship of this discharge to the tinnitus?

6. *Diplacusis.** Is this symptom constant or intermittent? What is its relationship to tinnitus?

Neurologic History. A brief neurologic history should also be obtained, with the focus on symptoms referable to the cranial nerves and brain stem pathways.

Family History. Is there a family history of hearing loss, diabetes or other metabolic disorder, or hypertension or other cardiovascular disorder?

Social and Occupational History. Is the patient frequently exposed to loud noises for occupational or recreational purposes? Can the patient remember one or more episodes of acoustic trauma associated with exposure to firearms, fireworks, or other loud noises? Has the patient ever had syphilis? Are there any conditions that subject the patient to stress or precipitate anxiety?

Drug History. Does the patient relate the onset of tinnitus to the use of any particular medication? Does he or she regularly use any medications known to precipitate tinnitus (Table 3)?

Significance of Information Obtained on the Medical History

The character of tinnitus may provide diagnostic clues as to its origin. Pulsating or humming tinnitus should suggest a vascular disorder, whereas rapid clicking sounds suggest neuromuscular dysfunction. High-pitched tinnitus is generally associated with cochlear, cochlear nerve, or central auditory disease. Low-pitched tinnitus is often associated with a disorder of the external auditory canal or middle ear, producing a conductive hearing loss; one exception to this observation is the low-pitched, roaring tinnitus classically associated with endolymphatic hydrops (Meniere's syndrome). Tinnitus that varies with respiration suggests a patulous eustachian tube.

The laterality of tinnitus is of obvious diagnostic value, strongly suggesting that the involved ear is the origin of the underlying pathologic process. Unilateral tinnitus is a "red flag" finding warranting a more extensive diagnostic evaluation, particularly with regard to the possibility of an acoustic tumor. Tinnitus originating in the middle of the head may suggest a generalized metabolic, toxic, or degenerative process. As noted previously, peripheral tinnitus often becomes imprinted in the central auditory pathways, and this possibility should be considered in assessing the diagnostic significance of tinnitus described as localized in the middle of the head. A patient's description of the severity of tinnitus is frequently of little diagnostic value but may provide insight into the emotional reaction and level of adjustment to this symptom. Severe tinnitus may suggest ototoxicity secondary to recent drug exposure. Interestingly, many adolescents and young adults who use mar-

*Sound (i.e. a tuning fork, music etc.) perceived as a different pitch in either ear. Diplacusis indicates cochlear dysfunction.

Table 3. DRUGS KNOWN TO INDUCE TINNITUS*

Anti-inflammatory agents	Salicylates Prednisolone Indomethacin (Indocin) Quinine Zomepirac (Zomax) Mefenamic acid (Ponstel) Tolmetin (Tolectin) Naproxen (Naprosyn)
Central nervous system agents	Aminophylline Caffeine Marijuana Tobacco Lithium Haloperidol (Haldol) Tricyclic antidepressants/monoamine oxidase inhibitors Levodopa
Antimicrobial agents	Aminoglycosides Sulfanilamides Tetracyclines Doxycycline (Vibramycin) Minocycline (Minocin) Dapsone Clindamycin (Cleocin) Metronidazole (Flagyl)
Cardiovascular agents	Beta-adrenergic blockers Digitalis
Organic solvents	Benzene Methyl alcohol
Diuretics	Ethacrynic acid (Edecrin) Furosemide (Lasix)

*Not an all-inclusive list.

ijuana note that their tinnitus becomes significantly more severe when using this drug in the presence of loud noise such as music.

The association of any of the other six cardinal symptoms of otologic dysfunction with tinnitus provides evidence that the underlying process originates in the ear or auditory pathways. Tinnitus associated with vertigo suggests endolymphatic hydrops or the presence of an acoustic tumor and is another "red flag" finding warranting more extensive evaluation. Aural fullness is often noted in the presence of endolymphatic hydrops but is more commonly associated with eustachian tube dysfunction with or without middle ear effusion. Diplacusis is most often associated with endolymphatic hydrops or other cochlear disorders.

Associated neurologic symptoms should suggest the presence of an acoustic tumor. Surprisingly, the common degenerative processes affecting the brain stem (e.g., multiple sclerosis) uncommonly produce tinnitus.

The vascular changes associated with diabetes and hypertension frequently produce tinnitus, and thus a family history of these disorders is of interest.

Noise-induced hearing loss is perhaps the most common cause of tinnitus, and consequently, prolonged noise exposure (occupational or recreational) or an episode of acoustic trauma is important. Syphilis, hypothyroidism, and disorders of glucose metabolism are rare but treatable causes of endolymphatic hydrops. Head injury and acoustic trauma are other possible causes of endolymphatic hydrops.

Drug ingestion is also a common cause of tinnitus.[6]

PHYSICAL EXAMINATION

After analyzing the history, the clinician performs a complete head and neck examination with emphasis on inspection of the external auditory canals, tympanic membranes, tuning fork tests (Weber and Rinne), and auscultation of the neck, mastoid, and temporal regions. If bruits are detected or if the patient describes tinnitus suggestive of a venous hum, the effect of jugular and/or carotid compression is determined. Blood pressure readings are obtained in each arm, and a brief neurologic examination (cranial nerves, Romberg's sign, cerebellar screening) is performed.

Significant features of physical examination are listed in Table 4.

DIAGNOSTIC STUDIES

Audiometric Testing

Each patient should undergo pure-tone audiometry even in the absence of a subjective hearing loss. Many cases of tinnitus are explained by

Table 4. SIGNIFICANT PHYSICAL FINDINGS IN TINNITUS

Physical Finding	Significance: Possible Cause(s)
Cerumen impaction or foreign body, external auditory canal; multiple exostoses or osteoma obstructing canal	May produce low-pitched tinnitus
Perforation of tympanic membrane with or without otorrhea	Chronic otitis media, traumatic perforation of tympanic membrane; low-pitched tinnitus
Dull, red or bulging, immobile tympanic membrane	Acute suppurative otitis media, otitis media with effusion; low-pitched tinnitus
Reddish hue or mass behind tympanic membrane	Glomus tumor, otosclerosis (Schwartze's sign), dehiscent jugular bulb
Lateralization (Weber test)	Conductive or sensorineural hearing loss
Negative result of Rinne test	Conductive hearing loss
Positive result of fistula test*	Perilymphatic fistula (trauma, infection)
Nystagmus	Vestibular dysfunction owing to acoustic tumor, endolymphatic hydrops, perilymphatic fistula, etc.
Spontaneous movement of tympanic membrane accompanied by tinnitus	Myoclonus (palatal, tensor tympani, stapedial); patulous eustachian tube (movement with respiration)
Audible bruit in neck, ear, or mastoid	Carotid stenosis, aneurysm, glomus tumor, arteriovenous malformation, aberrant carotid artery, dehiscent jugular bulb, persistent stapedial artery
Tinnitus decreases with jugular compression	Venous hum
Tinnitus decreases with carotid compression	Carotid stenosis (atherosclerosis), aneurysm, aberrant carotid artery

*Vertigo *and* nystagmus on pneumomassage with pneumatic otoscope.

asymptomatic high-frequency hearing losses that are unnoticed because the speech frequencies are minimally affected. Additional audiometric evaluation depends on the results of the initial pure-tone screen as well as findings of the history and physical examination.

Conductive hearing loss is often the explanation for low-pitched tinnitus, whereas sensorineural hearing loss is most often associated with high-pitched tinnitus. An exception to this generalization is the low-pitched, roaring tinnitus associated with endolymphatic hydrops (Meniere's syndrome).

Individuals with sensorineural hearing loss should undergo an audiometric battery designed to determine the "site of lesion" (i.e., cochlear or retrocochlear), including the speech reception threshold test and speech discrimination score, impedance audiometry, short increment sensitivity index (SISI), and tone decay tests.

Asymmetric hearing loss or the presence of an abnormally low speech discrimination score in one ear warrants a search for a retrocochlear mass (i.e., acoustic neuroma, cerebellopontine angle meningioma or epidermoid tumor). Audiometric tests indicated in this search include impedance audiometry (for assessment of the stapedius reflex thresholds), tone decay, Békésey audiometry, and brain stem evoked response audiometry.

Low-frequency sensorineural hearing loss should arouse suspicion of endolymphatic hydrops (Meniere's syndrome), and the effect of diuretic agents (i.e., oral glycerol) on the hearing threshold level and speech discrimination score should be determined (the "glycerol test"). Patients with unilateral hearing loss and/or retrocochlear findings on "site of lesion" testing should also undergo electronystagmography for evaluation of the vestibular system.

Audiometric techniques for matching the frequency and intensity of tinnitus are currently available, but because their primary indication is obtaining information for use in treatment of this condition, they are not discussed.

Diagnostic Imaging

The major indication for radiographic examination is audiometric findings suggestive of a retrocochlear mass. Plain x-rays of the petrous pyramid detect 80 to 85 per cent of such masses, and this accuracy rate is improved with use of polytomography. CT scanning with infusion of iodine is indicated if an acoustic tumor is suspected; if results are negative, 4 cc of oxygen are instilled into the subarachnoid space in order to enhance visualization of the internal auditory canals, enabling detection of small intercanalicular tumors.

In objective tinnitus of the pulsatile type, particularly in cases with an audible bruit, polytomography is indicated to assess the vascular structures in the temporal bone (jugular bulb and carotid artery). Angiography or venography is indicated if further evaluation of these structures is required.

Laboratory Studies

History, physical examination, audiometric studies, and diagnostic imaging provide sufficient information for diagnosis of tinnitus in the majority of patients. On occasion, however, laboratory studies are indicated. These include a complete blood count (anemia) as well as fluorescent treponemal antibody absorption test, measurements of triiodothyronine and thyroxine, and a glucose tolerance test (to rule out treatable causes of endolymphatic hydrops). Blood lipid studies may be indicated in the hypertensive patient complaining of tinnitus.

ASSESSMENT

In evaluating tinnitus, the first step is localization of its origin. Is it otologic or nonotologic? If otologic, does the tinnitus arise in the external canal, middle ear, cochlea-auditory nerve, or central auditory pathways? If nonotologic, is the cause neuromuscular or vascular? Next, the underlying pathophysiologic disorder is defined. Categorization of possible etiologies according to their pathologic mechanisms (inflammatory, neoplastic, degenerative, vascular, etc.) as in Tables 1 and 2 is helpful in this determination.

Constellations of Findings

The diagnostic process is initiated by information obtained from the history and its focus is progressively refined on the basis of data yielded by physical examination and ancillary studies. Rarely does the entire battery of audiometric, radiographic, and laboratory studies require completion, because the results of basic screening examinations allow placement of findings into certain constellations that are associated with the majority of causes of tinnitus. The extent of diagnostic evaluation is individualized, depending upon the index of suspicion raised by various findings encountered along the diagnostic pathway. Utilization of "red flag" findings facilitates decisions regarding procurement of various studies (Table 5). A summary of the most common constellations of findings that characterize disorders commonly associated with tinnitus follows.

Table 5. "RED FLAG" FINDINGS IN TINNITUS

History	Unilateral tinnitus
	Fluctuating hearing loss
	Sudden hearing loss
	Vertigo
Physical examination	Bruits
	Neurologic signs
	Red mass behind tympanic membrane
	Positive result of fistula test
Audiometry	Unilateral hearing loss
	Unusually low speech discrimination score
	Stapedius reflex decay or absence (impedance audiometry)
Diagnostic imaging	Asymmetry of internal auditory canals
	Enlargement/erosion of jugular foramen
	Enlargement/erosion of carotid canal
	Erosion of temporal bone

Noise-Induced Hearing Loss. Perhaps the most common cause of tinnitus, particularly in men, tinnitus associated with noise-induced hearing loss is described as high-pitched and ringing. In its initial stages, tinnitus is noted only following noise exposure but it becomes more persistent as the degree of cochlear damage secondary to noise exposure increases. Eventually the tinnitus becomes constant. It is most often bilateral but may be unilateral. Unilateral symptoms suggest an episode of acoustic trauma. Unilateral tinnitus in association with noise-induced hearing loss is also common in a recreational hunter, in whom the same ear is always closer to the barrel of a rifle, as well as in a pilot or copilot, whose left or right ear is continually exposed to engine noise.

Physical findings are generally normal except for results of the tuning fork tests. If hearing loss is more marked in one ear, the Weber test lateralizes to the better-hearing ear. The Rinne test result is positive. Pure-tone audiometry demonstrates a high-frequency sensorineural hearing loss. Initially a characteristic notch appears at 4,000 Hertz, but as the hearing loss becomes progressive, the notch widens into both lower and higher frequencies and then disappears. Speech discrimination is characteristically diminished, especially in the presence of background noise. The short increment sensitivity index (SISI) is usually positive and tone decay testing is negative, consistent with a cochlear lesion. Temporal bone radiographs of the internal auditory canals obtained in cases of asymmetric hearing loss show no abnormalities.

Presbycusis. This condition is also characterized by high-pitched tinnitus, which is often described as ringing. The tinnitus may be constant or intermittent, unilateral or bilateral. Physical findings are generally normal except for tuning fork test results, which show a sensorineural hearing loss.

Pure-tone audiometry demonstrates a sensorineural hearing loss that is frequently more severe in the high frequencies but may be flat. The speech discrimination score is usually diminished if high-frequency sensorineural hearing loss is present but may be normal or near normal in association with a flat sensorineural hearing loss. The SISI test is generally positive and tone decay testing is negative, consistent with a cochlear lesion. Temporal bone radiographs obtained in cases of unilateral asymmetric hearing loss show no abnormalities.

Endolymphatic Hydrops (Meniere's Syndrome). This disorder is characterized by an intermittent, low-pitched, roaring tinnitus, which in most cases (85 per cent) is unilateral. Classically, tinnitus is associated with vertigo and hearing loss, but in some cases tinnitus may be an isolated phenomenon or may be associated only with fluctuating hearing loss. Fluctuating symptoms—hearing loss, tinnitus, and vertigo—are the hallmark of endolymphatic hydrops. Physical findings are normal except for tuning fork test results, which indicate sensorineural hearing loss. Early in the disease process, results of both tuning fork tests and pure-tone audiometry may be normal during asymptomatic periods. As the condition progresses, however, sensorineural hearing loss characterized by a greater involvement in the low frequencies develops. The speech discrimination score is generally normal in early cases but may be markedly decreased as the condition progresses. The SISI test is positive and tone decay testing is negative, consistent with a cochlear lesion. Screening radiographs of the internal auditory canal show no abnormalities.

Otosclerosis. Tinnitus associated with otosclerosis is variable in pitch and may be intermittent or constant. Physical findings are usually normal except for the tuning fork test results, which show a conductive hearing loss. In rare cases, a retrotympanic reddish hue is visible as the result of vascular proliferation in the middle ear (Schwartze's sign). Audiometric examination shows a conductive hearing loss, which is usually bilateral but more marked in one ear. The speech discrimination score is normal. Impedance audiometry shows decreased compliance of the middle ear. The stapedius reflexes are absent or show elevated thresholds. Routine mastoid radiographs are normal, but on occasion, polytomography demonstrates involvement of the cochlea (cochlear otosclerosis).

Acoustic Tumor. Unilateral tinnitus is often the initial symptom of a cerebellopontine angle tumor. It is usually high-pitched and may be constant or intermittent. As the tumor enlarges, tinnitus often becomes more bothersome and is accompanied by hearing loss and/or vertigo. Although physical examination may yield neurologic signs in patients with large tumors, findings are often normal with small tumors, as are pure-tone audiometry results. The earliest audiometric finding is often absence or decay of the stapedius reflexes, detected on impedance audiometry. Brain stem evoked response audiometry also allows early detection of acoustic tumors. The classic audiometric finding in retrocochlear lesions is the speech discrimination score, which is diminished out of proportion to the hearing threshold level. The SISI test is negative and tone decay testing is positive. Electronystagmography usually shows vestibular hypofunction on the involved side. Temporal bone radiographs frequently show asymmetry of the internal auditory canals, a finding confirmed on polytomography. CT scanning performed with infusion of iodine or oxygen often reveals small intercanalicular tumors not visualized on routine radiographs.

Ototoxic Drugs. Tinnitus associated with ototoxicity is usually high-pitched and is often described as loud. The tinnitus may be constant or intermittent and is almost always bilateral. Physical findings are usually normal except for nystagmus in the presence of concomitant vestibular dysfunction. Pure-tone audiometry generally shows a high-frequency sensorineural hearing loss, which initially may be confined to frequencies above 4,000 Hertz. Speech discrimination varies with the degree of hearing loss. The SISI test is positive and tone decay testing is negative, consistent with a cochlear lesion. Temporal bone radiographs show no abnormalities.

Head Injury. The features of the tinnitus associated with head injury depends on the mechanism of injury, and thus tinnitus may be low-pitched or high-pitched. Commonly, findings are similar to those in noise-induced hearing loss (cochlear concussion). If a perilymphatic fistula is present (rupture of the round or oval windows), the findings are similar to those in endolymphatic hydrops. Occasionally, head trauma results in perforation of the tympanic membrane or ossicular dislocation, in which case a conductive hearing loss with its characteristic tinnitus ensues. Whiplash injuries of the cervical region may produce high-pitched tinnitus, which typically appears 7 to 10 days following cervical injury.

Sudden Sensorineural Hearing Loss. The features of the tinnitus associated with this symptom depend upon the type of insult responsible for the hearing loss. The underlying pathophysiologic process is usually related to vascular insult or viral infection of the cochlea or spiral ganglion. A spontaneous perilymphatic fistula must also be considered, the symptoms of which are suggestive of endolymphatic hydrops. In such cases result of the fistula test is positive (vertigo and nystagmus precipitated by pneumomassage of the tympanic membrane with a pneumatic otoscope). Otherwise the physical findings are normal, except for the tuning fork test results, which show a sensorineural hearing loss. The results of pure-tone audiometry vary according to the pathophysiologic process. Speech discrimination is usually decreased. The SISI test is usually positive and tone decay testing is negative. Temporal bone radiographs usually show no abnormalities, except for the rare case of a cerebellopontine tumor producing sudden sensorineural hearing loss as a result of vascular compression. Vestibular abnormalities often accompany sensorineural hearing loss.

External Canal Obstruction. Tinnitus is usually described as low-pitched and roaring, similar to the sound produced by placing a sea shell over the auricle. Physical examination reveals the cause of obstruction (cerumen, foreign body, exostosis, etc.). Results of tuning fork tests are consistent with a conductive hearing loss. Pure-tone audiometry confirms the presence of a conductive hearing loss, and other audiometric test results are normal.

Middle Ear Inflammation. Tinnitus is usually low-pitched but may be pulsatile in cases of acute inflammation. Examination shows the presence of acute or chronic inflammation, and tuning fork and audiometric tests confirm a conductive hearing loss. Radiographic appearance is consistent with acute or chronic inflammation of the middle ear or mastoid.

Glomus Tumor. Pulsatile tinnitus is the hallmark of this uncommon disorder. In early cases the physical findings are often normal, but as the tumor enlarges a reddish mass may be noted behind the tympanic membrane. As the mass enlarges and erodes the ossicular chain, a conductive hearing loss is demonstrated by tuning fork tests and pure-tone audiometry. Impedance audiometry often shows pulsatile movement of the tympanic membrane. Standard temporal bone films often show no abnormalities, but as the tumor enlarges, bone erosion is noted. Venography defines the extent of tumor.

Arteriovenous Malformation, Aneurysm of the Internal Carotid Artery, or Aberrant Internal Carotid Artery. These disorders are characterized by a pulsatile tinnitus and frequently manifest as an audible bruit over the ear, mastoid, or temporal region. Other than this bruit, physical findings are often unremarkable, as are tuning fork test and pure tone audiometry results. Temporal bone x-rays and/or polytomograms are often suggestive of the presence of such abnormalities, but angiography is required for documentation.

Patulous Eustachian Tube. This disorder is characterized by intermittent tinnitus that is synchronous with respiration. Tinnitus is usually more marked in the upright position, gradually disappearing when the patient lies down. It is often temporarily diminished by vigorous sniffing or snorting. This condition is more common in women and is frequently associated with weight loss, pregnancy, and use of oral contraceptives. Physical findings are usually normal. On occasion, movement of the tympanic membrane synchronous with respiration is noted, and it may be documented by impedance audiometry. Pure-tone audiometry results are normal.

Myoclonus (Palatal, Tensor Tympani, Stapedius). These disorders are characterized by intermittent, clicking tinnitus produced by tetanic contraction of the palatal or middle ear muscles. The precise etiology of these disorders is unknown, but stapedius myoclonus is often associated with disease of the facial nerve (e.g., hemifacial spasm, early Bell's palsy) and may be precipitated by loud noises. Palatal myoclonus should arouse suspicion of a brain stem lesion, but associated neurologic evidence is often lacking. Physical findings are usually normal, although on occasion clonic movements of the palate and/or tympanic membrane synchronous with the bursts of tinnitus are noted. Results of audiometry are normal.

Significance of Tinnitus

In evaluating the patient with tinnitus, the physician should remember that in most cases, this symptom is associated with one of the otologic disorders, most of which are benign and nonprogressive. The physician should be aware, however, that tinnitus may be a symptom of serious underlying disease and should maintain a high index of suspicion regarding cardinal symptoms and signs of such conditions.

REFERENCES

1. Pulec J, Hodell S, Anthony P. Tinnitus: diagnosis and treatment. Ann Otol Rhinol Laryngol 1978;87:821–33.
2. Vernon JA. Tinnitus masking. Ciba Found Symp 1981;85:236–56.
3. Fowler EP. Head noises in normal and disordered ears. Arch Otolaryngol 1944;39:498–503.
4. Fowler EP. The illusion of loudness of tinnitus. Ann Otol Rhinol Laryngol 1942;52:275–85.
5. House PR. Personality of the tinnitus patient. Ciba Found Symp 1981;85:193–9.
6. Brown RD, Penny JE, Hanley CM, et al. Ototoxic drugs and noise. Ciba Found Symp 1981;85:151–65.

TREMOR

E. WAYNE MASSEY □ JANICE M. MASSEY

□ SYNONYMS: Trembling, quivering

BACKGROUND

Tremor, the most common of all involuntary movement disorders, is defined as oscillatory movements produced by contractions of reciprocally innervated antagonistic muscles. This innervation causes rhythmical movements that occur at rest or during activity with abatement during sleep. Tremor is pathologic when it impairs an individual's function.[1]

The classification of tremor is based chiefly on whether it occurs during the resting state *(resting tremor)* or during voluntary activity *(action tremor).* Other variables important in classifying tremors include amplitude, frequency, rhythm, anatomic localization, the influence of various physiologic and psychologic factors, and the response to treatment.[2] Tremor occurring at rest is typically associated with Parkinson's disease or related conditions. Action tremors may be subdivided into *postural tremor,* most prominent during maintenance of a sustained antigravity posture such as outstretched arms or abducted shoulder and flexed elbow ("wing-beating" position); *contraction tremor,* which is evident during an isometric contraction such as making a fist; and *intention tremor,* which is produced by a dynamic goal-directed performance of the limb such as finger-to-nose movement. Action tremors are characteristically seen in patients with essential tremors and accentuated physiologic tremors or with lesions in the dentatorubrothalamic pathway.

CLINICAL CHARACTERISTICS OF TREMOR

Tremor may be classified according to etiology as: physiologic, essential, parkinsonian, cerebellar, or neuropathic.

Table 1. CAUSES OF PHYSIOLOGIC TREMOR

Stress	Anxiety
	Fright
	Fatigue
Endocrine	Thyrotoxicosis
	Hypoglycemia
	Pheochromocytoma
Drugs	Epinephrine
	Isuprel
	Caffeine
	Theophylline and other catecholamine-like agents
	Levodopa
	Amphetamines
	Lithium
	Tricyclic antidepressants
	Phenothiazines
	Butyrophenones
	Thyroid hormone
	Hypoglycemic agents
	Adrenocorticosteroids
Toxins	Mercury
	Lead
	Arsenic
	Bismuth
	Carbon monoxide
	Methyl bromide
	Monosodium glutamate
	Sodium valproate
Miscellaneous	Alcohol withdrawal
	Action tremor with parkinsonism

Physiologic Tremor

Most normal asymptomatic persons manifest a low-amplitude, high-frequency tremor which is evident when amplified by the placing of a sheet of paper on the outstretched hands. The frequency of the tremor varies from 6 to 12 Hertz (Hz). It is slower in children and in elderly individuals (Table 1).

Electromyography shows poorly synchronized activity, which, with increased muscle contraction and other enhancing factors, develops into rhythmic bursts of discharges reflecting increased synchronization of motor units. Peripheral beta-adrenergic receptors appear to play a significant role in determining the amplitude of physiologic tremor.[3] The exact location of the receptors and their possible relation to muscle spindles is not known.[4]

Many of the accentuated physiologic tremors respond readily to propranolol. In fact, the response of tremor to propranolol may be used to classify tremors into one of the two categories.[2] Tremors that respond immediately after intravenous or intra-arterial administration (for example, accentuated physiologic tremors) are assumed to be mediated via peripheral beta-adrenergic receptors, and those that respond only after long-term oral therapy (for example, essential tremors) are assumed to be of central origin. In addition, physiologic tremor is also modified by the mechanical properties of the body segment, force of contraction, and passive body vibration produced by cardiac activity.[1] These mechanical factors combined with the synchronizing influence of the spinal reflex arc result in accentuated physiologic tremor.

Essential Tremor

Essential tremor may be hereditary (autosomal dominant) or sporadic; may be associated with various movement disorders, such as parkinsonism, torsion dystonia, and spasmodic torticollis; may be associated with migraine and senility; and may be exacerbated by alcohol. Persons of all ages may be affected. During the chronic course there may be intermittent fluctuations and plateaus. In general, frequency tends to diminish and amplitude to increase with age. Essential tremor is characteristically present during maintenance of a position and is usually of flexion-extension type, as opposed to the supination-pronation movement of the parkinsonian tremor. At rest, like the parkinsonian tremor, it usually localizes to the fingers and hands initially, but in contrast to the parkinsonian tremor, the essential tremor is of higher frequency (7 to 12 Hz) and tends to progress proximally. When fully developed, it usually involves the head and neck (titubation), manifested as lateral displacement or vertical displacement. Tremor involving the jaw, tongue, or voice is also seen.[5] Occasionally, essential tremor actually begins in the head or neck, a feature that should differentiate it from the tremor associated with Parkinson's disease.

Essential tremor may be isolated to the head, chin, hand, or even voice (Table 2).[6] It is most prominent in the upper extremities and is exacerbated with activity. Associated neuropsychiatric signs have been described, including rigidity, dystonia, adductor spastic dysphonia, tic, habit spasms, and intellectual impairment. Associated features include family history of tremor, alcohol intake, and migraine.[6] Isolated vocal tremor may occur, although it usually accompanies head and

Table 2. SITE OF TREMOR IN 131 PATIENTS

Site	Number of Patients
Hands only	66
Head only	15
Legs only	1
Voice only	4
Head, hands, and voice (equal)	2
Head and hands	23
Head and voice	5
Hands and voice	14
Head, voice, and chin	1

(From Massey EW, Paulson FW. Essential vocal tremor response to therapy (abstract). Neurology 1982;32:A113.)

neck titubation. The clinical characteristics in patients with isolated vocal tremor are similar to those with other types of essential tremor, except that spastic dysphonia may occur.[7] Respiratory tremor is likely a similar phenomenon.[8]

Essential tremor is exacerbated by attempted voluntary control and by emotional and physical stress. Tremor of the hands characteristically increases in amplitude with handwriting and when bringing food or liquid to the mouth, which may force the patient to drink with a straw. The amplitude diminishes with rest, mental concentration, and the use of alcohol or oral propranolol.[9, 10, 11] The failure of intra-arterial injection of either propranolol or alcohol to suppress essential tremor suggests that, in contrast to physiologic tremor, central rather than peripheral mechanisms are involved. This suggestion is further supported by the observation that differentiation techniques of ischemia or procaine block do not reduce the tremor, whereas ventrolateral thalamotomy does. Although the central origin of essential tremor has been generally accepted, the few reported neuropathologic studies failed to reveal any specific abnormalities.[12, 13]

Electromyographic recording of essential tremor usually shows bursts of activity occurring simultaneously in the antagonistic muscles. However, in less than 10 per cent of patients, the electromyographic recording shows a pattern of alternating burst discharges. This small group of patients with "alternating" essential tremor may eventually develop parkinsonian features.[14] Although both parkinsonian and essential tremors may occur within the same family or the same patient, there is sufficient evidence to suggest that essential tremor is directly linked to Parkinson's disease. Both are common diseases. Patients with essential tremor are frequently misdiagnosed as having Parkinson's disease, even though they do not have rigidity, bradykinesia, and postural instability. The phenomenon of cogwheeling on passive movement, which accentuates a tremor, may, however, be present.

As mentioned, essential tremor has been reported in association with various toxic and neurologic conditions. Some patients with spasmodic torticollis have essential tremor, which may interfere with their function.[15] Essential tremor may be genetically linked with certain hereditary peripheral neuropathies.[16] It is often seen in patients with migraine. However, common diseases can occur simultaneously by chance alone.

Parkinsonian Tremor

The typical parkinsonian tremor, causes of which are listed in Table 3, is described as a tremor at rest with a frequency of 3 to 7 Hertz. However,

Table 3. CAUSES OF PARKINSONIAN TREMOR

Causes of secondary tremor	Postencephalitis
	Toxins
	Phenothiazines
	Reserpine
	Carbon monoxide
	Manganese
	Carbon disulfide
	Tumor
	Trauma
	Vascular disease
	Metabolic disease
	Hypoparathyroidism
	Chronic hepatocerebral degeneration
Heterogeneous disorders with parkinsonian features	Striatonigral degeneration
	Olivopontocerebellar atrophy
	Progressive supranuclear palsy
	Shy-Drager disease
	Wilson's disease
	Huntington's disease
	Normal-pressure hydrocephalus

when the patient is truly relaxed or asleep, the tremor actually disappears, although it may transiently reappear during the rapid eye movement phase of sleep. As with other involuntary movements, factors such as emotional stress and mental concentration may exacerbate the tremor, whereas sudden emotional or physical distraction may transiently suppress it. The typical resting "pill-rolling" tremor usually begins asymmetrically in the fingers and thumb and progresses to pronation-supination of the forearm and flexion-extension of the wrists or hands. Parkinsonian tremor is characteristically most pronounced in the distal extremities. The lips, tongue, jaw, and face may also become involved, but active tremor of the head is rare. Head tremor, especially if unaccompanied by rigidity, bradykinesia, postural instability, shuffling gait, flexed posture, micrographia, and other parkinsonian features, should suggest the diagnosis of essential tremor. Marked rigidity may mask the tremor, and only after improvement in the rigidity may the resting tremor become evident.

Hoehn and Yahr[17] have suggested that parkinsonian patients in whom tremor is the initial manifestation of disease have an overall better prognosis than do those who present with other features such as rigidity and bradykinesia. There appears to be a correlation between the degree of bradykinesia evident clinically and the degree of dopamine and homovanillic acid deficiency in the caudate nucleus at postmortem examination, whereas the severity of tremor is paralleled by a corresponding deficiency of homovanillic acid in the globus pallidum.

Of the four cardinal symptoms of parkinsonism (tremor, bradykinesia, rigidity, and postural instability), tremor and postural instability can sometimes be resistant to levodopa therapy. The addition of an anticholinergic agent may effectively reduce the parkinsonian tremor in such a situation.

Parkinsonian tremor is induced by alternate contractions of antagonistic muscles ("mirror movements"). The corticospinal pathway is probably important in mediating descending volleys from the somatomotor cortex to the alpha motor neurons to produce the characteristic tremor. This probability is supported by the finding that rostral pyramidal tract lesions abolish the parkinsonian tremor. During volitional movement, the increasing innervation results in fusion of motor unit discharges and desynchronization with consequent suppression of the tremor. On the other hand, mental stress or a vibration of a tendon augments the amplitude of the tremor. The latter suggests that group Ia primary spindle afferent feedback may modify parkinsonian tremor, but such input is not essential for the production of the tremor. Hagbarth and colleagues[18] have shown that in parkinsonian tremor, as in normal voluntary alternating movement, the group Ia afferent fibers discharge during relaxation and contraction phases (fusimotor activation), suggesting that the normal alpha-gamma linkage is preserved. Thus, the tremor is centrally programmed and is not critically dependent on peripheral sensory feedback. Dorsal rhizotomy does not abolish the tremor in parkinsonian patients.[19, 20]

In addition to the characteristic tremor at rest, a significant action tremor may be observed in parkinsonian patients. Isometric muscle contraction, such as clenching the fist, results in a tremor in which electromyographic recording shows synchronous contraction of antagonistic muscles. This action tremor persists after ischemic block of group Ia afferent fibers. Therefore, this tremor, like an accentuated physiologic tremor, does not depend on the integrity of the stretch reflex arc. Lance and associates[21] have correlated the frequency of the cogwheel phenomenon elicited by a passive movement of the limb with the frequency of this action tremor instead of the tremor at rest.

Studies of monkeys with experimental lesions have suggested that the essential lesion in parkinsonian resting tremor involves the ascending nigrostriatal dopaminergic pathway, the rubrotegmentospinal fibers, and the rubroolivodentatorubral loop that normally modifies the input into the ventrolateral nucleus of the thalamus.[2]

Cerebellar Tremor

Patients with cerebellar lesions manifest both intention and postural tremors with a frequency of 3 to 5 Hz. Causes of cerebellar tremor include: cerebellar degenerations and atrophies; multiple sclerosis; Wilson's disease; drugs, such as phenytoin, barbiturates, lithium, alcohol, mercury, and 5-fluorouracil; hereditary sensory neuropathy (Dejerine-Sottas disease); midbrain ("rubral") tremor; and cerebellar and cerebellofugal trauma and lesions.

Cerebellar tremor should be distinguished from cerebellar ataxia, which results in an irregular, nonpatterned incoordination. *Ataxic tremor* is used to describe a disorder of movement in which ataxia and tremor coexist. Holmes[22] suggested that cerebellar tremor is related to accompanying hypotonia, fatigue, and inability to maintain muscles in fixation. Others contend that the loss of check coupled with delay in muscular contraction plays an essential role in the production of the cerebellar tremor.[2] The loss of modulating control as a result of the cerebellar deficit apparently leads to inappropriate feedback of corrections to the motor cortex. This instability of the suprasegmental loop may be modified by addition of weight to the limb, which tends to reduce tremor amplitude.[23]

Neuropathic Tremor

Tremor associated with certain hereditary neuropathies—Landry-Guillain-Barré syndrome, chronic recurrent polyneuropathy, and Charcot-Marie-Tooth (Roussy-Levy) disease—is well-recognized. Recently, patients have been reported with action-fast frequency tremors in conjunction with acquired polyneuropathies. It has been suggested that a loss of proprioceptive input is primarily responsible for this tremor.[24]

ASSESSMENT

After clinically differentiating the specific type of tremor (Table 4), the physician can choose the appropriate therapy. In addition to being given compassionate understanding and encouragement, the tremulous patient needs to be motivated to avoid social withdrawal. Learning to cope with

Table 4. CLINICAL ASSESSMENT OF TREMOR

Tremor Type	Frequency (Hz)	Occurrence			
		Rest	*Intention*	*Contraction*	*Postural*
Physiologic	6–12	Rare	Occasional	Occasional	Usual
Essential	6–11	Rare	Occasional	Common	Often
Cerebellar	3–5	Rare	Usual	Occasional	Often
Parkinsonian	3–12	Usual	Occasional	Rare	Often

various emotional stresses may prevent the stress-related exacerbations of the tremor. Frequently, mild anti-anxiety agents such as benzodiazepines may help diminish some of the stress-induced tremors. Such agents or even beta-blockers may be taken prophylactically, for example, before an important meeting or public speech or preceding other potentially stressful situations.

Patients with parkinsonian tremor often obtain some relief from the antiparkinsonian medications, such as various anticholinergic agents, amantadine, levodopa, and levodopa-carbidopa combinations. Although these medications have an ameliorating effect on the parkinsonian tremor at rest, they do not reduce, and may actually exacerbate, the parkinsonian action tremor. This action tremor, which responds favorably to propranolol therapy, has features of accentuated physiologic tremor. Five to 10 per cent of patients with Parkinson's disease also have essential tremor.[25, 26]

Patients with essential tremor often find significant relief after drinking a glass of wine or some liquor, but this practice should not be encouraged indiscriminately because it can lead to alcohol abuse.[27] Several studies have clearly shown the beneficial effects of propranolol.[3, 10, 11] Although it may be quite effective in smaller doses, 320 mg of propranolol a day or more may be needed to achieve the desired effects. In patients who have congestive heart failure or asthma or are prone to hypoglycemia, propranolol should be used only with great caution. Metoprolol, a selective $beta_1$ antagonist, can be of benefit in these patients.[28, 29, 30] Beta-blocking agents like propranolol are also helpful for certain accentuated physiologic tremors, such as those associated with stage fright.

The technique of triaxial accelerometry promises to be a simple, accurate, and reproducible method that allows a quantitative analysis of tremor in three dimensions.[31]

Despite the recent advances in our understanding of tremors, many forms of tremor remain unclassified, and their mechanisms are only speculative.

REFERENCES

1. Jankovic J, Fahn S. Physiologic and pathologic tremors. Ann Intern Med 1980;93:460–5.
2. Fahn S. Differential diagnosis of tremors. Med Clin North Am 1972;56:1363–75.
3. Young RR, Growdon JH, Shahani BT. Beta-adrenergic mechanisms in action tremor. N Engl J Med 1975;293:950–3.
4. Banker BQ, Girvin JP. The ultrastructural features of the mammalian muscle spindle. J Neuropathol Exp Neurol 1971;30:155–95.
5. Brown JF, Simonson J. Organic voice tremor. Neurology 1963;13:520–5.
6. Massey EW, Paulson GW. Essential vocal tremor response to therapy (abst). Neurology 1982;32:A113.
7. Aronson AE, Hartman DE. Adductor spastic dysphonia as a sign of essential vocal tremor. J Speech Hear Disor 1981;46:52–8.
8. Hachinski VC, Thomsen IV, Buch NH. The nature of primary vocal tremor. Canad J Neurol 1975;195:195–6.
9. Growdon JH, Shahani BT, Young RR. The effect of alcohol on essential tremor. Neurology (Minneap) 1975;25:259–62.
10. Winkler GF, Young RR. Efficacy of chronic propranolol therapy in action tremors of the familial, senile or essential varieties. N Engl J Med 1974;290:984–8.
11. McAllister RG, Markesbery WR, Ware RW, Howell SM. Suppression of essential tremor by propranolol: correlation effect with drug plasma levels and intensity of beta-adrenergic blockade. Ann Neurol 1977;1:160–6.
12. Cooper IS. Heredofamilial tremor abolition by chemothalamectomy. Arch Neurol 1962;7:129–31.
13. Herskovits E, Blackwood W. Essential (familial, hereditary) tremor: a case report. J Neurol Neurosurg Psychiatry. 1969;32:509–11.
14. Shahani BT, Young RR. Action tremors: a clinical neurophysiological review. Prog Clin Neurophysiol 1978;5:129–37.
15. Couch JR. Dystonia and tremor in spasmodic torticollis. Adv Neurol 1976;14:245–58.
16. Salisach P. Charcot-Marie-Tooth disease associated with "essential tremor." J Neurol Sci 1976;28:17–40.
17. Hoehn M, Yahr MD. Parkinsonism: onset, progression, and mortality. Neurology (Minneap) 1967;17:427–42.
18. Hagbarth KE, Lofstedt L, Aquilonius SM. Muscle spindle activity in alternating tremor of Parkinsonism and in clonus. J Neurol Neurosurg Psychiatry 1975;38:636–41.
19. Pollock LJ, Davis l. Muscle tone in parkinsonian states. Arch Neurol Psychiatry 1931;23:303–19.
20. Ohye CR, Bouchard L, Larochelle L, Nashold B. Effect of dorsal rhizotomy on postural tremor in the monkey. Exp Brain Res 1970;10:140–50.
21. Lance JW, Schwab RS, Peterson EA. Action tremor and the cogwheel phenomenon in Parkinson's disease. Brain 1963;86:95–110.
22. Holmes G. The cerebellum of man. Brain 1939;62:1–30.
23. Vilis T, Hore J. Effects of changes in mechanical state of limb on cerebellar intention tremor. J Neurophysiol 1977;40:1214–24.
24. Adams RD, Shahani BT, Young RR. Tremor in association with polyneuropathy. Trans Am Neurol Assoc 1972;97:44–8.
25. Shahani BT, Young RR. Physiological and pharmacological aids in the differential diagnosis of tremor. J Neurol Neurosurg Psychiatry 1976;39:772–83.
26. Schwab RS, Young RR. Non-resting tremor in Parkinson's disease. Trans Am Neurol Assoc 1971;96:305–7.
27. Massey EW, Paulson GW. Cause and effect in "alcoholic tremor." Am J Psychiatry 1978;135:1572.
28. Britt CW Jr, Peters BH. Metoprolol for essential tremor (letter). N Engl J Med 1979;301:331.
29. Riley T, Pleet AB. Metoprolol tartrate for essential tremor. N Engl J Med 1979;301:663.
30. Ljung O. Treatment of essential tremor with metoprolol. N Engl J Med 1979;301:1005.
31. Jankovic J, Frost JD. Quantitative assessment of parkinsonian and essential tremor: clinical application of triaxial accelerometry (abstract). Neurology (Minneap) 1980;30:393.

UNCONSCIOUS PATIENT

JOHN E. HOCUTT, JR.

☐ SYNONYMS: Comatose, impaired consciousness, insensible, impaired responsiveness, stupor

BACKGROUND

Definition

Coma is a deep state of unconsciousness in which the patient is unable to make more than a few basic reflex responses to noxious stimulation.[1] It represents a life threatening complication of central nervous system disease, injury, or metabolic derangement.[2,3] An accurate and speedy systematic approach to diagnosis is required to optimize appropriate treatment of this condition.

Immediate Considerations

The unconscious patient represents one of the few true medical emergencies. The damage from many causes of coma is progressive; the longer the patient remains untreated, the worse is the prognosis. Therefore, the history-taking, physical examination, and initial steps of treatment should be performed simultaneously. Table 1 summarizes the most urgent steps to be taken.

An airway must be insured and ventilatory support provided first. Cardiac rhythm should then be checked and monitored as necessary. Appropriate antidysrhythmic treatment is administered immediately to stabilize cardiac output and maintain an adequate blood pressure. An IV line is inserted for the emergency administration of medications and fluids. Simultaneously, blood is drawn for a complete blood count, electrolyte and BUN measurements, alcohol and drug screen, calcium determination, Dextrostix test, blood sugar analysis, and measurement of arterial blood gases.[1] Then, 50 ml of 50 per cent dextrose (1 ampule) is given by IV push (2 ml/kg in a child) with a dextrose continuous infusion to follow. Delay in giving glucose if a patient is hypoglycemic may increase the likelihood of permanent brain damage.[4] Thiamine, 100 mg IV, is also given if alcohol-induced coma is suspected (Wernicke's encephalopathy).[5,6] If narcotic poisoning is at all possible, give naloxone (Narcan), 0.01 mg/kg or 0.4 mg IV, and repeat as needed. If any improvement in the patient's state of consciousness is observed, naloxone should be repeated several times; extremely high doses are necessary for propoxyphene (Darvon) overdose. Fortunately, naloxone does not cause respiratory depression or interfere with circulation, as do other narcotic antagonists.[1,7,8] Another urgent diagnostic treatment is the administration of physostigmine, 1–2 mg IV slowly, for the possibility of overdose of an anticholinergic, antihistamine, or tricyclic antidepressant. The dose is repeated if any sign of improvement is noted. Careful attention to the cardiac rhythm is necessary when administering physostigmine because of its potential for causing dysrhythmias. Poisoning from an unknown agent unresponsive to naloxone and/or physostigmine directs one to the physical examination for additional clues to the type of drug ingested. Finally, a Foley catheter is inserted to monitor urine flow and a urine specimen is sent for measurements of sugar, ketones, and albumin, and a drug screen. Now, with the results from this diagnostic treatment in mind, the physician should proceed to the history.

Table 1. URGENT INITIAL MEASURES FOR THE UNCONSCIOUS PATIENT

1. Airway: Insure patency.
2. Breathing: Provide ventilatory support with oxygen.
3. Cardiac rhythm: Stabilize.
4. Insert IV line; stabilize and support patient.
5. Lab tests: Order CBC, electrolytes, BUN, alcohol level, drug screen, Ca^{++}, Dextrostix, blood sugar analysis, and arterial blood gases.
6. Dextrose: Give 50 ml of 50% dextrose with IV push (2 ml/kg for a child).
7. Give naloxone, 0.4 mg (0.01 mg/kg), IV push and repeat p.r.n.
8. Give physostigmine, 1–2 mg IV slowly.
9. Look for signs of meningitis.
10. Give (if appropriate): thiamine, 100 mg IV; hydrocortisone, 100 mg IV push; L-thyroxine, 200–500 μg IV bolus.
11. Look for signs of cerebellar hemorrhage.
12. Proceed with a thorough work-up as described in the remainder of the chapter.

HISTORY

The history must be obtained from friends, relatives, or available medical records. Another source of information is the person(s) who found or was with the patient at the time of losing consciousness. Also, some clues may be provided by the patient: a Medic Alert tag, a card in the wallet, medication, a suicide note, a physician's prescription in the patient's belongings, or an ID badge indicating the patient works with items potentially dangerous to health can each provide vital information.

If narcotic poisoning is strongly suspected, one

should continue to repeat the naloxone doses. Gastric lavage should also be performed and the contents sent for drug screen.

One should ask whoever is available about a history of trauma, other medications, poisoning, infection, seizures, diabetes, depression, and recent events in the patient's life.

A history or possibility of trauma should direct the physician to the physical examination. Medication ingestion or possible poisoning leads to toxicologic treatment using the available historical information and results of the physical examination. A history of seizures could mean that the patient is postictal, but a thorough history and physical examination as well as supportive care are still vital.

Suspicion that the patient is diabetic mandates prompt evaluation of the blood for glucose level. A Chemstrip test with a drop of the patient's blood is done immediately, to avoid delaying treatment until the serum blood sugar test results are available. A very high blood sugar level with sugar but not ketones in the urine demands immediate treatment for nonketotic hyperglycemic coma. A thorough evaluation of the patient should continue, in order to rule out the possibility of concurrent contributing or causative factors. Hypoglycemia has already been covered by the immediate initiation of dextrose infusion. Any resulting improvement indicates that the dextrose infusion should be continued.

Depression or recent emotional trauma guides one back to the possibility that poisoning may be causing a metabolic comatose state. Every effort should be made to determine the drugs and poisons to which the patient had access. One should make a thorough search for self-inflicted injury.

A history of rapidly progressive loss of consciousness preceded by vertigo, headache, and ataxia suggests a cerebellar hemorrhage. Early recognition of this subtentorial cause of coma is rarely achieved, but complete recovery is possible if the cause is recognized early.[4, 9] Most other subtentorial causes of coma have a very poor prognosis.[4]

PHYSICAL EXAMINATION

General Examination. Once the patient's airway, cardiac rhythm, and vital signs are attended to, one should perform a thorough search for signs of trauma, bleeding, needle marks, and infection. The ears, nose, and mouth should be checked for blood or cerebrospinal fluid (CSF) drainage (clear, usually Dextrostix-positive). If blood is found, a skull fracture with cerebral hemorrhage must be ruled out. CSF leakage is diagnostic of a serious fracture and definite central nervous system (CNS) injury.

The patient's mouth, body, and clothes should be quickly inspected for the characteristic odors of alcohol or petroleum and nonpetroleum distillates. Acetone breath is suggestive of ketoacidosis, whereas fetor hepaticus indicates hepatic encephalopathy.[1, 4]

Extremes of temperature (rectal) will require immediate treatment while the diagnostic evaluation proceeds. Table 2 lists common causes of altered temperature in the unconscious patient. Hyperthermia most likely indicates infection or salicylate intoxication or overdose, but it may also be from heat stroke or anticholinergic poisoning. Hypothermia is seen with barbiturate, ethanol, narcotic, phenothiazine, and tricyclic antidepressant overdose.

The patient's respiratory pattern may indicate the level of consciousness and suggest a cause for coma. A normal, regular, even breathing pattern suggests a very light coma, hysteria, or a postictal state. Slow regular breathing indicates a deeper level of coma, possibly from poisoning or metabolic abnormalities. Cheyne-Stokes breathing is a regular, gradual, alternating pattern of hyperventilation and apnea indicating bilateral cerebral hemispheric dysfunction and an even deeper level

Table 2. CAUSES OF TEMPERATURE ALTERATION IN THE UNCONSCIOUS PATIENT

Hypothermia	Excess cold exposure
	Severe infection (especially in the elderly)
	Metabolic disorders
	Hypopituitarism
	Myxedema
	Uremia
	Poisoning from
	Barbiturates
	Chloral hydrate
	Ethanol (acute)
	Methaqualone
	Narcotics
	Phenothiazines
	Tetracyclines
	Tricyclic antidepressants
	Cardiovascular or septic shock
Hyperthermia	Delirium tremens
	Heat stroke
	Infection*
	Sepsis
	Meningitis
	Poisoning from
	Amphetamines
	Anticholinergic agents
	Methanol
	Nicotine
	Paraldehyde
	Salicylates*
	Succinylcholine
	Thyroid storm

*Most common causes.

(Adapted from Hocutt JE Jr. Emergency medicine: a quick reference for primary care. New York: ARCO Publishing, 1982:281. With permission.)

of coma. Causes include profound metabolic poisoning, diffusely increased intracranial pressure (ICP), severe cardiopulmonary disease, and morphine poisoning. Regular, rapid, deep respirations (or Kussmaul breathing) occurs with acidosis, diabetes, uremia, some pulmonary disorders, and midline or high pontine lesions producing central neurogenic hyperventilation. Ataxic irregular breathing (cluster breathing) indicates pontine and medullar involvement and often signifies impending apnea.[1, 6, 10, 11, 12]

Asterixis (hepatic flap) is characteristic of liver failure, uremia, and chronic obstructive lung disease. Coma from structural CNS lesions rarely causes tremor, asterixis, myoclonus, or seizures.[4]

Skin Examination. Examination of the skin can yield several clues to the cause of coma. Cyanosis indicates hypoxia, and cherry-red color suggests carbon monoxide poisoning. Multiple bruises indicate multiple injuries or internal bleeding. Marked pallor also suggests internal bleeding. A maculopapular hemorrhagic rash may signify the presence of meningococcal meningitis, Rocky Mountain spotted fever, or staphylococcal endocarditis or sepsis.[13] Jaundice points to liver failure. Evidence of a necrotizing spider bite like that of *Loxosceles reclusa* (brown recluse) may range from a shallow skin infarct to a large blue, necrotic, recessed skin infarct; anuria and coma associated with a necrotic spider bite are diagnostic of systemic loxoscelism.[14]

Head and Neck Examination. Head and neck trauma are to be considered as possible causes for the patient's loss of consciousness. One must carefully inspect and palpate the scalp, neck, and face for any evidence of trauma. Battle's sign (hemorrhagic, boggy mastoid) and blood behind the eardrum, which indicate a basilar skull fracture, should be sought.[4] One should be especially careful when examining the neck to maintain proper cervical alignment. Any question of injury to the head or neck requires skull films and a cross-table lateral cervical spine film, which must include all seven cervical vertebrae. In addition, the neck and head must be stabilized prior to any movement.

A patient with a stiff neck, especially with an accompanying fever, merits a lumbar puncture to rule out meningitis and subarachnoid hemorrhage. Whenever possible, a CT head scan is requested before the spinal tap is done to rule out excessively increased intracranial pressure (ICP) from a hemorrhage or tumor. If the spinal tap must be done and increased ICP is at all possible, a thin (22-gauge) needle should be used. Elicitation of Brudzinski's (passive neck flexion producing leg flexion) and Kernig's (resisted leg extension from 90 degrees of hip flexion because of nuchal irritation) signs indicate nuchal irritation and require that meningitis and subarachnoid hemorrhage be ruled out.

Table 3. CAUSES OF MYDRIASIS IN THE UNCONSCIOUS PATIENT

Brain death
Severe hypoxia
Poisoning from
Antihistamines
Atropine
Barbiturates
Carbon monoxide
Cocaine
Cyanide
Ethyl alcohol
Glutethimide
Nicotine
Parasympatholytics
Phenothiazines
Sympathomimetics
Tricyclic antidepressants
Third nerve lesions (complete)

(Adapted from Hocutt JE Jr. Emergency medicine: a quick reference for primary care. New York: ARCO Publishing, 1982:281. With permission.)

Eye Examination

Pupils. The pupils should be evaluated for asymmetry or marked constriction or dilatation. Asymmetry may indicate local trauma or cerebral herniation but is normal in some people. Fixed, dilated pupils (mydriasis) have several causes (Table 3). If cyanosis is seen with mydriasis, cyanide poisoning must be considered. Pink skin in association with mydriasis indicates that carbon monoxide poisoning may be the cause of the loss of consciousness. Fixed and midposition (4–6 mm) pupils implies a midbrain lesion or severe glutethimide or atropine overdose.[12] Late supratentorial herniation can cause such a midbrain lesion from compression, producing fixed and immobile pupils.

Pinpoint pupils (miosis) in an unconscious patient most commonly indicate narcotic poisoning. Immediate diagnostic treatment with naloxone as described above is indicated. Other causes of miosis are listed in Table 4. True pinpoint pupils, less than 1 mm in diameter, are "pinpoint pontine

Table 4. CAUSES OF MIOSIS IN THE UNCONSCIOUS PATIENT

Poisoning from
Anticholinesterase inhibitors (carbamate insecticides, organic phosphates)
Caffeine
Chloral hydrate
Mushrooms
Narcotics*
Nicotine
Parasympathomimetics
Propoxyphene (Darvon)
Sympatholytics
Pontine lesion or trauma

*Most common cause.

(Adapted from Hocutt JE Jr. Emergency medicine: a quick reference for primary care. New York: ARCO Publishing, 1982:280. With permission.)

pupils." A pontine lesion interfering with the sympathetic fibers in the pons but not involving the pupiloconstrictor fibers from higher in the brain stem will produce unopposed pupillary constriction. Absence of corneal reflexes is also suggestive of pontine damage.[12] One should keep in mind that narcotic poisoning can also cause the pupils to constrict to less than 1 mm in diameter. Ordinarily, miosis from other toxins is not so severe.[1, 3] Some pupil reactivity is usually noted in metabolic encephalopathy.

Fundi. The fundi are evaluated for signs of papilledema, hemorrhage, and diabetic or uremic retinitis. Bleeding noted on funduscopic examination in an unconscious patient may mean there is additional CNS hemorrhage from hypertension, stroke, or trauma. Papilledema usually indicates increased intracranial pressure, which may have several causes, including trauma, brain abscess, tumor, stroke, hypertensive encephalopathy, and CSF obstruction. Other signs of increased ICP include a progressively decreasing level of consciousness, newly developing focal neurologic signs, dilating pupils, and a decreasing pulse rate with an increasing blood pressure (Cushing's phenomenon). If increased ICP is suspected, mild hyperventilation will cause a respiratory alkalosis, immediately lowering the ICP. An increase in the level of consciousness may then be evident.

Cardiac Examination. Dysrhythmias, depending on the age of the patient, suggest either poisoning, overdose, or cardiac disease. The younger the patient, the more likely the cause is to be an overdose of tricyclic antidepressant. Depression occurs at any age, and one must always consider such an overdose as a cause for dysrhythmias in any unconscious patient. Certainly, cardiac disease can also cause significant hypoxia, producing abnormalities in rhythm that lead to coma. Other causes of severe dysrhythmias include low-voltage electrical injury (less than 350 volts), digitalis toxicity, electrolyte abnormalities, and sick sinus syndrome.[1]

Abdominal Examination. The abdomen is carefully examined for rigidity, which may represent peritonitis or intra-abdominal bleeding. Infection and shock should be considered as causes for both rigidity and coma.

Neurologic Examination

Focal Signs. A thorough neurologic examination is obviously very important. Focal neurologic signs are sought first. They may indicate a cerebrovascular accident (CVA), CNS trauma with hemorrhage, brain abscess, or tumor. Asymmetric movements or posturing can help localize the site of CNS injury. Asymmetric reflex responses to noxious stimuli also point to focal CNS disease, as do unequal pupil size, deviation of both eyes to one side, and a unilateral Babinski sign (extensor response to the plantar reflex).

Level of Consciousness. The level of consciousness should be assessed first in general terms—i.e., alert, drowsy, stuporous, unresponsive. The stuporous stage is further described by the responses to stimuli. Specific description of the patient's behavior when stimulated is the most accurate way to record the level of consciousness.[15] Meaningful and appropriate gestures indicate a very light coma. Decorticate posturing (forced flexion of the upper limbs and extension of the lower limbs) indicates that the cerebral cortex is further suppressed. Decerebrate posturing (extension of all limbs) means that the brain stem is deeply involved.[10] A total absence of responses places the patient very close to death.[4] Prognosis can be relatively objectively evaluated using the Glasgow Coma Scale, which is discussed under "Assessment."

Brain Stem Herniation. Drifting or weakness of the limbs on one side indicates a contralateral lesion in the cerebral cortex. As the problem increases, bilateral motor signs will develop, leading to decorticate posturing in response to stimulation. At this point, stimulation of the feet produces a symmetric upcurling of the toes (normal Babinski response), and the pupils still appear normal. A further increase in ICP compresses the hypothalamus and interrupts the sympathetic nervous system. At this point, the pupils lose the ability to dilate but can still react to light. Respirations may become irregular (Cheyne-Stokes respirations) because of the loss of fine tuning that is controlled by the cerebral cortex. As the upper brain stem becomes involved, the third nerve and motor pathways are blocked. The pupils become fixed and dilated, decerebrate posturing occurs, and further interruption of respirations may develop. Once the medulla and pons are involved, pulse and blood pressure are markedly abnormal, respirations are ataxic, and the patient is totally flaccid.[4] Response to elicitation of the oculocephalic reflex (doll's-eye reflex) will be negative; an intact pons and midbrain would produce conjugate deviation of the eyes in response to rapid head turning (positive response).

Caloric stimulation of the oculovestibular reflex will evaluate pons and midbrain function in the comatose patient. Iced-water stimulation of the ear canal and tympanic membrane will produce conjugate ipsilateral deviation of the eyes in a patient with an intact pons and midbrain. A normal oculovestibular reflex response is impossible for the patient with a pontine lesion that has impaired pontine function.[11]

Eye Findings. Metabolic coma is suggested by brain stem findings with relative sparing of the pupil responses. Severe overdoses can produce the miosis and mydriasis described previously, but less severe metabolic encephalopathy can produce decerebrate posturing, markedly reduced and abnormal breathing, and tremors with fairly normal pupil responses.[3, 15] Barbiturates and phenytoin (Dilantin) are the only reported common intoxicating drugs that affect ocular movements while leaving pupillary reactions relatively intact.[13]

The corneomandibular reflex is tested by stimulating the cornea on one side and noting mandibular (lower jaw) movement to the opposite side. A positive response in a comatose patient suggests that a structural lesion exists or brain stem herniation is occurring. Possibilities include a major hemorrhage or infarct or significantly increased ICP. With normal ICP, the reflex is absent, for example, in the patient with a metabolic cause of coma.[16]

Corneal reflexes are tested and caloric stimulation is done to evaluate pontine function. An intact pons will allow normal corneal reflexes and response to caloric stimulation.[10, 12] Asymmetry in corneal reflex response indicates an interruption in the afferent fifth or efferent seventh cranial nerve contralateral to the side on which the reflex is absent.

An isolated third nerve palsy with a fixed, dilated pupil and ptosis associated with a rapidly deepening coma indicates brain stem herniation from a lateral cortical lesion or compression. Early diagnosis and treatment are life-saving.

Nystagmus may be a nonspecific sign of CNS irritation or may even be normal. The direction of nystagmus may indicate the side of an irritative or ablative lesion. Cerebellar hemorrhage usually produces nystagmus with forced deviation of gaze opposite to the side of the hematoma.[15] Metabolic causes of nystagmus most commonly include poisoning by barbiturates, carbamazepine, ethanol, phencyclidine, diphenylhydantoin, primidone, and sedatives. Phencyclidine can produce a combination horizontal and vertical nystagmus.

Hysteria. Signs of hysterical coma include resistance to opening of the eyelids, intentional movements, brisk pupil responses, normal muscle tone and deep tendon reflexes, and rapid resolution of deep coma.[17]

DIAGNOSTIC STUDIES

Laboratory Studies

The first laboratory study performed is a dipstick test for blood glucose level estimation. An extremely low blood sugar level indicates hypoglycemia, whereas a very high level may indicate hyperglycemic ketotic or nonketotic coma. Results of the complete blood count, and serum blood sugar, electrolyte, and BUN determinations, which are performed on a blood specimen drawn immediately before the 50 per cent glucose IV infusion was started, should be available promptly and may indicate hemorrhage, infection, electrolyte abnormality, hypoglycemia, or hyperglycemia. Most of the laboratory tests performed in the unconscious patient are listed in Table 5.

Examination of the CSF is indicated if the cause of unconsciousness is undetermined and the intracranial pressure is not increased.[1, 17] If there is any chance of increased ICP, a thin (22-gauge) needle should be used. The lumbar puncture is especially important in the comatose patient who experienced dizziness, vertigo, ataxia, or a severe headache just prior to the onset of coma. Subarachnoid hemorrhage, subdural hematoma, and meningitis should be ruled out. The fluid extracted should be analyzed for cell count, protein and glucose levels, and presence of bacteria and other organisms. A concurrent blood sugar determination is helpful in interpreting the CSF glucose level.

Focal neurologic findings associated with several red blood cells in the CSF suggest that an intracerebral hemorrhage has occurred. Focal neurologic findings associated with white blood cells and bacteria in the CSF indicate a brain abscess is likely.

Imaging

A computed tomography (CT) scan of the brain is extremely helpful in many ways. It can help diagnose with certainty life-threatening intracerebral and cerebellar hemorrhages. It can also help the clinician determine how safe a lumbar puncture will be in a particular patient by accurately determining the presence or absence of increased ICP. A CT scan also frequently saves time and money by expediting the work-up in diagnostically difficult comatose states. It is particularly helpful in detecting acute intracranial bleeding, brain abscesses, and tumors. CT scanning should not be relied on, however, to detect chronic subdural hematomas, because the blood clot may resolve into a fluid that is isodense with brain on a CT scan.[15]

X-rays of the skull and cervical spine should be taken when there is any suggestion of trauma to these areas. Basilar skull fractures and high cervical fractures are important to find as soon as possible. The finding of calcified pineal gland that is shifted to one side suggests a space-occupying lesion on the other.

Electrocardiogram

An electrocardiogram (ECG) or cardiac monitoring may reveal a dysrhythmia or a problem that can produce significant dysrhythmias such as a myocardial infarction, pericarditis, sick sinus syndrome, or other conduction defect. The presence

Table 5. LABORATORY TESTS USEFUL IN COMA

Test	Indicated Cause(s) of Coma
Complete blood count (CBC)	Hemorrhage Infection Thiamine, B_{12}, or niacin deficiency
Electrolyte determinations	Hyponatremia Inappropriate ADH (antidiuretic hormone) secretion Hypernatremia Diabetes insipidus Severe dehydration

Blood sugar level	Hypoglycemia
	  Diabetes mellitus
	  Addisonian crisis
	  Myxedema coma
	  Wernicke's encephalopathy
	Ketoacidosis
	Nonketotic hyperosmolar hyperglycemic coma

Blood urea nitrogen (BUN) and creatinine concentrations	Uremia
Ammonia and potassium levels	Hepatic coma
Arterial blood gas analysis	Hypoxia Hypercapnia
Urinalysis	Infection Hyperglycemia Poisoning
CSF analysis	Meningitis Intracerebral hemorrhage Tumor Subarachnoid hemorrhage
Lactic dehydrogenase (LDH), SGOT, alkaline phosphatase, and creatinine phosphokinase (CPK) levels	Liver failure Cardiac damage Trauma
Gastric lavage and examination of aspirate	Poisoning Overdose GI bleeding
Calcium determination	Hypercalcemia Hypocalcemia (most frequently with cancer)
Cortisol level	Addisonian crisis
T_3 and T_4 levels and free thyroxine index (FTI)	Myxedema coma
Blood smear examination	Malaria

(Adapted from Hocutt JE Jr. Emergency medicine: a quick reference for primary care. New York: ARCO Publishing, 1982:95.)

of any of these findings suggest that hypoxia may be the cause of the patient's unconsciousness.

Additional Studies

Additional laboratory tests of blood and urine will need to be performed if the cause of coma is not yet evident. One of the most common causes of unexplained coma is drug overdose. Frequently, ingestion of several drugs contributes to the unconsciousness of a single patient. Samples of blood, urine, and gastric contents should be sent for drug content analysis along with any pertinent historical information.[18] Major organ function (kidney, liver, lung, pancreas) should be evaluated, and consideration should be given to the possibility of Reye's syndrome in the patient less than 18 years old who has recently had influenza or chicken pox, ingested aspirin, or been exposed to insecticide spraying.[19, 20] Malarial blood smears should be ordered in malarial districts.[13]

ASSESSMENT

Glasgow Coma Scale

The Glasgow Coma Scale can provide information regarding the prognosis of coma. Depending on the score first determined and the rapidity of change in the score, important and relatively accurate prognostic information can be deduced. The absolute objective score on the coma scale is determined by evaluating the best eye-opening, motor, and verbal response that the patient can ex-

Table 6. GLASGOW COMA SCALE

Activity	Response	Score
Eye opening	Spontaneous	4
	To verbal command	3
	To pain	2
	None	1
Motor response		
To verbal command	Obeys	6
To painful stimulus*	Localizes pain	5
	Flexion-withdrawal	4
	Flexion abnormal (decorticate rigidity)	3
	Extension (decerebrate rigidity)	2
	None	1
Verbal response†	Oriented and converses	5
	Disoriented and converses	4
	Inappropriate words	3
	Incomprehensible sounds	2
	None	1
Total	3–15	

*Apply to two sites: first the fingertip and then the supraorbital notch.

†Arouse patient with painful stimulus if necessary.

(Adapted slightly from Gennarelli TA. A new perspective on a coma scale. Emerg Med 1982;14:87. With permission.)

hibit (Table 6).[21, 22, 23] Interpreting the total score in light of important physical findings such as marked pupil inequality greater than 1 mm) and severe head trauma leads to even better accuracy.

Severe focal trauma has the worst prognosis for each level on the coma scale, whereas depressant drug overdose (e.g., alcohol or barbiturates) has the best. The longer the period of coma and the faster the decrease in level of consciousness, the worse the prognosis. A drop of two or three points should prompt urgency in diagnosis and treatment.[21]

First Diagnostic Considerations

The very first causes of coma to be ruled out are, in order: hypoxia, life-threatening dysrhythmia, hypoglycemia, meningitis, and cerebellar hemorrhage (see Table 1). The ABCs of cardiopulmonary resuscitation (CPR) will enable the physician to immediately diagnose and begin correction of the first two causes. If hypoglycemia is suspected, a blood specimen is drawn, and a dextrose infusion is started as soon as the IV line is inserted. Primarily because of ease of diagnosis and treatment, narcotic poisoning is the next cause considered in most cases by means of immediate injection of naloxone. There have been isolated cases of non–narcotic-induced coma responding to IV naloxone.[24] Physostigmine is also given at this time if there is any possibility of anticholinergic, antihistamine, or tricyclic antidepressant overdose.[1] A response to physostigmine is diagnostic of poisoning with one of these agents until proven otherwise (Table 7).

If Addisonian crisis is a possibility, giving 100 mg of hydrocortisone in IV push after 50 per cent dextrose and 5 per cent dextrose in normal saline may lighten the level of coma. Such a response should make one look for concurrent hypotension, hyponatremia, hyperkalemia, hypoglycemia, and a low plasma cortisol level to confirm the diagnosis.[1, 3] If myxedema coma is a possibility, 50 ml of 50 per cent dextrose is given IV, followed by 5 per cent dextrose in normal saline, 100 mg hydrocortisone IV push, and 200 to 500 μg of L-thyroxine in an IV bolus. Rapid movement may be noted with light coma.

The patient with a headache, fever, and a stiff neck—especially in the presence of Kernig's and/or Brudzinski's sign—is presumed to have meningitis or CNS hemorrhage until proven otherwise. Immediate CT scan and lumbar puncture are man-

Table 7. THERAPEUTIC AGENTS WHOSE ADMINISTRATION MAY BE DIAGNOSTIC IN THE UNCONSCIOUS PATIENT

Agent	Dosage	Possible Diagnosis with Positive Response
Dextrose	50 ml of 50% dextrose in IV push (2 ml/kg in a child)	Hypoglycemia
Naloxone	0.4 mg IV push (0.01 mg/kg/dose)	Narcotic poisoning
Physostigmine	1–2 mg IV slowly	Tricyclic antidepressant, antihistamine, or anticholinergic poisoning
Thiamine	100 mg IV	Wernicke's encephalopathy
Hydrocortisone	100 mg IV push	Adrenal crisis Myxedema coma
L-Thyroxine	200–500 μg IV bolus	Myxedema coma
Oxygen	Mask or ventilator	Hypoxia

datory. If one obtains the history of vertigo, ataxia, and dizziness in addition to the headache for the unconscious patient with a stiff neck and fever, prompt consultation with a neurosurgeon is indicated.[4, 9]

Head and neck trauma are usually obvious if contributing to the patient's coma, but the physician is cautioned to avoid assuming that there is no other cause. People who take overdoses and then drive motor vehicles are prone to multiple causes of unconsciousness.

Focal Versus Nonfocal Neurologic Signs

At this point in the evaluation, if the cause of coma is still undiagnosed, the patient should be given basic life support, and the physician should try to identify any focal neurologic signs. A metabolic encephalopathy is less likely to produce focal findings and often relatively spares pupillary responses. CNS lesions, on the other hand, usually produce focal or asymmetric signs. While waiting for results of the laboratory work, the physician should concentrate diagnostic efforts in the appropriate direction.

Absence of focal neurologic or physical signs and normal CT scan and spinal fluid findings indicate a metabolic coma due to poisoning, overdose, hypoglycemia, ketotic or nonketotic coma, Addisonian crisis, electrolyte disturbance, hypertensive encephalopathy, hypoxia, uremia, hepatic failure, or myxedema. If the spinal fluid findings are abnormal and focal signs are not evident, analysis of the fluid should help discern the cause; meningitis, encephalitis, and hemorrhage are most likely. Chronic subdural hematomas often do not cause focal signs or spinal fluid abnormalities.

Focal neurologic findings usually indicate trauma, cerebrovascular accident, brain abscess, or CNS tumor. The CT scan is often very helpful in making the diagnosis.

Therapeutic versus Diagnostic Considerations

Increased intracranial pressure with signs of impending or active CNS herniation require treatment even at the expense of interrupting diagnostic measures. Extreme hyperthermia or hypothermia similarily requires immediate corrective care (see Table 1). Finally, a notable decrease in level of consciousness is a grave prognostic sign and mandates immediate heroic treatment measures before the diagnosis is confirmed.

REFERENCES

1. Hocutt JE Jr. Emergency medicine: a quick reference for primary care. New York: ARCO Publishing, 1982:91–6.
2. Caronna JJ. Diagnosis: the comatose patient. Hos Med 1980;16:37–48.
3. Plum F, Posner J. Diagnosis of stupor and coma. 2nd ed. Philadelphia: FA Davis, 1978.
4. Edmeads J. Assessing the comatose patient. Emerg Med 1982;14:71–80.
5. Goldfrank LR. A vitamin for an emergency. Emerg Med 1982;14:113–4.
6. Sabin TD. The differential diagnosis of coma. N Engl J Med 1974;290:1062–4.
7. Martin WR. Naloxone. Ann Intern Med 1976;85:765–8.
8. Rappolt RT, Gay GR. NAGD regimen for the coma of drug-related overdoses. Clin Toxicol 1980;16:395–6.
9. Ott KH, Kase CS, Ojemann RG, Mohr JP. Cerebellar hemorrhage: diagnosis and treatment. Arch Neurol 1974;31:160–7.
10. Adams RD, Victor M. Coma and related disorders of consciousness. In: Principles of neurology. New York: McGraw-Hill, 1977;200–9.
11. Denny-Brown D, Dawson DM, Tyler HR. The patient in coma. In: Handbook of neurological examination and case recording. 3rd ed. Cambridge, Mass: Harvard University Press, 1982;63–9.
12. Weiner HL, Levitt LP. Coma. In: Neurology for the house officer. 2nd ed. Baltimore: Williams & Wilkins, 1978;40–4.
13. Adams RD. Coma and related disturbances of consciousness. In: Isselbacher KJ, Adams RD, Braunwald E, Petersdorf RG, Wilson JD, eds. Harrison's principles of internal medicine. 9th ed. New York: McGraw-Hill, 1980;114–21.
14. Anderson PC. Necrotizing spider bites. Am Fam Phys 1982;26:198–203.
15. Sabin TD. Coma and the acute confusional state in the emergency room. Med Clin North Am 1981;65:15–32.
16. Guberman A. A reflex to test in coma. Emerg Med 1983;15:115–9.
17. White HH. When you're faced with an unconscious patient. Med Times 1980;108:27–31.
18. Benjamin SP. Clinical laboratory coma profile. Drug Therapy 1976;6:7–11.
19. Jarvis DA. And the unconscious child. Emerg Med 1980;12:45–52.
20. Starko KM, Ray CG, Dominguez LB, Stromberg WL, Woodall DF. Reye's syndrome and salicylate use. Pediatrics 1980;66:859–64.
21. Gennarelli TA. A new perspective on a coma scale. Emerg Med 1982;14:86–93.
22. Young B, Rapp FP, Norton JA, Haack D, Tibbs PA, Bean JR. Early prediction of outcome in head-injured patients. J Neurosurg 1981;54:300–3.
23. Dean JM, Kaufman ND. Prognostic indicators in pediatric near-drowning: the Glasgow Coma Scale. Crit Care Med 1981;9:536–9.
24. Finkelstein M, Bayne LH, Rango RE. Nonspecific arousal with naloxone. Can Med Assoc J 1980;123:33–5.

URINARY INCONTINENCE

L. KEITH LLOYD

☐ SYNONYMS: Enuresis, stress incontinence

BACKGROUND

Urinary incontinence is the involuntary loss of urine either through the urethra or through an abnormal opening between the urinary tract and the body surface. It is properly a symptom or sign and not a diagnosis unto itself, because it may be caused by a variety of abnormalities. Urinary incontinence has a broad range of severity, and as with many symptoms, the patient's perception of its severity is the major determinant in seeking medical care. It is perhaps as much a social as a medical problem, because incontinence alone does not usually result in serious disease. It may, however, be associated with rash or skin breakdown, particularly in the bedridden and debilitated. Although generally not a serious medical problem, incontinence can be psychologically devastating for both the patient and family members. It may result in withdrawn or reclusive behavior as the patient attempts to avoid situations that are socially embarrassing. Conversely, incontinence may be associated with various psychological abnormalities.[1,2]

Although urinary incontinence is a relatively common problem, the exact incidence is difficult to estimate. An epidemiologic study found the prevalence of recognized urinary incontinence in a community to be about 1 per cent.[3] A postal survey in the same community showed "unrecognized" incontinence in 8 per cent of the women and 3.3 per cent of the men. Of patients older than 65 years, it is estimated that 10 to 20 per cent of those in the general community and up to 50 per cent of those in nursing homes suffer from urinary incontinence.[4] Loss of urine or feces is a major reason for admission of the elderly into nursing homes. In the nursing home population, approximately 75 per cent of incontinent patients are female. In every age range except preadolescence, in which enuresis is more common in boys,[5] the incidence of incontinence is much greater in females.[3] This difference would seem to be related principally to the structural differences in the male and female urethra, the assaults of childbirth and sexual intercourse, and alterations in hormonal milieu to which the lower urinary tract of the female is subjected.

Normal Urinary Control

Proper assessment and diagnosis of the etiology of urinary incontinence requires a basic understanding of the normal continence mechanisms. At its simplest level, normal urinary control requires an anatomically intact urinary tract with a compliant, responsive bladder and urethra under control of the cortical inhibitory centers. Learned control of micturition begins at about the age of 2½ to 3 years in this country. Voluntary initiation of micturition usually occurs by age 3½ to 4, and the child can usually void at will with any bladder volume by age 6 or 7. Day and night control is present in 90 per cent of children by age 9.[5] The vast majority of the remainder will gain normal volitional control by the time puberty is completed. Loss of this cortical inhibitory ability is a major cause of incontinence in the elderly.[3,4]

Bladder and urethral relationships are shown in Figure 1. The bladder is a storage vessel that in the adult can normally accommodate up to 500 ml of urine while maintaining a low intravesical pressure. The functional urethra is about 4 cm long in both males and females, and during storage it maintains an active closure as a result of smooth

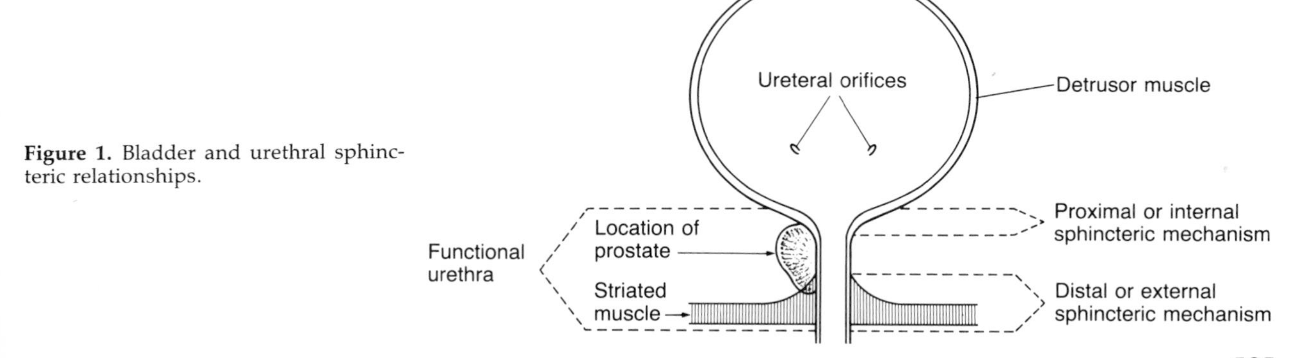

Figure 1. Bladder and urethral sphincteric relationships.

muscle, periurethral striated muscle, elastic fibers, and blood vessels.[6] A proximal urethral mechanism sometimes called the internal sphincter lies at the junction of bladder and urethra and is composed principally of smooth muscle. A distal or external sphincter mechanism, located about 2 to 3 cm distal to the bladder neck, is composed of both smooth and striated muscle. The striated muscle is most responsive to voluntary control and initially contracts in response to a command to stop voiding. Either sphincter mechanism alone is capable of providing adequate urinary control, although generally, both are better-defined and more functionally capable in the male. With loss of either sphincter mechanism, then, the male is more likely to retain normal urinary control than the female.[7]

Increases in intravesical pressure, whether passive (due to intra-abdominal pressure increase) or active (due to uncontrolled detrusor contraction), do not result in urinary incontinence as long as intraurethral pressure is maintained at a higher level. Intraurethral pressure may be maintained by intrinsic tone, by transmission of intra-abdominal pressure increases to the proximal urethra, and by active contraction. Urinary incontinence therefore occurs when intravesical pressure exceeds intraurethral pressure because of anatomic alterations in the urethrovesical anatomy, lack of proper neural control of urethral and bladder muscle, or both.

Smooth muscle of the bladder and urethra is rich in cholinergic nerve endings, whereas that of the bladder neck and proximal urethra is rich in adrenergic nerve endings, principally the alpha sympathetic type.[8] This dual innervation of bladder and urethra should be remembered particularly in relation to drugs that might exert alpha-antagonist effects and precipitate or worsen urinary incontinence.

Types of Incontinence

Urinary incontinence may be classified into several types depending upon history, physical findings, and results of laboratory tests. Such categorization is helpful in arriving at the proper diagnosis and instituting appropriate therapy. A working classification of incontinence is shown in Table 1. Historical and physical examination data will allow classification of the majority of patients presenting with incontinence. Often, however, symptoms can be misleading, and a variety of functional tests may be required to arrive at a precise diagnosis. Specific features of the various types of incontinence are discussed later.

Table 1. TYPES OF URINARY INCONTINENCE

Urge incontinence	Loss of urine associated with a strong desire to void
Stress incontinence	Loss of urine associated with increased intra-abdominal pressure in absence of detrusor activity
Overflow incontinence	Loss of urine when bladder is overfilled and urine dribbles out in small amounts at frequent intervals
Reflex incontinence	Loss of urine associated with abnormal reflex activity in absence of usual sensation of need to void
True or total incontinence	Loss of urine almost continuously with little or no accumulation in bladder
Extraurethral incontinence	Loss of urine through abnormal connection of urinary tract to body surface

Causes of Urinary Incontinence

Table 2 is a list of causes of urinary incontinence. Congenital anatomic defects and gross neurologic abnormalities are usually easily diagnosed, although careful investigation may be required to determine optimal treatment. The most common causes of urinary incontinence are stress incontinence in the middle-aged or elderly female, uninhibited bladder in the elderly male or female, and primary or secondary enuresis in the preadolescent. Multiple factors or diagnoses may contribute to urinary incontinence in the same individual. Careful history and physical examination and a few simple tests will allow a working diagnosis to be made in the majority of patients.[9]

HISTORY

Severity of incontinence often has little relationship to the severity of symptoms. Some patients tolerate an amazing amount of incontinence for long periods, and others seek medical attention at the first signs of small amounts of urinary loss. A careful history usually allows a general categorization of the type of incontinence involved and directs subsequent examinations to arrive at the proper diagnosis and treatment.

History of the Present Illness. Initial queries should allow assessment of the incontinence and any associated urologic or neurologic disturbance. How long has the incontinence been present? How severe is it? Does the patient have to employ special protection such as pads or other devices?

Table 2. CAUSES OF URINARY INCONTINENCE

	Congenital Causes	Acquired Causes
Urethral incontinence	Myelomeningocele Sacral agenesis Primary enuresis	Anatomic Stress incontinence Traumatic urethral injury Surgical urethral injury Simple prostatectomy Radical prostatectomy Transurethral resection of posterior urethral valves Y-V plasty of bladder neck Posterior urethral stricture repair Outflow obstruction with overflow incontinence Prostatic enlargement Bladder neck contracture Urethral stricture Neural-mediated Spinal cord trauma or tumors Degenerative neurologic disease Urgency incontinence Sensory Inflammatory Idiopathic Tumor Motor (uninhibited bladder) Secondary enuresis
Extraurethral incontinence	Bladder exstrophy Epispadias Ectopic ureter Patent urachus	Vesicovaginal fistula Ureterovaginal fistula

Is the incontinence intermittent or continuous? Continuous incontinence is suggestive of an extraurethral abnormality such as urinary fistula[10] or may be associated with severe loss of urethral function. Intermittent incontinence may occur in small amounts or may consist of large gushes of urine. *Enuresis* is the term applied to sudden uncontrolled voiding, and although it is often taken to mean simple bedwetting, it can occur in the day or night and should be appropriately termed diurnal or nocturnal enuresis, respectively. This type of incontinence is usually seen in children or the elderly and is due to lack of cortical inhibition of the micturition reflex.

If incontinence occurs in smaller amounts, is it related to activity or is it associated with a desire to void? If related to activity, does it take vigorous physical activity or can it be precipitated by change of position or mild coughing? Activity-related incontinence, or stress incontinence, can be due to involuntary detrusor contractions or impaired sphincteric activity. It is difficult to distinguish them on the basis of historical data alone,[11] but an associated history of urinary frequency and urgency is suggestive of involuntary detrusor activity.

Are there associated urinary tract symptoms? Urinary frequency and urgency suggest involuntary detrusor activity but may also indicate associated urinary tract infection. Burning with urination and pelvic, low back, and perineal pain may signify urinary tract infection. Hematuria may be associated with either urinary tract infection or urothelial tumors, and its presence, especially in older patients (over 45 years), merits careful urologic investigation. Are there any symptoms of urethral obstruction, such as decreased size and force of stream, hesitancy, intermittency, and terminal dribbling?

Important associated symptoms relating to bowel control, sexual function, and lower extremity function should be sought. Motor and sensory innervation to the bladder is principally from sacral cord segments 2, 3, and 4. These segments also supply innervation to the lower bowel and the genitalia. An impairment of sexual function, change in bowel habit, or fecal incontinence would suggest the possibility of sacral or distal spinal cord neuropathy as a cause of incontinence. Likewise, any abnormality that affects the spinal cord, causing neurological impairment of bladder function, may also affect the lower extremities, resulting in weakness, spasticity, or impaired sensation.

Previous Medical History. Important features here relate to previous urinary or genital tract disease or neurologic disease. Of particular importance are surgical procedures on the urethra in the male such as prostatectomy and urethral stricture repair. Relevant procedures in the female are any gynecologic operation such as hysterectomy (simple or radical) or anterior vaginal repair, and previous surgical treatment of urinary incontinence. Onset of continuous urinary leakage 1 to 4 weeks after hysterectomy is almost certainly due to vesicovaginal fistula. Has the patient ever undergone radiation therapy for pelvic or genital tumors? Radiation therapy can result in tissue damage that may not appear or become symptomatic until many years later.

Has there been any previous neurologic disease or surgery? Surgery for lumbar disc disease suggests the possibility of neurologic bladder dysfunction. Any intracranial procedure may result in some impairment of cortical inhibitory activity. Is there any history of diabetes?

Family History. This aspect is probably of significance only in childhood enuresis. A history of bedwetting or delayed urinary control in parents or siblings of a child with bedwetting is common and suggests the same benign disorder in the patient.[5]

Drug History. Any drug that possesses autonomic activity (either agonist or inhibitor) can affect lower urinary tract function. Particular classes of drugs to note are antihypertensives, psychotropic agents, antihistamine-decongestants, and gastrointestinal drugs. Obtaining the drug history is particularly important in the elderly patient, who may be taking multiple drugs that may have an additive effect.

PHYSICAL EXAMINATION

Physical examination is directed toward the genitourinary system, but some general evaluation is necessary to fully assess the patient's complaints and is also helpful in directing therapeutic options.

Assessment of mental status is valuable in determining whether urinary loss may be based on impaired cortical inhibition, because there is some correlation between the two.[4] Evaluation of general mobility is also helpful, particularly in the elderly; transient lack of mobility, such as that due to fracture or arthritis, often precipitates incontinence in the elderly.[4]

Abdominal examination will disclose obvious abnormalities such as bladder exstrophy. Drops of urine and periumbilical inflammation will be seen in patent urachus, although this is a rare disorder. Palpation for bladder distension is helpful to identify patients with urinary retention and overflow incontinence.

Examination of the external genitalia in the male is often not helpful other than to note erythema and excoriation as a result of incontinence. Epididymal induration is suggestive of urinary tract infection particularly in the elderly. The patient should be asked to cough, to determine whether urinary leakage occurs with increased intra-abdominal pressure. If leakage is present, is it just a small amount (stress incontinence) or does coughing precipitate full voiding? Examination of the prostate will disclose prostatic enlargement due to benign hyperplasia or carcinoma, although size of the prostate does not necessarily correlate with degree of outflow obstruction.

Examination of the external genitalia in the female allows assessment of vaginal tissues for hormonal effect. Atrophic vaginitis, manifested by thin, shiny, erythematous, and friable mucosa, may be a precipitating or aggravating factor in the postmenopausal female. Is cystocele, rectocele, or uterine prolapse present? Presence or absence of these abnormalities gives some idea of the integrity of pelvic supporting tissues. The physician should ask the patient to cough or strain while examining the vagina to see if the urethra and bladder base are well-supported. A large vesicovaginal fistula may be seen easily on vaginal speculum examination, although detection of smaller fistulas may require special measures. Urethra and bladder base should be palpated to see whether any tenderness is present, which would suggest bladder inflammation. The urethra can be stripped with the examining finger to ascertain whether any purulent material is expressed, as with urethral diverticulum.

The female patient should be asked to cough with the bladder partially full while the urethra is examined for incontinence. The Bonney test is performed by elevating the anterior vaginal wall with the index and middle fingers, taking care not to compress the urethra. If this maneuver prevents leakage during coughing and leakage resumes on release of anterior elevation, a presumptive diagnosis of anatomic stress incontinence is made. Many false-positive results occur, however, and some investigators believe that the Bonney test adds little to the evaluation.[11]

Neurologic Examination. In addition to general neurologic examination, certain features have special relevance to urinary tract dysfunction. The lower extremities should be examined for strength and sensation. Deep tendon reflexes and Babinski reflex should be checked for the presence of suprasacral long tract signs.

Perineal and genital sensations to pinprick and light touch give a measure of the integrity of sacral cord segments 2, 3, and 4. These sensations are mediated through the pudendal nerve and do not correlate perfectly with impaired bladder function, but their integrity does give a reasonable estimate of spinal cord function in these dermatomes. Anal tone and volitional control of anal contraction also allow assessment of the sacral cord segments. Anal reflex and bulbocavernosus reflex may be elicited by scratching the perianal skin and compressing the glans penis or clitoris. If the sacral reflex arc is intact, the anal sphincter will contract. It should be remembered, however, that the bulbocavernosus reflex is normally absent in a significant portion of the population.

DIAGNOSTIC STUDIES

Urinalysis

Microscopic examination of the urine should be done in all patients to ascertain presence of urinary tract infection or hematuria. Urine culture and sensitivity tests should be performed if there is a history of urinary tract infection, symptoms suggesting infection, or abnormal urinalysis results.

Residual Urine Determination

Measurement of the bladder residual volume immediately after voiding is helpful in assessing patients in whom outflow obstruction is suspected and in the elderly, in whom the history may be poor and the incidence of obstructive problems is somewhat higher. The patient is asked to empty the bladder, and immediately afterward, a small (12–14F) catheter is passed per urethra and the residual volume is determined. It should normally be less than 30 ml. Urine obtained at this time may be used for culture and sensitivity determination.

Imaging

Excretory urography (intravenous pyelography [IVP]) should be performed in any patient (1) with suspicion of outflow obstruction, (2) with a history of urinary tract infection, or (3) with continuous incontinence, particularly when onset followed recent surgery. Patients with overt neurologic disease of the bladder may have abnormalities on IVP, such as ureteral dilatation or pyelocaliectasis, which would have some influence on therapeutic decisions. Ureterovaginal fistula may be demonstrated, or the usually associated ureteral obstruction may be evident. In incontinence secondary to ectopic ureter, IVP may show a duplicated collecting system[12] or the "drooping lily" appearance of the lower pole collecting system if the ectopic upper system is functioning poorly.

Cystography may be performed alone or in conjunction with urinary pressure-flow studies. The cystogram may demonstrate a vesicovaginal fistula or reflux into the lower collecting system of a complete duplication (ectopic ureter). Lateral films taken during straining or bearing down may show descent of the bladder base and proximal urethra, as may be seen in anatomic stress incontinence. Competence of the distal mechanism (external sphincter area) can be assessed by asking the patient to stop voiding and observing the "milking-back" of contrast in the normal, proximal urethra.[7, 11]

Cystoscopy

Endoscopic examination of the bladder and urethra often provides valuable information to assist in diagnosis and management. Residual urine determination can be made at the same time if it was not done previously or if a redetermination is desired.

The bladder mucosa may show evidence of chronic inflammation such as erythema or cystitis cystica. Trabeculation, cellules, and diverticula may be seen in association with outflow obstruction or neurologic bladder dysfunction. Vesicovaginal fistula may be detected; it is most commonly seen just above the interureteric ridge. Incidental mucosal lesions may occasionally be found.

The urethra should be examined for evidence of previous surgical procedures at the vesical outlet, surgical or traumatic injury to the external sphincter area, and urethral stricture. Rigidity or fixation of the periurethral tissues secondary to prior surgery, injury, or irradiation may be discovered. An ectopic orifice can be sought, although these are generally quite difficult to visualize.

Dye Tests

In some cases when vesicovaginal fistula or ureterovaginal fistula is suspected but not located by speculum, endoscopic, or radiographic examination, intravenous administration of indigo carmine and/or intravesical instillation of indigo carmine or milk allows visualization of the fistula.[10] A gauze sponge placed in the vagina will show whether leakage is per urethra or from a fistula higher in the vaginal vault.

Urodynamic Testing

Modern methods of urodynamic testing permit accurate functional evaluation of the detrusor and urethral mechanisms.[7, 11, 13, 14] Such testing is essential in the evaluation and management of neurologic bladder dysfunction and complicated incontinence. The level of testing required depends in part on the disorder and in part on the preferences of the investigator. The various types of testing available are reviewed briefly.

Urinary flow rate is a basic screening examination that gives an overall measure of detrusor and urethral function. Peak urinary flow, average flow, and appearance of the curve all may be helpful, although peak flow is generally considered the single most useful parameter.[15] Flow will vary in relation to voided volume, sex, and age.[15, 16] Electromyography (EMG) of the striated external sphincter may be added to determine whether there is appropriate relaxation during voiding.[17] Females with impaired urethral resistance and anatomic stress incontinence may have very high peak flow rates.

Urethral pressure profiles measure intraurethral pressures and may be performed either as a static measurement of resistance[18] or as part of dynamic testing during pressure-flow studies.[13] These measurements have not proved as helpful as initially anticipated but are useful in the overall assessment and management of complicated bladder-urethral dysfunction.

Cystometrography, probably the most useful test of bladder function, may be performed in a variety of ways. Important measurements are: functional bladder capacity, sensation perceived during bladder filling, presence or absence of uninhibited bladder contractions, presence or absence of the normal contractile response to bladder filling, and the patient's ability to suppress this response. EMG of the external sphincter may be combined with cystometrography to establish whether there is appropriate relaxation of the striated periurethral muscle during bladder contraction. Simultaneous measurement of rectal (intra-abdominal) pressure permits distinction between intravesical pressure increases that are detrusor-mediated and those that are secondary to increases in general intra-abdominal pressure during cough, laugh, or straining to void. In evaluation of the incontinent patient, the functional bladder capacity and presence of uninhibited or hyperactive detrusor responses are the most important features to discern.[11]

Cystometrography may be combined with radiography by the use of a contrast agent for bladder filling. Simultaneous measurements of intra-abdominal and intraurethral pressures and urinary flow rate and EMG of the external sphincter may be utilized for a comprehensive investigation of bladder and urethral function.[11, 13] Although such comprehensive testing is not necessary in all patients, it may be valuable in assessing patients with complicated disorders of micturition.

ASSESSMENT

It can be seen from the preceding discussion that a wide variety of tests are available for assessing the incontinent patient. The level of testing required depends upon the clinical situation and is guided by the history and physical findings. A brief discussion of the most common causes of urinary incontinence may help place this in perspective. Childhood enuresis, female stress incontinence, and incontinence in the elderly are the most common situations the practitioner will be called upon to evaluate and treat.

Some degree of enuresis may be present in up to 10 per cent of children as late as age 9.[4] In the past, these children often received thorough urologic investigation, although recent studies clearly show such an approach to be unnecessary unless there is associated urinary tract infection or symptoms of obstruction.[19, 20] A rational program of management can then be based upon results of history, physical examination, and urinalysis for most patients.

Female stress incontinence remains a somewhat problematic area. Stress incontinence may be a symptom, a sign, or a condition.[21] Historical data may be misleading[11]; the best results of therapy are usually achieved through careful and detailed examination, including urinalysis, radiography, cystourethroscopy, and urodynamic assessment.[13] Previously failed incontinence surgery and significant symptoms of urgency and frequency are especially important indicators of the need for detailed evaluation.[22] Patients with such features are perhaps best served by referral to special centers.

Urinary incontinence in the elderly is most often due to cortical inhibition impairment or urethral sphincter incompetence.[9, 23] Level of evaluation in these patients is also highly dependent on the clinical situation. Often, bedfast patients and those with severe cortical functional impairment are best treated simply, with catheters or incontinence aids, rather than being subjected to extensive investigation. In less severely impaired patients, a logical and stepwise assessment allows adequate management with a minimum of expensive and invasive testing.[9] Following the steps outlined in this chapter should enable one to arrive at an accurate diagnosis and rational plan of management for most patients.

REFERENCES

1. Frewen WK. An objective assessment of the unstable bladder of psychosomatic origin. Br J Urol 1978;50:246–9.
2. Berg I, Fielding D, Meadow R. Psychiatric disturbance, urgency, and bacteriuria in children with day and night wetting. Arch Dis Child 1977;52:651–7.
3. Fenely RCL, Shepherd AM, Powell PH, Blannin J. Urinary incontinence: prevalence and needs. Br J Urol 1979;51:493–6.
4. Ouslander JG, Kane RL, Abrass IB. Urinary incontinence in elderly nursing home patients. JAMA 1982;248:1194–8.
5. Doleys, DM, Dolce JJ. Toilet training and enuresis. Pediatr Clin North 1982;29:297–313.
6. Gosling J. The structure of the bladder and urethra in relation to function. Urol Clin North Am 1979;6:31–8.

7. Turner-Warwick RT. Observations on the function and dysfunction of the sphincter and detrusor mechanisms. Urol Clin North Am 1979;6:13–30.
8. Elbadawi A. Neuromorphologic basis of vesico-urethral function: I. Histochemistry, ultra-structure, and function of intrinsic nerves of the bladder and urethra. Neurourol Urodynam 1982;1:3–50.
9. Hilton P, Stanton SL. Algorithmic method for assessing urinary incontinence in elderly women. Br Med J 1981;282:940–2.
10. Goodwin WE, Scardino PT. Vesicovaginal and ureterovaginal fistulas: a summary of 25 years of experience. J Urol 1980;123:370–4.
11. Stanton SL. Preoperative investigation and diagnosis. Clin Obstet Gynecol 1978;21:705–24.
12. Zornow DH. Embryology of urinary incontinence. Urology 1977;10:293–300.
13. McGuire EJ, Lytton B, Pepe V, Kohorn EI. Stress urinary incontinence. Obstet Gynecol 1976;47:255–64.
14. Mayo ME, Ansell JS. Urodynamic assessment of incontinence after prostatectomy. J Urol 1979;122:60–1.
15. Drach GW, Layton T, Bottacini MR. A method of adjustment of male peak urinary flow rate for varying age and volume voided. J Urol 1982;128:960–2.
16. Siroky MB, Olsson CA, Krane RJ. The flow rate nomogram: I. Development. J Urol 1979;122:665–8.
17. Kaplan WE, Firlit CF, Schoenberg HW. The female urethral syndrome: external sphincter spasm as etiology. J Urol 1980;124:48–9.
18. Brown M, Wickham J. The urethral pressure profile. Br J Urol 1969;41:211–6.
19. Redman JF, Seibert JJ. The uroradiographic evaluation of the enuretic child. J Urol 1979;122:799–801.
20. Kass EJ, Diokno AC, Montealegre A. Enuresis: principles of management and result of treatment. J Urol 1979;121:794–6.
21. Bates P, Bradley WE, Glen E, et al. The standardization of terminology of lower urinary tract function. J Urol 1979;121:551–4.
22. Stanton SL, Cardozo L, Williams JE, Ritchie D, Allan V. Clinical and urodynamic features of failed incontinence surgery in the female. Obstet Gynecol 1978;51:515–20.
23. Vetter NJ, Jones DA, Victor CR. Urinary incontinence in the elderly at home. Lancet 1981;2:1275–7.

URTICARIA, CHRONIC

M. ELIZABETH ARCHER □ JOSEPH L. JORIZZO

□ SYNONYMS: Hives, welts, nettle rash

BACKGROUND

Definitions

Urticaria is a vascular reaction clinically characterized by evanescent, circumscribed, raised, erythematous areas of edema involving the superficial portion of the dermis. These areas, called wheals, are usually pruritic. Individual wheals arise suddenly and most often resolve within 24 hours.

Angioedema is the deeper reaction that occurs when the edematous process extends through the dermis and into the subcutaneous or submucosal tissue. Angioedema occurs most commonly on the face and extremities and often with urticaria, although either can occur alone. In a study of 554 patients with angioedema or urticaria, 40 per cent had urticaria alone, 11 per cent had angioedema alone, and 49 per cent had both.

Urticaria is usually defined as chronic when it occurs daily and persists for more than 4 weeks. Akers and Naversen,[2] however, also consider urticaria that occurs 4 days of the week for more than 8 weeks to be chronic.

Incidence

Persons of any sex, race, age, or occupation can be affected by urticaria. An estimate has been made that 15 to 20 per cent of the population are affected by urticaria at some time during their lives.[3] The incidence is 0.11 per cent in males and 0.14 per cent in females. Acute urticaria occurs most often in young adults, and chronic urticaria in middle-aged women.[5]

Pathogenesis

Urticaria may have a variety of causes and may be mediated by immunologic as well as nonimmunologic factors. The mechanisms underlying urticaria are not entirely known, but the final common pathway is thought to involve activation of mast cells and basophilic leukocytes. When these cells are activated, they release mediator substances that increase vascular permeability. With this increase, plasma leaks into the dermis and the wheals of urticaria result.

One immunologic mechanism in urticaria is immediate, or type I, hypersensitivity reaction, the central element of which is IgE antibodies. IgE is produced by B lymphocytes and plasma cells in response to antigens, including proteins, polysaccharides, and haptens. Once IgE is formed, it can bind to mast cells and basophils by means of Fc receptors. Then, upon stimulation by the antigen, in which the antigen bridges at least two of the IgE molecules on the mast cells or basophils, numerous biologically active products are released from the mast cells or basophils. These products are discussed later. (The biochemical mechanisms governing the release of the mediators has been reviewed in detail.)[3, 6, 7]

Urticaria may be caused by immunologic mechanisms that do not require IgE.[6] The interaction of antigens with IgG or IgM can activate the classic complement cascade and produce the anaphylatoxins C3a and C5a, which on their own can cause the release of histamine from mast cells and basophils. The alternative pathway of the complement cascade may result in mast cell degranulation via C3a and C5a after activation with agents such as endotoxins, venoms, and inulin.[5]

Circulating immune complex, or type III, hypersensitivity reactions are responsible for some cases of urticaria, such as urticarial vasculitis. Immune complexes are aggregations of antigen, antibody, and complement formed in the circulation or tissue. These immune complexes can interact with blood vessel walls and other tissues and can cause tissue damage through the activation of complement and the influx of neutrophils, resulting in a characteristic histopathologic appearance called leukocytoclastic vasculitis.[6]

In addition to immunologic mechanisms, a variety of chemicals can release histamine from mast cells and basophils by direct pharmacologic mechanisms that are thought not to involve immunologic processes.[6] These chemicals include amines, codeine, morphine, curare, quinine, thiamine, aspirin, and the newer nonsteroidal anti-inflammatory agents.

Physical agents such as heat, cold, light, and vibration may also cause histamine release and urticaria. The release of histamine and other mediators in the physical urticarias may occur by immunologic or nonimmunologic means or a combination of both.[6, 7]

Once mast cells and basophils are activated, a variety of mediators are released that may cause urticaria. Histamine and slow-reacting substance of anaphylaxis (SRS-A) both cause a relaxation of vascular smooth muscle and an increase in vascular permeability. SRS-A also causes prostaglandins to be generated, and arachidonic acid metabolites, such as the prostaglandins and leukotrienes, increase vascular permeability, have effects on smooth muscle contraction, and enhance chemotaxis of eosinophils and neutrophils. Eosinophil chemotactic factor of anaphylaxis (ECF-A), ECF-oligopeptides, lipid chemotactic factors, and high-molecular-weight neutrophil chemotactic factor (HMW-NCF) are all mast cell and basophil products that cause chemotactic attraction or deactivation of eosinophils or neutrophils.[7]

Histology

The histopathologic features of an individual wheal usually include: edema of the dermis, dilation and engorgement of blood vessels, and a mild polymorphous, perivascular infiltrate composed mainly of lymphocytes and a few eosinophils.[9] These findings are most evident in the middle and upper parts of the dermis in urticaria. In angioedema, the primary involvement is in the lower dermis and subcutaneous tissue.[9]

The histopathologic appearance of urticaria secondary to vasculitis differs from that of other urticarias. Urticarial vasculitis is characterized histologically by endothelial swelling of the blood vessel wall, leukocytoclasis (breaking up of neutrophils), fibrinoid deposits in and around the blood vessel walls, extravasation of red blood cells, and a perivascular leukocytic infiltrate.[9]

HISTORY

In most patients, determining the underlying cause of urticaria is difficult, and without a careful history, it is impossible. A complete history of the present illness, review of systems, family history, social history, and medication history are necessary in every case of chronic urticaria.

In obtaining a history of the present illness, it is helpful to ask how long individual wheals last in order to separate urticaria from dermatologic conditions that mimic urticaria. Urticarial wheals usually resolve within 2 to 4 hours, and to fit the definition, individual lesions must not last for more than 24 hours.

It is important to discover whether the patient has observed an association between the onset of urticaria and any other factor. Specifically, one should ask about all medications being used by the patient, including vitamins, contraceptives, laxatives, and salicylates. It is also important to inquire about recent infections. Occult urinary tract infections, tooth abscesses, and sinusitis can cause urticaria. If the urticaria is seasonal, pollens are a possible etiology. Patients should be asked about symptoms indicative of serum sickness, such as fever, arthralgias, arthritis, and myalgias, which would suggest then the possibility of urticaria secondary to circulating immune complexes (serum sickness with urticaria or urticarial vasculitis).

Table 1. SOME CAUSES OF URTICARIA

Infections	Bacterial Dental abscess Sinusitis Otitis Cholecystitis Pneumonitis Cystitis Hepatitis Vaginitis Fungal Tinea Candida Other Scabies Helminth Protozoa Trichomonas
Drugs and chemicals	Salicylates Indomethacin and other, newer nonsteroidal anti-inflammatory agents Opiates Radiocontrast material Penicillin (medication, milk, blue cheese) Sulfonamides Sodium benzoate Cosmetics Douches Ear or eye drops Insulin Menthol (cigarettes, toothpaste, iced tea, hand cream, lozenges, candy) Tartrazine (vitamins, birth control pills, antibiotics, TDC yellow #5)
Foods	Nuts Berries Fish Seafood Bananas Grapes Tomatoes Eggs Cheese
Inhalants	Animal danders Pollen
Contactants	Wool Silk Occupational exposure Potatoes Antibiotics Cosmetics Dyes Hair spray Nail polish Mouthwash Toothpaste Perfumes Hand cream Soap Insect repellent
Endocrinopathies	Hyperthyroidism Menstruation Hormones
Physical stimuli	Dermatographism Light Pressure Heat Cold Water Vibration
Systemic diseases	Rheumatic fever Juvenile rheumatoid arthritis Leukemia Lymphoma Collagen vascular disease
Familial disorders	Hereditary angioedema Muckle-Wells syndrome

Inquiry should be made about each of the possible causes of chronic urticaria listed in Table 1. Having a questionnaire available to give to a patient with urticaria may facilitate uncovering the cause, because often a patient will not consider something as a possible cause or will not be able to remember exposure to a substance unless reminded. For instance, patients who deny taking medications may be taking vitamins or other over-the-counter preparations that they do not consider important.

PHYSICAL EXAMINATION

A complete physical examination may reveal systemic signs associated with urticaria or systemic causes of urticaria. The clinical signs and symptoms occur soon after exposure to an appropriate antigen in immunologic urticaria, so it is especially important to examine the patient as soon as possible, although prompt examination is equally important for nonimmunologic urticaria.

Physical examination of the skin will reveal an erythematous wheal of localized dermal edema. The wheals may vary in size from papules less than 1 cm in diameter to large plaques. The lesions may coalesce and form annular or geographic configurations; they are generally pruritic, so excoriations and (rarely) even secondary infection may be present.

At times, patients are not aware of the transitory nature of the individual wheals. Asking a patient to draw a line around a wheal and then to observe it a few hours later will help to confirm whether or not it lasts for less than 24 hours and, therefore, represents true urticaria. Urticaria can appear suddenly and may resolve within a few hours, or new lesions can continue to appear.[5]

Dermatographism is a linear wheal that appears when the skin has been stroked with a firm object, such as a fingernail or pen top. The wheal usually fades within 30 minutes. This sign is often observed on physical examination of a patient with urticaria, but it has an incidence of 4.2 per cent in the general population.[5] Eliciting dermatographism is a useful means of monitoring the adequacy of antihistamine therapy in urticaria patients. Antihistamines can be increased to the point where no urticarial wheal is produced by skin stroking.

Urticaria may be accompanied by systemic signs and symptoms, stemming either from urticarial involvement of viscera or from an indirect effect of the systemic release of chemicals such as histamine and acetylcholine.[5] Wheals of the deeper type, known as angioedema, may occur with involvement of mucous membranes, tongue, soft palate, pharynx, and even larynx. This involvement may give rise to signs of hoarseness and respiratory difficulty. Anorexia, abdominal pain, and gastrointestinal bleeding may be seen as the result of swelling of the mucous membranes in the stomach and intestines. Headaches, flushing, and increased salivation may also be observed. Occasionally, neurologic complications have been reported as a consequence of urticaria.[7] Cerebral edema may result in coma, mental confusion, hemiparesis, headaches, and convulsions. Hypotension, syncope, shock, and anuria may be seen, especially in acute urticaria associated with anaphylaxis.

A search should be made for physical signs of systemic diseases that can cause urticaria. A careful check for signs of infection such as maxillary tenderness, costovertebral angle tenderness, poor dentition, vaginal discharge, and tinea pedis is useful. The patient should be examined for signs of serum sickness such as arthritis, lymphadenopathy, and hepatomegaly as well as purpura within the urticarial lesions. These findings support a diagnosis of urticaria mediated by circulating immune complexes, such as serum sickness with urticaria or urticarial vasculitis.

ASSESSMENT: CAUSES OF URTICARIA

After the initial history and physical examination, the cause of the urticaria must be investigated. In acute urticaria a specific cause may be found 80 per cent of the time, but in chronic urticaria, only 20 per cent of the time.[6] Further evaluation should be done in stages and should be guided by what is learned from the history and physical examination. Table 2 lists the types of urticaria.

Table 2. TYPES OF URTICARIA

Immunologic urticaria IgE-dependent	Atopic diathesis Antigen sensitivity Physical urticaria Symptomatic dermatographism Delayed dermatographism Pressure urticaria Solar urticaria Cold urticaria Heat urticaria Cholinergic urticaria Aquagenic urticaria Vibratory angioedema
Complement-mediated	Hereditary angioedema Acquired angioedema
Possible circulating immune complex mechanism	Urticarial vasculitis Reaction to blood products Serum sickness
Nonimmunologic urticaria	Urticaria due to direct mast cell releasing agents Urticaria due to agents that alter arachidonic acid metabolism
Idiopathic urticaria	

Numerous laboratory tests could be done to evaluate urticaria. To perform all of the tests, however, would be too costly and is usually unrewarding. The tests are chosen on the basis of the history and physical findings. A "shotgun" approach should be avoided. Laboratory tests that may help confirm causes of urticaria are listed in Table 3.

If individual lesions persist for longer than 24 hours and if symptoms and signs of serum sickness are present, then a biopsy specimen should be taken of an urticarial lesion. Biopsy of one of these lesions may show a form of vasculitis (leukocytoclastic vasculitis) that would be compatible

Table 3. LABORATORY TESTS THAT MAY BE HELPFUL IN EVALUATION OF URTICARIA

Complete blood count with differential counts
Erythrocyte sedimentation rate
VDRL test
Hepatitis B surface antigen assay
Monospot test (mononucleosis-heterophile test)
T_3 resin uptake and T_4 level
Antinuclear antibody test
C3 and C4 tests
Antistreptolysin titer
Urinalysis
Vaginal smear
Stool specimen examination for ova and parasites
Sinus radiographs
Dental radiographs
Skin biopsy
Other specific tests as directed by history and physical examination

with a diagnosis of urticarial vasculitis.[10] This is an important distinction, because the treatment and prognosis of urticarial vasculitis are different from those of the usual chronic urticaria.[10] Some additional laboratory data tests that might be performed in patients with urticarial vasculitis include: C3, C4, and antinuclear antibody tests, determination of erythrocyte sedimentation rate, and urinalysis.

Immunologic Urticarias

IgE-Dependent Urticarias

Atopic Diathesis

Patients with a personal or family history of eczema, allergic rhinitis, or asthma have a higher incidence of urticaria and angioedema, although the skin disorders seldom accompany an exacerbation of any of these conditions.[6]

Antigen Sensitivity

Hundreds of substances are capable of causing a type I (immediate) hypersensitivity reaction that can result in urticaria. Occasionally, a patient will recognize a relationship between a specific substance and episodes of urticaria. When a specific cause is suspected but cannot be isolated by the patient, food diaries, elimination diets, scratch testing, therapeutic trials, and oral challange tests can be helpful.

Food allergy may be responsible for only 5 per cent of cases of urticaria, but when it is suspected, a food diary may be helpful.[2] The patient is told to record everything ingested, including medications, as well as the days when urticaria appears. The onset of episodes of urticaria may be correlated with exposure to specific substances, which can then be eliminated from the patient's diet.

Some physicians prefer elimination diets to food diaries, although the two can often be combined effectively. A variety of food elimination diets are available. Patients with a history of penicillin allergy should be given a pencillin-free diet, excluding milk, milk products, wines, beer, and frozen turkey.[2] Patients with a history of aspirin or salicylate allergy should be given a salicylate-free diet. Noid and associates[11] have described a diet free of salicylate, tartrazine, benzoic acid, and azo dye that may be used. Akers and Naversen[2] use a "rare-food" diet, which eliminates penicillin, molds, yeasts, salicylates, and food additives and which consists of green tea, water, cane sugar, sea salt, whole rice, and one meat that is eaten only rarely (lamb, duck, rabbit, or frog legs). If a food is the culprit, improvement should be seen by the fifth day of the elimination diet. If no improvement occurs after 7 days, causes other than food must be sought. If a patient remains free of urticaria after 7 days, a single food can be added every 48 hours provided that urticaria does not recur. If urticaria does recur, that food must be eliminated and then reintroduced after a 5-day interval to confirm the observation.[6]

Scratch testing with inhalants and food allergens is seldom recommended by dermatologists because the procedure has proved unreliable in evaluating urticaria patients.[12] Small and associates[12] found that some of their patients had skin reactivity to multiple agents but a specific diagnosis of food or inhalant allergy could not be correlated with a positive skin test result.[12]

Akers and Naversen[2] have summarized a series of therapeutic trials for occult bacterial infections, occult dermatophytosis, inapparent scabies, amebic infestations, trichomonal infections, yeast allergy, and dermatitis herpetiformis.[2] An improvement during a therapeutic trial suggests a possible cause. We favor accurate diagnosis, however, rather than arbitrary experimental therapy.

Oral challenge tests may also be helpful when a specific substance is suspected, but such challenges are done when the urticaria is under control. Akers and Naversen[2] have summarized the guidelines for a 13-day test battery. They test tartrazine, benzoate, food dyes, yeast extract, and aspirin. Extreme caution should be exercised in the performance of oral challenge tests, because urticarial reactions may be severe. Challenge testing should be performed only under the supervision of a physician because of the risk of anaphylactic reactions.

Physical Urticarias

Physical urticarias are a subgroup of chronic urticarias (accounting for 7 to 17 per cent of all cases)[13] in which lesions are induced by various physical stimuli (see Table 2). Some forms of physical urticaria are IgE-dependent, as confirmed by passive transfer experiments, but the mechanism of others remains unknown.

The physical urticarias are distinguished from other forms of chronic urticaria by frequent occurrence in young adults, short duration of lesions, restriction of the lesions to areas of physical stimuli, a tendency of lesions not to occur at night, inducibility by physical stimuli, and general unresponsiveness to systemic corticosteroid therapy.[13]

Symptomatic Dermatographism. Dermatographism appears as an exaggerated, transient, wheal and flare response after firm stroking of the skin. The back is the most responsive area. Symptomatic dermatographism describes the state in patients who complain of generalized pruritus.[7] Patients experience episodes of itching and they rub or scratch the skin, which then develops urticarial wheals at the traumatized sites. A positive dermatographism test result alone is not sufficient for a diagnosis of symptomatic dermatographism, because normal persons may have dermatographism. Both the history and physical findings and a positive provocation test result are required for the diagnosis to be made. It is not unusual for patients to have persistent positive test results for dermatographism but to become symptomatic only episodically.[13]

Delayed Dermatographism. In this form of urticaria, a normal triple response of Lewis, or a dermatographic response, may occur after a dermatographic stimulus but will resolve in 20 to 30 minutes. Then, after 1 to 8 hours, deep, painful, discontinuous wheals develop at the dermatographic test site and last perhaps 24 to 48 hours. The diagnosis of delayed dermatographism is made on clinical grounds, is substantiated by the appearance of a delayed and persistent wheal after testing, and must be differentiated from that of pressure urticaria.

Pressure Urticaria. Pressure urticaria is characterized by the development of deep, tender wheals 3 to 12 hours after the local application of pressure.[13] The wheals persist for 8 to 24 hours. Two notable features of affected patients are that they are young and that they do not develop the early lesions seen in delayed dermatographism. Any skin site can be affected, but certain activities predispose specific body areas to develop lesions. Wheals may develop on the hands after clapping, on the feet after walking, or on the buttocks after sitting.[13] Refractory periods of up to 7 days have been observed after resolution of lesions.[15] Patients may be unaware of the association between pressure and urticaria because of the delayed onset of the lesions. A diagnostic test for pressure urticaria is performed by placing a weight (8 kg, 4 cm in diameter) on the thigh for 10 to 20 minutes and then examining the site 4 and 8 hours afterwards for signs of urticaria.[13]

Solar Urticaria. Solar urticaria may occur as a primary disease or in association with other diseases such as porphyria cutanea tarda, systemic lupus erythematosus, and erythropoietic protoporphyria.[14] Solar urticaria is manifested by the prompt formation of a pruritic wheal at the site of exposure to the appropriate wavelengths of light. Affected patients will experience wheals within 5 minutes after exposure to electromagnetic waves or to ultraviolet or visible light. The wheals persist for 15 minutes to 3 hours, and their severity correlates with the duration and intensity of light exposure.[13]

Phototesting is an important part of the evaluation of patients with solar urticaria. This procedure can be performed in an office with a hot quartz lamp or outdoors with natural sunlight, with and without a window glass filter to separate the effects of ultraviolet-A (UVA) and ultraviolet-B (UVB) radiation (the glass filters out UVA). Most patients have lesions induced by UVB (290 nm); others are sensitive to UVA (320–400 nm).[13] Solar urticaria needs to be differentiated from polymorphic light eruption (PMLE), the lesions of which occur hours or days after exposure to light rather than within minutes. Also, they last for longer than 24 hours, whereas lesions of solar urticaria resolve within several hours.

Cold Urticaria. Cold urticaria may be seen secondary to underlying disease such as cryoglobulinemia, cryofibrinogenemia, cold hemolysis, crystalglobulinemia, connective tissue diseases, paroxysmal cold hemoglobinuria of syphilis, and hematopoietic malignancies.[3] Cold urticaria also occurs in an acquired and familial form.

Essential, acquired cold urticaria is the most common type of cold urticaria. Young adults are most often affected, and the onset often follows a systemic disturbance, emotional stress, viral illness, or multiple insect bites.[13] Patients develop wheals at the sites of cold contact within minutes of rewarming. The wheals last for 1 to 2 hours and have been associated with bronchospasm, angioedema, hypotension, and flushing and have even been associated with death by drowning.[13] Provocative testing with an ice cube or by immersing the patient's arm in cold water will help to make the diagnosis of essential cold urticaria.

Familial cold urticaria is a rare autosomal-dominant form of cold urticaria. Patients develop burning wheals 30 minutes to 3 hours after exposure to cold wind (rather than cold contact). The wheals may persist for 48 hours and may be accompanied by tremor, fever, and headache, and leukocytosis may be discovered on hematologic examination.[13] Provocative testing is done by exposing half of the patient's body in a cold room for 20 to 30 minutes. Caution must be used because life-threatening reactions are possible.

Heat Urticaria. Heat urticaria is one of the rarest forms of physical urticaria. The patient (usually female) develops pruritic wheals within 5 minutes after contact with a hot object at the site of contact. The wheals may last up to 1 hour and may be associated with nausea, diarrhea, abdominal cramps, and dizziness. Provocative testing is done by filling a metal beaker with water that has been warmed to a temperature of 50 to 55°C and applying it to the skin for 5 minutes.[13] The site is then observed for wheal development. Solar and cholinergic urticaria should be excluded by performing the appropriate diagnostic tests.

Cholinergic Urticaria. Cholinergic urticaria, one of the most common physical urticarias, usually occurs in young adults and is characterized by 3-mm pruritic wheals surrounded by a large flare reaction. The lesions develop within 20 minutes after the onset of perspiration and last 30 minutes to one hour.[15] In severe cases, wheals may be accompanied by nausea, vomiting, abdominal cramps, wheezing, diarrhea, salivation, and headaches.[13, 15] The onset may be precipitated by exercise, warm temperatures, emotional stress, and spicy foods, all of which raise the body temperature and stimulate the sweat glands. A provocative test may be done by having the patient exercise until sweating is induced.

Aquagenic Urticaria. Aquagenic urticaria is a rare physical urticaria manifested by follicular pruritic wheals at the site of water contact. The exposure time required to induce lesions varies from 3 to 30 minutes.[13] The eruption is similar to that of cholinergic urticaria, which should be excluded by provocative testing. A diagnostic test for aquagenic urticaria consists of applying water compresses to the patient's back and maintaining the temperature at 35°C with a hot water bottle applied to the compresses.[13]

Vibratory Angioedema. Vibratory angioedema is an extremely rare form of physical urticaria, which develops in a localized area within 5 minutes of vibrating stimuli. An autosomal dominant mode of inheritance had been reported.[13] Provocative stimuli is done by applying vibratory stimuli to the forearm.

Complement-Mediated Urticarias

Hereditary Angioedema

Hereditary angioedema is the most common form of angioedema that is associated with either a qualitative or quantitative C1 esterase inhibitor (C1INH) deficiency.[16] It is an autosomal dominant disease, but lack of a family history does not exclude the diagnosis. It is manifested by urticaria, which most commonly affects the face or extremities. The swelling may persist for 24 to 48 hours but always subsides within 72 hours. It may be accompanied by edema of the upper respiratory tract, which can progress to asphyxiation,[17] as well as edema of the gastrointestinal tract, which causes abdominal pain, vomiting, and diarrhea. These symptoms may occur simultaneously or separately. The reasons for the episodic attacks remain unclear.

Laboratory findings disclose absence of the C1 inhibitor. As a result of the uninhibited C1 activity, reduced levels of C4 and C2 may be found during clinical attacks, although the C3 level is usually normal.[17] Histamine concentrations in urine are increased during attacks of hereditary angioedema because of activation of the mast cells and basophils by C3a.

Acquired Angioedema

Acquired angioedema, with an acquired deficiency of C1INH, is less common than the hereditary form. Sporadic cases have been reported with lymphoproliferative disorders, monoclonal gammopathy, systemic lupus erythematosus, and rectal enoplasia.[16] In the acquired form, other family members are not found to have abnormalities of C1INH levels. In addition to decreased C4 and C1INH levels, patients have reduced C1 and C1q, features that help to differentiate it from the hereditary form.

Circulating Immune Complex–Mediated Urticarias

Urticarial Vasculitis

Two features are required for diagnosis of urticarial vasculitis: a clinical picture of urticaria and the histologic changes of leukocytoclastic vasculitis. (The histologic features of leukocytoclastic vasculitis have been discussed.)

Patients with urticarial vasculitis present a wide variety of clinical, laboratory, and immunopathologic abnormalities. The cutaneous findings are usually described as painful, urticaria-like lesions that persist for 24 to 72 hours. They may resolve and leave residual purpura and pigmentation. Some patients also have erythema multiforme–like lesions, Raynaud's phenomenon, livedo reticularis, or photosensitivity.[13]

Affected patients often have extracutaneous features suggestive of multisystem disease.[12] Arthralgias and arthritis are the most common extracutaneous manifestations of urticarial vasculitis, but abdominal pain, adenopathy, fever, asthma, conjunctivitis, myositis, and renal and neurologic dysfunction may also be encountered. Urticarial vasculitis was originally reported as a "lupus-like syndrome" because of its similarities to systemic lupus erythematosus.[18]

Laboratory tests have revealed an elevated erythrocyte sedimentation rate in almost all patients.[12] Other findings may include hypocomplementemia, with depressed levels of CH50 and/or C1q, C2, and C1.[10, 12, 18] Direct immunofluorescence examination of cutaneous lesions of urticarial vasculitis has revealed immunoglobulin and complement deposited in blood vessel walls. In some patients examination of biopsy specimens (as by the "lupus band test") has also revealed immunoglobulin or complement at the dermoepidermal junction. Also, circulating immune complexes may be detected by standard in vitro assays.[13]

According to diagnostic schemes currently in use, patients with urticarial vasculitis have been divided into two groups. Patients who are less severely affected have chronic urticaria, minimal systemic disease, normal complement levels, some serologic and immunologic findings suggestive of vasculitis, and mild histologic changes of leukocytoclastic vasculitis.[18] Severe cases have been called "hypocomplementemic vasculitis," "unusual SLE-related syndrome," and "urticaria with vasculitis."[19] These patients, with chronic urticaria and additional cutaneous findings, have multisystem disease and a high incidence of hypocomplementemia as well as increased serologic and immunopathologic findings suggestive of systemic vasculitis.[19] Further studies of patients with urticarial vasculitis should help to determine whether this spectrum of findings represents a specific immune complex disease or a nonspecific reaction pattern caused by a number of etiologic agents.

Serum Sickness

Serum sickness represents a type III, circulating immune complex, hypersensitivity reaction. It occurs 7 to 12 days after exposure to heterologous proteins, certain drugs, or viral, bacterial, or parasitic infection.[8] The introduction of a foreign protein initiates the synthesis of a specific antibody, usually IgG. These soluble antigen-antibody complexes circulate and may be deposited in various tissues, especially in blood vessel walls.

Serum sickness is manifested by fever, urticaria, lymphadenopathy, myalgias, arthralgias, and arthritis. The urticaria is often preceded by pruritus and erythema. The symptoms usually last 4 to 5 days and are self-limited.

Reaction to Blood Products

Urticaria may occur after exposure to whole blood, serum, or immunoglobulin, because of transfusion to the recipient of donor IgE that is directed toward an antigen to which the recipient was exposed. More commonly, an antigen in the donor blood product may be transfused into a sensitized recipient. Urticaria can also occur after transfusion of IgG, in which immune complexes are formed and complement is activated.

Nonimmunologic Urticarias

Urticaria Due to Direct Mast Cell Releasing Agents

Histamine-releasing agents include quinine, opiates, curare, atropine, hydralazine, thiamine, alcohol, radiographic contrast material, and antibiotics such as polymyxin B and chlortetracycline.[6, 14] Shellfish, snake venom, jellyfish, and bacterial toxins can also cause histamine release.[14] Benzoic acid, which is present in fruit drinks, jelly, gelatin, and cheeses, may also release histamine from mast cells and basophils.

Urticaria Due to Agents That May Alter Arachidonic Acid Metabolism

Urticaria may occur after exposure to aspirin and other nonsteroidal anti-inflammatory agents, although the mechanism is not entirely clear. One theory is that these agents block the cyclooxygenase pathway of arachidonic acid metabolism but increase the lipooxygenase pathway products, which may mediate urticaria.[14, 19]

Idiopathic Urticaria

The cause of urticaria/angioedema may remain unknown in more than 80 per cent of patients, even after careful evaluation.[13] Most patients appear to be in good health with no significant systemic disease. In 50 per cent of patients, the urticaria will resolve in 6 months. Of the patients who continue to have urticaria after 6 months, 40 per cent have active disease for 10 years.

DIFFERENTIAL DIAGNOSIS

Urticaria and angioedema are usually easily recognized because of their episodic and transitory appearance.[20] Other conditions may occasionally appear urticarial. Urticaria pigmentosa, which is due to mast-cell infiltration of the skin, may appear as pigmented macules and papules and then become urticarial after the lesions are rubbed (Darier's sign). It is more common in children, as is papular urticaria, which is a consequence of the bites of fleas, bedbugs, and other insects. Small wheals develop in crops after insect bites and persist for several days. Erythema multiforme may also be urticarial, but generally the lesions are papulovesciular or bullous eruptions or are of the typical target type. Bullous pemphigoid is an autoimmune bullous disease in which, occasionally, urticarial lesions may dominate the clinical picture.

REFERENCES

1. Champion RH, Roberts SOB, Carpenter RG, Roger JH. Urticaria and Angio-oedema: a review of 554 patients. Br J Dermatol 1969;81:588–97.
2. Akers WA, Naversen DN. Diagnosis of chronic urticaria. Int J Dermatol 1978;17:616–27.
3. Monroe EW, Jones HE. Urticaria: an update review. Arch Dermatol 1977;113:80–90.
4. Hellgren L. The prevalence of urticaria in the total population. Acta Allergol 1972;27:236–40.
5. Maize JC. Urticaria. In: Demis DJ, Dobson RL, McGuire J, eds. Clinical dermatology. Philadelphia: Harper & Row, 1982; Section 7-9:1–13.
6. Soter NA, Wasserman SI. Urticaria/angioedema. A consideration of pathogenesis of clinical manifestations. Int J Dermatol 1979;18:517–32.

7. Warin RP, Champion RH. Urticaria. 1st ed. London: WB Saunders, 1974:15–36.
8. Dahl MV. Clinical immunodermatology. 1st ed. Chicago: Year Book, 1981:5.
9. Lever WF, Schaumburg-Lever G. Histopathology of the skin. 5th ed. Philadelphia: JB Lippincott, 1975:133.
10. Soter NA. Chronic urticaria as a manifestation of necrotizing venulitis. N Engl J Med 1977;296:1440–2.
11. Noid HE, Schulze TW, Winkelmann RK. Diet plan for patients with salicylate-induced urticaria. Arch Dermatol 1974;109:866–9.
12. Small P, Barrett D, Champlin E. Chronic urticaria and vasculitis. Ann Allergy 1982;48:172–4.
13. Jorizzo JL, Smith EB. The physical urticarias. Arch Dermatol 1982;118:194–201.
14. Guin JD. Treatment of urticaria. Med Clin North Am 1982;66:831–49.
15. Lawrence CM, Jorizzo JL, Kobza-Black A, Coutts A, Greaves MW. Cholinergic urticaria with associated angio-oedema. Br J Dermatol 1982;105:543–50.
16. Chiu JT. Familial angioedema associated with C_1 esterase-inhibitor deficiency: a new genetic variant of hereditary angioedema. JAMA 1982;247:1734–6.
17. Brasher GW, Starn JC, Hall FF, Spiekerman AM. Complement component analysis in angioedema: diagnostic value. Arch Dermatol 1975;111:1140–2.
18. Monroe EW. Urticarial vasculitis: an updated review. J Am Acad Dermatol 1981;5:88–95.
19. Gammon WR, Wheeler CE Jr. Urticarial vasculitis: report of a case and review of the literature. Arch Dermatol 1979;115:76–80.
20. Schneider SB, Atkinson JP. Urticaria and angioedema. In: Fitzpatrick TB, Eisen AZ, Wolff K, Freedburg IM, Austen KF, eds. Update one: dermatology in general medicine. New York: McGraw-Hill, 1982;63–67.

VERTIGO

ROBERT A. GOLDENBERG

□ SYNONYMS: Dizziness, lightheadedness, falling out, fuzziness, blurred vision, feeling faint, imbalance, staggering, nausea

BACKGROUND

Vertigo is a sensation of rotatory movement. *Dizziness* is everything else. These definitions of vertigo and dizziness deliberately oversimplify the multiple complaints of a patient who presents with a balance disorder. Often, after taking such a history, the physician will be as dizzy as the patient.

Why this oversimplification? Vertigo almost always indicates vestibular disease, i.e., an abnormality of the labyrinth of the inner ear. Dizziness generally suggests nonvestibular disease of a neurologic, metabolic, or visual etiology. Therefore, this relationship of vertigo to inner ear disease can readily be utilized when taking the history. For a full understanding of the symptoms of vertigo and dizziness, the basic physiology of the entire balance system must be understood.[1] The term vestibular system was taken from *labyrinthine vestibule.* This vestibule is the connection between the semicircular canals and the cochlea. The three semicircular canals are arranged in three mutually perpendicular planes. Each canal ends in an ampula near the vestibule. The hollow bony semicircular canals, vestibule, and connecting cochlear duct are filled with perilymph. Perilymph is thought to be an ultrafiltrate of cerebrospinal fluid and is in direct continuity with the subarachnoid space.

Within these bony canals lies a series of membranous cavities known as the endolymphatic system, which floats in the perilymph fluid and is an entirely closed system. It is filled with endolymph, which is probably secreted by cells within the labyrinth itself. The three main endolymphatic cavities are the utricle and semicircular canals, the saccule and cochlear duct, and the endolymphatic sac and duct. The utricle, saccule, and semicircular canals house the main receptor organs for the sense of motion and position (Fig. 1).

Normal equilibrium is a state of symmetry between the right and left vestibular systems as they function to maintain a proper relationship between the individual and the environment.[2] The vestibular end-organs at rest are constantly discharging signals to the central nervous system. When stimulated, the semicircular canals respond to radial acceleration. The utricle and saccule respond to linear displacement. Obviously, if one of the vestibular end-organs is diseased and is sending asymmetric signals to the central nervous system, the body will interpret them as motion even though it is at rest (Fig. 2).

Nystagmus results from ocular muscle movement in response to head motion involving acceleration of the endolymph in each labyrinthine system.[3] The direction of nystagmus may be horizontal, vertical, diagonal, or rotatory, depending

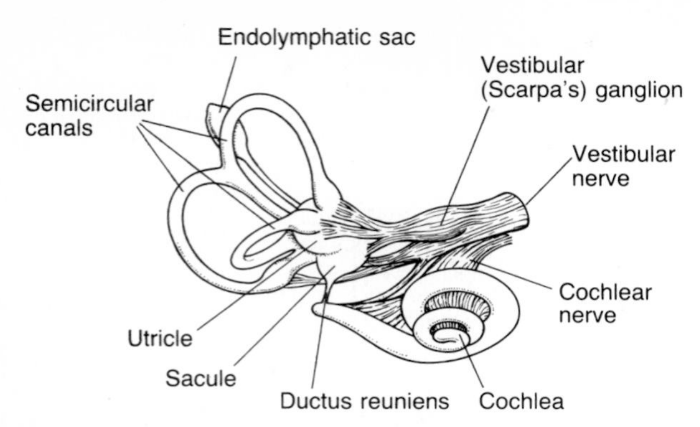

Figure 1. The cochleovestibular system.

on the stimulation involved. Nystagmus is therefore a measure of inner ear function and is used both clinically and in laboratory testing to document inner ear disease.

The orientation role of the vestibular labyrinth is linked to a unified coordinating mechanism consisting of both labyrinths, the vestibular nerves, central ocular pathways, spinal cord, cerebellum, medial longitudinal fasciculus, red nucleus, thalamus, hypothalamus, and cerebellar cortex. The role of the medial longitudinal fasciculus is most important, because its fibers connect with the vestibular pathways leading to eye muscle nuclei as well as other cranial nerves and anterior horn cells of the spinal cord, which supply extremity musculature (Fig. 3).

The interaction between vestibular symmetry, visual stabilization, and central nervous system responses will enable the body to maintain a normal upright posture and balance of movement. Obviously, an abnormality of any one of the three components will lead to a balance disorder. A continued awareness of this interrelationship enables the physician to make an accurate diagnosis in a patient presenting with a balance disturbance.

HISTORY

Very few presenting symptoms demand the skills of history taking as much as a disturbance of the sense of balance. One of the best initial means of approaching a patient with multiple complaints is to decide whether the disease is peripheral or central in origin. *Peripheral disease* is defined as a disorder affecting the vestibular end-organ. *Central disease* is defined as a disorder originating from higher neural pathways within the central nervous system or another non-neural condition such as a metabolic, visual, circulatory, or functional abnormality.

With very few exceptions, peripheral disease has vertigo as its primary symptom. Vertigo has been defined as a hallucination or sensation of rotatory motion. It makes no difference whether the room is spinning and the patient is still or vice versa. Peripheral disease may also create a state of imbalance or unsteadiness in some cases. This state is still a sensation or hallucination and is not, in fact, real; it must not be confused with ataxia, which is primarily of cerebellar origin.

Central disease generally has dizziness as a primary complaint. Description of dizziness may include such words as lightheadedness, syncope, falling out spells, giddiness, blurred vision, nausea, eyespots, and lethargy. The key factor is a lack of rotatory sensation.

Associated symptoms of hearing loss or tinnitus suggest that the cause may be an inner ear disorder. Because of the intimate relationship between the hearing and balance mechanisms of the inner ear, a condition that affects one will often affect

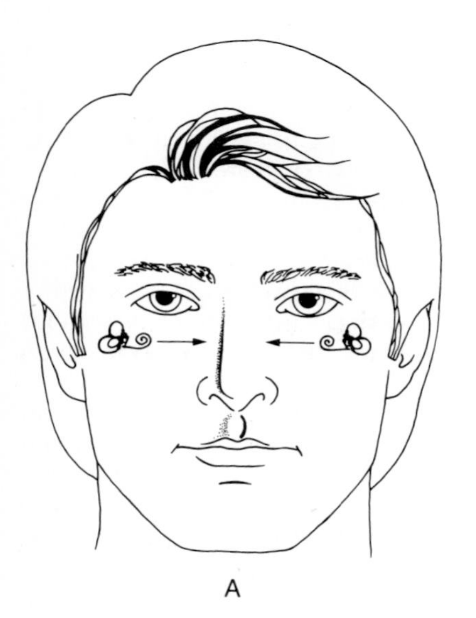

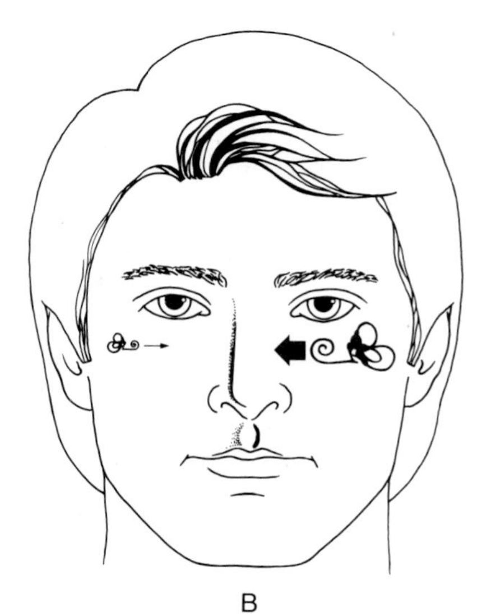

Figure 2. Vestibular function. *A,* Equal input yields normal balance. *B,* Unequal input (asymmetrical signals) to the nervous system are interpreted as rotary motion (hallucination of rotation).

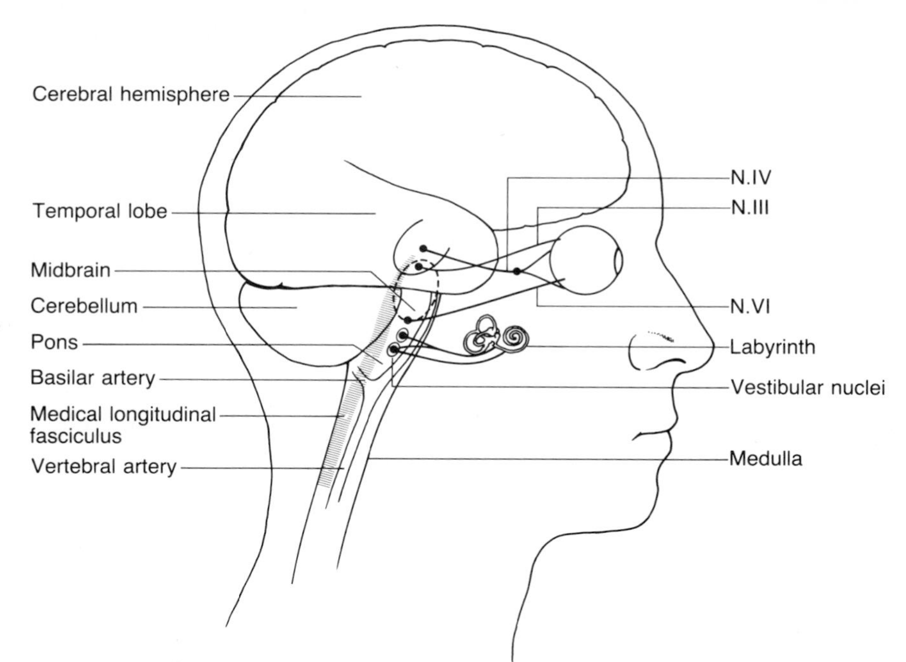

Figure 3. Peripheral and central pathways for vertigo.

the other, especially when symptoms are unilateral, indicating that one ear is the source of the problem. Peripheral disease may be bilateral, however, so this observation is not always the case.

A detailed description of symptoms must include duration, constant or episodic nature, gradual or abrupt onset, and whether there is a progression of severity. What makes the symptoms better or worse (including positional change, medication, and activity)? Is there a history of trauma? Do any dietary habits, medications, or allergies predate this condition? Complete family, social, and previous histories should, obviously, be taken in order to evaluate any coexisting or hereditary disease. A basic review of systems is essential to make certain there is no other abnormality that might be causing or aggravating the condition.

A recommended method of history taking is to allow the patient to develop the symptom complex in his or her own words (the physician interrupting only when absolutely necessary to keep the patient on a relevant course). Although this method may lengthen the initial evaluation, it is very important to let the patient describe the symptoms without being asked leading questions. In the course of verbalizing what may seem to be a vast array of complaints, the patient often articulates a key word that will be critical to the diagnosis. Direct questioning may be necessary to elaborate specific local symptoms that may contribute to the disorder.

After the patient has described the symptoms without interruption and there has been a complete review of systems and questioning about other relevant history, the physician should ask the patient again to describe the symptoms in one simple word without using the word dizziness. This one basic word may provide that key concept that will lead the examiner to distinguish between vertigo and dizziness.

The examiner should be very suspicious of a patient who uses sophisticated medical terminology or certain "buzz words." A patient who complains specifically of "episodic vertigo" may have read extensively on the condition of Meniere's disease and may be giving misleading clues to the examining physician.

At the completion of the history, the examiner should have one or more specific diagnoses in mind. The physical examination and laboratory findings are therefore only confirmatory. As is true with many other conditions, if the physician is unable to make a diagnosis on the basis of the history, he or she probably will be unable to make a diagnosis at all.

PHYSICAL EXAMINATION

Patients with vestibular disease generally lack specific physical findings. However, thorough physical evaluation is essential to accurate diagnosis; vertigo due to a perforated tympanic membrane or glomus tumor of the middle ear can be easily missed if the tympanic membrane is not directly visualized. There are always anecodotal reports of a severe cerumen impaction against the tympanic membrane causing vertigo that subsides immediately upon its removal in the office.

A standard otolaryngologic examination is performed, including examination of the ears, nose, throat, nasopharynx, and larynx and palpation of the neck. Funduscopic examination, auscultation for carotid and temporoparietal bruits, and palpation of the temporomandibular joint should be done. A neurologic examination is performed, including cranial nerve testing, tests of cerebellar function, and a Romberg test. Simply having the patient walk several times around a stationary object will give the examiner good clues as to the type and validity of the balance complaints. Similar information is gathered from watching a patient walk down the hallway and return.

Tuning fork tests or simple voice tests for hearing done in the office may be helpful to determine whether or not any hearing loss exists to confirm the existence of this problem. Observation for spontaneous nystagmus and the use of simple caloric irrigation may also document labyrinthine disease. Hearing loss or nystagmus may be very subtle; the basic office tests may be misleading and must be used with clinical judgment.

DIAGNOSTIC STUDIES

Many specialized and sophisticated tests have been developed to aid in evaluation of a patient with vertigo. Audiometry has reached a very high level of sophistication.[4] The pure-tone audiogram, word discrimination test, impedance audiogram, specific site of lesion testing, and auditory brainstem response (ABR) are routine methods of localizing a lesion along the auditory pathway. Obviously, such testing is beyond the expertise of a nonspecialist and must be performed and/or interpreted by qualified practitioners. Thorough audiometric evaluation is probably one of the more critical tests used to determine whether an inner ear problem exists.

Electronystagmography (ENG) is the basic laboratory test for evaluating a patient with balance complaints.[5] Surface electrodes placed around the eye record the action potential of the ocular muscles. This method is much more sensitive than simple observation of nystagmus even with specialized magnifying glasses. Although the ENG must not be overinterpreted and although it must be used only to support clinical judgment, it is often very helpful in localizing specific types of lesions.

The ENG consists of at least three separate tests. The first test is a central battery that records pendular tracking, gaze nystagmus, saccadic movement, spontaneous nystagmus, vertical nystagmus, and optokinetic nystagmus. Abnormal results in this portion of the ENG suggest central or nonlabyrinthine disease. The second part of the test examines positional nystagmus. The classic Dix-Hallpike provocation test is usually performed, and strict criteria are applied to make the diagnosis of positional vertigo. The third portion of the test is the caloric evaluation of inner ear function. Water or air (slightly above and below body temperature) is used to elicit a response from each labyrinth. Bilaterally equal responses are indicative of equally functioning labyrinths, and the result is interpreted as normal. The caloric test result is abnormal if one can demonstrate hypoactivity; the hypoactive ear is generally the diseased ear.

There are other, quite sophisticated means of measuring the static end-organs and semicircular canals. Testing may be done on a torsion swing, in a centrifuge rotational chair, or with other specialized equipment. Such testing is generally reserved for research or occasional difficult diagnostic problems.

X-rays of the petrous portion of the temporal bone complete the basic evaluation of the inner ear. By means of the standard radiographic techniques available in all institutions, structures such as the internal auditory canal, semicircular canals, and cochlea can easily be visualized. Polytomography of the temporal bone, when available, increases the definition of these structures. Computed tomography (CT scanning) has revolutionized diagnostic protocols for patients with neurologic complaints. CT scanning may be used with positive contrast myelography, air cisternography, or high-resolution techniques. It is hoped that advances in CT scanning techniques may eventually eliminate the need for more conventional radiographic evaluation. Arteriography, venography, and digitalized angiography, used when indicated, may also facilitate diagnosis.

Although electrocardiography and electroencephalography are not done routinely in the evaluation of a patient with vertigo, they are useful in some patients with seizure disorders or cardiac arrythmias. Selected blood studies may aid in ruling out metabolic or systemic factors. Evaluation may include a complete blood count, urinalysis, 5-hour glucose tolerance test, thyroid battery, lipid profile, and serologic evaluation.

In summary, the basic, routine evaluation of inner ear function consists of audiometry, ENG, and inner ear x-ray, which allow evaluation of the architectural structure of the inner ear as well as the function of the cochlear and vestibular systems. Further tests are ordered as required.

ASSESSMENT: CAUSES OF VERTIGO

The evaluation of a patient with vertigo depends on an organized, systematic, thorough approach to the information obtained through history, physical evaluation, and laboratory tests. In order to accomplish this, the physician must have a mental checklist of primary diseases that can cause this symptom. The following diseases are the more common causes of vertigo and dizziness.

Meniere's Disease

Meniere's disease manifests principally as episodic vertigo, which may last hours or days and often is severe enough to confine the patient to bed or resting positions. Such confinement is often a necessity in the treatment of acute attacks. Following the acute attack, there may be a period of *imbalance* or *unsteadiness* which takes several days to subside. Vertigo may be associated with other vegetative symptoms such as diaphoresis, palpitation, nausea, vomiting, blurred vision, and shortness of breath.

Fluctuant hearing loss is the second important finding in this disease. During the acute exacerbation of the attack, hearing seems to decrease; as the acute attack subsides, the hearing may improve. There is an uncommon variant of this disease, known as Lermoyez's syndrome, in which the opposite process occurs: The patient has a sustained loss of hearing, but during an attack the hearing actually improves. The hearing loss is generally a low-frequency one. Aural pressure or fullness may also occur with the hearing loss.

Tinnitus is the third important finding. Classically it is roaring and quite severe. The tinnitus is worse during attacks of vertigo and may subside between attacks.

The disease usually affects middle-aged patients; however, its occurrence in children as well as in very elderly patients has been reported. There is a sudden onset of symptoms that usually last hours to days, followed by intermittent periods of remission. The disease is commonly unilateral, but both ears may be involved in up to 40 per cent of the cases studied.[6]

The natural course of Meniere's disease is one of acute exacerbations with periods of remission. As the disease progresses, the attacks become more frequent, have less warning, and become more disabling. Over many years the inner ear may become totally nonfunctional or "burn itself out." At the time of this natural labyrinthectomy, there may be no further vertigo but there is also no hearing.

On physical examination there are seldom any findings of diagnostic significance. Nystagmus may be noted, particularly during an acute attack. No abnormalities of the tympanic membrane are found, and the remainder of the ear, nose, and throat examination is normal. Audiometric evaluation usually documents a low-frequency hearing loss of variable severity. The ENG usually shows the involved ear to be hypoactive. Radiographic evaluation generally is nonrevealing.

It is important to note that there are two variants of Meniere's disease. In the first—cochlear hydrops—hearing fluctuates in an episodic manner (confirmed audiometrically) but there is no vertigo associated with it. In the second—endolymphatic hydrops—there is episodic vertigo (generally confirmed by a hypoactive labyrinth on the involved site) but no loss of hearing is demonstrated. These two variants account for much of the confusion about Meniere's disease that has led to errors in diagnosis in past years. Keeping this in mind, one should make a diagnosis of Meniere's disease only when the classic triad—episodic vertigo, fluctuant hearing loss, and tinnitus—exists.

Acute Labyrinthitis

If a patient presents with an acute onset of vertigo without auditory symptoms, the clinician usually makes a diagnosis of "acute labyrinthitis." Bacterial labyrinthitis, associated with otitis media, is quite serious and often leads to meningitis; fortunately it is very uncommon. Inflammation of the labyrinth may be associated with a viral problem such as mumps, flu-like symptoms, or upper respiratory tract infection. However, most of these cases of "viral labyrinthitis" are probably not true labyrinthine lesions but inflammation of the eustachian tube, changes in intratympanic pressure, or vestibular neuronitis. Therefore, such a diagnosis is incorrect and should be generally avoided. "Acute labyrinthitis," in North America, is often the term erroneously used to describe the condition of vestibular neuronitis.

Vestibular Neuronitis

An acute onset of severe vertigo without auditory symptoms, frequently following a viral upper respiratory tract infection, is the presenting symptom of vestibular neuronitis.[7] Spontaneous nystagmus is usually present, caloric studies may show a hypoactive labyrinth on the involved side, and auditory test results are normal. The disease usually is self-limiting; there may be several recurrent episodes with decreasing frequency for up to one year.

Histopathologic changes have been described in the central and peripheral neurons of Scarpa's ganglion (vestibular nerve) as well as in the semicircular canals and utricle.[8]

One problem with this diagnosis is that the symptoms are nonspecific and may represent early signs of other labyrinthine or CNS lesions. Full evaluation and long-term follow-up of affected patients is therefore advised.

Benign Paroxysmal Positional Vertigo

The clinical picture of benign paroxysmal positional vertigo (BPPV) consists of acute vertigo brought on by changes in position. There is no associated hearing loss or tinnitus. Abrupt changes of head position or posture cause transitory vertigo that lasts for very brief periods (seconds to minutes).

In a classic demonstration of this condition (also called cupulolithiasis),[9] placing the diseased ear in a dependent position causes vertigo and removing the diseased ear from that position causes a cessation of symptoms. This particular and common form of positional vertigo may result from the deflection of the cupula of the posterior semicircular canal by the otoconia when the head is placed in the critical position. In this condition, symptoms may often be elicited when the patient turns from one side to the other in bed.

The diagnosis of BPPV must be confirmed by the classic Dix-Hallpike provocation test performed during ENG,[10] according to four essential criteria:

1. There must be a delay in the onset of nystagmus after the head is placed in the causal position.
2. The nystagmus must fatigue.
3. The symptom of vertigo must occur at the same time the nystagmus is noted.
4. Nystagmus must be present toward the involved ear.

BPPV is generally self-limiting, with vertigo and nystagmus disappearing in a matter of months; symptoms may last up to a year. It is most important in making this diagnosis to be certain that no other etiology exists.

Chronic Otitis Media

Long-standing infection of the middle ear and mastoid may cause a condition that aggravates the labyrinthine system. A simple perforation of the tympanic membrane may cause asymmetry of middle ear pressure and thus vertigo. Fluid in the middle ear, particularly when only one ear is involved, may also alter middle ear pressure and cause vertigo as well. A lateral semicircular fistula is actually an erosion of bone over the lateral semicircular canal caused by chronic mastoiditis or cholesteatoma formation; the fistula occurs in a chronically infected ear and creates vertigo that may be quite incapacitating. Otorrhea is always a disturbing symptom in a patient with vertigo, and thorough examination of the middle ear is always required in these cases.

Other Middle Ear Diseases

Any involvement of the middle ear may cause pressure against the labyrinth. In most cases, vertigo is accompanied by hearing loss or tinnitus. A glomus tumor (tympanicum or jugulare) may cause vertigo that is usually associated with pulsatile tinnitus and hearing loss. Malignant or benign tumors of the external or middle ear may cause vertigo by pressure. A tumor of the inner ear, base of skull, or infratemporal fossa will generally cause other symptoms with associated neurologic findings.

Temporal Bone Fractures

Fractures of the temporal bone are the most common fractures of the skull. They tend to follow one of two general pathways, because of the architecture of the temporal bone, and they produce relatively predictable clinical effects.

Longitudinal fractures account for approximately 80 per cent of cases and usually result from a blow to the side of the head. Often a rupture of the tympanic membrane is associated, with blood in the middle ear and a cerebrospinal fluid (CSF) otorrhea. There is generally bleeding from the external auditory canal; hearing loss is of the conductive type. Facial nerve injury may occur but usually is delayed and is transient. There is normally no vertigo or nystagmus.

Transverse fractures of the temporal bone account for approximately 20 per cent of cases. The hearing loss is usually neural; bleeding from the external canal, a tympanic membrane perforation, or cerebrospinal fluid leak rarely occurs. There usually is blood in the middle ear, and approximately half the cases cause an immediate and permanent injury to the facial nerve. Vertigo is severe and may last many months, until relief occurs by normal compensatory mechanisms; occasionally it is a permanent disability. Radiographic diagnosis is often difficult, and tomography may be required. Audiometry, with or without vestibular testing, is of some value to assess the extent of labyrinthine or cochlear damage.

Labyrinthine Concussion

A history of vertigo following head injury associated with loss of consciousness but not causing a basal skull fracture is highly suggestive of a condition known as labyrinthine concussion. Vertigo and imbalance may be permanent if there has been actual destruction of the end-organ or nerve. A mild concussion, defined as simple edema or bruising of the end-organ, will result in self-limiting symptoms that abate with time.[11]

This condition must be distinguished from the cervical vertigo of whiplash injury. Care must be taken in documenting these conditions, as they are often accompanied by disability of medicolegal magnitude. An ENG performed on such patients many times shows depressed caloric responses or some positional nystagmus.[12] Labyrinthine concussion generally subsides within 12 to 18 months.

Perilymph Fistula

The patient who experiences sudden vertigo associated with trauma may have a perilymph fistula.[13] Barotrauma such as from SCUBA diving, sneezing, nose blowing, or airplane descent is often implicated. The trauma may also be a direct blow to the ear or previous otologic surgery. Otoscopic findings are negative but a fistula test result is positive. This test is performed by introducing air into the external auditory canal under direct pressure with a pneumatic otoscope. Extreme vertigo, observable nystagmus, or both are immediately experienced by the patient. The history is often identical to that of vestibular neuronitis, but there is a definite preceding trauma. Hearing is often totally depressed (sensorineural loss), and an ENG will show markedly abnormal responses.

Syphilis

Syphilis, the great imitator, can produce vertigo. It may be associated with a history of hearing loss and tinnitus that may be indistinguishable from Meniere's disease. However, instead of the episodic attacks, as in Meniere's disease, equilibrium and imbalance are more common presenting symptoms. The condition is bilateral vestibular end-organ disease. ENG may show definite and marked abnormalities. Positive results of the VDRL and fluorescent treponemal antibody tests (FTA) are diagnostic. In some cases colloidal gold analysis of spinal fluid is required. This diagnosis is rewarding, because syphilis is one of the causes of nerve deafness that may be reversed with medical treatment.

Acoustic Neuroma

A high index of suspicion is the key element in making the early diagnosis of an acoustic neuroma. Any of the symptoms described thus far in this chapter may be attributed to an acoustic neuroma; presenting symptoms can mimic those of Meniere's disease exactly. Abnormalities of cranial nerve V or VII on the involved side should immediately raise the index of suspicion. Cerebellar signs and papilledema are late findings that may indicate a larger tumor.

In the diagnostic evaluation of a patient with vertigo who has a total or severe one-sided hearing loss, an extremely poor discrimination score on audiometric evaluation, a unilateral severely depressed caloric response on ENG, an abnormal auditory brain-stem response (ABR), or an asymmetry of the internal auditory canal by x-ray evaluation would immediately lead one to further evaluation techniques. ABR may be the most sensitive early indicator of this condition.[14] If any of these features are detected or if the index of suspicion still remains high, CT scanning with or without air cisternography should be performed. Early diagnosis is particularly important because of the difficulty in management and poor prognosis of larger tumors.

In our experience, unilateral tinnitus has been the single most common symptom associated with an acoustic neuroma. Should this symptom exist in a patient with concurrent vertigo, a full evaluation for such a lesion must be accomplished.

Drug Ototoxicity

Several antibiotics, diuretics, and chemotherapeutic agents have vestibulotoxic properties (Table 1). These are usually associated with ototoxic symptoms; loss of hearing accompanies the vestib-

Table 1. OTOTOXIC AGENTS

Chemicals	Carbon monoxide
	Mercury
	Oil of chenopodium
	Tobacco
	Gold
	Lead
	Arsenic
	Analine dyes
	Alcohol
Drugs	
Antibiotics	Streptomycin
	Neomycin
	Gentamicin
	Viomycin
	Phenacetin
	Chloramphenicol
	Dihydrostreptomycin
	Kanamycin
	Vancomycin
	Ristocetin
	Polymyxin
	Tobramycin
	Amikacin
Diuretics	Ethacrynic acid
	Furosemide
Miscellaneous	Salicylates
	Hexadimethrine
	Quinine
	Nitrogen mustard

ular findings. Aminoglycosides are particularly damaging to vestibular and cochlear sensory cells. Toxicity is definitely related to plasma concentration levels. Streptomycin, gentamicin, and neomycin are common offenders. Furosemide is especially noted to cause severe vertigo.[15]

Traumatic Perforation of the Tympanic Membrane

Traumatic rupture of the tympanic membrane produced by cotton-tipped applicators, hairpins, other foreign bodies, or external trauma may produce vertigo. This generally is associated with a concomitant hearing loss, the severity of which is directly related to the extent of the middle and inner ear damage in addition to the tympanic membrane defect itself. Visual examination of the tympanic membrane is diagnostic in these cases.

Herpes Zoster Oticus

Herpes zoster oticus (Ramsay Hunt syndrome) is a viral inflammation of the geniculate ganglion in the petrous portion of the temporal bone. The usual symptoms are severe otalgia and seventh nerve paralysis. Vertigo, hearing loss, and tinnitus may also be severe presenting symptoms. Classically, small herpetic eruptions around the auricle are noted. These generally follow the distribution of cranial nerve VII.

Motion Sickness

The vertigo of motion sickness is characterized by extreme nausea and vomiting accompanied by pallor, cold sweats, headache, hyperventilation, and anxiety. It is the presence of these vestibular symptoms that separates motion sickness from dysequilibrium. The underlying factor in all provocative motion sickness is that of sensory rearrangement in which information to the vestibular receptors is artificially distorted by unusual stimuli.[16]

Cerebrovascular Disease

Cerebrovascular disease generally causes symptoms of dizziness only infrequently. However, vertigo may be the most common symptom in insufficiency of basilar-vertebral artery circulation. If this vertigo is episodic or sudden in onset, it is commonly thought that the patient is suffering from a peripheral labyrinthine disturbance.

Vertigo occurs when there is a drop in blood flow through the vessels supplying the vestibular nuclei and fibers in the brain stem.[17] Drop attacks, in which the patient falls abruptly without losing consciousness, are characteristic of basilar artery disease and invariably are due to a decrease in the blood flow to the vestibular system. Occlusive disease of the extracranial vessels is present in about 50 per cent of subjects with basilar-vertebral artery symptoms. It is important to note that about half the patients with vertebral artery stenosis also demonstrate carotid stenosis in the neck. A subclavian steal syndrome (stenosis or occlusion of the proximal subclavian artery with retrograde flow through the vertebral artery) has been found in about 3 per cent of the subjects with symptoms of basilar artery insufficiency.

Vertigo is also the most common symptom in insufficiency of the basilar-vertebral arterial system. It is present as part of a complex of symptoms that can be easily recognized as arising from the brain stem and is rarely an isolated symptom; the vertigo is often accompanied by vomiting and slurred speech. Hearing loss and tinnitus rarely are basilar-vertebral artery symptoms; this fact may aid greatly in the differential diagnosis. Evaluation of the patient with transient symptoms should include consideration of factors that may predispose to cerebrovascular disease. Arteriography is the only definitive method of localizing a vascular lesion; when the diagnosis is not in doubt, the purpose of the procedure is to seek surgically correctable extracranial vascular stenosis.

Multiple Sclerosis

Vertigo is the presenting symptom of multiple sclerosis in approximately 10 per cent of patients; it eventually occurs during the course of the disease in approximately one-third of patients. Abrupt-onset, severe rotatory or vertical vertigo may be associated with nausea, vomiting, and severe prostration, suggesting labyrinthine disease. More often, the patient complains of unsteadiness, milder degrees of imbalance, or positional vertigo.

Nystagmus is almost invariably demonstrated in patients with multiple sclerosis.[18] Horizontal nystagmus is most common, but a significant number of patients also show vertical or rotatory nystagmus, which points to a pathologic process of the brain stem. Bilateral internuclear ophthalmoplegia is virtually pathognomonic of multiple sclerosis. It is recognized when the adducting eye (third nerve) is weak or shows no movement at all, while the abducting eye (sixth nerve) moves normally. A coarse nystagmus may be displayed during ENG, probably owing to an involvement of the vestibular nuclei. This finding generally indicates an interruption of the medial longitudinal fasciculus, which when bilateral is almost always caused by a demyelinating disorder. Asynchronous eye movements, especially with overshooting the mark on lateral gaze, may also be suggestive of multiple sclerosis.

The onset usually is between 20 and 40 years of age. There are absolutely no diagnostic laboratory criteria, and the diagnosis is essentially a clinical one. Elevated CSF gamma globulin levels or an elevated midzone colloidal gold curve may be the only laboratory finding.

Neurologic Conditions

A variety of neurologic conditions may manifest as vertigo. Intracranial tumors other than an acoustic neuroma may cause vertigo; there may be other lesions in the cerebellopontine angle such as a meningioma, hemoangioma, and arachnoid cyst. Other intracranial tumors, arteriovenous malformations, and intracranial aneurysms should also be included in the differential diagnosis.

Vertigo may be present in migraine headaches. Typically the attacks are preceded by an aura, often with scotomas, rarely with hemianopsia. Dysarthria, ataxia, paresthesias, diplopia, or the visual field disturbances already described may accompany the vertigo. When the vertigo is followed by a severe throbbing occipital headache accompanied by vomiting, the condition is diagnosed. After falling asleep, the patient usually awakens pain-free and without any residual neurologic or otologic problems. A family history is positive in about half of the patients.

Vestibular epilepsy occurs from a lesion in the temporal lobe of the cortex. Vertigo is the principal manifestation of the seizure. Lesions include tumors, arteriovenous malformations, small cerebral infarcts, and post-traumatic scars. The vertigo may be severe and may be associated with nausea and vomiting. Auditory hallucinations may accompany the vestibular symptoms. There is usually an aura, and the majority of affected patients may progress to classic grand mal seizure patterns at some period in life. The electroencephalographic pattern is abnormal in the majority of cases, although a normal pattern does not exclude the diagnosis of vestibular epilepsy.

Temporomandibular Joint Neuralgia

Temporomandibular joint neuralgia (Costen's syndrome) is classically described as dizziness, tinnitus, and temporomandibular joint (TMJ) tenderness. Direct palpation of the joint elicits marked tenderness on opening and closing of the mandible. Spasm of the pterygoid muscles may be palpated intraorally. TMJ x-rays are often diagnostic. A therapeutic trial of dental occlusion therapy or a bite plane may be diagnostic.

Medications

Asking the patient which medications he or she is currently taking may be the single most important question in the history. Drug ingestion is an often-overlooked but very important cause of vertigo. Tranquilizers, mood elevators, muscle relaxants, and antihypertensive medications are the most common drugs that may have vertigo as a side effect; this obviously is not a true ototoxicity. Often the decision to use a particular drug must be weighed against the severity and type of its side effects.

Hyperventilation

Anxiety attacks causing hyperventilation may be a common cause of vertigo. An accurate history will usually determine this diagnosis and will easily distinguish it from other causes of vertigo. Many times the initial psychological impression of such a patient may be helpful. A useful diagnostic test is accomplished by performing an electronystagmogram while asking the patient to hyperventilate. In some cases, the ENG result will be abnormal, with nystagmus and central disfigurations recorded.

Miscellaneous Disorders

Orthostatic hypotension may be a cause of vertigo, although often its presenting symptoms are syncope and lightheadedness; obviously, measuring the sitting, standing, and lying blood pressures will aid in the diagnosis. Cataracts may cause vertigo because of decreased visual acuity. Thyroid dysfunction and reactive hypoglycemia are thought by some clinicians to be a cause of vertigo, but the issue is somewhat controversial. Diabetic neuropathy, particularly a retinopathy causing decreased visual function, definitely may create a situation of imbalance. Cardiac arrhythmias can cause a certain degree of lightheadedness.

Functional Vertigo

Functional vertigo is essentially a diagnosis of exclusion. It should be made only after exhaustion of all other diagnostic possibilities and competent psychiatric evaluation.

WHEN TO REFER

One of the most important questions a primary care physician can consider is when to refer a patient with a particular symptom complex. Although all the findings described in the section on assessment are helpful in differential diagnosis, certain findings are warning signs of serious disease that may require more immediate referral.

A patient with vertigo who has an associated *facial paralysis or weakness, severe headaches, diplopia, or ataxia* should be referred immediately for further evaluation. If the *vertigo itself persists beyond 4 weeks*, referral is also indicated. Symptomatic treatment for these conditions alone may mask a more significant problem.

REFERENCES

1. Altmann F. Otologic aspects of vertigo. Med Sci 1966; Feb: 43–49.
2. Goodhill V. Ear: diseases, deafness, dizziness. Hagerstown, Maryland: Harper & Row, 1979; 218–9.
3. Aschan, G, Bergstedt M, Stahle J. Nystagmography; recording of nystagmus in clinical neuro-otological examination. Acta Otolaryngol 1956; (Suppl 129):1–103.
4. Martin F. Introduction to audiology. Englewood Cliffs, NJ: Prentice-Hall, 1975.
5. Ruben W. Electronystagmography. Arch Otolaryngol 1969;89:9–21.
6. Morrison AW. The surgery of vertigo: saccus drainage for idiopathic endolymphatic hydrops. J Laryngol Otol 1976;90:87–93.
7. Clemis JD, Becker GW. Vestibular neuronitis. Otolaryngol Clin North Am 1973;6:139–155.
8. Morganstein KM, Seung HI. Vestibular neuronitis. Laryngoscope 1971;81:131–9.
9. Schuknecht HF. Cupulolithiasis. Arch Otolaryngol 1969;90:765–78.
10. Dix MR, Hallpike CS. The pathology, symptomatology and diagnosis of certain common disorders of the vestibular system. Proc Roy Soc Med 1952;45:341–54.
11. Barber HO. Head injury: audiological and vestibular findings. Ann Otol 1969;78:239–52.
12. Woods WW, Compare WE. Electronystagmography in cervical injuries. Int Surg 1969;51:251–8.
13. Goodhill V, Harris I, Brockman SJ, et al. Sudden deafness and labyrinthine window ruptures. Ann Otol Rhinol Laryngol 1973;82:2–12.
14. Selters W, Brackman D. Acoustic tumor detection with brainstem electrical response audiometry. Arch Otolaryngol 1977;103:181–7.
15. Schwartz H, David DS, Riggio RR, et al. Ototoxicity induced by furosemide. N Engl J Med 1970;282:1413–4.
16. Reason JT, Brand JJ. Motion sickness. London: Academic, 1975.
17. Burns RA. Basilar-artery insufficiency as a cause of vertigo. Otolaryngol Clin North Am 1973;6:287–300.
18. Noffsinger D, Olsen W, Carhart R, et al. Auditory and vestibular aberrations in multiple sclerosis. Acta Otolaryngol [Suppl] (Stockh) 1972;303:7–57.

VISUAL FIELD DEFECTS

JOHN E. CARTER

BACKGROUND

Visual field evaluation is critical in assessing the patient presenting with a chief complaint of visual loss. Characterization of the visual field defect enables the physician to establish the location of the lesion and formulate a clinical diagnosis or perform diagnostic procedures that will be likely to have a positive yield. There are many techniques for examining the fields of vision, but evaluation at the bedside or in the office of the primary care physician usually involves confrontation testing, which is not as sensitive as formal perimetry in detecting and characterizing subtle visual field defects. Formal perimetry will be necessary in some situations, such as persistent visual complaints in a patient in whom no abnormalities can be detected by confrontation techniques. However, confrontation testing is a means of rapid evaluation without special apparatus and with little sacrifice in sensitivity. The majority of neurologic visual field defects can be detected and often adequately characterized by confrontation testing, especially if the visual symptoms are present at the time of the examination.

Visual Field Representation Within the Visual System

In general, neurologic visual field defects conform to a limited set of patterns. These are altitudinal field defects, central scotomas, bitemporal hemianopias, and homonymous hemianopias. The character of each of these patterns corresponds to the organization of the nerve fibers at the location of the lesion causing the visual field defect. Therefore, evaluation revolves around several important landmarks within the visual fields.

The horizontal meridian from 0 to 180 degrees passes through the fixation point and the blind spot. The vertical meridian from 90 to 270 degrees passes through the fixation point. The blind spot is centered about 15 degrees from the fixation point in the temporal visual field. Central vision constitutes the area of fixation and up to 30 degrees around fixation.

The Horizontal Meridian

The first level at which grouping of visual elements occurs in such a way as to create specific visual field defects is the nerve fiber layer of the retina carrying axons of the ganglion cells to the optic nerve head. Because these fibers must swing above and below the macular region to reach the optic nerve head, the visual pathways within the eye are effectively split into superior and inferior halves (Fig. 1).

The vascular supply of the retina also follows this pattern. The central retinal artery divides into superior and inferior divisions, which like the nerve fibers have an arcuate pattern and supply their respective superior and inferior halves of the retina. The central retinal artery provides very little blood to the optic nerve head itself. Instead, the disc receives its blood supply from short penetrating arterioles derived from the posterior ciliary arteries, which also supply the choroidal circulation. Therefore the optic nerve head also has a segmental blood supply, and vascular injury here will produce a discrete visual field defect whose location is related to the group of nerve fiber bundles that have been damaged.

This characteristic distribution of the nerve fibers and the blood supply within the eye provides virtually certain localization of altitudinal visual field defects (Fig. 2). An altitudinal visual field defect lies in one vertical half of the visual field of one eye with a sharp border at the horizontal meridian and is caused by a lesion within the eye. If it is within the nasal field it should cross the vertical meridian and extend toward or "point to" the blind spot. If it is within the temporal field it will once again "point to" the blind spot rather than extending past the blind spot toward fixation.

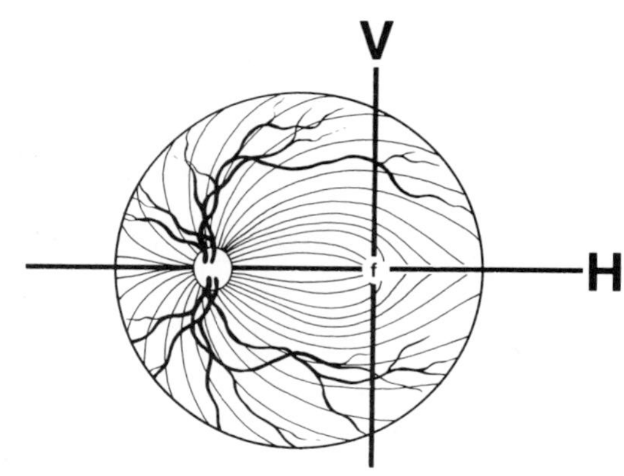

Figure 1. Illustration of the arcuate pattern of nerve fiber layer axons and the retinal arteries and veins. *F*, fovea. *H* and *V*, the horizontal meridian and vertical meridian superimposed on the retina, respectively.

Central Vision

Ganglion cell axons from the retina enter the optic nerve head in an orderly fashion. Those from the papillomacular bundle that carry macular or central visual information enter the temporal aspect of the disc. As they progress proximally they assume a more central location within the optic nerve. Clinically, the optic nerve behaves as though it were primarily a channel for central

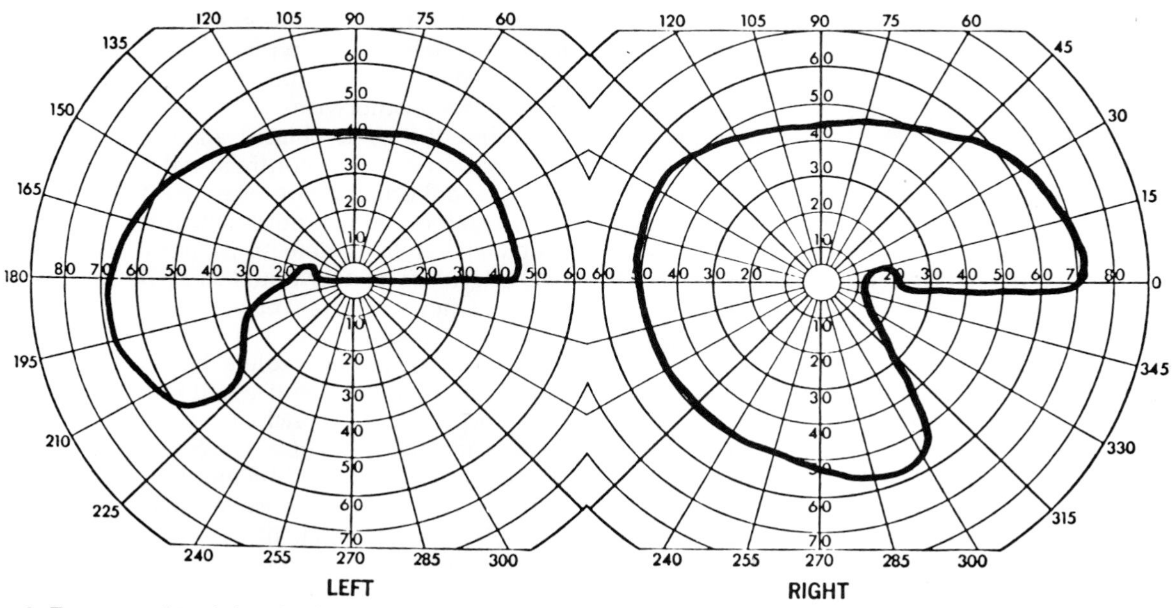

Figure 2. Two examples of altitudinal visual field defects that may be due to ischemic optic neuropathy or occlusion of a branch of the central retinal artery. On the left, the more common pattern extends from the nasal quadrant across the vertical meridian into the temporal quadrant. On the right there is a "quadrantanopia," but the blind spot, not fixation, is the focal point. In these and subsequent visual field illustrations, the patient sees everywhere inside the enclosed area except where a solid area indicates a scotoma such as the blind spot.

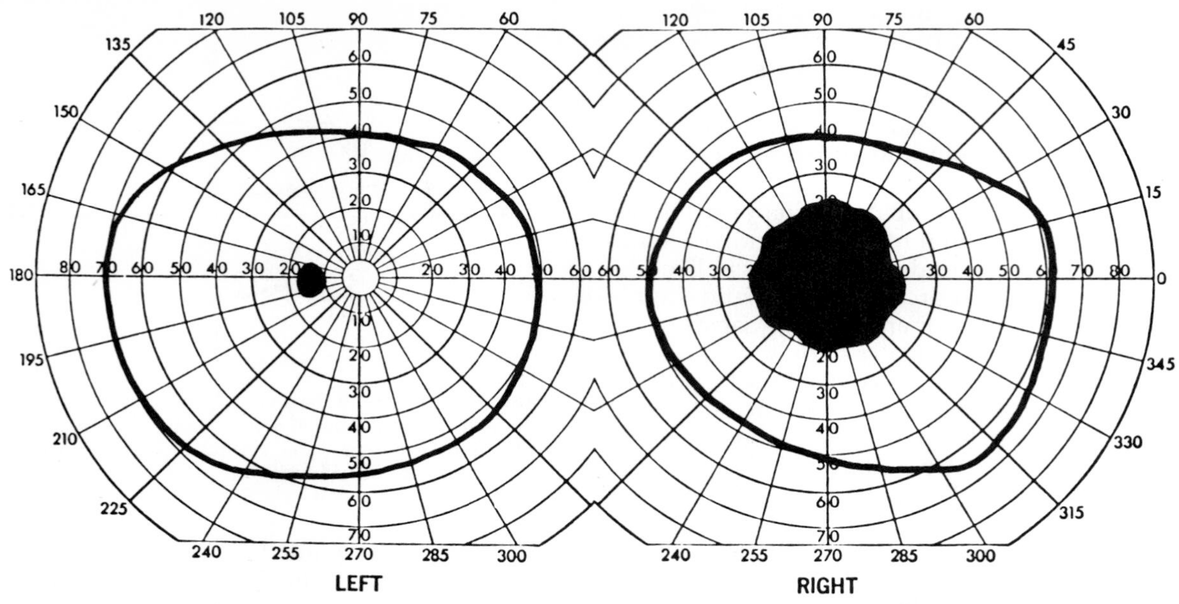

Figure 3. A central scotoma indicates the presence of a lesion of the optic nerve.

visual information. Therefore lesions of the optic nerve produce some combination of the following: loss of visual acuity, diminished color perception, diminished brightness of the visual environment, defective pupillary reaction to light, and visual field defects. The visual field defect usually consists of a depression of central vision in a central or centrocecal scotoma (Fig. 3).

The Vertical Meridian

At the chiasm all visual axons become segregated into crossed and uncrossed systems. At this level the visual system becomes functionally divided by a vertical line through the fixation point. This functional division at the vertical meridian enables one to localize lesions to the chiasm or to the retrochiasmal visual pathways in the optic tracts, visual radiations, or visual cortex.

The great majority of lesions affecting the optic chiasm are neoplastic,[1] although vascular, demyelinating, and traumatic lesions are seen occasionally. Lesions at the chiasm commonly produce the classic bitemporal hemianopia (Fig. 4). However, the chiasm is not an isolated structure and may be affected in conjunction with the optic nerve or optic tract in the case of a laterally placed lesion.

Some decussating fibers swing anteriorly to the junction of the opposite optic nerve and chiasm as they cross (Fig. 5). A lesion at this point produces symptoms and signs of an optic nerve lesion on that side. However, careful testing along the superior or inferior aspect of the vertical meridian will reveal a temporal field defect in the opposite eye (Fig. 6). This is referred to as a junctional scotoma. A more posteriorly and laterally situated lesion affecting the optic tract and chiasm may produce homonymous field defects in both eyes with the addition of a temporal field defect in the appropriate eye. In fact, most cases of optic tract visual field defects have extensive involvement of the chiasmal region with impaired visual acuity and central vision loss in at least one of the eyes.[2] Occasionally a chiasmal lesion will produce a temporal field defect in one eye only. A monocular temporal field defect with a sharp border at the vertical meridian should be considered chiasmal until proven otherwise.

Behind the optic chiasm all fibers carry visual information from the contralateral visual field, and fibers from both eyes are present. With rare exception, retrochiasmal lesions will produce homonymous visual field defects in both eyes. Certain characteristics of the visual field defects may indicate where in the retrochiasmal pathways a lesion is situated.

In the case of a complete homonymous hemianopia involving the entire half visual field in both eyes, no localizing conclusions can be drawn beyond the diagnosis of a retrochiasmal lesion on the contralateral side. Incomplete homonymous hemianopias provide more localizing information. Within the optic tract, fibers from corresponding regions of the two retinas are not closely grouped together. Therefore, visual field defects from optic tract lesions are characteristically incongruous; that is, the borders of the visual field defects are not the same in the two eyes (Fig. 7).

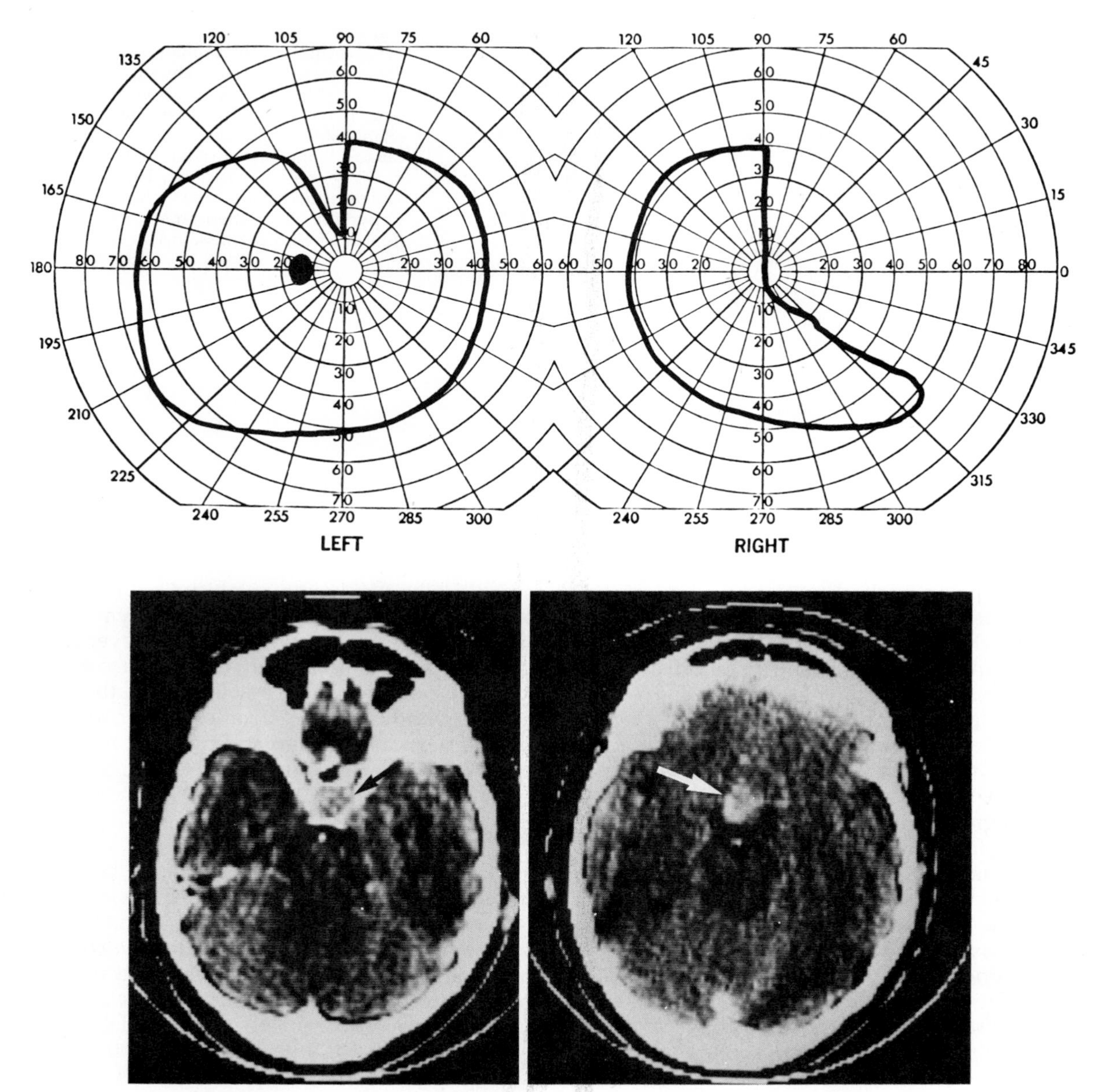

Figure 4. Bitemporal hemianopias are frequently incongruous, as in this case, and indicate a lesion of the optic chiasm. *Top*, Visual field illustrations. *Bottom*, CT scans showing pituitary tumor inside an enlarged sella turcica and extending upwards into the suprasellar cistern.

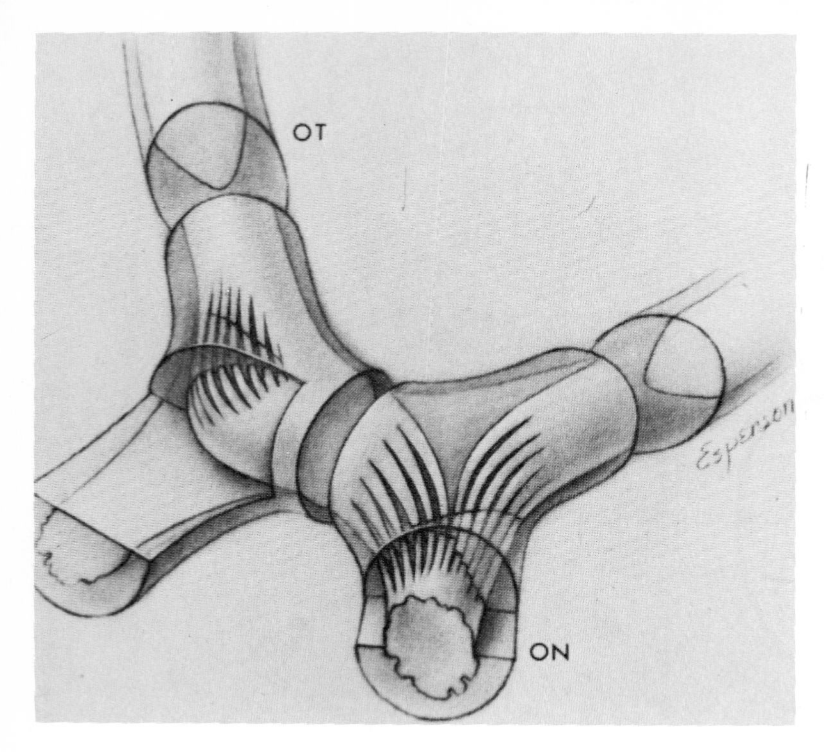

Figure 5. Crossed and uncrossed macular projections through the primate chiasm. Note that fibers crossing in the chiasm swing slightly anteriorly toward the junction of the opposite optic nerve *(ON)* and chiasm. Because of these relationships, laterally situated lesions may cause a "junctional scotoma," as seen in Figure 6. OT = optic tract. (From Hoyt WF, Luis O: The primate chiasm. Arch Ophthalmol 70:69–85. Copyright 1963, American Medical Association. Reprinted with permission.)

After synapsing in the lateral geniculate, visual fibers stream laterally into the parietal and temporal lobes. Here also, retinal correspondence of adjacent axons is not great, and field defects may be incongruous. Temporal lobe lesions produce the classic "pie in the sky" defect consisting of homonymous defects along the vertical meridian in the superior visual fields (Fig. 8). The visual radiations extend up into the parietal lobe to a variable degree. When parietal lobe lesions produce visual field defects, they should involve the inferior visual fields, although they often erode the lateral aspect of the visual field (Fig. 9), instead of beginning along the vertical meridian as temporal lobe visual field defects characteristically do in the superior field. As the radiations approach the visual cortex, fibers from homologous areas of the two retinas come together so that lesions in the occipital region cause congruous visual field defects (Fig. 10).

The calcarine cortex is divided into a superior bank and an inferior bank. The superior bank receives information from the inferior visual field, and the inferior bank receives information from the superior visual field. A very discrete lesion may occasionally affect only the superior or inferior bank, producing a true quadrantanopia in which the vertical meridian and horizontal meridian form the two borders of the visual field defect (Fig. 11). This should not be confused with the retinal lesion producing an altitudinal field defect, because it will be a congruous homonymous hemianopia. Even in a patient with one eye, the two lesions should not be confused, because an occipital lobe quadrantanopia will respect the vertical meridian and "point to" fixation rather than crossing the vertical meridian and pointing to the blind spot (compare Fig. 2 and Fig. 11).

Macular Sparing

Macular sparing is a homonymous hemianopia in which a small area, 5 to 10 degrees, or fixation is spared in the defective visual field. When the visual field is mapped on the calcarine cortex, the most peripheral field is represented in the depths of the interhemispheric fissure, whereas the macular representation is most superficial and may extend outside the interhemispheric fissure onto the surface of the occipital pole. If the entire calcarine cortex is damaged, macular sparing will not occur. Macular sparing is occasionally seen with vascular lesions in the distributions of the posterior cerebral artery. The most distal branches of the middle cerebral artery may supply blood to the occipital pole, thereby sparing a portion of the calcarine cortex that subserves macular function (Fig. 12). Macular sparing is best demonstrated and most helpful when formal quantitative perimetry is being used.

Text continued on page 558

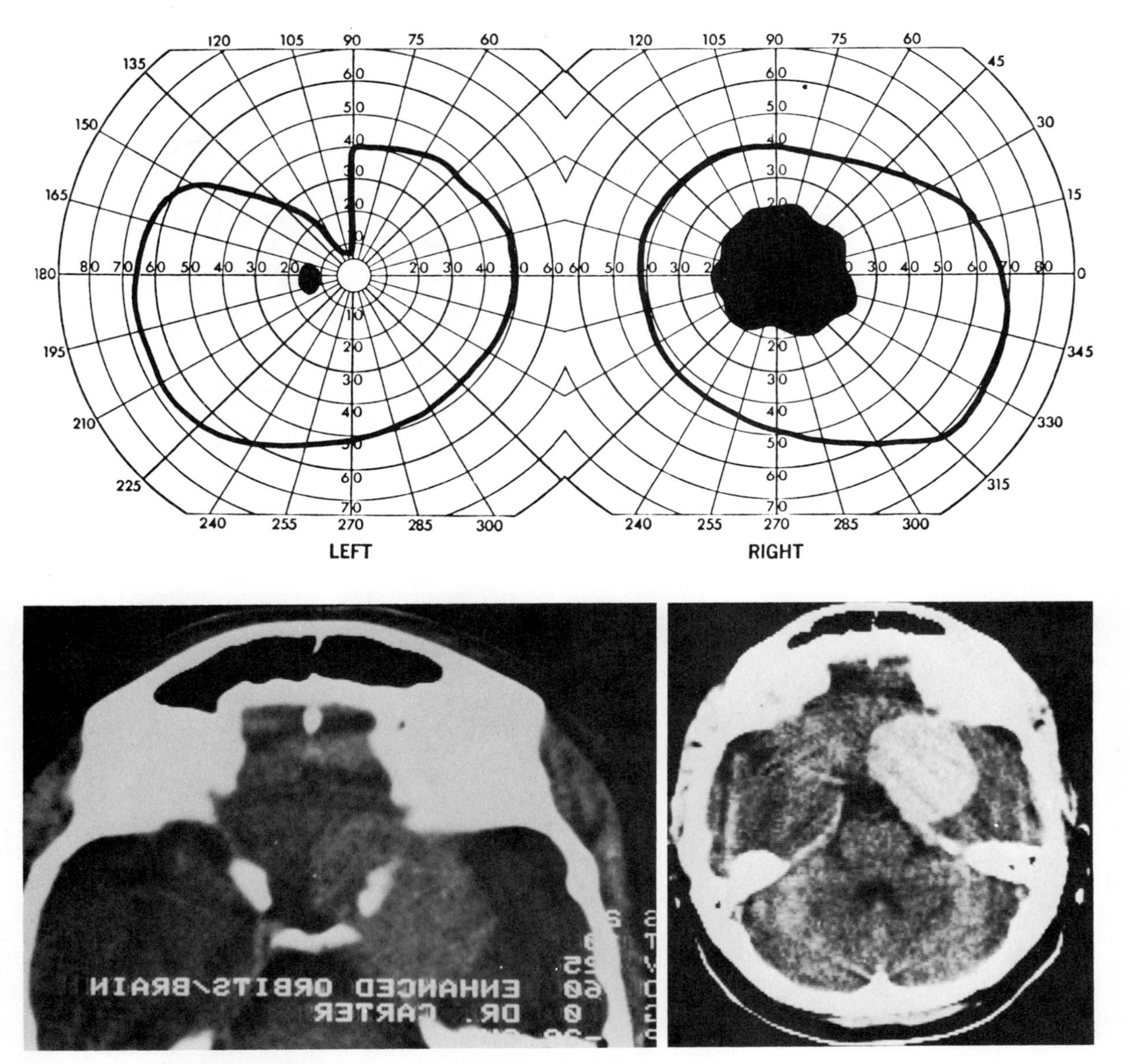

Figure 6. *Top,* Visual field illustration of a junctional scotoma consists of a central scotoma in the visual field of one eye and a temporal visual field defect in the other eye. This condition indicates an intracranial lesion involving the optic chiasm on the side of the central scotoma. *Bottom,* CT scans showing a large meningioma arising from the sphenoid ridge, extending into both the anterior and middle cranial fossas and involving the right optic nerve and chiasm. The chief complaint was visual loss in the right eye, but questioning revealed symptoms of seizure activity in the temporal lobe.

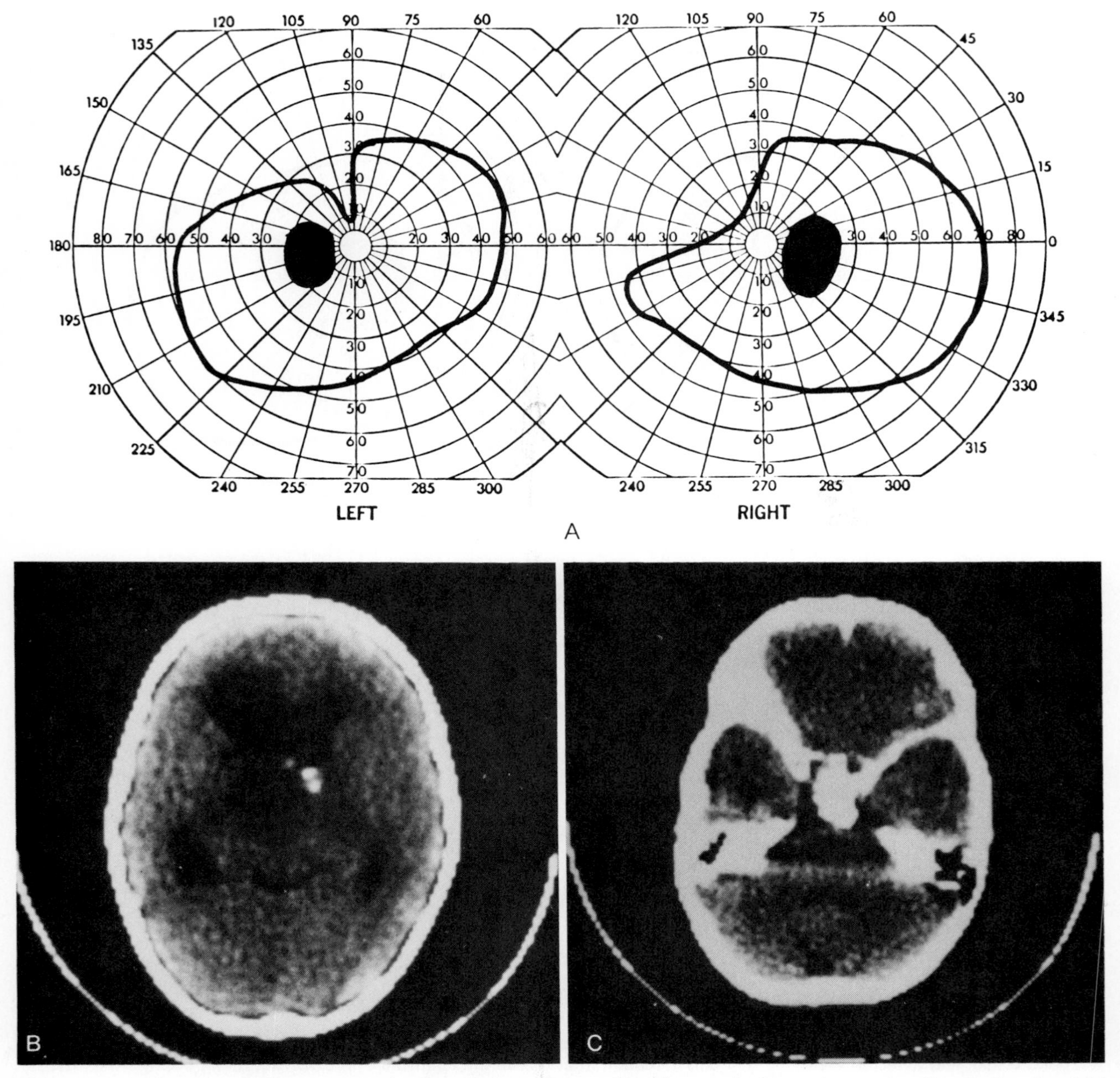

Figure 7. *A,* An incongruous homonymous hemianopia in an 8 year old with a craniopharyngioma primarily affecting the right optic tract. Papilledema produced enlarged blind spots. *B* and *C,* CT scans demonstrate a lesion with extensive calcifications in the suprasellar cisterns and a round cystic component in the higher cut, just left of the midline, obliterating the third ventricle and obstructing cerebrospinal flow out of the lateral ventricles.

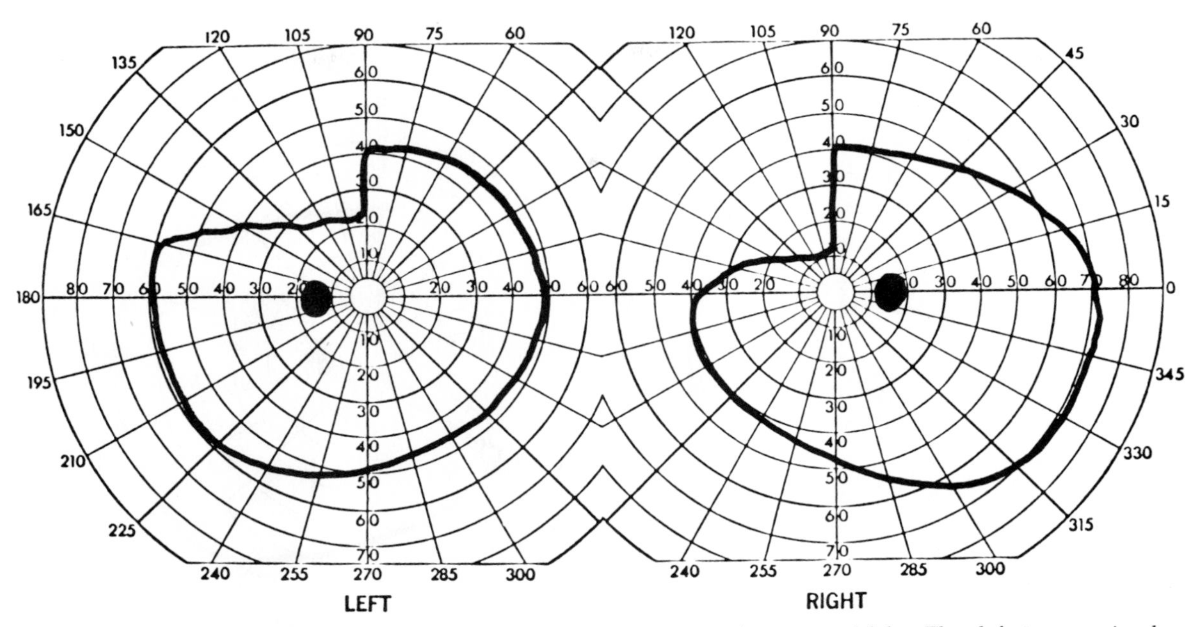

Figure 8. Mildly incongruous homonymous hemianopia due to a lesion in the temporal lobe. The defect moves in along the vertical meridian but will not cause an exact quadrantanopia, which is seen only with an occipital lobe lesion, as shown in Figure 11.

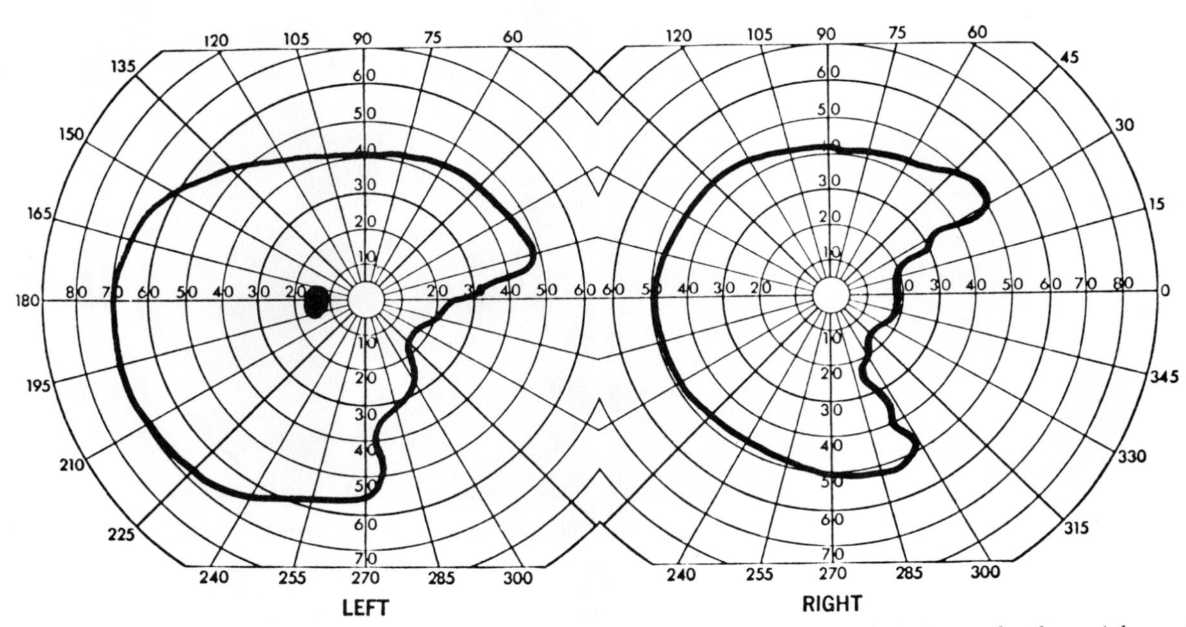

Figure 9. Incongruous homonymous hemianopia due to a lesion in the parietal lobe. An early lesion erodes the periphery of the inferior visual field without forming a sharp margin at the vertical meridian. If it is a progressive lesion, it will finally reach but not cross the vertical meridian.

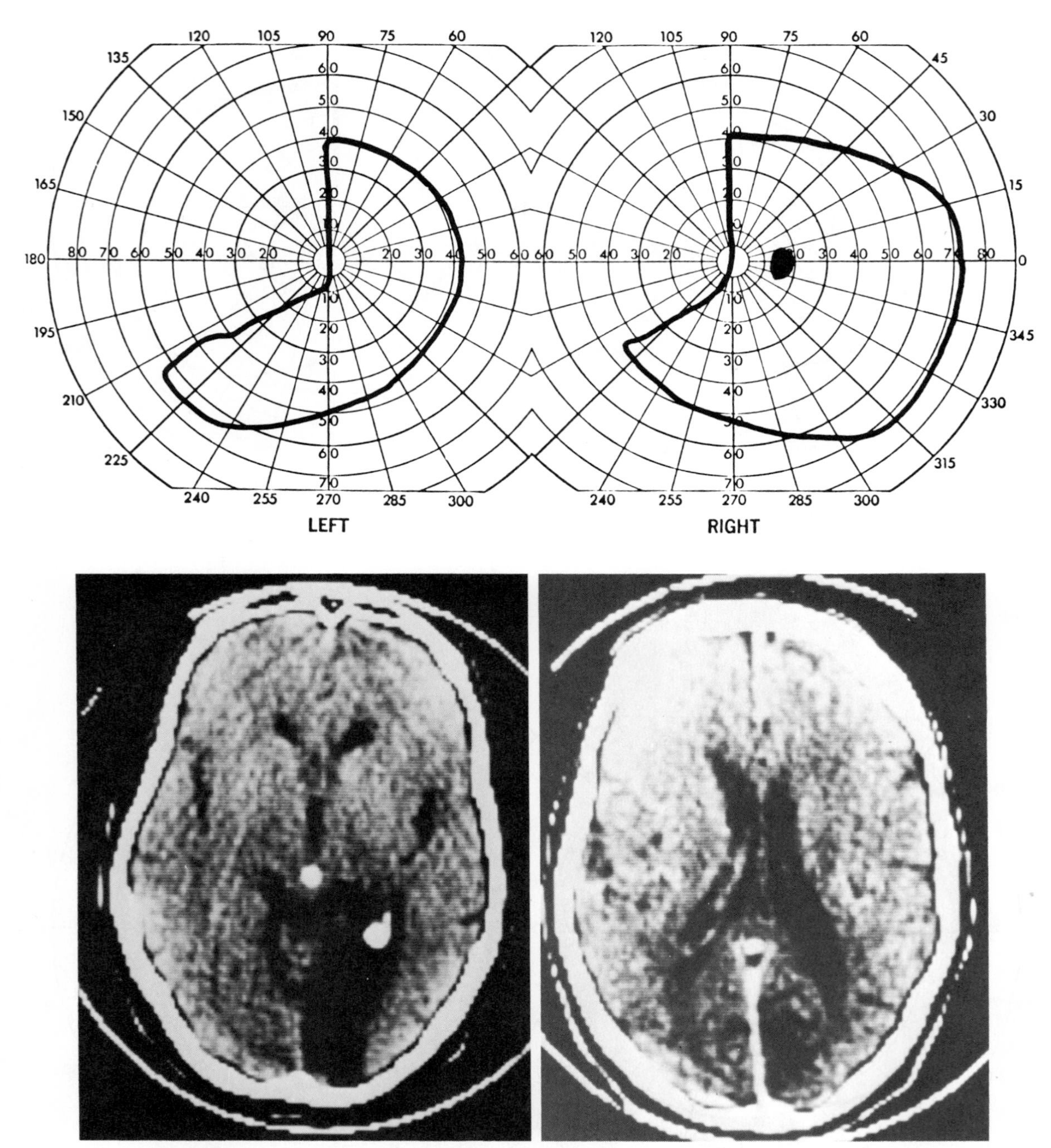

Figure 10. A congruous homonymous hemianopia due to a lesion of the occipital lobe. Whatever the size of the field defect, it should be identical in the two eyes if it is caused by an occipital lobe lesion. *Top,* visual field illustrations. *Bottom,* CT scans showing infarction of part of the occipital lobe on the right. The higher level *(right)* is less involved, and part of the inferior field is therefore preserved.

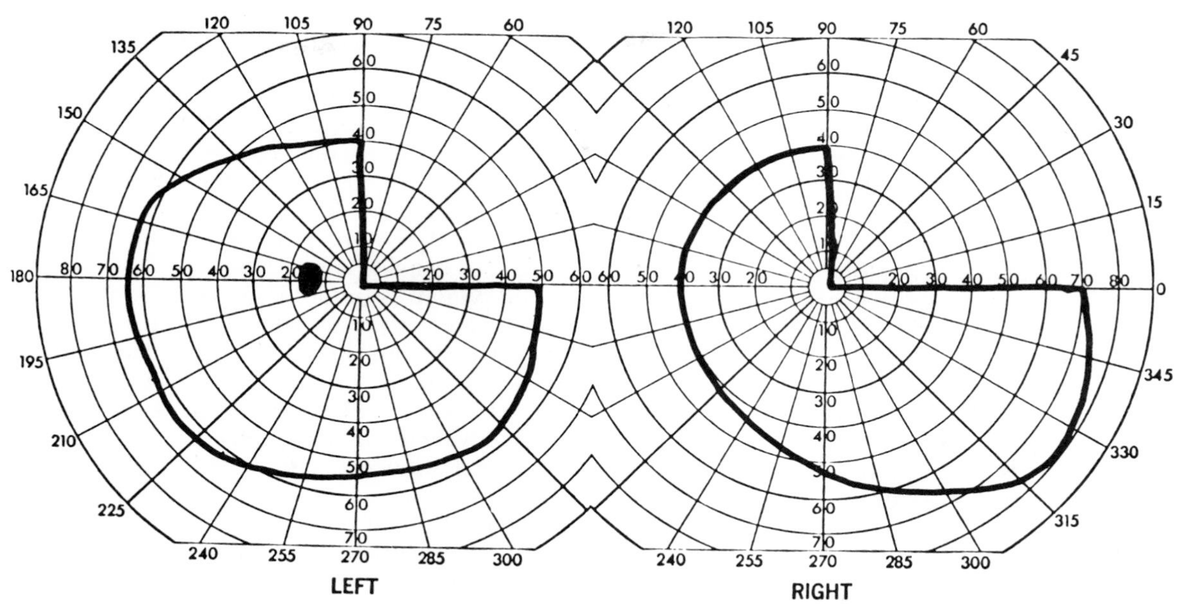

Figure 11. An infarction of either superior or inferior bank of the calcarine cortex produces a precise quadrantanopia that is homonymous and points to fixation.

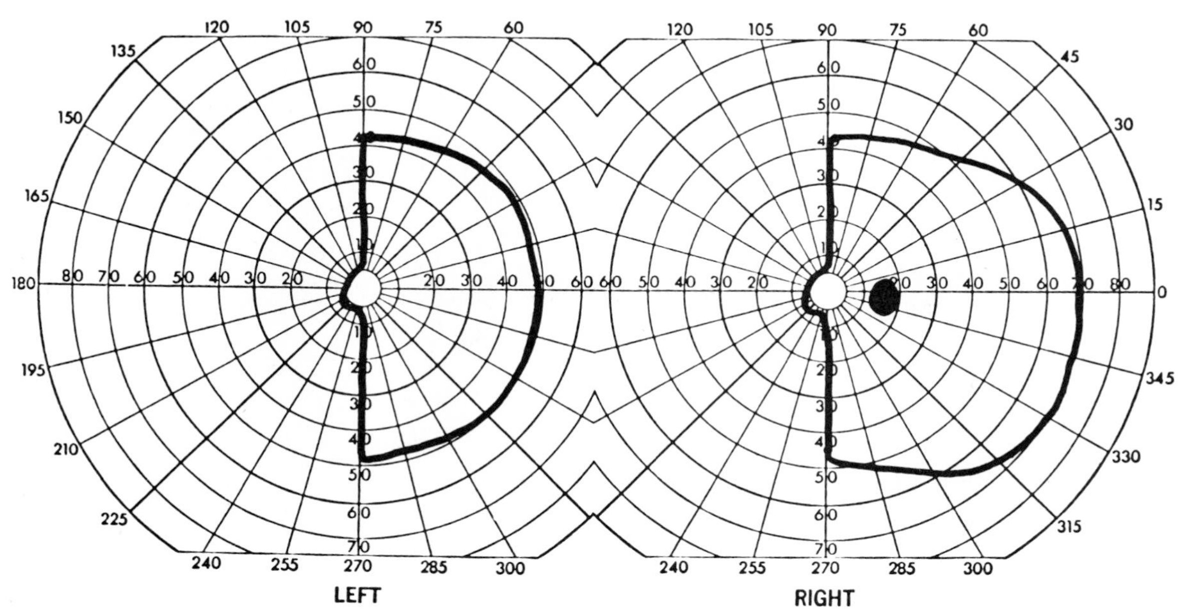

Figure 12. Macular sparing. Occlusion of the posterior cerebral artery may produce a complete homonymous hemianopia sparing only a few degrees of central vision, which is represented at the occipital pole and supplied by distal branches of the middle cerebral artery.

HISTORY

The character of a visual field defect provides the localization of the responsible lesion. The nature of that lesion is most likely to be provided by a carefully taken history. The patients under consideration here should complain of loss of vision of some type. The physician must clarify this complaint. What does the patient mean by "blurred vision"? Is it throughout the visual field or in one specific area? Are the symptoms in one or both eyes? What happens when each eye is covered individually? What did the patient first notice? A film over the eye, dirty glasses, looking through a fog? An observant patient may report changes in the color of objects or difficulty with traffic lights or tuning a color TV. Bumping into objects on one side may lead to an awareness of a difficulty seeing to that side.

The temporal profile of an illness is most helpful when determining the nature of the disease. The patient should be asked when he or she first became aware of the problem. Difficulty establishing this point often means that a slowly progressive lesion is present. Sudden onset, on the other hand, implies a vascular cause. It is important, however, to determine how the patient first noticed the visual loss. For example, if the patient happened to cover one eye and suddenly became aware of visual loss in the other eye, the loss is often interpreted as an acute change by the patient when in fact it may have been there for some time. How long did it take the deficit to become maximal? Is it improving, stable, or continuing to worsen? If the visual loss is intermittent, how often does it occur and are there any factors that seem to precipitate it? Figure 13 provides a graphic representation of the temporal profile of the major processes causing visual loss.

The patient should be questioned regarding the presence of any associated symptoms during the presence of visual loss. Pain or headache, diplopia, weakness or incoordination, and sensory disturbances are all important. Both formed and unformed visual hallucinations are common in patients experiencing visual disturbances. Patients may be reluctant to complain of hallucinations because of perceived psychiatric implications. Reassurance followed by specific questions regarding visual hallucinations may be surprisingly productive.

The previous medical history is of importance

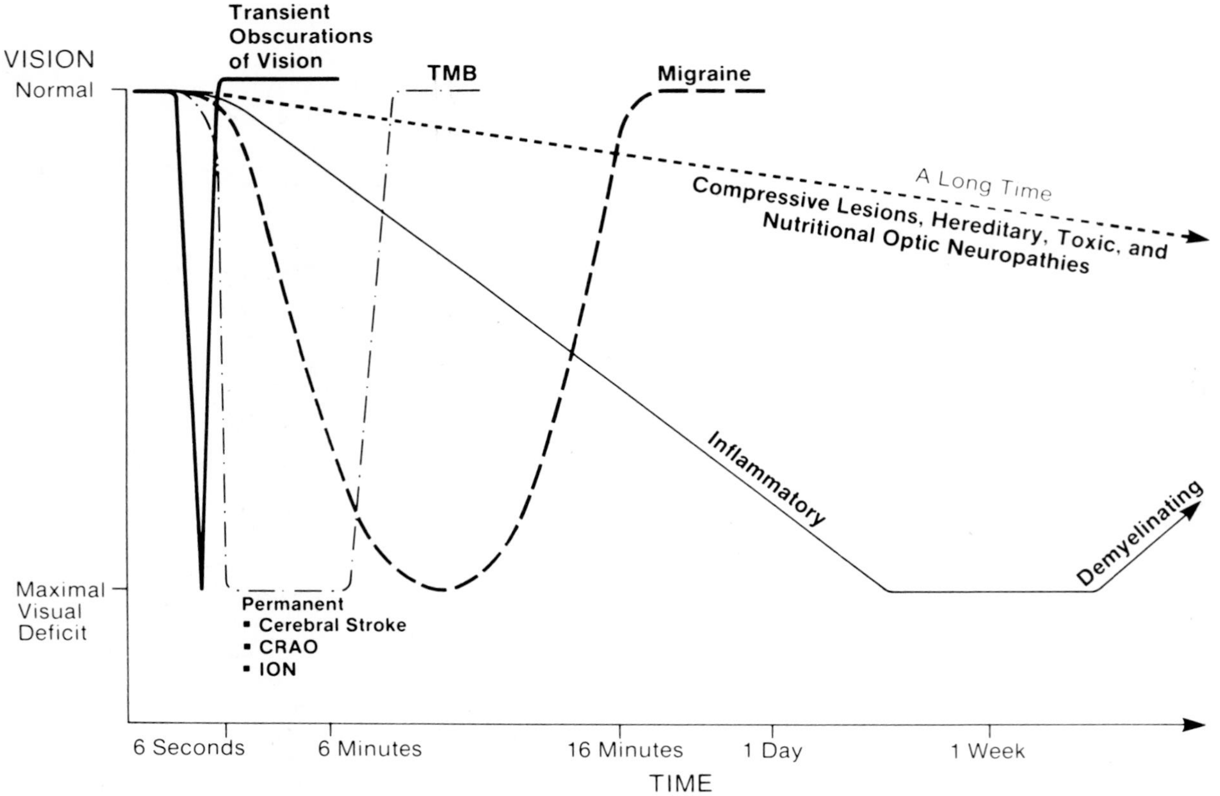

Figure 13. The temporal profile of visual loss produced by various pathologic processes affecting the visual system. *TMB*, transient monocular blindness; *TIA*, transient (cerebral) ischemic attack; *CRAO*, central retinal artery occlusion; *ION*, ischemic optic neuropathy. Specific inflammatory processes (infections, sarcoidosis, systemic lupus erythematosus) may not have as good a prognosis for recovery as idiopathic demyelinating lesions such as those of multiple sclerosis.

to document previous neurologic or visual disturbances that may relate to the present illness and to determine whether there are any systemic illnesses that might contribute to the present illness. A list of the patient's medications should be included.

The family history is also of importance because a number of conditions that cause visual disturbances may be familial.

PHYSICAL EXAMINATION

Visual Acuity

Although not usually thought of as such, visual acuity is simply a measure of the sensitivity of the most central part of the visual field. Even a best-corrected visual acuity of 20/25 implies the presence of a central scotoma. Therefore, in any patient complaining of visual loss the visual acuity should be checked, preferably with a Snellen chart or at least with a near-vision card. This check should be done with the patient's glasses on and may be further checked by having the patient view the material through a pin hole.

Because half of the visual field is adequate for a visual acuity of 20/20, the central scotoma implied by a diminished visual acuity indicates some process anterior to the chiasm. Two additional visual acuity tests, neither requiring the sophisticated equipment found in ophthalmologists' offices, can help distinguish between the three common causes of impaired acuity—amblyopia, retinopathy, and optic neuropathy. These two tests are the light stress test and the neutral density filter test.

In the light stress test, the patient's visual acuity is first determined.[3] Then a penlight is shined in the patient's eye for 10 seconds. Following this, the patient will have a decrease in visual acuity which should return to its prestress level within 1 minute. In retinal diseases, the return to the prestress level takes longer than 1 minute.

In the neutral density filter test, the patient views the reading chart through a neutral density filter (Kodak #96, ND 2.00). In patients with amblyopia, the visual acuity is unchanged. In normals and patients with retinal disease, the visual acuity may be decreased by two lines, for example, from 20/30 to 20/50. In patients with optic neuropathy, the visual acuity shows a dramatic decrease of several lines, perhaps from 20/30 to 20/80 or 20/100.

Color Vision and Pupillary Reactions

Although disturbances of color vision may be seen with hemispheric lesions, the presence of a disturbance in color vision is most helpful in diagnosing an optic neuropathy in the patient with diminished acuity. Ishihara and American Optical color plates are most commonly used. Symmetric impairment may be due to a congenital color vision defect, and other parts of the examination are required to separate congenital from acquired color vision defects. Asymmetric performance on color vision tests always indicates the presence of an optic neuropathy.

The pupillary reaction to light is also important in determining the presence of optic nerve disease. Mild defects consist of initial constriction followed by a redilation (pupillary escape) despite the continued presence of the light stimulus. In unilateral disease, the defect is most easily seen with the swinging penlight test (Fig. 14). This test consists of shining the light in the normal eye, the pupil of which will constrict; the consensual response will result in constriction of the pupil in the abnormal eye. Quickly swinging the penlight to the affected eye will result in partial redilation of both pupils owing to the defective response in the eye that is now being stimulated. Returning the penlight to the normal eye will again produce a distinct constriction.

Visual Field Testing

Amsler Grid

A simple and effective method of testing for the presence of central and paracentral scotomas uses

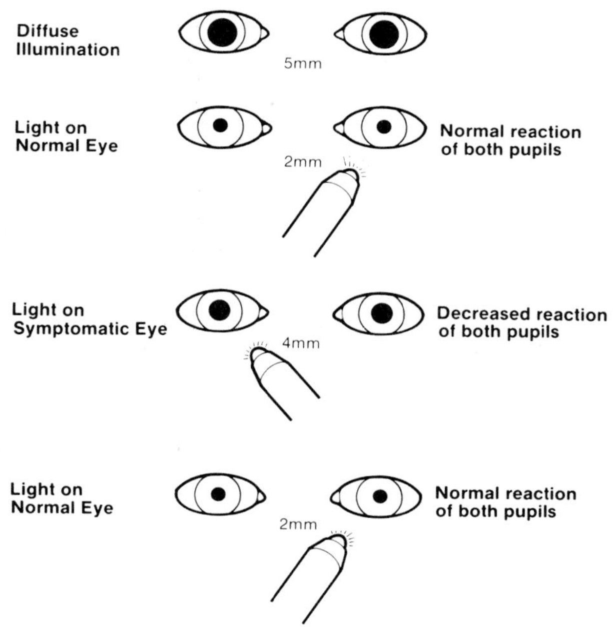

Figure 14. The swinging flashlight test is useful in an asymmetric optic nerve disturbance. Light in the symptomatic eye does produce some constriction but not as much as in the normal eye. When the flashlight is quickly moved from the normal eye to the symptomatic eye, both pupils dilate instead of remaining constricted.

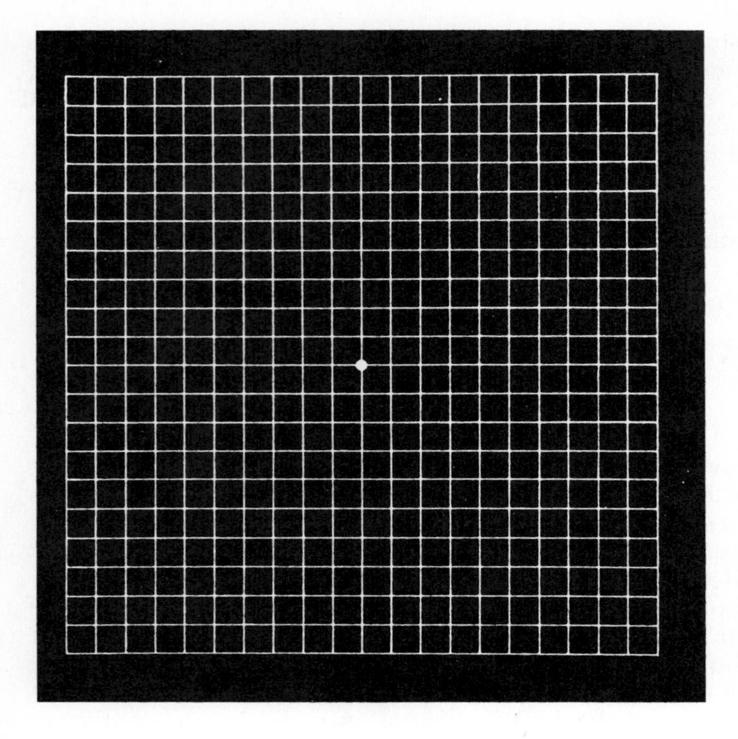

Figure 15. An Amsler grid.

the Amsler Grid (Fig. 15). The patient is told to look at the center dot of the grid and is then asked whether he or she can see all four corners and all four sides. The patient is asked whether all the lines appear straight or if any lines appear wavy or otherwise distorted. The patient is given a copy of the chart on which to draw the defect he or she sees.

Confrontation Visual Field Testing

Confrontation testing is generally performed with the examiner seated in front of the subject and utilizes two kinds of comparisons. In one, the patient's response to a visual stimulus is compared to the examiner's presumably normal responses. In the second, the patient is requested to compare a visual stimulus in the two eyes or in two areas of the visual field in the same eye.

A variety of stimuli have been used in comparing the patient's and the examiner's visual fields. Hand waving and finger wiggling are the most common but the least sensitive. The larger or more intense the stimulus, the more dense a visual field defect must be to be detected. Straight pins with heads of colored plastic from 3 to 5 mm in diameter are easily found at fabric stores and make excellent stimuli for field testing. The pins may be stuck into the head of an eraser on a pencil for more convenient manipulation. The examiner sits directly across from the patient and moves the target in a plane perpendicular to the line of vision and equidistant from the patient and the examiner. The patient covers up one eye and the examiner closes his or her own eye opposite the occluded eye of the patient. The patient may fixate on the examiner's open eye, allowing the examiner to monitor the patient for eye movements. If the target is midway between examiner and patient, then the visual fields in the two eyes should be equal, allowing the examiner's normal fields to serve as a standard against which to judge the patient's fields. The patient must clearly understand that he or she is to respond only to the target bead and not to the pencil or examiner's hand or other objects. This method of confrontation field testing should always begin with a demonstration of the patient's blind spot. If this cannot be done, something is wrong with the patient's understanding of the instructions, and the validity of the remainder of the test is questionable. This method of testing is most reliable in retrochiasmal visual field defects, which tend to be more dense than prechiasmal visual field defects. However, altitudinal field defects from ischemic optic neuropathy or retinal arterial occlusions may also be quite dense. The most important areas to explore are the vertical and horizontal meridians. The examiner should proceed from outside the visual field toward the center just beside the meridian being examined. When the patient responds, the opposite side of the same meridian is immediately explored for comparison. A step-off at one of the horizontal meridians implies retinal vascular disease, whereas a step-off at one of the vertical meridians implies chiasmal or retrochiasmal disease. A single determination of the edge of the peripheral field midway between the vertical and horizontal meridians in each quadrant is usually sufficient if no defects have been found along the vertical and horizontal meridia. Sometimes a central scotoma may also be plotted with this technique. A red target is most useful in this situation. The examiner begins at the center of the field and moves the target out with instructions for the patient to respond when the target becomes red or more clearly red or brighter red.

In finger counting, the examiner extends both arms and raises one to several fingers on each hand in each of the two fields being compared (Fig. 16). Simultaneous presentation of the stimuli increases the test's sensitivity, because mildly impaired visual processing in one field may be further impaired by the occurrence of visual processing at the same time in another field. This is common with parietal lobe disturbances, which may produce no overt visual field defect even with formal perimetry and yet exhibit extinction of the stimuli in the contralateral field on double simultaneous stimulation of left and right visual fields. Finger counting may also be the best technique for young children. Even if they are unable to count the fingers, they may be able to imitate the examiner with their own fingers.

The remainder of the confrontation techniques involve the patient's subjective color comparison between the eyes or between a suspected impaired field and a normal field in the same eye.[4, 5] Red is most commonly used, and the red bottle caps on mydriatic solutions in the ophthalmologist's office are a popular choice. It is important for both patient and physician to understand what comparison is desired. In a defective area of field, an object may appear dull and when it is moved into a normal area it may be described as brighter by the patient. However, in a defective field, the color may appear to be more washed out and lighter and, when moved into a normal area of visual field, may be described as darker by the patient. It may be best to ask the patient to tell the examiner when the object appears to be most truly red or to give the patient something to compare it to. I ask patients to tell me when the red object appears to be most like the red that they expect to see on a fire engine.

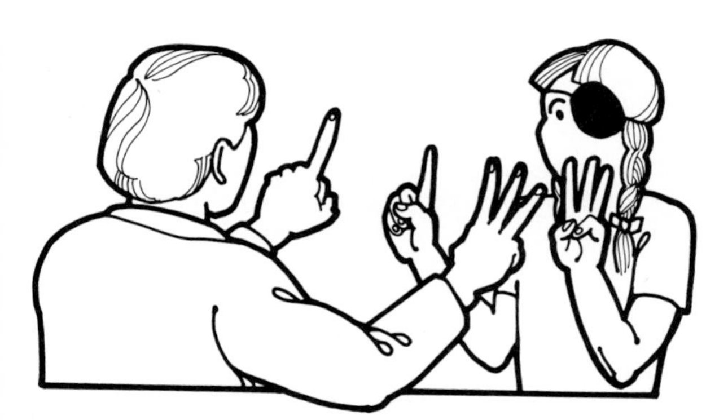

Figure 16. Finger counting visual fields. The patient may state the total or imitate the examiner.

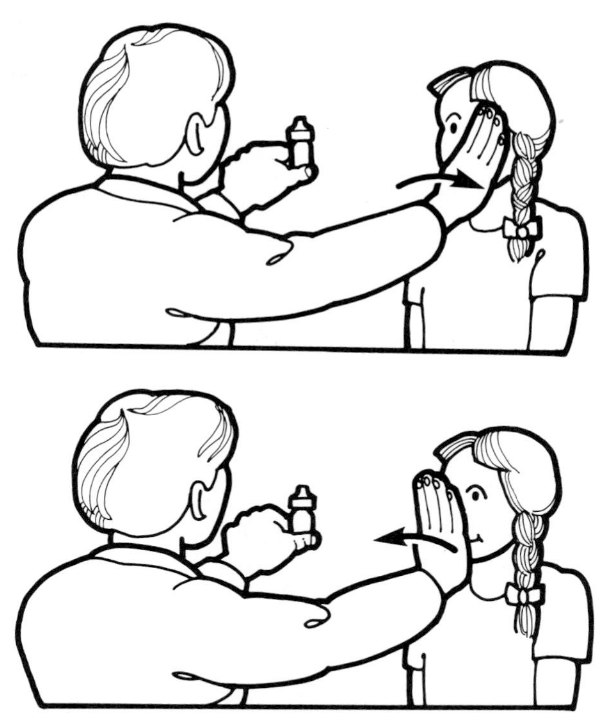

Figure 17. Comparison of color saturation in the two eyes.

When a central scotoma is suspected, the red target may be held up while one of the patient's eyes is occluded by the examiner (Fig. 17). The examiner then occludes the eyes alternatively and asks whether there is any difference in the redness.

The remainder of color comparison testing will be performed in one eye at a time. Two red objects are presented on either side of a meridian for the patient to compare (Fig. 18). Thus, comparisons are made between: the upper nasal and upper temporal quadrants, the lower nasal and lower temporal quadrants, the upper and lower quadrants on the temporal side, and the upper and lower quadrants on the nasal side. When testing is completed, a simple charting method can be utilized to record the presence of an altitudinal, bitemporal, or homonymous field defect if color desaturation abnormalities are present (Fig. 19).

ASSESSMENT

Once the character of the visual field defect has been determined, the history and other information can be used to establish a differential diagnosis and proceed to appropriate diagnostic tests or therapy.

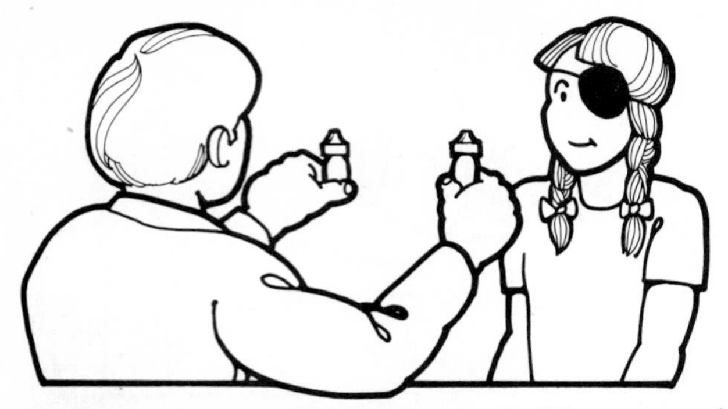

Figure 18. Comparison of color saturation in different parts of the visual field of one eye.

Altitudinal Field Defects

The patient presenting with visual loss and an altitudinal field defect (see Fig. 2) may have either ischemic optic neuropathy or occlusion of one of the branches of the central retinal artery. These two diagnoses have very different implications for further diagnostic evaluation. Distinguishing between them is possible owing to the characteristic appearance of the fundus in each.

Ischemic Optic Neuropathy

Ischemic optic neuropathy consists of an infarction of a segment of the optic disc or of the entire optic nerve head. The characteristic fundus appearance is that of a normal retina with a swollen optic disc. The swelling is characteristically pale, lacking the hyperemia seen with optic neuritis or papilledema (Fig. 20). However, the area of pale swelling may include only a segment of the disc, which will be in the opposite vertical quadrant from the visual field defect (Fig. 21). In this case, the remainder of the disc may exhibit secondary swelling with hyperemia similar to that of other causes of disc edema.

The natural history of ischemic optic neuropathy has been well described by Boghen and Glaser.[6] This condition may be idiopathic or may be caused by temporal arteritis.

Patients with temporal arteritis are almost always more than 70 years old, although occasionally the disease develops in younger patients. Other symptoms of temporal arteritis, such as progressively worsening headaches, jaw claudication, polymyalgia rheumatica, night sweats or fever of unknown etiology, and anemia, may be relatively mild or may not have been recognized. It is common for the diagnosis of temporal arteritis to be made because of an episode of ischemic optic neuropathy. Because 65 per cent of patients who present with ischemic optic neuropathy due to temporal arteritis in one eye will experience visual loss in the other eye, often within 24 hours and usually within the first week,[7, 8] it is very important to make this diagnosis during the patient's initial visit. A history suggestive of temporal arteritis should prompt initiation of therapy with steroids pending a temporal artery biopsy. In a patient with ischemic optic neuropathy but no other symptoms of temporal arteritis, the erythrocyte sedimentation rate should be determined at the time of the visit. If the rate is higher than 40 mm/hr, it may be appropriate to start the patient on steroids pending temporal artery biopsy.

The majority of patients with nonarteritic ischemic optic neuropathy are between 55 and 70 years old, although they may be as young as 40 years. These patients are generally healthy, except that hypertension is present in up to 50 per cent and diabetes is common.[6, 9] Boghen and Glaser[6] found no association with carotid atherosclerotic disease and indicated that carotid arteriography was not necessary in these patients. This condition seldom occurs a second time in the same eye, but 20 to 40 per cent of the patients with ischemic optic neuropathy have a subsequent episode in the other eye.

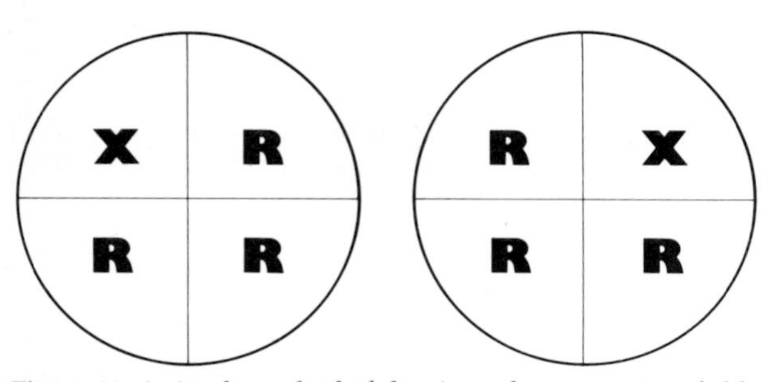

Figure 19. A simple method of charting color comparison fields. In this example the abnormal area in each eye *(X)* is in the superior temporal quadrant, indicating the bitemporal field defect of a chiasmal lesion.

Central Retinal Artery Occlusive Disease

Occlusion of the central retinal artery or one of its branches results in infarction of the retina, giving a milky opaque appearance to the retina owing to retinal edema (Fig. 22*A*). The optic disc itself is not involved, but the retinal edema may extend onto the surface of the disc, blurring the disc margins. If the macular region is involved, a classic cherry red spot will be seen (see Fig. 22*A*).

Occlusion of the central retinal artery or its branches may be caused by either small vessel atherosclerotic disease of the ophthalmic or central retinal artery or by embolic occlusion, most commonly from the carotid artery. A complete central retinal artery occlusion infarcting the entire retina in an older patient is very likely to be due to atherosclerotic disease in the retrobulbar portion

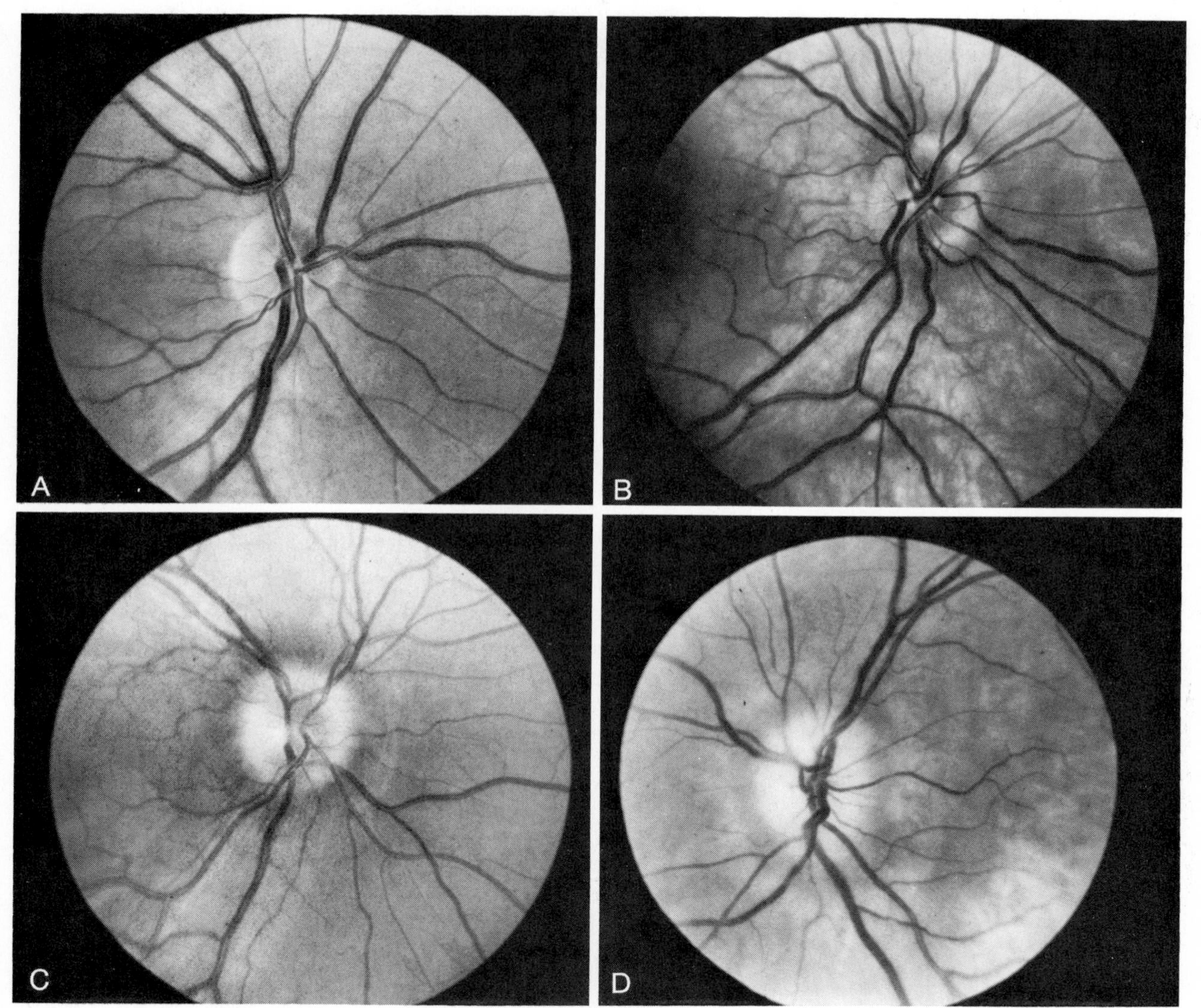

Figure 20. Optic disc swelling from three different causes. *A,* A normal disc for comparison. Note that the temporal quadrant is normally lighter in color than the remaining quadrants but is still well vascularized. *B,* Papilledema. The peripapillary nerve fiber layer is opacified and pale in comparison with the rest of the fundus, but the middle of the disc is still well vascularized and even hyperemic. *C,* Optic neuritis may be indistinguishable from the early stages of papilledema such as that in *B,* but the presence of visual loss suggests that optic neuritis is the correct diagnosis. *D,* Ischemic optic neuropathy may look like optic neuritis, but the more characteristic appearance is seen here. The optic disc is swollen, but the absence of the normal vascularity makes the entire disc pale.

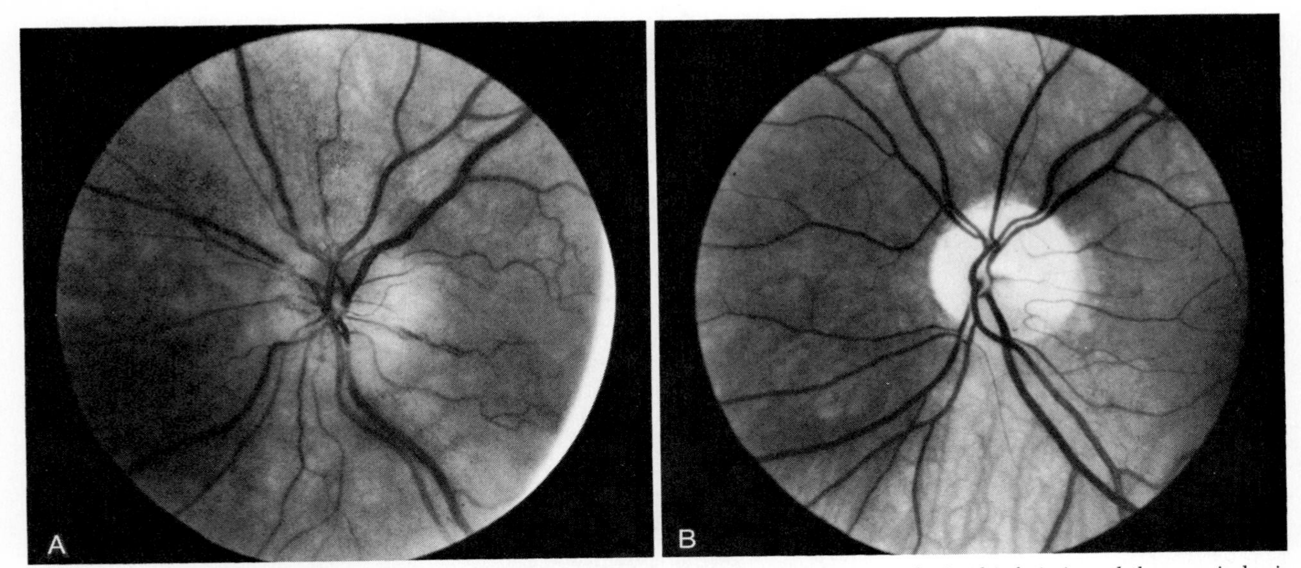

Figure 21. *A,* In ischemic optic neuropathy one area may be swollen and pale, as seen right (and inferior), and the remainder is swollen but well vascularized. The infarcted area of disc is the pale area, and the altitudinal field defect will be opposite this area, superior in this case. *B,* After the acute swelling has resolved and optic atrophy is evident, the segment of optic disc that was not infarcted remains well vascularized and healthy in appearance, as seen in the inferior quadrant in the disc illustrated. This pattern identifies the cause of the optic atrophy as ischemic optic neuropathy rather than central retinal artery occlusion.

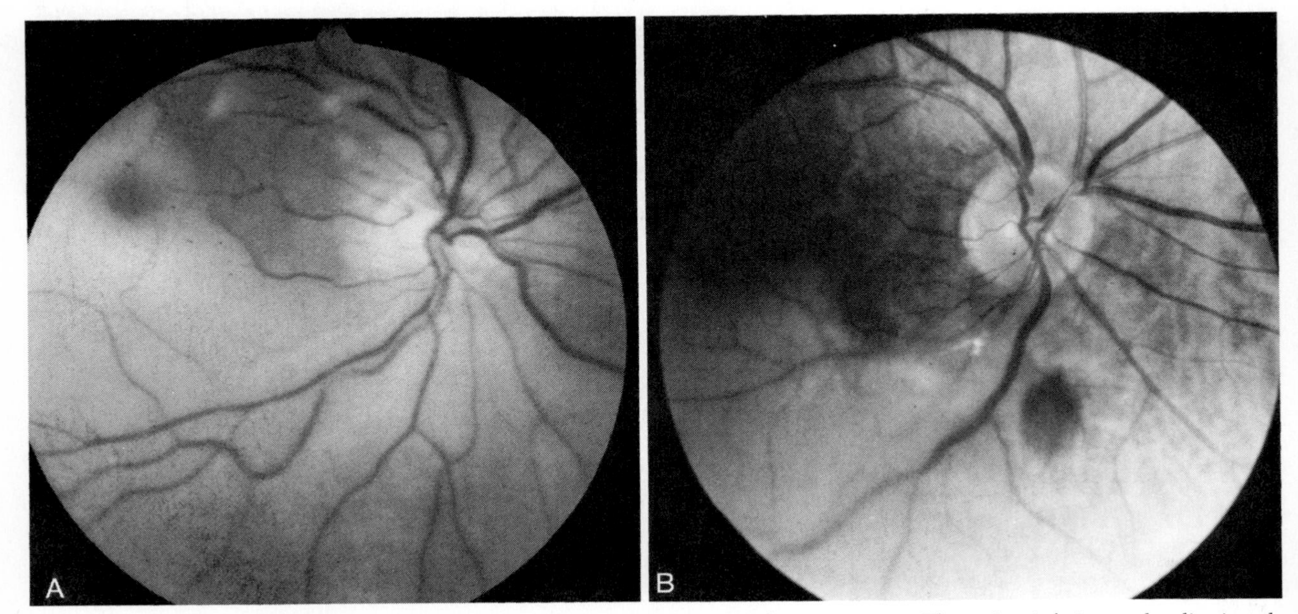

Figure 22. *A,* Central retinal artery occlusion due to an embolus that is no longer present. The retina inferior to the disc is pale and infarcted. The macular area is involved to the left of the disc, producing a cherry red spot. Although the superior retina looks better, the pale areas represent patchy retinal infarction and indicate that the superior retina is also ischemic. *B,* Occlusion of an inferior branch of the central retinal artery by an embolus that is still occluding the artery. The retina distal to the occlusion is pale and edematous.

of the central retinal artery. However, careful inspection of the retinal arteries may reveal embolic material, in which case diagnostic efforts should be aimed at locating the source of the embolus in the heart or extracranial vasculature in hopes of preventing cerebral infarction. Embolic material may fragment and move out of the retinal vasculature, leaving no direct evidence of its presence. However, branch occlusions of the central retinal artery circulation are almost always due to emboli (Fig. 22*B*). Therefore, altitudinal visual field defects due to retinal infarctions can be presumed to be due to an embolus and to have the same diagnostic implications as the presence of a visible embolus.

Altitudinal Visual Field Defects and Optic Atrophy

Occasionally a patient will present with an altitudinal visual field defect and optic atrophy. This combination indicates that the episode of visual loss occurred some time ago. In both ischemic optic neuropathy and branch retinal artery occlusion, the end result after resolution of the acute edematous changes will be optic atrophy. Figure 21*B* shows an optic disc in which one inferior quadrant still contains healthy, well-vascularized optic nerve tissue. This is a segment of optic nerve head that was unaffected during an earlier episode of ischemic optic neuropathy. In the absence of this characteristic change, it may be very difficult to tell whether the optic atrophy was due to ischemic optic neuropathy or retinal arterial occlusion. Retinal artery caliber may become quite narrow following either of these conditions. More sophisticated diagnostic procedures such as electroretinography may distinguish between the two.

Central Scotomas

In the patient with visual loss in whom an afferent package defect—that is, loss of visual acuity, decreased color vision, central scotoma, and diminished pupillary reaction to light—is found, there is probably a process affecting the optic nerve in the orbit, in the optic canal, or intracranially. The nature of the process is best determined by the patient's history.

Optic neuritis may involve the optic nerve head, producing visible disc edema, or may involve the retrobulbar portion of the optic nerve, producing symptoms and signs without visible fundus abnormalities. Characteristically there is decreasing vision, which may develop very rapidly but usually progresses over several days to a week. The visual loss may remain unchanged for several days, but usually by the end of 2 weeks, vision begins to improve. The large majority of patients experience good visual recovery.[1] In patients less than 20 years of age, optic neuritis is commonly bilateral. The majority of cases occur in the age group from 20 to 40 years old and are unilateral. An aching pain in or around the eye is common and is likely to be worse during eye movements. Most optic neuritis is idiopathic, but it is occasionally caused by contiguous inflammation of the meninges, orbit, or paranasal sinuses and may also be caused by syphilis, sarcoidosis, tuberculosis, and cryptococcosis. It is occasionally seen with systemic arteritides such as systemic lupus erythematosus. If there is no evidence of a systemic inflammatory disease or inflammation in structures along the course of the optic nerve, a patient with a presumed diagnosis of idiopathic optic neuritis may be followed expectantly. If the expected return of visual function begins within 2 to 3 weeks of the onset, radiologic studies such as CT scanning may not be necessary. Although steroids continue to be widely used in the treatment of idiopathic optic neuritis, there is no evidence that they change the ultimate outcome of optic neuritis, whereas in some cases of neoplastic optic nerve compression, the visual function may be improved temporarily, thus delaying the correct diagnosis. Therefore, I prefer not to use steroids in an initial episode of optic neuritis.

Compressive lesions of the optic nerve may be due to neoplastic or aneurysmal mass lesions and are generally unilateral. Diffuse infiltrative lesions of various causes, including sarcoidosis, lymphomas, and leukemias, may affect one or both nerves in the orbit or intracranially. Meningeal carcinomatosis frequently affects the optic nerves. CT scanning and examination of the cerebrospinal fluid are the primary diagnostic procedures for these conditions. Insidious and slowly progressive bilateral loss of vision (Table 1) with central sco-

Table 1. DIFFERENTIAL DIAGNOSIS OF INSIDIOUSLY PROGRESSIVE BILATERAL VISUAL LOSS

Toxic optic neuropathy	Heavy metals Chloroquine Ethambutol Isoniazid Streptomycin Digitalis Chlorpropamide Antabuse Chloramphenicol Placidyl
Nutritional optic neuropathy	Vitamin B_{12} deficiency Thiamine deficiency
Hereditary optic atrophies	
Demyelinating disease	
Dysthyroid optic neuropathy	
Macular dystrophies	
Atypical glaucoma	

tomas suggests toxic or nutritional optic neuropathy or hereditary optic atrophy.[1]

Bitemporal Visual Field Defects

Bitemporal field defects and junctional scotomas as well as most optic tract lesions are due to mass lesions somewhere in the suprasellar region.[1, 2] CT scanning is the primary diagnostic procedure and should provide information on which to base further diagnostic studies.

Homonymous Hemianopias

Major incongruity in the visual fields is indicative of an optic tract lesion. However, isolated optic tract lesions are seldom responsible for visual symptomatology. Most instances of optic tract involvement in patients with visual symptoms involve other structures in the chiasmal region, producing a mixture of field defects.[6] As in bitemporal visual field defects, mass lesions cause the great majority of optic tract syndromes.

Homonymous hemianopias due to lesions in the visual radiations or the occipital lobe will be caused by stroke or neoplasm in most instances. The temporal profile of the visual loss (see Fig. 13), associated symptoms such as visual hallucinations or seizures, and CT scanning should provide accurate information about the nature of the lesion.

Intermittent Visual Loss

Many patients experience intermittent visual symptoms and have no visual loss or visual field defects at the time of their examination. The temporal profile of their visual loss (see Fig. 13) should provide the information necessary to establish a diagnosis. Visual loss lasting for a few seconds is most likely to be seen with papilledema and to lead the physician to an evaluation of increased intracranial pressure. Transient monocular blindness (amaurosis fugax) with sudden loss of vision persisting for 5 to 10 minutes should lead to consideration of carotid vascular disease if the patient is in the correct age range. The presence of an arterial embolus provides further substantiation of a carotid atherosclerotic lesion. Visual loss that builds up over a period of 15 minutes in one visual field or occasionally in one eye should suggest migraine and may be seen without the headache on some occasions in patients with classic migraine. Similar episodes and other neurologic defects with a more gradual buildup and no headache occasionally occur in older patients who had migraine at a younger age,[12] but it is difficult to be certain that these patients do not have carotid vascular disease without performing an arteriogram.

QUANTITATIVE (FORMAL) PERIMETRY

Just as there are occasional patients with color desaturation or loss of brightness in one visual field who have normal visual fields on formal perimetry, some patients have subtle visual field defects that are demonstratable only at the perimeter. Therefore, any patient who has persistent visual complaints with no abnormalities on routine examination should have formal perimetry to define the visual disturbance.

Although confrontation visual field testing is effective in detection of many visual field defects, it is not a quantitative procedure. A number of situations occur in which serial quantitative visual field evaluations are necessary in managing the condition. Glaucoma is the most common ophthalmic condition in which this is true, but several neurologic conditions also require serial visual field evaluations. The major morbidity of pseudotumor cerebri is the visual loss that occurs in 10 to 25 per cent of patients;[13–15] as in glaucoma, the field defects often begin in the periphery and progress insidiously. By the time the patient notices loss of acuity there may be little of the peripheral vision field remaining. Patients with pituitary adenomas who are undergoing medical therapy and those who have received surgical treatment (and may subsequently have chiasmatic arachnoiditis or herniations of the chiasm into the empty sella turcica) should have serial quantitative perimetry examinations as part of continuing care.

REFERENCES

1. Glaser JS. Neuro-ophthalmology. Hagerstown, Md: Harper and Row, 1978: 91–104, 135.
2. Savino PJ, Paris M, Schatz NJ, Orr LS, Corbett JJ. Optic tract syndrome: a review of 21 patients. Arch Ophthalmol 1978;96:656–63.
3. Glaser JS, Savino PJ, Sumers KD, McDonald SA, Knighton RW. The photostress recovery test: a practical adjunct in the clinical assessment of visual function. Am J Ophthalmol 1977;83:255–60.
4. Frisen L. A versatile color confrontation test for the central visual field. A comparison with quantitative perimetry. Arch Ophthalmol 1973;89:3–9.
5. Trobe JO, Acosta PC, Krischer JP, Trick GL. Confrontation visual field techniques in the detection of anterior visual pathway lesions. Ann Neurol 1981;10:28–34.
6. Boghen DR, Glaser JS. Ischemic optic neuropathy: the clinical profile and natural history. Brain 1975;98:689–708.
7. Hollenhorst RW, Brown JR, Wagener HP, Shick RM. Neurologic aspects of temporal arteritis. Neurology 1960;10:490–98.
8. Meadows SP. Temporal or giant cell arteritis. Proc Roy Soc Med 1966;59:329–333.
9. Ellenberger C, Keltner JL, Burde RM. Acute optic neuropathy in older patients. Arch Neurol 1973;28:182–5.

10. Hollenhorst RW. Embolic retinal phenomena. In: Burde RM, Glaser JS, Hollenhorst RW, et al, eds. Symposium on neuro-ophthalmology. Transactions of the New Orleans Academy of Ophthalmology. St. Louis: CV Mosby, 1976;168–90.
11. Cohen M, Lessell S. A prospective study of the risk of developing multiple sclerosis in uncomplicated optic neuritis. Neurol 1979;29:208–13.
12. Fisher CM. Late-life migraine accompaniments as a cause of unexplained transient ischemic attacks. Can J Neurol Sci 1980;7:9–17.
13. Boddie HG, Banna M, Bradley WG. "Benign" intracranial hypertension. Brain 1974;97:313–26.
14. Rush JA. Pseudotumor cerebri. Clinical profile and visual outcome in 63 patients. Mayo Clin Proc 1980;55:541–6.
15. Corbett JJ, Savino PJ, Thompson HS, et al. Visual loss in pseudotumor cerebri: 57 patients followed 5 to 41 years and a profile of 14 patients with permanent severe visual loss. Arch Neurol 1982;39:461–74.

WEIGHT LOSS

DAVID E. SWEE □ FRANK C. SNOPE

□ SYNONYMS: Wasting, marasmus, cachexia

BACKGROUND

In approaching the diagnoses that underlie the finding of weight loss, one has to consider the period of time during which the loss was incurred as well as the degree of loss in terms of both absolute weight loss and percentage lost. Owing to the natural variability of body weight in the normal adult, most authorities would classify medically important weight loss as being, at minimum, a 5 per cent reduction of *usual* (not ideal) body weight over 6 months.[1] However, significant weight loss over a shorter time, especially in younger adults, also can be considered pathologic (such as seen in anorexia nervosa or athletic overconditioning).[2] Certainly, in the young child or infant, a one-day loss of 5 per cent body weight may be enough to lead to hospitalization. And although not necessarily always presenting with weight loss, the young child's "failure to thrive" may also lead to hospitalization.[3]

Many patients lose weight, but most of them are cycling between weight gain and weight loss in a constant effort to be thin. It has been argued that such cycling should be considered potentially dangerous to health. Regardless, this chapter focuses on the problem of weight loss that is of an *involuntary* or pathologic nature.

Although weight gain is a common complaint of patients seeing family physicians, and obesity is even a more common diagnosis, weight loss is much less frequently noted as a problem and, of course, should never be recorded as a diagnosis.[4] Patients are slow to complain of weight loss because it is often a happy event and it is rarely troubling or dramatically disturbing, in contrast to symptoms such as headaches and hematuria. The patient is more likely to report weight loss when the reduction has been overly rapid (by whatever standard the patient uses), when it is associated with other constitutional symptoms (e.g., malaise or fever), or when the patient finally considers himself or herself as "underweight." One has only to observe that less than 20 per cent of the population is underweight, and less than 10 per cent is significantly (greater than 10 per cent) underweight, to recognize why weight loss is so rarely troubling to patients.[5]

Indeed, more often than not, it is the physician rather than the patient who first notices the weight loss. In a recent survey of selected older adults with involuntary weight loss, only one-third of the patients had complained of weight loss.[1] The other two-thirds were identified by documenting the loss or by appropriate observations during physical examination. In the Virginia study of patient problems, weight loss by itself was ranked as the 142nd most common "diagnosis," accounting for approximately 0.1 per cent of all diagnoses.[6]

Causes of Weight Loss

The causes of weight loss are manifold. Because it is a generalized systemic effect, it can be found in connection with any prolonged or severe illness. Weight is considered to be controlled by the balance between calories acquired and calories expended. Thus, weight loss is produced by deficiencies of intake and assimilation on the one hand, or by extraordinary losses, usually by means of increased metabolism, on the other. The patient's appetite can be increased, normal (usually classified with increased), or decreased.

In the category of increased metabolism, hyperthyroidism is a classic example. In fact, weight loss may even precede such findings as tachycardia, nervousness, excessive perspiration, fine tremor, exophthalmos, and thyroid enlargement.[7] Diabetes mellitus is another condition involving increased metabolism in which weight loss may be the presenting symptom, especially in the young. Both diabetes and hyperthyroidism can present with weight loss in conjunction with an *increased* appetite, certainly a dramatic association.

However, most high metabolic states are associated with a decrease in appetite. Fever by itself can cause weight loss. For each degree of temperature rise (Fahrenheit), the basal metabolic rate increases 7 per cent. Chronic infections likewise lead to increased metabolism and weight loss. In children, many chronic illnesses can lead to poor growth and even outright weight loss. Cardiac disease in infants is a classic example, in which weight loss is often due to the combined causes of increased metabolism and decreased assimilation (e.g., difficulty eating secondary to dyspnea). Congestive heart failure in adults may present with weight gain secondary to edema, but also may present with weight loss for the same reasons as those in infants. In adults presenting with weight loss, however, physicians most commonly think of cancer as the probable cause. A recent survey demonstrated that of the patients who were ultimately found to have a physical cause for their illness, 25 per cent had cancer.[1] Even if the cancer does not cause difficulties of absorption or digestion of food, it may produce weight loss by increasing the metabolic processes of the patient.[8]

Difficulties with assimilation include both inadequate digestion and inadequate absorption leading to weight loss. In cystic fibrosis in infancy, weight loss in spite of large food intake can be an early symptom. Conditions that lead to malabsorption are multiple. Causes can be classified as defects in intraluminal hydrolysis or solubilization (e.g., pancreatic insufficiency), mucosal abnormality (e.g., Vitamin B_{12} malabsorption, celiac disease, Crohn's disease), lymphatic obstruction (e.g., tuberculosis, lymphadenitis), or infection (e.g., tropical sprue). Of course, some conditions have multiple causes (e.g., radiation enteritis), some remain unexplained (e.g., carcinoid syndrome), and some are iatrogenic (e.g., drug-induced as with cholestyramine).[9]

Finally, deficiency of intake may be the primary cause of weight loss. Almost any profound psychological illness can lead to a decreased intake, as in anxiety or depression. By definition, anorexia nervosa appears with a loss of at least 25 per cent of the patient's body weight.[10] This condition has become of increasing concern as its actual prevalence, which is approximately 1 in 200 young teenage females, becomes known.[11] It is classically associated with amenorrhea, constipation, hypotension, bradycardia, and hypothermia.[12]

Any major physical illness that leads to inanition and loss of interest in food can certainly lead to decreased intake and weight loss. Malignancy, uremia, chronic infections, cardiac conditions, and inflammatory conditions are among this group. Likewise, addiction to alcohol, drugs, or tobacco may lead to decreased food intake. Mechanical causes, such as advanced crippling leading to poor ability to prepare meals as well as difficulties at the oral level (e.g., lack of dentures), may decrease food intake. In the elderly, protein calorie malnutrition is a common finding. Malabsorption has some role to play in this syndrome, but diseases of the oral cavity, poor dentition, and poor activity states also are important causes.[13]

HISTORY

Information concerning the onset of the involuntary weight loss, whether it is sudden or subtle, as well as its progression, should be obtained. If the patient states that the weight loss has been voluntary, further exploration of efforts to lose weight, including special diets and changes in activity, will be important. Information concerning changes in the patient's clothing size can help objectify the amount of weight loss.[14] Knowing how long the patient was at his or her previous weight is as useful as knowing at what rate the weight was lost. It sometimes is helpful to recall weights in conjunction with important events in the patient's life, such as holidays, birthdays, and special events.

In general, a complete nutritional history, including diet previous to the weight change, eating habits, and expectations concerning appropriate weight, should be elicited. Whether or not the patient has retained his or her appetite is also helpful although not definitive. Any major concurrent diseases and changes in status are, of course, of immediate importance. Specifically, symptoms referable to the gastrointestinal tract are particularly important.

Questions regarding the patient's general health and well-being will help direct further investigations. Thus, a report of recurrent fevers should lead the questioner to ask about exposure to other infected persons and about pulmonary symptomatology. Likewise the report of diarrhea and abdominal discomfort will lead the questioner to ask about travel, eating exposure, and associated findings such as melena, blood, or mucus. Changes in energy level may lead to questions regarding the endocrine system or the emotional well-being of the patient.

As a general rule, it is helpful to get as full an understanding of the patient's social and family situation as possible. This support system provides the background within which the patient is eating and losing weight; it also may be part of the cause of the patient's problem. Questions regarding the patient's relationship with immediate family as well as co-workers are appropriate. Questions about body image and ideal body weight are also important in this regard.

Drug history can be especially useful in patients with weight loss. Is the patient an alcoholic? Has the patient been utilizing ilicit drugs? Is the patient a heavy smoker? Previous medical history might include information regarding gastrointestinal illness in childhood as well as previous episodes of weight loss or failure to gain. Is weight loss a typical response to stress for the patient, or is this an unusual occurrence?

A list of selected conditions in which weight loss is a prominent symptom is found in Table 1.[15] As can be seen, even patients with classic conditions, such as hyperthyroidism, do not always note weight loss. Even fewer patients will describe weight loss early in their presentation. For example, although 59 per cent of patients with systemic lupus erythematosus will develop weight loss, only 6 per cent complain of this on initial presentation. Also, although not all patients will complain of weight loss, many may exhibit it on physical examination. Table 2 highlights the frequency of weight loss in cancer patients in the 6 months prior to diagnosis.[8]

Table 1. FREQUENCY OF WEIGHT LOSS IN SELECTED DISEASES

Disease	Frequency (%)
Addison's disease	100
Giardiasis	63
Hyperthyroidism	60
Systemic lupus erythematosus	59
Hepatitis, alcoholic	58
Crohn's disease	51
Hemochromatosis	51
Multiple myeloma	48
Cirrhosis, Laennec's	46
Lung abscess	45
Liver abscess, amebic	42
Subacute bacterial endocarditis	36
Sarcoidosis	32
Duodenal ulcer	31
Diverticulitis	23
Parathyroiditis	17
Pheochromocytoma	14
Urolithiasis	7

(Data from Perlroth MG, Weiland DJ. Fifty diseases—fifty diagnoses. Copyright © 1981 by Year Book Medical Publishers, Inc., Chicago. Used by permission.)

Table 2. FREQUENCY OF WEIGHT LOSS IN CANCER PATIENTS

	Weight Loss in the Previous 6 Months (%)*			
Type of Cancer	*0*	*0–5*	*5–10*	*> 10*
Favorable non-Hodgkin's lymphoma†	69	14	8	10
Breast	64	22	8	6
Acute nonlymphocytic leukemia	61	27	8	7
Sarcoma	60	21	11	7
Unfavorable non-Hodgkin's lymphoma‡	52	20	13	15
Colon	46	26	14	14
Prostate	44	28	18	10
Lung, small cell	43	23	20	14
Lung, non–small cell	39	25	21	15
Pancreas§	17	29	28	26
Nonmeasurable gastric	17	21	32	30
Measurable gastric	13	20	29	38
Total	46	22	17	15

*Data shown are percentages of line total in each weight loss category.

†The favorable non-Hodgkin's lymphoma protocol includes nodular lymphocytic well-differentiated, nodular lymphocytic poorly differentiated, nodular mixed, nodular histiocytic, and diffuse lymphocytic well-differentiated.

‡The unfavorable non-Hodgkin's lymphoma protocol includes diffuse lymphocytic poorly differentiated, diffuse mixed, diffuse histiocytic, diffuse undifferentiated, and mycosis fungoides.

§Data for pancreatic cancer are weight loss in previous two months.

(Adapted from Dewys WD, Begg C, Lavin PT. Prognostic effect of weight loss prior to chemotherapy in cancer patients. Am J Med 1980; 69:491–7. With permission.)

High-Payoff Queries

1. *How much weight have you lost exactly? Has there been a change in your clothing sizes?* One survey demonstrated that half of the patients who claimed to have lost weight in fact had not and suggested that answers to these two questions could exclude these patients.[1] Another survey has found that remembered weight is close to actual previous weight in the majority of patients.[16] Thus, asking patients how much they weighed previously and how much they weigh now in order to determine actual weight loss is a useful technique. Likewise, asking about changes in clothing size, e.g. belt size, can be useful.

2. *Do you have any GI upsets, such as vomiting and diarrhea?* Any diseases of the gastrointestinal tract are especially suspect when it comes to symptoms and signs of weight loss. Such symptoms usually lead to a further exploration of the whole area of malabsorption as well as chronic illnesses with secondary effects on the gastrointestinal system.

3. *Has your appetite changed? Have you noticed any changes in your activities, energy, strength, or interest*

in activities? This series of questions is important in exploring both the patient's psychological status (e.g., depressed patients are likely to have a decreased appetite, decreased energy and strength, and loss of interest in activities), as well as the effects of chronic illness (e.g., hepatitis classically manifests as decreased appetite as well as decreased strength, energy, and interest in activities).

4. *What changes have occurred in your diet? What was it like before the weight loss and what is it like now?* Certainly, a dietary history is essential in assessing actual weight loss. This history should include not only food but also alcohol, drugs, and smoking.

5. *Do you have a major illness? Has it worsened in this period of weight loss?* Certainly any patient with a major chronic illness who undergoes significant change of status may experience weight loss, and patients themselves may be able to report this correlation. In addition, important symptomatology associated with a major illness such as pneumonia (e.g., cough) may be essential to the ultimate diagnosis. Specific questions regarding the presence of a febrile illness, cancer of the lungs or gastrointestinal tract, or cardiovascular disease may be especially helpful in this regard.

PHYSICAL EXAMINATION

Physical examination plays a key role in the evaluation of the patient with the complaint of weight loss. Marton and colleagues[1] recently studied 91 patients with involuntary weight loss. They found that 59 patients had a physical cause for the loss, and that in 55 the cause was clinically evident on the initial evaluation. Because of the vague nature of weight loss as a symptom, the physical examination becomes crucial in determining whether weight loss is, in fact, present and in detecting its underlying cause.

In conducting the physical assessment for the evaluation of weight loss, the examiner will be guided in large part by the subjective findings and the age and sex of the patient. However, certain *general* principles apply to all cases with this presenting complaint:

1. Although self-reported weights are quite useful for epidemiologic purposes,[17] they may not be helpful in evaluating an individual case. It is much simpler and more accurate if a reported weight loss can be judged against a previous data base. It is therefore incumbent upon physicians to weigh patients regularly when they are seen for routine periodic evaluations or when they present with other complaints.

2. A critical observation of the patient's appearance is of value in evaluting weight loss. For example, the patient with thyrotoxicosis and weight loss may appear different to the examiner from an individual with an underlying malignancy and weight loss. The examiner can determine by inspection whether the patient appears ill, whether there is evidence of loss of adipose tissue or increased anxiety, whether there is weakness while walking or rising from sitting position, and whether there are changes in skin color.

3. The question of whether weight loss is secondary to diminished intake or increased metabolism, if not answered by the historical data, may be obvious on physical examination. The distinction between a malignancy with its associated weight loss and a disease such as thryotoxicosis should be obvious on physical examination.

4. If objective data on weight loss are not available, it is helpful to question the patient regarding changes in clothing size, belt size, and shoe size.

5. The examiner should keep in mind simple reasons for weight loss. One should never forget, for instance, that older individuals who lack teeth may have difficulty eating and may lose weight as a consequence.

Physical Findings and Their Significance

In their study of 91 patients in inpatient and outpatient settings, Marton and colleagues[1] found that 24 had no apparent cause of weight loss and eight had psychiatric causes. Of the 59 cases in which a physical cause could be found, 18 were due to cancer and 13 to gastrointestinal problems. Table 3 shows the breakdown of causes for weight loss of all the patients in this study. It is clear from these findings that emphasis in the physical assessment should be placed on an evaluation of

Table 3. CAUSES OF WEIGHT LOSS IN STUDY PATIENTS

Diagnosis	Patients*(n = 91) Number	%
No physical cause found (n = 32)		
No apparent cause	24	26
Psychiatric	8	9
Physical cause found (n = 59)		
Cancer	18	19
Gastrointestinal	13	14
Cardiovascular	8	9
Nutritional/alcoholic	7	8
Pulmonary	5	6
Endocrine/metabolic	4	4
Infectious	3	3
Granulomatous/inflammatory	2	2
Drug-induced	2	2
Neurologic	2	2

*Percentage figures add up to more than 100 because several patients had more than one diagnosis. All percentages refer to the total 91 patients.

(Modified from Marton KI, Sox HC, Krupp JR. Involuntary weight loss: diagnostic and prognostic significance. Ann Intern Med 1981; 95:568–74. Used with permission.)

the patient's psychological and emotional state. The primary care physician is in an excellent position to make this evaluation in view of his or her long-standing relationship with the patient and knowledge of the patient's environment.

The key elements in examination of the patient for the presence of malignancy include: (1) examination of the skin for pallor, icterus, abnormal growth, rashes, and evidence of hemorrhage, (2) the search for abnormal masses, those most readily accessible to physical examination being enlargement of the lymph glands, enlargement of the thyroid gland, masses of the abdomen and pelvis, organomegaly and masses of the external genitalia, and (3) identification of localized neurologic findings that can be useful in detecting occult malignancies of the neurologic system.

Careful examination of the gastrointestinal system is critical in the evaluation of weight loss. In the mouth, the condition of the teeth, the presence or absence of mass lesions, and the patency of the oropharynx are significant observations. Examination of the neck is important in distinguishing enlargement of nodes or other masses that may impinge on swallowing mechanisms. The abdominal examination may reveal the presence of hyperactive bowel sounds or a tender palpable bowel, aiding in the diagnosis of a malabsorption syndrome. The importance of the digital rectal examination in revealing masses and occult blood cannot be overstressed.

Other examinations that may prove useful will emphasize body systems highlighted by historical data. Inasmuch as weight loss has a serious prognostic significance, a careful general physical examination is indicated in all cases of documented weight loss.[18]

DIAGNOSTIC STUDIES

As with the physical assessment, laboratory tests should be keyed to symptoms and physical findings. However, in the study of Marton and colleagues,[1] the most commonly seen abnormalities were found on chest x-rays (41 per cent), blood chemistry tests (22 per cent), blood count (14 per cent), and urinalysis (3 per cent). It can be recommended that all patients whose cause for weight loss is not immediately apparent should have a chest x-ray, a multi-channel screening analysis (which includes liver and thyroid function studies), a complete blood count, and a urinalysis. The abnormalities most likely to be discovered in performing these tests are: evidence of pulmonary masses or adenopathy, heart failure, abnormal liver function values, anemia, and glycosuria.

Because gastrointestinal illnesses account for a significant proportion of weight loss cases, laboratory examination of the gastrointestinal (GI) tract may be essential in selected patients. The upper gastrointestinal series is probably the single most useful of the more specialized tests, particularly if it is combined with a small bowel series. Malignant disease of the various portions of the GI tract, duodenal and gastric ulcers, sprue syndromes, and inflammation of the bowel are apparent on gastrointestinal radiographs. The use of endoscopy, biopsy, and various organ scanning procedures should be reserved for the more difficult diagnostic problems.

The search for occult malignant disease utilizing the clinical laboratory and radiography may touch on all of the body systems. Of particular help may be bone scanning in the search for metastatic disease of the breast and prostate and sigmoidoscopy with a flexible sigmoidoscope in the patient with weight loss and blood in the stool.

Diabetes mellitus and thyrotoxicosis are the most common metabolic abnormalities resulting in weight loss. As a consequence, thyroid function studies and glucose tolerance tests may be useful in individuals whose symptoms suggest either of these illnesses.

ASSESSMENT

Weight loss is a challenging symptom because its associated prognosis can be either quite good or quite bad. Many individuals who present with weight loss have either no illness or an emotional or psychological problem, so the prognosis for continued life in this group is obviously good. On the other hand, those individuals who manifest an organic cause generally have serious, if not life-threatening illness. As a consequence, the physician must treat the symptom seriously and follow the patient carefully over time if a cause is not apparent early in the course.

Constellations of Findings

Since weight loss can be associated with any major illness, a listing of associated findings has to be broad in scope. In general, fatigue, inanition, and loss of appetite accompany all but a few causes of weight loss, the classic exceptions being diabetes mellitus and thyrotoxicosis. The following areas are typical of the broad range of findings possible with this condition.

Emotional Causes of Weight Loss. Anorexia nervosa is the classic syndrome in this category. More commonly, weight loss as a consequence of emotional problems is seen in individuals in stressful life situations who become anxious or depressed. Weight loss is then associated with decreased appetite and with signs and symptoms of anxiety or depression.

Gastrointestinal Disorders. A combination of weight loss, abdominal pain, and change in bowel habits should make the physician alert to this group of problems. Depending on the location of the lesion, nausea, vomiting, and increased flatulence may also be part of the clinical constellation.

Diabetes Mellitus. A combination of increased food and water intake and polyuria in the face of weight loss almost certainly points to this problem.

Thyrotoxicosis. In the classic form of this disease, weight loss is associated with tremulousness, increased sweating, exophthalmos, increased food intake, enlarged thyroid gland, and hyper-reflexia.

Malignancy in the Absence of Other Major Signs and Symptoms. Weight loss and anorexia are most commonly secondary to malignancy of the gastrointestinal tract, pancreas, or liver, to a lymphoma, or to leukemia.

Table 4. ATTRIBUTE RULE

Attribute	Score
Less than 20 pack-years of smoking	+3
No decrease in activities due to fatigue	+5
Patient complaints of nausea/vomiting	−3
Recent improvement in appetite	−2
Cough that has recently changed	−1
Findings on physical examination suggesting physical cause of weight loss	−1
Correction factor*	+8
Total	1–16

*Used to make all possible results occur as "positive" numbers.

(From Marton KI, Sox HC, Krupp JR. Involuntary weight loss: diagnostic and prognostic significance. Ann Intern Med 1981; 95:568–74. Used with permission.)

Diagnostic Approach

Table 3 lists the common causes of weight loss. The most important first step in the work-up is to determine whether there is an underlying organic cause for this finding. Fortunately, the history and physical examination usually provide sufficient clues to make this determination. Marton and colleagues have determined the following factors to be of primary importance for differentiating between organic and nonorganic causes: (1) smoking status, (2) level of activity (changed or unchanged), (3) presence of nausea and vomiting, (4) change in appetite, (5) change in cough, and (6) physical findings consistent with organic causes of weight loss. Thus, the non-smoking patient who maintains usual physical activity is unlikely to have a physical cause for weight loss. On the other hand, the patient with nausea or vomiting or recent appetite improvement or changes in cough is more likely to have a physical cause of weight loss. Using their data, the researchers developed an "attribute rule," as seen in Table 4. Their data showed that no patients with a score of 12 or greater had a physical cause for weight loss, and that using a score of 9 as a cut-off was most effective. Hence, 57 out of 59 patients with physical causes for weight loss had a score of less than 9, and the other two patients had causes obvious on physical examination. In addition, only nine out of 32 patients without physical causes of their weight loss had a score of less than 9. Thus, sensitivity was 97 per cent, specificity was 72 per cent, and the positive predicted value in their population was 85 per cent.

Once the determination has been made that a physical cause is likely, then a careful follow-up of those clues elicited from the history and physical examination should be accomplished. A combination of appropriate laboratory testing plus watchful waiting should be the rule. However, there is some concern about delaying too long if the clinician has sufficient suspicion about underlying physical causes, especially when those suspicions center on malignancy. It has been shown that the effect of any weight loss on median cancer survival is severe.[8] Also, prognosis in the geriatric age group, regardless of cause, is less than optimal.[18] Thus, the quickest determination of the underlying cause is most appropriate.

Because of the large percentage of patients without underlying organic causes, the physician often must make a diagnosis of "functional" weight loss. Of course, the assessment should not stop here but should continue into further investigation of the environmental stresses and strains upon an affected person, including functioning at work and in significant relationships. Any unusual statements concerning the patient's body image should be fully explored, and evidence of significant depression should likewise be investigated in depth.

In the end, the diagnosis of weight loss is not a true diagnosis. It is merely a reflection of an underlying problem with many possible causes. Once the clues from the history, physical examination, and laboratory studies have been gathered, the diagnosis is usually readily apparent. Weight loss is not benign whether caused by emotional factors such as anorexia nervosa or by underlying physical illness. Patients with weight loss deserve the most careful attention and management.

REFERENCES

1. Marton KI, Sox HC, Krupp JR. Involuntary weight loss: diagnostic and prognostic significance. Ann Intern Med 1981;95:568–74.
2. Smith NJ. Excessive weight loss and food aversion in athletes simulating anorexia nervosa. Pediatrics 1980;66:139–42.

3. Cupoli JM, Hallock JA, Barness LA. Failure to thrive. In: Gluck L, ed. Current problems in pediatrics. Chicago: Year Book Medical Publishers, 1980;1–43.
4. National ambulatory medical care survey of visits to general and family physicians, January 1974–December 1974. Rockville, Maryland: National Center for Health Statistics. Monthly Vital Statistics Report 1976;25:1–8.
5. Schoenborn CA, Danchik KM. Health practices among adults: United States, 1977. Hyattsville, Maryland: National Center for Health Statistics. Advance data 1980; No. 64, November 4.
6. Marsland DW, Wood M, Mayo F. A data bank for patient care, curriculum and research in family practice: 526,196 patient problems. Part I: Rank order of diagnoses by frequency. Part II: Diagnoses by disease categories by age/sex distribution. J Fam Pract 1976;3:37–68.
7. Hart FD. Loss of weight. In: French's index of differential diagnosis. 11th ed. Chicago: John Wright & Sons, 1979.
8. Dewys WD, Begg C, Lavin PT, et al. Prognostic effect of weight loss prior to chemotherapy in cancer patients. Am J Med 1980;69:491–7.
9. Glickman RM. Malabsorption. Pathophysiology and diagnosis. In: Wyngaarden JB, Smith LH Jr, eds. Cecil textbook of medicine. 16th ed. Philadelphia: WB Saunders, 1982;678–90.
10. Klibanski A. Anorexia nervosa. Prim Care 1981;8:19–31.
11. Crisp AH, Palmer RL, Kalucy RS. How common is anorexia nervosa? A prevalence study. Br J Psychiatr 1976; 128:549–54.
12. Warren MP, Vande Wiele RL. Clinical and metabolic features of anorexia nervosa. Am J Obstet Gynecol 1973;117:435–49.
13. Gambert SR, Guansing AR. Protein-calorie malnutrition in the elderly. J Am Geriatr Soc 1980;28:272–5.
14. Winfield RA. Weight loss and the belt. Ann Intern Med 1973;79:910.
15. Perlroth MG, Weiland DJ. Fifty diseases—fifty diagnoses. Chicago: Year Book Medical Publishers, 1981.
16. Morgan DB, Path MRC, Hill GL, Burkinshaw L. The assessment of body weight loss from a single measurement of body weight: the problems and limitations. Am J Clin Nutr 1980;33:2101–5.
17. Stunkard AJ, Albaum JM. The accuracy of self-reported weights. Am J Clin Nutr 1981;34:1593–9.
18. Kent S. Body weight and life expectancy. Geriatrics 1982;37:149–57.

INDEX

Note: Page numbers referring to illustrations are in *italic* type. Page numbers followed by (t) indicate tables.